AF708784

Principles of Heating, Ventilating and Air Conditioning

A Textbook with Design Data Based on the
1997 ASHRAE Handbook—Fundamentals

Ronald H. Howell
University of South Florida

Harry J. Sauer, Jr.
University of Missouri—Rolla

William J. Coad
McClure Engineering Associates

American Society of Heating, Refrigerating and Air-Conditioning Engineers, Inc.
1791 Tullie Circle NE, Atlanta, Georgia 30329 http://www.ashrae.org

Copyright © 1998 by the American Society of Heating, Refrigerating and Air-Conditioning Engineers, Inc. All rights reserved.

No part of this book may be reproduced without permission in writing from ASHRAE, except by a reviewer who may quote brief passages or reproduce illustrations in a review with appropriate credit: nor may any part of this book be reproduced, stored in a retrieval system, or transmitted in any form or by any means—electronic, photocopying, recording, or other—without permission in writing from ASHRAE.

ASHRAE has compiled this publication with care, but ASHRAE has not investigated, and ASHRAE expressly disclaims any duty to investigate, any product, service, process, procedure, design, or the like that may be described herein. The appearance of any technical data or editorial material in this publication does not constitute endorsement, warranty, or guaranty by ASHRAE of any product, service, process, procedure, design, or the like. ASHRAE does not warrant that the information in this publication is free of errors. The user assumes the entire risk of the use of any information in this publication.

Comments, criticism, and suggestions regarding the subject matter are invited. Any errors or omissions in the data should be brought to the attention of the editor.

ISBN 1-883413-56-7

Edited by Robert A. Parsons
Typography by Nancy F. Thysell

CONTENTS

Part I General Concepts

Part II HVAC Systems

Part III HVAC Equipment

Appendices

Index

PREFACE

Principles of Heating, Ventilating, and Air-Conditioning a textbook based on the 1997 *ASHRAE Handbook—Fundamentals,* should provide an attractive text for air-conditioning courses at engineering colleges and technical institutes. The text has been developed to give broad and current coverage of the heating, ventilation, and air conditioning field when combined with the 1997 *ASHRAE Handbook—Fundamentals.* The book should prove most suitable as a textbook and subsequent reference book for (a) undergraduate engineering courses in the general field of HVAC, (b) similar courses at technical institutes, (c) continuing education and refresher short courses for engineers, and (d) adult education courses for non-engineers. It contains more material than can normally be covered in a one-semester course. However, several different single-semester or shorter courses can be easily planned by merely eliminating the chapters and/or parts which are least applicable to the objectives of the particular course. This text will also readily aid in self-instruction of the 1997 *ASHRAE Handbook—Fundamentals* by engineers wishing to develop their competence in the HVAC&R field.

Although numerous references are made to the other *ASHRAE Handbook* volumes, sufficient material has been included from these to make this text complete enough for various courses in the HVAC&R field. The material covered for various audiences in regular university courses, technical institute courses, and short courses can and will vary greatly. The supplement needed to be complete to satisfy all of these anticipated uses and needs. Toward this end, the following major sections are included:

Part I	General Concepts, Chapter 1-10
Part II	Air-Conditioning Systems, Chapters 11-16
Part III	HVAC&R Equipment, Chapters 17-19

Although the 1997 *ASHRAE Handbook—Fundamentals* is published in an SI edition, which uses international units, and an inch-pound (I-P) edition, this single version of *Principles of Heating, Ventilating, and Air-Conditioning* is designed to serve both the I-P and SI editions of *Fundamentals.* For the most part, the sample tables and figures are taken from the I-P edition, but illustrative and home problems are provided in both systems of units. A set of appropriate SI tables and figures follows each chapter.

The major changes in the edition of *Principles of Heating, Ventilating, and Air-Conditioning* include the weather data in a new format, a complete restructuring on the systems part, and a chapter on hydronic system design. Also, the inclusion of a new, third author brings the perspective of a system designer.

January 1998

Ronald H. Howell
Harry J. Sauer, Jr.
William J. Coad

Chapter 1

BACKGROUND

This chapter provides a brief background on the heating, ventilating, air conditioning, and refrigeration (HVAC&R) field and industry, including the early history and some significant developments. An introduction to a few basic concepts is included along with suggestions for further reading.

1.1 Introduction

The primary function of a heating, ventilating and air-conditioning (HVAC) system is either (1) the generation and maintenance of comfort for occupants in a conditioned space; or (2) the supplying of a set of environmental conditions (high temperature and high humidity; low temperature and high humidity, etc.) for a process or product within a space. Human comfort design conditions are quite different than the conditions required in textile mills or for grain storage and vary depending on such things as the time of year and the activity and clothing levels of the occupants.

If improperly sized equipment or the wrong type of equipment is used, the desired environmental conditions usually will not be met. Furthermore, improperly selected and/or sized equipment normally requires excess power and/or energy and may have a higher initial cost.

The following details should be considered to properly design an air-conditioning system:

1. The location, elevation, and orientation of the structure so that the effects of the weather (wind, sun, and precipitation) on the building air-conditioning load can be anticipated.
2. The building size (wall area, roof area, glass area, floor area, and so forth).
3. The building shape (L-shaped, A-shaped, rectangular, etc.), which influences equipment location, type of heating and air conditioning system used, and duct or piping locations.
4. The space use characteristics. Will there be different users (office, bank, school, dance studios, etc.) of the space from year to year? Will there be different concurrent requirements from the tenants? Will there be night setback of the temperature controller or intermittent use of the building's facilities?
5. The type of material (wood, masonry, metal, and so forth) used in the construction of the building. What is the expected quality of the construction?
6. The type of fenestration (light transmitting partition) used, its location in the building, and how it might be shaded. Is glass heat absorbing, reflective, colored, etc.?
7. The types of doors (sliding, swinging, revolving) and windows (sealed, wood or metal frames, etc.) used. What is their expected use? This will determine the amount of infiltration air.
8. The expected occupancy for the space and the time schedule of this occupancy.
9. Type and location of lighting. Types of appliances and electrical machinery in the space and their expected use.
10. Location of electric, gas, and water services. These services should be integrated with the locations of the heating and air-conditioning duct, piping, and equipment.
11. Ventilation requirements for the structure. Does it require 100% outdoor air, a given number of cfm per person, or a given number of cfm per square foot of floor area?
12. Local and/or national codes relating to ventilation and gas, and/or electric piping.
13. Outside design temperatures and wind velocities for the location.
14. The environmental conditions that are maintained. Will fluctuations of these conditions with load be detrimental to the purpose served by the structure?
15. The heating and cooling loads (also consider the moisture load, air contaminants, and noise).
16. The type of heating and air-conditioning system to be used in the structure. Is it forced air, circulated water, or direct expansion? Will it be a multizone, single zone, reheat, variable air volume, or another type of system? What method of control will be used?
17. The heating and cooling equipment size that will maintain the inside design conditions for the selected outside design condition. Electric heat or fossil fuel? Mechanical vapor compression or absorption chiller?
18. The advantages and disadvantages of oversizing and undersizing the equipment as applied to the structure. Survey any economic tradeoffs to be made. Should a different type of unit be installed in order to reduce operating costs? Should a more sophisticated control system be used to give more exact control of humidity and temperature or should an on-off cycle be used? Fuel economy as related to design will become an even more important factor in system selection and operation.
19. What is the estimated annual energy usage?

In general, no absolute rules dictate correct selections or specifications for each of the above items, so only engineering estimates or educated guesses can be made. However, estimates must be based on sound fundamental principles and concepts. This book presents a basic philosophy of environmental control as well as the basic concepts of design. These ideas relate directly to the ASHRAE Handbook Series: 1994 Refrigeration, 1995 HVAC Applications, 1996 HVAC Systems and Equipment, and most directly to the 1997 Fundamentals.

1.2 Historical Notes

Knowing something of the past helps in understanding current design criteria and trends. As in other fields of technology, the accomplishments and failures of the past affect current and future design concepts. The following paragraphs consist mainly of edited excerpts from *ASHRAE Journal* articles: "A History of Heating" by John W. James, "The History of Refrigeration" by Willis R. Woolrich, and "Milestones in Air Conditioning" by Walter A. Grant, with additional information obtained from ASHRAE's Historical Committee. These excerpts provide a synopsis of the history of environmental control.

Obviously, the earliest form of heating was the open fire. The addition of a chimney to carry away combustion byproducts was the first important step in the evolution of heating systems. By the time of the Romans, there was sufficient knowledge of ventilation to allow for the installation of ventilating and panel heating in baths. Leonardo da Vinci had invented a ventilating fan by the end of the 15th century. Robert Boyle's law was established in 1659; John Dalton's in 1800. In 1775, Dr. William Cullen made ice by pumping a vacuum in a vessel of water. A few years later, Benjamin Franklin wrote his treatise on Pennsylvania fireplaces, detailing their construction, installation, and operation.

Although warming and ventilating techniques had greatly improved by the 19th century, manufacturers were unable to exploit these techniques because:

1. Data available on such subjects as transmission coefficients, air and water friction in pipes, and brine and ammonia properties were sparse and unreliable.
2. Neither set design conditions nor reliable psychrometric charts existed.
3. A definitive rational theory that would permit performance calculation and prediction of results had not yet been developed.
4. Little was known about physical, thermodynamic, and fluid dynamic properties of air, water, brines, and refrigerants.
5. No authoritative information existed on heat transmission involving combustion, conduction, convection, radiation, evaporation, and condensation.
6. No credible performance information for manufactured equipment was available.

Thanks to Thomas Edison, the first electric power plant opened in New York in 1882, making it possible for the first time to have an inexpensive source of energy for residential and commercial buildings.

Furnaces

By 1894, the year the American Society of Heating and Ventilating Engineers (ASH&VE) was born, central heating was fairly well developed. The basic heat sources were warm air furnaces and boilers. The combustion chambers of the first warm air furnaces were made of cast iron. Circulation in a gravity warm air furnace system is caused by the difference in air density in the many parts of the system. As the force of combustion is small, the system was designed to allow air to circulate freely. The addition of fans (circa 1899) to furnace systems provided a mechanical means of air circulation. Other additions to the modern furnace include cooling systems, humidification apparatuses, air distributors, and air filters. Another important step for the modern heating industry was the conversion of furnaces from coal to oil and gas, and from manual to automatic firing.

Steam Systems

James Watt developed the first steam heating system in 1770. However, the first real breakthrough in design did not occur until the early 1900s when circulation problems in these systems were improved with the introduction of a fluid-operated thermostatic trap.

From 1900 to 1925, two-pipe steam systems with thermostatic traps at the outlet of each radiator and at drip points in the piping gained wide acceptance. In smaller buildings, gravity systems were commonly installed to remove condensate. For larger systems, boiler return traps and condensate pumps with receivers were used. By 1926, the vacuum return line system was perfected for installation in large and moderate size buildings.

Hot water heating systems were developed in parallel with steam systems. As mentioned before, the first hot water heating system was the gravity system. In 1927, the circulator, which forced water through the system, was added to two-pipe heating systems. A few years later, a diverting tee was added to the one-pipe system, allowing for forced circulation.

During the 1930s, radiators and convectors were commonly concealed by enclosures, shields, and cabinets. In 1944, the baseboard radiator was developed. Baseboard heating improved comfort conditions as it reduced floor-to-ceiling temperature stratification.

Unit heaters and unit ventilators are two other forms of convection heating developed in the 1920s. Unit heaters were available in suspended and floor types and were classified according to the heating medium used (e.g., steam, hot water, electricity, gas, oil, or coal combustion). In addition to the heating element and fan, unit ventilators were often equipped with an air filter. Many designs provided air recirculation and were equipped with a separate outdoor air connection.

Panel heating, another form of heat distribution, was developed in the 1920s. In panel heating, a fluid such as hot water, steam, air, or electricity, circulates through distribution units embedded in the building components.

Early Refrigeration

Early forms of refrigeration included the use of snow, pond and lake ice, chemical mixture cooling to form freezing baths, and the manufacture of ice by evaporative and radiation cooling of water on clear nights.

By the 18th century, certain mixtures were known to lower temperatures. One such mixture, calcium chloride and snow, was introduced for commercial use. This particular mixture made possible a temperature down to −27°F (−33°C). In Great Britain, machines using chemical mixtures to produce low temperatures were introduced. However, by the time these machines were ready for commercial exploitation, mechanical ice-making processes had been perfected to such an extent that chemical mixture freezing was rendered obsolete except for such batch processes as ice cream making.

Mechanical and Chemical Refrigeration

In 1748, in Scotland, Dr. William Cullen and Joseph Black lectured on the latent heat of fusion and evaporation and "fixed air" (later identified as carbon dioxide). These discoveries served as the foundation on which modern refrigeration is based.

In 1851, Dr. John Gorrie, was granted U.S. Patent No. 8080 for a refrigeration machine that produced ice and refrigerated air with compressed air in an open cycle. Also in 1851, Ferdinand Carre' designed the first ammonia absorption unit.

In 1853, Professor Alexander Twining of New Haven, Connecticut, produced 1600 lb of ice a day with a doubleacting vacuum and compression pump that used sulfuric ether as the refrigerant.

Daniel L. Holden improved the Carre' machine by designing and building reciprocating compressors. These compressors were applied to ice making, brewing, and meat packing. In 1872, David Boyle developed an ammonia compression machine that produced ice.

Until 1880, mechanical refrigeration was primarily used to make ice and preserve meat and fish. Notable exceptions were the use of these machines in the United States, Europe, and Australia for beer making, oil dewaxing, and wine cooling. At this time, comfort air cooling was obtained by ice or by chilling machines that made use of either lake or manufactured ice.

History of ASHRAE

The American Society of Heating and Ventilating Engineers (ASHVE) was formed in New York City in 1894 with the objectives of conducting research, developing standards, holding technical meetings, and publishing technical articles in journals and handbooks. Its scope was limited to the fields of heating and ventilating for commercial and industrial applications, with secondary emphasis on residential heating. Years later the Society's name was changed to the American Society of Heating and Air-Conditioning Engineers (ASHAE) to recognize the increasing importance of air conditioning.

In 1904, the American Society of Refrigerating Engineers (ASRE) was organized and headquartered at the American Society of Mechanical Engineers (ASME). The new Society had 70 charter members and was the only engineering group in the world that confined its activities to refrigeration, which at that time consisted mainly of ammonia systems.

In 1905, ASME established 288,000 Btu in 24 hrs as the commercial ton of refrigeration (within the United States). In the same year, the New York Stock Exchange was cooled by refrigeration. In 1906, Stuart W. Cramer coins the term "air conditioning."

The First International Congress on Refrigeration was organized in Paris in 1908 and a delegation of 26 was sent from the United States. Most of the participants were members of ASRE.

ASHAE and ASRE merged in 1959, creating the American Society of Heating, Refrigerating and Air-Conditioning Engineers.

Figure 1-1 depicts ASHRAE's history. ASHRAE celebrated its Centennial Year during society year 1994-95. In commemoration of the centennial, two books on the history of ASHRAE and of the HVAC industry were published, *Proclaiming the Truth* and *Heat and Cold: Mastering the Great Indoors*.

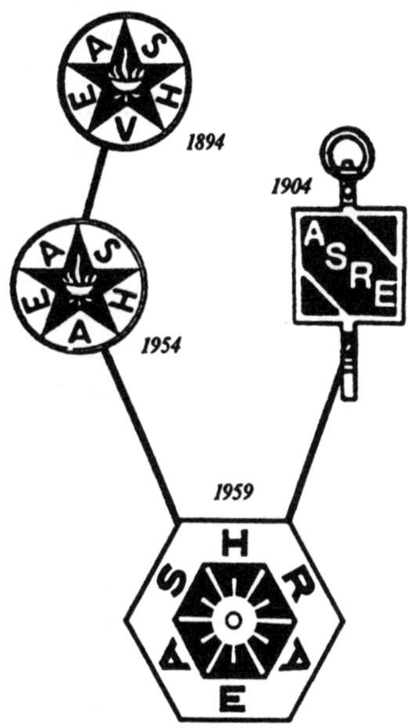

Figure 1-1 Background of ASHRAE

Willis H. Carrier

Willis H. Carrier (1876-1950) has often been referred to as the "Father of Air Conditioning." His analytical and practical accomplishments contributed greatly to the development of the refrigeration industry.

Carrier graduated from Cornell University in 1901 and was employed by the Buffalo Forge Company. He realized that satisfactory refrigeration could not be installed due to the inaccurate data that was available. By 1902, he developed formulas to optimize forced-draft boiler fans, conducted tests and developed multirating performance tables on indirect pipe coil heaters, and set up the first research laboratory in the heating and ventilating industry.

In 1902, Carrier was asked to solve the problem faced by the lithographic industry of poor color register caused by weather changes. Carrier's solution was to design, test, and install at the Sackett-Wilhelms Lithographing Company of Brooklyn a scientifically engineered, year-round air-conditioning system that provided heating, cooling, humidifying, and dehumidifying.

By 1904, Carrier had adapted atomizing nozzles and developed eliminators for air washers to control dew-point temperature by heating or cooling a system's recirculated water. Soon after this development, over 200 industries were using year-round air conditioning.

At the 1911 ASME meeting, Carrier presented his paper, "Rational Psychrometric Formulae," which related dry-bulb, wet-bulb, and dew-point temperatures of air, as well as its sensible, latent, and total heat load, and set forth the theory of adiabatic saturation. The formulas and psychrometric chart presented in this paper became the basis for all fundamental calculations used by the air-conditioning industry.

By 1922, Carrier's centrifugal refrigeration machine, together with the development of nonhazardous, low-pressure refrigerants, made water chilling for large and medium-size commercial and industrial applications both economical and practical. A conduit induction system for multiroom buildings, was invented in 1937 by Carrier and his associate, Carlyle Ashley.

Comfort Cooling

Although comfort air-cooling systems had been built as of the 1890s, no real progress was made in mechanical air cooling until after the turn of the century. At that time, several scientifically designed air-conditioning plants were installed in buildings. One such installation included a theater in Cologne, Germany. In 1902, Alfred Wolff designed a 400-ton system for the New York Stock Exchange. Installed in 1902, this system was in operation for 20 years. The Boston Floating Hospital, in 1908, was the first hospital to be equipped with modern air conditioning. Mechanical air cooling was installed in a Texas church in 1914. In 1922, Grauman's Metropolitan Theater, the first air conditioned movie theater, opened in Los Angeles. The first office building designed with and built for comfort air-conditioning specifications was the Milam Building, in San Antonio, Texas, which was completed in 1928. Also in 1928, the Chamber of the House of Representatives became air conditioned. The Senate became air conditioned the following year and in 1930, the White House and the Executive Office Building were air conditioned.

The system of air bypass control, invented in 1924 by L. Logan Lewis, solved the difficult problem of humidity control under varying load. By the end of the 1920s, the first room air conditioner was introduced by Frigidaire. Other important inventions of the 1920s include lightweight extended surface coils and the first unit heater and cold diffuser.

Thomas Midgley, Jr. developed the halocarbon refrigerants in 1930. These refrigerants were found to be safe and economical for the small reciprocating compressors used in commercial and residential markets. Manufacturers were soon producing mass market room air conditioners that used Refrigerant 12.

Fluorinated refrigerants were also applied to centrifugal compression, which required only half the number of impellers for the same head as chlorinated hydrocarbons. Space and materials were saved when pressure-formed extended-surface tubes in shell-and-tube exchangers were introduced by Walter Jones. This invention was an important advance for centrifugal and reciprocating equipment.

Other achievements of the 1930s included:

1. The first residential lithium bromide absorption machine was introduced in 1931 by Servel.
2. In 1931, Carrier marketed steam ejector cooling units for railroad passenger cars.
3. As of the mid-1930s, General Electric introduced the heat pump; the electrostatic air cleaner was put out by Westinghouse; Charles Neeson of Airtemp invented the high-speed radial compressor; and W.B. Connor discovered that odors could be removed by using activated carbon.

With the end of World War II, air-conditioning technology advanced rapidly. Among the advances were air-source heat pumps, large lithium-bromide water chillers, automobile air conditioners, rooftop heating and cooling units, small, outdoor-installed ammonia absorption chillers, air purifiers, a vapor cycle aircraft cabin cooling unit, and a large capacity Lysholm rotary compressor.

Improvements on and expansions of products that already existed include:

- dual-duct central systems for office buildings
- change from open to hermetic compressors from the smallest reciprocating units to large capacity centrifugals
- resurgence of electric heating in all kinds of applications
- use of heat pumps to reclaim heat in large buildings
- application of electrostatic cleaners to residences
- self-contained variable volume air terminals for multiple interior rooms
- increasing use of total energy systems for large buildings and clusters of buildings
- larger sizes of centrifugals, now over 5000 tons in a single unit
- central heating and cooling plants for shopping centers, colleges, and apartment and office building complexes

In the late 1940s and into the early 1950s, development work continued on unitary heat pumps for residential and small commercial installations. These factory engineered and assembled units, like conventional domestic boilers, could be easily and cheaply installed in the home or small commercial businesses by engineers. In 1952, heat pumps were placed on the market for mass consumption.

Early heat pumps lacked the durability needed to withstand winter temperatures. Low winter temperatures placed severe stress on the components of these heat pumps (compressors, reversing valves, and control hardware).

Improvements in the design of heat pumps has continued. Improved designs included more reliable compressors and lubricating systems, improved reversing valves, and refined control systems.

In 1987, the United Nations Montreal Protocol for protecting the earth's ozone layer was signed, establishing the phase-out schedule for the production of CFC refrigerants. CFC production in the U.S. ended December 31, 1995.

1.3 Building Energy Use

Energy is generally used in buildings to perform functions of heating, lighting, mechanical drives, cooling, and special applications. A typical breakdown of the relative energy use in a commercial building is given as Figure 1-2.

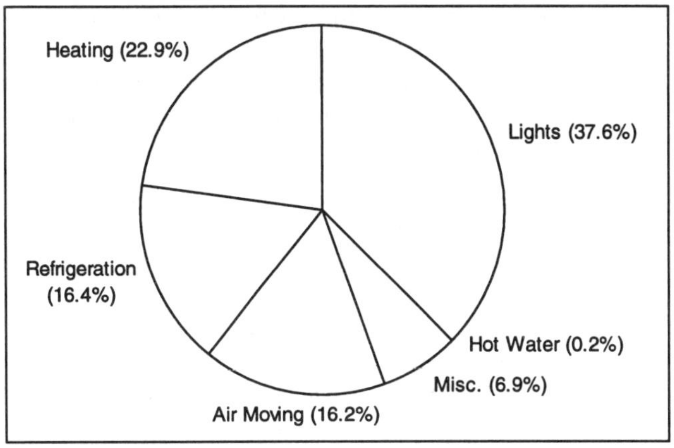

Figure 1-2 Energy Use in a Commercial Building

Energy is available in limited forms, such as electricity, fossil fuels, and solar energy, and these energy forms must be converted within a building to serve the end use of the various functions. A degradation of energy is associated with any conversion process. In energy conservation efforts, two avenues of approach were taken: (1) reducing the amount of use and/or (2) reducing conversion losses. For example, the furnace that heats a building produces unusable and toxic flue gas that must be vented to the outside and in this process some of the energy is lost. Table 1-1 presents typical values for building heat losses and gains at design conditions for mid-America climate. Actual values will vary significantly with climate and building construction.

The efficient use of energy in buildings can be achieved by implementing (1) optimum energy designs, (2) well-developed energy use policies, and (3) dedicated management backed up by a properly trained and motivated operating staff. Optimum energy conservation is attained when the least amount of energy is used to achieve a desired result. If this is not fully realizable, the next best method is to move excess energy from where it is not wanted to where it can be used or stored for future use, which generally results in a minimum expenditure of new energy. If possible, a system should be designed so that it cannot heat and cool the same locations simultaneously.

Table 1.1 Typical Building Design Heat Losses or Gains

	Air Conditioning		Heating	
Building Type	**ft^2/ton**	**m^2/kW**	**Btu/h·ft^3**	**W/m^3**
Apartment	450	12	4.5	45
Bank	250	7	3.0	30
Department Store	250	7	1.0	10
Dormitories	450	12	4.5	45
House	700	18	3.0	30
Medical Center	300	8	4.5	45
Night Club	250	7	3.0	30
Office Interior	350	9	3.0	30
Exterior	275	7	3.0	30
Post Office	250	7	3.0	30
Restaurant	250	7	3.0	30
Schools	275	7	3.0	30
Shopping Center	250	7	3.0	30

ASHRAE *Standard* 90.1-1989, "Energy Efficient Design of New Buildings Except Low-Rise Residential Buildings," and the 100 series standards, "Energy Conservation in Existing Buildings," provide minimum guidelines for energy conservation design and operation. They incorporate these types of energy standards: (1) prescriptive, which specifies the materials and methods for design and construction of buildings; (2) system performance, which sets requirements for each component, system, or subsystem within a building; and (3) building energy, which considers the performance of the building as a whole. In this last type, a design goal is set for the annual energy requirements of the entire building on basis such as Btu/ft^2 per year (GJ/m^2 per year). Any combination of materials, systems, and operating procedures can be applied, as long as design energy usage does not exceed the building's annual energy budget goal.

This approach allows greater flexibility while promoting the goals of energy efficiency. It also allows and encourages the use of innovative techniques and the development of new methods for saving energy. Means for its implementation are still being developed. They are different for new and for existing buildings; in both cases, an accurate data base is required as well as an accurate, verifiable means of measuring consumption.

As energy prices have risen, more sophisticated schemes for reducing energy consumption have been conceived. Included in such schemes are: cogeneration, energy management systems (EMS), direct digital control (DDS), daylighting, closed water-loop heat pumps, variable air volume (VAV) systems, variable frequency drives, thermal storage, dessicant dehumidication, and heat recovery in commercial and institutional buildings and industrial plants.

As detailed in a 1992 Department of Energy Report, "Commercial Buildings Consumption and Expenditures, 1989," more than seventy percent of the commercial-industrial-institutional (C-I-I) buildings recently built in the United States made use of energy conservation measures for heating and cooling.

The type of building and its use strongly affects the energy use as shown in Table 1-2.

Table 1.2 Annual Energy Use Per Unit Floor Area

Building Type	Annual Energy Use kWh/ft²
Assembly	18.7
Education	25.5
Food Sales	51.5
Health Care	64.0
Lodging	38.8
Mercantile	24.8
Office	30.5
Warehouse	16.9
Vacant	6.9
All Buildings	26.7

Heating and air-conditioning systems that are simple in design and of the proper size for a given building generally have relatively low maintenance and operating costs. For optimum results, as much inherent thermal control as is economically possible should be built into the basic structure. Such control might include materials with high thermal properties, insulation, and multiple or special glazing and shading devices. The relationship between the shape, orientation, and air-conditioning requirement of a building should also be considered. Since the exterior load may vary from 30 to 60% of the total air-conditioning load when the fenestration (light transmitting) area ranges from 25 to 75% of the floor area, it may be desirable to minimize the perimeter area. For example, a rectangular building with a 4-to-1 aspect ratio requires substantially more refrigeration than a square building with the same floor area.

When a structure is characterized by several exposures and multipurpose use, especially with wide load swings and noncoincident energy use in certain areas, multiunit or unitary systems may be considered for sych areas, but not necessarily for the entire building. The benefits of transferring heat absorbed by cooling from one area to other areas, processes, or services that require heat may enhance the selection of such systems.

Buildings in the U.S. consume roughly $220 billion worth of energy each year, according to the U.S. Department of Energy (DOE). Buildings account for 36% of all the energy used in the U.S., and 66% of all the electricity used. Beyond economics, energy use in the buildings sector has significant implications for our environment. Emissions related to building energy use account for 35% of carbon dioxide emissions, 47% of sulfur dioxide emissions, and 22% of nitrogen oxide emissions.

The Energy Policy Act of 1992 (EPACT) required all states to review their building energy codes, and certify to the Secretary of Energy by October 24, 1994, that they met the provisions of EPACT. For commercial buildings, EPACT specifies that new commercial construction must meet or exceed, by that date, ASHRAE/IES *Standard* 90.1-89.

1.4 Conceptualizing an HVAC System

An important tool for the HVAC design engineer is the ability to develop a quick overview or "concept" of the magnitude of the project at hand. Toward this goal, the industry has developed a number of "rules of thumb," some more accurate than others. As handy as they might be, these approximations must be treated as just that—approximations.

Tables 1-1 and 1-2 are examples of such rules-of-thumb, providing data for a quick estimate of heating and cooling equipment sizes and of building energy use, requiring knowledge only of the size and intended use of the building. Other rules-of-thumb include using a face velocity of 500 FPM in determining the face area for a cooling coil, the use of 400 CFM/ton for estimating the required cooling airflow rate, the use of 2.5 gpm/ton for determining the water flow rate through the cooling coil and chiller unit, using 1.2 CFM/sq ft of gross floor area for estimating the required conditioned airflow rate for comfort cooling, and the estimation of 1 kW/ton as the power requirement for air conditioning. Table 1-3 provides very approximate data related to the cost of HVAC equipment and systems.

Table 1.3 Capital Cost Estimating Factors

Cooling Systems
- $1,000/installed ton of cooling

Heating Systems
- $2/CFM of installed heating

Fans/Ducting
- $3/CFM for installed supply air handlers
- $1/CFM for installed exhaust fans
- $2/CFM for installed duct work

Complete Hvac Systems
- $1.50/CFM for rooftop units
- $4/CFM for field erected units

The material presented in this book will enable the reader to validate appropriate rules as well as to improve upon these approximations for the final design.

1.5 Problems

1.1 Estimate whether ice will form on a clear night when ambient air temperature is 45°F (7.2°C), if the water is placed in a shallow pan in a sheltered location where the convective heat transfer coefficient is 0.5 Btu/h·ft²·°F [2.8 W/(m²·K)].

1.2 Obtain a sketch or drawing of Gorrie's refrigeration machine and describe its operation.

1.3 Plot the history of the annual energy use per square foot of floor space for nonresidential buildings and predict the values for the years 2000 and 2010.

1.4 Estimate the size of cooling and heating equipment that is needed for a new bank building in middle America that is 140 ft by 220 ft by 12 ft high (42.7 m by 67 m by 3.7 m high).

1.5 Estimate the size of heating and cooling equipment that will be needed for a residence in middle America that is 28 ft by 78 ft by 8 ft high (8.5 m by 23.8 m by 2.4 m high).

1.6 Estimate the initial cost of the complete HVAC system (heating, cooling, and air moving) for an office building, 40 ft by 150 ft by 10 ft high (12.2 m by 45.7 m by 3.1 m high).

1.7 Estimate the annual operating cost for the building in Problem 1.6 if all-electric with electricity priced at a flat rate of 8 cents per kWh.

1.6 Bibliography

ASHRAE. 1994. *Refrigeration*. ASHRAE, Atlanta, GA.

ASHRAE. 1995. *HVAC Applications*. ASHRAE, Atlanta, GA.

ASHRAE. 1996. *HVAC Systems and Equipment*. ASHRAE, Atlanta, GA.

ASHRAE. 1997. *Fundamentals*. ASHRAE, Atlanta, GA.

ASHRAE. 1995. *Proclaiming the Truth*. ASHRAE, Atlanta, GA.

Coad, W.J. 1997. Designing for Tomorrow, *Heating/Piping/Air Conditioning*, February.

Donaldson, B. and B. Nagengast. 1995. *Heat and Cold: Mastering the Great Indoors*. ASHRAE, Atlanta, GA.

Downing, R. 1984. Development of Chlorofluorocarbon Refrigerants. *ASHRAE Transactions* 90(2).

Faust, F.H. 1992. The Merger of ASHAE and ASRE: The Author Presents An Overview on Events Leading up to ASHRAE's Founding. *ASHRAE Insights* 7(5).

Ivanovich, M.G. 1997. HVAC&R and the Internet: Where to Go, *Heating/Piping/Air Conditioning*, May.

Nagengast, B.A. 1988. A historical look at CFC refrigerants. *ASHRAE Journal* 30(11).

Nagengast, B.A. 1993. The 1920s: The first realization of public air conditioning. *ASHRAE Journal* 35(1).

Nelson, L.W. 1989. Residential comfort: A historical look at early residential HVAC systems. *ASHRAE Journal* 31(1).

Woolrich, W.R. 1969. The History of Refrigeration; 220 Years of Mechanical and Chemical Cold: 1748-1968. *ASHRAE Journal* 33(7).

Chapter 2

THERMODYNAMICS AND PSYCHROMETRICS

This chapter reviews the principles of thermodynamics, evaluates thermodynamic properties, and applies thermodynamics and psychrometrics to air-conditioning and refrigeration processes and systems. Greater details on thermodynamics, particularly relating to the Second Law and irreversibility, is found in Chapter 1, 1997 *Handook—Fundamentals*. Details on psychrometric properties can be found in Chapter 6 of the 1997 *Handbook—Fundamentals*.

2.1 Fundamental Concepts and Principles

2.1.1 Thermodynamics

Thermodynamics is the science devoted to the study of energy, its transformations, and its relation to status of matter. Since every engineering operation involves an interaction between energy and materials, the principles of thermodynamics can be found in all engineering activities.

Thermodynamics may be considered the description of the behavior of matter in equilibrium and its changes from one equilibrium state to another. The important concepts of thermodynamics are energy and entropy; the two major principles of thermodynamics are called the first and second laws of thermodynamics. The first law of thermodynamics deals with energy. The idea of energy represents the attempt to find an invariant in the physical universe, something that remains constant in the midst of change. The second law of thermodynamics explains the concept of entropy; e.g., every naturally occurring transformation of energy is accompanied somewhere by a loss in the availability of energy for future performance of work.

The German physicist, Rudolf Clausius (1822-1888), devised the concept of entropy to quantitatively describe the loss of available energy in all naturally occurring transformations. Although the natural tendency is for heat to flow from a hot to a colder body with which it is in contact, corresponding to an increase in entropy, it is possible to make heat flow from a colder body to a hot body, as is done every day in a refrigerator. However, this does not take place naturally or without effort exerted somewhere.

According to the fundamental principles of thermodynamics, the energy of the world stays constant and the entropy of the world increases without limit. If the essence of the first principle in everyday life is that one cannot get something for nothing, the second principle emphasizes that every time one does get something, the opportunity to get that something in the future is reduced by a measurable amount, until ultimately, there will be no more "getting." This "heat death," envisioned by Clausius, will be a time when the universe reaches a level temperature; and though the total amount of energy will be the same as ever, there will be no means of making it available, as entropy will have reached its maximum value.

Like all sciences, the basis of thermodynamics is experimental observation. Findings from these experimental observations have been formalized into basic laws. In the sections that follow, these laws and their related thermodynamic properties will be presented and applied to various examples. These examples should give the student an understanding of the basic concepts and an ability to apply these fundamentals to thermodynamic problems. It is not necessary to memorize numerous equations, for problems are best solved by applying the definitions and laws of thermodynamics.

Thermodynamic reasoning is always from the general law to the specific case, i.e., the reasoning is deductive rather than inductive. To illustrate the elements of thermodynamic reasoning, the analytical processes may be divided into two steps:

1. The idealization or substitution of an analytical model for a real system. This step is taken in all engineering sciences. Therefore, skill in making idealizations is an essential part of the engineering art.
2. The second step, unique to thermodynamics, is the deductive reasoning from the first and second laws of thermodynamics.

These steps involve: (a) an energy balance, (b) a suitable properties relation, and (c) accounting for entropy changes.

2.1.2 System and Surroundings

Most applications of thermodynamics require the definition of a system and its surroundings. A system can be an object, any quantity of matter, or any region of space selected for study and set apart (mentally) from everything else, which then becomes the surroundings. The systems of interest in thermodynamics are finite, and the point of view taken is macroscopic rather than microscopic. No account is taken of the detailed structure of matter, and only the coarse characteristics of the system, such as its temperature and pressure, are regarded as thermodynamic coordinates.

Everything external to the system is the surroundings, and the system is separated from the surroundings by the system boundaries. These boundaries may be either movable or fixed; either real or imaginary.

2.1.3 Properties and State

A property of a system is any observable characteristic of the system. The more common thermodynamic properties are temperature, pressure, specific volume or density, internal energy, enthalpy, and entropy.

The state of a system is its condition or configuration described in sufficient detail so that one state may be distinguished from all other states. A listing of a sufficient number of independent properties constitutes a complete definition of the state of a system.

The state may be identified or described by observable, macroscopic properties such as temperature, pressure, and density. Each property of a substance in a given state has only one value; this property always has the same value for a given state, regardless of how the substance arrived at that state. In fact, a property can be defined as any quantity that depends on the state of the system and is independent of the path (i.e., the prior history) by which the system arrived at that given state. Conversely, the state is specified or described by its properties.

The state of a macroscopic system is the condition of the system as characterized by the values of its properties. This chapter directs attention to **equilibrium states**, with equilibrium used in its generally accepted context—the equality of forces, or the state of balance. In future discussion, the term *state* refers to an equilibrium state unless otherwise noted. The concept of equilibrium is important, as it is only in an equilibrium state that thermodynamic properties have meaning. A system is in thermodynamic equilibrium if it is incapable of finite, spontaneous change to another state without a finite change in the state of the surroundings.

Included in the many types of equilibria are thermal, mechanical, and chemical. A system in thermal equilibrium is at the same temperature as the environment and the temperature is the same throughout. A system in mechanical equilibrium has no part accelerating ($\Sigma F = 0$) and the pressure within the system is the same as in the environment. A system in chemical equilibrium does not tend to undergo a chemical reaction; the matter in the system is said to be inert.

Any property of a thermodynamic system has a fixed value in a given equilibrium state, regardless of how the system arrives at that state. Therefore, the change that occurs in the value of a property when a system is altered from one equilibrium state to another is always the same. This is true regardless of the method used to bring about a change between the two end states. The converse of this statement is equally true. If a measured quantity always has the same value between two given states, that quantity is a measure of the change in a property. This latter assertion is useful in connection with the conservation of energy principle introduced in the next section.

The uniqueness of a property value for a given state can be described mathematically in the following manner. The integral of an exact differential dY is given by:

$$\int_1^2 dY = Y_2 - Y_1 = \Delta Y$$

Thus the value of the integral depends solely on the initial and final states. Likewise, the change in the value of a property depends only on the end states. Hence the differential change dY in a property Y is an exact differential. Throughout this text, the infinitesimal variation of a property will be identified by the differential symbol d preceding the property symbol. For example, the infinitesimal change in the pressure p of a system is given by dp. The finite change in a property is denoted by the symbol Δ (capital delta), for example, Δp. The change in a property value ΔY always represents the final value minus the initial value. This convention must be kept in mind.

The symbol δ is used instead of the usual differential operator d as a reminder that some quantities depend on the process and are not a property of the system. δQ represents only a small quantity of heat, not a differential. δm represents only a small quantity of matter.

The same qualifications for δ hold in the case of thermodynamic work. As there is no exact differential dW, small quantities of W similar in magnitude to differentials are expressed as δW.

2.1.4 Processes and Cycles

A process is a change in state which can be defined as *any change in the properties of a system.* A process is described in part by the series of states passed through by the system. Often, but not always, some interaction between the system and surroundings occurs during a process; the specification of this interaction completes the description of the process.

Describing a process typically involves specifying the initial and final equilibrium states, the path (if identifiable), and the interactions which take place across the boundaries of the system during the process. The following terms define special processes:

isobaric or **constant pressure**—process wherein the pressure does not change;

isothermal—process that occurs at constant temperature;

isometric—process with constant volume;

adiabatic—process in which no heat is transferred to or from the system;

isentropic—process with no change in entropy.

A **cycle** is a process, or more frequently, a series of processes wherein the initial and final states of the system are identical. Therefore, at the conclusion of a cycle, all the properties have the same value they had at the beginning.

2.1.5 Reversibility

All naturally occurring changes or processes are irreversible. Like a clock, they tend to run down and cannot rewind themselves without other changes in the surroundings occurring. Familiar examples are the transfer of heat with a finite temperature difference, the mixing of two gases, a waterfall, and a chemical reaction. *All of the above changes can be reversed, however.* Heat can be transferred from a region of low temperature to one of higher temperature; gas can be separated into its components; water can be forced to flow uphill. The important point is that these things can be done *only at the expense of some other system*, which itself becomes run down.

A process is reversible if its direction can be reversed at any stage by an infinitesimal change in external conditions. If a connected series of equilibrium states is considered, each representing only an infinitesimal displacement from the adjacent one, but with the overall result a finite change, then a reversible process exists.

All actual processes can be made to approach a reversible process by a suitable choice of conditions; but like the absolute zero of temperature, the strictly reversible process is only a concept that aids in the analysis of problems. The approach of actual processes to this ideal limit can be made almost as close as is desired. However, the closeness of approach is generally limited by economic factors rather than physical ones. The truly reversible process would require an infinite time for completion. The sole reason for the concept of the reversible process is to establish a standard for the comparison of actual processes. The reversible process is one that gives the maximum accomplishment, i.e., yields the greatest amount of work or requires the least amount of work to bring about a given change. It gives the maximum efficiency toward which to strive, but which will never be equalled. The reversible process is the standard for judging the efficiency of an actual process.

Since the reversible process represents a succession of equilibrium states, each only a differential step from its neighbor, the reversible process can be represented as a continuous line on a state diagram (*p-v*, *T-s*, etc.). The irreversible process cannot be so represented. The terminal states and general direction of change can be noted, but the complete path of change is an indeterminate, irreversible process and cannot be drawn as a line on a thermodynamic diagram.

Irreversibilities always lower the efficiencies of processes. Their effect is identical to that of friction, which is one cause of irreversibility. Conversely, no process more efficient than a reversible process can be imagined. The reversible process represents a standard of perfection that cannot be exceeded because:

1. It places an upper limit on the work that may be obtained for a given work-producing process;
2. It places a lower limit on the work input for a given work-requiring process.

2.1.6 Conservation of Mass

From relativistic considerations, mass m and energy E are related by the well-known equation:

$$E = mc^2$$

where c = velocity of light.

This equation shows that the mass of a system does change when its energy changes. However, for other than nuclear reactions, the change is quite small and even the most accurate chemical balance cannot detect the change in mass. Thus, conservation of mass and conservation of energy are treated as separate laws in basic thermodynamics.

The mass rate of flow of a fluid passing through a cross-sectional area A is:

$$m = AV/v \tag{2-1}$$

where V is the average velocity of the fluid in a direction normal to the plane of the area A, and v is the specific volume of the fluid. For steady flow with fluid entering a system at a section 1 and leaving at a section 2,

$$m_1 = m_2 = A_1V_1/v_1 = A_2V_2/v_2$$

This is the continuity equation of steady flow. It can readily be extended to any number of system inlets and outlets and is used in nearly all energy analyses.

2.2 Properties of a Substance

2.2.1 Specific Volume and Density

The specific volume of a substance v is the volume per unit mass. The density of a substance ρ is the mass per unit volume, and is therefore the reciprocal of the specific volume. Specific volume and density are intensive properties in that they are independent of the size of the system.

2.2.2 Pressure

When dealing with liquids and gases, we ordinarily speak of *pressure*; in solids we speak of *stresses*. The pressure in a fluid at rest at a given point is the same in all directions. Pressure is defined as the normal component of force per unit area.

Absolute pressure is the quantity of interest in most thermodynamic investigations. Most pressure and vacuum gages, however, read the difference between absolute pressure and the atmospheric pressure existing at the gage (Figure 2-1).

2.2.3 Temperature

Because temperature is difficult to define, equality of temperature is defined instead. Two bodies have **equality of temperature** if no change in any observable property occurs when they are in thermal communication.

The **zeroth law of thermodynamics** states that when two bodies have equality of temperature with a third body, they in turn have equality of temperature with each other. Since this fact is not derivable from other laws, and since in the logical presentation of thermodynamics it precedes the first and second laws of thermodynamics, it has been called the zeroth law of thermodynamics. This law is the basis of temperature measurement. Every time a body has equality of temperature with a thermometer, it is said that the body has the temperature read on the thermometer. The problem remains, however, of relating temperatures that might be read on different thermometers, or that are obtained when different temperature-measuring devices are used, such as thermocouples and resis-

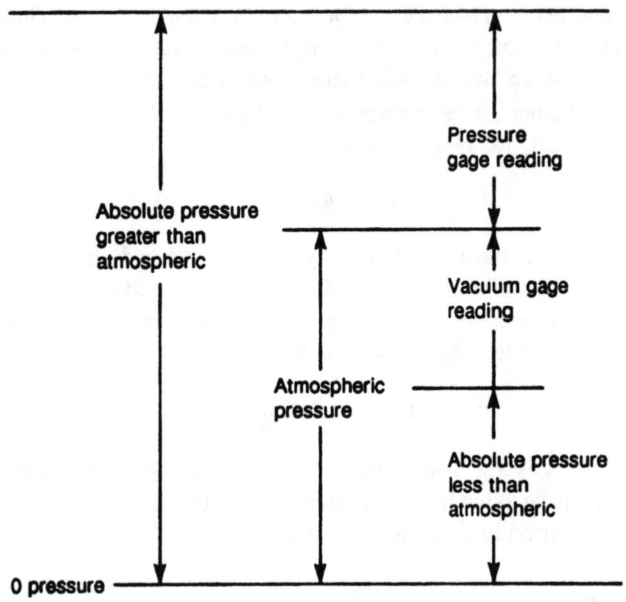

Fig. 2-1 Terms Used in Pressure Measurement

tance thermometers. The need for a standard scale for temperature measurements is apparent.

Fahrenheit and **Celsius** are two commonly used temperature measuring scales. The Celsius scale was formerly called the Centigrade scale.

In this text, the abbreviations °F and °C denote the Fahrenheit and Celsius scales, respectively. The symbols t and T are both used in the literature for temperature on all temperature scales. Unfortunately, little uniformity exists with nomenclature in engineering.

The absolute scale related to the Celsius scale is referred to as the Kelvin scale and is designated K. For SI units, the degree sign is not used with the Kelvin scale. The relation between the SI temperature scales is:

$$K = °C + 273.15$$

The absolute scale related to the Fahrenheit scale is referred to as the Rankine scale and is designated °R. The relation between these scales is:

$$°R = °F + 459.67$$

2.2.4 Internal Energy

Internal energy refers to the energy possessed by a material due to the motion and/or position of the molecules. This form of energy may be divided into two parts: (1) kinetic internal energy, which is due to the velocity of the molecules; and (2) potential internal energy, which is due to the attractive forces existing between molecules. Changes in the average velocity of molecules are indicated by temperature changes of the system; variations in relative distance between molecules are denoted by changes in phase of the system.

The symbol U designates the internal energy of a given mass of a substance. Following the convention used with other extensive properties, the symbol u designates the internal energy per unit mass. As in the case of specific volume, u can represent specific internal energy.

2.2.5 Enthalpy

In analyzing specific types of processes, certain combinations of thermodynamic properties, which are therefore also properties of the substance undergoing the change of state, are frequently encountered. One such combination is $U + pV$. It is convenient to define a new extensive property, called *enthalpy*:

$$H = U + pV$$

or, per unit mass:

$$h = u + pv \tag{2-2}$$

As in the case of internal energy, specific enthalpy can be referred to as h, and total enthalpy H. However, both may be called enthalpy, since the context makes it clear which is meant.

2.2.6 Entropy

Entropy S is a measure of the molecular disorder or of the probability of a given state. The more disordered a system, the greater is its entropy; conversely, an orderly or unmixed configuration is one of low entropy.

By applying the theory of probability to molecular systems, Boltzmann showed a simple relationship between the entropy of a given system of molecules and the probability of its occurrence. This relationship is given as:

$$S = k \ln W$$

where k is the Boltzmann constant and W is the thermodynamic probability.

Since entropy is the property used in quantifying the Second Law of Thermodynamics, additional discussion from a classical thermodynamic viewpoint will be presented when the 2nd Law is covered.

2.2.7 Specific Heats

The constant-volume specific heat and the constant-pressure specific heat are useful functions for thermodynamic calculations—particularly for gases.

The constant-volume specific heat c_v is defined by the relation:

$$c_v = (\partial u / \partial T)_v \tag{2-3}$$

The constant-pressure specific heat c_p is defined by the relation:

$$c_v = (\partial h / \partial T)_p \tag{2-4}$$

Note that each of these quantities is defined in terms of properties. Thus, the constant-volume and constant-pressure specific heats are thermodynamic properties of a substance.

2.2.8 Dimensions and Units

The fundamental and primitive concepts which underlie all physical measurements and all properties are: time, length, mass, absolute temperature, electric current, and amount of substance. Arbitrary scales of measurement must be established for these primary dimensions, with each scale divided into specific units of size. The internationally accepted base units for the six quantities are as follows:

length	metre (m)
mass	kilogram (kg)
tim	second (s)
electric current	ampere (A)
thermodynamic temperature	kelvin (K)
amount of substance	mole (mol)

Each of these has a precise definition according to international agreement. They form the basis for the SI from the French document, *Le Système International d'Unités* (*SI*), or International System of Units.

The mass of a system is often given by stating the number of moles it contains. A mole is the mass of a chemical species equal numerically to its molecular mass. Thus, a kilogram mole of oxygen (O_2) contains 32 kilograms. In addition, the number of molecules in a kilogram mole is the same for all substances. This is also true for a gram mole, and in this case the number of molecules is Avogadro's number, equal to 6.0225×10^{23} molecules.

Many derived units are important in thermodynamics. Examples are force, pressure, and density. Force is determined through Newton's second law of motion, $F = ma$, and has the basic unit kg·m/s^2. The SI unit for this composite set is the newton (N). Pressure is defined as force per unit area (N/m^2), called the pascal (Pa); and density is mass per unit volume (kg/m^3).

The U.S. customary engineering system of units also recognizes the second as the basic unit of time, and the ampere as the unit of current. However, absolute temperature is measured in degrees Rankine (°R). The foot (ft) is the usual unit of length and the pound mass (lb_m) is the unit of mass. The molar unit is the pound mole. ASHRAE calls this system the inch-pound (I-P) unit system.

The unit of force, the pound force (lb_f), is defined without reference to Newton's second law, so this law must be written to include a dimensional proportionality constant:

$$F = ma/g_c$$

where g_c is the proportionality constant. In the I-P system, the proportionality constant is:

$$g_c = 32.174\ (lb_m/lb_f)(ft/s^2)$$

The unit of density is lb_m/ft^3, and the unit of pressure is lb_f/ft^2 or lb_f/in^2, often written psi. Pressure gages usually measure pressure relative to atmospheric pressure. The term **absolute pressure** is often used to distinguish thermodynamic (actual) pressure (psia) from gage (relative) pressure (psig).

In SI units, the proportionality constant g_c in Newton's law is unity or:

$$g_c = 1\ (kg/N)(m/s^2)$$

In this book, all equations that derive from Newton's law carry the constant g_c.

2.2.9 Pure Substance

A pure substance is one that has a homogeneous and invariable chemical composition. It may exist in more than one phase, but the chemical composition is the same in all phases. Thus, liquid water, a mixture of liquid water and water vapor (steam), or a mixture of ice and liquid water are all pure substances, for every phase has the same chemical composition. On the other hand, a mixture of liquid air and gaseous air is not a pure substance, since the composition of the liquid phase is different from that of the vapor phase.

Sometimes a mixture of gases is considered a pure substance as long as there is no change of phase. Strictly speaking, this is not true. A mixture of gases, such as air, exhibits some of the characteristics of a pure substance as long as there is no change of phase.

Consider as a system that water is contained in the piston-cylinder arrangement of Figure 2-2. Suppose that the piston maintains a pressure of 14.7 lb_f/in (101.3 kPa) in the cylinder containing H_2O, and that the initial temperature is 59°F (15°C). As heat is transferred to the water, the temperature increases appreciably, the specific volume increases slightly, and the pressure remains constant. When the temperature reaches 212°F (100°C), additional heat transfer results in a change of phase. That is, some of the liquid becomes vapor, and during this process both the temperature and pressure remain constant, while the specific volume increases considerably. When the last drop of liquid has vaporized, further heat transfer results in an increase in both temperature and specific volume of the vapor.

Saturation temperature designates the temperature at which vaporization takes place at a given pressure; this pressure is called the *saturation pressure* for the given temperature. Thus for water at 212°F (100°C), the saturation pressure is 14.7 lb_f/in^2 (101.3 kPa), and for water at 14.7 lb_f/in^2 (101.3 kPa), the saturation temperature is 212°F (100°C).

If a substance exists as liquid at the saturation temperature and pressure, it is called saturated liquid. If the temperature of the liquid is lower than the saturation temperature for the existing pressure, it is called a subcooled liquid (implying that the temperature is lower than the saturation temperature for the given pressure) or a compressed liquid (implying that the pressure is greater than the saturation pressure for the given temperature).

When a substance exists as part liquid and part vapor at the saturation temperature, its quality is defined as the ratio of the mass of vapor to the total mass. The quality may be considered as an intensive property, and it has the symbol x. Quality has meaning only when the substance is in a saturated state, i.e., at saturation pressure and temperature.

If a substance exists as vapor at the saturation temperature, it is called **saturated vapor**. (Sometimes the term dry satu-

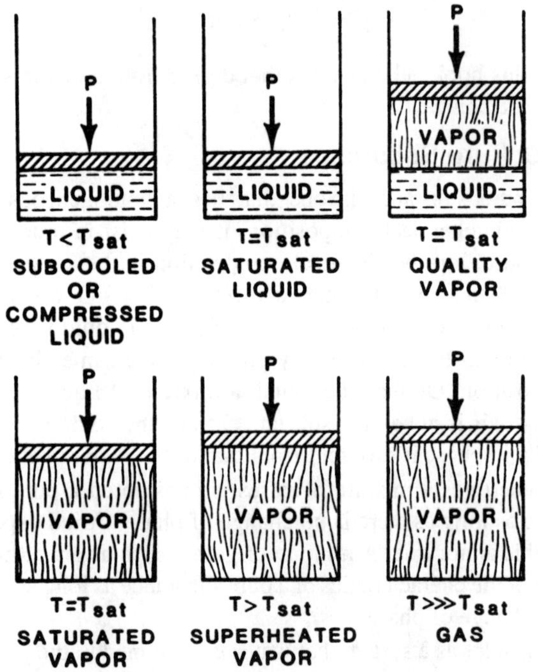

Fig. 2-2 Thermodynamic Fluid States

rated vapor is used to emphasize that the quality is 100%.) When the vapor is at a temperature greater than the saturation temperature, it is said to exist as superheated vapor. The pressure and temperature of superheated vapor are independent properties because the temperature may increase while the pressure remains constant. Actually, gases are highly superheated vapors.

The entire range of phases is summarized by Figure 2-3, which shows how the solid, liquid, and vapor phases may exist together in equilibrium. Along the sublimation line, the solid and vapor phases are in equilibrium, along the fusion line, the solid and liquid phases are in equilibrium, and along the vaporization line, the liquid and vapor phases are in equilibrium. The only point at which all three phases may exist in equilibrium is the triple point. The vaporization line ends at the critical point because there is no distinct change from the liquid phase to the vapor phase above the critical point.

Consider a solid in state A, Figure 2-3. When the temperature is increased while the pressure (which is less than the triple point pressure) is constant, the substance passes directly from the solid to the vapor phase. Along the constant pressure line EF, the substance first passes from the solid to the liquid phase at one temperature, and then from the liquid to the vapor phase at a higher temperature. Constant-pressure line CD passes through the triple point, and it is only at the triple point that the three phases may exist together in equilibrium. At a pressure above the critical pressure, such as GH, there is no sharp distinction between the liquid and vapor phases.

One important reason for introducing the concept of a pure substance is that the state of a simple compressible pure substance is defined by two independent properties. This means, for example, if the specific volume and temperature

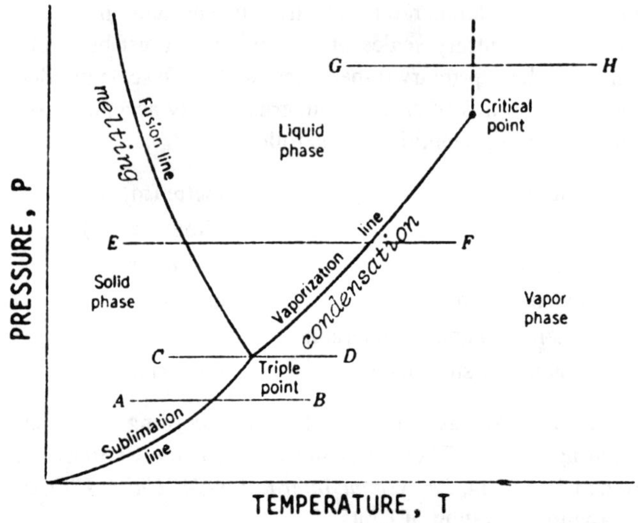

Fig. 2-3 The Pure Substance

of superheated steam are specified, the state of the steam is determined.

To understand the significance of the term **independent property**, consider the saturated-liquid and saturated-vapor states of a pure substance. These two states have the same pressure and the same temperature, but are definitely not the same state. Therefore, in a saturation state, pressure and temperature are not independent properties. Two independent properties such as pressure and specific volume, or pressure and quality, are required to specify a saturation state of a pure substance.

Thus, a mixture of gases, such as air, has the same characteristics as a pure substance, as long as only one phase is present. The state of air, which is a mixture of gases of definite composition, is determined by specifying two properties as long as it remains in the gaseous phase, and in this regard, air can be treated as a pure substance.

2.2.10 Tables and Graphs of Thermodynamic Properties

Tables of thermodynamic properties of many substances are available, and they all generally have the same form. This section refers to the tables for H_2O and R-134a, as well as their respective Mollier diagrams, the *h-s* chart for steam, and the *p-h* diagram for R-134a.

Table 3 in Chapter 6 of the 1997 *Handbook—Fundamentals* gives thermodynamic properties of water at saturation and is reproduced in part as Table 2-1 on the following pages. In Table 2-1, the first two columns after the temperature give the corresponding saturation pressure in pounds force per square inch and in inches of mercury. The next three columns give specific volume in cubic feet per pound mass. The first of these gives the specific volume of the saturated liquid v_f; the third column gives the specific volume of saturated vapor v_g. The difference between these two values, $v_g - v_f$, represents the increase in specific volume when the state changes from saturated liquid to saturated vapor, and is designated v_{fg}.

Table 2-1 Thermodynamic Properties of Water

(Table 3, Chapter 6, 1997 *Handbook—Fundamentals*)

Temp. t, °F	Absolute Pressure p psi	Absolute Pressure p in. Hg	Specific Volume, ft³/lb Sat. Solid/Liq. v_i	Specific Volume Evap. v_{ig}	Specific Volume Sat. Vapor v_g	Enthalpy, Btu/lb Sat. Solid/Liq. h_i	Enthalpy Evap. h_{ig}	Enthalpy Sat. Vapor h_g	Entropy, Btu/lb·°F Sat. Solid/Liq. s_i	Entropy Evap. s_{ig}	Entropy Sat. Vapor s_g	Temp., °F
−80	0.000116	0.000236	0.01732	1953234	1953234	−193.50	1219.19	1025.69	−0.4067	3.2112	2.8045	−80
−79	0.000125	0.000254	0.01732	1814052	1814052	−193.11	1219.24	1026.13	−0.4056	3.2029	2.7972	−79
−78	0.000135	0.000275	0.01732	1685445	1685445	−192.71	1219.28	1026.57	−0.4046	3.1946	2.7900	−78
−77	0.000145	0.000296	0.01732	1566663	1566663	−192.31	1219.33	1027.02	−0.4036	3.1964	2.7828	−77
−76	0.000157	0.000319	0.01732	1456752	1456752	−191.92	1219.38	1027.46	−0.4025	3.1782	2.7757	−76
−75	0.000169	0.000344	0.01733	1355059	1355059	−191.52	1219.42	1027.90	−0.4015	3.1701	2.7685	−75
−74	0.000182	0.000371	0.01733	1260977	1260977	−191.12	1219.47	1028.34	−0.4005	3.1619	2.7615	−74
−73	0.000196	0.000399	0.01733	1173848	1173848	−190.72	1219.51	1028.79	−0.3994	3.1539	2.7544	−73
−72	0.000211	0.000430	0.01733	1093149	1093149	−190.32	1219.55	1029.23	−0.3984	3.1459	2.7475	−72
−71	0.000227	0.000463	0.01733	1018381	1018381	−189.92	1219.59	1029.67	−0.3974	3.1379	2.7405	−71
−70	0.000245	0.000498	0.01733	949067	949067	−189.52	1219.63	1030.11	−0.3963	3.1299	2.7336	−70
−69	0.000263	0.000536	0.01733	884803	884803	−189.11	1219.67	1030.55	−0.3953	3.1220	2.7267	−69
−68	0.000283	0.000576	0.01733	825187	825187	−188.71	1219.71	1031.00	−0.3943	3.1141	2.7199	−68
−67	0.000304	0.000619	0.01734	769864	769864	−188.30	1219.74	1031.44	−0.3932	3.1063	2.7131	−67
−66	0.000326	0.000664	0.01734	718508	718508	−187.90	1219.78	1031.88	−0.3922	3.0985	2.7063	−66
−65	0.000350	0.000714	0.01734	670800	670800	−187.49	1219.82	1032.32	−0.3912	3.0907	2.6996	−65
−64	0.000376	0.000766	0.01734	626503	626503	−187.08	1219.85	1032.77	−0.3901	3.0830	2.6929	−64
−63	0.000404	0.000822	0.01734	585316	585316	−186.67	1219.88	1033.21	−0.3891	3.0753	2.6862	−63
−62	0.000433	0.000882	0.01734	548041	547041	−186.26	1219.91	1033.65	−0.3881	3.0677	2.6730	−62
−61	0.000464	0.000945	0.01734	511446	511446	−185.85	1219.95	1034.09	−0.3870	3.0601	2.6730	−61
−60	0.000498	0.001013	0.01734	478317	478317	−185.44	1219.98	1034.54	−0.3860	3.0525	2.6665	−60
−59	0.000533	0.001086	0.01735	447495	447495	−185.03	1220.01	1034.98	−0.3850	3.0449	2.6600	−59
−58	0.000571	0.001163	0.01735	418803	418803	−184.61	1220.03	1035.42	−0.3839	3.0374	2.6535	−58
−57	0.000612	0.001246	0.01735	392068	392068	−184.20	1220.06	1035.86	−0.3829	3.0299	2.6470	−57
−56	0.000655	0.001333	0.01735	367172	367172	−183.78	1220.09	1036.30	−0.3819	3.0225	2.6406	−56
−55	0.000701	0.001427	0.01735	343970	343970	−183.37	1220.11	1036.75	−0.3808	3.0151	2.6342	−55
−54	0.000750	0.001526	0.01735	322336	322336	−182.95	1220.14	1037.19	−0.3798	3.0077	2.6279	−54
−53	0.000802	0.001632	0.01735	302157	302157	−182.53	1220.16	1037.63	−0.3788	3.0004	2.6216	−53
−52	0.000857	0.001745	0.01735	283335	283335	−182.11	1220.18	1038.07	−0.3778	2.9931	2.6153	−52
−51	0.000916	0.001865	0.01736	265773	265773	−181.69	1220.21	1038.52	−0.3767	2.9858	2.6091	−51
−50	0.000979	0.001992	0.01736	249381	249381	−181.27	1220.23	1038.96	−0.3757	2.9786	2.6029	−50
−49	0.001045	0.002128	0.01736	234067	234067	−180.85	1220.25	1039.40	−0.3747	2.9714	2.5967	−49
−48	0.001116	0.002272	0.01736	219766	219766	−180.42	1220.26	1039.84	−0.3736	2.9642	2.5906	−48
−47	0.001191	0.002425	0.01736	206398	206398	−180.00	1220.28	1040.28	−0.3726	2.9570	2.5844	−47
−46	0.001271	0.002587	0.01736	193909	193909	−179.57	1220.30	1040.73	−0.3716	2.9499	2.5784	−46
−45	0.001355	0.002760	0.01736	182231	182231	−179.14	1220.31	1041.17	−0.3705	2.9429	2.5723	−45
−44	0.001445	0.002943	0.01736	171304	171304	−178.72	1220.33	1041.61	−0.3695	2.9358	2.5663	−44
−43	0.001541	0.003137	0.01737	161084	161084	−178.79	1220.34	1042.05	−0.3685	2.9288	2.5603	−43
−42	0.001642	0.003343	0.01737	151518	151518	−177.86	1220.36	1042.50	−0.3675	2.9218	2.5544	−42
−41	0.001749	0.003562	0.01737	142566	142566	−177.43	1220.37	1042.94	−0.3664	2.9149	2.5485	−41
−40	0.001863	0.003793	0.01737	134176	134176	−177.00	1220.38	1043.38	−0.3654	2.9080	2.5426	−40
−39	0.001984	0.004039	0.01737	126322	126322	−176.57	1220.39	1043.82	−0.3644	2.9011	2.5367	−39
−38	0.002111	0.004299	0.01737	118959	118959	−176.13	1220.40	1044.27	−0.3633	2.8942	2.5309	−38
−37	0.002247	0.004574	0.01737	112058	112058	−175.70	1220.40	1044.71	−0.3623	2.8874	2.5251	−37
−36	0.002390	0.004866	0.01738	105592	105592	−175.26	1220.41	1045.15	−0.3613	2.8806	2.5193	−36
−35	0.002542	0.005175	0.01738	99522	99522	−174.83	1220.42	1045.59	−0.3603	2.8738	2.5136	−35
−34	0.002702	0.005502	0.01738	93828	93828	−174.39	1220.42	1046.03	−0.3592	2.8671	2.5078	−34
−33	0.002872	0.005848	0.01738	88489	88489	−173.95	1220.43	1046.48	−0.3582	2.8604	2.5022	−33
−32	0.003052	0.006213	0.01738	83474	83474	−173.51	1220.43	1046.92	−0.3572	2.8537	2.4965	−32
−31	0.003242	0.006600	0.01738	78763	78763	−173.07	1220.43	1047.36	−0.3561	2.8470	2.4909	−31
−30	0.003443	0.007009	0.01738	74341	74341	−172.63	1220.43	1047.80	−0.3551	2.8404	2.4853	−30
−29	0.003655	0.007441	0.01738	70187	70187	−172.19	1220.43	1048.25	−0.3541	2.8338	2.4797	−29
−28	0.003879	0.007898	0.01739	66282	66282	−171.74	1220.43	1048.69	−0.3531	2.8272	2.4742	−28
−27	0.004116	0.008380	0.01739	62613	62613	−171.30	1220.43	1049.13	−0.3520	2.8207	2.4687	−27
−26	0.004366	0.008890	0.01739	59161	59161	−170.86	1220.43	1049.57	−0.3510	2.8142	2.4632	−26
−25	0.004630	0.009428	0.01739	55915	55915	−170.41	1220.42	1050.01	−0.3500	2.8077	2.4577	−25
−24	0.004909	0.009995	0.01739	52861	52861	−169.96	1220.42	1050.46	−0.3489	2.8013	2.4523	−24
−23	0.005203	0.010594	0.01739	49986	49986	−169.51	1220.41	1050.90	−0.3479	2.7948	2.4469	−23
−22	0.005514	0.011226	0.01739	47281	47281	−169.07	1220.41	1051.34	−0.3469	2.7884	2.4415	−22
−21	0.005841	0.011892	0.01740	44733	44733	−168.62	1220.40	1051.78	−0.3459	2.7820	2.4362	−21
−20	0.006186	0.012595	0.01740	42333	42333	−168.16	1220.39	1052.22	−0.3448	2.7757	2.4309	−20
−19	0.006550	0.013336	0.01740	40073	40073	−167.71	1220.38	1052.67	−0.3438	2.7694	2.4256	−19
−18	0.006933	0.014117	0.01740	37943	37943	−167.26	1220.37	1053.11	−0.3428	2.7631	2.4203	−18
−17	0.007337	0.014939	0.01740	35934	35934	−166.81	1220.36	1053.55	−0.3418	2.7568	2.4151	−17
−16	0.007763	0.015806	0.01740	34041	34041	−166.35	1220.34	1053.99	−0.3407	2.7506	2.4098	−16
−15	0.008211	0.016718	0.01740	32256	32256	−165.90	1220.33	1054.43	−0.3397	2.7444	2.4046	−15
−14	0.008683	0.017678	0.01741	30572	30572	−165.44	1220.31	1054.87	−0.3387	2.7382	2.3995	−14

Table 2-1 Thermodynamic Properties of Water (*Continued*)

(Table 3, Chapter 6, 1997 *Handbook—Fundamentals*)

	Absolute Pressure p		Specific Volume, ft³/lb			Enthalpy, Btu/lb			Entropy, Btu/lb·°F			
Temp. t, °F	psi	in. Hg	Sat. Solid/Liq. v_i	Evap. v_{ig}	Sat. Vapor v_g	Sat. Solid/Liq. h_i	Evap. h_{ig}	Sat. Vapor h_g	Sat. Solid/Liq. s_i	Evap. s_{ig}	Sat. Vapor s_g	Temp., °F
−13	0.009179	0.018689	0.01741	28983	28983	−164.98	1220.30	1055.32	−0.3377	2.7320	2.3943	−13
−12	0.009702	0.019753	0.01741	27483	27483	−164.52	1220.28	1055.76	−0.3366	2.7259	2.3892	−12
−11	0.010252	0.020873	0.01741	26067	26067	−164.06	1220.26	1056.20	−0.3356	2.7197	2.3841	−11
−10	0.010830	0.022050	0.01741	24730	24730	−163.60	1220.24	1056.64	−0.3346	2.7136	2.3791	−10
−9	0.011438	0.023288	0.01741	23467	23467	−163.14	1220.22	1057.08	−0.3335	2.7076	2.3740	−9
−8	0.012077	0.024590	0.01741	22274	22274	−162.68	1220.20	1057.53	−0.3325	2.7015	2.3690	−8
−7	0.012749	0.025958	0.01742	21147	21147	−162.21	1220.18	1057.97	−0.3315	2.6955	2.3640	−7
−6	0.013456	0.027396	0.01742	20081	20081	−162.75	1220.16	1058.41	−0.3305	2.6895	2.3591	−6
−5	0.014197	0.028906	0.01742	19074	19074	−161.28	1220.13	1058.85	−0.3294	2.6836	2.3541	−5
−4	0.014977	0.030493	0.01742	18121	18121	−160.82	1220.11	1059.29	−0.3284	2.6776	2.3492	−4
−3	0.015795	0.032159	0.01742	17220	17220	−160.35	1220.08	1059.73	−0.3274	2.6717	2.3443	−3
−2	0.016654	0.033908	0.01742	16367	16367	−159.88	1220.05	1060.17	−0.3264	2.6658	2.3394	−2
−1	0.017556	0.035744	0.01742	15561	15561	−159.41	1220.02	1060.62	−0.3253	2.6599	2.3346	−1
0	0.018502	0.037671	0.01743	14797	14797	−158.94	1220.00	1061.06	−0.3243	2.6541	2.3298	0
1	0.019495	0.039693	0.01743	14073	14073	−158.47	1219.96	1061.50	−0.3233	2.6482	2.3249	1
2	0.020537	0.041813	0.01743	13388	13388	−157.99	1219.93	1061.94	−0.3223	2.6424	2.3202	2
3	0.021629	0.044037	0.01743	12740	12740	−157.52	1219.90	1062.38	−0.3212	2.6367	2.3154	3
4	0.022774	0.046369	0.01743	12125	12125	−157.05	1219.87	1062.82	−0.3202	2.6309	2.3107	4
5	0.023975	0.048813	0.01743	11543	11543	−156.57	1219.83	1063.26	−0.3192	2.6252	2.3060	5
6	0.025233	0.051375	0.01743	10991	10991	−156.09	1219.80	1063.70	−0.3182	2.6194	2.3013	6
7	0.026552	0.054059	0.01744	10468	10468	−155.62	1219.76	1064.14	−0.3171	2.6138	2.2966	7
8	0.027933	0.056872	0.01744	9971	9971	−155.14	1219.72	1064.58	−0.3161	2.6081	2.2920	8
9	0.029379	0.059817	0.01744	9500	9500	−154.66	−1219.68	−1065.03	−0.3151	−2.6024	−2.2873	9
10	0.030894	0.062901	0.01744	9054	9054	−154.18	1219.64	1065.47	−0.3141	2.5968	2.2827	10
11	0.032480	0.066131	0.01744	8630	8630	−153.70	1219.60	1065.91	−0.3130	2.5912	2.2782	11
12	0.034140	0.069511	0.01744	8228	8228	−153.21	1219.56	1066.35	−0.3120	2.5856	2.2736	12
13	0.035878	0.073047	0.01745	7846	7846	−152.73	1219.52	1066.79	−0.3110	2.5801	2.2691	13
14	0.037696	0.076748	0.01745	7483	7483	−152.24	1219.47	1067.23	−0.3100	2.5745	2.2645	14
15	0.039597	0.080621	0.01745	7139	7139	−151.76	1219.43	1067.67	−0.3089	2.5690	2.2600	15
16	0.041586	0.084671	0.01745	6811	6811	−151.27	1219.38	1068.11	−0.3079	2.5635	2.2556	16
17	0.043666	0.088905	0.01745	6501	6501	−150.78	1219.33	1068.55	−0.3069	2.5580	2.2511	17
18	0.045841	0.093332	0.01745	6205	6205	−150.30	1219.28	1068.99	−0.3059	2.5526	2.2467	18
19	0.048113	0.097960	0.01745	5924	5924	−149.81	1219.23	1069.43	−0.3049	2.5471	2.2423	19
20	0.050489	0.102796	0.01746	5657	5657	−149.32	1219.18	1069.87	−0.3038	2.5417	2.2379	20
21	0.052970	0.107849	0.01746	5404	5404	−148.82	1219.13	1070.31	−0.3028	2.5363	2.2335	21
22	0.055563	0.113128	0.01746	5162	5162	−148.33	1219.08	1070.75	−0.3018	2.5309	2.2292	22
23	0.058271	0.118641	0.01746	4932	4932	−147.84	1219.02	1071.19	−0.3008	2.5256	2.2248	23
24	0.061099	0.124398	0.01746	4714	4714	−147.34	1218.97	1071.63	−0.2997	2.5203	2.2205	24
25	0.064051	0.130408	0.01746	4506	4506	−146.85	1218.91	1072.07	−0.2987	2.5149	2.2162	25
26	0.067133	0.136684	0.01747	4308	4308	−146.35	1218.85	1072.50	−0.2977	2.5096	2.2119	26
27	0.070349	0.143233	0.01747	4119	4119	−145.85	1218.80	1072.94	−0.2967	2.5044	2.2077	27
28	0.073706	0.150066	0.01747	3940	3940	−145.35	1218.74	1073.38	−0.2956	2.4991	2.2035	28
29	0.077207	0.157195	0.01747	3769	3769	−144.85	1218.68	1073.82	−0.2946	2.4939	2.1992	29
30	0.080860	0.164632	0.01747	3606	3606	−144.35	1218.61	1074.26	−0.2936	2.4886	2.1951	30
31	0.084669	0.172387	0.01747	3450	3450	−143.85	1218.55	1074.70	−0.2926	2.4834	2.1909	31
32	0.088640	0.180474	0.01747	3302	3302	−143.35	1218.49	1075.14	−0.2915	2.4783	2.1867	32
32*	0.08865	0.18049	0.01602	3302.07	3302.09	−0.02	1075.15	1075.14	0.0000	2.1867	2.1867	32
33	0.09229	0.18791	0.01602	3178.15	3178.16	0.99	1074.59	1075.58	0.0020	2.1811	2.1832	33
34	0.09607	0.19559	0.01602	3059.47	3059.49	2.00	1074.02	1076.01	0.0041	2.1756	2.1796	34
35	0.09998	0.20355	0.01602	2945.66	2945.68	3.00	1073.45	1076.45	0.0061	2.1700	2.1761	35
36	0.10403	0.21180	0.01602	2836.60	2836.61	4.01	1072.88	1076.89	0.0081	2.1645	2.1726	36
37	0.10822	0.22035	0.01602	2732.13	2732.15	5.02	1072.32	1077.33	0.0102	2.1590	2.1692	37
38	0.11257	0.22919	0.01602	2631.88	2631.89	6.02	1071.75	1077.77	0.0122	2.1535	2.1657	38
39	0.11707	0.23835	0.01602	2535.86	2535.88	7.03	1071.18	1078.21	0.0142	2.1481	2.1623	39
40	0.12172	0.24783	0.01602	2443.67	2443.69	8.03	1070.62	1078.65	0.0162	2.1426	2.1589	40
41	0.12654	0.25765	0.01602	2355.22	2355.24	9.04	1070.05	1079.09	0.0182	2.1372	2.1554	41
42	0.13153	0.26780	0.01602	2270.42	2270.43	10.04	1069.48	1079.52	0.0202	2.1318	2.1521	42
43	0.13669	0.27831	0.01602	2189.02	2189.04	11.04	1068.92	1079.96	0.0222	2.1265	2.1487	43
44	0.14203	0.28918	0.01602	2110.92	2110.94	12.05	1068.35	1080.40	0.0242	2.1211	2.1454	44
45	0.14755	0.30042	0.01602	2035.91	2035.92	13.05	1067.79	1080.84	0.0262	2.1158	2.1420	45
46	0.15326	0.31205	0.01602	1963.85	1963.87	14.05	1067.22	1081.28	0.0282	2.1105	2.1387	46
47	0.15917	0.32407	0.01602	1894.71	1894.73	15.06	1066.66	1081.71	0.0302	2.1052	2.1354	47
48	0.16527	0.33650	0.01602	1828.28	1828.30	16.06	1066.09	1082.15	0.0321	2.1000	2.1321	48
49	0.17158	0.34935	0.01602	1764.44	1764.46	17.06	1065.53	1082.59	0.0341	2.0947	2.1288	49
50	0.17811	0.36263	0.01602	1703.18	1703.20	18.06	1064.96	1083.03	0.0361	2.0895	2.1256	50
51	0.18484	0.37635	0.01602	1644.25	1644.26	19.06	1064.40	1083.46	0.0381	2.0843	2.1224	51
52	0.19181	0.39053	0.01603	1587.64	1587.65	20.07	1063.83	1083.90	0.0400	2.0791	2.1191	52

*Extrapolated to represent metastable equilibrium with undercooled liquid.

Table 2-1 Thermodynamic Properties of Water (*Continued*)
(Table 3, Chapter 6, 1997 *Handbook—Fundamentals*)

Temp.	Absolute Pressure p		Specific Volume, ft³/lb			Enthalpy, Btu/lb			Entropy, Btu/lb·°F			Temp.,
			Sat. Solid/Liq.	Evap.	Sat. Vapor	Sat. Solid/Liq.	Evap.	Sat. Vapor	Sat. Solid/Liq.	Evap.	Sat. Vapor	
t, °F	psi	in. Hg	v_f	v_{fg}	v_g	h_f	h_{fg}	h_g	s_f	s_{fg}	s_g	°F
53	0.19900	0.40516	0.01603	1533.22	1533.24	21.07	1063.27	1084.34	0.0420	2.0740	2.1159	53
54	0.20643	0.42029	0.01603	1480.89	1480.91	22.07	1062.71	1084.77	0.0439	2.0689	2.1128	54
55	0.21410	0.43591	0.01603	1430.61	1430.62	23.07	1062.14	1085.21	0.0459	2.0637	2.1096	55
56	0.22202	0.45204	0.01603	1382.19	1382.21	24.07	1061.58	1085.65	0.0478	2.0586	2,1064	56
57	0.23020	0.46869	0.01603	1335.65	1335.67	25.07	1061.01	1086.08	0.0497	2.0536	2.1033	57
58	0.23864	0.48588	0.01603	1290.85	1290.87	26.07	1060.45	1086.52	0.0517	2.0485	2.0002	58
59	0.24735	0.50362	0.01603	1247.76	1247.78	27.07	1059.89	1086.96	0.0536	2.0435	2.0971	59
60	0.25635	0.52192	0.01604	1206.30	1206.32	28.07	1059.32	1087.39	0.0555	2.0385	2.0940	60
61	0.26562	0.54081	0.01604	1166.38	1166.40	29.07	1058.76	1087.83	0.0575	2.0334	2.0909	61
62	0.27519	0.56029	0.01604	1127.93	1127.95	30.07	1058.19	1088.27	0.0594	2.0285	2.0878	62
63	0.28506	0.58039	0.01604	1090.94	1090.96	31.07	1057.63	1088.70	0.0613	2.0235	2.0848	63
64	0.29524	0.60112	0.01604	1055.32	1055.33	32.07	1057.07	1089.14	0.0632	2.0186	2.0818	64
65	0.30574	0.62249	0.01604	1020.98	1021.00	33.07	1056.50	1089.57	0.0651	2.0136	2.0787	65
66	0.31656	0.64452	0.01604	987.95	987.97	34.07	1055.94	1090.01	0.0670	2.0087	2.0758	66
67	0.32772	0.66724	0.01605	956.11	956.12	35.07	1055.37	1090.44	0.0689	2.0039	2.0728	67
68	0.33921	0.69065	0.01605	925.44	925.45	36.07	1054.81	1090.88	0.0708	1.9990	2.0698	68
69	0.35107	0.71478	0.01605	895.86	895.87	37.07	1054.24	1091.31	0.0727	1.9941	2.0668	69
70	0.36328	0.73964	0.01605	867.34	867.36	38.07	1053.68	1091.75	0.0746	1.9893	2.0639	70
71	0.37586	0.76526	0.01605	839.87	839.88	39.07	1053.11	1092.18	0.0765	1.9845	2.0610	71
72	0.38882	0.79164	0.01606	813.37	813.39	40.07	1052.55	1092.61	0.0783	1.9797	2.0580	72
73	0.40217	0.81883	0.01606	787.85	787.87	41.07	1051.98	1093.05	0.0802	1.9749	2.0552	73
74	0.41592	0.84682	0.01606	763.19	763.21	42.06	1051.42	1093.48	0.0821	1.9702	2.0523	74
75	0.43008	0.87564	0.01606	739.42	739.44	43.06	1050.85	1093.92	0.0840	1.9654	2.0494	75
76	0.44465	0.90532	0.01606	716.51	726.53	44.06	1050.29	1094.35	0.0858	1.9607	2.0465	76
77	0.45966	0.93587	0.01607	694.38	794.40	45.06	1049.72	1094.78	0.0877	1.9560	2.0437	77
78	0.47510	0.96732	0.01607	673.05	673.06	46.06	1049.16	1095.22	0.0896	1.9513	2.0409	78
79	0.49100	0.99968	0.01607	652.44	652.46	47.06	1048.59	1095.65	0.0914	1.9466	2.0380	79
80	0.50736	1.03298	0.01607	632.54	632.56	48.06	1048.03	1096.08	0.0933	1.9420	2.0352	80
81	0.52419	1.06725	0.01608	613.35	613.37	49.06	1047.46	1096.51	0.0951	1.9373	2.0324	81
82	0.54150	1.10250	0.01608	594.82	594.84	50.05	1046.89	1096.95	0.0970	1.9327	2.0297	82
83	0.55931	1.13877	0.01608	576.90	576.92	51.05	1046.33	1097.38	0.0988	1.9281	2.0269	83
84	0.57763	1.17606	0.01608	559.63	559.65	52.05	1045.76	1097.81	0.1006	1.9235	2.0242	84
85	0.59647	1.21442	0.01609	542.93	542.94	53.05	1045.19	1098.24	0.1025	1.9189	2.0214	85
86	0.61584	1.25385	0.01609	526.80	526.81	54.05	1044.63	1098.67	0.1043	1.9144	2.0187	86
87	0.63575	1.29440	0.01609	511.21	511.22	55.05	1044.06	1099.11	0.1061	1.9098	2.0160	87
88	0.65622	1.33608	0.01609	496.14	496.15	56.05	1043.49	1099.54	0.1080	1.9053	2.0133	88
89	0.67726	1.37892	0.01610	481.60	481.61	57.04	1042.92	1099.97	0.1098	1.9008	2.0106	89
90	0.69889	1.42295	0.01610	467.52	467.53	58.04	1042.36	1100.40	0.1116	1.8963	2.0079	90
91	0.72111	1.46820	0.01610	453.91	453.93	59.04	1041.79	1100.83	0.1134	1.8918	2.0053	91
92	0.74394	1.51468	0.01611	440.76	440.78	60.04	1041.22	1101.26	0.1152	1.8874	2.0026	92
93	0.76740	1.56244	0.01611	428.04	428.06	61.04	1040.65	1101.69	0.1170	1.8829	2.0000	93
94	0.79150	1.61151	0.01611	415.74	415.76	62.04	1040.08	1102.12	0.1188	1.8785	1.9973	94
95	0.81625	1.66189	0.01612	403.84	403.86	63.03	1039.51	1102.55	0.1206	1.8741	1.9947	95
96	0.84166	1.71364	0.01612	392.33	392.34	64.03	1038.95	1102.98	0.1224	1.8697	1.9921	96
97	0.86776	1.76678	0.01612	381.20	381.21	65.03	1038.38	1103.41	0.1242	1.8653	1.9895	97
98	0.89456	1.82134	0.01612	370.42	370.44	66.03	1037.81	1103.84	0.1260	1.8610	1.9870	98
99	0.92207	1.87736	0.01613	359.99	360.01	67.03	1037.24	1104.26	0.1278	1.8566	1.9844	99
100	0.95031	1.93485	0.01613	349.91	349.92	68.03	1036.67	1104.69	0.1296	1.8523	1.9819	100
101	0.97930	1.99387	0.01613	340.14	340.15	69.03	1036.10	1105.12	0.1314	1.8479	1.9793	101
102	1.00904	2.05443	0.01614	330.69	330.71	70.02	1035.53	1105.55	0.1332	1.8436	1.9768	102
103	1.03956	2.11667	0.01614	321.53	321.55	71.02	1034.95	1105.98	0.1349	1.8393	1.9743	103
104	1.07088	2.18034	0.01614	312.67	312.69	72.02	1034.38	1106.40	0.1367	1.8351	1.9718	104
105	1.10301	2.24575	0.01615	304.08	304.10	73.02	1033.81	1106.83	0.1385	1.8308	1.9693	105
106	1.13597	2.31285	0.01615	295.76	295.77	74.02	1033.24	1107.26	0.1402	1.8266	1.9668	106
107	1.16977	2.38168	0.01616	287.71	287.73	75.01	1032.67	1107.68	0.1420	1.8223	1.9643	107
108	1.20444	2.45226	0.01616	279.91	279.92	76.01	1032.10	1108.11	0.1438	1.8181	1.9619	108
109	1.23999	2.52464	0.01616	272.34	272.36	77.01	1031.52	1108.54	0.1455	1.8139	1.9594	109
110	1.27644	2.59885	0.01617	265.02	265.03	78.01	1030.95	1108.96	0.1473	1.8097	1.9570	110
111	1.31381	2.67494	0.01617	257.91	257.93	79.01	1030.38	1109.39	0.1490	1.8055	1.9546	111
112	1.35212	2.75293	0.01617	251.02	251.04	80.01	1029.80	1109.81	0.1508	1.8014	1.9521	112
113	1.39138	2.83288	0.01618	244.36	244.38	81.01	1029.23	1110.24	0.1525	1.7972	1.9497	113
114	1.43162	2.91481	0.01618	237.89	237.90	82.00	1028.66	1110.66	0.1543	1.7931	1.9474	114
115	1.47286	2.99878	0.01619	231.62	231.63	83.00	1028.08	1111.09	0.1560	1.7890	1.9450	115
116	1.51512	3.08481	0.01619	225.53	225.55	84.00	1027.51	1111.51	0.1577	1.7849	1.9426	116
117	1.55842	3.17296	0.01619	219.63	219.65	85.00	1026.93	1111.93	0.1595	1.7808	1.9402	117
118	1.60277	3.26327	0.01620	213.91	213.93	86.00	1026.36	1112.36	0.1612	1.7767	1.9379	118
119	1.64820	3.35577	0.01620	208.36	208.37	87.00	1025.78	1112.78	0.1629	1.7726	1.9356	119
120	1.69474	3.45052	0.01620	202.98	202.99	88.00	1025.20	1113.20	0.1647	1.7686	1.9332	120

Table 2-1 Thermodynamic Properties of Water (*Continued*)

(Table 3, Chapter 6, 1997 *Handbook—Fundamentals*)

	Absolute Pressure p		Specific Volume, ft³/lb			Enthalpy, Btu/lb			Entropy, Btu/lb·°F			
Temp. t, °F	psi	in. Hg	Sat. Solid/Liq. v_f	Evap. v_{fg}	Sat. Vapor v_g	Sat. Solid/Liq. h_f	Evap. h_{fg}	Sat. Vapor h_g	Sat. Solid/Liq. s_f	Evap. s_{fg}	Sat. Vapor s_g	Temp., °F
121	1.74240	3.54755	0.01621	197.76	197.76	89.00	1024.63	1113.62	0.1664	1.7645	1.9309	121
122	1.79117	3.64691	0.01621	192.69	192.69	90.00	1024.05	1114.05	0.1681	1.7605	1.9286	122
123	1.84117	3.74863	0.01622	187.78	187.78	90.99	1023.47	1114.47	0.1698	1.7565	1.9263	123
124	1.89233	3.85282	0.01622	182.98	182.99	91.99	1022.90	1114.89	0.1715	1.7525	1.9240	124
125	1.94470	3.95945	0.01623	178.34	178.36	92.99	1022.32	1115.31	0.1732	1.7485	1.9217	125
126	1.99831	4.06860	0.01623	173.85	173.86	93.99	1021.74	1115.73	0.1749	1.7445	1.9195	126
127	2.05318	4.18032	0.01623	169.47	169.49	94.99	1021.16	1116.15	0.1766	1.7406	1.9172	127
128	2.10934	4.29465	0.01624	165.23	165.25	95.99	1020.58	1116.57	0.1783	1.7366	1.9150	128
129	2.16680	4.41165	0.01624	161.11	161.12	96.99	1020.00	1116.99	0.1800	1.7327	1.9127	129
130	2.22560	4.53136	0.01625	157.11	157.12	97.99	1019.42	1117.41	0.1817	1.7288	1.9105	130
131	2.28576	4.65384	0.01625	153.22	153.23	98.99	1018.84	1117.83	0.1834	1.7249	1.9083	131
132	2.34730	4.77914	0.01626	149.44	149.46	99.99	1018.26	1118.25	0.1851	1.7210	1.9061	132
133	2.41025	4.90730	0.01626	145.77	145.78	100.99	1017.68	1118.67	0.1868	1.7171	1.9039	133
134	2.47463	5.03839	0.01627	142.21	142.23	101.99	1017.10	1119.08	0.1885	1.7132	1.9017	134
135	2.54048	5.17246	0.01627	138.74	138.76	102.99	1016.52	1119.50	0.1902	1.7093	1.8995	135
136	2.60782	5.30956	0.01627	135.37	135.39	103.98	1015.93	1119.92	0.1919	1.7055	1.8974	136
137	2.67667	5.44975	0.01628	132.10	132.12	104.98	1015.35	1120.34	0.1935	1.7017	1.8952	137
138	2.74707	5.59308	0.01628	128.92	128.94	105.98	1014.77	1120.75	0.1952	1.6978	1.8930	138
139	2.81903	5.73961	0.01629	125.83	125.85	106.98	1014.18	1121.17	0.1969	1.6940	1.8909	139
140	2.89260	5.88939	0.01629	122.82	122.84	107.98	1013.60	1121.58	0.1985	1.6902	1.8888	140
141	2.96780	6.04250	0.01630	119.90	119.92	108.98	1013.01	1122.00	0.2002	1.6864	1.8867	141
142	3.04465	6.19897	0.01630	117.05	117.07	109.98	1012.43	1122.41	0.2019	1.6827	1.8845	142
143	3.12320	6.35888	0.01631	114.29	114.31	110.98	1011.84	1122.83	0.2035	1.6789	1.8824	143
144	3.20345	6.52229	0.01631	111.60	111.62	111.98	1011.26	1123.24	0.2052	1.6752	1.8803	144
145	3.28546	6.68926	0.01632	108.99	109.00	112.98	1010.67	1123.66	0.2068	1.6714	1.8783	145
146	3.36924	6.85984	0.01632	106.44	106.45	113.98	1010.09	1124.07	0.2085	1.6677	1.8762	146
147	3.45483	7.03410	0.01633	103.96	103.98	114.98	1009.50	1124.48	0.2101	1.6640	1.8741	147
148	3.54226	7.21211	0.01633	101.55	101.57	115.98	1008.91	1124.89	0.2118	1.6603	1.8721	148
149	3.63156	7.39393	0.01634	99.21	99.22	116.98	1008.32	1125.31	0.2134	1.6566	1.8700	149
150	3.72277	7.57962	0.01634	96.93	96.94	117.98	1007.73	1125.72	0.2151	1.6529	1.8680	150
151	3.81591	7.76925	0.01635	94.70	94.72	118.99	1007.14	1126.13	0.2167	1.6492	1.8659	151
152	3.91101	7.96289	0.01635	92.54	92.56	119.99	1006.55	1126.54	0.2184	1.6455	1.8639	152
153	4.00812	8.16061	0.01636	90.44	90.46	120.99	1005.96	1126.95	0.2200	1.6419	1.8619	153
154	4.10727	8.36247	0.01636	88.39	88.41	121.99	1005.37	1127.36	0.2216	1.6383	1.8599	154
155	4.20848	8.56854	0.01637	86.40	86.41	122.99	1004.78	1127.77	0.2233	1.6346	1.8579	155
156	4.31180	8.77890	0.01637	84.45	84.47	123.99	1004.19	1128.18	0.2249	1.6310	1.8559	156
157	4.41725	8.99360	0.01638	82.56	82.58	124.99	1003.60	1128.59	0.2265	1.6274	1.8539	157
158	4.52488	9.21274	0.01638	80.72	80.73	125.99	1003.00	1128.99	0.2281	1.6238	1.8519	158
159	4.63472	9.43637	0.01639	78.92	78.94	126.99	1002.41	1129.40	0.2297	1.6202	1.8500	159
160	4.7468	9.6646	0.01639	77.175	77.192	127.99	1001.82	1129.81	0.2314	1.6167	1.8480	160
161	4.8612	9.8974	0.01640	75.471	75.488	128.99	1001.22	1130.22	0.2330	1.6131	1.8461	161
162	4.9778	10.1350	0.01640	73.812	73.829	130.00	1000.63	1130.62	0.2346	1.6095	1.8441	162
163	5.0969	10.3774	0.01641	72.196	72.213	131.00	1000.03	1131.03	0.2362	1.6060	1.8422	163
164	5.2183	10.6246	0.01642	70.619	70.636	132.00	999.43	1131.43	0.2378	1.6025	1.8403	164
165	5.3422	10.8768	0.01642	69.084	69.101	133.00	998.84	1131.84	0.2394	1.5989	1.8383	165
166	5.4685	11.1340	0.01643	67.587	67.604	134.00	998.24	1132.24	0.2410	1.5954	1.8364	166
167	5.5974	11.3963	0.01643	66.130	66.146	135.00	997.64	1132.64	0.2426	1.5919	1.8345	167
168	5.7287	11.6638	0.01644	64.707	64.723	136.01	997.04	1133.05	0.2442	1.5884	1.8326	168
169	5.8627	11.9366	0.01644	63.320	63.336	137.01	996.44	1133.45	0.2458	1.5850	1.8308	169
170	5.9993	12.2148	0.01645	61.969	61.986	138.01	995.84	1133.85	0.2474	1.5815	1.8289	170
171	6.1386	12.4983	0.01646	60.649	60.666	139.01	995.24	1134.25	0.2490	1.5780	1.8270	171
172	6.2806	12.7874	0.01646	59.363	59.380	140.01	994.64	1134.66	0.2506	1.5746	1.8251	172
173	6.4253	13.0821	0.01647	58.112	58.128	141.02	994.04	1135.06	0.2521	1.5711	1.8233	173
174	6.5729	13.3825	0.01647	56.887	56.904	142.02	993.44	1135.46	0.2537	1.5677	1.8214	174
175	6.7232	13.6886	0.01648	55.694	55.711	143.02	992.83	1135.86	0.2553	1.5643	1.8196	175
176	6.8765	14.0006	0.01648	54.532	54.549	144.02	992.23	1136.26	0.2569	1.5609	1.8178	176
177	7.0327	14.3186	0.01649	53.397	53.414	145.03	991.63	1136.65	0.2585	1.5575	1.8159	177
178	7.1918	14.6426	0.01650	52.290	52.307	146.03	991.02	1137.05	0.2600	1.5541	1.8141	178
179	7.3539	14.9727	0.01650	51.210	51.226	147.03	990.42	1137.45	0.2616	1.5507	1.8123	179
180	7.5191	15.3091	0.01651	50.155	50.171	148.04	989.81	1137.85	0.2632	1.5473	1.8105	180
181	7.6874	15.6518	0.01651	49.126	49.143	149.04	989.20	1138.24	0.2647	1.5440	1.8087	181
182	7.8589	16.0008	0.01652	48.122	48.138	150.04	988.60	1138.64	0.2663	1.5406	1.8069	182
183	8.0335	16.3564	0.01653	47.142	47.158	151.05	987.99	1139.03	0.2679	1.5373	1.8051	183
184	8.2114	16.7185	0.01653	46.185	46.202	152.05	987.38	1139.43	0.2694	1.5339	1.8034	184
185	8.3926	17.0874	0.01654	45.251	45.267	153.05	986.77	1139.82	0.2710	1.5306	1.8016	185
186	8.5770	17.4630	0.01654	44.339	44.356	154.06	986.16	1140.22	0.2725	1.5273	1.7998	186
187	8.7649	17.8455	0.01655	43.448	43.465	155.06	985.55	1140.61	0.2741	1.5240	1.7981	187
188	8.9562	18.2350	0.01656	42.579	42.595	156.07	984.94	1141.00	0.2756	1.5207	1.7963	188
189	9.1510	18.6316	0.01656	41.730	41.746	157.07	984.32	1141.39	0.2772	1.5174	1.7946	189

Table 2-1 Thermodynamic Properties of Water (*Continued*)

(Table 3, Chapter 6, 1997 *Handbook—Fundamentals*)

Temp.	Absolute Pressure p		Specific Volume, ft³/lb			Enthalpy, Btu/lb			Entropy, Btu/lb·°F			Temp.,
			Sat. Solid/Liq.	Evap.	Sat. Vapor	Sat. Solid/Liq.	Evap.	Sat. Vapor	Sat. Solid/Liq.	Evap.	Sat. Vapor	
t, °F	psi	in. Hg	v_f	v_{fg}	v_g	h_f	h_{fg}	h_g	s_f	s_{fg}	s_g	°F
190	9.3493	19.0353	0.01657	40.901	40.918	158.07	983.71	1141.78	0.2787	1.5141	1.7929	190
191	9.5512	19.4464	0.01658	40.092	40.108	159.08	983.10	1142.18	0.2803	1.5109	1.7911	191
192	9.7567	19.8648	0.01658	39.301	39.317	160.08	982.48	1142.57	0.2818	1.5076	1.7894	192
193	9.9659	20.2907	0.01659	38.528	38.544	161.09	981.87	1142.95	0.2834	1.5043	1.7877	193
194	10.1788	20.7242	0.01659	37.774	37.790	162.09	981.25	1143.34	0.2849	1.5011	1.7860	194
195	10.3955	21.1653	0.01660	37.035	37.052	163.10	980.63	1143.73	0.2864	1.4979	1.7843	195
196	10.6160	21.6143	0.01661	36.314	36.331	164.10	980.02	1144.12	0.2880	1.4946	1.7826	196
197	10.8404	22.0712	0.01661	35.611	35.628	165.11	979.40	1144.51	0.2895	1.4914	1.7809	197
198	11.0687	22.5361	0.01662	34.923	34.940	166.11	978.78	1144.89	0.2910	1.4882	1.7792	198
199	11.3010	23.0091	0.01663	34.251	34.268	167.12	978.16	1145.28	0.2926	1.4850	1.7776	199
200	11.5374	23.4904	0.01663	33.594	33.610	168.13	977.54	1145.66	0.2941	1.4818	1.7759	200
201	11.7779	23.9800	0.01664	32.951	32.968	169.13	976.92	1146.05	0.2956	1.4786	1.7742	201
202	12.0225	24.4780	0.01665	32.324	32.340	170.14	976.29	1146.43	0.2971	1.4755	1.7726	202
203	12.2713	24.9847	0.01665	31.710	31.726	171.14	975.67	1146.81	0.2986	1.4723	1.7709	203
204	12.5244	25.5000	0.01666	31.110	31.127	172.15	975.05	1147.20	0.3002	1.4691	1.7693	204
205	12.7819	26.0241	0.01667	30.523	30.540	173.16	974.42	1147.58	0.3017	1.4660	1.7677	205
206	13.0436	26.5571	0.01667	29.949	29.965	174.16	973.80	1147.96	0.3032	1.4628	1.7660	206
207	13.3099	27.0991	0.01668	29.388	29.404	175.17	973.17	1148.34	0.3047	1.4597	1.7644	207
208	13.5806	27.6503	0.01669	28.839	28.856	176.18	972.54	1148.72	0.3062	1.4566	1.7628	208
209	13.8558	28.2108	0.01669	28.303	28.319	177.18	971.92	1149.10	0.3077	1.4535	1.7612	209
210	14.1357	28.7806	0.01670	27.778	27.795	178.19	971.29	1149.48	0.3092	1.4503	1.7596	210
212	14.7096	29.9489	0.01671	26.763	26.780	180.20	970.03	1150.23	0.3122	1.4442	1.7564	212
214	15.3025	31.1563	0.01673	25.790	25.807	182.22	968.76	1150.98	0.3152	1.4380	1.7532	214
216	15.9152	32.4036	0.01674	24.861	24.878	184.24	967.50	1151.73	0.3182	1.4319	1.7501	216
218	16.5479	33.6919	0.01676	23.970	23.987	186.25	966.23	1152.48	0.3212	1.4258	1.7469	218
220	17.2013	35.0218	0.01677	23.118	23.134	188.27	964.95	1153.22	0.3241	1.4197	1.7438	220
222	17.8759	36.3956	0.01679	22.299	22.316	190.29	963.67	1153.96	0.3271	1.4136	1.7407	222
224	18.5721	37.8131	0.01680	21.516	21.533	192.31	962.39	1154.70	0.3301	1.4076	1.7377	224
226	19.2905	39.2758	0.01682	20.765	20.782	194.33	961.11	1155.43	0.3330	1.4016	1.7347	226
228	20.0316	40.7848	0.01683	20.045	20.062	196.35	959.82	1156.16	0.3359	1.3957	1.7316	228
230	20.7961	42.3412	0.01684	19.355	19.372	198.37	958.52	1156.89	0.3389	1.3898	1.7287	230
232	21.5843	43.9461	0.01686	18.692	18.709	200.39	957.22	1157.62	0.3418	1.3839	1.7257	232
234	22.3970	45.6006	0.01688	18.056	18.073	202.41	955.92	1158.34	0.3447	1.3780	1.7227	234
236	23.2345	47.3060	0.01689	17.446	17.463	204.44	954.62	1159.06	0.3476	1.3722	1.7198	236
238	24.0977	49.0633	0.01691	16.860	16.877	206.46	953.31	1159.77	0.3505	1.3664	1.7169	238
240	24.9869	50.8738	0.01692	16.298	16.314	208.49	952.00	1160.48	0.3534	1.3606	1.7140	240
242	25.9028	52.7386	0.01694	15.757	15.774	210.51	950.68	1161.19	0.3563	1.3548	1.7111	242
244	26.8461	54.6591	0.01695	15.238	15.255	212.54	949.35	1161.90	0.3592	1.3491	1.7083	244
246	27.8172	56.6364	0.01697	14.739	14.756	214.57	948.03	1162.60	0.3621	1.3434	1.7055	246
248	28.8169	58.6717	0.01698	14.259	14.276	216.60	946.70	1163.29	0.3649	1.3377	1.7026	248
250	29.8457	60.7664	0.01700	13.798	13.815	218.63	945.36	1163.99	0.3678	1.3321	1.6998	250
252	30.9043	62.9218	0.01702	13.355	13.372	220.66	944.02	1164.68	0.3706	1.3264	1.6971	252
254	31.9934	65.1391	0.01703	12.928	12.945	222.69	942.68	1165.37	0.3735	1.3208	1.6943	254
256	33.1135	67.4197	0.01705	12.526	12.147	226.73	939.99	1166.72	0.3764	1.3153	1.6691	256
258	34.2653	69.7649	0.01707	12.123	12.140	226.76	939.97	1166.73	0.3792	1.3097	1.6889	258
260	35.4496	72.1760	0.01708	11.742	11.759	228.79	938.61	1167.40	0.3820	1.3042	1.6862	260
262	36.6669	74.6545	0.01710	11.376	11.393	230.83	937.25	1168.08	0.3848	1.2987	1.6835	262
264	37.9180	77.2017	0.01712	11.024	11.041	232.87	935.88	1168.74	0.3876	1.2932	1.6808	264
266	39.2035	79.8190	0.01714	10.684	10.701	234.90	934.50	1169.41	0.3904	1.2877	1.6781	266
268	40.5241	82.5078	0.01715	10.357	10.374	236.94	933.12	1170.07	0.3932	1.2823	1.6755	268
270	41.8806	85.2697	0.01717	10.042	10.059	238.98	931.74	1170.72	0.3960	1.2769	1.6729	270
272	43.2736	88.1059	0.01719	9.737	9.755	241.03	930.35	1171.38	0.3988	1.2715	1.6703	272
274	44.7040	91.0181	0.01721	9.445	9.462	243.07	928.95	1172.02	0.4016	1.2661	1.6677	274
276	46.1723	94.0076	0.01722	9.162	9.179	245.11	927.55	1172.67	0.4044	1.2608	1.6651	276
278	47.6794	97.0761	0.01724	8.890	8.907	247.16	926.15	1173.31	0.4071	1.2554	1.6626	278
280	49.2260	100.2250	0.01726	8.627	8.644	249.20	924.74	1173.94	0.4099	1.2501	1.6600	280
282	50.8128	103.4558	0.01728	8.373	8.390	251.25	923.32	1174.57	0.4127	1.2448	1.6575	282
284	52.4406	106.7701	0.01730	8.128	8.146	253.30	921.90	1175.20	0.4154	1.2396	1.6550	284
286	54.1103	110.1695	0.01731	7.892	7.910	255.35	920.47	1175.82	0.4182	1.2343	1.6525	286
288	55.8225	113.6556	0.01733	7.664	7.681	257.40	919.03	1176.44	0.4209	1.2291	1.6500	288
290	57.5780	117.2299	0.01735	7.444	7.461	259.45	917.59	1177.05	0.4236	1.2239	1.6476	290
292	59.3777	120.8941	0.01737	7.231	7.248	261.51	916.15	1177.66	0.4264	1.2187	1.6451	292
294	61.2224	124.6498	0.01739	7.026	7.043	263.56	914.69	1178.26	0.4291	1.2136	1.6427	294
296	63.1128	128.4987	0.01741	6.827	6.844	265.62	913.24	1178.86	0.4318	1.2084	1.6402	296
298	65.0498	132.4425	0.01743	6.635	6.652	267.68	911.77	1179.45	0.4345	1.2033	1.6378	298
300	67.0341	136.4827	0.01745	6.450	6.467	269.74	910.30	1180.04	0.4372	1.1982	1.6354	300

The specific volume of a substance having a given quality can be found by using the definition of quality. **Quality** is defined as the ratio of the mass of vapor to total mass of liquid plus vapor when a substance is in a saturation state. Consider a mass of 1 kg having a quality x. The specific volume is the sum of the volume of the liquid and the volume of the vapor. The volume of the liquid is $(1 - x)v_f$, and the volume of the vapor is xv_g. Therefore, the specific volume v is:

$$v = xv_g + (1 - x)v_f \quad (2\text{-}5)$$

Since $v_f + v_{fg} = v_g$, Equation (2-5) can also be written in the following form:

$$v = v_f + xv_{fg} \quad (2\text{-}6)$$

The same procedure is followed for determining the enthalpy and the entropy for quality conditions:

$$h = xh_g + (1 - x)h_f \quad (2\text{-}7)$$

$$s = xs_g + (1 - x)s_f \quad (2\text{-}8)$$

Internal energy can then be obtained from the definition of enthalpy as $u = h - pv$.

If the substance is a compressed or subcooled liquid, the thermodynamic properties of specific volume, enthalpy, internal energy, and entropy are strongly temperature dependent (rather than pressure dependent). If compressed liquid tables are unavailable, they may be approximated by the corresponding values for saturated liquid (v_f, h_f, u_f, and s_f) at the existing temperature.

In the superheat region, thermodynamic properties must be obtained from superheat tables or a plot of the thermodynamic properties, called a Mollier diagram (Figure 2-4).

The thermodynamic and transport properties of the refrigerants used in vapor compression systems are found in similar tables typified by Table 2-2, which is a section of the R-134a property tables from Chapter 19 of the 1997 *Handbook—Fundamentals*. However, for these refrigerants the common Mollier plot is the *p-h* diagram as illustrated in Figure 2-5.

For fluids used in absorption refrigeration systems, the thermodynamic properties are commonly found on a different type of plot—the enthalpy-concentration diagram, as illustrated in Figure 2-6 for aqua-ammonia and in Figure 2-7 for lithium-bromide/water.

2.2.11 Property Equations for Ideal Gases

An ideal gas is defined as a gas at sufficiently low density so that intermolecular forces are negligible. As a result, an ideal gas has the equation of state:

$$pv = RT \quad (2\text{-}9)$$

For an ideal gas, the internal energy is a function of temperature only, which means that regardless of the pressure, an ideal gas at a given temperature has a certain definite specific internal energy u.

The relation between the internal energy u and the temperature can be established by using the definition of constant-volume specific heat given by:

$$c_v = (\partial u/\partial T)_v$$

Since the internal energy of an ideal gas is not a function of volume, an ideal gas can be written as:

$$c_v = du/dT$$

$$du = c_v\, dt \quad (2\text{-}10)$$

This equation is always valid for an ideal gas regardless of the kind of process considered.

From the definition of enthalpy and the equation of state of an ideal gas, it follows that:

$$h = u + pv = u + RT$$

Since R is a constant and u is a function of temperature only, the enthalpy h of an ideal gas is also a function of temperature only.

The relation between enthalpy and temperature is found from the constant pressure specific heat as defined by:

$$c_p = (\partial h/\partial T)_p$$

Since the enthalpy of an ideal gas is a function of the temperature only, and is independent of the pressure, it follows that:

$$c_p = dh/dT$$

$$dh = c_p\, dT \quad (2\text{-}11)$$

This equation is always valid for an ideal gas regardless of the kind of process considered.

Entropy, however, remains a function of both temperature and pressure, and is given by the equation:

$$ds = c_p(dT/T) - R(dp/p) \quad (2\text{-}12)$$

where c_p is frequently treated as being constant.

The ratio of heat capacities is often denoted by:

$$k = c_p/c_v \quad (2\text{-}13)$$

and is a useful quantity in calculations for ideal gases. Ideal gas values for some common gases are listed in Table 2-3.

No real gas exactly satisfies these equations over any finite range of temperature and pressure. However, all real gases approach ideal behavior at low pressures, and in the limit as $p_i \rightarrow 0$ do in fact meet the above requirements.

Thus, in solving problems, ideal behavior is assumed in two cases. First, at very low pressures, ideal gas behavior can be assumed with good accuracy, regardless of the temperature. Second, at temperatures that are double the critical temperature or above (the critical temperature of nitrogen is 126 K), ideal gas behavior can be assumed with good accuracy to pressures of at least 1000 lb_f/in^2 (7000 kPa). In the superheated vapor region, when the temperature is less than twice the critical temperature and the pressure is above a very

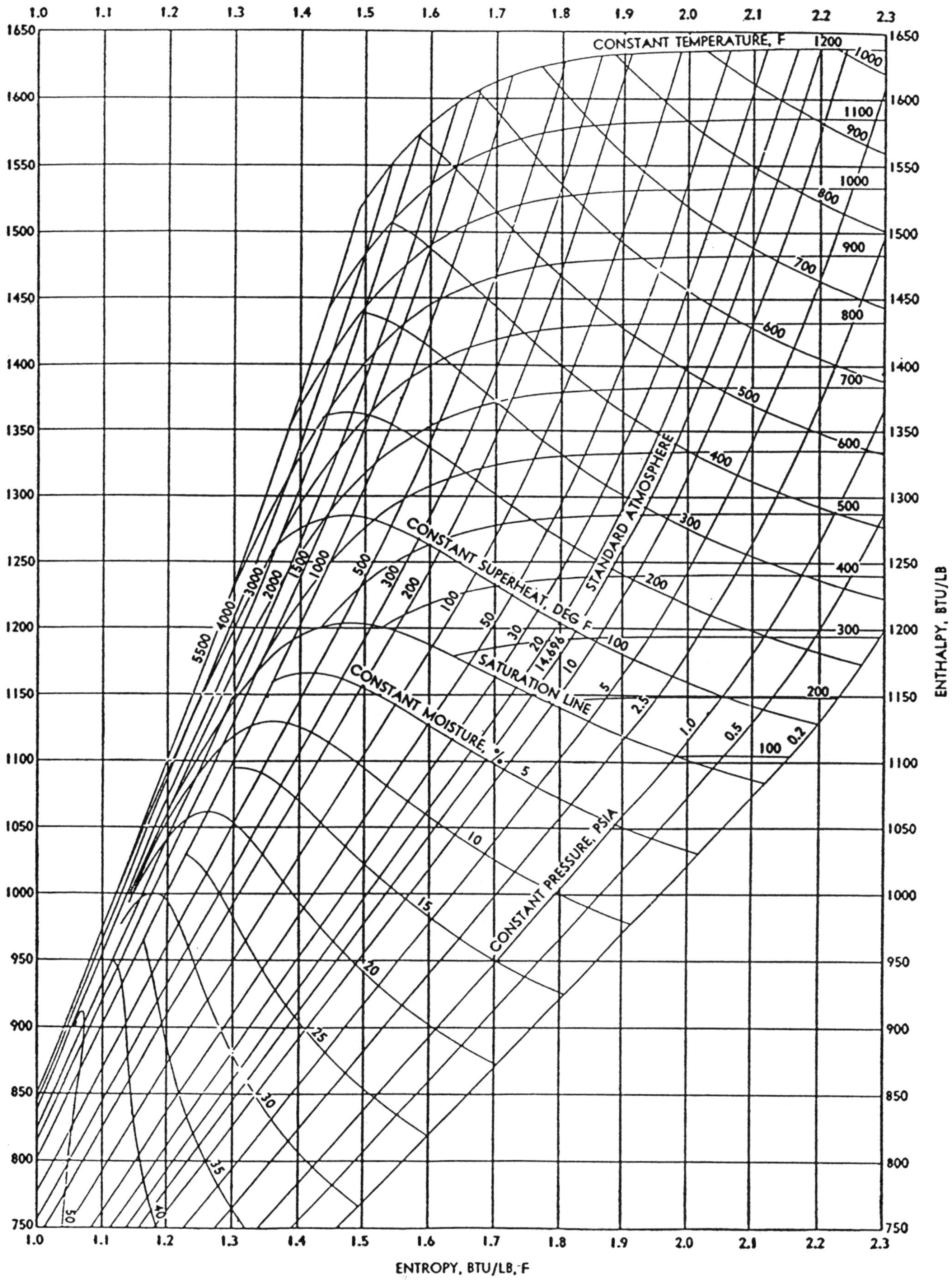

Fig. 2-4 Mollier (h,s) Diagram for Steam

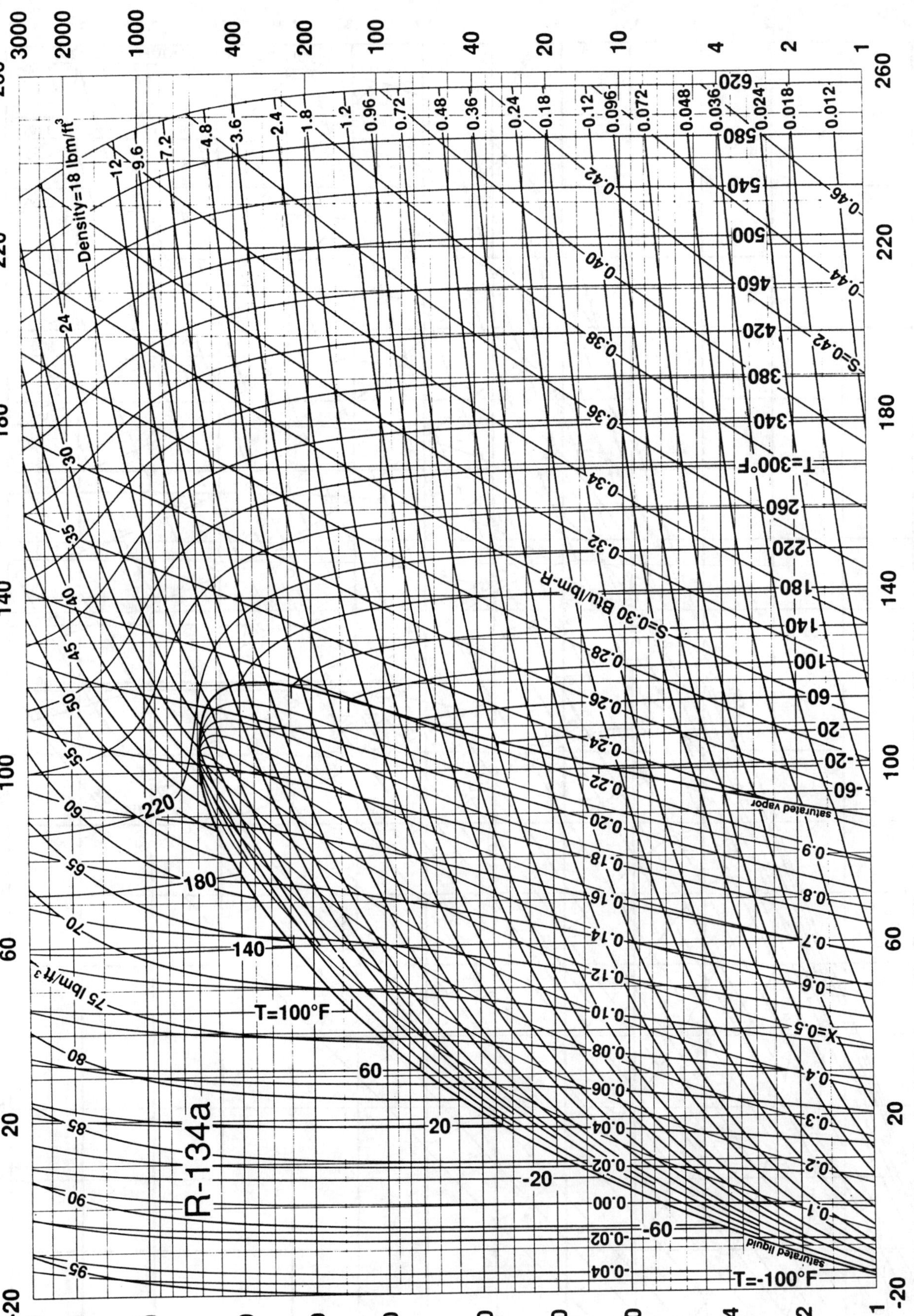

Fig. 2-5 Mollier (p-h) Diagram for Refrigerant 134a

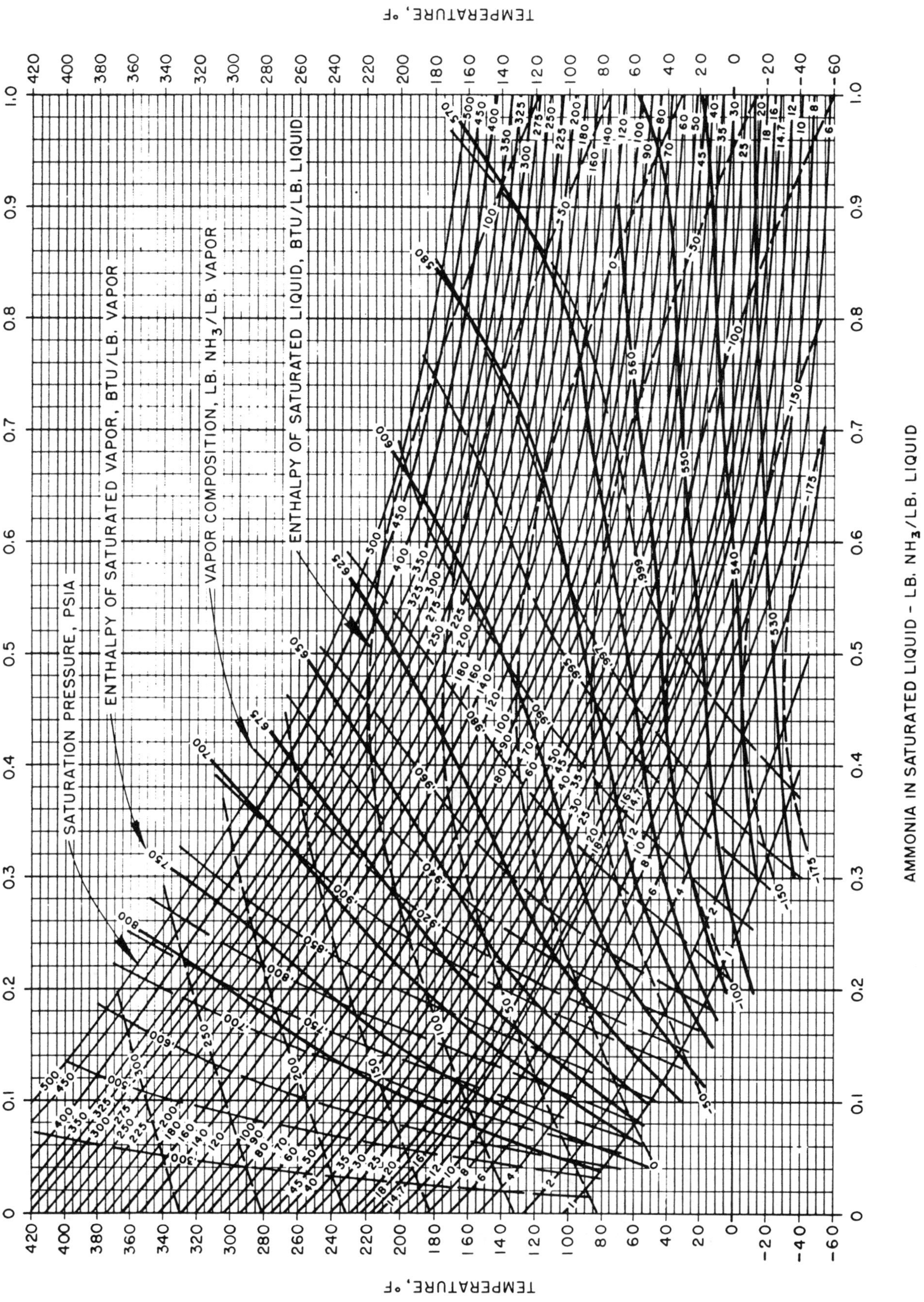

Fig. 2-6 Enthalpy-Concentration Diagram for Aqua-Ammonia

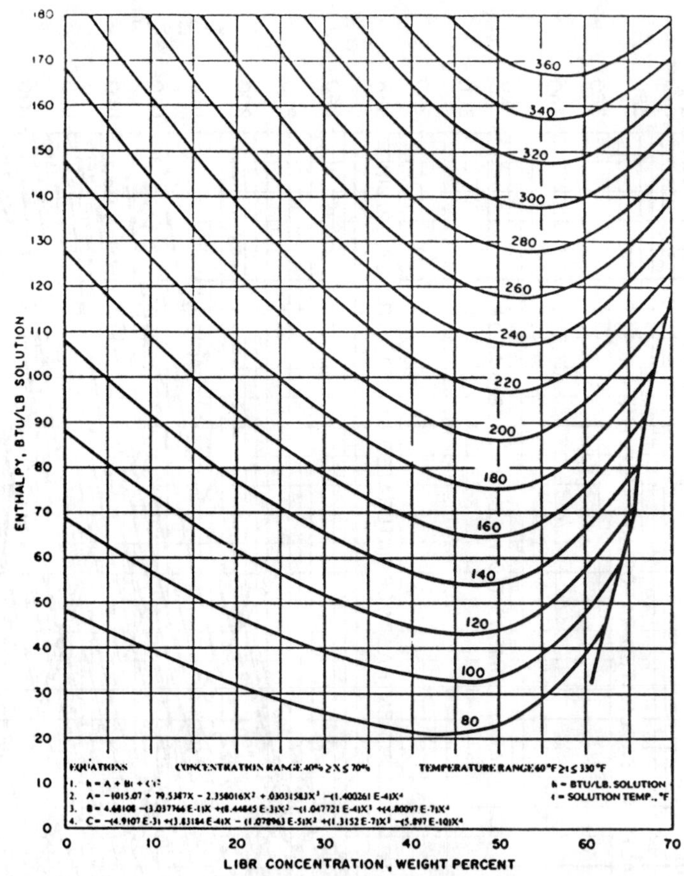

EQUATIONS

1. t = At′ + B
2. t′ = (t − B)/A
3. A = −2.00755 + .16976X − (3.133362 E-3)X² +(1.97668 E-5)X³
4. B = 321.128 − 19.322X + .374382X² −(2.0637 E-3)X³
5. $\text{Log}_{10} P = C + D/(t' + 459.72) + E/(t' + 459.72)^2$

6. $t' = \dfrac{-2E}{D + [D^2 - 4E(C - \log_{10} P]^{0.5}} - 459.72$

TEMP. RANGE (REFRIGERANT) $0 \geq t' \leq 230$ F
TEMP. RANGE (SOLUTION) $40 \geq t \leq 350$ °F
CONCENTRATION RANGE $.45\% \geq X \leq 70\%$

C = 6.21147
D = −2886.373
E = −337269.46
t′ = REFRIGERANT TEMP. °F
t = SOLUTION TEMP. °F
X = PERCENT LIBR
P = PSIA

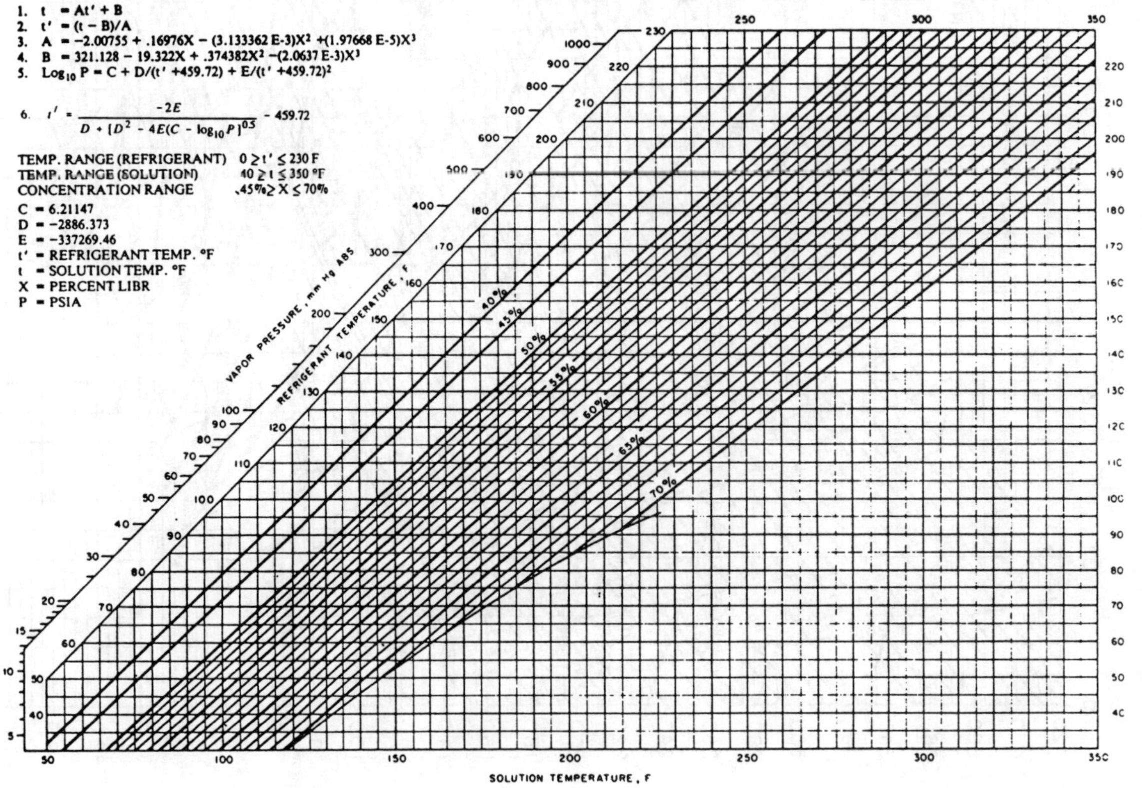

Fig. 2-7 Enthalpy-Concentration and Equilibrium Charts for Li-Br/Water

Table 2-2 Refrigerant 134a Properties of Saturated Liquid and Saturated Vapor

(Chapter 19, 1997 *Handbook—Fundamentals*)

Temp,* °F	Pressure, psia	Density, lb/ft³ Liquid	Volume, ft³/lb Vapor	Enthalpy, Btu/lb Liquid	Enthalpy, Btu/lb Vapor	Entropy, Btu/lb·°F Liquid	Entropy, Btu/lb·°F Vapor	Specific Heat c_p, Btu/lb·°F Liquid	Specific Heat c_p, Btu/lb·°F Vapor	c_p/c_v Vapor	Velocity of Sound, ft/s Liquid	Velocity of Sound, ft/s Vapor	Viscosity, lb_m/ft·h Liquid	Viscosity, lb_m/ft·h Vapor	Thermal Cond, Btu/h·ft·°F Liquid	Thermal Cond, Btu/h·ft·°F Vapor	Surface Tension, dyne/cm	Temp,* °F
−153.94a	0.057	99.34	564.85	32.989	80.235	0.09154	0.27880	0.2740	0.1397	1.1628	3723.	416.	5.289	0.0160	—	—	28.15	−153.94
−150.00	0.072	98.95	449.29	31.902	80.783	0.08801	0.27588	0.2776	0.1409	1.1615	3670.	418.	4.913	0.0163	—	—	27.76	−150.00
−140.00	0.130	97.98	259.15	29.093	82.190	0.07908	0.26903	0.2837	0.1438	1.1583	3552.	424.	4.117	0.0168	—	—	26.78	−140.00
−130.00	0.222	97.01	155.69	26.238	83.618	0.07029	0.26294	0.2870	0.1467	1.1554	3448.	430.	3.497	0.0173	—	—	25.81	−130.00
−120.00	0.367	96.05	97.027	23.359	85.066	0.06169	0.25752	0.2886	0.1497	1.1528	3352.	436.	3.006	0.0179	—	—	24.86	−120.00
−110.00	0.586	95.09	62.509	20.467	86.531	0.05330	0.25270	0.2895	0.1527	1.1507	3261.	441.	2.613	0.0184	—	—	23.92	−110.00
−100.00	0.906	94.13	41.496	17.569	88.011	0.04513	0.24842	0.2900	0.1559	1.1489	3173.	446.	2.292	0.0190	—	—	22.99	−100.00
−90.00	1.363	93.17	28.303	14.665	89.504	0.03717	0.24462	0.2906	0.1591	1.1475	3087.	451.	2.028	0.0195	0.0721	—	22.08	−90.00
−80.00	1.997	92.21	19.783	11.755	91.005	0.02940	0.24125	0.2913	0.1624	1.1466	3001.	456.	1.808	0.0200	0.0706	—	21.17	−80.00
−75.00	2.396	91.73	16.680	10.297	91.759	0.02559	0.23972	0.2917	0.1641	1.1463	2959.	458.	1.712	0.0203	0.0699	—	20.73	−75.00
−70.00	2.859	91.25	14.138	8.837	92.514	0.02182	0.23827	0.2922	0.1658	1.1462	2916.	460.	1.623	0.0206	0.0691	—	20.28	−70.00
−65.00	3.393	90.77	12.045	7.374	93.270	0.01809	0.23691	0.2928	0.1676	1.1461	2874.	462.	1.542	0.0209	0.0684	—	19.84	−65.00
−60.00	4.006	90.28	10.310	5.907	94.026	0.01440	0.23563	0.2935	0.1694	1.1462	2832.	464.	1.466	0.0212	0.0677	0.00405	19.40	−60.00
−55.00	4.707	89.80	8.8656	4.437	94.783	0.01075	0.23443	0.2943	0.1712	1.1465	2790.	466.	1.396	0.0214	0.0669	0.00423	18.96	−55.00
−50.00	5.505	89.31	7.6569	2.963	95.539	0.00713	0.23331	0.2951	0.1731	1.1468	2747.	468.	1.331	0.0217	0.0662	0.00440	18.52	−50.00
−45.00	6.409	88.82	6.6405	1.484	96.295	0.00355	0.23225	0.2960	0.1750	1.1473	2705.	470.	1.271	0.0220	0.0654	0.00457	18.09	−45.00
−40.00	7.429	88.32	5.7819	0.000	97.050	0.00000	0.23125	0.2970	0.1769	1.1479	2663.	471.	1.215	0.0223	0.0647	0.00473	17.66	−40.00
−35.00	8.577	87.83	5.0533	1.489	97.804	0.00352	0.23032	0.2981	0.1789	1.1487	2621.	473.	1.163	0.0225	0.0639	0.00489	17.23	−35.00
−30.00	9.862	87.33	4.4325	2.984	98.556	0.00701	0.22945	0.2992	0.1810	1.1497	2579.	474.	1.113	0.0228	0.0632	0.00505	16.81	−30.00
−25.00	11.297	86.82	3.9014	4.484	99.306	0.01048	0.22863	0.3004	0.1831	1.1508	2536.	476.	1.068	0.0231	0.0625	0.00521	16.38	−25.00
−20.00	12.895	86.32	3.4452	5.991	100.054	0.01392	0.22786	0.3017	0.1852	1.1521	2494.	477.	1.024	0.0234	0.0617	0.00536	15.96	−20.00
−15.00	14.667	85.81	3.0519	7.505	100.799	0.01733	0.22714	0.3031	0.1874	1.1535	2452.	478.	0.984	0.0237	0.0610	0.00550	15.54	−15.00
−14.92b	14.696	85.80	3.0462	7.529	100.811	0.01739	0.22713	0.3031	0.1874	1.1535	2451.	478.	0.983	0.0237	0.0610	0.00551	15.54	−14.92
−10.00	16.626	85.29	2.7116	9.026	101.542	0.02073	0.22647	0.3045	0.1897	1.1552	2410.	479.	0.946	0.0240	0.0602	0.00565	15.13	−10.00
−5.00	18.787	84.77	2.4161	10.554	102.280	0.02409	0.22584	0.3060	0.1920	1.1570	2367.	480.	0.910	0.0243	0.0595	0.00579	14.71	−5.00
0.00	21.162	84.25	2.1587	12.090	103.015	0.02744	0.22525	0.3075	0.1943	1.1590	2325.	481.	0.876	0.0245	0.0588	0.00593	14.30	0.00
5.00	23.767	83.72	1.9337	13.634	103.745	0.03077	0.22470	0.3091	0.1968	1.1613	2283.	481.	0.843	0.0248	0.0580	0.00607	13.89	5.00
10.00	26.617	83.18	1.7365	15.187	104.471	0.03408	0.22418	0.3108	0.1993	1.1637	2240.	482.	0.813	0.0251	0.0573	0.00621	13.48	10.00
15.00	29.726	82.64	1.5630	16.748	105.192	0.03737	0.22370	0.3126	0.2018	1.1664	2198.	482.	0.784	0.0254	0.0565	0.00635	13.08	15.00
20.00	33.110	82.10	1.4101	18.318	105.907	0.04065	0.22325	0.3144	0.2045	1.1694	2155.	482.	0.756	0.0257	0.0558	0.00649	12.67	20.00
25.00	36.785	81.55	1.2749	19.897	106.617	0.04391	0.22283	0.3162	0.2072	1.1726	2113.	482.	0.730	0.0260	0.0550	0.00662	12.27	25.00
30.00	40.768	80.99	1.1550	21.486	107.320	0.04715	0.22244	0.3182	0.2100	1.1761	2070.	482.	0.705	0.0263	0.0543	0.00676	11.87	30.00
35.00	45.075	80.42	1.0484	23.085	108.016	0.05038	0.22207	0.3202	0.2129	1.1799	2027.	482.	0.681	0.0267	0.0536	0.00690	11.48	35.00
40.00	49.724	79.85	0.9534	24.694	108.705	0.05359	0.22172	0.3223	0.2159	1.1841	1985.	482.	0.658	0.0270	0.0528	0.00704	11.08	40.00
45.00	54.732	79.26	0.8685	26.314	109.386	0.05679	0.22140	0.3244	0.2190	1.1886	1942.	481.	0.636	0.0273	0.0521	0.00718	10.69	45.00
50.00	60.116	78.67	0.7925	27.944	110.058	0.05998	0.22110	0.3267	0.2222	1.1935	1899.	481.	0.615	0.0276	0.0513	0.00732	10.30	50.00
55.00	65.895	78.07	0.7243	29.586	110.722	0.06316	0.22081	0.3290	0.2255	1.1988	1856.	480.	0.595	0.0280	0.0506	0.00746	9.91	55.00
60.00	72.087	77.46	0.6630	31.239	111.376	0.06633	0.22054	0.3314	0.2289	1.2046	1813.	479.	0.576	0.0283	0.0499	0.00761	9.53	60.00
65.00	78.712	76.84	0.6077	32.905	112.019	0.06949	0.22028	0.3339	0.2325	1.2109	1770.	477.	0.557	0.0286	0.0491	0.00776	9.15	65.00
70.00	85.787	76.21	0.5577	34.583	112.652	0.07264	0.22003	0.3366	0.2363	1.2178	1726.	476.	0.539	0.0290	0.0484	0.00791	8.77	70.00
75.00	93.333	75.57	0.5125	36.274	113.272	0.07578	0.21979	0.3393	0.2402	1.2252	1683.	474.	0.522	0.0294	0.0476	0.00806	8.39	75.00
80.00	101.37	74.91	0.4715	37.978	113.880	0.07892	0.21957	0.3422	0.2444	1.2334	1640.	472.	0.505	0.0297	0.0469	0.00822	8.02	80.00
85.00	109.92	74.25	0.4343	39.697	114.475	0.08205	0.21934	0.3453	0.2487	1.2424	1596.	470.	0.489	0.0301	0.0462	0.00838	7.65	85.00
90.00	119.00	73.57	0.4004	41.430	115.055	0.08518	0.21912	0.3485	0.2533	1.2522	1552.	468.	0.473	0.0305	0.0454	0.00855	7.28	90.00
95.00	128.63	72.87	0.3694	43.179	115.619	0.08830	0.21890	0.3519	0.2582	1.2630	1509.	466.	0.458	0.0309	0.0447	0.00872	6.91	95.00
100.00	138.83	72.16	0.3411	44.943	116.166	0.09142	0.21868	0.3555	0.2633	1.2748	1465.	463.	0.443	0.0313	0.0439	0.00890	6.55	100.00
105.00	149.63	71.43	0.3153	46.725	116.694	0.09454	0.21845	0.3594	0.2689	1.2880	1421.	460.	0.428	0.0318	0.0432	0.00908	6.20	105.00
110.00	161.05	70.68	0.2915	48.524	117.203	0.09766	0.21822	0.3635	0.2748	1.3026	1376.	457.	0.414	0.0322	0.0425	0.00926	5.84	110.00
115.00	173.11	69.91	0.2697	50.343	117.690	0.10078	0.21797	0.3680	0.2812	1.3189	1332.	454.	0.400	0.0327	0.0417	0.00946	5.49	115.00
120.00	185.84	69.12	0.2497	52.181	118.153	0.10391	0.21772	0.3728	0.2881	1.3372	1288.	450.	0.387	0.0332	0.0410	0.00965	5.15	120.00
125.00	199.25	68.31	0.2312	54.040	118.591	0.10704	0.21744	0.3781	0.2957	1.3577	1243.	446.	0.374	0.0338	0.0403	0.00986	4.80	125.00
130.00	213.38	67.47	0.2141	55.923	119.000	0.11018	0.21715	0.3839	0.3040	1.3810	1198.	442.	0.361	0.0343	0.0395	0.01007	4.47	130.00
135.00	228.25	66.60	0.1983	57.830	119.377	0.11333	0.21683	0.3903	0.3133	1.4075	1153.	437.	0.348	0.0349	0.0388	0.01029	4.13	135.00
140.00	243.88	65.70	0.1836	59.764	119.720	0.11650	0.21648	0.3974	0.3236	1.4379	1108.	432.	0.335	0.0356	0.0380	0.01052	3.81	140.00
145.00	260.31	64.77	0.1700	61.727	120.024	0.11968	0.21609	0.4053	0.3353	1.4731	1062.	427.	0.323	0.0363	0.0373	0.01075	3.48	145.00
150.00	277.57	63.80	0.1574	63.722	120.284	0.12288	0.21566	0.4144	0.3486	1.5143	1017.	421.	0.311	0.0370	0.0366	0.01100	3.17	150.00
155.00	295.69	62.78	0.1455	65.752	120.495	0.12611	0.21517	0.4247	0.3640	1.5630	971.	416.	0.298	0.0378	0.0358	0.01125	2.86	155.00
160.00	314.69	61.72	0.1345	67.823	120.650	0.12938	0.21463	0.4368	0.3821	1.6213	924.	409.	0.286	0.0387	0.0351	0.01151	2.55	160.00
165.00	334.62	60.60	0.1241	69.939	120.739	0.13268	0.21400	0.4511	0.4036	1.6921	877.	403.	0.274	0.0397	0.0343	0.01178	2.26	165.00
170.00	355.51	59.42	0.1144	72.106	120.753	0.13603	0.21329	0.4683	0.4299	1.7798	829.	396.	0.262	0.0407	0.0336	0.01206	1.97	170.00
175.00	377.40	58.16	0.1052	74.335	120.677	0.13945	0.21247	0.4896	0.4627	1.8908	781.	388.	0.249	0.0420	0.0329	0.01235	1.69	175.00
180.00	400.34	56.80	0.0965	76.636	120.493	0.14295	0.21151	0.5168	0.5048	2.0354	731.	380.	0.237	0.0434	0.0321	0.01265	1.41	180.00
185.00	424.37	55.33	0.0881	79.027	120.175	0.14655	0.21037	0.5527	0.5612	2.2309	680.	372.	0.224	0.0450	0.0314	0.01296	1.15	185.00
190.00	449.55	53.70	0.0801	81.534	119.684	0.15029	0.20901	0.6031	0.6406	2.5087	627.	363.	0.211	0.0469	—	—	0.90	190.00
195.00	475.95	51.86	0.0723	84.196	118.963	0.15423	0.20733	0.6794	0.7612	2.9338	572.	353.	0.197	0.0493	—	—	0.67	195.00
200.00	503.64	49.70	0.0646	87.088	117.906	0.15847	0.20519	0.8100	0.9673	3.6640	514.	343.	0.182	0.0523	—	—	0.45	200.00
205.00	532.72	47.00	0.0566	90.368	116.289	0.16326	0.20226	1.0906	1.4042	5.2174	450.	331.	0.164	0.0566	—	—	0.25	205.00
210.00	563.34	43.03	0.0474	94.548	113.411	0.16933	0.19750	—	—	—	378.	316.	0.142	0.0639	—	—	0.09	210.00
213.85c	588.27	32.04	0.0312	103.775	103.775	0.18128	0.18128	∞	∞	∞	0.	0.	—	—	∞	∞	0.00	213.85

*temperatures are on the ITS−90 scale a = triple point b = normal boiling point c = critical point

Table 2-3 Properties of Gases

Gas	Chemical Formula	Relative Molecular Mass	R, ft·lb$_f$/lb$_m$°R	c_p, Btu/lb$_m$°R	c_p, kJ/kg·K	c_v, Btu/lb$_m$°R	c_v, kJ/kg·K	k
Air	—	28.97	53.34	0.240	1.0	0.171	0.716	1.400
Argon	Ar	39.94	38.66	0.125	0.523	0.075	0.316	1.667
Carbon Dioxide	CO_2	44.01	35.10	0.203	0.85	0.158	0.661	1.285
Carbon Monoxide	CO	28.01	55.16	0.249	1.04	0.178	0.715	1.399
Helium	He	4.003	386.0	1.25	5.23	0.753	3.153	1.667
Hydrogen	H_2	2.016	766.4	3.43	14.36	2.44	10.22	1.404
Methane	CH_4	16.04	96.35	0.532	2.23	0.403	1.69	1.32
Nitrogen	N_2	28.016	55.15	0.248	1.04	0.177	0.741	1.400
Oxygen	O_2	32.000	48.28	0.219	0.917	0.157	0.657	1.395
Steam	H_2O	18.016	85.76	0.445	1.863	0.335	1.402	1.329

low value (e.g., atmospheric pressure), the deviation from ideal gas behavior may be considerable. In this region, tables of thermodynamic properties or charts for a particular substance should be used.

2.2.12 Mixtures

A large number of thermodynamic problems involve mixtures of different pure substances. A pure substance is a substance which is homogeneous and unchanging in chemical composition. Homogeneous mixtures of gases that do not react with each other are therefore pure substances, and the properties of such mixtures can be determined, correlated, and either tabulated or fitted by equations just like the properties of any other pure substance. This work has been done for common mixtures such as air and certain combustion products, but, as an unlimited number of mixtures is possible, properties of all of them cannot be determined experimentally and tabulated. Thus, it is important to be able to calculate the properties of any mixture from the properties of its constituents. Such calculations are discussed in this section, first for gas mixtures and then for gas-vapor mixtures.

Since individual gases can often be approximated as ideal gases, the study of mixtures of ideal gases and their properties is of considerable importance. Each constituent gas in a mixture has its own pressure called the **partial pressure** of the particular gas. The Gibbs-Dalton law states that in a mixture of ideal gases, the pressure of the mixture is equal to the sum of the partial pressures of the individual constituent gases. In equation form:

$$p_m = p_a + p_b + p_c \qquad (2\text{-}14)$$

where p_m is the total pressure of the mixture of gases a, b, and c, and p_a, p_b, and p_c are the partial pressures. In a mixture of ideal gases, the partial pressure of each constituent equals the pressure that constituent would exert if it existed alone at the temperature and volume of the mixture.

Generally, in gas mixtures, each constituent gas behaves as though the other gases were not present; each gas occupies the total volume of the mixture at the temperature of the mixture and the partial pressure of the gas. Thus, if V_m is the volume of the mixture, then the volume of each component is also V_m, or:

$$V_m = V_a = V_b = V_c \qquad (2\text{-}15)$$

However, the volume of a mixture of ideal gases equals the sum of the volumes of its constituents if each existed alone at the temperature and pressure of the mixture. This property is known as **Amagat's law, Leduc's law**, or the **law of additive volumes**. Like Dalton's law, it is strictly true only for ideal gases, but holds approximately for real-gas mixtures, even those in some ranges of pressure and temperature where $p_v = RT$ is inaccurate. When the temperature of a real-gas mixture is well above the critical temperatures of all its constituents, the additive volume law is usually more accurate than the additive pressure law.

For ideal-gas mixtures, volumetric analyses are frequently used. The volume fraction is defined as:

$$\text{Volume fraction of A} = \frac{V_a(p_m, T_m)}{V_m}$$

$$= \frac{\text{Volume of A existing alone at } p_m, T_m}{\text{Volume of mixture at } p_m, T_m}$$

Note that in a gas mixture, each constituent occupies the total volume; thus volume fraction is not defined as the ratio of a constituent volume to the mixture volume because this ratio is always unity.

Avogadro's law goes on to state, *equal volumes of ideal gases held under exactly the same temperature and pressure have equal numbers of molecules.* If T_m is the temperature of the mixture:

$$T_m = T_a = T_b = T_c \qquad (2\text{-}16)$$

for the temperature relationship.

The analysis of a gas mixture based on mass is called a **gravimetric analysis**. It is based on the fact that the mass of a mixture equals the sum of the masses of its constituents:

$$m_m = m_a + m_b + m_c \qquad (2\text{-}17)$$

where the subscript m refers to the mixture and the subscripts *a, b*, and *c* refer to individual constituents of the mixture. The ratio m_a/m_m is called the mass fraction of constituent *a*.

The total number of moles in a mixture is defined as the sum of the number of moles of its constituents:

$$N_m = N_a + N_b + N_c \quad (2\text{-}18)$$

The mole fraction x is defined as N/N_m, and:

$$M_m = x_a M_a + x_b M_b + x_c M_c \quad (2\text{-}19)$$

where M_m is called the apparent (or average) molecular weight of the mixture. The second part of the Gibbs-Dalton law can be taken as a basic definition:

$$U_m = U_a + U_b + U_c \quad (2\text{-}20)$$

$$H_m = H_a + H_b + H_c \quad (2\text{-}21)$$

$$S_m = S_a + S_b + S_c \quad (2\text{-}22)$$

Remember that the constituent entropies here must be evaluated at the temperature and volume of the mixture or at the mixture temperature and the constituent partial pressures. The entropy of any constituent at the volume and temperature of the mixture (and hence at its partial pressure) is greater than its entropy when existing at the pressure and temperature of the mixture (and hence at its partial volume).

Consider the constituents as perfect gases:

$$R_m = (m_a R_a + m_b R_b + m_c R_c)/m_m \quad (2\text{-}23)$$

$$c_{vm} = (m_a c_{va} + m_b c_{vb} + m_c c_{vc})/m_m \quad (2\text{-}24)$$

$$c_{pm} = (m_a c_{pa} + m_b c_{pb} + m_c c_{pc})/m_m \quad (2\text{-}25)$$

2.2.13 Psychrometrics: Moist Air Properties

Consider a simplification of the problem involving a mixture of ideal gases that is in contact with a solid or liquid phase of one of the components. The most familiar example is a mixture of air and water vapor in contact with liquid water or ice, such as the problems encountered in air conditioning or drying. This, and a number of similar problems can be analyzed simply and with considerable accuracy if the following assumptions are made:

1. The solid or liquid phase contains no dissolved gases.
2. The gaseous phase can be treated as a mixture of ideal gases.
3. When the mixture and the condensed phase are at a given pressure and temperature, the equilibrium between the condensed phase and its vapor is not influenced by the presence of the other component. This means that when equilibrium is achieved, the partial pressure of the vapor equals the saturation pressure corresponding to the temperature of the mixture.

If the vapor is at the saturation pressure and temperature, the mixture is referred to as a **saturated mixture**. For an air-water vapor mixture, the term **saturated air** is used.

Psychrometrics is the science involving thermodynamic properties of moist air and the effect of atmospheric moisture on materials and human comfort. As it applies in this text, the definition is broadened to include the method of controlling the thermal properties of moist air.

When moist air is considered to be a mixture of independent, perfect gases, dry air, and water vapor, each is assumed to obey the perfect gas equation of state:

$$\text{Dry air: } p_a V = n_a RT$$

$$\text{Water vapor: } p_w V = n_w RT$$

where

p_a = partial pressure of dry air
p_w = partial pressure of water vapor
V = total mixture volume
n_a = number of moles of dry air
n_w = number of moles of water vapor
R = universal gas constant (8.31441 J/g-mol·K or 1545.32 ft-lb$_f$ / lb-mol·°R)
T = absolute temperature

The mixture also obeys the perfect gas equation:

$$pV = nRT \text{ or } (p_a + p_w)V = (n_a + n_w)RT$$

Dry-bulb temperature t is the temperature of air as registered by an ordinary thermometer.

Thermodynamic wet-bulb temperature t^* is the temperature at which water (liquid or solid), by evaporating into moist air at a given dry-bulb temperature t and humidity ratio W, can bring the air to saturation adiabatically at the same temperature t^*, while the pressure p is maintained constant. Figure 2-8 may be used as a schematic representation of the adiabatic saturation process, where the leaving air is saturated and at a temperature equal to that of the injected water. A device used in place of the adiabatic saturator is the psychrometer.

The psychrometer consists of two thermometers or other temperature-sensing elements, one of which has a wetted cotton wick covering the bulb (Figure 2-9). When the wet bulb is placed in an airstream, water may evaporate from the wick. The equilibrium temperature the water eventually reaches is called the **wet-bulb temperature**. This process is not one of adiabatic saturation which defines the thermodynamic wet-bulb temperature, but is one of simultaneous heat and mass transfer from the wet bulb. Fortunately, the corrections applied to wet-bulb thermometer readings to obtain the thermodynamic wet-bulb temperature are usually small.

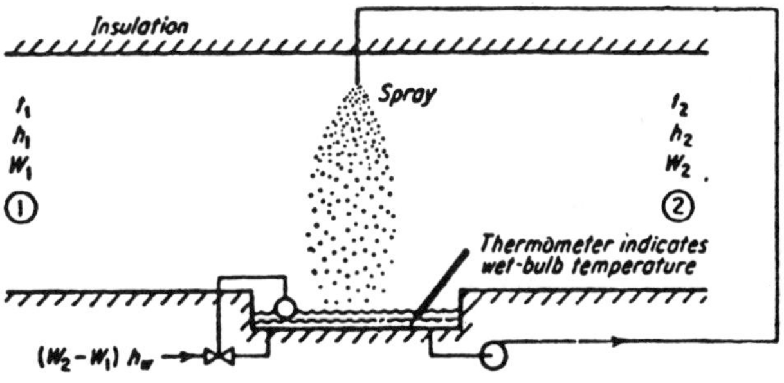

Fig. 2-8 Adiabatic Saturator

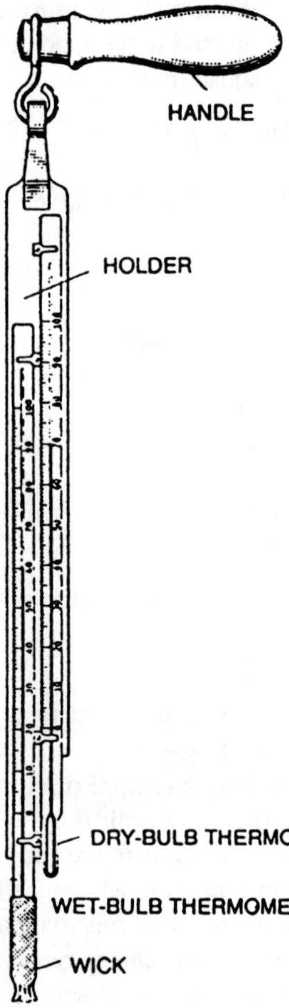

Fig. 2-9 Sling Psychrometer

Humidity ratio W of a given moist air sample is defined as the ratio of the mass of water vapor to the mass of dry air contained in the sample:

$$W = m_w/m_a$$
$$W = 0.62198p_w/(p-p_w) \tag{2-26}$$

$$W = \frac{(2501 - 2.381t^*)W_s^* - (t - t^*)}{2501 + 1.805t - 4.186t^*} \tag{2-27a}$$

where t and t^* are in °C.

In inch-pound units:

$$W = \frac{(1093 - 0.556t^*)W_s^* - 0.240(t - t^*)}{1093 + 0.444t - t^*} \tag{2-27b}$$

where t and t^* are in °F.

The term W_s* indicates the humidity ratio if saturated at the wet bulb temperature.

Degree of saturation μ is the ratio of the actual humidity ratio W to the humidity ratio W_s of saturated air at the same temperature and pressure.

$$\mu = \left.\frac{W}{W_s}\right|_{t,p} \tag{2-28}$$

Relative humidity ϕ is the ratio of the mole fraction of water vapor xw in a given moist air sample to the mole fraction xws in an air sample which is saturated at the same temperature and pressure:

$$\phi = \left.\frac{x_w}{x_{ws}}\right|_{t,p} \qquad \phi = \left.\frac{p_w}{p_{ws}}\right|_{t,p} \tag{2-29}$$

The term p_{ws} is the saturation pressure of water vapor at the given temperature t.

Dew-point temperature t_d is the temperature of moist air which is saturated at the same pressure p and has the same humidity ratio W as that of the given sample of moist air. It corresponds to the saturation temperature (Column 1) of Table 2-1 for the vapor pressure found in Column 2. As an alternate to using the table, equations have been formulated for the relationship.

For 0 to 70°C:

$$t_d = -35.957 - 1.8726a + 1.1689a^2 \tag{2-30a}$$

and for −60 to 0°C:

$$t_d = -60.45 + 7.0322a + 0.3700a^2 \tag{2-30b}$$

with t_d in °C and $a = \ln p_w$, with p_w in pascals.

For the temperature range of 32 to 150°F:

$$t_d = 79.047 + 30.5790a + 1.8893a^2 \tag{2-31a}$$

and for temperatures below 32°F:

$$t_d = 71.98 + 24.873a + 0.8927a^2 \tag{2-31b}$$

where t_d is the dew-point temperature in °F and $a = \ln p_w$, with p_w the water vapor partial pressure (in. Hg).

The volume v of a moist air mixture is expressed in terms of a unit mass of dry air, with the relation $p = p_a + p_w$, or:

$$v = R_aT/(p - p_w) \tag{2-32}$$

The enthalpy of a mixture of perfect gases is equal to the sum of the individual partial enthalpies of the components. The enthalpy of moist air is then:

$$h = h_a + Wh_g$$

where h_a is the specific enthalpy for dry air and h_g is the specific enthalpy for saturated water vapor at the temperature of the mixture. Approximately:

$$h_a = t \text{ (kJ/kg)} \tag{2-33}$$

$$h_g = 2501 + 1.805t \text{ (kJ/kg)} \tag{2-34}$$

Table 2-4 Thermodynamic Properties of Moist Air at Standard Pressure

(Table 2, Chapter 6, 1997 *Handbook—Fundamentals*)

Temp. t, °F	Humidity Ratio, lb_w/lb_{da} W_s	Volume, ft^3/lb dry air v_a	v_{as}	v_s	Enthalpy, Btu/lb dry air h_a	h_{as}	h_s	Entropy, Btu/(lb dry air) · °F s_a	s_{as}	s_s	Condensed Water: Enthalpy, Btu/lb h_w	Condensed Water: Entropy, Btu/lb·°F s_w	Condensed Water: Vapor Press., in. Hg p_s	Temp., °F
−80	0.0000049	9.553	0.000	9.553	−19.221	0.005	−19.215	−0.04594	0.00001	−0.04592	−193.45	−0.4067	0.000236	−80
−79	0.0000053	9.579	0.000	9.579	−18.980	0.005	−18.975	−0.04531	0.00002	−0.04529	−193.06	−0.4056	0.000255	−79
−78	0.0000057	9.604	0.000	9.604	−18.740	0.006	−18.734	−0.04468	0.00002	−0.04466	−192.66	−0.4046	0.000275	−78
−77	0.0000062	9.629	0.000	9.629	−18.500	0.007	−18.493	−0.04405	0.00002	−0.04403	−192.27	−0.4036	0.000296	−77
−76	0.0000067	9.655	0.000	9.655	−18.259	0.007	−18.252	−0.04342	0.00002	−0.04340	−191.87	−0.4025	0.000319	−76
−75	0.0000072	9.680	0.000	9.680	−18.019	0.007	−18.011	−0.04279	0.00002	−0.04277	−191.47	−0.4015	0.000344	−75
−74	0.0000078	9.705	0.000	9.705	−17.778	0.008	−17.770	−0.04217	0.00002	−0.04215	−191.07	−0.4005	0.000371	−74
−73	0.0000084	9.731	0.000	9.731	−17.538	0.009	−17.529	−0.04155	0.00002	−0.04152	−190.68	−0.3994	0.000400	−73
−72	0.0000090	9.756	0.000	9.756	−17.298	0.010	−17.288	−0.04093	0.00003	−0.04090	−190.27	−0.3984	0.000430	−72
−71	0.0000097	9.781	0.000	9.782	−17.057	0.010	−17.047	−0.04031	0.00003	−0.04028	−189.87	−0.3974	0.000463	−71
−70	0.0000104	9.807	0.000	9.807	−16.806	0.011	−16.817	−0.03969	0.00003	−0.03966	−189.47	−0.3963	0.000498	−70
−69	0.0000112	9.832	0.000	9.832	−16.577	0.012	−16.565	−0.03907	0.00003	−0.03904	−189.07	−0.3953	0.000536	−69
−68	0.0000120	9.857	0.000	9.858	−16.336	0.013	−16.324	−0.03846	0.00003	−0.03843	−188.66	−0.3943	0.000576	−68
−67	0.0000129	9.883	0.000	9.883	−16.096	0.013	−16.083	−0.03785	0.00004	−0.03781	−188.26	−0.3932	0.000619	−67
−66	0.0000139	9.908	0.000	9.908	−15.856	0.015	−15.841	−0.03724	0.00004	−0.03720	−187.85	−0.3922	0.000665	−66
−65	0.0000149	9.933	0.000	9.934	−15.616	0.015	−15.600	−0.03663	0.00004	−0.03659	−187.44	−0.3912	0.000714	−65
−64	0.0000160	9.959	0.000	9.959	−15.375	0.017	−15.359	−0.03602	0.00005	−0.03597	−187.04	−0.3901	0.000766	−64
−63	0.0000172	9.984	0.000	9.984	−15.117	0.018	−15.135	−0.03541	0.00005	−0.03536	−186.63	−0.3891	0.000822	−63
−62	0.0000184	10.009	0.000	10.010	−14.895	0.019	−14.876	−0.03481	0.00005	−0.03476	−186.22	−0.3881	0.000882	−62
−61	0.0000198	10.035	0.000	10.035	−14.654	0.021	−14.634	−0.03420	0.00006	−0.03415	−185.81	−0.3870	0.000945	−61
−60	0.0000212	10.060	0.000	10.060	−14.414	0.022	−14.392	−0.03360	0.00006	−0.03354	−185.39	−0.3860	0.001013	−60
−59	0.0000227	10.085	0.000	10.086	−14.174	0.024	−14.150	−0.03300	0.00006	−0.03294	−184.98	−0.3850	0.001086	−59
−58	0.0000243	10.111	0.000	10.111	−13.933	0.025	−13.908	−0.03240	0.00007	−0.03233	−184.57	−0.3839	0.001163	−58
−57	0.0000260	10.136	0.000	10.137	−13.693	0.027	−13.666	−0.03180	0.00007	−0.03173	−184.15	−0.3829	0.001246	−57
−56	0.0000279	10.161	0.000	10.162	−13.453	0.029	−13.424	−0.03121	0.00008	−0.03113	−183.74	−0.3819	0.001333	−56
−55	0.0000298	10.187	0.000	10.187	−13.213	0.031	−13.182	−0.03061	0.00008	−0.03053	−183.32	−0.3808	0.001427	−55
−54	0.0000319	10.212	0.001	10.213	−12.972	0.033	−12.939	−0.03002	0.00009	−0.02993	−182.90	−0.3798	0.001526	−54
−53	0.0000341	10.237	0.001	10.238	−12.732	0.035	−12.697	−0.02943	0.00009	−0.02934	−182.48	−0.3788	0.001632	−53
−52	0.0000365	10.263	0.001	10.263	−12.492	0.038	−12.454	−0.02884	0.00010	−0.02874	−182.06	−0.3778	0.001745	−52
−51	0.0000390	10.288	0.001	10.289	−12.251	0.041	−12.211	−0.02825	0.00011	−0.02814	−181.64	−0.3767	0.001865	−51
−50	0.0000416	10.313	0.001	10.314	−12.011	0.043	−11.968	−0.02766	0.00011	−0.02755	−181.22	−0.3757	0.001992	−50
−49	0.0000445	10.339	0.001	10.340	−11.771	0.046	−11.725	−0.02708	0.00012	−0.02696	−180.80	−0.3747	0.002128	−49
−48	0.0000475	10.364	0.001	10.365	−11.531	0.050	−11.481	−0.02649	0.00013	−0.02636	−180.37	−0.3736	0.002272	−48
−47	0.0000507	10.389	0.001	10.390	−11.290	0.053	−11.237	−0.02591	0.00014	−0.02577	−179.95	−0.3726	0.002425	−47
−46	0.0000541	10.415	0.001	10.416	−11.050	0.056	−10.994	−0.02533	0.00015	−0.02518	−179.52	−0.3716	0.002587	−46
−45	0.0000577	10.440	0.001	10.441	−10.810	0.060	−10.750	−0.02475	0.00016	−0.02459	−179.10	−0.3705	0.002760	−45
−44	0.0000615	10.465	0.001	10.466	−10.570	0.064	−10.505	−0.02417	0.00017	−0.02400	−178.67	−0.3695	0.002943	−44
−43	0.0000656	10.491	0.001	10.492	−10.329	0.068	−10.261	−0.02359	0.00018	−0.02342	−178.24	−0.3685	0.003137	−43
−42	0.0000699	10.516	0.001	10.517	−10.089	0.073	−10.016	−0.02302	0.00019	−0.02283	−177.81	−0.3675	0.003343	−42
−41	0.0000744	10.541	0.001	10.543	−9.849	0.078	−9.771	−0.02244	0.00020	−0.02224	−177.38	−0.3664	0.003562	−41
−40	0.0000793	10.567	0.001	10.568	−9.609	0.083	−9.526	−0.02187	0.00021	−0.02166	−176.95	−0.3654	0.003793	−40
−39	0.0000844	10.592	0.001	10.593	−9.368	0.088	−9.280	−0.02130	0.00022	−0.02107	−176.52	−0.3644	0.004039	−39
−38	0.0000898	10.617	0.002	10.619	−9.128	0.094	−9.034	−0.02073	0.00024	−0.02049	−176.08	−0.3633	0.004299	−38
−37	0.0000956	10.643	0.002	10.644	−8.888	0.100	−8.788	−0.02016	0.00025	−0.01991	−175.65	−0.3623	0.004575	−37
−36	0.0001017	10.668	0.002	10.670	−8.648	0.106	−8.541	−0.01959	0.00027	−0.01932	−175.21	−0.3613	0.004866	−36
−35	0.0001081	10.693	0.002	10.695	−8.407	0.113	−8.294	−0.01902	0.00028	−0.01874	−174.78	−0.3603	0.005175	−35
−34	0.0001150	10.719	0.002	10.721	−8.167	0.120	−8.047	−0.01846	0.00030	−0.01816	−174.34	−0.3529	0.005502	−34
−33	0.0001222	10.744	0.002	10.746	−7.927	0.128	−7.799	−0.01790	0.00032	−0.01758	−173.90	−0.3582	0.005848	−33
−32	0.0001298	10.769	0.002	10.772	−7.687	0.136	−7.551	−0.01733	0.00034	−0.01699	−173.46	−0.3572	0.006214	−32
−31	0.0001379	10.795	0.002	10.797	−7.447	0.145	−7.302	−0.01677	0.00036	−0.01641	−173.02	−0.3561	0.006601	−31
−30	0.0001465	10.820	0.003	10.822	−7.206	0.154	−7.053	−0.01621	0.00038	−0.01583	−172.58	−0.3551	0.007009	−30
−29	0.0001555	10.845	0.003	10.848	−6.966	0.163	−6.803	−0.01565	0.00040	−0.01525	−172.14	−0.3541	0.007442	−29
−28	0.0001650	10.871	0.003	10.873	−6.726	0.173	−6.553	−0.01510	0.00043	−0.01467	−171.70	−0.3531	0.007898	−28
−27	0.0001751	10.896	0.003	10.899	−6.486	0.184	−6.302	−0.01454	0.00045	−0.01409	−171.25	−0.3520	0.008381	−27
−26	0.0001858	10.921	0.003	10.924	−6.245	0.195	−6.051	−0.01399	0.00048	−0.01351	−170.81	−0.3510	0.008890	−26
−25	0.0001970	10.947	0.003	10.950	−6.005	0.207	−5.798	−0.01343	0.00051	−0.01293	−170.36	−0.3500	0.009428	−25
−24	0.0002088	10.972	0.004	10.976	−5.765	0.220	−5.545	−0.01288	0.00054	−0.01235	−169.92	−0.3489	0.009995	−24
−23	0.0002214	10.997	0.004	11.001	−5.525	0.233	−5.292	−0.01233	0.00057	−0.01176	−169.47	−0.3479	0.010594	−23
−22	0.0002346	11.022	0.004	11.027	−5.284	0.247	−5.038	−0.01178	0.00060	−0.01118	−169.02	−0.3469	0.011226	−22
−21	0.0002485	11.048	0.004	11.052	−5.044	0.261	−4.783	−0.01123	0.00063	−0.01060	−168.57	−0.3459	0.011893	−21
−20	0.0002632	11.073	0.005	11.078	−4.804	0.277	−4.527	−0.01069	0.00067	−0.01002	−168.12	−0.3448	0.012595	−20
−19	0.0002786	11.098	0.005	11.103	−4.564	0.293	−4.271	−0.01014	0.00071	−0.00943	−167.67	−0.3438	0.013336	−19
−18	0.0002950	11.124	0.005	11.129	−4.324	0.311	−4.013	−0.00960	0.00075	−0.00885	−167.21	−0.3428	0.014117	−18
−17	0.0003121	11.149	0.006	11.155	−4.084	0.329	−3.754	−0.00905	0.00079	−0.00826	−166.76	−0.3418	0.014939	−17
−16	0.0003303	11.174	0.006	11.180	−3.843	0.348	−3.495	−0.00851	0.00083	−0.00768	−166.30	−0.3407	0.015806	−16
−15	0.0003493	11.200	0.006	11.206	−3.603	0.368	−3.235	−0.00797	0.00088	−0.00709	−165.85	−0.3397	0.016718	−15
−14	0.0003694	11.225	0.007	11.232	−3.363	0.390	−2.973	−0.00743	0.00093	−0.00650	−165.39	−0.3387	0.017679	−14
−13	0.0003905	11.250	0.007	11.257	−3.123	0.412	−2.710	−0.00689	0.00098	−0.00591	−164.93	−0.3377	0.018690	−13
−12	0.0004128	11.276	0.007	11.283	−2.882	0.436	−2.447	−0.00635	0.00103	−0.00532	−164.47	−0.3366	0.019754	−12
−11	0.0004362	11.301	0.008	11.309	−2.642	0.460	−2.182	−0.00582	0.00109	−0.00473	−164.01	−0.3356	0.020873	−11

Table 2-4 Thermodynamic Properties of Moist Air at Standard Pressure (*Continued*)

(Table 2, Chapter 6, 1997 *Handbook—Fundamentals*)

Temp. t, °F	Humidity Ratio, lb_w/lb_{da} W_s	Volume, ft^3/lb dry air			Enthalpy, Btu/lb dry air			Entropy, Btu/(lb dry air) · °F			Condensed Water Enthalpy, Btu/lb	Condensed Water Entropy, Btu/lb·°F	Condensed Water Vapor Press., in. Hg	Temp., °F
		v_a	v_{as}	v_s	h_a	h_{as}	h_s	s_a	s_{as}	s_s	h_w	s_w	p_s	
−10	0.0004608	11.326	0.008	11.335	−2.402	0.487	−1.915	−0.00528	0.00115	−0.00414	−163.55	−0.3346	0.022050	−10
−9	0.0004867	11.351	0.009	11.360	−2.162	0.514	−1.647	−0.00475	0.00121	−0.00354	−163.09	−0.3335	0.023289	−9
−8	0.0005139	11.377	0.009	11.386	−1.922	0.543	−1.378	−0.00422	0.00127	−0.00294	−162.63	−0.3325	0.024591	−8
−7	0.0005425	11.402	0.010	11.412	−1.681	0.574	−1.108	−0.00369	0.00134	−0.00234	−162.17	−0.3315	0.025959	−7
−6	0.0005726	11.427	0.010	11.438	−1.441	0.606	−0.835	−0.00316	0.00141	−0.00174	−161.70	−0.3305	0.027397	−6
−5	0.0006041	11.453	0.011	11.464	−1.201	0.640	−0.561	−0.00263	0.00149	−0.00114	−161.23	−0.3294	0.028907	−5
−4	0.0006373	11.478	0.012	11.490	−0.961	0.675	−0.286	−0.00210	0.00157	−0.00053	−160.77	−0.3284	0.030494	−4
−3	0.0006722	11.503	0.012	11.516	−0.721	0.712	−0.008	−0.00157	0.00165	0.00008	−160.30	−0.3274	0.032160	−3
−2	0.0007088	11.529	0.013	11.542	−0.480	0.751	0.271	−0.00105	0.00174	0.00069	−159.83	−0.3264	0.033909	−2
−1	0.0007472	11.554	0.014	11.568	−0.240	0.792	0.552	−0.00052	0.00183	0.00130	−159.36	−0.3253	0.035744	−1
0	0.0007875	11.579	0.015	11.594	0.0	0.835	0.835	0.00000	0.00192	0.00192	−158.89	−0.3243	0.037671	0
1	0.0008298	11.604	0.015	11.620	0.240	0.880	1.121	0.00052	0.00202	0.00254	−158.42	−0.3233	0.039694	1
2	0.0008742	11.630	0.016	11.646	0.480	0.928	1.408	0.00104	0.00212	0.00317	−157.95	−0.3223	0.041814	2
3	0.0009207	11.655	0.017	11.672	0.721	0.978	1.699	0.00156	0.00223	0.00380	−157.47	−0.3212	0.044037	3
4	0.0009695	11.680	0.018	11.699	0.961	1.030	1.991	0.00208	0.00235	0.00443	−157.00	−0.3202	0.046370	4
5	0.0010207	11.706	0.019	11.725	1.201	1.085	2.286	0.00260	0.00247	0.00506	−156.52	−0.3192	0.048814	5
6	0.0010743	11.731	0.020	11.751	1.441	1.143	2.584	0.00311	0.00259	0.00570	−156.05	−0.3182	0.051375	6
7	0.0011306	11.756	0.021	11.778	1.681	1.203	2.884	0.00363	0.00635	0.00272	−155.57	−0.3171	0.054060	7
8	0.0011895	11.782	0.022	11.804	1.922	1.266	3.188	0.00414	0.00286	0.00700	−155.09	−0.3161	0.056872	8
9	0.0012512	11.807	0.024	11.831	2.162	1.332	3.494	0.00466	0.00300	0.00766	−154.61	−0.3151	0.059819	9
10	0.0013158	11.832	0.025	11.857	2.402	1.402	3.804	0.00517	0.00315	0.00832	−154.13	−0.3141	0.062901	10
11	0.0013835	11.857	0.026	11.884	2.642	1.474	4.117	0.00568	0.00330	0.00898	−153.65	−0.3130	0.066131	11
12	0.0014544	11.883	0.028	11.910	2.882	1.550	4.433	0.00619	0.00347	0.00966	−153.17	−0.3120	0.069511	12
13	0.0015286	11.908	0.029	11.937	3.123	1.630	4.753	0.00670	0.00364	0.01033	−152.68	−0.3110	0.073049	13
14	0.0016062	11.933	0.031	11.964	3.363	1.714	5.077	0.00721	0.00381	0.01102	−152.20	−0.3100	0.076751	14
15	0.0016874	11.959	0.032	11.991	3.603	1.801	5.404	0.00771	0.00400	0.01171	−151.71	−0.3089	0.080623	15
16	0.0017724	11.984	0.034	12.018	3.843	1.892	5.736	0.00822	0.00419	0.01241	−151.22	−0.3079	0.084673	16
17	0.0018613	12.009	0.036	12.045	4.084	1.988	6.072	0.00872	0.00439	0.01312	−150.74	−0.3069	0.088907	17
18	0.0019543	12.035	0.038	12.072	4.324	2.088	6.412	0.00923	0.00460	0.01383	−150.25	−0.3059	0.093334	18
19	0.0020515	12.060	0.040	12.099	4.564	2.193	6.757	0.00973	0.00482	0.01455	−149.76	−0.3049	0.097962	19
20	0.0021531	12.085	0.042	12.127	4.804	2.303	7.107	0.01023	0.00505	0.01528	−149.27	−0.3038	0.102798	20
21	0.0022592	12.110	0.044	12.154	5.044	2.417	7.462	0.01073	0.00529	0.01602	−148.78	−0.3028	0.107849	21
22	0.0023703	12.136	0.046	12.182	5.285	2.537	7.822	0.01123	0.00554	0.01677	−148.28	−0.3018	0.113130	22
23	0.0024863	12.161	0.048	12.209	5.525	2.662	8.187	0.01173	0.00580	0.01753	−147.79	−0.3008	0.118645	23
24	0.0026073	12.186	0.051	12.237	5.765	2.793	8.558	0.01223	0.00607	0.01830	−147.30	−0.2997	0.124396	24
25	0.0027339	12.212	0.054	12.265	6.005	2.930	8.935	0.01272	0.00636	0.01908	−146.80	−0.2987	0.130413	25
26	0.0028660	12.237	0.056	12.293	6.246	3.073	9.318	0.01322	0.00665	0.01987	−146.30	−0.2977	0.136684	26
27	0.0030039	12.262	0.059	12.321	6.486	3.222	9.708	0.01371	0.00696	0.02067	−145.81	−0.2967	0.143233	27
28	0.0031480	12.287	0.062	12.349	6.726	3.378	10.104	0.01420	0.00728	0.02148	−145.31	−0.2956	0.150066	28
29	0.0032984	12.313	0.065	12.378	6.966	3.541	10.507	0.01470	0.00761	0.02231	−144.81	−0.2946	0.157198	29
30	0.0034552	12.338	0.068	12.406	7.206	3.711	10.917	0.01519	0.00796	0.02315	−144.31	−0.2936	0.164631	30
31	0.0036190	12.363	0.072	12.435	7.447	3.888	11.335	0.01568	0.00832	0.02400	−143.80	−0.2926	0.172390	31
32	0.0037895	12.389	0.075	12.464	7.687	4.073	11.760	0.01617	0.00870	0.02487	−143.30	−0.2915	0.180479	32
32*	0.003790	12.389	0.075	12.464	7.687	4.073	11.760	0.01617	0.00870	0.02487	0.02	0.0000	0.18050	32
33	0.003947	12.414	0.079	12.492	7.927	4.243	12.170	0.01665	0.00905	0.02570	1.03	0.0020	0.18791	33
34	0.004109	12.439	0.082	12.521	8.167	4.420	12.587	0.01714	0.00940	0.02655	2.04	0.0041	0.19559	34
35	0.004277	12.464	0.085	12.550	8.408	4.603	13.010	0.01763	0.00977	0.02740	3.05	0.0061	0.20356	35
36	0.004452	12.490	0.089	12.579	8.648	4.793	13.441	0.01811	0.01016	0.02827	4.05	0.0081	0.21181	36
37	0.004633	12.515	0.093	12.608	8.888	4.990	13.878	0.01860	0.01055	0.02915	5.06	0.0102	0.22035	37
38	0.004820	12.540	0.097	12.637	9.128	5.194	14.322	0.01908	0.01096	0.03004	6.06	0.0122	0.22920	38
39	0.005014	12.566	0.101	12.667	9.369	5.405	14.773	0.01956	0.01139	0.03095	7.07	0.0142	0.23835	39
40	0.005216	12.591	0.105	12.696	9.609	5.624	15.233	0.02004	0.01183	0.03187	8.07	0.0162	0.24784	40
41	0.005424	12.616	0.110	12.726	9.849	5.851	15.700	0.02052	0.01228	0.03281	9.08	0.0182	0.25765	41
42	0.005640	12.641	0.114	12.756	10.089	6.086	16.175	0.02100	0.01275	0.03375	10.08	0.0202	0.26781	42
43	0.005863	12.667	0.119	12.786	10.330	6.330	16.660	0.02148	0.01324	0.03472	11.09	0.0222	0.27831	43
44	0.006094	12.692	0.124	12.816	10.570	6.582	17.152	0.02196	0.01374	0.03570	12.09	0.0242	0.28918	44
45	0.006334	12.717	0.129	12.846	10.810	6.843	17.653	0.02244	0.01426	0.03669	13.09	0.0262	0.30042	45
46	0.006581	12.743	0.134	12.877	11.050	7.114	18.164	0.02291	0.01479	0.03770	14.10	0.0282	0.31206	46
47	0.006838	12.768	0.140	12.908	11.291	7.394	18.685	0.02339	0.01534	0.03873	15.10	0.0302	0.32408	47
48	0.007103	12.793	0.146	12.939	11.531	7.684	19.215	0.02386	0.01592	0.03978	16.10	0.0321	0.33651	48
49	0.007378	12.818	0.152	12.970	11.771	7.984	19.756	0.02433	0.01651	0.04084	17.10	0.0341	0.34937	49
50	0.007661	12.844	0.158	13.001	12.012	8.295	20.306	0.02480	0.01712	0.04192	18.11	0.0361	0.36264	50
51	0.007955	12.869	0.164	13.033	12.252	8.616	20.868	0.02528	0.01775	0.04302	19.11	0.0381	0.37636	51
52	0.008259	12.894	0.171	13.065	12.492	8.949	21.441	0.02575	0.01840	0.04415	20.11	0.0400	0.39054	52
53	0.008573	12.920	0.178	13.097	12.732	9.293	22.025	0.02622	0.01907	0.04529	21.11	0.0420	0.40518	53
54	0.008897	12.945	0.185	13.129	12.973	9.648	22.621	0.02668	0.01976	0.04645	22.11	0.0439	0.42030	54
55	0.009233	12.970	0.192	13.162	13.213	10.016	23.229	0.02715	0.02048	0.04763	23.11	0.0459	0.43592	55
56	0.009580	12.995	0.200	13.195	13.453	10.397	23.850	0.02762	0.02122	0.04884	24.11	0.0478	0.45205	56
57	0.009938	13.021	0.207	13.228	13.694	10.790	24.484	0.02808	0.02198	0.05006	25.11	0.0497	0.46870	57
58	0.010309	13.046	0.216	13.262	13.934	11.197	25.131	0.02855	0.02277	0.05132	26.11	0.0517	0.48589	58
59	0.010692	13.071	0.224	13.295	14.174	11.618	25.792	0.02901	0.02358	0.05259	27.11	0.0536	0.50363	59

*Extrapolated to represent metastable equilibrium with undercooled liquid.

Table 2-4 Thermodynamic Properties of Moist Air at Standard Pressure (*Continued*)

(Table 2, Chapter 6, 1997 *Handbook—Fundamentals*)

Temp. t, °F	Humidity Ratio, lb_w/lb_{da} W_s	Volume, ft^3/lb dry air v_a	v_{as}	v_s	Enthalpy, Btu/lb dry air h_a	h_{as}	h_s	Entropy, Btu/(lb dry air) · °F s_a	s_{as}	s_s	Condensed Water: Enthalpy, Btu/lb h_w	Condensed Water: Entropy, Btu/lb · °F s_w	Condensed Water: Vapor Press., in. Hg p_s	Temp., °F
60	0.011087	13.096	0.233	13.329	14.415	12.052	26.467	0.02947	0.02442	0.05389	28.11	0.0555	0.52193	60
61	0.011496	13.122	0.242	13.364	14.655	12.502	27.157	0.02994	0.02528	0.05522	29.12	0.0575	0.54082	61
62	0.011919	13.147	0.251	13.398	14.895	12.966	27.862	0.03040	0.02617	0.05657	30.11	0.0594	0.56032	62
63	0.012355	13.172	0.261	13.433	15.135	13.446	28.582	0.03086	0.02709	0.05795	31.11	0.0613	0.58041	63
64	0.012805	13.198	0.271	13.468	15.376	13.942	29.318	0.03132	0.02804	0.05936	32.11	0.0632	0.60113	64
65	0.013270	13.223	0.281	13.504	15.616	14.454	30.071	0.03178	0.02902	0.06080	33.11	0.0651	0.62252	65
66	0.013750	13.248	0.292	13.540	15.856	14.983	30.840	0.03223	0.03003	0.06226	34.11	0.0670	0.64454	66
67	0.014246	13.273	0.303	13.577	16.097	15.530	31.626	0.03269	0.03107	0.06376	35.11	0.0689	0.66725	67
68	0.014758	13.299	0.315	13.613	16.337	16.094	32.431	0.03315	0.03214	0.06529	36.11	0.0708	0.69065	68
69	0.015286	13.324	0.326	13.650	16.577	16.677	33.254	0.03360	0.03325	0.06685	37.11	0.0727	0.71479	69
70	0.015832	13.349	0.339	13.688	16.818	17.279	34.097	0.03406	0.03438	0.06844	38.11	0.0746	0.73966	70
71	0.016395	13.375	0.351	13.726	17.058	17.901	34.959	0.03451	0.03556	0.07007	39.11	0.0765	0.76567	71
72	0.016976	13.400	0.365	13.764	17.299	18.543	35.841	0.03496	0.03677	0.07173	40.11	0.0783	0.79167	72
73	0.017575	13.425	0.378	13.803	17.539	19.204	36.743	0.03541	0.03801	0.07343	41.11	0.0802	0.81882	73
74	0.018194	13.450	0.392	13.843	17.779	19.889	37.668	0.03586	0.03930	0.07516	42.11	0.0821	0.84684	74
75	0.018833	13.476	0.407	13.882	18.020	20.595	38.615	0.03631	0.04062	0.07694	43.11	0.0840	0.87567	75
76	0.019491	13.501	0.422	13.923	18.260	21.323	39.583	0.03676	0.04199	0.07875	44.10	0.0858	0.90533	76
77	0.020170	13.526	0.437	13.963	18.500	22.075	40.576	0.03721	0.04339	0.08060	45.10	0.0877	0.93589	77
78	0.020871	13.551	0.453	14.005	18.741	22.851	41.592	0.03766	0.04484	0.08250	46.10	0.0896	0.96733	78
79	0.021594	13.577	0.470	14.046	18.981	23.652	42.633	0.03811	0.04633	0.08444	47.10	0.0914	0.99970	79
80	0.022340	13.602	0.487	14.089	19.222	24.479	43.701	0.03855	0.04787	0.08642	48.10	0.0933	1.03302	80
81	0.023109	13.627	0.505	14.132	19.462	25.332	44.794	0.03900	0.04945	0.08844	49.10	0.0951	1.06728	81
82	0.023902	13.653	0.523	14.175	19.702	26.211	45.913	0.03944	0.05108	0.09052	50.10	0.0970	1.10252	82
83	0.024720	13.678	0.542	14.220	19.943	27.120	47.062	0.03988	0.05276	0.09264	51.09	0.0988	1.13882	83
84	0.025563	13.703	0.561	14.264	20.183	28.055	48.238	0.04033	0.05448	0.09481	52.09	0.1006	1.17608	84
85	0.026433	13.728	0.581	14.310	20.424	29.021	49.445	0.04077	0.05626	0.09703	53.09	0.1025	1.21445	85
86	0.027329	13.754	0.602	14.356	20.664	30.017	50.681	0.04121	0.05809	0.09930	54.09	0.1043	1.25388	86
87	0.028254	13.779	0.624	14.403	20.905	31.045	51.949	0.04165	0.05998	0.10163	55.09	0.1061	1.29443	87
88	0.029208	13.804	0.646	14.450	21.145	32.105	53.250	0.04209	0.06192	0.10401	56.09	0.1080	1.33613	88
89	0.030189	13.829	0.669	14.498	21.385	33.197	54.582	0.04253	0.06392	0.10645	57.09	0.1098	1.37893	89
90	0.031203	13.855	0.692	14.547	21.626	34.325	55.951	0.04297	0.06598	0.10895	58.08	0.1116	1.42298	90
91	0.032247	13.880	0.717	14.597	21.866	35.489	57.355	0.06810	0.04340	0.11150	59.08	0.1134	1.46824	91
92	0.033323	13.905	0.742	14.647	22.107	36.687	58.794	0.04384	0.07028	0.11412	60.08	0.1152	1.51471	92
93	0.034433	13.930	0.768	14.699	22.347	37.924	60.271	0.04427	0.07253	0.11680	61.08	0.1170	1.56248	93
94	0.035577	13.956	0.795	14.751	22.588	39.199	61.787	0.04471	0.07484	0.11955	62.08	0.1188	1.61154	94
95	0.036757	13.981	0.823	14.804	22.828	40.515	63.343	0.04514	0.07722	0.12237	63.08	0.1206	1.66196	95
96	0.037972	14.006	0.852	14.858	23.069	41.871	64.940	0.04558	0.07968	0.12525	64.07	0.1224	1.71372	96
97	0.039225	14.032	0.881	14.913	23.309	43.269	66.578	0.04601	0.08220	0.12821	65.07	0.1242	1.76685	97
98	0.040516	14.057	0.912	14.969	23.550	44.711	68.260	0.04644	0.08480	0.13124	66.07	0.1260	1.82141	98
99	0.041848	14.082	0.944	15.026	23.790	46.198	69.988	0.04687	0.08747	0.13434	67.07	0.1278	1.87745	99
100	0.043219	14.107	0.976	15.084	24.031	47.730	71.761	0.04730	0.09022	0.13752	68.07	0.1296	1.93492	100
101	0.044634	14.133	1.010	15.143	24.271	49.312	73.583	0.04773	0.09306	0.14079	69.07	0.1314	1.99396	101
102	0.046090	14.158	1.045	15.203	24.512	50.940	75.452	0.04816	0.09597	0.14413	70.06	0.1332	2.05447	102
103	0.047592	14.183	1.081	15.264	24.752	52.621	77.373	0.04859	0.09897	0.14756	71.06	0.1349	2.11661	103
104	0.049140	14.208	1.118	15.326	24.993	54.354	79.346	0.04901	0.10206	0.15108	72.06	0.1367	2.18037	104
105	0.050737	14.234	1.156	15.390	25.233	56.142	81.375	0.04944	0.10525	0.15469	73.06	0.1385	2.24581	105
106	0.052383	14.259	1.196	15.455	25.474	57.986	83.460	0.04987	0.10852	0.15839	74.06	0.1402	2.31297	106
107	0.054077	14.284	1.236	15.521	25.714	59.884	85.599	0.05029	0.11189	0.16218	75.06	0.1420	2.38173	107
108	0.055826	14.309	1.279	15.588	25.955	61.844	87.799	0.05071	0.11537	0.16608	76.05	0.1438	2.45232	108
109	0.057628	14.335	1.322	15.657	26.195	63.866	90.061	0.05114	0.11894	0.17008	77.05	0.1455	2.52473	109
110	0.059486	14.360	1.367	15.727	26.436	65.950	92.386	0.05156	0.12262	0.17418	78.05	0.1473	2.59891	110
111	0.061401	14.385	1.414	15.799	26.677	68.099	94.776	0.05198	0.12641	0.17839	79.05	0.1490	2.67500	111
112	0.063378	14.411	1.462	15.872	26.917	70.319	97.237	0.05240	0.13032	0.18272	80.05	0.1508	2.75310	112
113	0.065411	14.436	1.511	15.947	27.158	72.603	99.760	0.05282	0.13434	0.18716	81.05	0.1525	2.83291	113
114	0.067512	14.461	1.562	16.023	27.398	74.964	102.362	0.05324	0.13847	0.19172	82.04	0.1543	2.91491	114
115	0.069676	14.486	1.615	16.101	27.639	77.396	105.035	0.05366	0.14274	0.19640	83.04	0.1560	2.99883	115
116	0.071908	14.512	1.670	16.181	27.879	79.906	107.786	0.05408	0.14713	0.20121	84.04	0.1577	3.08488	116
117	0.074211	14.537	1.726	16.263	28.120	82.497	110.617	0.05450	0.15165	0.20615	85.04	0.1595	3.17305	117
118	0.076586	14.562	1.784	16.346	28.361	85.169	113.530	0.05492	0.15631	0.21122	86.04	0.1612	3.26335	118
119	0.079036	14.587	1.844	16.432	28.601	87.927	116.528	0.05533	0.16111	0.21644	87.04	0.1629	3.35586	119
120	0.081560	14.613	1.906	16.519	28.842	90.770	119.612	0.05575	0.16605	0.22180	88.04	0.1647	3.45052	120
121	0.084169	14.638	1.971	16.609	29.083	93.709	122.792	0.05616	0.17115	0.22731	89.04	0.1664	3.54764	121
122	0.086860	14.663	2.037	16.700	29.323	96.742	126.065	0.05658	0.17640	0.23298	90.03	0.1681	3.64704	122
123	0.089633	14.688	2.106	16.794	29.564	99.868	129.432	0.05699	0.18181	0.23880	91.03	0.1698	3.74871	123
124	0.092500	14.714	2.176	16.890	29.805	103.102	132.907	0.05740	0.18739	0.24480	92.03	0.1715	3.85298	124
125	0.095456	14.739	2.250	16.989	30.045	106.437	136.482	0.05781	0.19314	0.25096	93.03	0.1732	3.95961	125
126	0.098504	14.764	2.325	17.090	30.286	109.877	140.163	0.05823	0.19907	0.25729	94.03	0.1749	4.06863	126
127	0.101657	14.789	2.404	17.193	30.527	113.438	143.965	0.05864	0.20519	0.26382	95.03	0.1766	4.18046	127
128	0.104910	14.815	2.485	17.299	30.767	117.111	147.878	0.05905	0.21149	0.27054	96.03	0.1783	4.29477	128
129	0.108270	14.840	2.569	17.409	31.008	120.908	151.916	0.21800	0.21810	0.27745	97.03	0.1800	4.41181	129

Table 2-4 Thermodynamic Properties of Moist Air at Standard Pressure (*Continued*)

(Table 2, Chapter 6, 1997 *Handbook—Fundamentals*)

Temp. t, °F	Humidity Ratio, lb_w/lb_{da} W_s	Volume, ft³/lb dry air			Enthalpy, Btu/lb dry air			Entropy, Btu/(lb dry air) · °F			Condensed Water Enthalpy, Btu/lb	Condensed Water Entropy, Btu/lb · °F	Condensed Water Vapor Press., in. Hg	Temp., °F
		v_a	v_{as}	v_s	h_a	h_{as}	h_s	s_a	s_{as}	s_s	h_w	s_w	p_s	
130	0.111738	14.865	2.655	17.520	31.249	124.828	156.076	0.05986	0.22470	0.28457	98.03	0.1817	4.53148	130
131	0.115322	14.891	2.745	17.635	31.489	128.880	160.370	0.06027	0.23162	0.29190	99.02	0.1834	4.65397	131
132	0.119023	14.916	2.837	17.753	31.730	133.066	164.796	0.06068	0.23876	0.29944	100.02	0.1851	4.77919	132
133	0.122855	14.941	2.934	17.875	31.971	137.403	169.374	0.06109	0.24615	0.30723	101.02	0.1868	4.90755	133
134	0.126804	14.966	3.033	17.999	32.212	141.873	174.084	0.06149	0.25375	0.31524	102.02	0.1885	5.03844	134
135	0.130895	14.992	3.136	18.127	32.452	146.504	178.957	0.06190	0.26161	0.32351	103.02	0.1902	5.17258	135
136	0.135124	15.017	3.242	18.259	32.693	151.294	183.987	0.06230	0.26973	0.33203	104.02	0.1919	5.30973	136
137	0.139494	15.042	3.352	18.394	32.934	156.245	189.179	0.06271	0.27811	0.34082	105.02	0.1935	5.44985	137
138	0.144019	15.067	3.467	18.534	33.175	161.374	194.548	0.06311	0.28707	0.35018	106.02	0.1952	5.59324	138
139	0.148696	15.093	3.585	18.678	33.415	166.677	200.092	0.06351	0.29602	0.35954	107.02	0.1969	5.73970	139
140	0.153538	15.118	3.708	18.825	33.656	172.168	205.824	0.06391	0.30498	0.36890	108.02	0.1985	5.88945	140
141	0.158643	15.143	3.835	18.978	33.897	177.857	211.754	0.06431	0.31456	0.37887	109.02	0.2002	6.04256	141
142	0.163748	15.168	3.967	19.135	34.138	183.754	217.892	0.06471	0.32446	0.38918	110.02	0.2019	6.19918	142
143	0.169122	15.194	4.103	19.297	34.379	189.855	224.233	0.06511	0.33470	0.39981	111.02	0.2035	6.35898	143
144	0.174694	15.219	4.245	19.464	34.620	196.183	230.802	0.06551	0.34530	0.41081	112.02	0.2052	6.52241	144
145	0.180467	15.244	4.392	19.637	34.860	202.740	237.600	0.06591	0.35626	0.42218	113.02	0.2068	6.68932	145
146	0.186460	15.269	4.545	19.815	35.101	209.550	244.651	0.06631	0.36764	0.43395	114.02	0.2085	6.86009	146
147	0.192668	15.295	4.704	19.999	35.342	216.607	251.949	0.06671	0.37941	0.44611	115.02	0.2101	7.03435	147
148	0.199110	15.320	4.869	20.189	35.583	223.932	259.514	0.06710	0.39160	0.45871	116.02	0.2118	7.21239	148
149	0.205792	15.345	5.040	20.385	35.824	231.533	267.356	0.06750	0.40424	0.47174	117.02	0.2134	7.39413	149
150	0.212730	15.370	5.218	20.589	36.064	239.426	275.490	0.06790	0.41735	0.48524	118.02	0.2151	7.57977	150
151	0.219945	15.396	5.404	20.799	36.305	247.638	283.943	0.06829	0.43096	0.49925	119.02	0.2167	7.76958	151
152	0.227429	15.421	5.596	21.017	36.546	256.158	292.705	0.06868	0.44507	0.51375	120.02	0.2184	7.96306	152
153	0.235218	15.446	5.797	21.243	36.787	265.028	301.816	0.06908	0.45973	0.52881	121.02	0.2200	8.16087	153
154	0.243309	15.471	6.005	21.477	37.028	274.245	311.273	0.06947	0.47494	0.54441	122.02	0.2216	8.36256	154
155	0.251738	15.497	6.223	21.720	37.269	283.849	321.118	0.06986	0.49077	0.56064	123.02	0.2233	8.56871	155
156	0.260512	15.522	6.450	21.972	37.510	293.849	331.359	0.07025	0.50723	0.57749	124.02	0.2249	8.77915	156
157	0.269644	15.547	6.686	22.233	37.751	304.261	342.012	0.07065	0.52434	0.59499	125.02	0.2265	8.99378	157
158	0.279166	15.572	6.933	22.505	37.992	315.120	353.112	0.07104	0.54217	0.61320	126.02	0.2281	9.21297	158
159	0.289101	15.598	7.190	22.788	38.233	326.452	364.685	0.07143	0.56074	0.63216	127.02	0.2297	9.43677	159
160	0.29945	15.623	7.459	23.082	38.474	338.263	376.737	0.07181	0.58007	0.65188	128.02	0.2314	9.6648	160
161	0.31027	15.648	7.740	23.388	38.715	350.610	389.325	0.07220	0.60025	0.67245	129.02	0.2330	9.8978	161
162	0.32156	15.673	8.034	23.707	38.956	363.501	402.457	0.07259	0.62128	0.69388	130.03	0.2346	10.1353	162
163	0.33336	15.699	8.341	24.040	39.197	376.979	416.175	0.07298	0.64325	0.71623	131.03	0.2362	10.3776	163
164	0.34572	15.724	8.664	24.388	39.438	391.095	430.533	0.07337	0.66622	0.73959	132.03	0.2378	10.6250	164
165	0.35865	15.749	9.001	24.750	39.679	405.865	445.544	0.07375	0.69022	0.76397	133.03	0.2394	10.8771	165
166	0.37220	15.774	9.355	25.129	39.920	421.352	461.271	0.07414	0.71535	0.78949	134.03	0.2410	11.1343	166
167	0.38639	15.800	9.726	25.526	40.161	437.578	477.739	0.07452	0.74165	0.81617	135.03	0.2426	11.3965	167
168	0.40131	15.825	10.117	25.942	40.402	454.630	495.032	0.07491	0.76925	0.84415	136.03	0.2442	11.6641	168
169	0.41698	15.850	10.527	26.377	40.643	472.554	513.197	0.07529	0.79821	0.87350	137.04	0.2458	11.9370	169
170	0.43343	15.875	10.959	26.834	40.884	491.372	532.256	0.07567	0.82858	0.90425	138.04	0.2474	12.2149	170
171	0.45079	15.901	11.414	27.315	41.125	511.231	552.356	0.07606	0.86058	0.93664	139.04	0.2490	12.4988	171
172	0.46905	15.926	11.894	27.820	41.366	532.138	573.504	0.07644	0.89423	0.97067	140.04	0.2506	12.7880	172
173	0.48829	15.951	12.400	28.352	41.607	554.160	595.767	0.07682	0.92962	1.00644	141.04	0.2521	13.0823	173
174	0.50867	15.976	12.937	28.913	41.848	577.489	619.337	0.07720	0.96707	1.04427	142.04	0.2537	13.3831	174
175	0.53019	16.002	13.504	29.505	42.089	602.139	644.229	0.07758	1.00657	1.08416	143.05	0.2553	13.6894	175
176	0.55294	16.027	14.103	30.130	42.331	628.197	670.528	0.07796	1.04828	1.12624	144.05	0.2569	14.0010	176
177	0.57710	16.052	14.741	30.793	42.572	655.876	698.448	0.07834	1.09253	1.17087	145.05	0.2585	14.3191	177
178	0.60274	16.078	15.418	31.496	42.813	685.260	728.073	0.07872	1.13943	1.21815	146.05	0.2600	14.6430	178
179	0.63002	16.103	16.139	32.242	43.054	716.524	759.579	0.07910	1.18927	1.26837	147.06	0.2616	14.9731	179
180	0.65911	16.128	16.909	33.037	43.295	749.871	793.166	0.07947	1.24236	1.32183	148.06	0.2632	15.3097	180
181	0.69012	16.153	17.730	33.883	43.536	785.426	828.962	0.07985	1.29888	1.37873	149.06	0.2647	15.6522	181
182	0.72331	16.178	18.609	34.787	43.778	823.487	867.265	0.08023	1.35932	1.43954	150.06	0.2663	16.0014	182
183	0.75885	16.204	19.551	35.755	44.019	864.259	908.278	0.08060	1.42396	1.50457	151.07	0.2679	16.3569	183
184	0.79703	16.229	20.564	36.793	44.260	908.061	952.321	0.08098	1.49332	1.57430	152.07	0.2694	16.7190	184
185	0.83817	16.254	21.656	37.910	44.501	955.261	999.763	0.08135	1.56797	1.64932	153.07	0.2710	17.0880	185
186	0.88251	16.280	22.834	39.113	44.742	1006.149	1050.892	0.08172	1.64834	1.73006	154.08	0.2725	17.4634	186
187	0.93057	16.305	24.111	40.416	44.984	1061.314	1106.298	0.08210	1.73534	1.81744	155.08	0.2741	17.8462	187
188	0.98272	16.330	25.498	41.828	45.225	1121.174	1166.399	0.08247	1.82963	1.91210	156.08	0.2756	18.2357	188
189	1.03951	16.355	27.010	43.365	45.466	1186.382	1231.848	0.08284	1.93221	2.01505	157.09	0.2772	18.6323	189
190	1.10154	16.381	28.661	45.042	45.707	1257.614	1303.321	0.08321	2.04412	2.12733	158.09	0.2787	19.0358	190
191	1.16965	16.406	30.476	46.882	45.949	1335.834	1381.783	0.08359	2.16684	2.25043	159.09	0.2803	19.4468	191
192	1.24471	16.431	32.477	48.908	46.190	1422.047	1468.238	0.08396	2.30193	2.38589	160.10	0.2818	19.8652	192
193	1.32788	16.456	34.695	51.151	46.431	1517.581	1564.013	0.08433	2.45144	2.53576	161.10	0.2834	20.2913	193
194	1.42029	16.481	37.161	53.642	46.673	1623.758	1670.430	0.08470	2.61738	2.70208	162.11	0.2849	20.7244	194
195	1.52396	16.507	39.928	56.435	46.914	1742.879	1789.793	0.08506	2.80332	2.88838	163.11	0.2864	21.1661	195
196	1.64070	16.532	43.046	59.578	47.155	1877.032	1924.188	0.08543	3.01244	3.09787	164.12	0.2880	21.6152	196
197	1.77299	16.557	46.580	63.137	47.397	2029.069	2076.466	0.08580	3.24914	3.33494	165.12	0.2895	22.0714	197
198	1.92472	16.583	50.636	67.218	47.638	2203.464	2251.102	0.08617	3.52030	3.60647	166.13	0.2910	22.5367	198
199	2.09975	16.608	55.316	71.923	47.879	2404.668	2452.547	0.08653	3.83275	3.91929	167.13	0.2926	23.0092	199
200	2.30454	16.633	60.793	77.426	48.121	2640.084	2688.205	0.08690	4.19787	4.28477	168.13	0.2941	23.4906	200

where t is the dry-bulb temperature, °C. The moist air enthalpy then becomes:

$$h = t + W(2501 + 1.805t) \text{ (kJ/kg dry air)} \quad (2\text{-}35)$$

In conventional (I-P) units:

$$h_a = 0.240t \text{ (Btu/lb)} \quad (2\text{-}36)$$

$$h_g = 1061 + 0.444t \text{ (Btu/lb)} \quad (2\text{-}37)$$

$$h = 0.240t + W(1061 + 0.444t) \text{ (Btu/lb)} \quad (2\text{-}38)$$

where t is the dry-bulb temperature, °F.

Table 2-4 is a tabulation of the thermodynamic properties of moist air at sea level standard atmospheric pressure. Table 2-5 shows variation of atmospheric pressure with altitude.

Table 2-5 Standard Atmospheric Data with Altitude
(Table 1, Chapter 6, 1997 *Fundamentals*)

		Pressure	
Altitude, ft	**Temperature, °F**	**in. Hg**	**psia**
−1000	62.6	31.02	15.236
−500	60.8	30.47	14.966
0	59.0	29.921	14.696
500	57.2	29.38	14.430
1000	55.4	28.86	14.175
2000	51.9	27.82	13.664
3000	48.3	26.82	13.173
4000	44.7	25.82	12.682
5000	41.2	24.90	12.230
6000	37.6	23.98	11.778
7000	34.0	23.09	11.341
8000	30.5	22.22	10.914
9000	26.9	21.39	10.506
10,000	23.4	20.58	10.108
15,000	5.5	16.89	8.296
20,000	−12.3	13.76	6.758
30,000	−47.8	8.90	4.371
40,000	−69.7	5.56	2.731
50,000	−69.7	3.44	1.690
60,000	−69.7	2.14	1.051

Data adapted from NASA (1976).

2.2.14 Psychrometric Chart

The ASHRAE psychrometric chart may be used to solve numerous process problems with moist air. Processes performed with air can be plotted on the chart for quick visualization, as well as for determining changes in significant properties such as temperature, humidity ratio, and enthalpy for the process. ASHRAE Psychrometric Chart No. 1 in I-P units is shown in Figure 2-10. Some of the basic air-conditioning processes are shown in Figure 2-11.

Sensible heating only (C) or *sensible cooling* (G) shows a change in dry-bulb temperature with no change in humidity ratio. For either sensible heat change process, the temperature changes but not the moisture content of the air.

Humidifying only (A) or *dehumidifying* only (E) shows a change in humidity ratio with no change in dry-bulb temperaturc. For these latent heat processes, the moisture content of the air is changed but not the temperature.

Cooling and dehumidifying (F) result in a reduction of both the dry-bulb temperature and the humidity ratio. Cooling coils generally perform this type of process.

Heating and humidifying (B) result in an increase of both the dry-bulb temperature and the humidity ratio.

Chemical dehumidifying (D) is a process in which moisture from the air is absorbed or adsorbed by a hygroscopic material. Generally, the process essentially occurs at constant enthalpy.

Evaporative cooling only (H) is an adiabatic heat transfer process in which the wet-bulb temperature of the air remains constant but the dry-bulb temperature drops as the humidity rises.

Adiabatic mixing of air at one condition with air at some other condition is represented on the psychrometric chart by a straight line drawn between the points representing the two air conditions (Figure 2-12).

2.3 Forms of Energy

2.3.1 Energy

Energy is the capacity for producing an effect. Thermodynamics is founded on the *law of conservation of energy*, which says that energy can neither be created nor destroyed. Heat and work are transitory forms of energy, losing their identity as soon as they are absorbed by the body or region to which they are delivered. Work and heat are not possessed by a system and, therefore, are not properties. Thus, if there is a net transfer of energy across the boundary from a system (as heat and/or work), from where did this energy come? The only answer is that it must have come from a store of energy in the given system. These stored forms of energy may be assumed to reside within the bodies or regions with which they are associated. In thermodynamics, accent is placed on the changes of stored energy rather than on absolute quantities.

2.3.2 Stored Forms of Energy

Energy may be stored in such forms as thermal (internal), mechanical, electrical, chemical, and atomic (nuclear).

Internal Energy, *U*. Internal (thermal) energy is the energy possessed by matter due to the motion and/or position of its molecules. This energy is comprised of two components: (1) kinetic internal energy—due to the velocity of the molecules and manifested by temperature; and (2) potential internal energy—due to the attractive forces existing between molecules and manifested by the phase of the system.

Potential Energy, P.E. Potential energy is the energy possessed by the system due to the elevation or position of the system. This potential energy is equivalent to the work required to lift the system from the arbitrary datum (0 elevation) to its elevation z in the absence of friction.

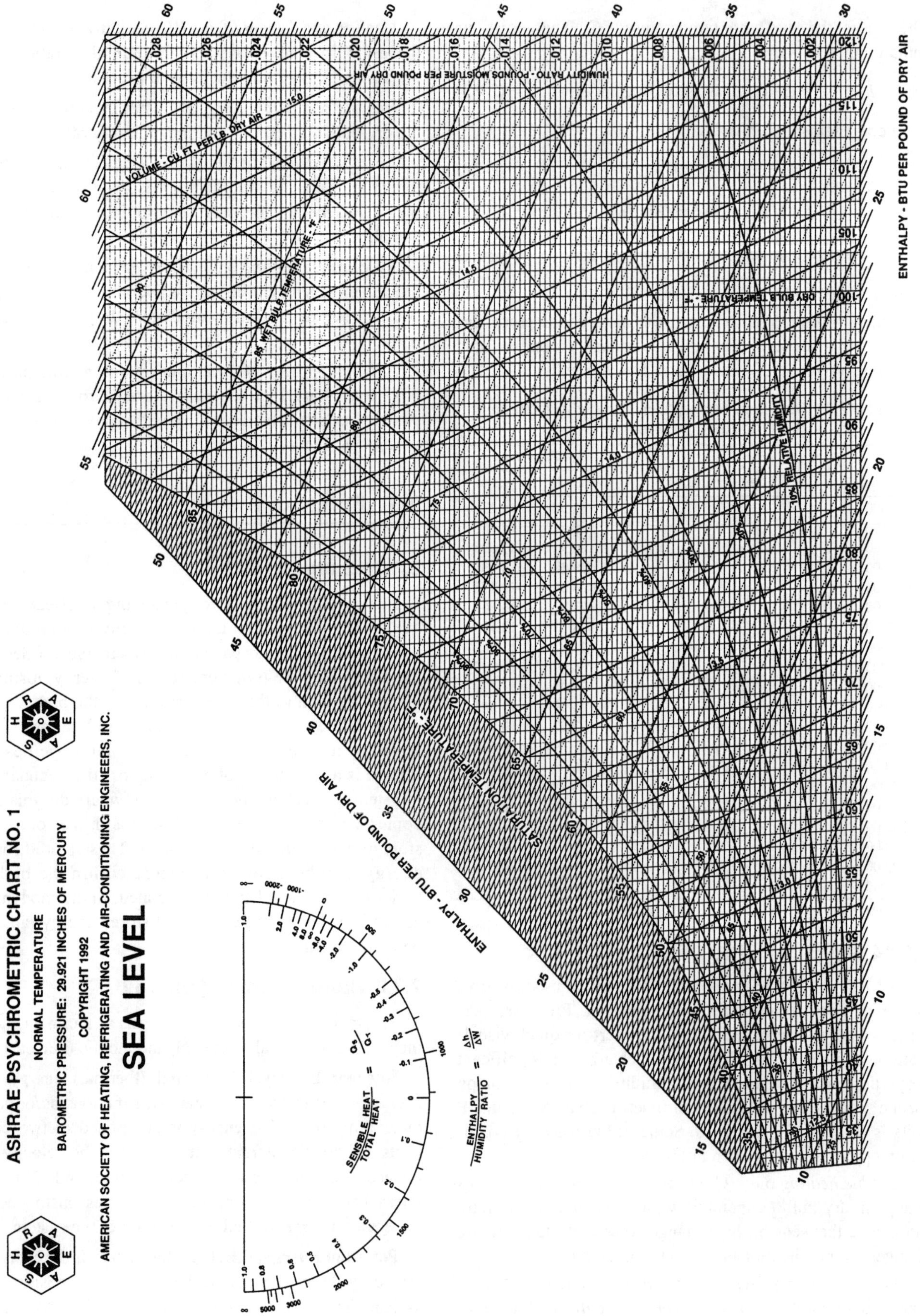

Fig. 2-10 ASHRAE Psychrometric Chart

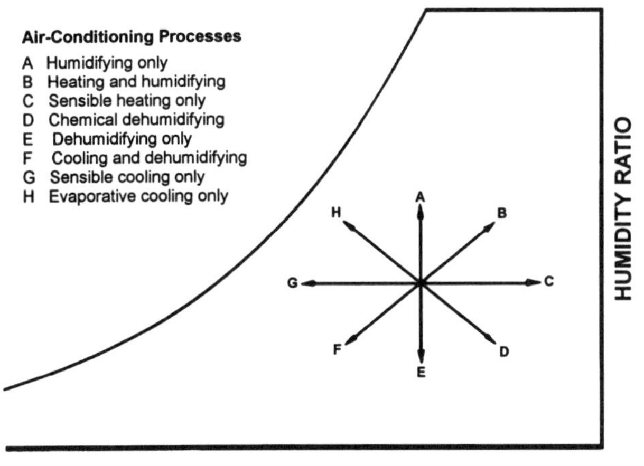

Fig. 2-11 Psychrometric Representations of Basic Air-Conditioning Process

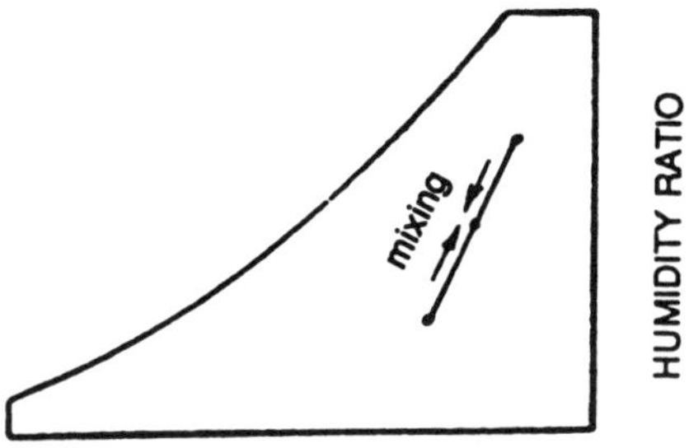

Fig. 2-12 Adiabatic Mixing

$$F = \frac{ma}{g_c} = \frac{mg}{g_c}$$

$$\text{P.E.} = W = \int_0^x F dx = \int_0^z m\frac{g}{g_c} dx = m\frac{g}{g_c} z \tag{2-39}$$

Kinetic Energy, K.E. Kinetic energy is the energy possessed by the system as a result of the velocity of the system. It is equal to the work that could be done in bringing to rest a system that is in motion, with a velocity V, in the absence of gravity.

$$F = \frac{ma}{g_c} = \frac{m}{g_c}\frac{dV}{dt} \tag{2-40}$$

Chemical Energy, E_c. Chemical energy is possessed by the system because of the arrangement of the atoms composing the molecules. Reactions that liberate energy are termed *exothermic* and those that absorb energy are termed *endothermic*.

$$\text{K.E.} = W = \int_0^x F\text{d}x = -\int_V^0 \frac{m}{g_c}\frac{\text{d}V}{\text{d}t}\text{d}x$$

$$= -\int_V^0 \frac{m}{g_c} V\text{d}v = \frac{mV^2}{2g_c}$$

Nuclear (Atomic) Energy, E_a. Nuclear energy is possessed by the system due to the cohesive forces holding the protons and neutrons together as the nucleus of the atom.

Stored energy is concerned with:

1. Molecules of the system (internal energy)
2. The system as a unit (kinetic and potential energy)
3. Arrangement of the atoms (chemical)
4. Nucleus of the atom (nuclear).

Molecular stored energy is associated with the relative position and velocity of the molecules; the total effect is called internal energy. Kinetic energy and potential energy are both forms of mechanical energy, and they can be converted readily and completely into work. Chemical, electrical, and atomic energy would be included in any accounting of stored energy; however, engineering thermodynamics frequently confines itself to systems not undergoing changes in these three forms of energy.

2.3.3 Transient Forms of Energy

Heat, Q. Heat is the mechanism by which energy is transferred across the boundary between systems by reason of the difference in temperature of the two systems, and always in the direction of the lower temperature. Being transitory, heat is not a property. It is redundant to speak of heat as being transferred, for the term *heat* signifies energy in transit. Nevertheless, in keeping with common usage, this text refers to heat as being transferred.

Although a body or system cannot contain heat, it is useful, when discussing many processes, to speak of heat received or heat rejected, so that the direction of heat transfer relative to the system is obvious. This should not be construed as treating heat as a substance.

Heat *transferred* to a system is considered to be positive, and *heat transferred* from a system, negative. Thus, positive heat represents energy transferred to a system, and negative heat represents energy transferred from a system. A process in which there is no heat transfer ($Q = 0$) is called an **adiabatic process**.

Work. Work is the mechanism by which energy is transferred across the boundary between systems by reason of the difference in pressure (or force of any kind) of the two systems, and is in the direction of the lower pressure.

If the total effect produced in the system can be reduced to the raising of a weight, then nothing but work has crossed the boundary. Work, like heat, is not possessed by the system, but occurs only as energy being transferred.

Work is, by definition, the energy resulting from a force having moved through a distance. If the force varies with distance x, work may be expressed as $\delta W = F\,dx$.

In thermodynamics, work is often done by a force distributed over an area, i.e., by pressure p acting through volume V, as in the case of fluid pressure exerted on a piston. In this event:

$$\delta W = p\,dV$$

where p is an external pressure exerted on the system.

Mechanical or shaft work W is the energy delivered or absorbed by a mechanism, such as a turbine, air compressor, or internal combustion engine. Shaft work can always be evaluated from the basic relation for work.

Power is the rate of doing work.

Work done *by* a system is considered positive; work done *on* a system is considered negative. The symbol W designates the work done by a system.

Work may be done on or by a system in a variety of ways. In addition to mechanical work and flow work (the types most frequently encountered in thermodynamics), work may be done due to surface tension, the flow of electricity, magnetic fields, and in other ways.

For nonflow processes, the form of mechanical work most frequently encountered is that done at the moving boundary of a system, such as the work done in moving the piston in a cylinder. It may be expressed in equation form for reversible processes as $W = \int pdV$. Generally, for the nonflow process, work can be expressed as:

$$W = \int pdv \ldots \qquad (2\text{-}41)$$

where the dots indicate other ways in which work can be done by or on the system.

The following section shows the derivation of a useful expression for the work of a frictionless steady-flow proc-ess. The derivation procedure is:

1. Make a free-body diagram of an element of fluid.
2. Evaluate the external forces on the free body.
3. Relate the sum of the external forces to the mass and acceleration of the free body.
4. Solve the resulting relation for the force by which work is done on the fluid.
5. Apply the definition of work as $\int Fds$. A free-body diagram is illustrated in Figure 2-13.

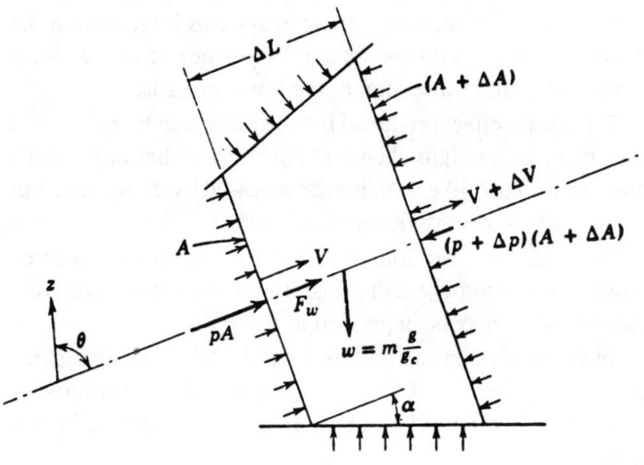

Fig. 2-13 Element of Fluid in Frictionless Steady Flow

Applying Newton's second law of motion, the sum of the external forces on the fluid element must equal ma/g_c. The mass of the element is $\rho(A + \Delta A/2)\Delta L$, and the acceleration is approximately $\Delta V/\Delta\tau$. Thus:

$$\Sigma F = \frac{ma}{g_c} = \frac{\rho}{g_c}\left(A + \frac{\Delta A}{2}\right)\Delta L\frac{\Delta V}{\Delta\tau}$$

The sum or resultant of the forces is:

$$\Sigma F = pA - (p + \Delta p)(A + \Delta A) - m\frac{g}{g_c}\cos\theta$$

$$+\left(p + \frac{\Delta p}{2}\right)\Delta A + F_W$$

$$= -A\Delta p - \frac{\Delta p\Delta A}{3} - m\frac{g}{g_c}\cos\theta + F_w$$

$$\text{Work}_{in} = F_w\Delta L = (\text{Volume})\Delta p + \frac{V\Delta V}{g_C} + \frac{g}{g_c}\Delta z$$

and per unit mass:

$$\text{Work}_{in} = v\Delta p + \frac{V\Delta V}{g_C} + \frac{g}{g_c}\Delta Z$$

Now, if ΔL is made to approach dL, then the other differences also approach differentials, and the work (per unit mass) done on the fluid in the distance dL is:

$$\delta\text{Work}_{in} = vdp + \frac{VdV}{g_c} + \frac{g}{g_c}dz \qquad (2\text{-}42)$$

or, for flow between sections a finite distance apart:

$$\text{Work}_{in} = \int vdp + \Delta\left(\frac{V^2}{2g_c}\right) + \frac{g}{g_c}\Delta z$$

This important relation shows the mechanical work done on a unit mass of fluid in a frictionless steady-flow process.

In addition to commonly encountering work done at a moving boundary in an **open system**, flow work must be considered. **Flow work** consists of the energy carried into or transmitted across the system boundary because of the work done by the fluid just outside the system on the adjacent fluid entering the system to force or push it into the system. Flow work also occurs as fluid leaves the system, this time by fluid in the system on the fluid just leaving the system. As an analogy, consider two people as particles of fluid, one in the doorway and one just outside. Flow work would be done by the person outside if he or she shoved the person in the doorway into the room (system).

$$\text{Flow work} = \int Fdx = \int pdAx, \qquad p = c$$

$$= p\int_0^v dV = pv \qquad (2\text{-}43)$$

where Flow work is per unit mass and v is the specific volume, or the volume displaced per unit mass.

This analysis shows that work must be done in causing fluid to flow into or out of a system. This work is called flow work. Such terms as flow energy and displacement energy are sometimes used.

2.4 First Law of Thermodynamics

The first law of thermodynamics is often called the *law of conservation of energy*. From the first law, it can be concluded that for any system, open or closed, there is an energy balance as:

Net amount of energy added to system	=	Net increase in stored energy of system

or:

Energy in − Energy out =
Increase in energy in system (2-44)

With both open and closed systems, energy can be added to or taken from the system by means of heat and work. In an open system, there is an additional mechanism for increasing or decreasing the stored energy of the system. When mass enters a system, the stored energy of the system is increased by the stored energy of the entering mass. The stored energy of a system is decreased whenever mass leaves the system because the mass leaving the system takes some stored energy with it. To distinguish this transfer of stored energy of mass crossing the system boundary from heat and work, consider:

	Stored energy of mass entering system	−	Stored energy of mass leaving system
+	Net energy added to system heat and work	=	Net increase in stored energy of system

The net exchange of energy between the system and its surroundings must be balanced by the change in energy of the system. Exchange of energy in transition includes either work or heat. However, what is meant by the energy of the system and the energy associated with any matter entering or leaving the system must be described further.

The energy E of the system is a property of the system and consists of all of the various forms in which energy is characteristic. These forms include potential energy (due to position), kinetic energy (due to any motion), electrical energy (due to charge), and so forth. Because work and heat are energy in transition and are not characteristic of the system, they are not included here.

All the energy of a system—exclusive of kinetic and potential energy—is called *internal energy*. The symbol for internal energy per unit mass is u. The symbol for internal energy contained in a mass of m pounds or kilograms is U. Each unit of mass flowing into or out of the system carries with it the energy characteristic of that unit of mass. This energy includes the internal energy u plus the kinetic and potential energy.

Work is always done on or by a system where fluid flows across the system boundary. Therefore, work in an energy balance for an open system is usually separated into two parts: (1) the work required to push a fluid into or out of the system; and (2) all other forms of work.

The work flow per unit mass crossing the boundary of a system is pv. If the pressure, specific volume, or both vary as a fluid flows across a system boundary, the flow work is calculated by integrating $\int pv\delta m$, where δm is an infinitesimal mass crossing the boundary. The symbol δm is used instead of dm because the amount of mass crossing the boundary is not a property. The mass within the system is a property, so the infinitesimal change in mass within the system is properly represented by dm.

Since the work term in an energy balance for an open system is usually separated into two parts, (1) flow work and (2) all other forms of work, the term work W without modifiers stands for all other forms of work except flow work, and the complete, two-word name is always used when referring to flow work.

An equation representing the first law can be written using the symbols defined for the general system of Figure 2-14. Referring to Figure 2-14, let δm_1 be the mass entering the system and δm_2 be the mass leaving. The first law in differential or incremental form becomes:

$$[\delta m(e + pv)]_{in} - [\delta m(e + pv)]_{out} + \delta Q - \delta W = dE \quad (2\text{-}45)$$

or,

$$\delta m_1\left(u_1 + p_1v_1 + \frac{V_1^2}{2g_c} + z_1\frac{g}{g_c}\right)$$

$$-\delta m_2\left(u_2 + p_2v_2 + \frac{V_2^2}{2g_c} + z_2\frac{g}{g_c}\right) + \delta Q - \delta W = dE$$

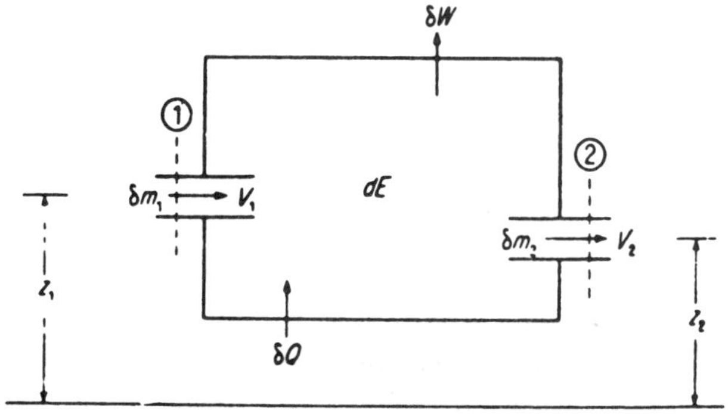

Fig. 2-14 Energy Flows in a General Thermodynamic System

where δQ and δW are the increments of work and heat, and dE is the differential change in the energy of the system. Because E or U (or e or u) are properties of the system, they are treated like any other property such as temperature, pressure, density, or viscosity.

The combination of properties $u + pv$ is also a property, which has been defined as enthalpy. The symbol H stands for the total enthalpy associated with a mass m; h stands for specific enthalpy, or enthalpy per unit mass. In equation form:

$$h = u + pv$$

In terms of enthalpy, the first law equation becomes:

$$\delta m_1\left(h_1 + \frac{V_1^2}{2g_c} + \frac{g}{g_c}z_1\right) - \delta m_2\left(h_2 + \frac{V_2^2}{2g_c} + \frac{g}{g_c}z_2\right) + \delta Q - \delta W = dE \tag{2-46}$$

or in integrated form:

$$\int_0^{m_1} \delta m_1\left(h_1 + \frac{V_1^2}{2g_c} + \frac{g}{g_c}z_1\right) - \int_0^{m_2} \delta m_2\left(h_2 + \frac{V_2^2}{2g_c} + \frac{g}{g_c}z_2\right) + \delta Q - \delta W = E_{final} - E_{initial} \tag{2-47}$$

or, if divided by the time interval $\Delta\tau$:

$$\frac{\delta m_1}{\Delta\tau}\left(h_1 + \frac{V_1^2}{2g_c} + \frac{g}{g_c}z_1\right) - \frac{\delta m_2}{\Delta\tau}\left(h_2 + \frac{V_2^2}{2g_c} + \frac{g}{g_c}z_2\right) + \frac{\delta Q}{\Delta\tau} - \frac{\delta W}{\Delta\tau} = \frac{dE}{\Delta\tau}$$

$$\Delta\tau \to 0, \quad \frac{\delta Q}{\Delta\tau} \to \dot{Q}, \quad \frac{\delta W}{\Delta\tau} \to \dot{W}$$

$$\frac{\delta m_1}{\Delta\tau} \to \dot{m}_1, \quad \frac{\delta m_2}{\Delta\tau} \to \dot{m}_2, \quad \frac{dE}{\Delta\tau} \to \frac{dE}{d\tau}$$

$$\dot{m}_1\left(h_1 + \frac{V_1^2}{2g_c} + \frac{g}{g_c}z_1\right) - \dot{m}_2\left(h_2 + \frac{V_2^2}{2g_c} + \frac{g}{g_c}z_2\right) + \dot{Q} - \dot{W} = \frac{dE}{d\tau} \tag{2-48}$$

where $\dot{Q}$ is heat flow and $\dot{W}$ is the work rate or power.

The most general case in which the prior integration of the first law is possible has the following conditions:

1. The properties of the fluids crossing the boundary remain constant at each point on the boundary.
2. The flow rate at each section where mass crosses the boundary is constant. (The flow rate cannot change as long as all properties, including velocity, remain constant at each point.)
3. All interactions with the surroundings occur at a steady rate.

Integration then yields:

$$\sum m_{in}\left(u + pv + \frac{V_1^2}{2g_c} + \frac{g}{g_c}z\right)_{in} - \sum m_{out}\left(u + pv + \frac{V_2^2}{2g_c} + \frac{g}{g_c}z\right)_{out} + Q - W = \left[m_f\left(u + \frac{V^2}{2g_c}z\right) - m_i\left(u + \frac{V^2}{2g_c}\right)_i\right]_{system} \tag{2-49}$$

A special case in engineering applications is the **steady-flow process**. In steady flow, all quantities associated with the system do not vary with time. Consequently:

$$\sum \dot{m}\left(h + \frac{V^2}{2g_c} + \frac{g}{g_c}z\right) - \sum \dot{m}\left(h + \frac{V^2}{2g_c} + \frac{g}{g_c}z\right) + \dot{Q} - \dot{W} = 0 \tag{2-50}$$

A second common application is the **closed-stationary system**, for which the first law equation reduces to:

$$Q - W = [m(u_f - u_i)]_{system} \tag{2-51}$$

Example 2.1 Nitrogen having a mass of 0.85 kg expands in an irreversible manner doing 572 J of work. The temperature of the nitrogen drops from 81°C to 34°C. Determine the heat transfer.

Solution:

First law for stationary closed system:

$$Q - W = m(u_f - u_i)$$

For gases:

$$U_f - U_i = mc_v(t_f - t_i)$$

$$Q - 572/1000 = 0.85(0.741)(34 - 81)$$

$$Q = -29.03 \text{ kJ } (-27.5 \text{ Btu})$$

Example 2.2 A tank having a volume of 40 ft³ is initially evacuated. This tank is connected to an air line. The air in this line has an internal energy of 80 Btu/lb, a pressure of 100 psia, and a specific volume of 32 ft³/lb. The valve is opened, the tank fills with air until the pressure is 100 psia, and then the valve is closed. The process takes place adiabatically, and kinetic and potential energies are negligible. Determine the final internal energy of the air in the tank in Btu/lb.

Solution:

First law:

$$m_{in}(u + pv)_{in} = m_f m_f$$

Conservation of mass:

$$m_f = m_{in}$$

$$(u + pv)_{in} = u_f = 80 + (100)(144)(32)/778$$

$$= 673 \text{ Btu/lb } (1565 \text{ kJ/kg})$$

2.5 Second Law of Thermodynamics

2.5.1 Second Law from Classical Thermodynamics

As a generality, the second law deals with the fact that many processes proceed only in one direction, and not in the opposite direction. Everyday examples include the fact that a cup of hot coffee cools to its surroundings, but the cooler surroundings never heat up the warmer cup of coffee; or the fact that the chemical energy in gasoline is used as a car is driven up a hill, but coasting down the hill does not restore the gasoline. The second law of thermodynamics is a formalized statement of such observations.

A system that undergoes a series of processes and returns to its initial state is said to go through a cycle. For the closed system undergoing a cycle, from the first law of thermodynamics:

$$\oint \delta Q = \oint \delta W$$

The symbol $\oint$ stands for the cyclical integral of the increment of heat or work. Any heat supplied to a cycling system must be balanced by an equivalent amount of work done by the system. Conversely, any work done on the cycling system gives off an equivalent amount of heat.

Many examples exist of work being completely converted into heat. However, a cycling system that completely converts heat into work has never been observed, although such complete conversion would not be a violation of the first law. The fact that heat cannot be completely converted into work is the basis for the second law of thermodynamics. The justification for the second law is based on empirical observations.

The second law has been stated in different ways; one is the *Kelvin-Planck statement* of the second law which states, *It is impossible for any cycling device to exchange heat with only a single reservoir and produce work.*

In this context, reservoir refers to a body whose temperature remains constant regardless of how much heat is added to or taken from it. In other words, the Kelvin-Planck statement says that heat cannot be continuously and completely converted into work; a fraction of the heat must be rejected to another reservoir at a lower temperature. The second law thus restricts the first law in relation to the way energy is transferred. Work can be continuously and completely converted into heat, but not vice versa.

If the Kelvin-Planck statement were not true and heat could be completely converted to work, heat might be obtained from a low-temperature source, converted into work, and the work converted back into heat in a region of higher temperature. The net result of this series of events would be the flow of heat from a low-temperature region to a high-temperature region with no other effect. This phenomenon has never been observed and is contrary to all experience.

The Clausius statement of the second law is, *No process is possible whose sole result is the removal of heat from a reservoir at one temperature and the absorption of an equal quantity of heat by a reservoir at a higher temperature.*

Two major consequences related to the Kelvin-Planck and Clausius statements of the second law are the limiting values for thermal efficiency of power systems operating on heat and for the coefficients of performance for heat pumps. In accordance with the Kelvin-Planck concept, the maximum possible thermal efficiency (work output/heat input) of a heat engine operating between temperature reservoirs at T_H and T_L is

$$\eta_{thermal,\ max} = [1 - T_L/T_H]\ 100$$

The maximum possible coefficient of performance for cooling (cooling effect/work input) is

$$COP_{c,max} = T_L/(T_H - T_L)$$

and the maximum possible coefficient of performance for heating (heating effect/work input) is

$$COP_{h,max} = T_H/(T_H - T_L)$$

2.5.2 Second Law from Statistical Thermodynamics

To help understand the significance of the second law of thermodynamics, consider the molecular nature of matter. Although a sample of a gas may be at rest, its molecules are not. Rather, they are in a state of continuous, random motion, with an average speed of the same order of magnitude as the speed of sound waves in the gas. For air, this is about 1100 ft/s (335 m/s) at room temperature. Some of the molecules move more rapidly than this and some more slowly.

Due to collisions with one another and with the walls of the containing vessel, the velocity of any one molecule is continually being changed in magnitude and direction. The number of molecules traveling in a given direction with a given speed, however, remains constant. If the gas as a whole is at rest, the molecular velocities are distributed randomly in any direction. From the standpoint of conservation of energy (the first law), molecules of a gas, flying about in all directions and with a wide range of speeds, could get together in a cooperative effort and simultaneously acquire a common velocity component in the same direction, although it is unexpected. Nevertheless, these phenomena have been observed and are described as fluctuations.

Hence, processes whose sole result is the flow of heat from a heat reservoir and the performance of an equivalent amount of work, do not occur with sufficient frequency or with objects of sufficient size to make them useful.

Thus, an accurate statement of the second law should replace the term *impossible* with *improbable*. Therefore, the second law is a statement of the improbability of the spontaneous passage of the system from a highly probable state (random or disordered) to one of lower probability.

2.5.3 Physical Meaning of Entropy

Entropy is a measure of the random mix or of the probability of a given state. The more completely shuffled any system is, the greater is its entropy; conversely, an orderly or unmixed configuration is one of low entropy. Thus, when a substance reaches a state in which all randomness disappears, it then has zero entropy.

In 1851, Rankine analytically demonstrated that the ratio of the heat exchanged in a reversible process to the temperature of the interaction defined a thermodynamic function that was not consumed in a reversible cycle. The following year, Clausius independently derived the same result, but identified the function as a property of a system, and designated it as the entropy.

The concept of energy serves as a measure of the quantity of heat, but entropy serves as a measure of its quality. Clausius also concluded that although the energy of the world is constant, the entropy increases to a maximum, due to the irreversible nature of real processes. This extreme represents a condition when there are no potential differ-ences in the universe.

In an irreversible process, the entropy of the universe is irretrievably increased, but no energy is lost. From the engineer's point of view, however, the opportunity to convert internal energy to mechanical energy is lost. An example is the mixing of hot and cold water from two reservoirs into a single reservoir. The internal energy of the system is the same before as after mixing, but at the end of the process, no heat can be withdrawn from the single reservoir to operate a cyclic machine. An engine could have been operated between the original hot and cold reservoirs, but once the reservoirs have come to the same temperature, this opporunity is lost.

Entropy is not conserved, except in reversible processes. When a beaker of hot water is mixed with a beaker of cold water, the heat lost by the hot water equals the heat gained by the cold water and energy is conserved. On the other hand, while the entropy of the hot water decreases, the entropy of the cold water increases a greater amount, and the total entropy of the system is greater at the end of the process than it is at the beginning. Where did this additional entropy come from? It was created in the process. Furthermore, once entropy has been created, it can never be destroyed. *Energy can neither be created nor destroyed*, states the first law of thermodynamics. *Entropy cannot be destroyed, but it can be created*, states the second law.

2.5.4 Entropy Equation of the Second Law of Thermodynamics

For the general case of an open system, the second law can be written:

$$dS_{system} = (\delta Q/T)_{rev} + \delta m_i s_i - \delta m_e s_e + dS_{irr} \qquad (2\text{-}52)$$

where

$\delta m_i s_i$ = entropy increase due to the mass entering
$\delta m_e s_e$ = entropy decrease due to the mass leaving
$\delta Q/T$ = entropy change due to reversible heat transfer between the system and surroundings
dS_{irr} = entropy created due to irreversibilities

The equation accounts for all the entropy changes in the system. Rearranging:

$$\delta Q = T[\delta m_e s_e - \delta m_i s_i) + dS_{sys} - dS_{irr}] \qquad (2\text{-}53)$$

In integrated form—subject to the restrictions that inlet and outlet properties, mass flow rates, and interactions with the surroundings do not vary with time—the general equation for the second law is:

$$(S_f - S_i)_{system} = \int_{rev} \delta Q/T + \Sigma(ms)_{in} - \Sigma(ms)_{out} + \Delta S_{produced} \qquad (2\text{-}54)$$

Example 2.3 A contact feedwater heater operates on the principle of mixing steam and water. Steam enters the heater at 100 psia and 98% quality. Water enters the heater at 100 psia, 80°F. As a result, 25,000 lb_m/h of water at 95 psia and 290°F leave the heater. No heat transfers between the heater and the surroundings. Evaluate each term in the general entropy equation for the second law.

Solution:

First law:

$$m_1 h_1 + m_2 h_2 - m_3 h_3 = 0$$

From Table 2-1:

$$h_1 = 298.61 + 0.98(889.2) = 1170$$

$$h_2 = 48.05$$

$$h_3 = 259.4 \text{ Btu/lb}$$

$$s_1 = 0.47439 + 0.98(1.1290) = 1.581$$

$$s_2 = 0.09325$$

$$s_3 = 0.4236 \text{ Btu/lb·°R}$$

$$m_1(1170) + (25000 - m_1)(48.05) = 25000(259.4)$$

$$m_1 = 4710 \text{ lb}_m\text{/h}; \quad m_2 = 20{,}290 \text{ lb}_m\text{/h}$$

Second law:

$$m_f s_f - m_i s_i = \int \delta Q/T + m_1 s_1 + m_2 s_2 - m_3 s_3 + \Delta S_{irr}$$

$$0 = 0 + 4710(1.581) + 20290(0.9325) - 25000(0.4236) + \Delta S_{irr}$$

$\Delta S_{irr} = 1150$

$$m_f s_f - m_i s_i = \int \delta Q/T + m_1 s_1 + m_2 s_2 - m_3 s_3 + \Delta S_{irr}$$

$$0 = 0 + 7450 + 2000 - 10600 + 1150$$

First Law of Thermodynamics (Energy Balance)

$$\sum m_{in}\left(u+\frac{Pv}{J}+\frac{V^2}{2g_cJ}+\frac{g}{g_c}\frac{z}{J}\right)_{in}$$

$$-\sum m_{out}\left(u+\frac{Pv}{J}+\frac{V^2}{2g_cJ}+\frac{g}{g_c}\frac{z}{J}\right)_{out}+Q-W$$

$$=\left[m_f\left(u+\frac{V^2}{2g_cJ}+\frac{g}{g_c}\frac{z}{J}\right)_f-m_i\left(u+\frac{V^2}{2g_cJ}+\frac{g}{g_c}\frac{z}{J}\right)_i\right]_{system}$$

Second Law of Thermodynamics (Availability)

General Equation:

$$(S_f-S_i)_{system}=\int_{rev}\frac{\delta Q}{T}+\sum(ms)_{in}$$

$$-\sum(ms)_{out}+\Delta S_{produced}$$

Mass Flow (Continuity)

$$m=\frac{AV}{v}=\rho AV$$

Perfect Gas Relations

$$Pv=RT;\ R=\frac{1544}{M};\ c_p-c_v=\frac{R}{J};\ K=\frac{c_p}{c_v}$$

$$\Delta h=h_2-h_1=\int_{T_1}^{T_2}c_pdT=c_p(T_2-T_1)$$

$$\Delta u=u_2-u_1=\int_{T_1}^{T_2}c_vdT=c_v(T_2-T_1)$$

$$\Delta s=s_2-s_1=\int_{T_1}^{T_2}c_p\frac{dT}{T}-\frac{R}{J}\ln\frac{P_2}{P_1}$$

$$=c_p\ln\frac{T_2}{T_1}-\frac{R}{J}\ln\frac{P_2}{P_1}\text{ or }c_v\ln\frac{T_2}{T_1}+\frac{R}{J}\ln\frac{v_2}{v_1}$$

Reversible Polytropic Processes

$$pv^n=C=p_1v_1^n=p_2v_2^n=\ldots$$

$$\frac{T_2}{T_1}=\left(\frac{P_2}{P_1}\right)^{\frac{n-1}{n}}=\left(\frac{v_2}{v_1}\right)^{n-1}$$

where, if

isentropic, $n=k$ constant volume, $n=\infty$

constant pressure, $n=0$

constant temperature, $n=1$ or for general case, $n=n$ as specified by problem

Definitions

Enthalpy, $h=u+Pv/J$

Work, $W=\int Fdx$

$=\int Pdv$ (reversible, closed system)

$=-\int vdP-\Delta ke-\Delta pe$ (reversible, steady flow system)

Fig. 2-15 Basic Equations of Thermodynamics

2.6 Third Law of Thermodynamics

In the late 1800s, Amontons found that a given volume of air, when heated or cooled, expands or contracts by the same amount for each degree of temperature change. He determined this change as about 1/240 of the gas volume at 0°C, which suggests that at −240°C, the volume becomes zero, and at still lower temperature, it has to become negative. Since this observation makes no sense, he concluded that an ultimate low temperature of absolute zero exists. Today, it is known that absolute zero is −273.15°C.

In 1889, Dewar approached absolute zero within 20°C. In 1906, Nernst formulated the third law of thermodynamics that states, *While absolute zero can be approached to an arbitrary degree, it can never be reached.* Postulates to this law conclude that it is not the energy, but the entropy that tends to zero, and that a residual amount of energy is left in any substance, even at absolute zero.

2.7 Basic Equations of Thermodynamics

Figure 2-15 contains the basic set of equations required for most applications of thermodynamics.

2.8 Thermodynamics Applied to Refrigeration

Continuous refrigeration can be accomplished by several processes. In most applications, and almost exclusively in the smaller power range, the vapor compression system (commonly termed the simple compression cycle) is used for the refrigeration process. However, absorption systems and steam-jet vacuum systems are being successfully used in many applications. In larger equipment, centrifugal systems are basically an adaptation of the compression cycle.

A larger number of working fluids (refrigerants) are used in vapor-compression refrigeration systems than in vapor power cycles. Ammonia and sulfur dioxide were first used as vapor-compression refrigerants. Today, the main refrigerants are the halogenated hydrocarbons. Two important considerations in selecting a refrigerant are the temperature at which refrigeration is desired and the type of equipment to be used.

Refrigerants used in most mechanical refrigeration systems are R-22, which boils at −41.4°F (−40.8°C), R-134a, which boils at −15.1°F (−26.2°C) at atmospheric pressure and R-123 with a boiling point of +82.2°F (+27.9°C) at atmospheric pressure. Past favorites of R-12 and R-11 are being phased out due to adverse effects on the ozone in the stratosphere.

The basic vapor compression cycle is illustrated in Figure 2-16. Cool, low-pressure liquid refrigerant enters the evaporator and evaporates. As it does so, it absorbs heat from another substance such as air or water, thereby accomplishing refrigeration. The refrigerant then leaves the evaporator as a cool, low-pressure gas and proceeds to the compressor. Here, its pressure and temperature are increased, and this hot, high-

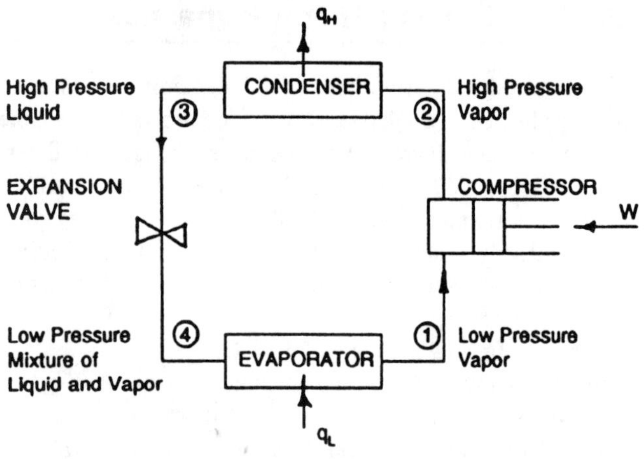

Fig. 2-16 Basic Vapor Compression Refrigeration Cycle

pressure gas is discharged to the condenser. In the condenser, the hot gas is condensed into a liquid. The condensing agent, air or water, is at a temperature lower than the refrigerant gas. This hot, high-pressure liquid flows from the condenser through the expansion valve to the evaporator. The expansion valve meters the liquid flow, reducing the hot, high-pressure liquid to a cool, low-pressure liquid as it enters the evaporator.

The basic refrigeration cycle is shown plotted on the Pressure-Enthalpy diagram as Figures 2-17. Subcooled liquid, at Point A, begins losing pressure as it goes through the metering valve, located at the point where the vertical liquid line meets the saturation curve. As it leaves the metering point, some of the liquid flashes into vapor and cools the liquid entering the evaporator at Point B. Notice that there is additional reduction in pressure from the metering point to Point B, but no change in enthalpy.

As it passes from Point B to C, the remaining liquid picks up heat and changes from a liquid to a gas but does not increase in pressure. Enthalpy, however, does increase. Superheat is added between Point C, where the vapor passes the saturation curve, and Point D.

As it passes through the compressor, Point D to E, the temperature and the pressure are markedly increased, as is the enthalpy, due to the heat of compression. Line E-F indicates that the vapor must be desuperheated within the condenser before it attains a saturated condition and begins condensing. Line F-G represents the change from vapor to liquid within the condenser. Line G-A represents subcooling within the liquid line or capillary tube, prior to flow through the metering device.

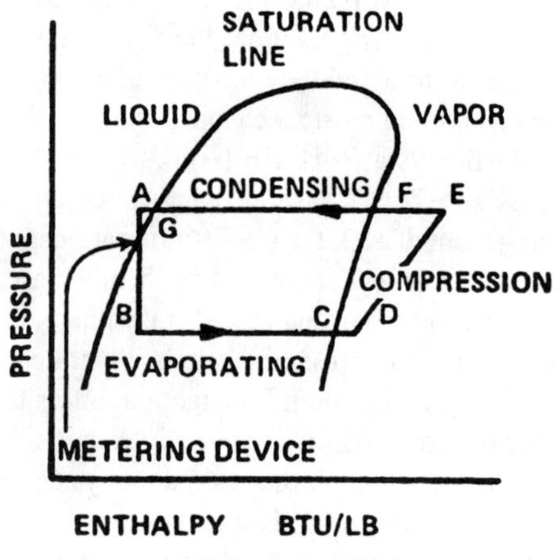

Fig. 2-17 Simplified Pressure-Enthalpy Plot

Note that the pressure remains essentially constant as the refrigerant passes through the evaporator, but due to superheat, its temperature is increased beyond the saturation point before it enters the compressor.

Likewise, the pressure remains constant as the refrigerant enters the condenser as a vapor and leaves as a liquid. While the temperature is constant through the condenser, it is reduced as the liquid is subcooled before entering the metering valve.

The change in enthalpy as the refrigerant passes through the evaporator is almost all latent heat since the temperature does not change appreciably.

Figure 2-18 provides a somewhat more completely labeled *p-h* diagram of the refrigeration cycle.

Applying the first law of thermodynamics to the vapor compression refrigeration system as a whole requires that the sum of all energy in must equal the sum of all energy out when the unit is operating at a steady state rate; hence:

$$Q_L + W = Q_H$$

The rate of heat being rejected at the condenser Q_H is numerically greater than the rate at which work is delivered to drive the compressor W and is also greater than the rate of heat absorption into the evaporator Q_L.

This relation shows that every refrigeration cycle operates as a heat pump. The household refrigerator absorbs a quantity of heat Q_L at a low temperature in the vicinity of the ice-making section (the evaporator) and rejects heat Q_H at a higher temperature to the air in the room. The rate of heat rejection Q_H is greater than the rate of absorption Q_L by the power input W to drive the compressor.

In air-conditioning applications the desired effect for cooling is the heat absorbed at the evaporator located inside the conditioned space. Heat is rejected through the condenser outside the conditioned space.

A heat pump uses this same basic cycle for heating. In this application, the condenser is located inside the building and the evaporator is located outside the building where it absorbs heat. Both modes of the cycle are in Figure 2-19.

Example 2.4 An R-134a air-conditioning unit contains a 1 hp (0.746 kW) motor and operates between pressures of 0.2 MPa (in evaporator) and 1.02 MPa (in condenser). Estimate the maximum cooling effect, in kW, that can be expected from this unit.

Solution:

$$COP = Q_i/W = Q_i/(Q_o - Q_i) = 1/[(Q_o/Q_i) - 1]$$

$$COP_{max} = 1/(T_o/T_i - 1)$$
$$= 1/(313/263 - 1) = 1/0.19 = 5.26$$

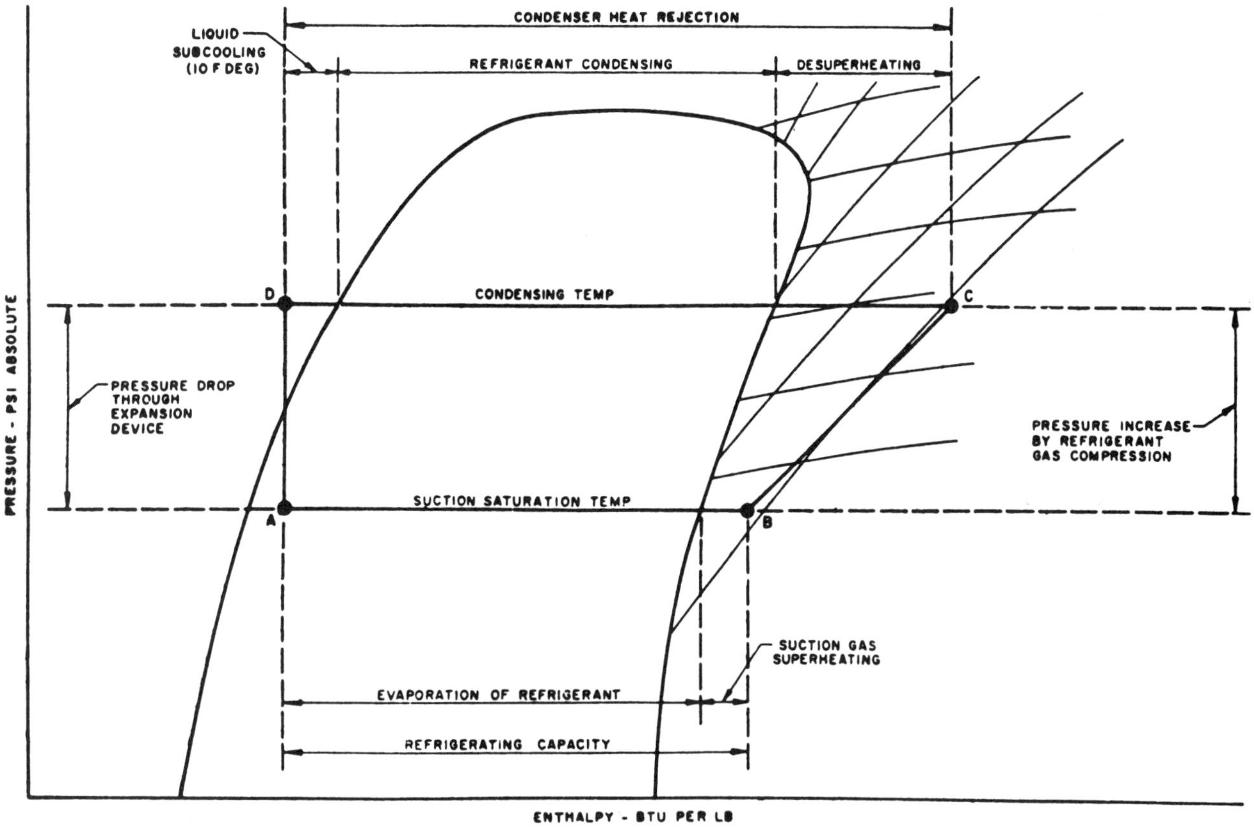

Fig. 2-18 Typical p-h Diagram for the Refrigeration Cycle

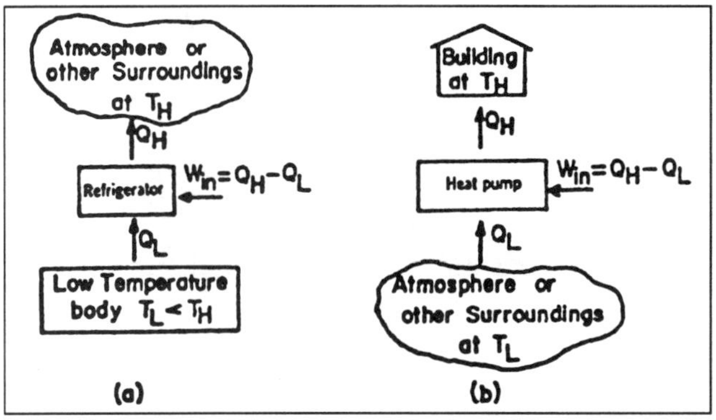

Fig. 2-19 Refrigeration Cycle (a) as Refrigerator, (b) as Heat Pump

$$Q_i = (\text{COP})W = 5.26(0.746)$$
$$= 3.92 \text{ kW } (13{,}400 \text{ Btu/h})$$

2.8.1 Energy Relations for the Basic Refrigeration Cycle

The first law of thermodynamics can be applied to each component of the system individually, since energy must be conserved at each of these, as well as for the entire system.

Compressor. The mass and major energy flows for a compressor are shown in Figure 2-20.

The rate of energy inflow must equal the rate of energy outflow during steady state operation; hence:

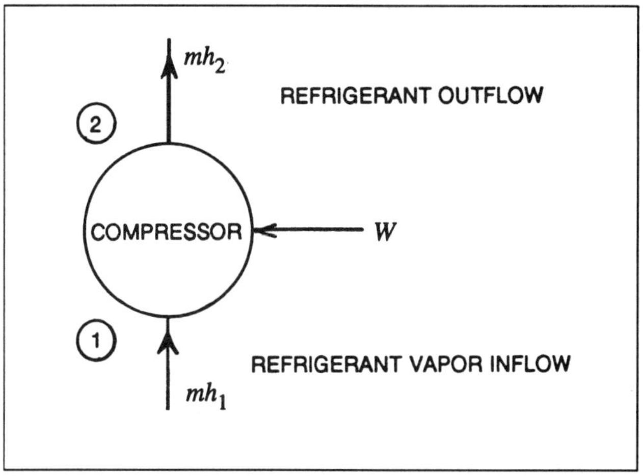

Fig. 2-20 Compressor Flows

$$mh_1 + W = mh_2$$

$$W = m(h_2 - h_1) \tag{2-55}$$

where

m = rate of refrigerant flow

h_1, h_2 = enthalpies of refrigerant at compressor inlet and outlet

Condenser. The mass and energy flow for a condenser are illustrated in Figure 2-21.

$$mh_2 = mh_3 + Q_R \quad \text{or} \quad Q_R = m(h_2 - h_3) \tag{2-56}$$

Typically, heat from the condensing refrigerant Q_R is rejected to another fluid. The Q_R leaving the condensing refrigerant must equal the heat absorbed by the fluid receiving it. Thus, from the viewpoint of the condenser cooling fluid:

$$Q_R = m_{fluid}(c_p)fluid(t_{out} - t_{in}) \qquad (2\text{-}57)$$

Expansion Device. An expansion device is essentially a flow restrictor—a small valve seat opening or a long length of small bore tubing—so neither work nor any significant amount of heat transfer occurs. Hence:

$$mh_3 = mh_4$$

or, dividing both sides by m gives:

$$h_3 = h_4 \qquad (2\text{-}58)$$

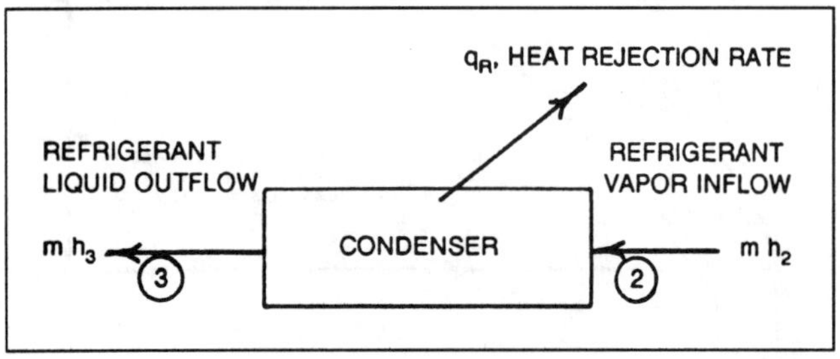

Fig. 2-21 Condenser Flows

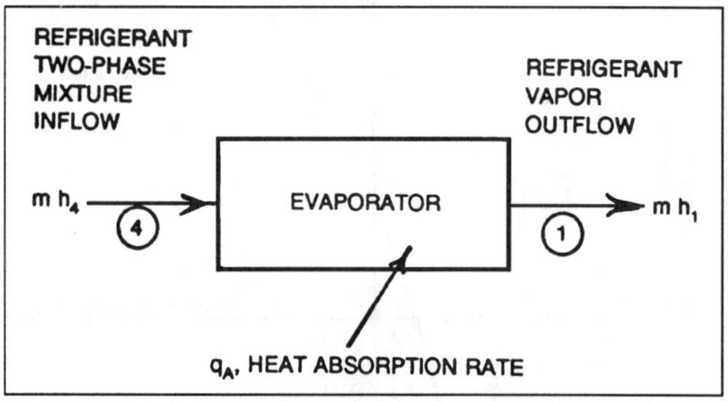

Fig. 2-22 Evaporator Flows

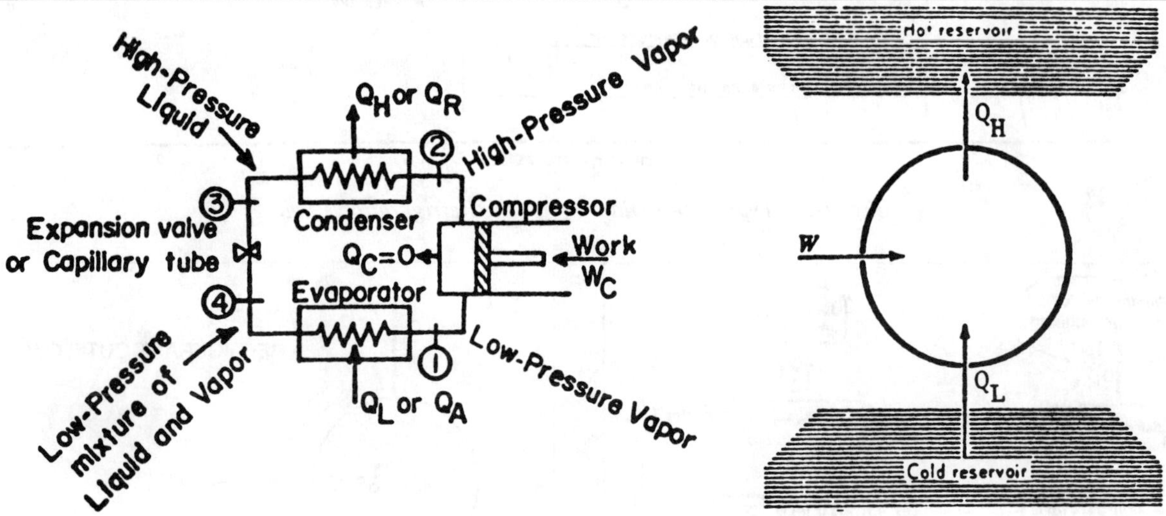

Compressor: $m(h_1 - h_2) + {}_1Q_2 - {}_1W_2 = 0 \qquad W_C = -{}_1W_2$

Condenser: $m(h_2 - h_3) + {}_2Q_3 = 0 \qquad Q_R = -{}_2Q_3$

Expansion Device: $h_3 - h_4 = 0$

Evaporator: $m(h_4 - h_1) + {}_4Q_1 = 0 \qquad Q_A = {}_4Q_1$

Overall: $Q_A + W_C = Q_C + Q_R$

or $({}_1Q_2 + {}_2Q_3 + {}_4Q_1) - ({}_1W_2) = 0$

Coefficient of Performance for Cooling:

$$\text{COP}_c = \frac{\text{Useful effect}}{\text{Input that costs}} = \frac{Q_L}{W} = \frac{1}{Q_H/Q_L - 1} \qquad \text{COP}_{c,max} = \frac{1}{T_H/T_L - 1}$$

Coefficient of Performance for Heating

$$\text{COP}_h = \frac{Q_h}{W} \qquad \text{COP}_{h,max} = \frac{1}{1 - T_L/T_H}$$

Fig. 2-23 The Vapor Compression System

Evaporator. Major mass and energy flows for an evaporator are shown in Figure 2-22.

$$mh_4 + Q_A = mh_1 \text{ or}$$

$$Q_A = m(h_1 - h_4) \tag{2-59}$$

Typically, the evaporator receives the heat flow quantity Q_A by heat transfer to it from another fluid—usually water or air. From the viewpoint of that other fluid

$$Q_A = m_{fluid}(c_p)_{fluid}(t_{in} - t_{out})_{fluid}$$

The results of applying the laws of thermodynamics to the basic vapor-compression refrigeration system are summarized in Figure 2-23.

Example 2.5 A window air conditioner using R-134A is rated at 24,000 Btu/h when operating between an evaporating temperature of 40°F and a condensing temperature of 125°F. A thermostatic expansion valve is used so that the refrigerant vapor leaving the evaporator is superheated by 20°F to safeguard against any liquid entering the compressor. If the compressor efficiency is 62%, determine the adiabatic discharge temperature from the compressor (°F) and the power input (kW). Show the cycle on the *p-h* diagram.

Solution:

Fig. 2-16 provides a sketch with notation for the cycle. Using the *p-h* diagram for R-134A, the following thermodynamic properties are found:

$p_H = 200$ psia (saturation pressure at 125°F)

$p_L = 50$ psia (saturation pressure at 40°F)

$h_3 = h_4 = h_{f@125°F} = 118$ Btu/lb

h_1 (50 psia, 60°F) = 176.8 Btu/lb

$s_1 = 0.420$

$h_{2,\,ideal}$ (200 psia, $s = 0.420$) = 189.7 Btu/lb

From first law, $m(h_1 - h_2) - W = 0$ for the compressor and, $m(h_4 - h_1) + q_L = 0$ for the evaporator.

Thus, $m(118 - 176.8) + 24000 = 0$, or

$$m = 408 \text{ lb/h}$$

The ideal compressor work is

$$W_i = 408(176.8 - 189.7) = -5265 \text{ Btu/h},$$

and the actual work using the compressor efficiency is

$$W_a = W_i/h = -5265/.62 = -8492 \text{ Btu/h or } 2.5 \text{ kW}$$

The actual enthalpy leaving the compressor can be determined using the efficiency as

$$h_{2a} = h(h_{2i} - h_1) + h_1 = 0.62(189.7 - 176.8) + 176.8 = 197.6 \text{ Btu/lb}$$

t_2 {200 psia, $h = 197.6$} = 180°F (adiabatic discharge)

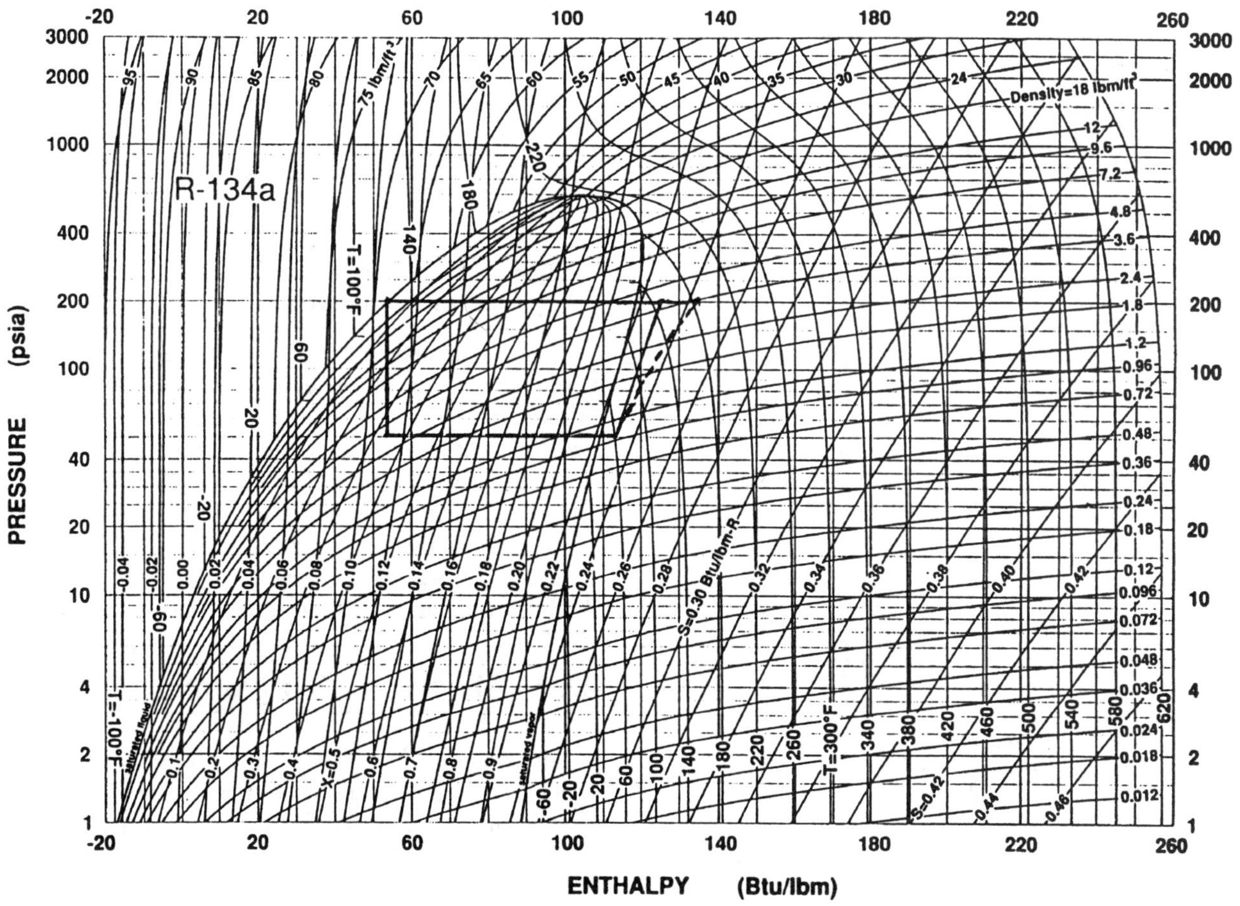

2.9 Applying Thermodynamics to Heat Pumps

A heat pump is a thermodynamic device that operates in a cycle requiring work; it transfers heat from a low-temperature body to a high-temperature body. The heat pump cycle is identical to a refrigeration cycle in principle, but differs in that the primary purpose of the heat pump is to *supply* heat rather than *remove* it from an enclosed space.

The heat pump cycle can be reversed to provide space cooling (Figure 2-24). A four-way valve switches the heat exchangers so that the indoor exchanger becomes the evaporator and the outdoor heat exchanger becomes the condenser.

The four basic components of a heat pump are the compressor, condenser, expansion device, and evaporator (Figure 2-16). The thermodynamic cycle for a heat pump is identical to the conventional vapor-compression refrigeration cycle (Figure 2-25).

Superheated refrigerant vapor with low pressure and temperature at state 1 is compressed to a much higher pressure and temperature at state 2. The high- pressure, high-temperature gas then passes through the condenser (indoor coil of a heat pump), where it gives up heat to the high-temperature environment, and changes from vapor to liquid at high pressure. At state 3, the refrigerant exits from the condenser

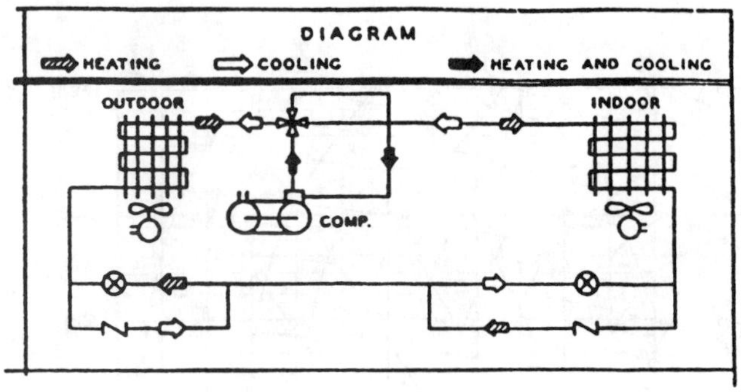

Fig. 2-24 Basic Heat Pump Cycle

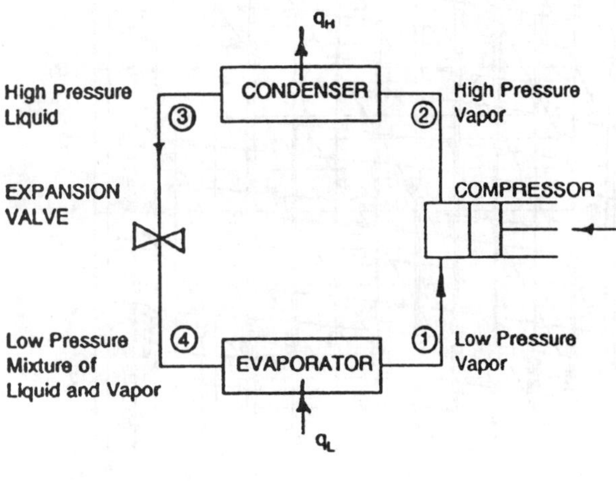

Fig. 2-25 Basic Heat Pump Components

(usually as a subcooled liquid). Next, the refrigerant passes through an expansion device where its pressure drops. This drop in pressure is accompanied by a drop in temperature such that the refrigerant leaves the expansion device and enters the evaporator (outdoor coil of a heat pump) as a low-pressure, low-temperature mixture of liquid and vapor at state 4. Finally, the refrigerant passes through the evaporator, where it picks up heat from the low-temperature environment, changes to all vapor, and exits at state 1.

An energy balance on the system shown in Figure 2-25 gives:

$$Q_H = Q_L + W$$

where

Q_H = heat energy rejected to the high-temperature environment
Q_L = heat energy taken from the low-temperature environment
W = input energy required to move Q_L from the low-temperature environment to the high-temperature environment

The coefficient of performance (COP) for heating equals the heat output divided by the work input:

$$\text{COP} = Q_H/W = (Q_L + W)/W$$

$$\text{COP} = 1 + Q_L/W \qquad (2\text{-}60)$$

The COP of a heat pump is always greater than one. That is, a heat pump always produces more heat energy than work energy consumed because a net gain of energy Q_L is transferred from the low-temperature to the high-temperature environment.

The heat pump is a reverse heat engine and is therefore limited by the Carnot cycle COP:

$$\text{COP}_{Carnot} = T_H/(T_H - T_L) \qquad (2\text{-}61)$$

where

T_L = low temperature in cycle
T_H = high temperature in cycle

The maximum possible COP for a heat pump maintaining a fixed temperature in the heated space is therefore a function of source temperature (Figure 2-26). However, any real heat transfer system must have finite temperature differences across the heat exchangers. The Carnot COP for a typical air-to-air heat pump, as well as the actual COP for the same heat pump, are illustrated in Figure 2-26. The difference between Carnot and actual COPs is due to the nature of real working fluids, flow losses, and compressor efficiency.

2.10 Absorption Refrigeration Cycle

Absorption refrigeration cycles are heat-operated cycles in which a secondary fluid, the absorbent, is used to absorb the primary fluid, gaseous refrigerant, that has been vaporized in the evaporator. The basic absorption cycle is shown in Fig. 2-27.

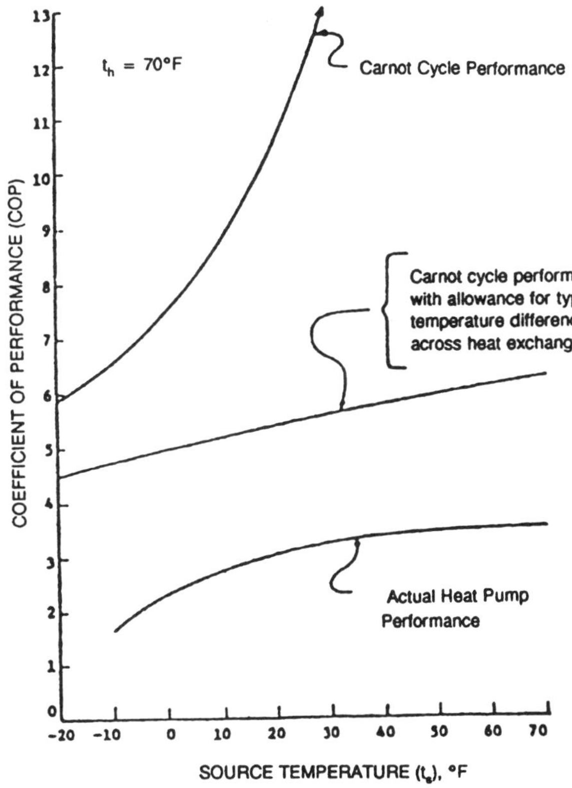

Fig. 2-26 Actual versus Ideal Heat Pump COPs

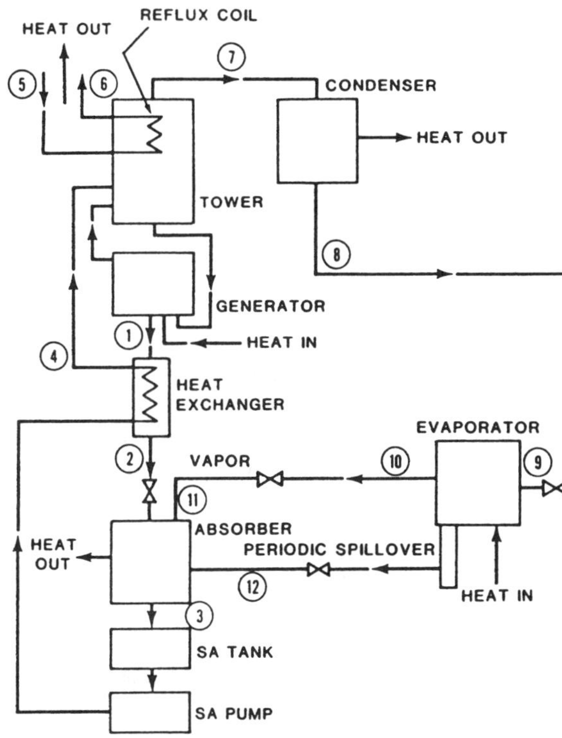

Fig. 2-27 The Basic Absorption Cycle

The low-pressure vapor leaving the evaporator enters the absorber where it is absorbed in the weak solution. Since the temperature is slightly above that of the surroundings, heat is transferred to the surroundings during this process. The strong solution is then pumped through a heat exchanger to the generator at a higher pressure and temperature. As a result of heat transfer, the refrigerant evaporates from the solution. The refrigerant vapor goes to the condenser (as in a vapor-compression system) and then to the expansion valve and evaporator. The weak solution is returned to the absorber through the heat exchanger.

The distinctive feature of the absorption system is that little work input is required because liquids (rather than vapors) are pumped. However, more equipment is involved in an absorption system than in the vapor-compression cycle. Thus, an absorption system is economically feasible only where a low-cost source of heat is available. Additional material on absorption systems is given in Chapter 18 with much greater details available in the 1997 *ASHRAE Handbook—Fundamentals*, Chapter 1, and in the 1994 *ASHRAE Handbook—Refrigeration*, Chapter 40.

2.11 Problems

2.1 Write the first law of thermodynamics in general integrated form.

2.2 Write the second law of thermodynamics in general integrated form.

2.3 Write the following perfect gas relations:

(a) the equation of state
(b) the equation for entropy change
(c) the equation for enthalpy change
(d) the equation for internal energy change

2.4 Write the continuity (mass flow) equation.

2.5 Write the equations for work for:

(a) a reversible, closed system
(b) a reversible, steady-flow system

2.6 Two pounds of air contained in a cylinder expand without friction against a piston. The pressure on the back side of the piston is constant at 200 psia. The air initially occupies a volume of 0.50 ft^3. What is the work done by the air in ft-lb$_f$ if the expansion continues until the temperature of the air reaches 100°F? [Ans: 45300 ft-lb$_f$]

2.7 Determine the specific volume, enthalpy, and entropy of 1 kg of R-134a at a saturation temperature of −5°C and a quality of 14%.

2.8 Saturated R-134a vapor at 42°C is superheated at constant pressure to a final temperature of 72°C. What is the pressure? What are the changes in specific volume, enthalpy, entropy, and internal energy?

2.9 A tank having a volume of 200 ft^3 contains saturated vapor (steam) at a pressure of 20 psia. Attached to this tank is a line in which vapor at 100 psia, 400°F flows. Steam from this line enters the vessel until the pressure is 100 psia. If there is no heat transfer from the tank and the heat capacity of the tank is neglected, calculate the mass of steam that enters the tank. [Ans: 24 lb_m]

2.10 Determine the heat required to vaporize 50 kg of water at a saturation temperature of 100°C.

2.11 The temperature of 150 kg of water is raised from 15 to 85°C by the addition of heat. How much heat is supplied?

2.12 Three cubic meters per second of water are cooled from 30 to 2°C. Compute the rate of heat transfer in kilojoules per second (kilowatts). [Ans: 351 000 kW]

2.13 Consider 10 lb_m of air that is initially at 14.7 psia, 100°F. Heat is transferred to the air until the temperature reaches 500°F. Determine the change of internal energy, the change in enthalpy, the heat transfer, and the work done for:

(a) a constant-volume process
(b) a constant-pressure process

2.14 The discharge of a pump is 10 ft above the inlet. Water enters at a pressure of 20 psia and leaves at a pressure of 200 psia. The specific volume of the water is 0.016 ft^3/lb. If there is no heat transfer and no change in kinetic or internal energy, what is the work per pound? [Ans: −0.546 Btu]

2.15 The discharge of a pump is 3 m above the inlet. Water enters at a pressure of 138 kPa and leaves at a pressure of 1380 kPa. The specific volume of the water is 0.001 m^3/kg. If there is no heat transfer and no change in kinetic or internal energy, what is the work per unit mass? [Ans: −30.7 J/kg]

2.16 Air is compressed in a reversible, isothermal, steady-flow process from 15 psia, 100°F to 100 psia. Calculate the work of compression per pound, the change of entropy, and the heat transfer per pound of air compressed.

2.17 Liquid nitrogen at a temperature of −240°F exists in a container, and both the liquid and vapor phases are present. The volume of the container is 3 ft^3 and the mass of nitrogen in the container has been determined as 44.5 lb_m. What is the mass of liquid and the mass of vapor present in the container?

2.18 A fan in an air-conditioning system is drawing 1.25 hp at 1760 rpm. The capacity through the fan is 0.85 m^3/s of 24°C air and the inlet and outlet ducts are 0.31 m in diameter. What is the temperature rise of the air due to this fan? [Ans: 0.9°C]

2.19 Air is contained in a cylinder. Initially, the cylinder contains 1.5 m^3 of air at 150 kPa, 20°C. The air is then compressed reversibly according to the relationship pv^n = constant until the final pressure is 600 kPa, at which point the temperature is 120°C. For this process determine:

(a) the polytropic exponent n
(b) the final volume of the air
(c) the work done on the air and the heat transfer

2.20 Water at 20°C is pumped from ground level to an elevated storage tank above ground level; the volume of the tank is 50 m^3. Initially, the tank contains air at 100 kPa, 20°C, and the tank is closed so that the air is compressed as the water enters the bottom of the tank. The pump is operated until the tank is three-quarters full. The temperature of the air and water remain constant at 20°C. Determine the work input to the pump.

2.21 A centrifugal pump delivers liquid oxygen to a rocket engine at the rate of 100 lb_m/s. The oxygen enters the pump as liquid at 15 psia and the discharge pressure is 500 psia. The density of liquid oxygen is 66.7 lb_m/ft^3. Determine the minmum size motor (in horsepower) to drive this pump. [Ans: 190.4 hp]

2.22 Air undergoes a steady-flow, reversible adiabatic process. The initial state is 200 psia, 1500°F, and the final pressure is 20 psia. Changes in kinetic and potential energy are negligible. Determine:

(a) final temperature
(b) final specific volume
(c) change in internal energy per lb_m
(d) change in enthalpy per lb_m
(e) work per lb_m

2.23 Air undergoes a steady-flow, reversible adiabatic process. The initial state is 1400 kPa, 815°C, and the final pressure is 140 kPa. Changes in kinetic and potential energy are negligible. Determine:

(a) final temperature
(b) final specific volume
(c) change in specific internal energy
(d) change in specific enthalpy
(e) specific work

2.24 A fan provides fresh air to the welding area in an industrial plant. The fan takes in outside air at 80°F and 14.7 psia at the rate of 1200 cfm with negligible inlet velocity. In the 10 ft^2 duct leaving the fan, air pressure is 1 psig. If the process is assumed to be reversible, adiabatic, determine the size motor needed to drive the fan. [Ans: W = 5.1 hp]

2.25 If the fan in the previous problem has an efficiency of 64% and is driven by a motor having an efficiency of 78%, determine the required power, kW.

2.26 A fan provides fresh air to the welding area in an industrial plant. The fan takes in outside air at 32.2°C and 101.4 kPa at the rate of 566 L/s with negligible inlet velocity. In the 0.93-m^2 duct leaving the fan, air pressure is 102 kPa. Determine the minimum size motor needed to drive the fan.

2.27 In an insulated feedwater heater, steam condenses at a constant temperature of 220°F. The feedwater is heated from 60 to 150°F at constant pressure.

(a) Assuming the specific heat at constant pressure of the feedwater is unity, how many Btu are absorbed by each pound in its passage through the heater? [Ans: 90 Btu/lb]
(b) What is the change in entropy of the condensing steam per pound of feedwater heated? [Ans: −0.1324]
(c) What is the change in entropy of 1 lb of feedwater as it passes through the heater? [Ans: +0.1595]
(d) What is the change in entropy of the combined system? Does this violate the second law? Explain. [Ans: +0.0271, No]

2.28 Steam at 124 kPa and 96% quality enters a radiator. The steam is condensed as it flows through the radiator and leaves as condensate at 88°C. If the radiator is to have a heating capacity of 1.85 kW, how many kilograms per hour steam must be supplied to the radiator?

2.29 Solve the following:

(a) Air at 50 psia and 90°F flows through a restriction in a 2-in. ID pipe. The velocity of the air upstream from the restriction is 450 fpm. If 58°F air is desired, what must the velocity downstream of the restriction be? Comment on this as a method of cooling.
(b) Air at 50 psia and 90°F flows through an insulated turbine at the rate of 1.6 lb_m/s. If the air delivers 11.5 hp to the turbine blades, at what temperature does the air leave the turbine?
(c) Air at 50 psia and 90°F flows through an insulated turbine at the rate of 1.6 lb_m/s to an exit pressure of 14.7 psia. What is the lowest temperature attainable at exit?

2.30 Liquid water at a pressure of 10 psia and a temperature of 80°F enters a 1-in. diameter tube at the rate of 0.8 ft/min. Heat is transferred to the water so that it leaves as saturated vapor at 9 psia. Determine the heat transfer per minute. [Ans: 95,800 Btu/min]

2.31 A refrigerator uses R-134a as the refrigerant and handles 200 lb_m/h. Condensing temperature is 110°F and evaporating temperature is 5°F. For a cooling effect of 11,000 Btu/h, determine the minimum size motor (hp) required to drive the compressor.

2.32 A heat pump is used in place of a furnace for heating a house. In winter, when the outside air temperature is 10°F, the heat loss from the house is 60,000 Btu/h if the inside is maintained at 70°F. Determine the minimum electric power required to operate the heat pump (in kW).

2.33 A heat pump is used in place of a furnace for heating a house. In winter, when the outside air temperature is −10°C, the heat loss from the house is 200 kW if the inside is maintained at 21°C. Determine the minimum electric power required to operate the heat pump. [Ans: 21.1 kW]

2.34 Refrigerant-134a vapor enters a compressor at 25 psia, 40°F, and the mass rate of flow is 5 lb_m/min. What is the smallest diameter tubing that can be used if the velocity of refrigerant must not exceed 20 ft/s?

2.35 An R-134a refrigerating system is operating with a condensing temperature of 86°F and evaporating temperature of 25°F. If the liquid line from the condenser is soldered to the suction line from the evaporator to form a simple heat exchanger, and if as a result of this saturated liquid leaving, the condenser is subcooled 6°F, how many degrees will the saturated vapor leaving the evaporator be superheated? (Use tables.)

2.36 Ammonia is heated in the evaporator of a refrigeration system from inlet conditions of 10°F, 10% quality, to saturated vapor. The pressure remains constant during the process. For each pound, determine the changes in enthalpy and volume. [Ans: 505 Btu/lb; 6.55 ft^3/lb]

2.37 For a compressor using R-134a with an evaporator temperature of 20°F and a condensing temperature of 80°F, calculate per ton of refrigeration:

(a) displacement
(b) mass flow
(c) horsepower required
(d) compare with values listed in Chapter 16 of the 1993 *Fundamentals.*

2.38 For a compressor using an R-22 system operating between 100°F condensing temperature and −10°F evaporator temperature, calculate per ton:

(a) displacement
(b) mass flow
(c) horsepower required
(d) compare with values given in Chapter 18 of the 1997 *Fundamentals.*

2.39 An industrial plant has available a 4-cylinder, 3-in. bore by 4-in. stroke, 800 rpm, single-acting compressor for use with R-134a. Proposed operating conditions for the compressor are 100°F condensing temperature and 40°F evaporating temperature. It is estimated that the refrigerant will enter the expansion valve as a saturated liquid, that vapor will leave the evaporator at a temperature of 45°F, and that vapor will enter the compressor at a temperature of 55°F. Assume a compressor-volumetric efficiency of 70%. Assume frictionless flow. Calculate the refrigerating capacity in tons for a system equipped with this compressor. Plot the cycle on the *p-h* diagram. [Ans: 12 tons]

2.40 A mechanical refrigerating system with R-134a is operating under such conditions that the evaporator pressure is 160 kPa and the liquid approaching the refrigerant control is at a temperature of 41°C. If the system has a capacity of 15 kW, determine:

(a) the refrigerating effect per kilogram of refrigerant circulated
(b) the mass flow rate in kilograms per second per kilowatt
(c) the volume flow rate in liters per second per kilowatt at the compressor inlet
(d) the total mass flow rate in kilograms per second

(e) the total volume flow rate in liters per second at the compressor inlet

2.41 A vapor-compression R-22 refrigeration system is being designed to provide 50 kW of cooling when operating between evaporating and condensing temperatures of 0°C and 34°C, respectively. The refrigerant leaving the condenser is subcooled 3 degrees and leaving the evaporator is superheated 5 degrees. Determine:

(a) ideal compressor discharge temperature, °C
(b) refrigerant flow rate, kg/s
(c) compressor motor size, kW
(d) COP for cooling
(e) compressor discharge temperature if compression efficiency is 60%

2.42 For a line of ammonia compressors, the actual volumetric efficiency is given by:

$$\eta_{va} = 94 - 6.1(p_d/p_s),\ \%$$

The compression efficiency is fairly constant at 82%. A compressor in this line has two cylinders, each having a 92-mm bore and a 74-mm stroke. The compressor has 4.5% clearance and operates at 28 r/s. The system is being selected for an air-conditioning unit and will therefore operate between an evaporating temperature of 0°C and a condensing temperature of 35°C. There is 5°C of subcooling in the condenser and 10°C of superheating in the evaporator. Sketch and label the system, including appropriate values for the thermodynamic properties, starting with state 1 at the compressor inlet. Determine:

(a) refrigerant flow rate [Ans: 0.0676 kg/s]
(b) refrigerating capacity [Ans: 77.5 kW]
(c) compressor motor size [Ans: 14.3 kW]
(d) compressor discharge temperature [Ans: 110°C]
(e) COP_c [Ans: 5.4]

2.43 An ammonia refrigerating system is operating with a condensing temperature of 30°C and an evaporating temperature of −4°C. For the ideal standard vapor compression cycle, determine:

(a) refrigerating effect
(b) COP

Sketch and label a *p-h* diagram showing values.

2.44 A single-cylinder R-22 compressor has a 50-mm bore, a 40-mm stroke, and operates at 1725 rpm. Clearance volume is 4%. Determine as close as possible the actual refrigerating capacity, kW, and the required motor size, in hp, if the compressor is used in a system operating between 10°C and 40°C, evaporating and condensing temperatures, respectively.

2.45 For the lithium-bromide/water absorption refrigeration system shown below, determine:

(a) heat required at generator per ton of cooling [Ans: 516 Btu/min]
(b) COP [Ans: 0.30]
(c) heat rejection ratio $(Q_{absorber} + Q_{condenser})/Q_{evaporator}$ [Ans: 3.58]

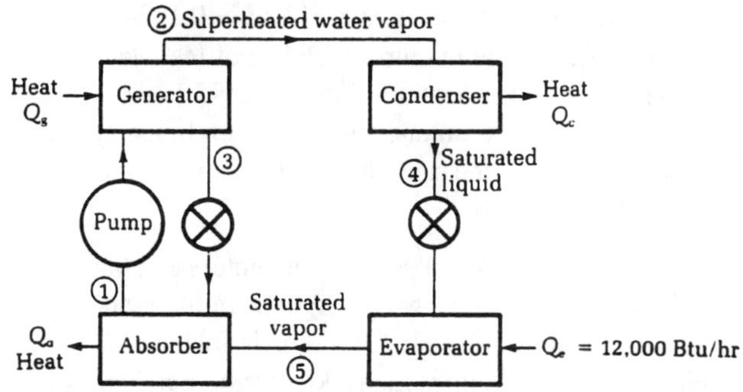

2.46 In the basic lithium-bromide water absorption system, the generator operates at 170°F while the evaporator is at 47°F. The absorbing temperature is 75°F and the condensing temperature is 88°F. Calculate the heat rejection ratio for these conditions.

2.47 For the aqua-ammonia absorption refrigeration system shown in the sketch below, complete the table of properties.

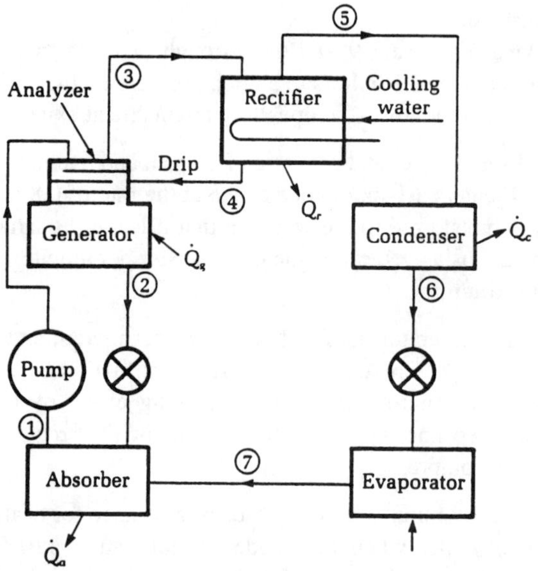

Point	*p*, psia	*t*, °F	*x*, lb NH_3/lb mix	*h*, Btu/lb
1		80		
2				
3	200	260		
4				
5		160		
6				
7	25	20		

2.48 Solar energy is to be used to warm a large collector plate. This energy will, in turn, be transferred as heat to a fluid within a heat engine, and the engine will reject energy as heat to the atmosphere. Experiments indicate that about 200 Btu/h·ft^2 of energy can be collected when the plate is operating at 190°F. Estimate the minimum collector area that will be required for a plant producing 1 kW of useful shaft power, when the atmospheric temperature is 70°F. [Ans: 92.7 ft^2]

2.49 What are the Seebeck, Peltier, Thomson, Joule, and Fourier effects? Which are reversible and which are irreversible?

2.50 A 20 ft by 12 ft by 8 ft (6.1 m by 3.6 m by 2.4 m) room contains an air-water vapor mixture at 80°F (26.7°C). The barometric pressure is standard and the partial pressure of the water vapor is measured to be 0.2 psia (1.38 kPa). Calculate:

(a) relative humidity
(b) humidity ratio
(c) dew-point temperature
(d) mass of water vapor contained in the room

2.51 Given room conditions of 75°F (23.9°C) dry bulb and 60% rh, determine for the air vapor mixture *without using* the psychrometric charts:

(a) humidity ratio
(b) enthalpy
(c) dew-point temperature
(d) specific volume
(e) degree of saturation

2.52 For the conditions of *Problem 2.51* (above), *using* the ASHRAE Psychrometric Chart, find:

(a) wet-bulb temperature [Ans: 65.2°F (18.4°C)]
(b) enthalpy [Ans: 30.2 Btu/lb$_m$ (70.2 J/g)]
(c) humidity ratio [Ans: 0.0112 lb/lb (0.0112 kg/kg)]

2.53 Using the ASHRAE Psychrometric Chart, complete the following table.

Dry Bulb, °F	Wet Bulb, °F	Dew Point, °F	Humidity W, lb/lb$_{air}$	Enthapy h, Btu/lb$_{air}$	Relative Humidity ϕ, %	Specific Volume v, ft^3/lb$_{air}$
85	60					
75		50				
				30	60	
	70		0.01143			
		82		50		

2.54 Using the ASHRAE Psychrometric Chart complete the following table:

Dry Bulb, °F	Wet Bulb, °F	Dew Point, °F	Humidity Ratio, lb$_v$/lb$_a$	Relative Humidity, %	Enthalpy, Btu/lb$_{air}$	Specific Volume, ft^3/lb$_{air}$
80						13.8
70	55					
100		70				
				40	40	
			0.01			13.8
	60	40				
40				20		
		60			30	
85			0.012			
80	80					

2.55 Complete the following table using the Psychrometric Chart.

Dry Bulb, °C	Wet Bulb, °C	Dew Point, °C	Humidity Ratio, kg/kg	Relative Humidity, %	Enthalpy, kJ/kg	Specific Volume, m^3/kg
26.5						0.86
21	13					
38		21				
				40	95	
			0.01			0.85
	16	4				
4				20		
		16			70	
30			0.012			
27	27					

2.56 Complete the following table.

Dry Bulb, °C	Wet Bulb, °C	Dew Point, °C	Humidity Ratio, kg/kg	Relative Humidity, %	Enthalpy, kJ/kg	Specific Volume, m^3/kg
32	24					
40					81	
		18		30		
			0.022			0.9
7	7					

2.57 Without using the psychrometric chart, determine the humidity ratio and relative humidity of an air-water vapor mixture with a dry-bulb temperature of 90°F and thermodynamic wet-bulb temperature of 78°F. The barometric pres-sure is 14.7 psia. Check your result using the psychrometric chart. [Ans: $W = 0.018$ lb/lb, relative humidity $\phi =$ 59%]

2.12 Bibliography

ASHRAE. 1994. *Refrigeration Handbook*, ASHRAE, Atlanta, GA

Look, D.C., Jr. and H.J. Sauer, Jr. 1986. *Engineering Thermodynamics.* PWS Engineering, Boston.

Sauer, H.J., Jr. and R.H. Howell. 1985. *Heat Pump Systems.* Wiley Interscience, New York.

SI Tables and Figures

Table 2-5 SI Standard Atmospheric Data with Altitude

(Table 1, Chapter 6, 1997 *Fundamentals*)

Altitude, m	Temperature, °C	Pressure, kPa
−500	18.2	107.478
0	15.0	101.325
500	11.8	95.461
1000	8.5	89.875
1500	5.2	84.556
2000	2.0	79.495
2500	−1.2	74.682
3000	−4.5	70.108
4000	−11.0	61.640
5000	−17.5	54.020
6000	−24.0	47.181
7000	−30.5	41.061
8000	−37.0	35.600
9000	−43.5	30.742
10000	−50	26.436
12000	−63	19.284
14000	−76	13.786
16000	−89	9.632
18000	−102	6.556
20000	−115	4.328

Data adapted from NASA (1976).

Table 2-1 SI Thermodynamic Properties of Water

(Table 3, Chapter 6, 1997 *Handbook—Fundamentals*)

Temp. t, °C	Absolute Pressure kPa p	Specific Volume, m³/kg Sat. Liquid v_i/v_f	Evap. v_{ig}/v_{fg}	Sat. Vapor v_g	Enthalpy, kJ/kg Sat. Liquid h_i/h_f	Evap. h_{ig}/h_{fg}	Sat. Vapor h_g	Entropy, kJ/(kg·K) Sat. Liquid s_i/s_f	Evap. s_{ig}/s_{fg}	Sat. Vapor s_g	Temp., °C
−60	0.00108	0.001082	90942.00	90942.00	−446.40	2836.27	2389.87	−1.6854	13.3065	11.6211	−60
−59	0.00124	0.001082	79858.69	79858.69	−444.74	2836.46	2391.72	−1.7667	13.2452	11.5677	−59
−58	0.00141	0.001082	70212.37	70212.37	−443.06	2836.64	2393.57	−1.6698	13.8145	11.5147	−58
−57	0.00161	0.001082	61805.35	61805.35	−441.38	2836.81	2395.43	−1.6620	13.1243	11.4623	−57
−56	0.00184	0.001082	54469.39	54469.39	−439.69	2836.97	2397.28	−1.6542	13.0646	11.4104	−56
−55	0.00209	0.001082	48061.05	48061.05	−438.00	2837.13	2399.12	−1.6464	13.0054	11.3590	−55
−54	0.00238	0.001082	42455.57	42455.57	−436.29	2837.27	2400.98	−1.6386	12.9468	11.3082	−54
−53	0.00271	0.001083	37546.09	37546.09	−434.59	2837.42	2402.83	−1.6308	12.8886	11.2578	−53
−52	0.00307	0.001083	33242.14	33242.14	−432.87	2837.55	2404.68	−1.6230	12.8309	11.2079	−52
−51	0.00348	0.001083	29464.67	29464.67	−431.14	2837.68	2406.53	−1.6153	12.7738	11.1585	−51
−50	0.00394	0.001083	26145.01	26145.01	−429.41	2837.80	2408.39	−1.6075	12.7170	11.1096	−50
−49	0.00445	0.001083	23223.69	23223.70	−427.67	2837.91	2410.24	−1.5997	12.6608	11.0611	−49
−48	0.00503	0.001083	20651.68	20651.69	−425.93	2838.02	2412.09	−1.5919	12.6051	11.0131	−48
−47	0.00568	0.001083	18383.50	18383.51	−424.27	2838.12	2413.94	−1.5842	12.5498	10.9656	−47
−46	0.00640	0.001083	16381.35	16381.36	−422.41	2838.21	2415.79	−1.5764	12.4949	10.9185	−46
−45	0.00721	0.001984	14612.35	14512.36	−420.65	2838.29	2417.65	−1.5686	12.4405	10.8719	−45
−44	0.00811	0.001084	13047.65	13047.66	−418.87	2838.37	2419.50	−1.5609	12.3866	10.8257	−44
−43	0.00911	0.001084	11661.85	11661.85	−417.09	2838.44	2421.35	−1.5531	12.3330	10.7799	−43
−42	0.01022	0.001084	10433.85	10433.85	−415.30	2838.50	2423.20	−1.5453	12.2799	10.7346	−42
−41	0.01147	0.001084	9344.25	9344.25	−413.50	2838.55	2425.05	−1.5376	12.2273	10.6897	−41
−40	0.01285	0.001084	8376.33	8376.33	−411.70	2838.60	2426.90	−1.5298	12.1750	10.6452	−40
−39	0.01438	0.001085	7515.86	7515.87	−409.88	2838.64	2428.76	−1.5221	12.1232	10.6011	−39
−38	0.01608	0.001085	6750.36	6750.36	−508.07	2838.67	1430.61	−1.5143	12.0718	10.5575	−38
−37	0.01796	0.001085	6068.16	6068.17	−406.24	2838.70	2432.46	−1.5066	12.0208	10.5142	−37
−36	0.02004	0.001085	5459.82	5459.82	−404.40	2838.71	2434.31	−1.4988	11.9702	10.4713	−36
−35	0.02235	0.001085	4917.09	4917.10	−402.56	2838.73	2436.16	−1.4911	11.9199	10.4289	−35
−34	0.02490	0.001085	4432.36	4432.37	−400.72	2838.73	2438.01	−1.4833	11.8701	10.3868	−34
−33	0.02771	0.001085	3998.71	3998.71	−398.86	2838.72	2439.86	−1.4756	11.8207	10.3451	−33
−32	0.03082	0.001086	3610.71	3610.71	−397.00	2838.71	2441.72	−1.4678	11.7716	10.3037	−32
−31	0.03424	0.001086	3263.20	3263.20	−395.12	2838.69	2443.57	−1.4601	11.7229	10.2628	−31
−30	0.03802	0.001086	2951.64	2951.64	−393.25	2838.66	2445.42	−1.4524	11.6746	10.2222	−30
−29	0.04217	0.001086	2672.03	2672.03	−391.36	2838.63	2447.27	−1.4446	11.6266	10.1820	−29
−28	0.04673	0.001086	2420.89	2420.89	−389.47	2838.59	2449.12	−1.4369	11.4790	10.1421	−28
−27	0.05174	0.001086	2195.23	2195.23	−387.57	2838.53	2450.97	−1.4291	11.5318	10.1026	−27
−26	0.05725	0.001087	1992.15	1992.15	−385.66	2838.48	2452.82	−1.4214	11.4849	10.0634	−26
−25	0.06329	0.001087	1809.35	1809.35	−383.74	2838.41	2454.67	−1.4137	11.4383	10.0246	−25
−24	0.06991	0.001087	1644.59	1644.59	−381.34	2838.34	2456.52	−1.4059	11.3921	9.9862	−24
−23	0.07716	0.001087	1495.98	1495.98	−379.89	2838.26	2458.37	−1.3982	11.3462	9.9480	−23
−22	0.08510	0.001087	1361.94	1361.94	−377.95	2838.17	2460.22	−1.3905	11.3007	9.9102	−22
−21	0.09378	0.001087	1240.77	1240.77	−376.01	2838.07	2462.06	−1.3828	11.2555	9.8728	−21
−20	0.10326	0.001087	1131.27	1131.27	−374.06	2837.97	2463.91	−1.3750	11.2106	9.8356	−20
−19	0.11362	0.001088	1032.18	1032.18	−372.10	2837.86	2465.76	−1.3673	11.1661	9.7988	−19
−18	0.12492	0.001088	942.46	942.47	−370.13	2837.74	2467.61	−1.3596	11.1218	9.7623	−18
−17	0.13725	0.001088	861.17	861.18	−368.15	2837.61	2469.46	−1.3518	11.0779	9.7261	−17
−16	0.15068	0.001088	787.48	787.49	−366.17	2837.47	2471.30	−1.3441	11.0343	9.6902	−16
−15	0.16530	0.001088	720.59	720.59	−364.18	2837.33	2473.15	−1.3364	10.9910	9.6546	−15
−14	0.18122	0.001088	659.86	659.86	−362.18	2837.18	2474.99	−1.3287	10.9480	9.6193	−14
−13	0.19852	0.001089	604.65	604.65	−360.18	2837.02	2476.84	−1.3210	10.9053	9.5844	−13
−12	0.21732	0.001089	554.45	554.45	−358.17	2836.85	2478.68	−1.3232	10.8629	9.5497	−12
−11	0.23774	0.001089	508.75	508.75	−356.15	2836.68	2480.53	−1.3055	10.8208	9.5153	−11
−10	0.25990	0.001089	467.14	467.14	−354.12	2836.49	2482.37	−1.2978	10.7790	9.4812	−10
−9	0.28393	0.001089	429.21	429.21	−352.08	2836.30	2484.22	−1.2901	10.7375	9.4474	−9
−8	0.30998	0.001090	394.64	394.64	−350.04	2836.10	2486.06	−1.2824	10.6962	9.4139	−8
−7	0.33819	0.001090	363.07	363.07	−347.99	2835.89	2487.90	−1.2746	10.6552	9.3806	−7
−6	0.36874	0.001090	334.25	334.25	−345.93	2835.68	2489.74	−1.2669	10.6145	9.3476	−6
−5	0.40176	0.001090	307.91	307.91	−343.87	2835.45	2491.58	−2.2592	10.4741	9.3149	−5
−4	0.43747	0.001090	283.83	283.83	−341.80	2835.22	2493.42	−1.2515	10.5340	9.2825	−4
−3	0.47606	0.001090	261.79	261.79	−339.72	2834.98	2495.26	−1.2438	10.4941	9.2503	−3
−2	0.51772	0.001091	241.60	241.60	−337.63	2834.72	2497.10	−1.2361	10.4544	9.2184	−2
−1	0.56267	0.001091	223.11	223.11	−335.53	2834.47	2498.93	−1.2284	10.4151	9.1867	−1
0	0.61115	0.001091	206.16	206.16	−333.43	2834.20	2500.77	−1.2206	10.3760	9.1553	0
0	0.6112	0.001000	206.141	206.143	−0.04	2500.81	2500.77	−0.0002	9.1555	9.1553	0
1	0.6571	0.001000	192.455	192.456	4.18	2498.43	2502.61	0.0153	9.1134	9.1286	1
2	0.7060	0.001000	179.769	179.770	8.39	2496.05	2504.45	0.0306	9.0716	9.1022	2
3	0.7580	0.001000	168.026	168.027	12.60	2493.68	2506.28	0.0459	9.0302	9.0761	3
4	0.8135	0.001000	157.137	157.138	16.81	2491.31	2508.12	0.0611	8.9890	9.0501	4
5	0.8725	0.001000	147.032	147.033	21.02	2488.94	2509.96	0.0763	8.9482	9.0244	5
6	0.9353	0.001000	137.653	137.654	25.22	2486.57	2511.79	0.0913	8.9077	8.9990	6
7	1.0020	0.001000	128.947	128.948	29.42	2484.20	2513.62	0.1064	8.8674	8.9738	7
8	1.0728	0.001000	120.850	120.851	33.62	2481.84	2515.46	0.1213	8.8273	8.9488	8
9	1.1481	0.001000	113.326	113.327	37.82	2479.47	2517.29	0.1362	8.7878	8.9245	9
10	1.2280	0.001000	106.328	106.329	42.01	2477.11	2519.12	0.1511	8.7484	8.8995	10
11	1.3127	0.001000	99.812	99.813	46.21	2474.74	2520.95	0.1659	8.7093	8.8752	11
12	1.4026	0.001001	93.743	93.744	50.40	2472.38	2522.78	0.1806	8.6705	8.8511	12

Table 2-1 SI Thermodynamic Properties of Water (*Continued*)
(Table 3, Chapter 6, 1997 *Handbook—Fundamentals*)

Temp. t, °C	Absolute Pressure kPa p	Specific Volume, m³/kg Sat. Liquid v_f	Evap. v_{fg}	Sat. Vapor v_g	Enthalpy, kJ/kg Sat. Liquid h_f	Evap. h_{fg}	Sat. Vapor h_g	Entropy, kJ/(kg·K) Sat. Liquid s_f	Evap. s_{fg}	Sat. Vapor s_g	Temp., °C
13	1.4978	0.001001	88.088	88.089	54.59	2470.02	2524.61	0.1953	8.6319	8.8272	13
14	1.5987	0.001001	82.815	82.816	58.78	2467.66	2526.44	0.2099	8.5936	3.8035	14
15	1.7055	0.001001	77.897	77.898	62.97	2465.30	2528.26	0.2244	8.5556	8.7801	15
16	1.8184	0.001001	73.307	73.308	67.16	2462.93	2530.09	0.2389	8.5178	8.7568	16
17	1.9380	0.001001	69.021	69.022	71.34	2460.57	2531.92	0.2534	8.4804	8.7338	17
18	2.0643	0.001002	65.017	65.018	75.53	2458.21	2533.74	0.2678	8.4431	8.7109	18
19	2.1978	0.001002	65.274	61.273	79.72	2455.85	2535.56	0.2821	8.4061	8.6883	19
20	2.3388	0.001002	57.774	57.773	83.90	2453.48	2537.38	0.2964	8.3694	8.6658	20
21	2.4877	0.001002	54.450	54.500	88.08	2451.12	2539.20	0.3107	8.3329	8.6436	21
22	2.6448	0.001002	51.433	51.434	92.27	2448.75	2541.02	0.3249	8.2967	8.6215	22
23	2.8104	0.001003	48.562	48.563	96.45	2446.39	2542.84	0.3390	8.2607	8.5996	23
24	2.9851	0.001003	45.872	45.873	100.63	2444.02	2544.65	0.3531	8.2249	8.5780	24
25	3.1692	0.001003	43.350	43.351	104.81	2441.66	2546.47	0.3672	8.1894	8.5565	25
26	3.3631	0.001003	40.985	40.986	108.99	2439.29	2548.28	0.3812	8.1541	8.5352	26
27	3.5673	0.001004	38.766	38.767	113.18	2436.92	2550.09	0.3951	8.1190	8.5141	27
28	3.7822	0.001004	36.682	36.683	117.36	2434.55	2551.90	0.4090	8.0842	8.4932	28
29	4.0083	0.001004	34.726	34.727	121.54	2432.17	2553.71	0.4229	8.0496	8.4724	29
30	4.2460	0.001004	32.889	32.889	125.72	2429.80	2555.52	0.4367	8.0152	8.4519	30
31	4.4959	0.001005	31.160	31.161	129.90	2427.43	2557.32	0.4505	7.9810	8.4315	31
32	4.7585	0.001005	29.535	29.536	134.08	2425.05	2559.13	0.4642	7.9471	8.4112	32
33	5.0343	0.001005	28.006	28.007	138.26	2422.67	2560.93	0.4779	7.9133	8.3912	33
34	5.3239	0.001006	26.567	26.568	142.44	2410.29	2562.73	0.4915	7.8790	8.3713	34
35	5.6278	0.001006	25.212	25.213	146.62	2417.91	2564.53	0.5051	7.8465	8.3516	35
36	5.9466	0.001006	23.935	23.936	150.80	2415.53	2566.33	0.5186	7.8134	8.3320	36
37	6.2810	0.001007	22.733	22.734	154.98	2413.14	2568.12	0.5321	7.7805	8.3127	37
38	6.6315	0.001007	21.599	21.600	159.16	2410.76	2569.91	0.5456	7.7479	8.2934	38
39	6.9987	0.001008	20.529	20.530	163.34	2408.37	2571.71	0.5590	7.7154	8.2744	39
40	7.3835	0.001008	19.520	19.521	167.52	2405.98	2573.50	0.5724	7.6831	8.2555	40
41	7.7863	0.001008	18.567	18.568	171.70	2403.58	2575.28	0.5857	7.6510	8.2367	41
42	8.2080	0.001009	17.667	17.668	175.88	2401.19	2577.07	0.5990	7.6191	8.2181	42
43	8.6492	0.001009	16.818	16.819	180.06	2398.79	2578.85	0.6122	7.5875	8.1997	43
44	9.1107	0.001010	16.014	16.015	184.24	2396.39	2580.63	0.6254	7.3560	8.1814	44
45	9.5932	0.001010	15.255	15.256	188.42	2393.99	2582.41	0.6386	7.5247	8.1632	45
46	10.0976	0.001010	14.537	14.538	192.60	2391.59	2584.19	0.6517	7.4936	8.1452	46
47	10.6246	0.001011	13.858	13.859	196.78	2389.18	2585.96	0.6648	7.4626	8.1274	47
48	11.1751	0.001011	13.214	13.215	200.97	2386.77	2587.74	0.6778	7.4319	8.1097	48
49	11.7500	0.001012	12.606	12.607	205.15	2384.36	2589.51	0.6908	7.4013	8.0921	49
50	12.3499	0.001012	12.029	12.029	209.33	2381.94	2591.27	0.7038	7.3709	8.0747	50
51	12.9759	0.001013	11.482	11.483	213.51	2379.53	2593.04	0.7167	7.3407	8.0574	51
52	13.6290	0.001013	10.964	10.965	217.70	2377.10	2594.80	0.7296	7.3107	8.0403	52
53	14.3100	0.001014	10.473	10.474	221.88	2374.68	2596.56	0.7424	7.2809	8.0233	53
54	15.0200	0.001014	10.001	10.008	226.06	2372.26	2598.32	0.7552	7.2512	8.0064	54
55	15.7597	0.001015	9.563	9.5663	230.25	2369.83	2600.07	0.7680	7.2217	7.9897	55
56	16.5304	0.001015	9.147	9.1468	234.43	2367.39	2601.82	0.7807	7.1924	7.9731	56
57	17.3331	0.001016	8.744	8.7489	238.61	2364.96	2603.57	0.7934	7.1632	7.9566	57
58	18.1690	0.001016	8.3690	8.3700	242.80	2362.52	2605.32	0.8061	7.1342	7.9403	58
59	19.0387	0.001017	8.0094	8.0114	246.99	2360.08	2607.06	0.8187	7.1054	7.9240	59
60	19.944	0.001017	7.6677	7.6697	251.17	2357.63	2608.80	0.8313	7.0767	7.9079	60
61	20.885	0.001018	7.3428	7.3438	255.36	2355.19	2610.54	0.8438	7.0482	7.8920	61
62	21.864	0.001018	7.0337	7.0347	259.54	2352.73	2612.28	0.8563	7.0198	7.8761	62
63	22.882	0.001019	6.7397	6.7407	263.73	2350.28	2614.01	0.8688	6.9916	7.8604	63
64	23.940	0.001019	6.4599	6.4609	267.92	2347.82	2615.74	0.8812	6.9636	7.8448	64
65	25.040	0.001020	6.1935	6.1946	272.11	2345.36	2617.46	0.8936	6.9357	7.8293	65
66	26.180	0.001020	5.9397	5.9409	276.30	2342.89	2619.19	0.9060	6.9080	7.8140	66
67	27.366	0.001021	5.6982	5.6992	280.49	2340.42	2620.90	0.9183	6.8804	7.7987	67
68	28.596	0.001022	5.4680	5.4690	284.68	2337.95	2622.62	0.9306	2.8530	7.7836	68
69	29.873	0.001022	5.2485	5.2495	288.87	2335.47	2624.33	0.9429	6.8257	7.7686	69
70	31.198	0.001023	5.0392	5.0402	293.06	2332.99	2626.04	0.9551	6.7986	7.7537	70
71	32.572	0.001023	4.8396	4.8407	297.25	2330.50	2627.75	0.9673	6.7716	7.7389	71
72	33.997	0.001024	4.6492	4.6502	301.44	2328.01	2629.45	0.9795	6.7448	7.7242	72
73	35.475	0.001025	4.4675	4.4685	305.63	2325.51	2631.15	0.9916	6.7181	7.7097	73
74	37.006	0.001025	4.2940	4.2951	309.83	2323.02	2632.84	1.0037	6.6915	7.6952	74
75	38.592	0.001026	4.1284	4.1294	314.02	2320.51	2634.53	1.0157	6.6651	7.6809	75
76	40.236	0.001026	3.9702	3.9712	318.22	2318.01	2636.22	1.0278	6.6389	7.6666	76
77	41.938	0.001027	3.8190	3.8201	322.41	2315.49	2637.90	1.0398	6.6127	7.6525	77
78	43.700	0.001028	3.6746	3.6756	326.61	2312.98	2639.58	1.0517	6.5867	7.6384	78
79	45.524	0.001028	3.5365	3.5375	330.81	2310.46	2641.26	1.0636	6.5609	7.6245	79
80	47.412	0.001029	3.4044	3.4055	335.00	2307.93	2642.93	1.0755	6.5351	7.6107	80

Table 2-1 SI Thermodynamic Properties of Water (*Continued*)

(Table 3, Chapter 6, 1997 *Handbook—Fundamentals*)

Temp. t, °C	Absolute Pressure kPa p	Specific Volume, m³/kg Sat. Liquid v_f	Evap. v_{fg}	Sat. Vapor v_g	Enthalpy, kJ/kg Sat. Liquid h_f	Evap. h_{fg}	Sat. Vapor h_g	Entropy, kJ/(kg·K) Sat. Liquid s_f	Evap. s_{fg}	Sat. Vapor s_g	Temp., °C
81	49.364	0.001030	3.2781	3.2792	339.20	2305.40	2644.60	1.0874	6.5095	7.5969	81
82	51.384	0.001030	3.1573	3.1583	343.40	2902.86	2646.26	1.0993	6.4841	7.5833	82
83	53.473	0.001031	3.0417	3.0427	347.60	2300.32	2647.92	1.1111	6.4587	7.5698	83
84	55.633	0.001032	2.9310	2.9320	351.80	2297.78	2649.58	1.1228	6.4335	7.5563	84
85	57.865	0.001032	2.8250	2.8260	356.01	2295.22	2651.23	1.1346	6.4084	7.5430	85
86	60.171	0.001033	2.7235	2.7245	350.21	2292.67	2652.88	1.1463	6.3834	7.5297	86
87	62.554	0.001034	2.6263	2.6273	364.41	2290.11	2654.52	1.1580	6.3586	7.5166	87
88	65.015	0.001035	2.5331	2.5341	368.62	2287.54	2656.16	1.1696	6.3339	7.5035	88
89	67.556	0.001035	2.4438	2.4448	372.82	2284.97	2657.79	1.1812	6.3093	7.4905	89
90	70.180	0.001036	2.3582	2.3592	377.03	2282.39	2659.42	1.1928	6.2848	7.4776	90
91	72.888	0.001037	2.2760	2.2771	381.24	2279.81	2661.04	1.2044	6.2605	7.4648	91
92	75.683	0.001037	2.1973	2.1983	385.45	2277.22	2662.66	1.2159	6.2362	7.4521	92
93	78.566	0.001038	2.1217	2.1228	389.66	2274.62	2664.28	1.2274	6.2121	7.4395	93
94	81.541	0.001039	2.0492	2.0502	393.87	2272.02	2665.89	1.2389	6.1881	7.4270	94
95	84.608	0.001040	1.9796	1.9806	398.08	2269.41	2667.49	1.2504	6.1642	7.4146	95
96	87.770	0.001040	1.9128	1.9138	402.29	2266.80	2669.09	1.2618	6.1404	7.4022	96
97	91.030	0.001041	1.8486	1.8496	406.51	2264.18	2670.69	1.2732	6.1168	7.3899	97
98	94.390	0.001042	1.7869	1.7880	410.72	2261.55	2672.28	1.2845	6.0932	7.3777	98
99	97.852	0.001044	1.7277	1.7287	414.94	2258.92	2673.86	1.2959	6.0697	7.3656	99
100	101.419	0.001044	1.6708	1.6718	419.16	2256.28	2675.44	1.3072	6.0464	7.3536	100
101	105.092	0.001044	1.6161	1.6171	423.38	2253.64	2677.02	1.3185	6.0232	7.3416	101
102	108.875	0.001045	1.5635	1.5645	427.60	2250.99	2678.58	1.3297	6.0000	7.3298	102
103	112.770	0.001046	1.5129	1.5139	431.82	2248.33	2680.15	1.3410	5.9770	7.3180	103
104	116.779	0.001047	1.4642	1.4652	436.04	2245.66	2681.71	1.3522	5.9541	7.3062	104
105	120.906	0.001047	1.4174	1.4184	440.27	2242.99	2683.26	1.3634	5.9313	7.2946	105
106	125.152	0.001048	1.3723	1.3734	444.49	2240.31	2684.80	1.3745	5.9086	7.2830	106
107	129.520	0.001049	1.3290	1.3300	448.72	2237.63	2686.35	1.3856	5.8860	7.2716	107
108	134.012	0.001050	1.2872	1.2883	452.95	2234.93	2687.88	1.3967	5.8635	7.2601	108
109	138.633	0.001051	1.2470	1.2481	457.18	2232.23	2689.41	1.4078	5.8410	7.2488	109
110	143.384	0.001052	1.2083	1.2093	461.41	2229.52	2690.93	1.4188	5.8187	7.2375	110
111	148.267	0.001052	1.1710	1.1720	465.64	2226.81	2692.45	1.4298	5.7965	7.2263	111
112	153.287	0.001053	1.1350	1.1361	469.88	2224.09	2693.96	1.4408	5.7744	7.2152	112
113	158.445	0.001054	1.1004	1.1015	474.11	2221.35	2695.47	1.4518	5.7524	7.2402	113
114	163.745	0.001055	1.0670	1.0681	478.35	2218.62	2696.97	1.4627	5.7304	7.1931	114
115	169.190	0.001056	1.0348	1.0359	482.59	2215.87	2698.46	1.4737	5.7086	7.1822	115
116	174.782	0.001057	1.0038	1.0048	486.83	2213.12	2699.95	1.4846	5.6868	7.1714	116
117	180.525	0.001058	0.9739	0.9749	491.07	2210.35	2701.43	1.4954	5.6652	7.1606	117
118	186.420	0.001059	0.9450	0.9460	495.32	2207.58	2702.90	1.5063	5.6436	7.1499	118
119	192.473	0.001059	0.9171	0.9182	499.56	2204.80	2704.37	1.5171	5.6221	7.1392	119
120	198.685	0.001060	0.8902	0.8913	503.81	2202.02	2705.83	1.5279	5.6007	7.1286	120
122	211.601	0.001062	0.8391	0.8402	512.31	2196.42	2706.73	1.5494	5.5582	7.1076	122
124	225.194	0.001064	0.7916	0.7927	520.82	2190.78	2711.60	1.5709	5.5160	7.0869	124
126	239.490	0.001066	0.7472	0.7483	529.33	2185.11	2714.44	1.5922	5.4742	7.0664	126
128	254.515	0.001068	0.7057	0.7068	537.86	2179.40	2717.26	1.6135	5.4326	7.0461	128
130	270.298	0.001070	0.6670	0.6681	546.39	2173.66	2720.05	1.6347	5.3914	7.0261	130
132	286.866	0.001072	0.6308	0.6318	554.93	2167.87	2722.80	1.6557	5.3505	7.0063	132
134	304.247	0.001074	0.5969	0.5979	563.48	2162.05	2725.53	1.6767	5.3099	6.9867	134
136	322.470	0.001076	0.5651	0.5662	572.04	2156.18	2728.22	1.6977	5.2697	6.9673	136
138	341.566	0.001078	0.5354	0.5364	580.60	2150.28	2730.88	1.7185	5.2296	6.9481	138
140	361.565	0.001080	0.5075	0.5085	589.18	2144.33	2733.51	1.7393	5.1899	6.9292	140
142	382.497	0.001082	0.4813	0.4824	597.76	2138.34	2736.11	1.7599	5.1505	6.9104	142
144	404.394	0.001084	0.4567	0.4578	606.36	2132.31	2738.67	1.7805	5.1113	6.8918	144
146	427.288	0.001086	0.4336	0.4347	614.97	2126.23	2741.19	1.8011	5.0724	6.8735	146
148	451.211	0.001088	0.4119	0.4130	623.58	2120.10	2743.68	1.8215	5.0338	6.8553	148
150	476.198	0.001091	0.3914	0.3925	632.21	2113.92	2746.13	1.8419	4.9954	6.8373	150
152	502.281	0.001093	0.3722	0.3733	640.85	2107.70	2748.55	1.8622	4.9573	6.8194	152
154	529.495	0.001095	0.3541	0.3552	649.50	2101.43	2750.93	1.8824	4.9194	6.8017	154
156	557.875	0.001097	0.3370	0.3381	658.16	2095.11	2753.27	1.9026	4.8817	6.7842	156
158	587.456	0.001100	0.3209	0.3220	666.83	2088.73	2755.57	1.9226	4.8443	6.7669	158
160	618.275	0.001102	0.3058	0.3069	675.52	2082.31	2757.82	1.9427	4.8070	6.7497	160
162	650.368	0.001104	0.2914	0.2925	684.22	2075.82	2760.04	1.9626	4.7701	6.7327	162
164	683.772	0.001107	0.2779	0.2790	692.93	2069.29	2762.22	1.9825	4.7333	6.7158	164
166	718.526	0.001109	0.2651	0.2662	701.65	2062.70	2764.35	2.0023	4.6967	6.6990	166
168	754.667	0.001112	0.2530	0.2541	710.39	2056.05	2766.44	2.0221	4.6603	6.6824	168
170	792.235	0.001114	0.2415	0.2427	719.14	2049.34	2768.48	2.0418	4.6242	6.6659	170
172	831.268	0.001117	0.2307	0.2318	727.91	2042.57	2770.48	2.0614	4.5882	6.6496	172
174	871.808	0.001119	0.2205	0.2216	736.69	2035.74	2772.43	2.0810	4.5524	6.6334	174
176	913.894	0.001122	0.2107	0.2119	745.48	2028.85	2774.33	2.1005	4.5168	6.6173	176
178	947.568	0.001125	0.2015	0.2026	754.29	2021.89	2776.19	2.1200	4.4813	6.6013	178
180	1002.871	0.001127	0.1928	0.1939	763.12	2014.87	2777.99	2.1394	4.4460	6.5854	180
182	1049.846	0.001130	0.1845	0.1856	771.96	2007.78	2779.74	2.1587	4.4109	6.5691	182
184	1098.535	0.001133	0.1766	0.1777	780.82	2000.63	2781.45	2.1780	4.3760	6.5540	184
186	1148.982	0.001136	0.1691	0.1703	789.69	1993.40	2783.10	2.1973	4.3412	6.5385	186
188	1201.230	0.001139	0.1620	0.1632	798.59	1986.11	2784.70	2.2165	4.3065	6.5230	188
190	1255.324	0.001141	0.1553	0.1564	807.50	1978.74	2786.24	2.2356	4.2720	6.5076	190
192	1311.309	0.001144	0.1488	0.1500	816.43	1971.30	2787.72	2.2547	4.2376	6.4924	192
194	1369.230	0.001147	0.1427	0.1439	825.37	1963.78	2789.15	2.2738	4.2034	6.4772	194
196	1429.133	0.001150	0.1369	0.1380	834.34	1956.19	2790.52	2.2928	4.1693	6.4621	196
198	1491.066	0.001153	0.1314	0.1325	843.32	1948.52	2791.83	2.3118	4.1353	6.4471	198
200	1555.074	0.001157	0.1261	0.1272	852.33	1940.76	2793.09	2.3307	4.1014	6.4321	200

Table 2-2 SI Refrigerant 134a Properties of Saturated Liquid and Saturated Vapor

(Chapter 19, 1997 *Handbook—Fundamentals*)

Temp.,* °C	Absolute Pressure, MPa	Density, kg/m³ Liquid	Volume, m³/kg Vapor	Enthalpy, kJ/kg Liquid	Enthalpy, kJ/kg Vapor	Entropy, kJ/(kg·K) Liquid	Entropy, kJ/(kg·K) Vapor	Specific Heat c_p, kJ/(kg·K) Liquid	Specific Heat c_p, kJ/(kg·K) Vapor	c_p/c_v Vapor	Velocity of Sound, m/s Liquid	Velocity of Sound, m/s Vapor	Viscosity, μPa·s Liquid	Viscosity, μPa·s Vapor	Thermal Cond, mW/(m·K) Liquid	Thermal Cond, mW/(m·K) Vapor	Surface Tension, mN/m	Temp.,* °C
−103.30a	0.00039	1591.2	35.263	71.89	335.07	0.4143	1.9638	1.147	0.585	1.163	1135.	127.	2186.6	6.63	—	—	28.15	−103.30
−100.00	0.00056	1581.9	25.039	75.71	337.00	0.4366	1.9456	1.168	0.592	1.161	1111.	128.	1958.2	6.76	—	—	27.56	−100.00
−90.00	0.00153	1553.9	9.7191	87.59	342.94	0.5032	1.8975	1.201	0.614	1.155	1051.	131.	1445.6	7.16	—	—	25.81	−90.00
−80.00	0.00369	1526.2	4.2504	99.65	349.03	0.5674	1.8585	1.211	0.637	1.151	999.	134.	1109.9	7.57	—	—	24.11	−80.00
−70.00	0.00801	1498.6	2.0528	111.78	355.23	0.6286	1.8269	1.215	0.660	1.148	951.	137.	879.6	7.97	125.8	—	22.44	−70.00
−60.00	0.01594	1471.0	1.0770	123.96	361.51	0.6871	1.8016	1.220	0.685	1.146	904.	139.	715.4	8.38	121.1	—	20.81	−60.00
−50.00	0.02948	1443.1	0.60560	136.21	367.83	0.7432	1.7812	1.229	0.712	1.146	858.	142.	594.3	8.79	116.5	7.12	19.22	−50.00
−40.00	0.05122	1414.8	0.36095	148.57	374.16	0.7973	1.7649	1.243	0.740	1.148	812.	144.	502.2	9.20	111.9	8.19	17.66	−40.00
−30.00	0.08436	1385.9	0.22596	161.10	380.45	0.8498	1.7519	1.260	0.771	1.152	765.	145.	430.4	9.62	107.3	9.16	16.13	−30.00
−28.00	0.09268	1380.0	0.20682	163.62	381.70	0.8601	1.7497	1.264	0.778	1.153	756.	145.	418.0	9.71	106.3	9.35	15.83	−28.00
−26.07b	0.10132	1374.3	0.19016	166.07	382.90	0.8701	1.7476	1.268	0.784	1.154	747.	146.	406.4	9.79	105.4	9.52	15.54	−26.07
−26.00	0.10164	1374.1	0.18961	166.16	382.94	0.8704	1.7476	1.268	0.785	1.154	747.	146.	406.0	9.79	105.4	9.53	15.53	−26.00
−24.00	0.11127	1368.2	0.17410	168.70	384.19	0.8806	1.7455	1.273	0.791	1.155	738.	146.	394.6	9.88	104.5	9.71	15.23	−24.00
−22.00	0.12160	1362.2	0.16010	171.26	385.43	0.8908	1.7436	1.277	0.798	1.156	728.	146.	383.6	9.96	103.6	9.89	14.93	−22.00
−20.00	0.13268	1356.2	0.14744	173.82	386.66	0.9009	1.7417	1.282	0.805	1.157	719.	146.	373.1	10.05	102.6	10.07	14.63	−20.00
−18.00	0.14454	1350.2	0.13597	176.39	387.89	0.9110	1.7399	1.286	0.812	1.159	710.	146.	363.0	10.14	101.7	10.24	14.33	−18.00
−16.00	0.15721	1344.1	0.12556	178.97	389.11	0.9211	1.7383	1.291	0.820	1.160	700.	147.	353.3	10.22	100.8	10.42	14.04	−16.00
−14.00	0.17074	1338.0	0.11610	181.56	390.33	0.9311	1.7367	1.296	0.827	1.162	691.	147.	344.0	10.31	99.9	10.59	13.74	−14.00
−12.00	0.18516	1331.8	0.10749	184.16	391.55	0.9410	1.7351	1.301	0.835	1.164	682.	147.	335.0	10.40	99.0	10.76	13.45	−12.00
−10.00	0.20052	1325.6	0.09963	186.78	392.75	0.9509	1.7337	1.306	0.842	1.166	672.	147.	326.3	10.49	98.0	10.93	13.16	−10.00
−8.00	0.21684	1319.3	0.09246	189.40	393.95	0.9608	1.7323	1.312	0.850	1.168	663.	147.	318.0	10.58	97.1	11.10	12.87	−8.00
−6.00	0.23418	1313.0	0.08591	192.03	395.15	0.9707	1.7310	1.317	0.858	1.170	654.	147.	309.9	10.67	96.2	11.28	12.58	−6.00
−4.00	0.25257	1306.6	0.07991	194.68	396.33	0.9805	1.7297	1.323	0.866	1.172	644.	147.	302.2	10.76	95.3	11.45	12.29	−4.00
−2.00	0.27206	1300.2	0.07440	197.33	397.51	0.9903	1.7285	1.329	0.875	1.175	635.	147.	294.7	10.85	94.3	11.62	12.00	−2.00
0.00	0.29269	1293.7	0.06935	200.00	398.68	1.0000	1.7274	1.335	0.883	1.178	626.	147.	287.4	10.94	93.4	11.79	11.71	0.00
2.00	0.31450	1287.1	0.06470	202.68	399.84	1.0097	1.7263	1.341	0.892	1.180	616.	147.	280.4	11.03	92.5	11.96	11.43	2.00
4.00	0.33755	1280.5	0.06042	205.37	401.00	1.0194	1.7252	1.347	0.901	1.183	607.	147.	273.6	11.13	91.6	12.13	11.14	4.00
6.00	0.36186	1273.8	0.05648	208.08	402.14	1.0291	1.7242	1.353	0.910	1.187	598.	147.	267.0	11.22	90.7	12.31	10.86	6.00
8.00	0.38749	1267.0	0.05284	210.80	403.27	1.0387	1.7233	1.360	0.920	1.190	588.	147.	260.6	11.32	89.7	12.48	10.58	8.00
10.00	0.41449	1260.2	0.04948	213.53	404.40	1.0483	1.7224	1.367	0.930	1.193	579.	146.	254.3	11.42	88.8	12.66	10.30	10.00
12.00	0.44289	1253.3	0.04636	216.27	405.51	1.0579	1.7215	1.374	0.939	1.197	569.	146.	248.3	11.52	87.9	12.84	10.02	12.00
14.00	0.47276	1246.3	0.04348	219.03	406.61	1.0674	1.7207	1.381	0.950	1.201	560.	146.	242.5	11.62	87.0	13.02	9.74	14.00
16.00	0.50413	1239.3	0.04081	221.80	407.70	1.0770	1.7199	1.388	0.960	1.206	550.	146.	236.8	11.72	86.0	13.20	9.47	16.00
18.00	0.53706	1232.1	0.03833	224.59	408.78	1.0865	1.7191	1.396	0.971	1.210	541.	146.	231.2	11.82	85.1	13.39	9.19	18.00
20.00	0.57159	1224.9	0.03603	227.40	409.84	1.0960	1.7183	1.404	0.982	1.215	532.	145.	225.8	11.92	84.2	13.57	8.92	20.00
22.00	0.60777	1217.5	0.03388	230.21	410.89	1.1055	1.7176	1.412	0.994	1.220	522.	145.	220.5	12.03	83.3	13.76	8.65	22.00
24.00	0.64566	1210.1	0.03189	233.05	411.93	1.1149	1.7169	1.420	1.006	1.226	512.	145.	215.4	12.14	82.4	13.96	8.38	24.00
26.00	0.68531	1202.6	0.03003	235.90	412.95	1.1244	1.7162	1.429	1.018	1.231	503.	144.	210.4	12.25	81.4	14.15	8.11	26.00
28.00	0.72676	1194.9	0.02829	238.77	413.95	1.1338	1.7155	1.438	1.031	1.238	493.	144.	205.5	12.36	80.5	14.35	7.84	28.00
30.00	0.77008	1187.2	0.02667	241.65	414.94	1.1432	1.7149	1.447	1.044	1.244	484.	143.	200.7	12.48	79.6	14.56	7.57	30.00
32.00	0.81530	1179.3	0.02516	244.55	415.90	1.1527	1.7142	1.457	1.058	1.251	474.	143.	196.0	12.60	78.7	14.76	7.31	32.00
34.00	0.86250	1171.3	0.02374	247.47	416.85	1.1621	1.7135	1.467	1.073	1.259	465.	142.	191.4	12.72	77.7	14.97	7.05	34.00
36.00	0.91172	1163.2	0.02241	250.41	417.78	1.1715	1.7129	1.478	1.088	1.267	455.	142.	186.9	12.84	76.8	15.19	6.78	36.00
38.00	0.96301	1154.9	0.02116	253.37	418.69	1.1809	1.7122	1.489	1.104	1.276	445.	141.	182.5	12.97	75.9	15.41	6.52	38.00
40.00	1.0165	1146.5	0.01999	256.35	419.58	1.1903	1.7115	1.500	1.120	1.285	436.	140.	178.2	13.10	75.0	15.64	6.27	40.00
42.00	1.0721	1137.9	0.01890	259.35	420.44	1.1997	1.7108	1.513	1.138	1.295	426.	140.	174.0	13.24	74.1	15.86	6.01	42.00
44.00	1.1300	1129.2	0.01786	262.38	421.28	1.2091	1.7101	1.525	1.156	1.306	416.	139.	169.8	13.38	73.1	16.10	5.76	44.00
46.00	1.1901	1120.3	0.01689	265.42	422.09	1.2185	1.7094	1.539	1.175	1.318	407.	138.	165.7	13.52	72.2	16.34	5.51	46.00
48.00	1.2527	1111.3	0.01598	268.49	422.88	1.2279	1.7086	1.553	1.196	1.331	397.	137.	161.7	13.67	71.3	16.59	5.26	48.00
50.00	1.3177	1102.0	0.01511	271.59	423.63	1.2373	1.7078	1.569	1.218	1.345	387.	137.	157.7	13.83	70.4	16.84	5.01	50.00
52.00	1.3852	1092.6	0.01430	274.71	424.35	1.2468	1.7070	1.585	1.241	1.360	377.	136.	153.8	13.99	69.5	17.10	4.76	52.00
54.00	1.4553	1082.9	0.01353	277.86	425.03	1.2562	1.7061	1.602	1.266	1.377	367.	135.	149.9	14.16	68.5	17.36	4.52	54.00
56.00	1.5280	1073.0	0.01280	281.04	425.68	1.2657	1.7051	1.621	1.293	1.395	358.	134.	146.1	14.33	67.6	17.63	4.28	56.00
58.00	1.6033	1062.8	0.01212	284.25	426.29	1.2752	1.7041	1.641	1.322	1.416	348.	133.	142.3	14.51	66.7	17.91	4.04	58.00
60.00	1.6815	1052.4	0.01146	287.49	426.86	1.2847	1.7031	1.663	1.354	1.438	338.	132.	138.6	14.71	65.8	18.19	3.81	60.00
62.00	1.7625	1041.7	0.01085	290.77	427.37	1.2943	1.7019	1.686	1.388	1.463	328.	131.	134.9	14.91	64.9	18.48	3.57	62.00
64.00	1.8464	1030.7	0.01026	294.08	427.84	1.3039	1.7007	1.712	1.426	1.490	318.	129.	131.2	15.12	63.9	18.78	3.34	64.00
66.00	1.9334	1019.4	0.00970	297.44	428.25	1.3136	1.6993	1.740	1.468	1.522	308.	128.	127.5	15.35	63.0	19.09	3.12	66.00
68.00	2.0234	1007.7	0.00917	300.84	428.61	1.3234	1.6979	1.772	1.515	1.557	298.	127.	123.9	15.59	62.1	19.40	2.89	68.00
70.00	2.1165	995.6	0.00867	304.29	428.89	1.3332	1.6963	1.806	1.567	1.597	287.	126.	120.3	15.85	61.2	19.72	2.67	70.00
72.00	2.2130	983.1	0.00818	307.79	429.10	1.3430	1.6945	1.846	1.626	1.642	277.	124.	116.7	16.12	60.3	20.05	2.46	72.00
74.00	2.3127	970.0	0.00772	311.34	429.23	1.3530	1.6926	1.890	1.693	1.695	267.	123.	113.1	16.41	59.3	20.39	2.24	74.00
76.00	2.4159	956.5	0.00728	314.96	429.27	1.3631	1.6905	1.941	1.770	1.757	256.	121.	109.4	16.73	58.4	20.74	2.03	76.00
78.00	2.5227	942.3	0.00686	318.65	429.20	1.3733	1.6881	2.000	1.861	1.830	246.	120.	105.8	17.08	57.5	21.09	1.83	78.00
80.00	2.6331	927.4	0.00646	322.41	429.02	1.3837	1.6855	2.069	1.967	1.917	235.	118.	102.1	17.46	56.6	21.46	1.63	80.00
85.00	2.9259	886.2	0.00550	332.27	427.91	1.4105	1.6775	2.313	2.348	2.231	207.	113.	92.7	18.59	54.3	22.41	1.15	85.00
90.00	3.2445	836.9	0.00461	343.01	425.48	1.4392	1.6663	2.766	3.064	2.832	178.	108.	82.6	20.15	—	—	0.72	90.00
95.00	3.5916	771.6	0.00374	355.43	420.60	1.4720	1.6490	3.961	4.942	4.424	145.	102.	70.9	22.59	—	—	0.33	95.00
100.00	3.9721	646.7	0.00265	374.02	407.08	1.5207	1.6093	—	—	—	105.	94.	53.0	28.86	—	—	0.03	100.00
101.03c	4.0560	513.3	0.00195	389.79	389.79	1.5593	1.5593	∞	∞	∞	0	0	—	—	∞	∞	0	101.03

*temperatures are on the ITS−90 scale a = triple point b = normal boiling point c = critical point

Table 2-4 SI Thermodynamic Properties of Moist Air at Standard Pressure

(Table 2, Chapter 6, 1997 *Handbook—Fundamentals*)

Temp. t, °C	Humidity Ratio, kg_w/kg_{da}	Volume, m^3/kg (dry air)			Enthalpy, kJ/kg (dry air)			Entropy, kJ/(kg·K) (dry air)			Condensed Water Enthalpy, kJ/kg	Condensed Water Entropy, kJ/(kg·K)	Condensed Water Vapor Pressure, kPa	Temp., °C
	W_s	v_a	v_{as}	v_s	h_a	h_{as}	h_s	s_a	s_{as}	s_s	h_w	s_w	p_s	
−60	0.0000067	0.6027	0.0000	0.6027	−60.351	0.017	−60.334	−0.2495	0.0001	−0.2494	−446.29	−1.6854	0.00108	−60
−59	0.0000076	0.6056	0.0000	0.6056	−59.344	0.018	−59.326	−0.2448	0.0001	−0.2447	−444.63	−1.6776	0.00124	−59
−58	0.0000087	0.6084	0.0000	0.6084	−58.338	0.021	−58.317	−0.2401	0.0001	−0.2400	−442.95	−1.6698	0.00141	−58
−57	0.0000100	0.6113	0.0000	0.6113	−57.332	0.024	−57.308	−0.2354	0.0001	−0.2353	−441.27	−1.6620	0.00161	−57
−56	0.0000114	0.6141	0.0000	0.6141	−56.326	0.028	−56.298	−0.2308	0.0001	−0.2306	−439.58	−1.6542	0.00184	−56
−55	0.0000129	0.6170	0.0000	0.6170	−55.319	0.031	−55.288	−0.2261	0.0002	−0.2260	−437.89	−1.6464	0.00209	−55
−54	0.0000147	0.6198	0.0000	0.6198	−54.313	0.036	−54.278	−0.2215	0.0002	−0.2214	−436.19	−1.6386	0.00238	−54
−53	0.0000167	0.6226	0.0000	0.6227	−53.307	0.041	−53.267	−0.2170	0.0002	−0.2168	−434.48	−1.6308	0.00271	−53
−52	0.0000190	0.6255	0.0000	0.6255	−52.301	0.046	−52.255	−0.2124	0.0002	−0.2122	−432.76	−1.6230	0.00307	−52
−51	0.0000215	0.6283	0.0000	0.6284	−51.295	0.052	−51.243	−0.2079	0.0002	−0.2076	−431.03	−1.6153	0.00348	−51
−50	0.0000243	0.6312	0.0000	0.6312	−50.289	0.059	−50.230	−0.2033	0.0003	−0.2031	−429.30	−1.6075	0.00394	−50
−49	0.0000275	0.6340	0.0000	0.6341	−49.283	0.067	−49.216	−0.1988	0.0003	−0.1985	−427.56	−1.5997	0.00445	−49
−48	0.0000311	0.6369	0.0000	0.6369	−48.277	0.075	−48.202	−0.1944	0.0004	−0.1940	−425.82	−1.5919	0.00503	−48
−47	0.0000350	0.6397	0.0000	0.6398	−47.271	0.085	−47.186	−0.1899	0.0004	−0.1895	−424.06	−1.5842	0.00568	−47
−46	0.0000395	0.6426	0.0000	0.6426	−46.265	0.095	−46.170	−0.1855	0.0004	−0.1850	−422.30	−1.5764	0.00640	−46
−45	0.0000445	0.6454	0.0000	0.6455	−45.259	0.108	−45.151	−0.1811	0.0005	−0.1805	−420.54	−1.5686	0.00721	−45
−44	0.0000500	0.6483	0.0001	0.6483	−44.253	0.121	−44.132	−0.1767	0.0006	−0.1761	−418.76	−1.5609	0.00811	−44
−43	0.0000562	0.6511	0.0001	0.6512	−43.247	0.137	−43.111	−0.1723	0.0006	−0.1716	−416.98	−1.5531	0.00911	−43
−42	0.0000631	0.6540	0.0001	0.6540	−42.241	0.153	−42.088	−0.1679	0.0007	−0.1672	−415.19	−1.5453	0.01022	−42
−41	0.0000708	0.6568	0.0001	0.6569	−41.235	0.172	−41.063	−0.1636	0.0008	−0.1628	−413.39	−1.5376	0.01147	−41
−40	0.0000793	0.6597	0.0001	0.6597	−40.229	0.192	−40.037	−0.1592	0.0009	−0.1584	−411.59	−1.5298	0.01285	−40
−39	0.0000887	0.6625	0.0001	0.6626	−39.224	0.216	−39.007	−0.1549	0.0010	−0.1540	−409.77	−1.5221	0.01438	−39
−38	0.0000992	0.6653	0.0001	0.6654	−38.218	0.241	−37.976	−0.1507	0.0011	−0.1496	−407.96	−1.5143	0.01608	−38
−37	0.0001108	0.6682	0.0001	0.6683	−37.212	0.270	−36.942	−0.1464	0.0012	−0.1452	−406.13	−1.5066	0.01796	−37
−36	0.0001237	0.6710	0.0001	0.6712	−36.206	0.302	−35.905	−0.1421	0.0014	−0.1408	−404.29	−1.4988	0.02005	−36
−35	0.0001379	0.6739	0.0001	0.6740	−35.200	0.336	−34.864	−0.1379	0.0015	−0.1364	−402.45	−1.4911	0.02235	−35
−34	0.0001536	0.6767	0.0002	0.6769	−34.195	0.375	−33.820	−0.1337	0.0017	−0.1320	−400.60	−1.4833	0.02490	−34
−33	0.0001710	0.6796	0.0002	0.6798	−33.189	0.417	−32.772	−0.1295	0.0018	−0.1276	−398.75	−1.4756	0.02772	−33
−32	0.0001902	0.6824	0.0002	0.6826	−32.183	0.464	−31.718	−0.1253	0.0020	−0.1233	−396.89	−1.4678	0.03082	−32
−31	0.0002113	0.6853	0.0002	0.6855	−31.178	0.517	−30.661	−0.1212	0.0023	−0.1189	−395.01	−1.4601	0.03425	−31
−30	0.0002346	0.6881	0.0003	0.6884	−30.171	0.574	−29.597	−0.1170	0.0025	−0.1145	−393.14	−1.4524	0.03802	−30
−29	0.0002602	0.6909	0.0003	0.6912	−29.166	0.636	−28.529	−0.1129	0.0028	−0.1101	−391.25	−1.4446	0.04217	−29
−28	0.0002883	0.6938	0.0003	0.6941	−28.160	0.707	−27.454	−0.1088	0.0031	−0.1057	−389.36	−1.4369	0.04673	−28
−27	0.0003193	0.6966	0.0004	0.6970	−27.154	0.782	−26.372	−0.1047	0.0034	−0.1013	−387.46	−1.4291	0.05175	−27
−26	0.0003533	0.6995	0.0004	0.6999	−26.149	0.867	−25.282	−0.1006	0.0037	−0.0969	−385.55	−1.4214	0.05725	−26
−25	0.0003905	0.7023	0.0004	0.7028	−25.143	0.959	−24.184	−0.0965	0.0041	−0.0924	−383.63	−1.4137	0.06329	−25
−24	0.0004314	0.7052	0.0005	0.7057	−24.137	1.059	−23.078	−0.0925	0.0045	−0.0880	−381.71	−1.4059	0.06991	−24
−23	0.0004762	0.7080	0.0005	0.7086	−23.132	1.171	−21.961	−0.0885	0.0050	−0.0835	−379.78	−1.3982	0.07716	−23
−22	0.0005251	0.7109	0.0006	0.7115	−22.126	1.292	−20.834	−0.0845	0.0054	−0.0790	−377.84	−1.3905	0.08510	−22
−21	0.0005787	0.7137	0.0007	0.7144	−21.120	1.425	−19.695	−0.0805	0.0060	−0.0745	−375.90	−1.3828	0.09378	−21
−20	0.0006373	0.7165	0.0007	0.7173	−20.115	1.570	−18.545	−0.0765	0.0066	−0.0699	−373.95	−1.3750	0.10326	−20
−19	0.0007013	0.7194	0.0008	0.7202	−19.109	1.729	−17.380	−0.0725	0.0072	−0.0653	−371.99	−1.3673	0.11362	−19
−18	0.0007711	0.7222	0.0009	0.7231	−18.103	1.902	−16.201	−0.0686	0.0079	−0.0607	−370.02	−1.3596	0.12492	−18
−17	0.0008473	0.7251	0.0010	0.7261	−17.098	2.092	−15.006	−0.0646	0.0086	−0.0560	−368.04	−1.3518	0.13725	−17
−16	0.0009303	0.7279	0.0011	0.7290	−16.092	2.299	−13.793	−0.0607	0.0094	−0.0513	−366.06	−1.3441	0.15068	−16
−15	0.0010207	0.7308	0.0012	0.7320	−15.086	2.524	−12.562	−0.0568	0.0103	−0.0465	−364.07	−1.3364	0.16530	−15
−14	0.0011191	0.7336	0.0013	0.7349	−14.080	2.769	−11.311	−0.0529	0.0113	−0.0416	−362.07	−1.3287	0.18122	−14
−13	0.0012262	0.7364	0.0014	0.7379	−13.075	3.036	−10.039	−0.0490	0.0123	−0.0367	−360.07	−1.3210	0.19852	−13
−12	0.0013425	0.7393	0.0016	0.7409	−12.069	3.327	−8.742	−0.0452	0.0134	−0.0318	−358.06	−1.3132	0.21732	−12
−11	0.0014690	0.7421	0.0017	0.7439	−11.063	3.642	−7.421	−0.0413	0.0146	−0.0267	−356.04	−1.3055	0.23775	−11
−10	0.0016062	0.7450	0.0019	0.7469	−10.057	3.986	−6.072	−0.0375	0.0160	−0.0215	−354.01	−1.2978	0.25991	−10
−9	0.0017551	0.7478	0.0021	0.7499	−9.052	4.358	−4.693	−0.0337	0.0174	−0.0163	−351.97	−1.2901	0.28395	−9
−8	0.0019166	0.7507	0.0023	0.7530	−8.046	4.764	−3.283	−0.0299	0.0189	−0.0110	−349.93	−1.2824	0.30999	−8
−7	0.0020916	0.7535	0.0025	0.7560	−7.040	5.202	−1.838	−0.0261	0.0206	−0.0055	−347.88	−1.2746	0.33821	−7
−6	0.0022811	0.7563	0.0028	0.7591	−6.035	5.677	−0.357	−0.0223	0.0224	−0.0000	−345.82	−1.2669	0.36874	−6
−5	0.0024862	0.7592	0.0030	0.7622	−5.029	6.192	1.164	−0.0186	0.0243	−0.0057	−343.76	−1.2592	0.40178	−5
−4	0.0027081	0.7620	0.0033	0.7653	−4.023	6.751	2.728	−0.0148	0.0264	−0.0115	−341.69	−1.2515	0.43748	−4
−3	0.0029480	0.7649	0.0036	0.7685	−3.017	7.353	4.336	−0.0111	0.0286	−0.0175	−339.61	−1.2438	0.47606	−3
−2	0.0032074	0.7677	0.0039	0.7717	−2.011	8.007	5.995	−0.0074	0.0310	−0.0236	−337.52	−1.2361	0.51773	−2
−1	0.0034874	0.7705	0.0043	0.7749	−1.006	8.712	7.706	−0.0037	0.0336	−0.0299	−335.42	−1.2284	0.56268	−1
0	0.0037895	0.7734	0.0047	0.7781	−0.000	9.473	9.473	0.0000	0.0364	0.0364	−333.32	−1.2206	0.61117	−0
0*	0.003789	0.7734	0.0047	0.7781	−0.000	9.473	9.473	0.0000	0.0364	0.0364	0.06	−0.0001	0.6112	0
1	0.004076	0.7762	0.0051	0.7813	1.006	10.197	11.203	0.0037	0.0391	0.0427	4.28	0.0153	0.6571	1
2	0.004381	0.7791	0.0055	0.7845	2.012	10.970	12.982	0.0073	0.0419	0.0492	8.49	0.0306	0.7060	2
3	0.004707	0.7819	0.0059	0.7878	3.018	11.793	14.811	0.0110	0.0449	0.0559	12.70	0.0459	0.7581	3
4	0.005054	0.7848	0.0064	0.7911	4.024	12.672	16.696	0.0146	0.0480	0.0627	16.91	0.0611	0.8135	4
5	0.005424	0.7876	0.0068	0.7944	5.029	13.610	18.639	0.0182	0.0514	0.0697	21.12	0.0762	0.8725	5
6	0.005818	0.7904	0.0074	0.7978	6.036	14.608	20.644	0.0219	0.0550	0.0769	25.32	0.0913	0.9353	6
7	0.006237	0.7933	0.0079	0.8012	7.041	15.671	22.713	0.0255	0.0588	0.0843	29.52	0.1064	1.0020	7
8	0.006683	0.7961	0.0085	0.8046	8.047	16.805	24.852	0.0290	0.0628	0.0919	33.72	0.1213	1.0729	8
9	0.007157	0.7990	0.0092	0.8081	9.053	18.010	27.064	0.0326	0.0671	0.0997	37.92	0.1362	1.1481	9
10	0.007661	0.8018	0.0098	0.8116	10.059	19.293	29.352	0.0362	0.0717	0.1078	42.11	0.1511	1.2280	10
11	0.008197	0.8046	0.0106	0.8152	11.065	20.658	31.724	0.0397	0.0765	0.1162	46.31	0.1659	1.3128	11
12	0.008766	0.8075	0.0113	0.8188	12.071	22.108	34.179	0.0433	0.0816	0.1248	50.50	0.1806	1.4026	12
13	0.009370	0.8103	0.0122	0.8225	13.077	23.649	36.726	0.0468	0.0870	0.1337	54.69	0.1953	1.4979	13

*Extrapolated to represent metastable equilibrium with undercooled liquid.

Table 2-4 SI Thermodynamic Properties of Moist Air at Standard Pressure (*Continued*)

(Table 2, Chapter 6, 1997 *Handbook—Fundamentals*)

Temp. t, °C	Humidity Ratio, kg_w/kg_{da} W_s	Volume, m^3/kg (dry air) v_a	v_{as}	v_s	Enthalpy, kJ/kg (dry air) h_a	h_{as}	h_s	Entropy, kJ/(kg·K) (dry air) s_a	s_{as}	s_s	Condensed Water: Enthalpy, kJ/kg h_w	Condensed Water: Entropy, kJ/(kg·K) s_w	Condensed Water: Vapor Pressure, kPa p_s	Temp., °C
14	0.010012	0.8132	0.0131	0.8262	14.084	25.286	39.370	0.0503	0.0927	0.1430	58.88	0.2099	1.5987	14
15	0.010692	0.8160	0.0140	0.8300	15.090	27.023	42.113	0.0538	0.0987	0.1525	63.07	0.2244	1.7055	15
16	0.011413	0.8188	0.0150	0.8338	16.096	28.867	44.963	0.0573	0.1051	0.1624	67.26	0.2389	1.8185	16
17	0.012178	0.8217	0.0160	0.8377	17.102	30.824	47.926	0.0607	0.1119	0.1726	71.44	0.2534	1.9380	17
18	0.012989	0.8245	0.0172	0.8417	18.108	32.900	51.008	0.0642	0.1190	0.1832	75.63	0.2678	2.0643	18
19	0.013848	0.8274	0.0184	0.8457	19.114	35.101	54.216	0.0677	0.1266	0.1942	79.81	0.2821	2.1979	19
20	0.014758	0.8302	0.0196	0.8498	20.121	37.434	57.555	0.0711	0.1346	0.2057	84.00	0.2965	2.3389	20
21	0.015721	0.8330	0.0210	0.8540	21.127	39.908	61.035	0.0745	0.1430	0.2175	88.18	0.3107	2.4878	21
22	0.016741	0.8359	0.0224	0.8583	22.133	42.527	64.660	0.0779	0.1519	0.2298	92.36	0.3249	2.6448	22
23	0.017821	0.8387	0.0240	0.8627	23.140	45.301	68.440	0.0813	0.1613	0.2426	96.55	0.3390	2.8105	23
24	0.018963	0.8416	0.0256	0.8671	24.146	48.239	72.385	0.0847	0.1712	0.2559	100.73	0.3531	2.9852	24
25	0.020170	0.8444	0.0273	0.8717	25.153	51.347	76.500	0.0881	0.1817	0.2698	104.91	0.3672	3.1693	25
26	0.021448	0.8472	0.0291	0.8764	26.159	54.638	80.798	0.0915	0.1927	0.2842	109.09	0.3812	3.3633	26
27	0.022798	0.8501	0.0311	0.8811	27.165	58.120	85.285	0.0948	0.2044	0.2992	113.27	0.3951	3.5674	27
28	0.024226	0.8529	0.0331	0.8860	28.172	61.804	89.976	0.0982	0.2166	0.3148	117.45	0.4090	3.7823	28
29	0.025735	0.8558	0.0353	0.8910	29.179	65.699	94.878	0.1015	0.2296	0.3311	121.63	0.4229	4.0084	29
30	0.027329	0.8586	0.0376	0.8962	30.185	69.820	100.006	0.1048	0.2432	0.3481	125.81	0.4367	4.2462	30
31	0.029014	0.8614	0.0400	0.9015	31.192	74.177	105.369	0.1082	0.2576	0.3658	129.99	0.4505	4.4961	31
32	0.030793	0.8643	0.0426	0.9069	32.198	78.780	110.979	0.1115	0.2728	0.3842	134.17	0.4642	4.7586	32
33	0.032674	0.8671	0.0454	0.9125	33.205	83.652	116.857	0.1148	0.2887	0.4035	138.35	0.4779	5.0345	33
34	0.034660	0.8700	0.0483	0.9183	34.212	88.799	123.011	0.1180	0.3056	0.4236	142.53	0.4915	5.3242	34
35	0.036756	0.8728	0.0514	0.9242	35.219	94.236	129.455	0.1213	0.3233	0.4446	146.71	0.5051	5.6280	35
36	0.038971	0.8756	0.0546	0.9303	36.226	99.983	136.209	0.1246	0.3420	0.4666	150.89	0.5186	5.9468	36
37	0.041309	0.8785	0.0581	0.9366	37.233	106.058	143.290	0.1278	0.3617	0.4895	155.07	0.5321	6.2812	37
38	0.043778	0.8813	0.0618	0.9431	38.239	112.474	150.713	0.1311	0.3824	0.5135	159.25	0.5456	6.6315	38
39	0.046386	0.8842	0.0657	0.9498	39.246	119.258	158.504	0.1343	0.4043	0.5386	163.43	0.5590	6.9988	39
40	0.049141	0.8870	0.0698	0.9568	40.253	126.430	166.683	0.1375	0.4273	0.5649	167.61	0.5724	7.3838	40
41	0.052049	0.8898	0.0741	0.9640	41.261	134.005	175.265	0.1407	0.4516	0.5923	171.79	0.5857	7.7866	41
42	0.055119	0.8927	0.0788	0.9714	42.268	142.007	184.275	0.1439	0.4771	0.6211	175.97	0.5990	8.2081	42
43	0.058365	0.8955	0.0837	0.9792	43.275	150.475	193.749	0.1471	0.5041	0.6512	180.15	0.6122	8.6495	43
44	0.061791	0.8983	0.0888	0.9872	44.282	159.417	203.699	0.1503	0.5325	0.6828	184.33	0.6254	9.1110	44
45	0.065411	0.9012	0.0943	0.9955	45.289	168.874	214.164	0.1535	0.5624	0.7159	188.51	0.6386	9.5935	45
46	0.069239	0.9040	0.1002	1.0042	46.296	178.882	225.179	0.1566	0.5940	0.7507	192.69	0.6517	10.0982	46
47	0.073282	0.9069	0.1063	1.0132	47.304	189.455	236.759	0.1598	0.6273	0.7871	196.88	0.6648	10.6250	47
48	0.077556	0.9097	0.1129	1.0226	48.311	200.644	248.955	0.1629	0.6624	0.8253	201.06	0.6778	11.1754	48
49	0.082077	0.9125	0.1198	1.0323	49.319	212.485	261.803	0.1661	0.6994	0.8655	205.24	0.6908	11.7502	49
50	0.086858	0.9154	0.1272	1.0425	50.326	225.019	275.345	0.1692	0.7385	0.9077	209.42	0.7038	12.3503	50
51	0.091918	0.9182	0.1350	1.0532	51.334	238.290	289.624	0.1723	0.7798	0.9521	213.60	0.7167	12.9764	51
52	0.097272	0.9211	0.1433	1.0643	52.341	252.340	304.682	0.1754	0.8234	0.9988	217.78	0.7296	13.6293	52
53	0.102948	0.9239	0.1521	1.0760	53.349	267.247	320.596	0.1785	0.8695	1.0480	221.97	0.7424	14.3108	53
54	0.108954	0.9267	0.1614	1.0882	54.357	283.031	337.388	0.1816	0.9182	1.0998	226.15	0.7552	15.0205	54
55	0.115321	0.9296	0.1713	1.1009	55.365	299.772	355.137	0.1847	0.9698	1.1544	230.33	0.7680	15.7601	55
56	0.122077	0.9324	0.1819	1.1143	56.373	317.549	373.922	0.1877	1.0243	1.2120	234.52	0.7807	16.5311	56
57	0.129243	0.9353	0.1932	1.1284	57.381	336.417	393.798	0.1908	1.0820	1.2728	238.70	0.7934	17.3337	57
58	0.136851	0.9381	0.2051	1.1432	58.389	356.461	414.850	0.1938	1.1432	1.3370	242.88	0.8061	18.1691	58
59	0.144942	0.9409	0.2179	1.1588	59.397	377.788	437.185	0.1969	1.2081	1.4050	247.07	0.8187	19.0393	59
60	0.15354	0.9438	0.2315	1.1752	60.405	400.458	460.863	0.1999	1.2769	1.4768	251.25	0.8313	19.9439	60
61	0.16269	0.9466	0.2460	1.1926	61.413	424.624	486.036	0.2029	1.3500	1.5530	255.44	0.8438	20.8858	61
62	0.17244	0.9494	0.2614	1.2109	62.421	450.377	512.798	0.2059	1.4278	1.6337	259.62	0.8563	21.8651	62
63	0.18284	0.9523	0.2780	1.2303	63.429	477.837	541.266	0.2089	1.5104	1.7194	263.81	0.8688	22.8826	63
64	0.19393	0.9551	0.2957	1.2508	64.438	507.177	571.615	0.2119	1.5985	1.8105	268.00	0.8812	23.9405	64
65	0.20579	0.9580	0.3147	1.2726	65.446	538.548	603.995	0.2149	1.6925	1.9074	272.18	0.8936	25.0397	65
66	0.21848	0.9608	0.3350	1.2958	66.455	572.116	638.571	0.2179	1.7927	2.0106	276.37	0.9060	26.1810	66
67	0.23207	0.9636	0.3568	1.3204	67.463	608.103	675.566	0.2209	1.8999	2.1208	280.56	0.9183	27.3664	67
68	0.24664	0.9665	0.3803	1.3467	68.472	646.724	715.196	0.2238	2.0147	2.2385	284.75	0.9306	28.5967	68
69	0.26231	0.9693	0.4055	1.3749	69.481	688.261	757.742	0.2268	2.1378	2.3646	288.94	0.9429	29.8741	69
70	0.27916	0.9721	0.4328	1.4049	70.489	732.959	803.448	0.2297	2.2699	2.4996	293.13	0.9551	31.1986	70
71	0.29734	0.9750	0.4622	1.4372	71.498	781.208	852.706	0.2327	2.4122	2.6448	297.32	0.9673	32.5734	71
72	0.31698	0.9778	0.4941	1.4719	72.507	833.335	905.842	0.2356	2.5655	2.8010	301.51	0.9794	33.9983	72
73	0.33824	0.9807	0.5287	1.5093	73.516	889.807	963.323	0.2385	2.7311	2.9696	305.70	0.9916	35.4759	73
74	0.36130	0.9835	0.5662	1.5497	74.525	951.077	1025.603	0.2414	2.9104	3.1518	309.89	1.0037	37.0063	74
75	0.38641	0.9863	0.6072	1.5935	75.535	1017.841	1093.375	0.2443	3.1052	3.3496	314.08	1.0157	38.5940	75
76	0.41377	0.9892	0.6519	1.6411	76.543	1090.628	1167.172	0.2472	3.3171	3.5644	318.28	1.0278	40.2369	76
77	0.44372	0.9920	0.7010	1.6930	77.553	1170.328	1247.881	0.2501	3.5486	3.7987	322.47	1.0398	41.9388	77
78	0.47663	0.9948	0.7550	1.7498	78.562	1257.921	1336.483	0.2530	3.8023	4.0553	326.67	1.0517	43.7020	78
79	0.51284	0.9977	0.8145	1.8121	79.572	1354.347	1433.918	0.2559	4.0810	4.3368	330.86	1.0636	45.5248	79
80	0.55295	1.0005	0.8805	1.8810	80.581	1461.200	1541.781	0.2587	4.3890	4.6477	335.06	1.0755	47.4135	80
81	0.59751	1.0034	0.9539	1.9572	81.591	1579.961	1661.552	0.2616	4.7305	4.9921	339.25	1.0874	49.3670	81
82	0.64724	1.0062	1.0360	2.0422	82.600	1712.547	1795.148	0.2644	5.1108	5.3753	343.45	1.0993	51.3860	82
83	0.70311	1.0090	1.1283	2.1373	83.610	1861.548	1945.158	0.2673	5.5372	5.8045	347.65	1.1111	53.4746	83
84	0.76624	1.0119	1.2328	2.2446	84.620	2029.983	2114.603	0.2701	6.0181	6.2882	351.85	1.1228	55.6337	84
85	0.83812	1.0147	1.3518	2.3666	85.630	2221.806	2307.436	0.2729	6.5644	6.8373	356.05	1.1346	57.8658	85
86	0.92062	1.0175	1.4887	2.5062	86.640	2442.036	2528.677	0.2757	7.1901	7.4658	360.25	1.1463	60.1727	86
87	1.01611	1.0204	1.6473	2.6676	87.650	2697.016	2784.666	0.2785	7.9128	8.1914	364.45	1.1580	62.5544	87
88	1.12800	1.0232	1.8333	2.8565	88.661	2995.890	3084.551	0.2813	8.7580	9.0393	368.65	1.1696	65.0166	88
89	1.26064	1.0261	2.0540	3.0800	89.671	3350.254	3439.925	0.2841	9.7577	10.0419	372.86	1.1812	67.5581	89
90	1.42031	1.0289	2.3199	3.3488	90.681	3776.918	3867.599	0.2869	10.9586	11.2455	377.06	1.1928	70.1817	90

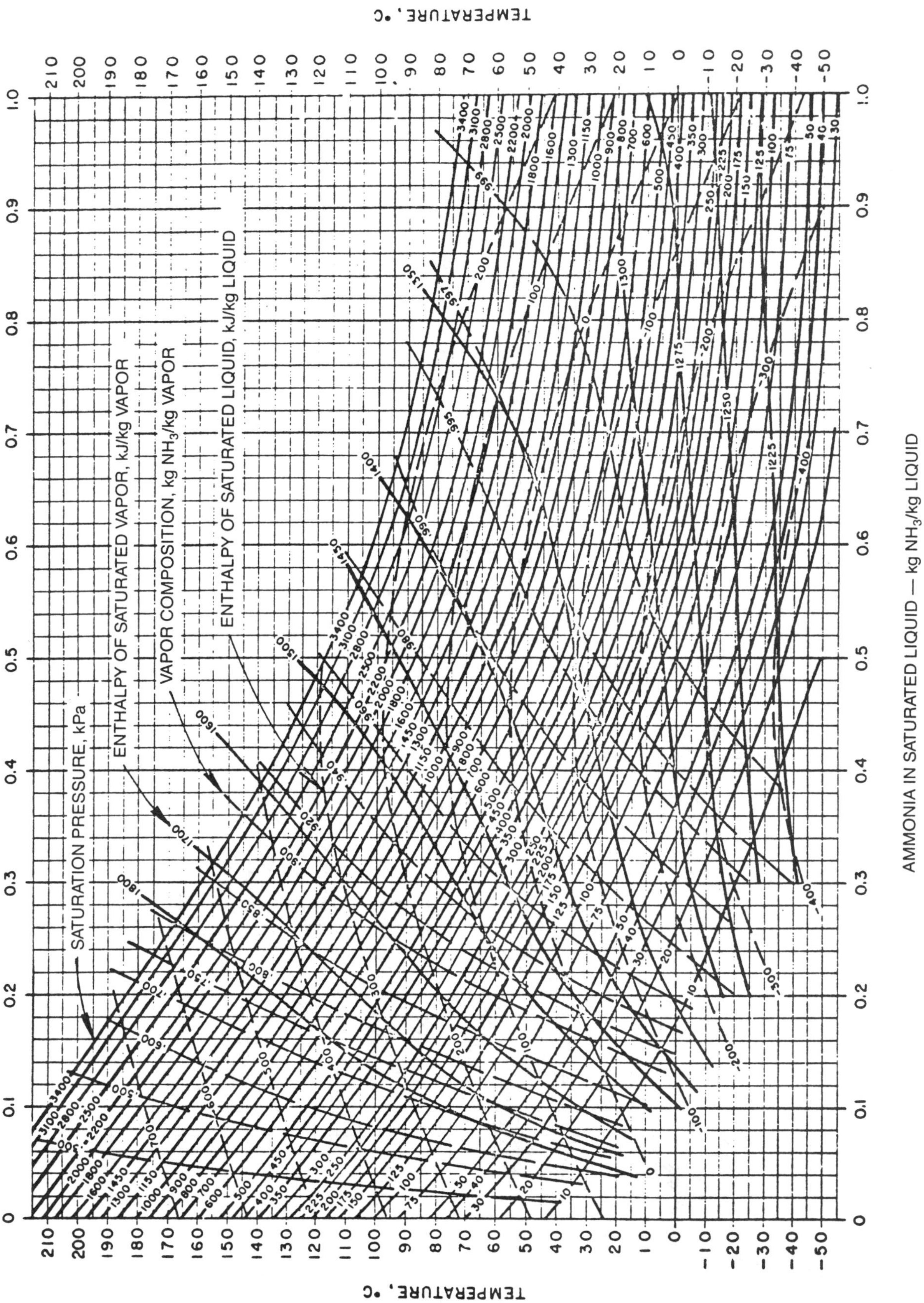

Fig. 2-6 SI Enthalpy-Concentration Diagram for Aqua-Ammonia

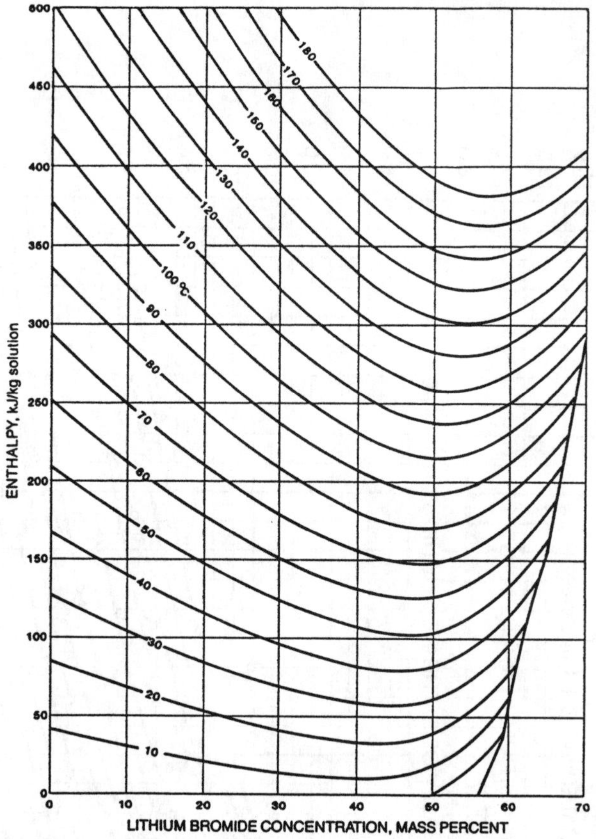

EQUATIONS CONCENTRATION RANGE $40 < X < 70\%$ LiBr TEMPERATURE RANGE $15 < t < 165°C$

$$h = \Sigma_0^4 A_n X^n + t\,\Sigma_0^4 B_n X^n + t^2 \Sigma_0^4 C_n X^n \text{ in kJ/kg, where } t = °C \text{ and } X = \%\text{LiBr}$$

$A_0 = -2024.33$	$B_0 = 18.2829$	$C_0 = -3.7008214$ E-2
$A_1 = 163.309$	$B_1 = -1.1691757$	$C_1 = 2.8877666$ E-3
$A_2 = -4.88161$	$B_2 = 3.248041$ E-2	$C_2 = -8.1313015$ E-5
$A_3 = 6.302948$ E-2	$B_3 = -4.034184$ E-4	$C_3 = 9.9116628$ E-7
$A_4 = -2.913705$ E-4	$B_4 = 1.8520569$ E-6	$C_4 = -4.4441207$ E-9

EQUATIONS

1. $t = \Sigma_0^3 B_n X^n + t' \Sigma_0^3 A_n X^n$ Solution Temp, °C
2. $t' = (t - \Sigma_0^3 B_n X^n)/\Sigma_0^3 A_n X^n$ Refrigerant Temp, °C
3. $\text{Log } P = C + D/T' + E/T'^2$ P = kPa; T' = K
4. $T' = \dfrac{-2E}{D + [D^2 - 4E(C - \log P)]^{0.5}}$

$A_0 = 2.007\,55$	$B_0 = 124.937$	$C = 7.05$
$A_1 = 0.169\,76$	$B_1 = -7.716\,49$	$D = -1596.49$
$A_2 = -3.133\,362$ E-03	$B_2 = 0.152\,286$	$E = -104\,095.5$
$A_3 = 1.976\,68$ E-05	$B_3 = -7.950\,90$ E-04	

RANGE: $-15 < t' < 110°C$
$5 < t < 175°C$
$45 < X < 70\%$ LiBr

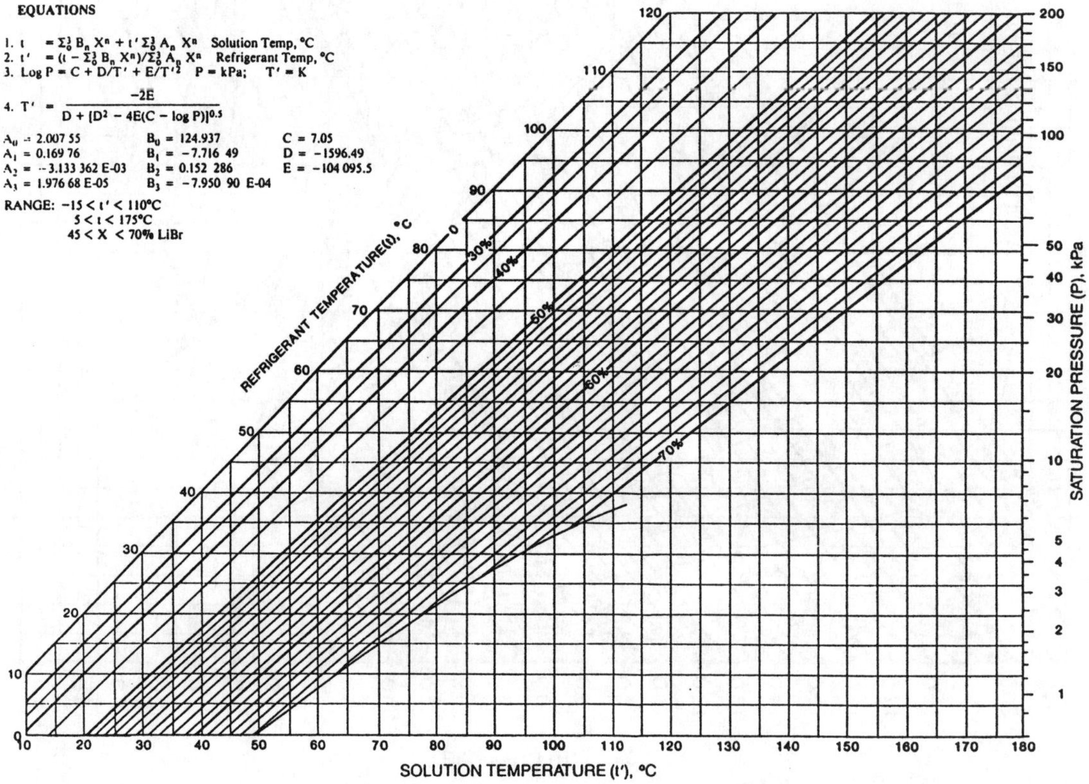

Fig. 2-7 SI Enthalpy-Concentration and Equilibrium Charts for Li-Br/Water

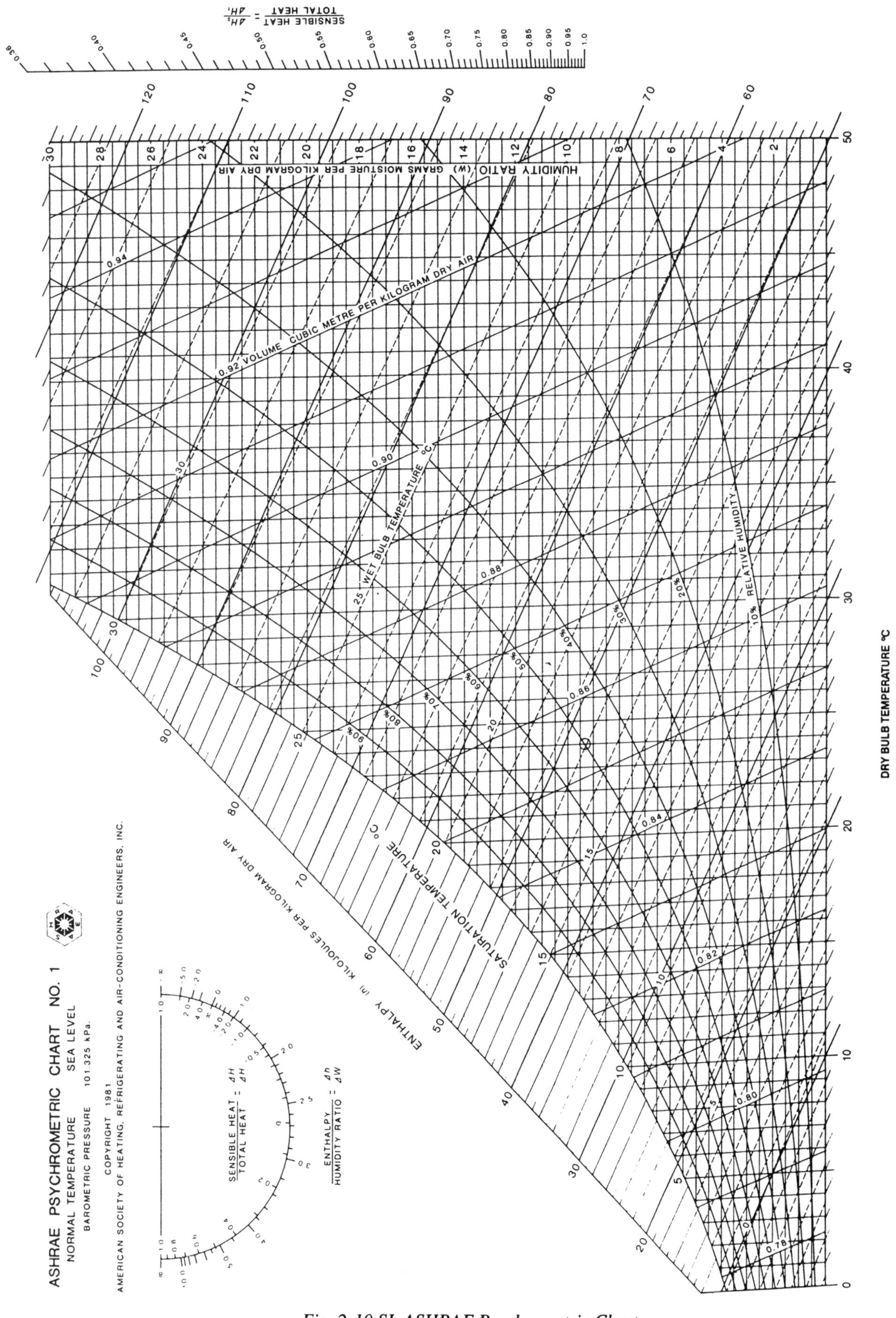

Fig. 2-10 SI ASHRAE Psychrometric Chart

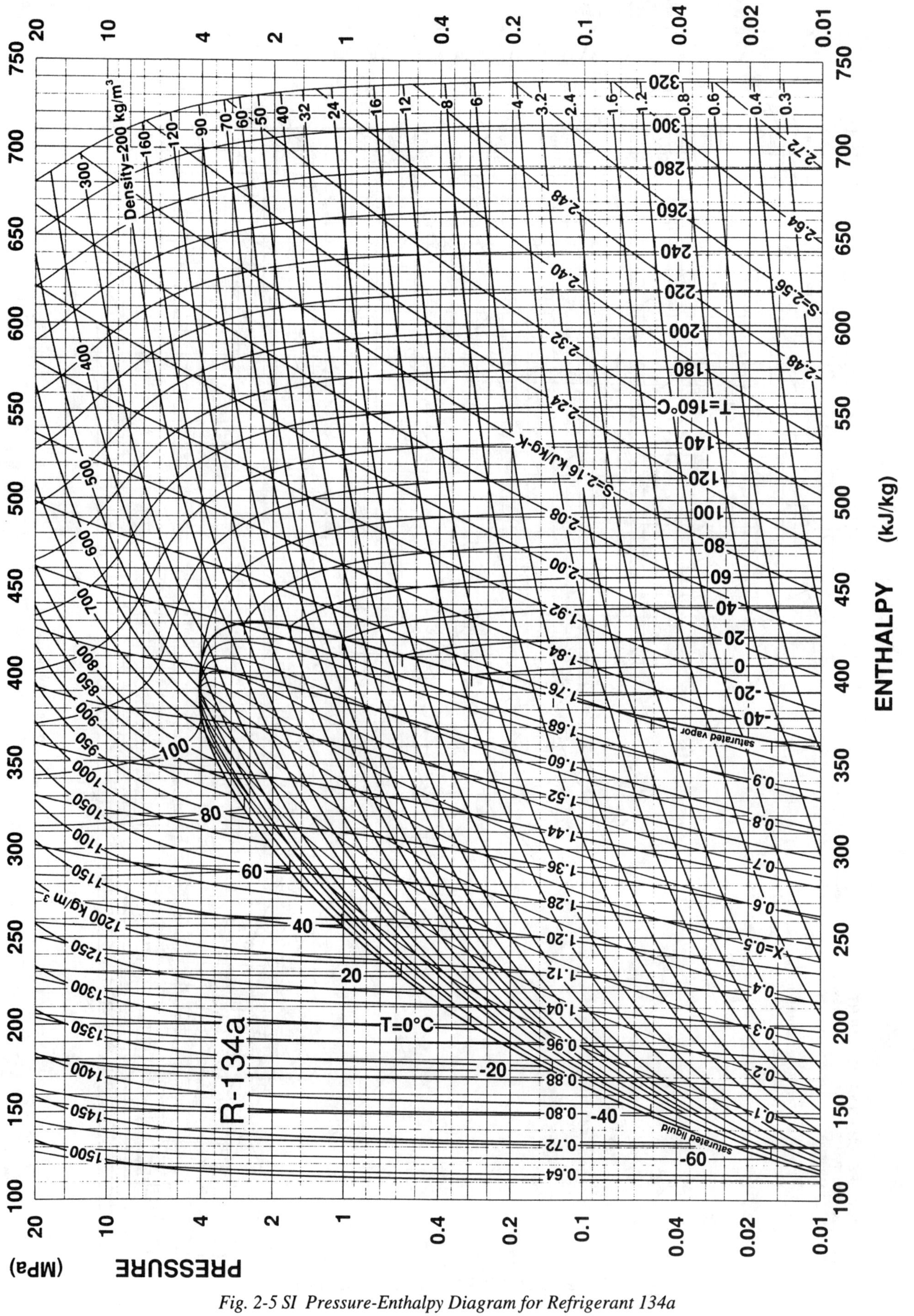

Fig. 2-5 SI Pressure-Enthalpy Diagram for Refrigerant 134a

Chapter 3

BASIC HVAC SYSTEM CALCULATIONS

This chapter illustrates the application of the principles of thermodynamics and psychrometrics to the various processes found in air-conditioning systems. It relates to material in Chapter 6 of the 1997 *ASHRAE Handbook—Fundamentals*.

3.1 Applying Thermodynamics to HVAC Processes

A simple but complete air-conditioning system is given schematically in Figure 3-1, which shows various space heat and moisture transfers. The symbol q_S represents a sensible heat transfer rate; the symbol m_w represents a moisture transfer rate. The symbol q_L designates the transfer of energy that accompanies moisture transfer and is given by $\Sigma m_w h_w$, where h_w is the specific enthalpy of the added (or removed) moisture. Solar radiation and internal loads are always gains upon the space. Heat transmission through solid construction components due to a temperature difference, as well as energy transfer because of infiltration, may represent a gain or a loss.

Note that the energy q_c and moisture m_c transfers at the conditioner cannot be determined from the space heat and moisture transfers alone. The effect of the outdoor ventilation air, as well as other system load components, must be included. The designer must recognize that items such as fan energy, duct transmission, roof and ceiling transmissions, heat from lights, bypass and leakage, type of return air system, location of main fans, and actual versus design room conditions are all related to one another, to component sizing, and to system arrangement.

The first law of thermodynamics (energy balance) and the conservation of mass (mass balance) are the basis for the analysis of moist air processes. The following sections demonstrate the application of these laws to specific HVAC processes.

In many air-conditioning systems, air is removed from the room, returned to the air-conditioning apparatus where it is reconditioned, and then supplied again to the room. In most systems, the return air from the room is mixed with outdoor air required for ventilation. A typical air-conditioning system and the corresponding psychrometric representation of the processes for cooling are illustrated in Figure 3-2. Outdoor air *o* is mixed with return air *r* from the room and enters the apparatus at condition *m*. Air flows through the conditioner and is supplied to the space *s*. The air supplied to the space picks up heat q_s and moisture m_w, and the cycle is repeated.

A typical psychrometric representation of the previous system operating under conditions of heating followed by humidification is given as Figure 3-3.

3.1.1 Absorption of Space Heat and Moisture Gains

The problem of air conditioning a space usually reduces to determining the quantity of moist air that must be supplied and the condition it must have to remove given amounts of energy and water from the space and be withdrawn at a specified condition. A space with incident rates of energy and moisture gains is shown in Figure 3-4. The quantity q_s denotes

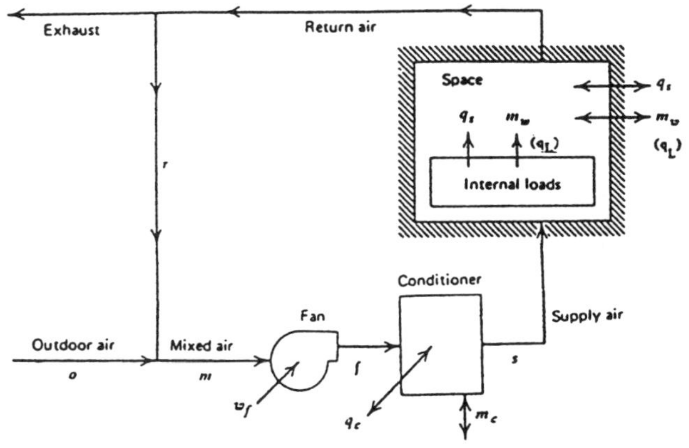

Fig. 3-1 Schematic of Air-Conditioning System

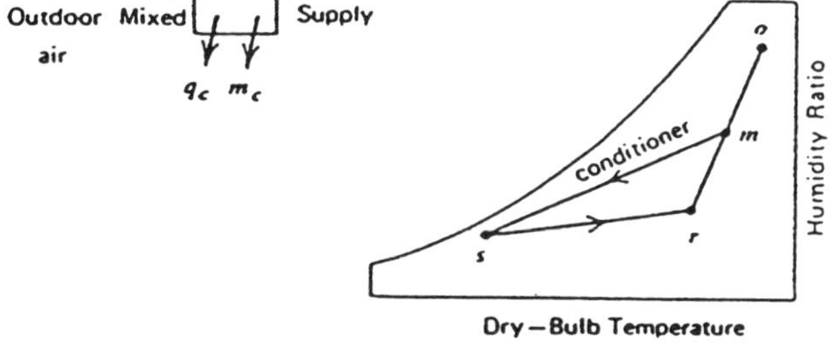

Fig. 3-2 Typical Air-Conditioning Cooling Processes

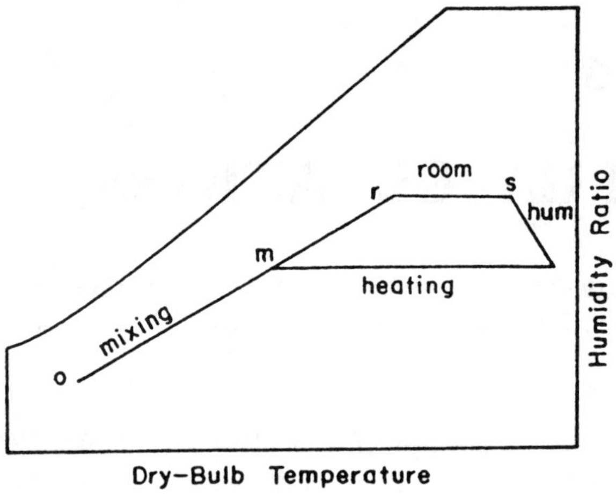

Fig. 3-3 Psychrometric Representation of Heating/ Humidifying Process

the net sum of all rates of heat gain upon the space arising from transfers through boundaries and from sources within the space. This gain, called **sensible heat gain**, involves the addition of energy alone, and does not include energy contributions due to the addition of water (or water vapor). The quantity m_w denotes the net sum of all rates of moisture gain upon the space arising from transfers through boundaries and from sources within the space. Each pound (kilogram) of moisture injected into the space adds an amount of energy equal to its specific enthalpy. A typical value of h_w is 1100 Btu/lb.

Assuming steady-state conditions, the governing equations are:

$$m_a h_1 + m_w h_w - m_a h_2 + q_s = 0 \qquad (3\text{-}1)$$

$$m_a W_1 + m_w = m_a W_2 \qquad (3\text{-}2)$$

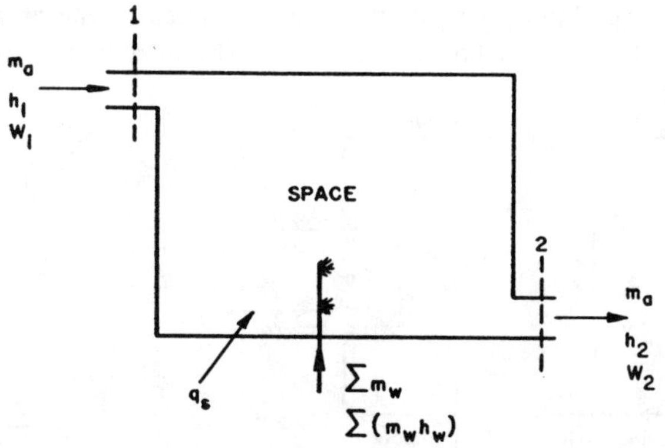

Fig. 3-4 Space HVAC Process

3.1.2 Heating or Cooling of Air

When air is heated or cooled without moisture loss or gain, the process yields a straight horizontal line on the psychrometric chart because the humidity ratio is constant. Such processes can occur when moist air flows through a heat exchanger (Figure 3-5).

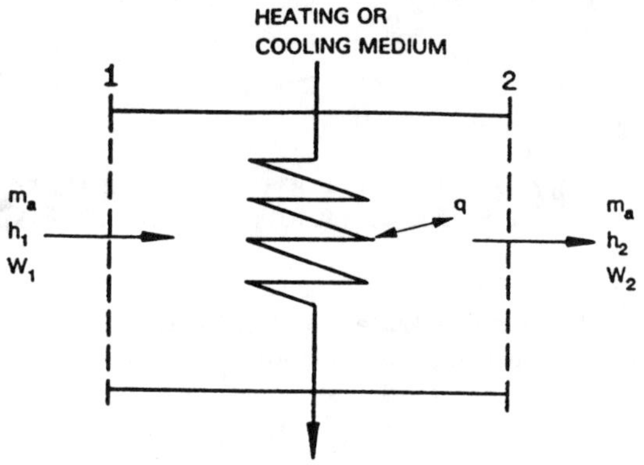

Fig. 3-5 Schematic Heating or Cooling Device

For steady-flow conditions, the governing equations are:

$$m_a h_1 - m_a h_2 + q = 0 \qquad (3\text{-}3)$$

$$W_2 = W_1 \qquad (3\text{-}4)$$

3.1.3 Cooling and Dehumidifying Air

When moist air is cooled to a temperature below its dew point, some of the water vapor condenses and leaves the air stream. A schematic cooling and dehumidifying device is shown in Figure 3-6.

Although the actual process path varies depending on the type of surface, surface temperature, and flow conditions, the heat and mass transfer can be expressed in terms of the initial and final states.

Although water may condense out at various temperatures ranging from the initial dew point to the final saturation temperature, it is assumed that condensed water is cooled to the final air temperature t_2 before it drains from the system. For the system shown in Figure 3-6, the steady-flow energy and material balance equations are:

$$m_a h_1 = m_a h_2 + q + m_w h_{w2} \qquad (3\text{-}5)$$

$$m_a W_1 = m_a W_2 + m_w \qquad (3\text{-}6)$$

Thus:

$$m_w = m_a (W_1 - W_2) \qquad (3\text{-}7)$$

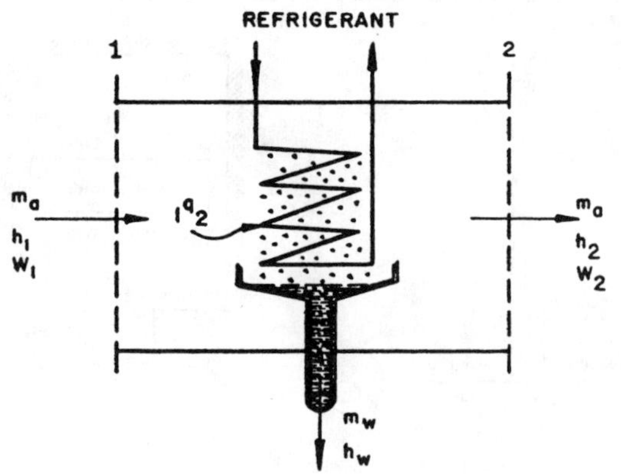

Fig. 3-6 Schematic Cooling and Dehumidifying Device

$$q = m_a[(h_1 - h_2) - (W_1 - W_2)h_{w_2}] \tag{3-8}$$

The cooling and dehumidifying process involves both sensible and latent heat transfer where sensible heat transfer is associated with the decrease in dry-bulb temperature and the latent heat transfer is associated with the decrease in humidity ratio. These quantities may be expressed as:

$$q_S = m_a c_p(t_1 - t_2) \tag{3-9}$$

$$q_L = m_a(W_1 - W_2)h_{fg} \tag{3-10}$$

Example 3-1. In a steady-flow process, a cooling and dehumidifying coil receives an air-water vapor mixture at 16 psia, 95°F, and 83% rh and discharges the air-water vapor mixture at 14.7 psia, 50°F, and 96% rh. The condensate leaves the unit at 50°F. Calculate the heat transfer per pound of dry air flowing through the unit.

Solution:

The first law of thermodynamics for a steady-state, steady-flow system is given by:

$${}_1\dot{Q}_2 + \left(\frac{V_1^2}{2g_c} + \frac{g}{g_c}z_1 + h_1\right)m_{a_1} = {}_1\dot{W}_2 + \left(\frac{V_2^2}{2g_c} + \frac{g}{g_c}z_2 + h_2\right)m_{a_2}$$

The continuity equation is:

$$m = A\rho V$$

For the air flowing through the apparatus this becomes:

$$m_{a_1} = m_{a_2} = m_a$$

For the water vapor this becomes:

$$m_{w_1} - m_{w_2} = m_{condensate}$$

Neglecting any kinetic or potential energy changes of the flowing fluid and noting that there is no mechanical work being done on or by the system, the First Law equation reduces to:

$${}_1\dot{Q}_2 = m_a(h_2 - h_1) + m_{concensate}h_{concensate}$$

and the enthalpy terms may be expanded, so that:

$$\frac{{}_1\dot{Q}_2}{m_a} = h_{a_2} - h_{a_1} + W_2h_{w_2} - W_1h_{w_1} + \frac{m_{condensate}}{m_a}h_{condensate}$$

With a mass balance on the water this becomes:

$$\frac{{}_1\dot{Q}_2}{m_a} = h_{a_2} - h_{a_1} + W_2h_{w_2} - W_1h_{w_1} + (W_1 - W_2)h_{condensate}$$

From Table 3, Chapter 6 of the 1997 *Handbook—Fundamentals*:

$$h_{w_2} = 1083.03 \text{ Btu/lb}$$

$$h_{w_1} = 1102.55 \text{ Btu/lb}$$

$$h_{condensate} = 18.06 \text{ Btu/lb}$$

W_1 and W_2 can be calculated:

$$p_{w_1} = \phi_1 p_{ws_1} = 0.83(0.8156) = 0.678 \text{ psia}$$

$$W_1 = 0.622p_{w_1}(p_1 - p_{w_1})$$
$$= 0.622 \times 0.678/(16 - 0.678) = 0.0275$$

$$p_{w_2} = 0.96(0.178) = 0.171 \text{ psia}$$

$$W_2 = 0.622p_{w_2}(p_2 - p_{w_2})$$
$$= 0.622 \times 0.171/(14.7 - 0.171) = 0.0073$$

Substituting into the energy equation:

$$\frac{{}_1\dot{Q}_2}{m_a} = 0.24(50 - 95) + 0.0073(1083.1) - 0.0275(1102.6)$$
$$+ (0.0275 - 0.0073)18.06$$
$$= -10.8 + 7.91 - 30.3 \div 0.36 = 32.8 \text{ Btu/lb}_{air}$$

3.1.4 Heating and Humidifying Air

A device to heat and humidify moist air is shown in Figure 3-7. This process is generally required during the cold months of the year. An energy balance on the device yields:

$$m_ah_1 + q + m_wh_w = m_ah_2 \tag{3-11}$$

and a mass balance on the water gives:

$$m_aW_1 + m_w = m_aW_2 \tag{3-12}$$

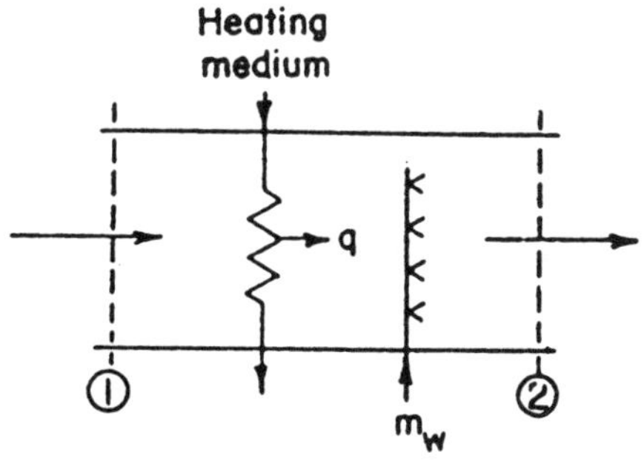

Fig. 3-7 Schematic Heating and Humidifying Device

3.1.5 Adiabatic Mixing of Two Streams of Air

A common process involved in air conditioning is the adiabatic mixing of two streams of moist air (Figure 3-8).

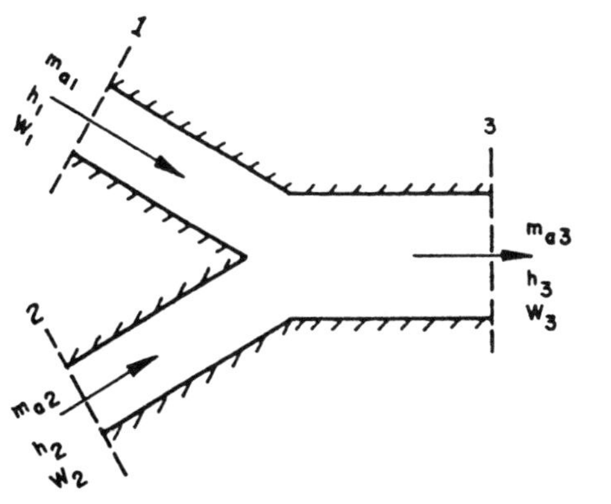

Fig. 3-8 Adiabatic Mixing of Two Streams of Moist Air

If the mixing is adiabatic, it must be governed by these three equations:

$$m_{a_1}h_1 + m_{a_2}h_2 = m_{a_3}h_3 \quad (3\text{-}13)$$

$$m_{a_1} + m_{a_2} = m_{a_3} \quad (3\text{-}14)$$

$$m_{a_1}W_1 + m_{a_2}W_2 = m_{a_3}W_3 \quad (3\text{-}15)$$

3.1.6 Adiabatic Mixing of Moist Air with Injected Water

Injecting steam or liquid water into a moist air stream to raise the humidity ratio of the moist air is a frequent air-conditioning process (Figure 3-9). If the mixing is adiabatic, the following equations apply:

$$m_a h_1 + m_w h_w = m_a h_2 \quad (3\text{-}16)$$

$$m_a W_1 + m_w = m_a W_2 \quad (3\text{-}17)$$

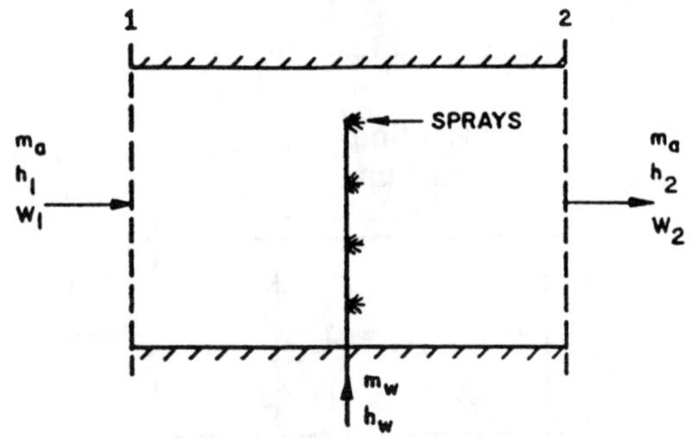

Fig. 3-9 Schematic Injection of Water into Moist Air

3.1.7 Moving Air

In all HVAC systems, a fan or blower is required to move the air. Under steady-flow conditions for the fan shown in Figure 3-10, the conservation equations are:

$$m_a h_1 - m_a h_2 - W_k = 0 \quad (3\text{-}18)$$

$$W_1 = W_2 \quad (3\text{-}19)$$

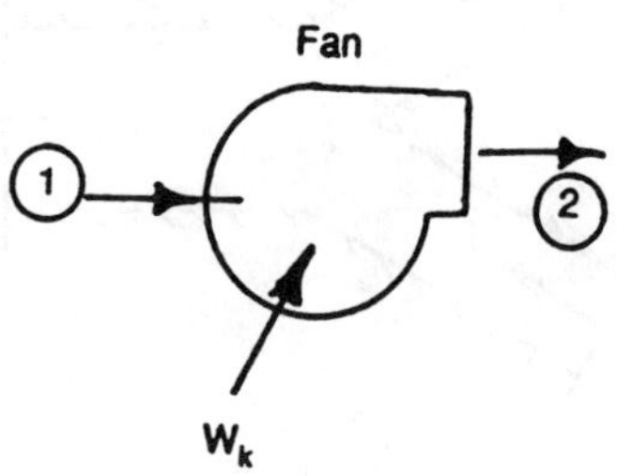

Fig. 3-10 Air Moving

3.1.8 Approximate Equations Using Volume Flow Rates

Since the specific volume of air varies appreciably with temperature, all calculations should be made with the mass of air instead of the volume. Nevertheless, volume values are required when selecting coils, fans, ducts, and other components.

In Chapter 6 of the 1997 *Handbook—Fundamentals*, basic calculations for air system loads, flow rates, and psychrometric representations are based on mass flow. Chapters 27 and 28 on load estimating give equations based on volumetric flow. These volumetric equations are commonly used and generally apply to most air systems.

One method of using volume while still including mass is to use volume values based on measurement at standard conditions. ASHRAE defines one standard condition as dry air at 20°C and 101.325 kPa (68°F and 14.7 psia). Under that condition the density of dry air is about 1.204 kg/m^3 (0.075 lb/ft^3) and the specific volume is 0.83 m^3/kg (13.3 ft^3/lb). Saturated air at 15°C (59.5°F) has about the same density or specific volume. Thus, in the range at which air usually passes through the coils, fans, ducts, and other equipment, its density is close to standard and is not likely to require correction.

When the actual volumetric airflow is desired at any particular condition or point, the corresponding specific volume is obtained from the psychrometric chart and the volume at standard conditions is multiplied by the ratio of the actual specific volume to the standard value of 0.83 (13.3). To illustrate, assume the outdoor airflow rate at ASHRAE standard conditions is 470 L/s (1000 cfm). The actual outdoor air condition is 35°C (95°F) dry bulb and 23.8°C (75°F) wet bulb [v = 0.89 m^3/kg (14.3 ft^3/lb)]. The actual volume flow rate at this condition would be 470 (0.89/0.83) = 500 L/s [1000(14.3/13.3) = 1080 cfm].

Air-conditioning design often requires the calculation of sensible, latent, and total energy gains as follow:

1. Sensible heat gain corresponding to the change of dry-bulb temperature for a given airflow (standard conditions). The sensible heat gain in watts (Btu/h) as a result of a difference in temperature Δt between the incoming air and leaving air flowing at ASHRAE standard conditions is:

$$q_s = Q(1.204)(1.00 + 1.872W)\Delta t \quad (3\text{-}20)$$

where

q_s = sensible heat gain, W
Q = airflow, L/s
1.204 = density of standard dry air, kg/m^3
1.00 = specific heat of dry air, kJ/(kg·K)
1.872 = specific heat of water vapor, kJ/(kg·K)
W = humidity ratio, mass of water per mass of dry air, kg/kg
Δt = temperature difference, °C

In I-P units:

$$q_s = Q(60)(0.075)(0.24 + 0.45W)\Delta t \quad (3\text{-}21)$$

where

q_s = sensible heat gain, Btu/h
Q = airflow, ft^3/min (cfm)
60 = minutes per hour
0.075 = density of dry air, lb/ft^3
0.24 = specific heat of dry air, Btu/lb·°F
0.45 = specific heat of water vapor, Btu/lb·°F
W = humidity ratio, pounds of water per pound of dry air
Δt = temperature difference, °F

Since $W \cong 0.01$ in many air-conditioning problems, the sensible heat gain may be approximated by:

$$q_s \approx 1.23Q\Delta t \text{ in which } Q \text{ is in L/s} \quad (3\text{-}22)$$

and in I-P units:

$$q_s \approx 1.10Q\Delta t \text{ in which } Q \text{ is in cfm} \quad (3\text{-}23)$$

2. Latent heat gain corresponding to the change of humidity ratio W for given airflow (standard conditions). The latent heat gain in watts (Btu/h) as a result of a difference in humidity ratio ΔW between the incoming and leaving air flowing at ASHRAE standard conditions is:

$$q_l = (\text{L/s})(1000)(0.001204)(2500)\Delta W \quad (3\text{-}24)$$

and in I-P units:

$$q_l = (\text{cfm})(60)(0.075)(1076)\Delta W \quad (3\text{-}25)$$

In Equations (3-24) and (3-25), respectively, 2500 kJ/kg (1076 Btu/lb) is the approximate energy content of the superheated water vapor at 23.8°C (75°F), less the energy content of water at 10°C (50°F). A temperature of 24°C (75°F) is a common design condition for the space and 10°C (50°F) is normal condensate temperature from cooling and dehumidifying coils. Combining the constants, the latent heat gain is:

$$q_l = 3010Q\Delta W \quad (3\text{-}26)$$

In I-P units:

$$q_l = 4840Q\Delta W \quad (3\text{-}27)$$

3. Total heat gain in watts (Btu/h) as a result of a difference in enthalpy Δh between the incoming and leaving air flowing at ASHRAE standard conditions is:

$$q = Q(1000)(0.001204)\Delta h \quad (3\text{-}28)$$

In I-P units:

$$q = Q(60)(0.075)\Delta h \quad (3\text{-}29)$$

If the product of the two constants is used as a single number, the total energy exchange is:

$$q = 4.33Q\Delta h \quad (3\text{-}30)$$

In I-P units:

$$q = 4.5Q\Delta h \quad (3\text{-}31)$$

The values 1.23 (1.10), 3010 (4840), and 4.33 (4.5) are useful in air-conditioning calculations for an atmospheric pressure of approximately 101.3 kPa (14.7 psia) and normal temperatures and moisture ratios. For other conditions, calculations should use more precise values. For frequent computations at other altitudes, it may be desirable to calculate appropriate values in the same manner. For example, at an altitude of 1500 m (5000 ft) with a pressure of 84.15 kPa (12.2 psia), appropriate values are 1.03 (0.92), 2500 (4020), and 3.59 (3.73), respectively.

Example 3-2. A hospital operating room is being designed to use the type of HVAC system shown in the following sketch. To avoid recirculating bacteria, 100% outside air is used. For summer operation, the air leaving the cooling coil and supplied to the space is at 55°F, 100% relative humidity. The summer design loads are: 37,500 Btu/h (sensible) and 8,800 Btu/h (latent). The indoor design temperature is 75°F. Outdoor design conditions are: 94°F (dry bulb) and 75°F (wet bulb). Atmospheric pressure is close to sea level standard of 14.7 psia. Neglecting the effect of the fan, determine the size of cooling unit required, Btu/h, and determine the relative humidity of the air leaving the operating room, %.

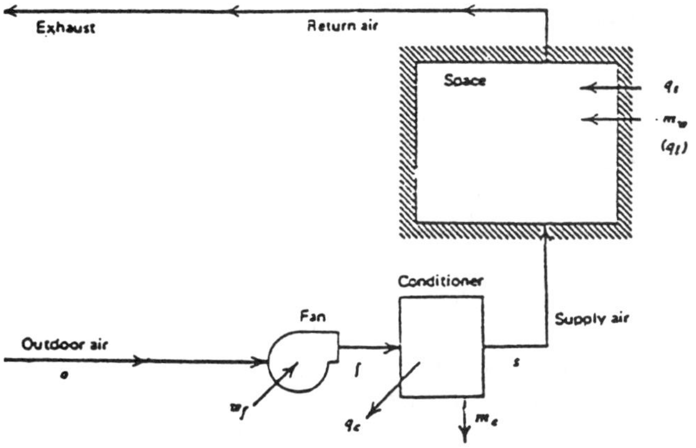

Solution:

Using either the psychrometric chart or corresponding psychrometric equations, the following properties are determined:

$$h_o = 38.4 \text{ Btu/lb};\ W_o = 0.0144 \text{ lb/lb}$$

$$h_s = 23.2 \text{ Btu/lb};\ W_s = 0.0092 \text{ lb/lb}$$

Using $Q_s = 0.244m_a(t_r - t_s)$

$$m_a = 37500/[0.244(75 - 55)] = 7680 \text{ lb/h}$$

A water vapor balance across the space may be written:

$$W_r = W_s + m_w/m_a$$

where: $m_w = Q_l/1100 = 8800/1100 = 8$ lb/h

Thus, $W_r = 0.0092 + 8/7680 = 0.01024$ lb/lb

At 75°F and 0.01024 lb/lb humidity ratio, the relative humidity is found to be 55%.

For the conditioner (cooling coil), the first law of thermodynamics may be written:

$$m_a[h_o - h_s - (W_o - W_s)] + Q_c = 0$$

$$7684\,[38.4 - 23.2 - (0.0144 - 0.0092)] + Q_c = 0$$

$Q_c = -115{,}900$ Btu/h

Alternately,

$$Q_c = Q[1.10\,(t_o - t_s) + 4840\,(W_o - W_s)]$$

where:

$$Q = m_a 13.33/60 = 7680(13.33/60) = 1706 \text{ cfm}$$

and:

$$Q_c = 1706\,[1.10(94 - 55) + 4840(0.0144 - 0.0092)]$$

$$= 116{,}100 \text{ Btu/h}$$

3.2 Single Path Systems

The simplest form of an all-air HVAC system is a single conditioner serving a single temperature control zone. The unit may be installed within, or remote from, the space it serves, and it may operate either with or without distributing ductwork. Well-designed systems can maintain temperature and humidity closely and efficiently and can be shut down when desired without affecting the operation of adjacent areas.

A single-zone system responds to only one set of space conditions. Its use is limited to situations where variations occur approximately uniformly throughout the zone served or where the load is stable; but when installed in multiple, it can handle a variety of conditions efficiently. Single-zone systems are used in such applications as small department stores, small individual shops in a shopping center, individual classrooms for a small school, and computer rooms. For example, a rooftop unit complete with a refrigeration system serving an individual space is a single-zone system. The refrigeration system, however, may be remote and serving several single-zone units in a larger installation.

A schematic of the single-zone central unit is shown in Figure 3-11. The return fan is necessary if 100% outdoor air is used for cooling purposes, but may be eliminated if air may be relieved from the space with very little pressure loss through the relief system. In general, a return air fan is needed if the resistance of the return air system (grilles and ductwork) exceeds 60 Pa (0.25 in. water gage).

Control of the single-zone system can be affected by on-off operation, varying the quantity of cooling medium providing reheat, face and bypass dampers, or a combination of these. The single-duct system with reheat satisfies variations in load by providing independent sources of heating and cooling. When a humidifier is included in the system, humidity control completely responsive to space needs is available. Since control is directly from space temperature and humidity, close regulation of the system conditions may be achieved. Single-duct systems without reheat offer cooling flexibility but cannot control summer humidity independent of temperature requirements.

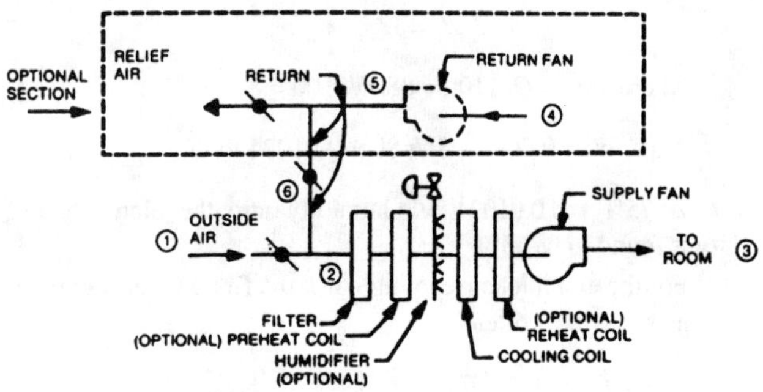

Fig. 3-11 Single-Duct System

3.3 Air-Volume Equations for Single-Path Systems

Basic equations for individual rooms (zones) are the same for all single-path systems. Air supplied to each room must be adequate to take care of each room's peak load conditions whether or not it occurs simultaneously in all rooms. The peak may be governed by sensible or latent room cooling loads, heating loads, outdoor air requirements, air motion, or exhaust.

Supply Air for Cooling:

$$(Q_{sRS1})^S = \frac{(q_{SR1})^S}{C_1(t_R - t_s)} \tag{3-32}$$

Supply Air for Dehumidification:

$$(Q_{sRL1})^S = \frac{(q_{LR1})^S}{C_2(W_R - W_s)} \tag{3-33}$$

Supply Air for Heating:

$$(Q_{sRS1})^W = \frac{(q_{SR1})^W}{C_1(t_s - t_R)} \tag{3-34}$$

where

$(Q_{sRS1})^S$ = summer room supply air volume required to satisfy peak sensible load of each room

$(Q_{sRL1})^S$ = summer room supply air volume required to satisfy peak latent load of each room

$(q_{SR1})^S$ = peak summer sensible room load for each room

$(q_{LR1})^S$ = peak summer latent room load for each room

$(Q_{sRS1})^W$ = winter room supply air volume required to satisfy peak heating load of each room

$(q_{SR1})^W$ = peak winter sensible room load (less any auxiliary heat) for each room

W_R = room humidity ratio

W_S = humidity ratio of dehumidified supply air

t_R = room air temperature

t_s = supply air temperature required to satisfy the summer or winter peak loads

C_1 = 1.23 (SI); 1.10 (IP)

C_2 = 3010 (SI); 4840 (IP)

Supply Air for Ventilation. Ventilation requirements, rather than sensible or latent loads, may govern when the supply air is deficient in any of the following ways:

1. If it does not contain adequate outdoor air, as determined by the outdoor ratio $X_o = Q_o/Q_s$, then, for such a room, supply air for outdoor air ventilation must be determined from the required room outdoor air Q_{oR} and:

$$Q_{sRv} = Q_{oR}/X_o \tag{3-35}$$

where

Q_{sRv} = room supply air required to satisfy ventilation requirements
Q_{oR} = minimum outdoor air required in a particular room
X_o = ratio of the system's total outdoor air to its total supply air that satisfies outdoor air requirements in most rooms

2. The supply air may not be adequate to serve as make-up for exhaust requirements in the room. In such cases, no return air comes from the room, and only conditioned supply air is assumed to be used as make-up (no supplementary ventilation supply system). This entire volume of make-up ventilation air would become an outdoor air burden to the system, in the form of a larger X_o distributed to all rooms, even though all the air supplied to this particular room is not outdoor air and:

$$Q_{sRv} = Q_{sR} \tag{3-36}$$

where

Q_{sR} = air exhausted or relieved from a room and not returned to the conditioned air system

3. If the desired rate of air change in the room is not satisfied, then supply air is determined as follows (in SI units):

$$Q_{sRv}\text{ (L/s)} = (\text{Room volume in m}^3) \times (\text{No. of air changes/hour})/3.6 \tag{3-37 SI}$$

and in I-P units:

$$Q_{sRv}\text{ (cfm)} = (\text{Room volume in ft}^3) \times (\text{No. of air changes/hour})/60 \tag{3-37 I-P}$$

4. If air movement, as measured by an area index instead of an air change index, is not satisfied, or:

$$Q_{sRv} = K \times [(\text{L/s})/\text{m}^2] \tag{3-38 SI}$$

$$Q_{sRv} = K \times (\text{cfm/ft}^2) \tag{3-38 I-P}$$

where K = a constant, greater or less than one.

Both the rate of air change and K are empirical values that vary according to designers' experiences and local building code requirements. For example, 5 air changes per hour in a room with a 12-ft (3.7-m) ceiling corresponds to 1 cfm/ft^2 (5 L/s·m^2), while the same air change rate with an 8-ft (2.4-m) ceiling is only 0.66 cfm/ft^2 (3.3 L/s·m^2). Physiologically, one may have no advantage over the other.

Case 1 is to be used when outdoor air Q_o governs, Cases 3 and 4 when air movement governs, and Case 2 when exhaust governs.

3.4 Psychrometric Representation of Single-Path Systems

The operation of a single path system is illustrated in Figure 3-12. Each state point is shown with corresponding nomenclature in the cycle diagram and in the summer and winter representations. Each change in temperature Δt or humidity ratio ΔW is a result of sensible or latent heat loss or gain q_S or q_L. The cycle diagram in Figure 3-12 shows the full symbol and subscript for each state, while psychrometric charts show only the corresponding state points. This section describes the flow paths in a typical single-duct, single-zone, draw-through system. In this illustration all return air is assumed to pass from the room through a hung- ceiling return air plenum.

In Figure 3-12, supply air CFM$_S$ at the fan discharge temperature t_{sf} in the summer mode absorbs transmitted supply duct heat q_{sd} and supply air fan velocity pressure energy q_{sfvp}, thereby raising the temperature to t_s. Room supply air absorbs room sensible and latent heat q_{SR} and q_{LR} along the room sensible heat factor (SHF) line **s-R**, reaching desired room state, t_R and W_R. Room (internal) sensible loads which determine CFMs are made up of:

1. Ceiling transmission c_{clg} (shown) from the hung ceiling above the room, and floor transmission q_D (not shown) from the floor deck below (the q_D shown is the heat gain to the hung ceiling from the roof deck above, not the floor deck below);
2. Direct light heat emissions to the room q_{lR} (without the direct light heat emission to the plenum q_{lp});
3. Transmissions q_{tran} from other surfaces such as walls, windows, etc.;
4. Appliance heat $(q_S)_{aux}$ and occupancy heat $(q_S)_{occ}$; and
5. Infiltration load $(q_S)_{inf}$ taken here as zero, with exfiltration air CFM$_{eR}$ shown instead.

The remaining air returned from the room (CFM$_s$ − CFM$_{er}$ = CFM$_R$) passes through the ceiling plenum along line **R-rp**, absorbing some ceiling heat q_{rp} while simultaneously retransmitting some of it back to the room q_{clg}. Air is picked up by the return duct system at t_{rp}, after passing through the ceiling at average temperature t_p.

Return volume CFM$_R$ picks up return duct transmissions q_{rd} and return fan heat gains q_{rf} (including both static and velocity energy) by the time it reaches the intake plenum entrance at t_r. CFM$_r$ may be less than CFM$_R$ if leakage occurs from the ducts or through the exhaust damper from the return air system. Mixing of outdoor air, CFM$_o$ at state o, with final return air occurs along process line **r-o** to mixture state m. Total system air CFM$_s$ passes through the cooling coil releasing the total sensible heat factor, SHR$_{cc}$ line **m-cc**, terminating

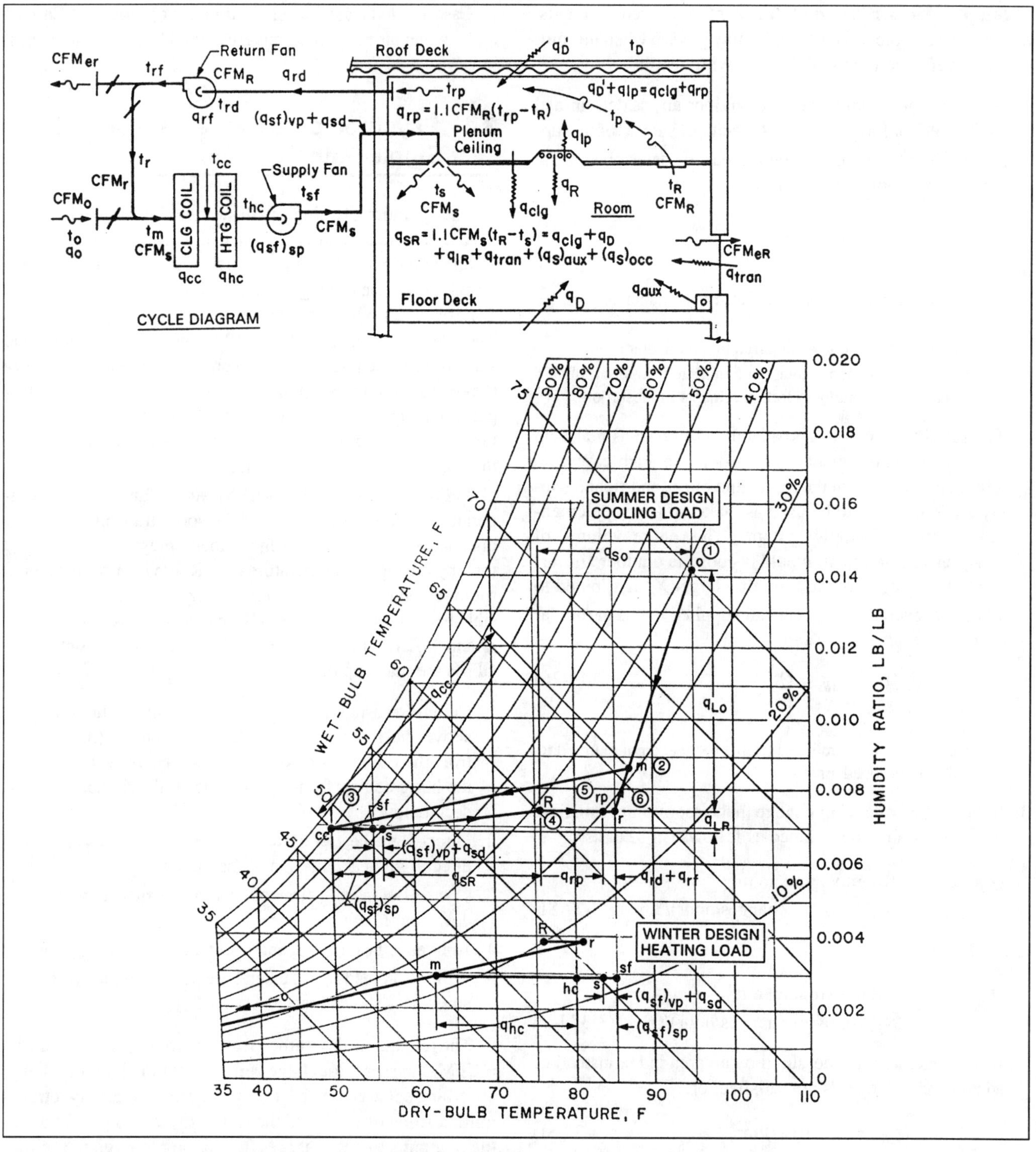

Fig. 3-12 Single-Duct, Single-Zone Cycle and Psychrometric Chart

in state *cc*. The temperature rise through the supply fan from $(q_{sf})_{sp}$ results in t_{sf}, which completes the cycle.

The winter cycle (Figure 3-12) is similar, except for the interposition of the heating coil energy q_{hc} added in process line **m-hc**; the deletion of the cooling coil action; and the temperature drop in process line **sf-s**, resulting from duct transmission losses q_{sd} instead of gains.

3.5 Sensible Heat Factor (Sensible Heat Ratio)

The **sensible heat factor** (SHF), also called the **sensible heat ratio** (SHR), is the ratio of the sensible heat for a process to the summation of the sensible and latent heat for the process. The sum of sensible and latent heat is also called the

total heat. On the ASHRAE Psychrometric Chart, values of sensible heat factors are given on the protractor as $\Delta H_s/\Delta H_T$, and they may be used to establish the process line for changes in the condition of the air across either the room or the conditioner on the psychrometric chart.

The supply air to a conditioned space must have the capacity to offset simultaneously both the room sensible and room latent heat loads. The room and the supply air conditions to the space may be plotted on the psychrometric chart and connected with a straight line called the room sensible heat factor line.

As air passes through the cooling coil of an air conditioner, the sensible heat factor line represents the simultaneous cooling and dehumidifying that occurs. If the cooling process involves removing only sensible and no latent heat, i.e., no moisture removal, the sensible heat factor line is horizontal and the sensible heat factor is 1.0. If 50% is sensible and 50% latent, the SHF is 0.5.

3.6 Problems

3.1 One of the many methods used for drying air is to cool the air below the dew point so that condensation or freezing of the moisture takes place. To what temperature must atmospheric air be cooled in order to have a humidity ratio of 0.000017 lb/lb (17 mg/kg)? To what temperature must this air be cooled if its pressure is 10 atm?

3.2 One method of removing moisture from atmospheric air is to cool the air so that the moisture condenses or freezes out. Suppose an experiment requires a humidity ratio of 0.0001. To what temperature must the air be cooled at a pressure of 0.1 kPa in order to achieve this humidity?

3.3 A room of dimensions 4 m by 6 m by 2.4 m contains an air-water vapor mixture at a total pressure of 100 kPa and a temperature of 25°C. The partial pressure of the water vapor is 1.4 kPa. Calculate:

(a) humidity ratio
(b) dew point
(c) total mass of water vapor in the room

3.4 The air conditions at the intake of an air compressor are 70°F (21.1°C), 50% rh, and 14.7 psia (101.3 kPa). The air is compressed to 50 psia (344.7 kPa), then sent to an intercooler. If condensation of water vapor from the air is to be prevented, what is the lowest temperature to which the air can be cooled in the intercooler?

3.5 Humid air enters a dehumidifier with an enthalpy of 21.6 Btu/lb_m of dry air and 1100 Btu/lb_m of water vapor. There are 0.02 lb_m of vapor per pound of dry air at entrance and 0.009 lb_m of vapor per pound of dry air at exit. The dry air at exit has an enthalpy of 13.2 Btu/lb_m, and the vapor at exit has an enthalpy of 1085 Btu/lb_m. Condensate leaves with an enthalpy of 22 Btu/lb_m. The rate of flow of dry air is 287 lb_m/min. Determine:

(a) the amount of moisture removed from the air (lbm/min)
(b) the rate of heat removal required

[Ans: 3.16 lb/min, −5860 Btu/min]

3.6 Air is supplied to a room from the outside, where the temperature is 20°F (−6.7°C) and the relative humidity is 60%. The room is to be maintained at 70°F (21.1°C) and 50% rh. How many pounds of water must be supplied per pound of air supplied to the room?

3.7 Air is heated to 80°F (26.7°C) without adding water, from 60°F (15.6°C) dry-bulb and 50°F (10°C) wet-bulb temperature. Use the psychrometric chart to find:

(a) relative humidity of the original mixture
(b) original dew-point temperature
(c) original humidity ratio
(d) initial enthalpy
(e) final enthalpy
(f) the heat added
(g) final relative humidity

3.8 Saturated air at 40°F (4.4°C) is first preheated and then saturated adiabatically. This saturated air is then heated to a final condition of 105°F (40.6°C) and 28% rh. To what temperature must the air initially be heated in the preheat coil?

[Ans: 101°F (37.8°C)]

3.9 Atmospheric air at 100°F (37.8°C) dry-bulb and 65°F (18.3°C) wet-bulb temperature is humidified adiabatically with steam. The supply steam contains 10% moisture and is at 16 psia (110.3 kPa). What is the dry-bulb temperature of the humidified air if enough steam is added to bring the air to 70% rh?

3.10 The summer design conditions in New Orleans, Louisiana, are 95°F (35°C) dry-bulb and 80°F (26.7°C) wet-bulb temperature. In Tucson, Arizona, the design conditions are 105°F (40.6°C) dry-bulb and 72°F (22.2°C) wet-bulb temperature. What is the lowest air temperature that could theoretically be attained in an evaporative cooler at the summer design conditions in these two cities?

3.11 Air at 29.92 in. Hg enters an adiabatic saturator at 80°F dry-bulb and 66°F wet-bulb temperature. Water is supplied at 66°F. Find (without using the psychrometric chart) the humidity ratio, degree of saturation, enthalpy, and specific volume of entering air.

[Ans: 0.014 lb/lb air, $\mu = 0.47$, h = 30.7 Btu/lb air, $v = 13.83$ ft^3/lb air]

3.12 An air-water vapor mixture enters an air-conditioning unit at a pressure of 150 kPa, a temperature of 30°C, and a relative humidity of 80%. The mass flow of dry air entering is 1 kg/s. The air-vapor mixture leaves the air-conditioning unit at 125 kPa, 10°C, 100% rh. The moisture condensed leaves at 10°C. Determine the heat transfer rate for the process.

3.13 Air at 40°C, 300 kPa, with a relative humidity of 35% is to be expanded in a reversible adiabatic nozzle. How low a pressure can the gas be expanded to if no condensation is to take place? What is the exit velocity at this condition?

3.14 By using basic definitions and Dalton's Law of partial pressure, show that:

$$v = R_a T/(p - p_w)$$

3.15 In an air-conditioning unit, 71,000 cfm at 80°F dry bulb, 60% rh, and standard atmospheric pressure, enter the unit. The air leaves the unit at 57°F dry bulb and 90% relative humidity. Calculate the following:

(a) cooling capacity of the air-conditioning unit, in Btu/h
(b) rate of water removal from the unit
(c) sensible heat load on the conditioner, in Btu/h
(d) latent heat load on the conditioner, in Btu/h
(e) the dew point of the air leaving the conditioner

3.16 Four pounds of air at 80°F (26.7°C) dry bulb and 50% rh are mixed with one pound of air at 50°F (15.6°C) and 50% rh. Determine:

(a) relative humidity of the mixture
(b) dew-point temperature of the mixture
[Ans: 52%, 56.2°F (13.5°C)]

3.17 Air is compressed from 85°F, 60% rh, 14.7 psia to 60 psia and then cooled in an intercooler before entering a second stage of compression. What is the minimum temperature to which the air can be cooled so that the condensation does not take place?

3.18 An air-water vapor mixture flowing at a rate of 4000 cfm (1890 L/s) enters a perfect refrigeration coil at 84°F (28.9°C) and 70°F (21.1°C) wet-bulb temperature. The air leaves the coil at 53°F (11.7°C). How many Btu/h of refrigeration are required?

3.19 Air at 40°F dry bulb and 35°F wet bulb is mixed with air at 100°F dry bulb and 77°F wet bulb in the ratio of 2 lb of cool air to 1 lb of warm air. Compute the resultant humidity ratio and enthalpy of the mixed air. [Ans: 0.007 lb/lb, 22.2 Btu/lb]

3.20 Outdoor air at 90°F (32.2°C) and 78°F (25.6°C) wet bulb is mixed with return air at 75°F (23.9°C) and 52% rh. There are 1000 lb (454 kg) of outdoor air for every 5000 lb (2265 kg) of return air. What are the dry- and wet-bulb temperatures for the mixed airstream?

3.21 In a mixing process of two streams of air, 10,000 cfm of air at 75°F and 50% rh mix with 4000 cfm of air at 98°F dry-bulb and 78°F wet-bulb temperature. Calculate the following conditions after mixing at atmospheric pressure:

(a) dry-bulb temperature
(b) humidity ratio
(c) relative humidity
(d) enthalpy
(e) dew-point temperature

3.22 Solve the following:

(a) Determine the humidity ratio and relative humidity of an air-water vapor mixture that has a dry-bulb temperature of 30°C, an adiabatic saturation temperature of 25°C, and a pressure of 100 kPa.
(b) Use the psychrometric chart to determine the humidity ratio and relative humidity of an air-water vapor mixture that has a dry-bulb temperature of 30°C, a wet-bulb temperature of 25°C, and a pressure of 100 kPa.
[Ans: 0.0183 kg/kg, 67%, 0.018 kg/kg, 67%]

3.23 An air-water vapor mixture at 100 kPa, 35°C, and 70% rh is contained in a 0.5 m^3 closed tank. The tank is cooled until the water just begins to condense. Determine the temperature at which condensation begins and the heat transfer for the process.

3.24 A room is to be maintained at 76°F and 40% rh. Supply air at 39°F is to absorb 100,000 Btu sensible heat and 35 lb of moisture per hour. How many pounds of dry air per hour are required? What should the dew-point temperature and relative humidity of the supply air be?
[Ans: 11,250 lb/h, 36°F, 90%]

3.25 Moist air enters a chamber at 40°F dry-bulb and 36°F wet-bulb temperature at a rate of 3000 cfm. In passing through the chamber, the air absorbs sensible heat at a rate of 116,000 Btu/h and picks up 83 lb/h of saturated steam at 230°F. Determine the dry-bulb and wet-bulb temperatures of the leaving air. [Ans: 74°F, 64°F]

3.26 In an auditorium maintained at a temperature not to exceed 77°F, and at a relative humidity not to exceed 55%, a sensible-heat load of 350,000 Btu and 1,000,000 grains of moisture per hour must be removed. Air is supplied to the auditorium at 67°F.

(a) How much air must be supplied, in lb/h?
(b) What is the dew-point temperature of the entering air, and what is its relative humidity?
(c) How much latent heat is picked up in the auditorium?
(d) What is the sensible heat ratio?

3.27 A meeting hall is maintained at 75°F dry bulb and 65°F wet bulb. The barometric pressure is 29.92 in. Hg. The space has a load of 200,000 Btu/h sensible, and 200,000 Btu/h latent. The temperature of the supply air to the space cannot be lower than 65°F dry bulb.

(a) How much air must be supplied, in lb/h?
(b) What is the required wet-bulb temperature of the supply air?
(c) What is the sensible heat factor?
[Ans: 81,970 lb/h, 58°F, 0.5]

3.28 A structure to be air conditioned has a sensible heat load of 20,000 Btu/h at a time when the total load is 100,000 Btu/h. If the inside state is to be at 80°F, 50% rh, is it possible to meet the load conditions by supplying air to the room at 100°F and

60% rh? If not, discuss the direction in which the inside state would be expected to move if such air were supplied.

3.29 A flow rate of 30,000 lb/h of conditioned air at 60°F and 85% rh enters a space that has a sensible load of 120,000 Btu/h and a latent load of 30,000 Btu/h.

(a) What are the dry- and wet-bulb temperatures in the space?
(b) If a mixture of 50% return air and 50% outdoor air at 98°F dry bulb and 77°F wet bulb enters the air conditioner, what is the refrigeration load?

3.30 An air-water vapor mixture enters a heater-humidifier unit at 5°C, 100 kPa, 50% rh. The flow rate of dry air is 0.1 kg/s. Liquid water at 10°C is sprayed into the mixture at the rate of 0.0022 kg/s. The mixture leaves the unit at 30°C, 100 kPa. Calculate:

(a) the relative humidity at the outlet
(b) the rate of heat transfer to the unit

[Ans: 91%, 7.94 kW]

3.31 A room is being maintained at 75°F and 50% rh. The outside air conditions are 40°F and 50% rh at this time. Return air from the room is cooled and dehumidified by mixing it with fresh ventilation air from the outside. The total airflow to the room is 60% outdoor and 40% return air by mass. Determine the temperature, relative humidity, and humidity content of the mixed air going to the room.

[Ans: 54.5°F, 58%, 0.00524 lb/lb]

3.32 A room with a sensible load of 20,000 Btu/h is maintained at 75°F and 50% rh. Outdoor air at 95°F and 80°F wet bulb was mixed with the room return air. The outdoor air, which is mixed, is 25% by mass of the total flow going to the conditioner. This air is then cooled and dehumidified by a coil and leaves the coil saturated at 50°F, which is on the condition line for the room. The air is then mixed with some room return air so that the temperature of the air entering the room is at 60°F. Find the following:

(a) the air-conditioning processes on the psychrometric chart
(b) ratio of latent to sensible load
(c) airflow rate
(d) the percent by mass of room return air mixed with air leaving the cooling coil

3.33 An air-water vapor mixture at 14.7 psia (101.5 kPa), 85°F (29.4°C), and 50% rh is contained within a 15 ft^3 (0.425 m^3) tank. At what temperature will condensation begin? If the tank and mixture are cooled an additional 15°F (8.3°C), how much water will condense from the mixture?

3.34 Air flowing at 1000 cfm and at 14.7 psia, 90°F, and 60% rh passes over a coil with a mean surface temperature of 40°F. A spray on the coil assures that the leaving air is saturated at the coil temperature. What is the required cooling capacity of the coil? [Ans: 9.3 tons]

3.35 An air-vapor mixture at 100°F (37.8°C) dry bulb contains 0.02 lb water vapor per pound of dry air (20 g/kg). The barometric pressure is 28.561 in. Hg (96.7 kPa). Calculate the relative humidity, dew-point temperature, and degree of saturation.

3.36 Air enters a space at 20°F and 80% rh. Within the space, sensible heat is added at the rate of 45,000 Btu/h and latent heat is added at the rate of 20,000 Btu/h. The conditions to be maintained inside the space are 50°F and 75% rh. What must the air exhaust rate (lb/h) from the space be to maintain a 50°F temperature? What must the air exhaust rate (lb/h) from the space to maintain a 75% rh be? Discuss the difference.

3.37 Moist air at a low pressure of 11 psia is flowing through a duct at a low velocity of 200 fpm. The duct is 1 ft in diameter and has negligible heat transfer to the surroundings. The dry-bulb temperature is 85°F and the wet-bulb temperature is 70°F. Calculate the following:

(a) humidity ratio, lb/lb
(b) dew-point temperature, °F
(c) relative humidity, %

[Ans: 0.0177 lb/lb, 52°F, 32%]

3.38 If an air compressor takes in moist air (at about 90% rh) at room temperature and pressure and compresses this to 120 psig (827 kPa) (and slightly higher temperature), would you expect some condensation to occur? Why? If yes, where would the condensation form? How would you remove it?

3.39 Does a sling psychrometer give an accurate reading of the adiabatic saturation temperature? Explain.

3.40 An air processor handles 2000 cfm of air with initial conditions of 50°F and 50% rh. The air is heated with a finned heat exchanger with 78 ft^2 of heat transfer surface area and a *UA* value of 210 Btu/h·°F.

Also, a steam spray system adds moisture to the air from saturated steam at 16 psia. The outlet air is at 100°F and 50% rh. Do the following:

(a) Show the processes on the psychrometric chart.
(b) Calculate the mass flow rate, lb/min.
(c) Calculate the pounds per minute of steam required.
(d) Calculate the heat added by the coil, Btu/min.

[Ans: 155 lb/min, 2.65 lb/min, 1900 Btu/min]

3.41 At an altitude of 5000 ft (1500 m), a sling psychrometer reads 80°F (26.7°C) and 67°F (19.4°C) wet bulb. Determine correct values of relative humidity and enthalpy from the chart. Compare these to the corresponding values for the same readings at sea level.

3.42 The average person gives off sensible heat at the rate of 250 Btu/h and perspires and respires about 0.27 lb/h of moisture. Estimate the sensible and latent load for a room with 25 people in it (the lights give off 9000 Btu/h). If the room conditions are to be 78°F and 50% rh, what flow rate of air would be required if the supply air came in at 63°F? What would be the supply air relative humidity?

3.43 A space in an industrial building has a winter sensible heat loss of 200,000 Btu/h and a negligible latent heat load (latent losses to outside are made up by latent gains within the space). The space is to be maintained precisely at 75°F and 50% rh. Due to the nature of the process, 100% outside air is required for ventilation. The outdoor air conditions can be taken as saturated air at 20°F. The amount of ventilation air is 7000 scfm and the air is to be preheated, humidified with an adiabatic saturator to the desired humidity, and then reheated. The temperature out of the adiabatic saturator is to be maintained at 60°F dry bulb. Determine the following:

(a) temperature of air entering the space to be heated, °F
(b) heat supplied to preheat coil, Btu/h
(c) heat supplied to reheat coil, Btu/h
(d) amount of water required for humidification, gpm

3.44 Using the SI psychrometric chart at standard atmospheric pressure, find:

(a) dew point and humidity ratio for air at 28°C dry bulb and 22°C wet bulb
(b) enthalpy and specific volume

3.45 Using the SI chart, find:

(a) moisture that must be removed in cooling air from 24°C dry bulb, 21°C wet bulb to 13°C dry bulb, saturated
(b) total, sensible, and latent heat removal for the process

3.46 An air-conditioned space has a sensible heat load of 200,000 Btu/h, a latent load of 50,000 Btu/h, and is maintained at 78°F dry bulb and 60% rh. On a mass basis, 25% outside air is mixed with return air. Outside air is at 95°F dry bulb and 76°F wet bulb. Conditioned air leaves the apparatus and enters the room at 60°F dry bulb. The fan must produce a pressure increase of 3.5 in. water to overcome the system pressure loss. Fan efficiency is estimated as 55%.

(a) Draw and label the schematic flow diagram for the complete system. (Hint: See Fig. 3-1)
(b) Complete the table below.
(c) Plot and draw all processes on a psychrometric chart.
(d) Specify the fan size, scfm, and fan motor rating, HP.
(e) Determine the size refrigeration unit needed, in Btu/h and tons.
(f) What percent of the required refrigeration is for (1) sensible cooling and (2) for dehumidification?
(g) What percent of the required refrigeration is due to the outside air load?

Point	Dry Bulb t, °F	ϕ, %	Enthalpy h, Btu/lb	W, lb/lb	m_a, lb/h	scfm	cfm
OA							
r							
m							
f							
s							

3.7 Bibliography

ASHRAE. 1996. Psychrometrics: Theory and Practice. Code 90162, ASHRAE, Atlanta, GA.

Goff, J.A. and S. Gratch. 1945. Thermodynamic properties of moist air. ASHVE *Transactions* 51:125.

Kusuda, T. 1970. Algorithms for psychrometric calculuations. NBS Publication BSS21 (January), Superintendent of Documents, U.S. Government Printing Office, Washington, D.C.

Chapter 4

DESIGN CONDITIONS

This chapter covers the selection, specification, and determination of the indoor and outdoor environmental conditions that are to be expected at "design time" or the conditions which will govern the sizing of the heating, cooling, and ventilating equipment. Additional details related to design conditions are provided in Chapters 8, 9, and 26 of the 1977 *ASHRAE Handbook—Fundamentals.*

4.1 Indoor Design Conditions

4.1.1 Physiological Principles

To design an environmental control system that is effective for comfort and health, the engineer must understand physiological principles. In its broadest sense, the term air conditioning implies control of any or all of the physical and chemical qualities of air. Herein, the definition of air conditioning pertains only to those conditions of air relating to health and comfort requirements of the occupants of the conditioned space.

Significant variations in the percentage composition of the normal constituents of air may make it unfit for human use. The presence of foreign materials classified as contaminants may also make air unfit. Air conditioning can control most climatological environmental factors for the service and comfort of people.

The objective of a comfort air-conditioning system is to provide a comfortable environment for the occupant or occupants of residential or commercial buildings. A comfortable environment is created by simultaneously controlling temperature, humidity, air cleanliness, and air distribution within the occupant's vicinity. These factors include mean radiant temperature, as well as air temperature, odor control, and control of the proper acoustic level within the occupant's vicinity.

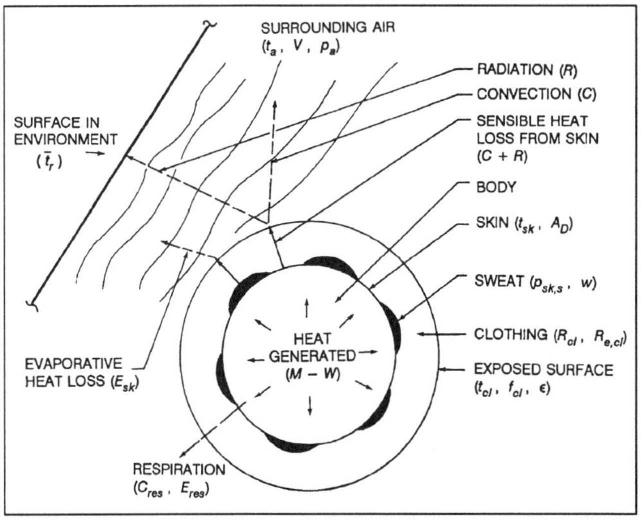

Fig. 4-1 Cylindrical Model of Body's Interaction with Environment

Both the air and surfaces of the enclosure surrounding the occupant are sinks for the metabolic heat emitted by the occupant (Fig. 4-1). Air circulates around the occupant and the surfaces. The occupant also exchanges radiant heat with the surrounding surfaces (i.e., glass and outside walls). Air is brought into motion within a given space thermally or by mechanical forces.

Both nude and clothed subjects feel comfortable at the same mean skin temperature of 91.5°F (33°C). The range of skin temperature within which no discomfort is experienced is about ±2.5°F (±1.4°C). The necessary criteria, indices, and standards for use where human occupancy is concerned are given in Chapter 8, "Thermal Comfort" and in Chapter 9, "Indoor Environmental Health," of the 1997 *ASHRAE Handbook—Fundamentals*.

The environmental indices used to evaluate the sensation of comfort for the human body are direct, rationally derived, and empirical indices, which include the following factors:

Direct Indices
- Dry-bulb temperature
- Dew-point temperature
- Wet-bulb temperature
- Relative humidity
- Air movement

Rationally Derived Indices
- Mean radiant temperature
- Operative temperature
- Humid operative temperature
- Heat stress index
- Index of skin wettedness

Empirical Indices
- Effective temperature
- Black globe temperature
- Corrected effective temperature
- Wet-bulb-globe temperature index
- Wind chill index

The **operative temperature** is the uniform temperature of a radiantly black enclosure in which an occupant exchanges the same amount of heat by radiation plus convection as in the actual nonuniform environment. Numerically, operative temperature is the average, weighted by respective heat transfer coefficients of the air and mean radiant temperatures. At air speeds of 0.4 m/s (80 fpm) or less and mean radiant temperature less than 50°C (120°F), operative temperature is approximately the simple average of the air and mean radiant temperatures.

Physiologists recognize that sensations of comfort and temperature may have different physiological and physical bases, thus each type should be considered separately. This dichotomy was recognized in the ANSI/ASHRAE *Standard* 55, where thermal comfort is defined as *"that state of mind which expresses satisfaction with the thermal environment."* In contrast, most current predictive charts are based on comfort defined as a sensation *"that is neither slightly warm nor slightly cool."*

Most research on comfort has been limited to lightly clothed, sedentary people. This research has proven sound since about 90% of people's indoor occupation and leisure time is spent at or near the sedentary activity level. The predictive methods to be described are all believed to be accurate depending upon the limitations stated. During physical activity, a change occurs in a person's physiology. Physiological thermal neutrality in the older (sedentary) sense does not exist. Some form of thermal regulation is always occurring during the sedentary condition. The same skin and body temperatures, if used as indices of comfort, prove false during moderate to heavy activity.

The main purpose of the HVAC system is to maintain comfortable indoor conditions for occupants. However, the purpose of load calculations is to obtain data for sizing the system components. In most cases, the system will rarely be set to operate at design conditions. Therefore, the use and occupancy of the space is a general consideration from the design temperature point of view. Later, when the energy requirements of the building are computed, the actual conditions in the space and outdoor environment (including internal heat gains) must be considered.

The indoor design temperature should be selected at the lower end of the acceptable temperature range so that the heating equipment will not be oversized. Even properly sized equipment usually operates under partial load, at reduced efficiency, most of the time; therefore, any oversizing aggravates this condition and lowers the overall system efficiency. A maximum design dry-bulb temperature of 72°F is recommended for most occupancies. The indoor design value of relative humidity should be compatible with a healthful environment and the thermal and moisture integrity of the building envelope. A maximum relative humidity of 30% is recommended for most situations.

The conscious mind appears to reach conclusions about thermal comfort and discomfort from direct temperature and moisture sensations from the skin, deep body temperatures, and the efforts necessary to regulate body temperatures. In general, comfort occurs when body temperatures are held within narrow ranges, skin moisture is low, and the physiological effort of regulation is minimized.

The ASHRAE thermal sensation scale with its numerical representation is:

+3	hot
+2	warm
+1	slightly warm
0	neutral
−1	slightly cool
−2	cool
−3	cold

The equations in Table 4-1 indicate that women are more sensitive to temperature and less sensitive to humidity than men. However, in general, about a 5.4°F change in temperature or a 0.44 psi change in water vapor pressure is necessary to change a thermal sensation vote by one unit or temperature category.

Table 4-1 Equations for Predicting Thermal Sensation (Y)[a,b]
(Table 9, Chapter 8, 1997 *Handbook—Fundamentals*)

Exposure Period, h	Sex	Regression Equations: t = dry-bulb temperature, °F; p = vapor pressure, psi
1.0	Male	$Y = 0.122t + 1.61p - 9.584$
	Female	$Y = 0.151t + 1.71p - 12.080$
	Combined	$Y = 0.136t + 1.71p - 10.880$
2.0	Male	$Y = 0.123t + 1.86p - 9.953$
	Female	$Y = 0.157t + 1.45p - 12.725$
	Combined	$Y = 0.140t + 1.65p - 11.339$
3.0	Male	$Y = 0.118t + 2.02p - 9.718$
	Female	$Y = 0.153t + 1.76p - 13.511$
	Combined	$Y = 0.135t + 1.92p - 11.122$

[a] *Y* values refer to the ASHRAE thermal sensation scale.
[b] For young adult subjects with sedentary activity and wearing clothing with a thermal resistance of approximately 0.5 clo, $\bar{t}_r \approx \bar{t}_a$ and air velocities are < 40 fpm.

4.1.2 Metabolic Rate

In choosing optimal conditions for comfort and health, the energy expended during the course of routine physical activities must be known, since body heat production increases in proportion to exercise intensity. Table 4-2 provides metabolic rates for various activities, on a per unit body surface area basis. The most useful measure of body surface area, proposed by DuBois, is described by:

$$A_D = 0.202 w^{0.425} h^{0.725} \tag{4-1}$$

where

A_D = body surface area, m²
w = mass of body, kg
h = height of body, m

An average size man has a mass of 70 kg (154 lb) and a height of 1.73 m (5 ft, 8 in.), so his body surface area is 1.8 m² (19.4 ft²).

In choosing optimal conditions for comfort and health, the rate of work done during routine physical activities must be known, because metabolic power increases in proportion to exercise intensity. Metabolic rate varies over a wide range, depending on the activity, the person, and the conditions under

Table 4-2 Metabolic Rates
(Table 4, Chapter 8, 1997 *Handbook—Fundamentals*)

	Btu/(h·ft²)	met[a]
Resting		
Sleeping	13	0.7
Reclining	15	0.8
Seated, quiet	18	1.0
Standing, relaxed	22	1.2
Walking (on level surface)		
2.9 ft/s (2 mph)	37	2.0
4.4 ft/s (3 mph)	48	2.6
5.9 ft/s (4 mph)	70	3.8
Office Activities		
Reading, seated	18	1.0
Writing	18	1.0
Typing	20	1.1
Filing, seated	22	1.2
Filing, standing	26	1.4
Walking about	31	1.7
Lifting/packing	39	2.1
Driving/Flying		
Car	18 to 37	1.0 to 2.0
Aircraft, routine	22	1.2
Aircraft, instrument landing	33	1.8
Aircraft, combat	44	2.4
Heavy vehicle	59	3.2
Miscellaneous Occupational Activities		
Cooking	29 to 37	1.6 to 2.0
Housecleaning	37 to 63	2.0 to 3.4
Seated, heavy limb movement	41	2.2
Machine work		
sawing (table saw)	33	1.8
light (electrical industry)	37 to 44	2.0 to 2.4
heavy	74	4.0
Handling 110 lb bags	74	4.0
Pick and shovel work	74 to 88	4.0 to 4.8
Miscellaneous Leisure Activities		
Dancing, social	44 to 81	2.4 to 4.4
Calisthenics/exercise	55 to 74	3.0 to 4.0
Tennis, singles	66 to 74	3.6 to 4.0
Basketball	90 to 140	5.0 to 7.6
Wrestling, competitive	130 to 160	7.0 to 8.7

[a]1 met = 18.4 Btu/(h·ft²)

which the activity is performed. Table 4-2 lists typical metabolic rates for an average adult (A_D = 19.6 ft²) for activities performed continuously. The highest power a person can maintain for any continuous period is approximately 50% of the maximal capacity to use oxygen (maximum energy capacity).

A unit used to express the metabolic rate per unit DuBois area is the met, defined as the metabolic rate of a sedentary person (seated, quiet): 1 met = 18.4 Btu/h·ft²) = 50 kcal/(h·m²). A normal, healthy man has a maximum capacity of approximately M_{act} = 12 met at age 20, which drops to 7 met at age 70. Maximum rates for women are about 30% lower. Long-distance runners and trained athletics have maximum rates as high as 20 met. An average 35 year-old that does not exercise has a maximum rate of about 10 met and activities with $M_{act} > 5$ met are likely to prove exhausting.

The metabolic activities of the body result almost completely in heat that must be continuously dissipated and regulated to prevent abnormal body temperatures. Insufficient heat loss leads to over-heating also called hyperthermia, and excessive heat loss results in body cooling also called hypothermia. Skin temperatures associated with comfort at sedentary activities are 91.5 to 93°F and decrease with increasing activity.

The heat produced by a resting adult is about 340 Btu/h. Because most of this heat is transferred to the environment through the skin, it is often convenient to characterize metabolic activity in terms of heat production per unit area of skin. For the resting person, this is about 18.4 Btu/h·ft² (50 kcal/(h·m²) (average person has a skin surface area of about 19.5 ft²) and is called 1 met. Higher metabolic rates are often described in terms of the resting rate. Thus, a person working at a metabolic rate five times the resting rate would have a metabolic rate of 5 met.

4.1.3 Clothing Level

Clothing insulation value may be expressed in clo units. In order to avoid confusion, the symbol *I* is used with the clo unit instead of the symbol *R*, normally used for thermal resistance per unit area. The relationship between the two is:

$$R = 0.88I \tag{4-2}$$

or 1.0 clo is equivalent to 0.88 ft²·h·°F/Btu. (0.155 m² K/w).

Often it is not possible to find an already measured clothing ensemble that matches the one in question. In this case, the ensemble insulation can be estimated from the insulation of individual garments. Table 4-3 gives a list of individual garments commonly worn. The insulation of an ensemble is estimated from the individual values using a summation formula

$$I_{cl} = \sum_i I_{clu,i} \tag{4-3}$$

The main source of inaccuracy is in determining the appropriate values for individual garments. Overall accuracies are on the order of ±25% if the tables are used carefully. Where $I_{clu,i}$ is the effective insulation of garment *i*, and I_{cl}, as before is the insulation for the entire ensemble.

4.1.4 Conditions for Thermal Comfort

Current and past studies are periodically reviewed to update ASHRAE *Standard* 55, "Thermal Environmental Conditions for Human Occupancy." This standard specifies conditions or comfort zones where 80% of sedentary or slightly active persons find the environment thermally acceptable.

The winter and summer comfort zones specified in ANSI/ASHRAE *Standard* 55 are given in Figure 4-2. The temperature ranges are appropriate for current seasonal clothing habits in the United States. Summer clothing is considered to be light slacks and a short-sleeved shirt or a comparable ensemble with an insulation value of 0.5 clo. Winter clothing is considered heavy slacks, long-sleeved shirt, and sweater or jacket with an insulation value of 0.9 clo. The temperature ranges are for sedentary and slightly active people.

The winter zone is for air speeds less than 0.15 m/s; the summer zone is for air movements less than 0.25 m/s. The standard allows the summer comfort zone to extend above 26°C if the average air movement is increased 0.275 m/s for each °C of temperature increase to a maximum temperature of 28°C and air movement of 0.8 m/s.

The temperature boundaries of the comfort zones in Figure 4-2 can be shifted −1°F (−0.6°C) per 0.1 clo for clothing levels other than 0.5 and 0.9. The zones can also be shifted lower for increased activity levels.

Thermal comfort conditions must be fairly uniform over the body to prevent local discomfort. The radiant temperature asymmetry should be less than 5°C in the vertical direction and 10°C in the horizontal direction. The vertical temperature difference between head and foot should not exceed 3°C.

Figure 4-2 applies generally to altitudes from sea level to 3000 m (10,000 ft), and to the most common indoor thermal environments in which mean radiant temperature is nearly equal to the dry-bulb air temperature and where the air velocity is less than 30 fpm in winter and 50 fpm in summer. For these cases, the thermal environment can be specified by operative temperature and humidity variables.

Comfort zones for other clothing levels can be approximated by decreasing the temperature borders of the zone by 1°F for each 0.1 clo increase in clothing insulation and vise-versa. Similarly, a zone's temperatures can be decreased by 2.5°F per met increase in activity above 1.2 met. The upper and lower humidity levels of the comfort zones are less precise. Low humidity can lead to drying of the skin and mucous surfaces. Comfort complaints about dry nose, throat, eyes, and skin occur in low humidity conditions, typically when the dew point is less than 32°F. In compliance with these and other discomfort observations, Standard 55 recommends that the dew point temperature of occupied spaces not be less than

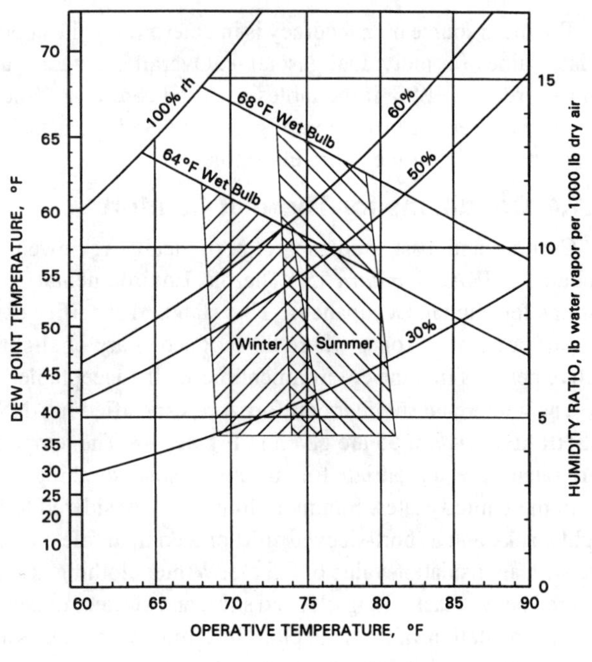

Fig. 4-2 ASHRAE Summer and Winter Comfort Zones
(Acceptable ranges of operative temperature and humidity for people in typical summer and winter clothing during primarily sedentary activity.)

35°F. In contrast, at high humidity levels too much skin moisture tends to increase discomfort, particularly skin moisture that is physiological in origin (water diffusion and perspiration). On the warm side of the comfort zone, the relative humidity should not exceed 60%.

Table 4-4 provides design criteria covering factors that apply to many different building types.

4.1.5 Adjustments for Clothing and/or Activity Levels

Activity. The indoor designated temperatures of Fig. 4-2 should be decreased when the average steady-state activity level of the occupants is higher than light, primarily sedentary (> 1.2 met).

This temperature can be calculated from the operative temperature at sedentary conditions with the following equation:

$$t_{i,active} = t_{i,sedentary} - 3(1 + \text{clo})(\text{met} - 1.2)(°\text{C}) \qquad (4\text{-}4)$$

$$t_{i,active} = t_{i,sedentary} - 5.4(1 + \text{clo})(\text{met} - 1.2)(°\text{F}) \qquad (4\text{-}5)$$

The equation is only appropriate between 1.2 and 3 met. The minimum allowable operative temperature for these activities is 15°C (59°F). The acceptable range (based on a 10% dissatisfaction criterion) will increase with activity and clothing. The ranges are approximately ±1.4°C (2.7°F) for 0.1 clo, ±2°C (3.5°F) for 0.5 clo, and ±3°C (5.4°F) for 0.9 clo.

Clothing. The temperatures of Fig. 4.2, after being corrected for activity level, can be corrected for clothing level using a decrease of 1°F for each 0.1 clo increase.

A wide range of environmental applications are covered by the ANSI/ASHRAE *Standard* 55. The comfort envelope defined by the standard applies only for sedentary and slightly active, normally clothed people at low air velocities, when the mean radiant temperature (MRT) equals the air temperature. For other clothing, activities, air temperatures, etc., the standard recommends use of Fanger's General Comfort Charts. Examples of these are shown in Figure 4-3.

Example 4-1: Determine the optimal comfort conditions for a conference room under summer conditions. Occupants wear light clothing (0.5 clo) during summer. Air movement is less than 0.1 m/s (20 fpm), MRT = air temperature, and summer rh = 70%.

Solution:

From Figure 4-3(a):
Air Temperature = MRT = 77°F (25°C)

Example 4-2: If, in winter, neither the air temperature nor the level of clothing for Example 4.1 change, what activity level must the occupant move up to in order to be comfortable?

Solution:

From Figure 4-3(b): Given conditions fall on comfort line, for approximately 1.25 met (standing, rather than sitting). The indoor conditions to be maintained within a building are the dry-bulb temperature and relative humidity of the air at the breathing line, 1 to 1.5 m (3 to 5 ft) above the floor, in an area that would indicate average conditions at that level and which would not be affected by abnormal or unusual heat gains or losses from the interior or exterior.

Table 4-3 Garment Insulation Values
(Table 8, Chapter 8, 1997 *Handbook—Fundamentals*)

Garment Description[a]	$I_{clu,i}$, clo[b]	Garment Description[a]	$I_{clu,i}$, clo[b]	Garment Description[a]	$I_{clu,i}$, clo[b]
Underwear		Long-sleeve, flannel shirt	0.34	Long-sleeve (thin)	0.25
Men's briefs	0.04	Short-sleeve, knit sport shirt	0.17	Long-sleeve (thick)	0.36
Panties	0.03	Long-sleeve, sweat shirt	0.34	**Dresses and skirts**[c]	
Bra	0.01	**Trousers and Coveralls**	0.06	Skirt (thin)	0.14
T-shirt	0.08	Short shorts	0.08	Skirt (thick)	0.23
Full slip	0.16	Walking shorts	0.15	Long-sleeve shirtdress (thin)	0.33
Half slip	0.14	Straight trousers (thin)	0.24	Long-sleeve shirtdress (thick)	0.47
Long underwear top	0.20	Straight trousers (thick)	0.28	Short-sleeve shirtdress (thin)	0.29
Long underwear bottoms	0.15	Sweatpants	0.30	Sleeveless, scoop neck (thin)	0.23
Footwear		Overalls	0.49	Sleeveless, scoop neck (thick), i.e., jumper	0.27
Ankle-length athletic socks	0.02	Coveralls			
Calf-length socks	0.03	**Suit jackets and vests (lined)**		**Sleepwear and Robes**	
Knee socks (thick)	0.06	Single-breasted (thin)	0.36	Sleeveless, short gown (thin)	0.18
Panty hose	0.02	Single-breasted (thick)	0.44	Sleeveless, long gown (thin)	0.20
Sandals/thongs	0.02	Double-breasted (thin)	0.42	Short-sleeve hospital gown	0.31
Slippers (quilted, pile-lined)	0.03	Double-breasted (thick)	0.48	Long-sleeve, long gown (thick)	0.46
Boots	0.10	Sleeveless vest (thin)	0.10	Long-sleeve pajamas (thick)	0.57
Shirts and Blouses		Sleeveless vest (thick)	0.17	Short-sleeve pajamas (thin)	0.42
Sleeveless, scoop-neck blouse	0.12	**Sweaters**		Long-sleeve, long wrap robe (thick)	0.69
Short-sleeve, dress shirt	0.19	Sleeveless vest (thin)	0.13	Long-sleeve, short wrap robe (thick)	0.48
Long-sleeve, dress shirt	0.25	Sleeveless vest (thick)	0.22	Short-sleeve, short robe (thin)	0.34

[a] "Thin" garments are made of light, thin fabrics worn in summer; "thick" garments are made of heavy, thick fabrics worn in winter.

[b] 1 clo = 0.880°F·ft²·h/Btu

[c] Knee-length

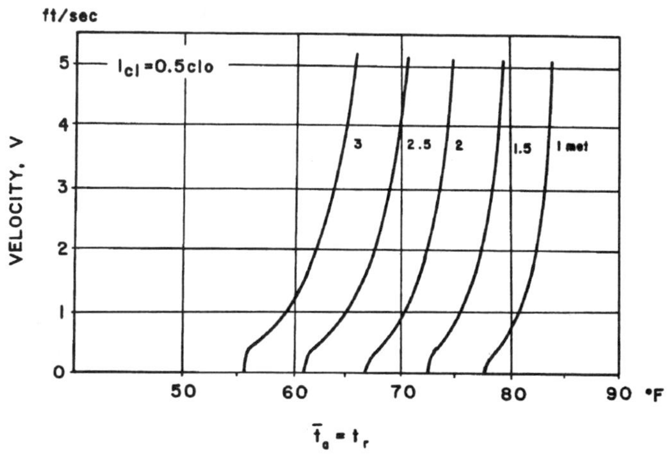

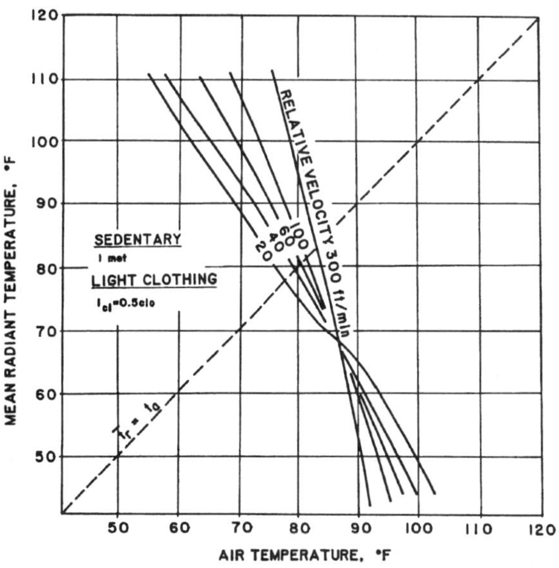

Fig. 4-3 Examples of Fanger's Charts
(Figs. 10 & 11, Chapter 8, 1997 ASHRAE Handbook—Fundamentals)

Table 4-4 General Design Criteria
(Table 1, Chapter 3, 1995 *Handbook—Applications*)

General Category	Specific Category	Inside Design Conditions		Air Movement	Circulation, Air Changes per Hour	Load Profile
		Winter	Summer			
Dining and Entertainment Centers	Cafeterias and Luncheonettes	70 to 74°F 20 to 30% rh	78°F[e] 50% rh	50 fpm at 6 ft above floor	12 to 15	Peak at 1 to 2 p.m. 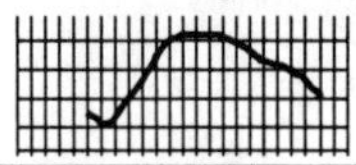
	Restaurants	70 to 74°F 20 to 30% rh	74 to 78°F 55 to 60% rh	25 to 30 fpm	8 to 12	Peak at 1 to 2 p.m. 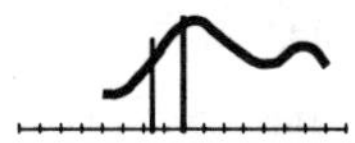
	Bars	70 to 74°F 20 to 30% rh	74 to 78°F 50 to 60% rh	30 fpm at 6 ft above floor	15 to 20	Peak at 5 to 7 p.m. 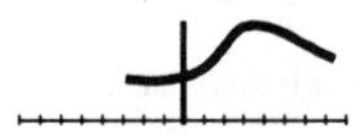
	Nightclubs	70 to 74°F 20 to 30% rh	74 to 78°F 50 to 60% rh	below 25 fpm at 5 ft above floor	20 to 30	Peak after 8 p.m., off from 2 a.m. to 4 p.m.
	Kitchens	70 to 74°F	85 to 88°F	30 to 50 fpm	12 to 15[h]	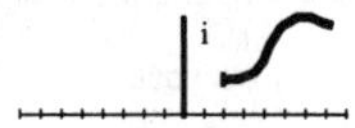
Office Buildings		70 to 74°F 20 to 30% rh	74 to 78°F 50 to 60% rh	25 to 45 fpm 0.75 to 2 cfm/ft^2	4 to 10	Peak at 4 p.m. 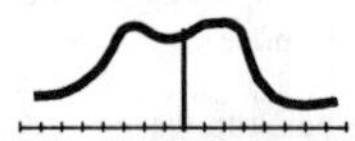
Libraries and Museums	Average	68 to 72°F 40 to 55% rh		below 25 fpm	8 to 12	Peak at 3 p.m. 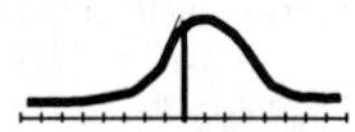
	Archival	See Special Considerations in the section on Libraries and Museums		below 25 fpm	8 to 12	Peak at 3 p.m. 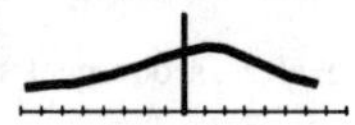
Bowling Centers		70 to 74°F 20 to 30% rh	75 to 78°F 50 to 55% rh	50 fpm at 6 ft above floor	10 to 15	Peak at 6 to 8 p.m. 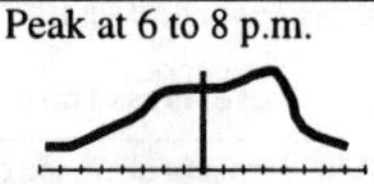
Communication Centers	Telephone Terminal Rooms	72 to 78°F 40 to 50% rh	72 to 78°F 40 to 50% rh	25 to 30 fpm	8 to 20	Varies with location and use
	Teletype Centers	70 to 74°F 40 to 50% rh	74 to 78°F 45 to 55% rh	25 to 30 fpm	8 to 20	Varies with location and use
	Radio and Television Studios	74 to 78°F 30 to 40% rh	74 to 78°F 40 to 55% rh	below 25 fpm at 12 ft above floor	15 to 40	Varies widely due to changes in lighting and people
Transportation Centers	Airport Terminals	70 to 74°F 20 to 30% rh	74 to 78°F 50 to 60% rh	25 to 30 fpm at 6 ft above floor	8 to 12	Peak at 10 a.m. to 9 p.m. 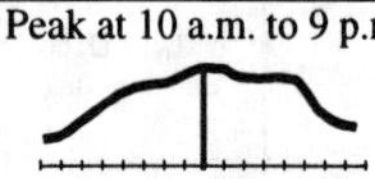
	Ship Docks	70 to 74°F 20 to 30% rh	74 to 78°F 50 to 60% rh	25 to 30 fpm at 6 ft above floor	8 to 12	Peak at 10 a.m. to 5 p.m. 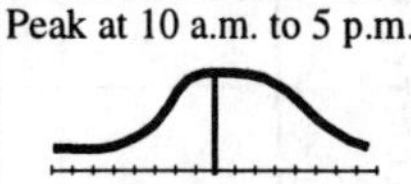
	Bus Terminals	70 to 74°F 20 to 30% rh	74 to 78°F 50 to 60% rh	25 to 30 fpm at 6 ft above floor	8 to 12	Peak at 10 a.m. to 5 p.m. 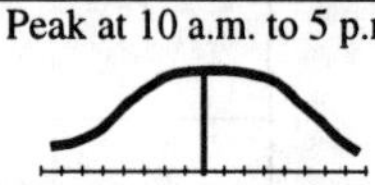
	Garages[l]	40 to 55°F	80 to 100°F	30 to 75 fpm	4 to 6 Refer to NFPA	Peak at 10 a.m. to 5 p.m. 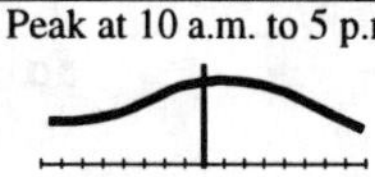
Warehouses		Inside design temperatures for warehouses often depend on the materials stored.			1 to 4	Peak at 10 a.m. to 3 p.m. 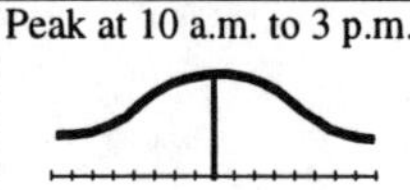

4.1.6 Moisture and Humidity

Too often, the behavior of moisture is given insufficient attention in building design and construction. Moisture is present as a vapor in all air and as absorbed moisture in most building materials. Problems involving moisture may arise from changes in moisture content, from the presence of excessive moisture, or from effects associated with its changes in state.

Water vapor originates from such activities as cooking, laundering, bathing, and people breathing and perspiring. Some typical values of moisture production are given in Table 4-5.

Exterior and interior building materials should allow vapor to pass five times more rapidly than materials inside the wall. Provided this condition is met, any moisture that may get into a wall will move on through it.

Selecting and applying humidification or dehumidification equipment involves considering both the environmental requirements of the occupancy or process and the limitations imposed by the thermal and permeable characteristics of the building enclosure. As these may not always be compatible, a compromise solution may be necessary, particularly in the case of existing buildings.

The environmental requirements for a particular occupancy or process may dictate a specific relative humidity, a required range of relative humidity, or certain limiting maximum or minimum values. The following classifications give guidance for most applications.

Human Comfort. The effect of relative humidity on human comfort has not been completely established. Nevertheless, humidity extremes are assumed to be undesirable and, for human comfort, relative humidities should be kept within a broad range of 30 to 70%.

Table 4-5 Moisture Production in Residences

Operation				Moisture	
				lb	(kg)
Floor mopping—80 ft^2 (7.4 m^2) kitchen				2.40	(1.09)
Clothes drying* (not vented)				26.40	(11.97)
Clothes washing*				4.33	(1.96)
Cooking (not vented)*	*From Food*		*From Gas*		
Breakfast	0.34	(0.16)	0.56 (0.25)	0.90	(0.41)
Lunch	0.51	(0.23)	0.66 (0.33)	1.17	(0.53)
Dinner	1.17	(0.53)	1.52 (0.69)	2.69	(1.22)
Bathing—shower				0.50	(0.23)
Bathing—tub				0.12	(0.05)
Dishwashing*					
Breakfast				0.20	(0.09)
Lunch				0.15	(0.07)
Dinner				0.65	(0.29)
Human Contribution—Adults					
When resting			Per hour	0.2	(0.09)
Working hard			Per hour	0.6	(0.27)
Average			Per hour	0.4	(0.18)
House plants			Per hour	0.04	(0.02)

*Based on family of four

Static Electricity. Electrostatic charges are generated when materials of high electrical resistance move against each other. Such charges may cause unpleasant sparks for people walking over carpets; difficulties in handling sheets of paper, fibers, and fabrics; objectionable clinging of dust to oppositely charged objects; or dangerous situations when explosive gases are present. Increasing the relative humidity of an environment tends to prevent the accumulation of such charges, but the optimum level of humidity depends to some extent on the materials involved. With many materials, relative humidities of 45% or more are usually required to reduce or eliminate electrostatic effects. Hospital operating rooms, where explosive mixtures of anesthetics are used, constitute a special and critical case in regard to electrostatic charges. A relative humidity of 50% or more is usually required and other special grounding arrangements and restrictions are imposed as to types of clothing the occupants wear. From a consideration of both comfort and safety, conditions of 72°F (22°C) and 55% rh are usually recommended in operating rooms.

Prevention and Treatment of Disease. Relative humidity has a significant effect on the control of airborne infection. At 50% rh, the mortality rate of certain organisms is highest (e.g., influenza virus loses much of its virulence). The mortality rate decreases both above and below this value. A relative humidity of 65% is regarded as optimum for nurseries for premature infants, while a value of 50% is suitable for full-terms and observational nurseries. In the treatment of allergic disorders, humidities well below 50% have proven satisfactory.

Visible Condensation. Condensation occurs on any interior surface when the dew point of the air in contact with it exceeds the surface temperature. The maximum permissible relative humidity that may be maintained without condensation is thus influenced by the thermal properties of the enclosure and the interior and exterior environment. In general, windows present the lowest surface temperature in most buildings and provide the best guide to permissible indoor humidity levels for no condensation (Table 4-6).

Concealed Condensation. The humidity level a building can tolerate without serious difficulties from concealed condensation may be much lower than indicated by visible condensation criteria. The migration of water vapor through the inner envelope by diffusion or air leakage brings it into contact with surfaces at temperatures approaching the outside

Table 4-6 Maximum Relative Humidity without Window Condensation

Natural Convection, Indoor Air at 23.3°C (74°F)		
Outdoor Temp., °C (°F)	Single Glazing	Double Glazing
4.4 (40)	39	59
−1.1 (30)	29	50
−6.7 (20)	21	43
−12.2 (10)	15	36
−17.8 (0)	10	30
−23.3 (−10)	7	26
−28.9 (−20)	5	21
−34.4 (−30)	3	17

temperature. Unless the building has been designed to eliminate or effectively reduce this possibility, the permissible humidity may be limited by the ability of the building enclosure to handle internal moisture rather than prevent the occurrence of moisture.

4.2 Outdoor Design Conditions: Weather Data

The climatic design conditions included in the 1997 *ASHRAE Handbook—Fundamentals* are those locations for which long-term hourly observations were available (at least 12 years). Consequently, many United States locations listed in previous versions are no longer listed because they lacked long-term data. The number of Canadian and international locations has increased significantly.

Design values of temperature and humidity have been updated from the 1993 *ASHRAE Handbook—Fundamentals*. The temperature and humidity conditions previously provided for at the 1, 2.5, and 5 percentile frequency of occurrence during summer months have been replaced by conditions corresponding to annual percentile values of 0.4, 1 and 2. Winter month conditions for 99 and 97.5 percentiles have been replaced by conditions based on annual percentiles of 99.6 and 99. This change was made in order to provide design conditions representing the same probability of occurrence anywhere, regardless of the seasonal distribution of extreme temperature and humidity. Previously, the summer and winter months used for the calculation of design conditions varied depending on location. For instance, summer design conditions for the United States were calculated over the four month period from June through September, whereas Canadian summer design conditions were based on only the month of July.

Values of ambient dry-bulb, dew-point, and wet-bulb temperature and wind speed corresponding to the various annual percentiles represent the value that is exceeded on average by the indicated percentage of the total number of hours in a year (8760). The 0.4%, 1.0%, 2.0%, and 5.0% values are exceeded on average 35,88,175, and 438 hours.

Two primary periods of record were used in the calculations. The values for the United States SAMSON and Canadian, CWEEDS locations are generally based on the period 1961-1993. DATSAV2 data were used for the 1991-1993 period for the SAMSON sites. The values for international locations and the rest of the United States, whose data were analyzed from the DATSAV2 files, are based on the period 1982 through 1993. DATSAV2 is a comprehensive database containing hourly observations for locations around the world collected from global telecommunications circuits. It is quality-controlled and archived by the Air Force Combat Climatology Center Operating Location A at Asheville, NC.

In the 1997 *ASHRAE Handbook—Fundamentals* design conditions for the United States appear in Tables 1A and 1B, for Canada in Tables 2A and 2B, and for international locations in Tables 3A and 3B. Information on station location, period analyzed, the heating design conditions, wind, mean annual extreme and standard deviation of minimum and maximum dry-bulb temperature, and mean daily temperature range are listed in Tables 1A, 2A, and 3A. Information on the design conditions for cooling and humidity control are provided in Tables 1B, 2B, and 3B.

The information provided in Tables 1A, 2A, and 3A are:

1. Name of the observing station as it appears in the data set from which it was abstracted, the World Meteorological Organization station number, latitude, longitude, elevation, standard pressure at elevation, and the period analyzed
2. Dry-bulb temperature corresponding to 99.6% and 99.0% annual cumulative frequency of occurrence (cold)
3. Wind speed corresponding to 1.0%, 2.5%, and 5.0% annual cumulative frequency of occurrence.
4. Wind speed corresponding to the 0.4% and 1.0% cumulative frequency of occurrence for the coldest month (lowest average dry-bulb temperature) at the location, and the mean coincident dry-bulb temperature
5. Mean wind speed coincident with the 99.6% dry-bulb temperature in Column 2 and 0.4% dry-bulb temperature from Column 2 of Tables 1B through 3B, and the wind direction most frequently occurring with the 99.6% and 0.4% dry-bulb temperatures (direction is reported in degrees true: 360 represents a north wind, 90 east, etc.)
6. Average of annual extreme maximum and minimum dry-bulb temperatures and standard deviations

Information provided in Tables 1B, 2B, and 3B includes:

1. Station name
2. Dry-bulb temperature corresponding to 0.4%, 1.0%, and 2.0% annual cumulative frequency of occurrence and the man coincident wet-bulb temperature (warm)
3. Wet-bulb temperature corresponding to 0.4%, 1.0%, and 2.0% annual cumulative frequency of occurrence and the mean coincident dry-bulb temperature
4. Dew-point temperature corresponding to 0.4%, 1.0%, and 2.0% annual cumulative frequency of occurrence and the mean coincident dry-bulb temperature and the humidity ratio (calculated for the dew-point temperature at the standard atmospheric pressure at the elevation of the station)
5. Mean daily range, which is the mean of the difference between daily maximum and minimum temperatures for the warmest month (highest average dry-bulb temperature)

The annual cumulative frequency of occurrences representing the design dry-bulb temperatures generally correspond to the seasonal design temperatures in the following fashion for locations in the mid-latitude, continental locations (characterized by a hot summer and cold winter). The 0.4% annual value is about the same as the 1% summer design temperature. The 1% annual values is about 1°F lower than the 2.5% summer design temperature in the 1993 *ASHRAE Handbook—Fundamentals*, and the 2% annual condition corresponds approximately to the 5% summer design temperature in the 1993 *ASHRAE Handbook—Fundamentals.*

Annual 99.6% and 99.0% design conditions represent a slightly colder condition than the previous cold season design temperatures, although there is considerable variability in this relationship from location to location.

Heating Design Conditions (Winter). The 99.6% and 99.0% design conditions in Column 2 in Tables 1A, 2A, and 3A are often used in sizing of heating equipment. In cold spells, dry-bulb temperatures below the design conditions can last for a week or more.

Cooling and Dehumidification Design Conditions (Summer). The 0.4%, 1.0%, and 2.0% dry-bulb temperatures and mean coincident wet-bulb temperatures in Column 2 of Tables 1B, 2B, and 3B often represent conditions on hot, mostly sunny days. These are useful for cooling applications, especially air-conditioning.

Mean Daily Range. The mean daily range is the mean difference between the daily maximum and minimum temperatures during the hottest month.

Design wind speeds in Column 3 of Tables 1A, 2A, and 3A are used for design of smoke management systems.

Columns 4 and 5 of Tables 1A, 2A, and 3A provide information useful for estimating peak loads accounting for infiltration. Column 4 provides extreme wind speeds only for the coldest month, with the mean coincident dry-bulb temperature. Column 5 provides the mean wind speed and direction coincident to the corresponding percentile design dry-bulb temperature.

Column 6 of Tables 1A, 2A, and 3A provides the mean and standard deviation of the annual extreme maximum and minimum dry-bulb temperatures. The probability of occurrence of very extreme conditions can be required for the operational design of equipment to ensure continuous operation and serviceability (regardless of whether the heating or cooling loads are being met). These values were calculated from the extremes of the hourly temperature observations.

Design conditions based on wet-bulb temperature in Column 3 of Tables 1B, 2B, and 3B represent extremes of the total sensible plus latent heat of outdoor air. This information is useful for cooling towers, evaporative coolers, and fresh air ventilation system design.

The design conditions based on dew-point temperatures in Column 4 of Tables 1B, 2B and 3B are directly related to extremes of humidity ratio, which represent peak moisture loads from the weather. Extreme dew-point conditions may occur on days with moderate dry-bulb temperatures resulting in high relative humidity. These values are especially useful for applications involving humidity control, such as desiccant cooling and dehumidification, cooling-based dehumidification, and fresh air ventilation systems.

Abbreviated versions of the climatic design tables from the 1997 *ASHRAE Handbook—Fundamentals* for the United States and Canada are provided as Table 4-7.

Minimum temperatures usually occur between 6:00 a.m. and 8:00 a.m. suntime on clear days when the daily range is greatest. For residential or other applications where the occupancy is continuous throughout the day, the recommended design temperatures apply. With commercial applications or other applications where occupancy is only during hours near the middle of the day, design temperatures above the recommended minimum may apply.

Maximum temperatures usually occur between 2:00 p.m. and 4:00 p.m. suntime with deviations on cloudy days when the daily range is less. Typically, the design dry-bulb temperatures should be used with the coincident wet-bulb temperatures in computing building cooling loads. For residential or other applications where the occupancy is continuous throughout the day, the recommended design temperatures apply. For commercial applications or other applications where occupancy is only during hours near the middle of the day, design temperatures below the recommended maximum might apply. In some cases, the peak occupancy load occurs before the effect of the outdoor maximum temperature has reached the space by conduction through the building mass. In other cases, the peak occupancy loads may be in months other than the three or four summer months when the maximum outdoor temperature is expected; here design temperatures from other months will apply.

When determining the heat loss for below grade components of a building (e.g., basement walls and floor), the average winter outdoor air temperature as well as the number of heating degree days (to base 65°F) are needed for the current ASHRAE loads methodology. Thus, Table 4-8 is provided. The heating load for the below grade structure also uses the amplitude of the ground temperature to determine the design ground surface temperature (see Chapter 6).

Although not a direct design criteria, another environmental index of general interest is the wind chill index. The wind chill index reliably expresses combined effects of temperature and wind on subjective discomfort. However, rather than using the numerical value of the wind chill index, meteorologists use an index derived from the WCI called the equivalent wind chill temperature. Table 4-9 shows a typical wind chill chart, expressed in equivalent wind chill temperature.

Table 4-7A Heating and Wind Design Conditions—United States

Selected data from Table 1A, Chapter 26, 1997 *ASHRAE Handbook—Fundamentals*

Station	WHO#	Lat. Deg. N	Long. Deg. W	Elev. ft	StdP, psia	Dates	Heating DB 99.6%	Heating DB 99%	Extreme Wind Speed, mph 1%	Extreme Wind Speed, mph 2.5%	Extreme Wind Speed, mph 5%	Coldest Month WS/MDB 0.4% WS	Coldest Month WS/MDB 0.4% MDB	Coldest Month WS/MDB 1% WS	Coldest Month WS/MDB 1% MDB	MWS/MWD to DB 99.6% MWS	MWS/MWD to DB 99.6% MWD	MWS/MWD to DB 0.4% MWS	MWS/MWD to DB 0.4% MWD	Annual Extreme Daily Mean DB Max.	Annual Extreme Daily Mean DB Min.	Annual Extreme Daily StdD DB Max.	Annual Extreme Daily StdD DB Min.
ALABAMA																							
Birmingham	722280	33.57	86.75	630	14.364	6193	18	23	19	17	15	20	41	18	42	7	340	9	320	98	9	3.3	6.4
Mobile	722230	30.68	88.25	220	14.579	6193	26	30	22	19	17	23	48	21	48	10	360	9	320	97	18	1.9	6.3
Montgomery	722260	32.30	86.40	203	14.588	6193	24	27	20	17	15	20	45	18	45	7	360	8	270	98	15	2.9	6.3
ALASKA																							
Anchorage Intl Aprt	702730	61.17	150.02	131	14.626	6193	−14	−9	22	19	17	23	18	19	18	4	10	8	290	77	−18	2.9	7.2
Fairbanks Intl Aprt	702610	64.82	147.87	453	14.457	6193	−47	−41	18	15	13	16	11	12	11	2	10	8	220	87	−48	3.8	7.8
ARIZONA																							
Phoenix Intl Airport	722780	33.43	112.02	1106	14.118	6193	34	37	19	16	14	17	59	14	58	5	90	9	270	114	30	2.2	4.6
Tucson	722740	32.12	110.93	2556	13.388	6193	31	34	24	21	18	24	56	21	56	7	140	12	300	108	25	2.8	4.0
ARKANSAS																							
Little Rock, AFB	723405	34.92	92.15	312	14.531	6193	16	21	20	18	16	20	42	18	42	9	360	9	200	101	10	3.8	6.2
CALIFORNIA																							
Fresno	723890	36.77	119.72	328	14.522	6193	30	32	17	15	13	17	53	14	52	4	90	9	290	107	26	2.2	3.8
Los Angeles	722950	33.93	118.40	105	14.640	6193	43	45	21	18	16	20	56	17	56	6	70	10	250	97	38	5.1	3.0
Sacramento, Metro	724839	38.70	121.58	23	14.683	6193	31	33	22	19	17	23	51	20	50	3	340	8	220	107	27	6.6	3.0
San Diego Intl Airport	722900	32.73	117.17	30	14.680	6193	44	46	18	16	15	20	59	16	60	3	70	10	310	95	39	6.4	4.4
San Francisco	724940	37.62	122.38	16	14.687	6193	37	39	29	26	23	27	53	22	52	5	160	13	300	94	33	4.3	3.0
San Jose Intl Airport	724945	37.37	121.93	56	14.666	8293	35	38	20	18	17	20	56	17	56	1	160	10	320	101	27	3.1	9.0
COLORADO																							
Colorado Springs	724660	38.82	104.72	6171	11.701	6193	−2	4	29	25	21	28	35	23	33	7	20	12	160	95	−9	2.0	6.9
Denver	724699	39.75	104.87	5331	12.076	8293	−3	3	24	21	18	25	39	21	40	6	180	9	160	97	−11	2.3	7.0
CONNECTICUT																							
Hartford, Brainard Fld	725087	41.73	72.65	20	14.685	6193	2	6	23	20	18	23	25	20	26	7	320	11	250	97	−6	2.4	5.7
DELAWARE																							
Wilmington	724089	39.68	75.60	79	14.654	6193	10	14	25	22	19	27	29	23	30	11	290	11	240	96	3	2.7	6.8
FLORIDA																							
Jacksonville Intl Airport	722066	30.40	81.42	16	14.687	8293	34	39	19	17	14	21	54	18	55	6	310	7	270	99	20	2.2	13.1
Miami Intl Airport	722020	25.82	80.28	13	14.688	6193	46	50	23	20	18	22	68	20	69	10	340	11	150	94	39	2.1	5.1
Orlando	722050	28.43	81.32	105	14.640	8293	37	42	20	18	16	21	66	19	65	8	330	9	290	96	29	1.6	6.5
Tallahassee	722140	30.38	84.37	69	14.659	6193	25	28	18	16	14	19	52	17	54	3	350	8	360	98	17	2.0	4.6
Tampa Intl Airport	722110	27.97	82.53	10	14.690	6193	36	40	19	17	15	21	59	19	59	8	20	10	270	95	29	1.2	4.8
GEORGIA																							
Atlanta	722190	33.65	84.42	1033	14.155	6193	18	23	22	19	17	23	37	21	36	12	320	9	300	96	9	3.5	7.3
Savannah	722070	32.13	81.20	49	14.669	6193	26	29	20	17	15	21	49	19	49	7	270	9	270	98	18	3.0	5.4
HAWAII																							
Honolulu	911820	21.35	157.93	16	14.687	6193	61	63	23	21	20	23	74	21	75	5	320	15	60	91	58	1.9	2.2
IDAHO																							
Boise	726810	43.57	116.22	2867	13.235	6193	2	9	24	21	18	22	37	19	37	6	130	11	320	103	−4	2.7	9.1
Pocatello	725780	42.92	112.60	4478	12.468	6193	−7	0	29	25	23	30	36	27	36	6	50	11	250	98	−15	2.3	9.1
ILLINOIS																							
Chicago, O'Hare Aprt	725300	41.98	87.90	673	14.342	6193	−6	−1	26	23	21	27	24	23	23	10	270	12	230	96	−12	2.8	6.5
Springfield	724390	39.85	89.67	614	14.373	6193	−4	2	25	23	21	27	25	24	27	10	270	12	230	97	−11	2.8	5.5
INDIANA																							
Fort Wayne	725330	41.00	85.20	827	14.262	6193	−4	2	25	23	20	27	19	24	22	10	250	12	230	95	−11	3.6	5.2
Indianapolis	724380	39.73	86.27	807	14.272	6193	−3	3	24	21	19	25	26	22	27	8	230	11	230	94	−10	2.8	6.8
IOWA																							
Cedar Rapids	725450	41.88	91.70	869	14.240	8293	−11	−5	25	22	20	29	12	26	14	10	300	11	180	96	−15	3.6	5.4
Des Moines	725460	41.53	93.65	965	14.190	6193	−9	−4	27	24	21	28	14	24	19	11	320	12	180	98	−15	3.4	5.1
KANSAS																							
Topeka	724560	39.07	95.62	886	14.231	6193	−2	4	25	22	20	25	28	22	29	9	320	12	180	100	−8	3.8	7.4
Wichita, Airport	724500	37.65	97.43	1339	13.998	6193	2	8	29	25	23	28	30	26	31	13	360	16	200	105	−4	2.9	6.3
KENTUCKY																							
Lexington	724220	38.03	84.60	988	14.179	6193	4	10	21	19	17	23	38	20	38	8	270	9	240	94	−4	3.5	8.3
Louisville	724230	38.18	85.73	489	14.438	6193	6	12	22	19	17	22	40	20	34	10	290	10	250	96	−1	3.1	7.9
LOUISIANA																							
Baton Rouge	722317	30.53	91.15	69	14.659	6193	27	30	20	18	16	21	48	19	49	8	360	8	270	97	20	2.2	5.4
New Orleans Intl Arpt	722310	29.98	90.25	30	14.680	6193	30	34	21	19	17	21	48	19	49	7	340	8	360	96	23	2.0	5.3
Shreveport	722480	32.47	93.82	259	14.558	6193	22	26	20	18	16	22	46	19	48	9	360	8	180	99	16	3.1	5.6
MAINE																							
Bangor	726088	44.80	68.83	194	14.593	8293	−7	−2	22	19	17	24	18	21	20	6	300	10	240	94	−16	2.9	5.9
Portland	726060	43.65	70.32	62	14.662	6193	−3	2	24	21	18	24	26	21	25	7	320	12	270	93	−13	3.6	5.5
MARYLAND																							
Baltimore, BWI Airport	724060	39.18	76.67	154	14.614	6193	11	15	24	21	19	25	31	22	31	10	290	11	280	97	4	2.9	5.8
MASSACHUSETTS																							
Boston	725090	42.37	71.03	30	14.680	6193	7	12	29	25	23	30	30	27	28	17	320	14	270	96	0	2.7	4.7
MICHIGAN																							
Detroit, Metro	725370	42.23	83.33	663	14.347	6193	0	5	27	23	21	28	28	24	27	11	240	13	230	95	−7	3.0	5.4

WMO = World Meteorological Organization number
Lat. = latitude Long. = longitude
Elev. = elevation, feet
StdP = standard pressure at station elevation, psia
DB = dry-bulb temperature, °F
WS = wind speed, mph

Table 4-7B Cooling and Dehumidification Design Conditions—United States

Selected data from Table 1B, Chapter 26, 1997 *ASHRAE Handbook—Fundamentals*

	Cooling DB/MWB						WB/MDB						DP/MDB and HR									
	0.4%		1%		2%		0.4%		1%		2%		0.4%			1%			2%			Range
Station	**DB**	**MWB**	**DB**	**MWB**	**DB**	**MWB**	**WB**	**MDB**	**WB**	**MDB**	**WB**	**MDB**	**DP**	**HR**	**MDB**	**DP**	**HR**	**MDB**	**DP**	**HR**	**MDB**	**of DB**
ALABAMA																						
Birmingham	94	75	92	75	90	74	78	89	77	88	76	87	75	135	83	74	131	82	73	127	81	18.7
Mobile	94	77	92	76	91	76	79	89	79	88	78	87	77	142	83	76	139	83	76	135	82	16.5
Montgomery	95	76	93	76	91	76	79	91	78	89	78	88	76	139	85	75	134	84	75	130	83	18.7
ALASKA																						
Anchorage, Intl Airport	71	59	68	57	65	56	60	69	58	66	57	63	56	68	62	55	64	61	53	61	60	12.6
Fairbanks, Intl Airport	81	61	77	59	74	58	63	77	61	74	59	71	58	72	65	56	68	64	54	64	63	18.6
ARIZONA																						
Phoenix, Intl Airport	110	70	108	70	106	70	76	97	75	96	74	95	71	118	82	69	111	84	67	104	85	23.0
Tucson	104	65	102	65	100	65	72	88	71	87	70	86	69	116	76	67	111	76	66	106	77	29.4
ARKANSAS																						
Little Rock, AFB	97	77	95	77	92	76	80	92	79	91	78	89	77	141	86	76	137	85	75	133	84	19.5
CALIFORNIA																						
Fresno	103	71	101	70	98	69	73	98	71	96	70	94	64	92	85	62	85	84	61	80	82	30.9
Los Angeles	85	64	81	64	78	64	70	78	69	76	68	75	67	99	75	66	95	73	65	92	72	10.9
Sacramento, Metro	100	69	97	69	94	68	72	96	70	94	69	91	62	84	82	61	79	80	59	76	78	33.3
San Diego, Intl Airport	85	67	81	67	79	67	73	79	71	78	70	77	70	111	77	68	104	76	67	99	74	8.9
San Francisco	83	63	78	62	74	61	64	79	63	75	62	72	59	76	67	58	73	66	57	71	65	16.7
San Jose Intl Airport	93	67	89	66	86	65	70	88	68	85	67	83	63	85	77	61	81	76	60	78	74	22.3
COLORADO																						
Colorado Springs	90	58	87	58	84	58	63	78	62	77	61	76	59	92	66	57	88	66	56	83	65	24.9
Denver	93	60	90	59	87	59	65	81	63	80	62	79	60	96	69	58	90	68	57	85	68	26.9
CONNECTICUT																						
Hartford, Brainard Field	91	73	88	72	85	70	76	87	74	84	73	82	81	228	71	79	216	70	78	207	0	20.9
DELAWARE																						
Wilmington	91	75	89	74	86	73	78	87	76	85	75	83	75	132	82	74	125	81	72	120	80	17.0
FLORIDA																						
JJacksonville Intl Airport	94	77	93	77	91	77	80	90	79	89	78	88	77	142	85	76	138	84	76	134	83	17.8
Miami, Intl Airport	91	77	90	77	89	77	80	87	79	87	78	86	78	144	83	77	141	83	76	138	82	11.4
Orlando	94	76	93	76	92	76	79	88	79	88	78	87	77	142	83	76	139	82	76	136	81	16.6
Tallahassee	95	77	93	76	91	76	80	89	79	88	78	87	77	142	83	76	138	82	76	135	82	18.5
Tampa, Intl Airport	92	77	91	77	90	77	80	88	79	88	78	87	78	144	85	77	140	84	76	137	83	15.0
GEORGIA																						
Atlanta	93	75	91	74	88	73	77	88	76	87	75	85	74	133	82	73	128	81	72	124	80	17.3
Savannah	95	77	93	76	91	76	79	90	78	89	78	87	77	139	84	76	135	83	75	132	82	17.5
HAWAII																						
Honolulu	89	73	88	73	87	73	76	84	75	84	74	84	74	125	80	72	120	80	71	116	79	12.2
IDAHO																						
Boise	96	63	94	63	91	62	66	90	64	89	63	87	58	79	72	55	72	71	53	67	71	30.3
Pocatello	93	61	90	60	87	59	64	84	62	83	61	82	57	83	70	55	76	70	53	70	69	32.1
ILLINOIS																						
Chicago, O'Hare Intl A	91	74	88	73	86	71	77	88	75	85	74	83	74	130	84	72	123	82	71	115	80	19.6
Springfield	93	76	91	75	88	74	79	89	77	88	76	85	76	139	86	75	132	84	73	125	82	19.4
INDIANA																						
Fort Wayne	90	74	88	73	85	71	77	86	75	84	74	82	74	131	83	72	124	81	71	117	79	19.9
Indianapolis	91	75	88	74	86	73	78	88	77	86	75	83	75	137	84	74	131	82	73	125	81	18.9
IOWA																						
Cedar Rapids	93	75	89	74	86	72	78	89	76	86	74	84	75	136	84	74	129	83	71	120	80	20.0
Des Moines	93	76	90	74	87	73	78	89	76	87	75	85	74	133	85	73	126	83	71	120	81	18.5
KANSAS																						
Topeka	96	75	93	75	90	75	79	90	78	89	76	88	76	139	87	74	132	85	73	126	83	20.3
Wichita, Airport	100	73	97	73	94	73	77	91	76	90	74	89	73	129	83	72	123	82	71	118	81	22.2
KENTUCKY																						
Lexington	91	74	89	73	86	72	77	87	75	86	74	83	74	130	83	72	124	81	71	120	80	18.4
Louisville	93	76	90	75	88	74	78	90	77	88	76	86	75	134	85	74	129	84	73	125	82	18.2
LOUISIANA																						
Baton Rouge	94	78	92	77	91	77	80	89	79	88	78	87	78	145	84	77	141	84	76	137	83	16.7
New Orleans, Intl A	93	79	92	78	90	78	81	90	80	88	80	87	79	151	86	78	146	85	77	142	84	15.5
Shreveport	97	77	95	77	93	76	79	91	79	90	78	89	76	139	84	76	135	83	75	132	83	19.1
MAINE																						
Bangor	87	71	84	69	81	67	73	83	71	81	69	77	70	111	78	68	104	75	67	99	73	20.5
Portland	86	71	83	70	80	68	74	83	72	80	70	77	71	114	79	69	107	76	67	101	74	18.7
MARYLAND																						
Baltimore, BWI Airport	93	75	91	74	88	73	78	88	76	86	75	85	75	132	83	74	125	81	72	120	80	18.8
MASSACHUSETTS																						
Boston	91	73	87	71	84	70	75	87	74	83	72	81	72	119	80	71	113	79	69	108	78	15.3
MICHIGAN																						
Detroit, Metro	90	73	87	72	84	70	76	86	74	84	73	81	73	125	83	71	118	80	70	111	78	20.4

MDB = mean coincident dry-bulb temperature, °F
MWB = mean coincident wet-bulb temperature, °F
MWS = mean coincident wind speed, mph
MWD = mean coincident wind direction, °
StdD = standard deviation
A = airport
HR = humidity ratio, grains/lb (dry air)
DP = dew-point temperature, °F

Table 4-7A Heating and Wind Design Conditions—United States (*Continued*)

Selected data from Table 1A, Chapter 26, 1997 *ASHRAE Handbook—Fundamentals*

									Extreme Wind			Coldest Month WS/MDB				MWS/MWD to DB				Annual Extreme Daily			
		Lat.	Long.	Elev.	StdP,		Heating DB		Speed, mph			0.4%		1%		99.6%		0.4%		Mean DB		StdD DB	
Station	WHO#	Deg. N	Deg. W	ft	psia	Dates	99.6%	99%	1%	2.5%	5%	WS	MDB	WS	MDB	MWS	MWD	MWS	MWD	Max.	Min.	Max.	Min.
Grand Rapids	726350	42.88	85.52	804	14.274	6193	0	5	25	22	20	26	25	23	24	8	180	13	240	93	−9	2.1	5.3
Sault Ste. Marie	727340	46.47	84.37	725	14.314	6193	−12	−7	23	20	18	24	19	21	18	7	90	10	230	89	−22	3.5	5.4
MINNESOTA																							
Duluth	727450	46.83	92.18	1417	13.958	6193	−21	−16	25	22	20	25	12	22	11	10	310	12	230	90	−28	2.8	4.7
Minneapolis-St. Paul	726580	44.88	93.22	837	14.257	6193	−16	−11	25	22	20	25	12	22	14	9	300	14	180	97	−22	3.5	5.4
MISSISSIPPI																							
Jackson	722350	32.32	90.08	331	14.520	6193	21	25	20	18	16	21	45	19	46	7	340	8	270	98	14	2.7	5.8
MISSOURI																							
Kansas City	724460	39.32	94.72	1024	14.160	6193	−1	4	26	23	20	26	34	23	33	10	320	13	190	100	−7	4.1	6.6
Springfield	724400	37.23	93.38	1270	14.034	6193	3	9	24	21	19	23	35	21	35	10	340	10	230	98	−4	3.5	6.4
St. Louis Intl Airport	724340	38.75	90.37	564	14.398	6193	2	8	26	23	20	26	26	23	27	12	290	11	240	99	−5	3.5	6.2
MONTANA																							
Billings	726770	45.80	108.53	3570	12.896	6193	−13	−7	28	24	22	30	25	27	30	10	230	10	240	99	−19	2.8	6.2
Great Falls Intl Arpt	727750	47.48	111.37	3658	12.854	6193	−19	−13	33	29	26	34	38	31	38	7	240	12	230	98	−25	3.2	7.4
NEBRASKA																							
Lincoln	725510	40.85	96.75	1188	14.076	8293	−7	−2	27	23	21	28	25	24	27	9	350	15	180	103	−11	6.5	8.1
Omaha, Eppley Arfld	725500	41.30	95.90	981	14.182	6193	−7	−2	26	23	20	27	21	23	17	10	340	12	180	100	−14	3.3	4.8
NEVADA																							
Las Vegas Intl Arpt	723860	36.08	115.17	2178	13.575	6193	27	30	30	26	23	25	48	22	49	7	250	12	230	111	21	2.2	4.7
Reno	724880	39.50	119.78	4400	12.505	6193	8	13	26	22	19	26	46	21	44	3	160	10	290	99	1	2.2	8.4
NEW HAMPSHIRE																							
Concord	726050	43.20	71.50	344	14.513	6193	−8	−2	23	20	17	23	20	20	21	4	320	10	230	95	−18	2.9	5.5
NEW JERSEY																							
Atlantic City	724070	39.45	74.57	66	14.661	6193	8	13	27	23	20	29	36	25	34	9	310	11	250	96	0	2.9	5.7
Newark	725020	40.70	74.17	30	14.680	6193	10	14	26	23	20	27	28	23	29	13	260	13	230	98	4	2.6	4.8
Trenton, McGuire AFB	724096	40.02	74.60	135	14.624	8293	11	15	22	19	17	23	31	21	31	8	330	8	240	97	2	2.2	5.2
NEW MEXICO																							
Albuquerque	723650	35.05	106.62	5315	12.084	6193	13	18	29	25	22	26	34	22	37	8	360	10	240	100	6	2.6	7.3
NEW YORK																							
Albany	725180	42.75	73.80	292	14.541	6193	−7	−2	24	22	19	23	20	20	22	5	300	10	230	95	−18	3.0	6.3
Buffalo	725280	42.93	78.73	705	14.325	6193	2	5	29	26	23	34	25	30	24	12	270	13	240	91	−6	2.3	5.3
New York, La Guardia	725030	40.77	73.90	30	14.680	8293	13	17	28	25	22	30	29	27	28	18	310	12	280	97	6	2.2	4.3
Rochester	725290	43.12	77.67	554	14.403	6193	1	5	27	23	21	29	22	26	21	10	230	12	250	93	−7	2.8	4.9
Syracuse	725190	43.12	76.12	407	14.481	6193	−3	2	26	22	20	28	20	25	21	7	90	11	250	93	−13	3.0	6.0
NORTH CAROLINA																							
Charlotte	723140	35.22	80.93	768	14.292	6193	18	23	20	17	15	20	44	18	45	6	50	9	240	97	10	2.9	6.0
Greensboro	723170	36.08	79.95	886	14.231	6193	15	19	19	17	15	20	40	18	40	7	290	8	230	96	7	2.7	5.0
Raleigh/Durham	723060	35.87	78.78	440	14.463	6193	16	20	21	18	16	21	42	19	43	8	360	9	240	96	9	2.9	5.3
NORTH DAKOTA																							
Fargo	727530	46.90	96.80	899	14.224	6193	−22	−17	31	27	24	32	7	28	7	8	180	14	160	98	−27	3.4	4.4
Grand Forks, AFB	727575	47.97	97.40	912	14.217	8293	−20	−16	27	24	21	30	9	26	13	7	290	13	180	98	−25	4.7	4.9
OHIO																							
Cincinnati, Lunken Fld	724297	39.10	84.42	482	14.441	8293	5	12	21	19	17	22	35	19	33	9	260	10	210	96	−3	3.2	9.4
Cleveland	725240	41.42	81.87	804	14.274	6193	1	6	26	23	20	27	28	24	28	12	230	12	230	93	−6	2.8	6.3
Columbus Intl Arpt	724280	40.00	82.88	817	14.267	6193	1	6	23	20	18	24	30	21	25	9	270	11	270	94	−6	2.6	7.1
Dayton Intl Airport	724290	39.90	84.20	1004	14.170	6193	−1	5	24	21	19	25	26	22	28	11	270	11	240	95	−8	2.9	7.0
OKLAHOMA																							
Oklahoma City, Rogers A	723530	35.40	97.60	1302	14.017	6193	9	15	29	25	23	29	33	26	37	15	360	13	180	103	4	3.4	4.9
Tulsa	723560	36.20	95.90	676	14.340	6193	9	14	25	23	21	24	46	22	40	11	360	12	180	103	3	3.6	5.6
OREGON																							
Eugene	726930	44.12	123.22	374	14.498	6193	21	26	20	18	16	22	46	19	45	8	360	12	360	99	16	3.7	7.9
Portland	726980	45.60	122.60	39	14.675	6193	22	27	25	21	18	28	37	25	39	13	120	11	340	99	18	4.4	6.0
PENNSYLVANIA																							
Philadelphia Intl Apt	724080	39.88	75.25	30	14.680	6193	11	15	24	21	19	26	31	23	30	12	290	11	230	96	5	2.8	5.6
Pittsburgh Intl Arpt	725200	40.50	80.22	1224	14.057	6193	2	7	25	21	19	26	24	23	25	10	260	11	230	93	−6	3.1	6.7
Wilkes-Barre/Scranton	725130	41.33	75.73	948	14.199	6193	2	7	20	18	16	21	26	19	25	8	230	11	220	92	−5	2.8	4.9
RHODE ISLAND																							
Providence	725070	41.73	71.43	62	14.662	6193	5	10	27	23	21	27	31	23	32	12	340	13	230	95	−2	3.7	5.0
SOUTH CAROLINA																							
Charleston	722080	32.90	80.03	49	14.669	6193	25	28	22	19	17	22	52	19	51	7	20	10	230	98	18	2.3	5.6
Columbia	723100	33.95	81.12	226	14.576	6193	21	24	20	17	15	20	48	18	49	5	220	9	240	100	13	3.1	5.6
SOUTH DAKOTA																							
Rapid City	726620	44.05	103.07	3169	13.089	6193	−11	−5	36	31	27	37	26	32	26	9	350	13	160	102	−17	3.4	5.4
Sioux Falls	726510	43.58	96.73	1427	13.953	6193	−16	−11	28	25	22	30	15	26	17	8	310	15	180	100	−23	4.1	4.9
TENNESSEE																							
Knoxville	723260	35.82	83.98	981	14.182	6193	13	19	21	18	15	21	48	19	45	7	50	8	250	95	4	3.0	7.8
Memphis	723340	35.05	90.00	285	14.544	6193	16	21	22	19	17	22	42	20	42	10	20	9	240	99	9	2.8	7.2
Nashville	723270	36.13	86.68	591	14.385	6193	10	16	22	19	17	22	46	20	42	8	340	9	230	97	1	3.3	7.8

WMO = World Meteorological Organization number   Elev. = elevation, feet   DB = dry-bulb temperature, °F
Lat. = latitude   Long. = longitude   StdP = standard pressure at station elevation, psia   WS = wind speed, mph

Table 4-7B Cooling and Dehumidification Design Conditions—United States (*Continued*)

Selected data from Table 1B, Chapter 26, 1997 *ASHRAE Handbook—Fundamentals*

	Cooling DB/MWB						WB/MDB						DP/MDB and HR									
	0.4%		1%		2%		0.4%		1%		2%		0.4%			1%			2%			Range
Station	DB	MWB	DB	MWB	DB	MWB	WB	MDB	WB	MDB	WB	MDB	DP	HR	MDB	DP	HR	MDB	DP	HR	MDB	of DB
Grand Rapids	89	73	86	71	84	70	76	85	74	83	72	81	73	126	81	71	118	79	70	112	77	20.7
Sault Ste. Marie	83	69	80	68	77	66	72	80	70	77	68	74	69	111	76	67	103	74	65	95	72	21.9
MINNESOTA																						
Duluth	84	69	81	67	78	65	72	81	69	78	67	75	68	110	77	66	102	75	64	94	72	20.2
Minneapolis-St. Paul	91	73	88	71	85	70	76	88	74	84	72	82	73	124	83	71	116	81	69	109	79	19.1
MISSISSIPPI																						
Jackson	95	77	93	76	92	76	80	90	79	89	78	88	77	142	84	76	138	83	75	134	82	19.2
MISSOURI																						
Kansas City	96	75	93	75	90	74	78	90	77	89	76	87	75	137	86	74	130	84	73	125	83	18.8
Springfield	95	74	92	74	89	74	78	89	76	88	75	86	74	134	84	73	128	83	72	124	81	20.8
St. Louis, Intl Airport	95	76	93	75	90	74	79	90	78	88	76	87	76	138	85	75	132	83	73	127	82	18.3
MONTANA																						
Billings	93	63	90	62	87	61	65	86	64	84	62	83	59	83	71	57	78	71	55	74	70	25.8
Great Falls, Intl Airport	92	61	88	60	85	59	64	84	62	82	61	81	57	81	69	55	74	67	53	69	66	27.2
NEBRASKA																						
Lincoln	97	74	94	74	91	73	78	90	76	89	75	87	75	136	84	73	130	83	71	121	82	22.3
Omaha, Eppley Airfield	95	75	92	75	89	73	78	90	77	88	75	86	75	136	85	73	128	84	72	121	82	19.9
NEVADA																						
Las Vegas, Intl Airport	108	66	106	66	103	65	71	95	70	93	69	93	65	102	79	63	92	81	60	84	85	24.8
Reno	95	61	92	60	90	59	63	87	62	86	60	85	56	77	69	53	69	69	50	63	68	37.3
NEW HAMPSHIRE																						
Concord	90	71	87	70	84	68	74	85	73	82	71	79	71	118	79	70	111	77	68	105	76	24.1
NEW JERSEY																						
Atlantic City	91	74	88	73	86	72	77	87	76	84	75	82	75	131	81	74	125	80	72	120	79	18.1
Newark	93	74	90	73	87	71	77	88	76	85	74	83	74	127	81	73	121	80	71	116	80	15.9
Trenton, McGuire AFB	93	75	90	74	87	73	78	89	76	87	75	84	75	132	83	74	127	82	72	118	80	18.9
NEW MEXICO																						
Albuquerque	96	60	93	60	91	60	65	83	64	82	64	81	61	98	68	60	93	69	58	89	69	25.4
NEW YORK																						
Albany	90	71	86	70	84	69	74	85	73	82	71	79	72	118	79	70	111	77	68	106	76	23.7
Buffalo	86	70	84	69	81	68	74	82	72	80	71	78	71	118	78	70	113	77	68	106	75	17.7
New York, La Guardia A	92	74	89	73	86	72	77	87	76	85	74	83	74	129	81	73	125	80	71	116	80	14.6
Rochester	89	73	86	71	83	70	75	85	74	82	72	80	73	123	81	71	116	79	69	109	77	20.1
Syracuse	88	72	85	71	83	70	75	85	73	82	72	80	72	120	80	70	113	78	69	107	77	20.3
NORTH CAROLINA																						
Charlotte	94	74	91	74	89	73	77	88	76	87	75	86	74	130	82	73	125	80	72	122	80	17.8
Greensboro	92	75	90	74	88	73	77	88	76	86	75	85	74	132	82	73	127	81	72	123	80	18.5
Raleigh/Durham	93	76	90	75	88	74	78	88	77	87	76	85	75	134	82	74	130	81	73	125	80	18.8
NORTH DAKOTA																						
Fargo	91	71	88	70	85	69	75	86	73	84	71	81	72	122	82	69	112	80	67	104	77	22.3
Grand Forks, AFB	91	71	88	69	85	68	75	86	72	83	70	80	71	118	81	69	109	78	67	101	76	22.9
OHIO																						
Cincinnati, Lunken Field	93	74	90	75	88	73	77	89	76	87	75	84	75	132	82	74	128	81	72	120	80	20.0
Cleveland	89	73	86	72	84	71	76	85	74	83	72	81	73	125	82	71	118	80	70	112	78	18.6
Columbus, Intl Airport	90	74	88	73	86	71	77	87	75	85	74	82	73	128	82	72	123	81	71	117	79	19.3
Dayton, Intl Airport	90	74	88	73	86	71	76	87	75	85	74	82	73	129	82	72	123	80	71	117	79	19.2
OKLAHOMA																						
Oklahoma City, W. Rogers	99	74	96	74	94	73	77	91	76	90	75	89	73	129	83	72	125	82	71	120	81	21.0
Tulsa	100	76	97	76	94	75	79	92	78	92	77	90	76	137	87	74	132	85	73	127	84	19.5
OREGON																						
Eugene	91	67	87	65	83	64	69	87	67	84	65	81	62	83	74	60	78	73	59	74	71	27.6
Portland	90	67	86	66	83	64	69	87	67	84	65	80	62	83	75	60	78	72	59	75	71	21.6
PENNSYLVANIA																						
Philadelphia, Intl Airport	92	75	89	74	87	73	78	88	77	86	75	84	75	132	83	74	126	81	73	121	80	17.7
Pittsburgh, Intl Airport	89	72	86	70	84	69	74	85	73	82	71	80	71	121	80	70	115	78	68	109	77	19.5
Wilkes-Barre/Scranton	88	71	85	70	83	69	74	83	73	81	71	79	71	120	79	70	115	77	69	109	76	18.8
RHODE ISLAND																						
Providence	89	73	86	71	83	70	76	85	74	82	73	80	73	124	80	72	118	78	70	112	77	17.4
SOUTH CAROLINA																						
Charleston	94	78	92	77	90	77	80	90	79	88	78	87	78	145	84	77	139	83	76	134	83	16.2
Columbia	96	76	94	75	92	74	78	90	77	89	77	87	75	134	82	75	130	81	74	127	81	19.9
SOUTH DAKOTA																						
Rapid City	95	65	91	65	88	64	70	85	68	84	67	82	65	104	76	63	98	75	61	92	73	25.3
Sioux Falls	94	73	90	72	87	71	76	89	75	87	73	84	73	127	84	71	119	82	69	112	80	22.1
TENNESSEE																						
Knoxville	92	74	90	74	87	73	77	88	76	86	75	85	74	131	82	73	127	81	72	123	80	18.1
Memphis	96	78	94	77	92	77	80	92	79	91	78	89	77	143	87	76	137	86	75	133	84	16.8
Nashville	94	76	92	75	90	74	78	89	77	88	76	86	75	134	83	74	130	82	73	126	81	19.1

MDB = mean coincident dry-bulb temperature, °F MWS = mean coincident wind speed, mph StdD = standard deviation HR = humidity ratio, grains/lb (dry air)
MWB = mean coincident wet-bulb temperature, °F MWD = mean coincident wind direction, ° A = airport DP = dew-point temperature, °F

Table 4-7A Heating and Wind Design Conditions—United States (*Continued*)

Selected data from Table 1A, Chapter 26, 1997 *ASHRAE Handbook—Fundamentals*

									Extreme Wind			Coldest Month WS/MDB				MWS/MWD to DB				Annual Extreme Daily			
		Lat.	Long.	Elev.	StdP,		Heating DB		Speed, mph			0.4%		1%		99.6%		0.4%		Mean DB		StdD DB	
Station	WHO#	Deg. N	Deg. W	ft	psia	Dates	99.6%	99%	1%	2.5%	5%	WS	MDB	WS	MDB	MWS	MWD	MWS	MWD	Max.	Min.	Max.	Min.
TEXAS																							
Dallas/Fort Worth Int'l A	722590	32.90	97.03	597	14.381	8293	17	24	26	23	21	26	46	24	47	13	350	10	170	103	14	3.1	8.3
El Paso	722700	31.80	106.40	3917	12.731	6193	21	25	25	21	18	24	51	21	49	5	20	8	180	104	14	3.3	6.1
Houston, Inter Airport	722430	29.97	95.35	108	14.638	6193	27	31	20	18	16	22	47	20	52	8	340	10	180	98	22	3.1	5.4
Lubbock Intl Airport	722670	33.65	101.82	3241	13.054	6193	11	17	30	26	23	30	43	27	44	12	0	14	160	102	4	2.6	5.6
San Antonio Intl A	722530	29.53	98.47	794	14.279	6193	26	30	22	19	17	23	43	20	45	10	350	10	160	100	19	2.9	5.2
UTAH																							
Ogden, Hill AFB	725755	41.12	111.97	4787	12.325	8293	6	11	22	19	17	22	27	19	28	9	110	6	190	96	1	2.9	6.3
Salt Lake City	725720	40.78	111.97	4226	12.586	6193	6	11	27	23	20	27	42	22	40	7	160	11	340	100	−3	1.9	6.7
VERMONT																							
Burlington	726170	44.47	73.15	341	14.515	6193	−11	−6	23	21	18	24	30	21	27	6	70	11	180	93	−19	2.7	5.6
Montpelier/Barre	726145	44.20	72.57	1165	14.087	8293	−10	−6	21	19	17	22	20	20	20	4	320	9	220	91	−18	3.6	5.9
VIRGINIA																							
Norfolk	723080	36.90	76.20	30	14.680	6193	20	24	25	22	20	26	40	23	40	12	340	12	230	97	14	2.8	5.4
Richmond	724010	37.50	77.33	177	14.602	6193	14	18	20	18	16	21	40	18	39	7	340	10	230	98	6	2.6	5.8
Washington, Natl A	724050	38.85	77.03	66	14.661	8293	15	20	23	20	18	24	34	21	35	11	340	11	170	99	8	2.5	6.8
WASHINGTON																							
Seattle Intl Airport	727930	47.45	122.30	449	14.458	6193	23	28	22	19	17	24	44	21	44	10	10	10	350	92	19	3.6	6.8
Spokane, Fairchild AFB	727855	47.62	117.65	2461	13.435	6193	1	7	27	23	20	28	39	25	38	7	50	9	240	98	−7	3.2	8.7
WEST VIRGINIA																							
Charleston	724140	38.37	81.60	981	14.182	6193	6	11	18	16	14	20	38	18	34	7	250	8	240	94	−2	2.8	6.7
WISCONSIN																							
Green Bay	726450	44.48	88.13	702	14.326	6193	−13	−8	25	22	20	25	19	22	18	10	270	12	200	93	−19	2.8	5.6
Madison	726410	43.13	89.33	866	14.241	6193	−11	−6	24	21	19	25	16	22	17	8	300	12	230	94	−18	3.2	6.0
Milwaukee	726400	42.95	87.90	692	14.332	6193	−7	−2	28	24	22	28	19	24	20	13	290	15	220	95	−12	3.2	6.7
WYOMING																							
Casper	725690	42.92	106.47	5289	12.096	6193	−13	−5	34	30	27	35	35	32	32	9	260	13	240	97	−22	2.2	8.4
Cheyenne, Warren AFB	725640	41.15	104.82	6142	11.714	6193	−7	0	34	29	26	38	36	33	34	10	290	13	290	92	−15	2.2	7.5

WMO = World Meteorological Organization number
Lat. = latitude
Long. = longitude
Elev. = elevation, feet
StdP = standard pressure at station elevation, psia
DB = dry-bulb temperature, °F
WS = wind speed, mph

Heating and Wind Design Conditions—Canada

Selected data from Table 2A, Chapter 26, 1997 *ASHRAE Handbook—Fundamentals*

									Extreme Wind			Coldest Month WS/MDB				MWS/MWD to DB				Annual Extreme Daily			
		Lat.	Long.	Elev.	StdP,		Heating DB		Speed, mph			0.4%		1%		99.6%		0.4%		Mean DB		StdD DB	
	WHO#	Deg. N	Deg. W	ft	psia	Dates	99.6%	99%	1%	2.5%	5%	WS	MDB	WS	MDB	MWS	MWD	MWS	MWD	Max.	Min.	Max.	Min.
ALBERTA																							
Calgary Intl A	718770	51.12	114.02	3556	12.90	6193	−22	−17	28	24	21	32	29	28	27	7	0	11	160	89	−28	2.7	5.6
Edmonton Intl A	711230	53.30	113.58	2372	13.48	6193	−28	−23	24	21	18	24	12	21	11	6	180	9	180	87	−36	3.1	8.1
BRITISH COLUMBIA																							
Vancouver Intl A	718920	49.18	123.17	7	14.69	6193	18	24	22	19	16	25	41	21	42	6	90	7	290	82	14	2.9	6.3
MANITOBA																							
Winnipeg Int'l A	718520	49.90	97.23	784	14.28	6193	−27	−23	29	25	23	30	5	26	5	7	320	13	180	94	−33	3.4	4.7
NEW BRUNSWICK																							
Saint John Airport	716090	45.32	65.88	358	14.51	6193	−9	−4	26	23	20	32	24	28	23	9	340	11	230	84	−18	4.0	4.7
NEWFOUNDLAND																							
St. John's Airport	718010	47.62	52.73	459	14.45	6193	3	7	37	33	29	41	24	37	25	17	290	17	250	82	−2	2.5	4.9
NORTHWEST TERRITORIES																							
Resolute Airport	719240	74.72	94.98	220	14.58	6393	−42	−40	39	34	30	42	−15	37	−18	9	320	12	110	55	−49	3.8	4.9
NOVA SCOTIA																							
Halifax Intl Airport	713950	44.88	63.50	476	14.44	6993	−2	2	27	23	20	30	26	27	26	11	320	12	200	87	−8	2.7	4.3
ONTARIO																							
London A	716230	94805	43.03	912	14.22	6193	−3	2	25	22	20	30	21	26	21	9	250	11	250	90	−11	3.4	5.6
Ottawa Int'l A	716280	45.32	75.67	374	14.50	6193	−13	−8	23	20	17	27	17	23	15	9	290	10	250	91	−19	2.7	5.0
Toronto Int'l A	716240	43.67	79.63	568	14.40	6593	−4	1	26	22	20	29	22	26	23	9	340	12	270	92	−11	2.9	5.6
PRINCE EDWARD ISLAND																							
Charlottetown A	717060	46.28	63.13	177	14.60	6193	−6	−2	24	22	20	35	17	29	18	13	270	12	230	85	−12	2.3	4.7
QUEBEC																							
Montreal Intl A	716270	45.47	73.75	118	14.63	6193	−12	−7	23	20	18	30	19	26	18	7	250	11	230	90	−19	2.3	4.5
Quebec A	717140	46.80	71.38	240	14.57	6193	−16	−11	24	21	19	30	13	26	11	10	250	12	250	89	−23	2.3	4.9
SASKATCHEWAN																							
Regina A	718630	50.43	104.67	1893	13.72	6193	−29	−24	30	27	23	34	8	29	10	9	270	14	180	96	−36	3.6	5.0
Saskatoon	718660	52.17	106.68	1654	13.84	6193	−31	−26	27	23	20	27	12	23	6	7	290	13	180	94	−37	3.8	5.9
YUKON TERRITORY																							
Whitehorse A	719640	60.72	135.07	2306	13.51	6193	−34	−31	23	20	18	28	17	24	15	2	340	8	140	83	−47	4.0	5.9

WMO = World Meteorological Organization number
Lat. = latitude
Long. = longitude
Elev. = elevation, feet
StdP = standard pressure at station elevation, psia
DB = dry-bulb temperature, °F
WS = wind speed, mph

Table 4-7B Cooling and Dehumidification Design Conditions—United States (*Continued*)

Selected data from Table 1B, Chapter 26, 1997 *ASHRAE Handbook—Fundamentals*

	Cooling DB/MWB						WB/MDB						DP/MDB and HR									Range
	0.4%		1%		2%		0.4%		1%		2%		0.4%			1%			2%			
Station	DB	MWB	DB	MWB	DB	MWB	WB	MDB	WB	MDB	WB	MDB	DP	HR	MDB	DP	HR	MDB	DP	HR	MDB	of DB
TEXAS																						
Dallas/Fort Worth, Intl A	100	74	98	74	96	74	78	92	77	91	76	90	75	132	82	74	130	82	73	126	81	20.3
El Paso	101	64	98	64	96	64	70	85	69	84	68	84	67	114	73	65	109	73	64	103	74	28.0
Houston, Intl Airport	96	77	94	77	92	77	80	90	79	89	79	88	78	144	83	77	141	83	76	137	83	18.2
Lubbock Intl Airport	97	67	95	67	93	67	73	87	72	86	71	85	69	120	77	68	115	76	67	111	76	22.1
San Antonio, Intl Airport	98	73	96	73	94	74	78	87	77	87	76	86	76	139	81	75	135	81	74	132	80	19.1
UTAH																						
Ogden, Hill AFB	93	61	90	60	87	60	65	83	64	81	62	81	60	91	72	57	83	73	55	77	73	22.0
Salt Lake City	96	62	94	62	92	61	66	85	65	85	64	85	60	92	73	58	84	73	56	77	73	27.7
VERMONT																						
Burlington	87	71	84	69	82	68	74	83	72	81	70	78	71	115	79	69	109	77	67	102	75	20.4
Montpelier/Barre	85	70	83	68	80	67	72	82	70	80	69	77	69	111	78	67	106	75	66	99	73	21.1
VIRGINIA																						
Norfolk	93	77	91	76	88	75	79	89	77	87	77	85	76	135	83	75	130	82	74	126	81	15.3
Richmond	94	76	92	75	89	74	79	90	78	88	76	86	76	137	84	75	131	82	74	126	81	19.1
Washington, National A	95	76	92	76	89	74	79	89	78	88	76	86	76	137	83	75	132	83	74	127	81	16.6
WASHINGTON																						
Seattle, Intl Airport	85	65	81	64	78	62	66	83	65	79	63	76	60	78	71	59	74	69	57	71	68	18.3
Spokane, Fairchild AFB	92	62	89	61	85	60	65	86	63	84	61	82	57	77	68	55	71	68	53	67	67	26.1
WEST VIRGINIA																						
Charleston	91	73	88	73	86	71	76	86	75	85	74	82	73	129	81	72	123	80	71	118	78	19.1
WISCONSIN																						
Green Bay	88	73	85	72	82	70	76	85	74	82	72	80	73	124	82	71	116	79	69	109	77	20.7
Madison	90	73	87	72	84	70	76	86	74	84	72	82	73	126	83	71	118	80	69	111	78	21.9
Milwaukee	89	74	86	72	83	70	76	86	74	83	72	81	73	127	83	71	119	80	70	111	78	16.6
WYOMING																						
Casper	92	59	89	58	86	58	62	81	61	80	60	79	57	85	66	55	78	66	53	73	65	30.4
Cheyenne, Warren AFB	87	58	85	57	82	57	62	77	61	76	60	75	58	90	66	56	85	65	55	80	64	25.7

MDB = mean coincident dry-bulb temperature, °F
MWB = mean coincident wet-bulb temperature, °F
MWS = mean coincident wind speed, mph
MWD = mean coincident wind direction, °
StdD = standard deviation
A = airport
HR = humidity ratio, grains/lb (dry air)
DP = dew-point temperature, °F

Cooling and Dehumidification Design Conditions—Canada

Selected data from Table 2B, Chapter 26, 1997 *ASHRAE Handbook—Fundamentals*

	Cooling DB/MWB						WB/MDB						DP/MDB and HR									Range
	0.4%		1%		2%		0.4%		1%		2%		0.4%			1%			2%			
Station	DB	MWB	DB	MWB	DB	MWB	WB	MDB	WB	MDB	WB	MDB	DP	HR	MDB	DP	HR	MDB	DP	HR	MDB	of DB
ALBERTA																						
Calgary Intl A	83	60	80	59	77	57	62	78	61	75	59	73	57	79	67	55	74	65	53	69	64	22.0
Edmonton Intl A	82	63	78	62	75	60	66	77	64	75	62	73	62	89	73	59	83	69	57	77	66	21.8
BRITISH COLUMBIA																						
Vancouver Intl A	76	65	74	64	71	62	66	75	64	72	63	70	62	83	71	61	79	70	60	76	68	14.0
MANITOBA																						
Winnipeg Intl A	87	68	84	67	81	66	72	82	70	80	68	78	68	107	78	66	99	75	64	92	73	20.5
NEW BRUNSWICK																						
Saint John A	78	65	75	64	72	62	68	75	66	72	64	69	66	96	71	64	90	69	62	84	66	16.9
NEWFOUNDLAND																						
St. John's A	76	65	73	64	70	63	68	73	66	71	64	68	66	98	71	64	92	69	62	85	67	15.7
NORTHWEST TERRITORIES																						
Resolute A	50	45	48	43	44	41	46	50	43	47	41	44	42	39	47	40	36	45	38	34	43	8.5
NOVA SCOTIA																						
Halifax Intl A	80	68	78	66	75	64	70	77	69	74	67	72	68	106	73	67	99	71	65	95	69	16.7
ONTARIO																						
London A	85	71	83	70	80	69	74	82	72	80	71	77	71	119	79	70	113	77	68	108	75	19.8
Ottawa Intl A	86	70	83	69	80	67	73	82	71	80	69	78	70	112	78	68	106	76	67	99	75	18.5
Toronto Intl A	87	71	84	70	81	68	74	83	72	80	70	78	71	116	79	69	110	77	68	104	75	20.2
PRINCE EDWARD ISLAND																						
Charlottetown A	79	69	77	67	74	65	71	77	69	74	67	72	68	105	75	67	99	72	65	94	71	15.1
QUEBEC																						
Montreal Intl A	85	71	83	70	80	68	74	82	72	80	70	77	70	112	79	69	106	77	67	101	75	17.6
Quebec A	84	70	80	68	78	66	73	80	70	77	68	75	70	111	77	68	103	75	66	95	73	19.1
SASKATCHEWAN																						
Regina A	89	64	85	64	82	62	68	82	66	80	64	78	63	92	75	61	85	71	59	79	69	23.6
Saskatoon	87	64	84	63	80	62	67	81	65	79	63	77	62	88	73	60	82	70	58	76	68	22.7
YUKON TERRITORY																						
Whitehorse A	77	57	73	55	69	53	58	73	56	70	55	67	52	62	61	50	58	59	48	55	58	20.9

MDB = mean coincident dry-bulb temperature, °F
MWB = mean coincident wet-bulb temperature, °F
MWS =mean coincident wind speed, mph
MWD = mean coincident wind direction, °
StdD = standard deviation
A = airport
HR = humidity ratio, grains/lb (dry air)
DP = dew-point temperature, °F

Table 4-8 Average Winter Temperature and Yearly Degree Days

(Table 3.5, ASHRAE Load Calculation Manual)

State	Station		Avg. Winter Temp.,[d] °F	Degree-Days Yearly Total
Ala.	Birmingham	A	54.2	2551
	Huntsville	A	51.3	3070
	Mobile	A	59.9	1560
	Montgomery	A	55.4	2291
Alaska	Anchorage	A	23.0	10864
	Fairbanks	A	6.7	14279
	Juneau	A	32.1	9075
	Nome	A	13.1	14171
Ariz.	Flagstaff	A	35.6	7152
	Phoenix	A	58.5	1765
	Tucson	A	58.1	1800
	Winslow	A	43.0	4782
	Yuma	A	64.2	974
Ark.	Fort Smith	A	50.3	3292
	Little Rock	A	50.5	3219
	Texarkana	A	54.2	2533
Calif.	Bakersfield	A	55.4	2122
	Bishop	A	46.0	4275
	Blue Canyon	A	42.2	5596
	Burbank	A	58.6	1646
	Eureka	C	49.9	4643
	Fresno	A	53.3	2611
	Long Beach	A	57.8	1803
	Los Angeles	A	57.4	2061
	Los Angeles	C	60.3	1349
	Mt. Shasta	C	41.2	5722
	Oakland	A	53.5	2870
	Red Bluff	A	53.8	2515
	Sacramento	A	53.9	2502
	Sacramento	C	54.4	2419
	Sandberg	C	46.8	4209
	San Diego	A	59.5	1458
	San Francisco	A	53.4	3015
	San Francisco	C	55.1	3001
	Santa Maria	A	54.3	2967
Colo.	Alamosa	A	29.7	8529
	Colorado Springs	A	37.3	6423
	Denver	A	37.6	6283
	Denver	C	40.8	5524
	Grand Junction	A	39.3	5641
	Pueblo	A	40.4	5462
Conn.	Bridgeport	A	39.9	5617
	Hartford	A	37.3	6235
	New Haven	A	39.0	5897
Del.	Wilmington	A	42.5	4930
D.C.	Washington	A	45.7	4224
Fla.	Apalachicola	C	61.2	1308
	Daytona Beach	A	64.5	879
	Fort Myers	A	68.6	442
	Jacksonville	A	61.9	1239
	Key West	A	73.1	108
	Lakeland	C	66.7	661
	Miami	A	71.1	214
	Miami Beach	C	72.5	141
Fla. (*Cont'd*)	Orlando	A	65.7	766
	Pensacola	A	60.4	1463
	Tallahassee	A	60.1	1485
	Tampa	A	66.4	683
	West Palm Beach	A	68.4	253
Ga.	Athens	A	51.8	2929
	Atlanta	A	51.7	2961
	Augusta	A	54.5	2397
	Columbus	A	54.8	2383
	Macon	A	56.2	2136
	Rome	A	49.9	3326
	Savannah	A	57.8	1819
	Thomasville	C	60.0	1529
Hawaii	Lihue	A	72.7	0
	Honolulu	A	74.2	0
	Hilo	A	71.9	0
Idaho	Boise	A	39.7	5809
	Lewiston	A	41.0	5542
	Pocatello	A	34.8	7033
Ill.	Cairo	C	47.9	3821
	Chicago (O'Hare)	A	35.8	6639
	Chicago (Midway)	A	37.5	6155
	Chicago	C	38.9	5882
	Moline	A	36.4	6408
	Peoria	A	38.1	6025
	Rockford	A	34.8	6830
	Springfield	A	40.6	5429
Ind.	Evansville	A	45.0	4435
	Fort Wayne	A	37.3	6205
	Indianapolis	A	39.6	5699
	South Bend	A	36.6	6439
Iowa	Burlington	A	37.6	6114
	Des Moines	A	35.5	6588
	Dubuque	A	32.7	7376
	Sioux City	A	34.0	6951
	Waterloo	A	32.6	7320
Kans.	Concordia	A	40.4	5479
	Dodge City	A	42.5	4986
	Goodland	A	37.8	6141
	Topeka	A	41.7	5182
	Wichita	A	44.2	4620
Ky.	Covington	A	41.4	5265
	Lexington	A	43.8	4683
	Louisville	A	44.0	4660
La.	Alexandria	A	57.5	1921
	Baton Rouge	A	59.8	1560
	Lake Charles	A	60.5	1459
	New Orleans	A	61.0	1385
	New Orleans	C	61.8	1254
	Shreveport	A	56.2	2184
Me.	Caribou	A	24.4	9767
	Portland	A	33.0	7511

[a]Data for United States cities from a publication of the United States Weather Bureau, *Monthly Normals of Temperature, Precipitation and Heating Degree Days*, 1962, are for the period 1931 to 1960 inclusive. These data also include information from the 1963 revisions to this publication, where available.

[b]Data for airport station, A, and city stations, C, are both given where available.

[c]Data for Canadian cities were computed by the Climatology Division, Department of Transport from normal monthly mean temperatures, and the monthly values of heating days data were obtained using the National Research Council computer and a method devised by H.C.S. Thom of the United States Weather Bureau. The heating days are based on the period from 1931 to 1960.

[d]For period October to April, inclusive.

Table 4-8 Average Winter Temperature and Yearly Degree Days (*Continued*)
(Table 3.5, ASHRAE Load Calculation Manual)

State	Station		Avg. Winter Temp.,[d] °F	Degree-Days Yearly Total
Md.	Baltimore	A	43.7	4654
	Baltimore	C	46.2	4111
	Frederick	A	42.0	5087
Mass.	Boston	A	40.0	5634
	Nantucket	A	40.2	5891
	Pittsfield	A	32.6	7578
	Worcester	A	34.7	6969
Mich.	Alpena	A	29.7	8506
	Detroit (City)	A	37.2	6232
	Detroit (Wayne)	A	37.1	6293
	Detroit (Willow Run)	A	37.2	6258
	Escanaba	C	29.6	8481
	Flint	A	33.1	7377
	Grand Rapids	A	34.9	6894
	Lansing	A	34.8	6909
	Marquette	C	30.2	8393
	Muskegon	A	36.0	6696
	Sault Ste. Marie	A	27.7	9048
Minn.	Duluth	A	23.4	10000
	Minneapolis	A	28.3	8382
	Rochester	A	28.8	8295
Miss.	Jackson	A	55.7	2239
	Meridian	A	55.4	2289
	Vicksburg	C	56.9	2041
Mo.	Columbia	A	42.3	5046
	Kansas	A	43.9	4711
	St. Joseph	A	40.3	5484
	St. Louis	A	43.1	4900
	St. Louis	C	44.8	4484
	Springfield	A	44.5	4900
Mont.	Billings	A	34.5	7049
	Glasgow	A	26.4	8996
	Great Falls	A	32.8	7750
	Havre	A	28.1	8700
	Havre	C	29.8	8182
	Helena	A	31.1	8129
	Kalispell	A	31.4	8191
	Miles City	A	31.2	7723
	Missoula	A	31.5	8125
Neb.	Grand Island	A	36.0	6530
	Lincoln	C	38.8	5864
	Norfolk	A	34.0	6979
	North Platte	A	35.5	6684
	Omaha	A	35.6	6612
	Scottsbluff	A	35.9	6673
	Valentine	A	32.6	7425
Nev.	Elko	A	34.0	7433
	Ely	A	33.1	7733
	Las Vegas	A	53.3	2709
	Reno	A	39.3	6332
	Winnemucca	A	36.7	6761
N.H.	Concord	A	33.0	7383
	Mt. Washington Obsv.		15.2	13817
N.J.	Atlantic City	A	43.2	4812
	Newark	A	42.8	4589
	Trenton	C	42.4	4980
N.M.	Albuquerque	A	45.0	4348
	Clayton	A	42.0	5158
	Raton	A	38.1	6228
	Roswell	A	47.5	3793
	Silver City	A	48.0	3705
N.Y.	Albany	A	34.6	6875
	Ablany	C	37.2	6201
	Binghamton	A	33.9	7286
	Binghamton	C	36.6	6451
	Buffalo	A	34.5	7062
N.Y. (*Cont'd*)	New York (Cent. Park)	C	42.8	4871
	New York (La Guardia)	A	43.1	4811
	New York (Kennedy)	A	41.4	5219
	Rochester	A	35.4	6748
	Schenectady	C	35.4	6650
	Syracuse	A	35.2	6756
N.C.	Asheville	C	46.7	4042
	Cape Hatterns		53.3	2612
	Charlotte	A	50.4	3191
	Greensboro	A	47.5	3805
	Raleigh	A	49.4	3393
	Wilmington	A	54.6	2347
	Winston-Salem	A	48.4	3595
N.D.	Bismarck	A	26.6	8851
	Devils Lake	C	22.4	9901
	Fargo	A	24.8	9226
	Williston	A	25.2	9243
Ohio	Akron-Canton	A	38.1	6037
	Cincinnati	C	45.1	4410
	Cleveland	A	37.2	6351
	Columbus	A	39.7	5660
	Columbus	C	41.5	5211
	Dayton	A	39.8	5622
	Mansfield	A	36.9	6403
	Sandusky	C	39.1	5796
	Toledo	A	36.4	6494
	Youngstown	A	36.8	6417
Okla.	Oklahoma City	A	48.3	3725
	Tulsa	A	47.7	3860
Ore.	Astoria	A	45.6	5186
	Burns	C	35.9	6957
	Eugene	A	45.6	4726
	Meacham	A	34.2	7874
	Medford	A	43.2	5008
	Pendleton	A	42.6	5127
	Portland	A	45.6	4635
	Portland	C	47.4	4109
	Roseburg	A	46.3	4491
	Salem	A	45.4	4486
Pa.	Allentown	A	38.9	5810
	Erie	A	36.8	6451
	Harrisburg	A	41.2	5251
	Philadelphia	A	41.8	5144
	Philadelphia	C	44.5	4486
	Pittsburgh	A	38.4	5987
	Pittsburgh	C	42.2	5053
	Reading	C	42.4	4945
	Scranton	A	37.2	6254
	Williamsport	A	38.5	5934
R.I.	Block Island	A	40.1	5804
	Providence	A	38.8	5954
S.C.	Charleston	A	56.4	2033
	Charleston	C	57.9	1794
	Columbia	A	54.0	2484
	Florence	A	54.5	2387
	Greenville-Spartenburg	A	51.6	2980
S.D	Huron	A	28.8	8223
	Rapid City	A	33.4	7345
	Sioux Falls	A	30.6	7839
Tenn.	Bristol	A	46.2	4143
	Chattanooga	A	50.3	3254
	Knoxville	A	49.2	3494
	Memphis	A	50.5	3232
	Memphis	C	51.6	3015
	Nashville	A	48.9	3578
	Oak Ridge	C	47.7	3817
Tex.	Abilene	A	53.9	2624
	Amarillo	A	47.0	3985
	Austin	A	59.1	1711
	Brownsville	A	67.7	600

Table 4-8 Average Winter Temperature and Yearly Degree Days (*Continued*)
(Table 3.5, ASHRAE Load Calculation Manual)

State	Station		Avg. Winter Temp.,[d] °F	Degree-Days Yearly Total
Tex. (*Cont'd*)	Corpus Christi	A	64.6	914
	Dallas	A	55.3	2363
	El Paso	A	52.9	2700
	Fort Worth	A	55.1	2405
	Galveston	A	62.2	1274
	Galveston	C	62.0	1235
	Houston	A	61.0	1396
	Houston	C	62.0	1278
	Laredo	A	66.0	797
	Lubbock	A	48.8	3578
	Midland	A	53.8	2591
	Port Arthur	A	60.5	1447
	San Angelo	A	56.0	2255
	San Antonio	A	60.1	1546
	Victoria	A	62.7	1173
	Waco	A	57.2	2030
	Wichita Falls	A	53.0	2832
Utah	Milford	A	36.5	6497
	Salt Lake City	A	38.4	6052
	Wendover	A	39.1	5778
Vt.	Burlington	A	29.4	8269
Va.	Cape Henry	C	50.0	3279
	Lynchburg	A	46.0	4166
	Norfolk	A	49.2	3421
	Richmond	A	47.3	3865
	Roanoke	A	46.1	4150
Wash.	Olympia	A	44.2	5236
	Seattle-Tacoma	A	44.2	5145
	Seattle	C	46.9	4424
	Spokane	A	36.5	6655
	Walla Walla	C	43.8	4805
	Yakima	A	39.1	5941
W.Va.	Charleston	A	44.8	4476
	Elkins	A	40.1	5675
	Huntington	A	45.0	4446
	Parkersburg	C	43.5	4754
Wisc.	Green Bay	A	30.3	8029
	La Crosse	A	31.5	7589
	Madison	A	30.9	7863
	Milwaukee	A	32.6	7635
Wyo.	Casper	A	33.4	7410
	Cheyenne	A	34.2	7381
	Lander	A	31.4	7870
	Sheridan	A	32.5	7680

Province	Station		Avg. Winter Temp.,[d] °F	Degree-Days Yearly Total
Alta.	Banff	C	—	10551
	Calgary	A	—	9703
	Edmonton	A	—	10268
	Lethbridge	A	—	8644
B.C.	Kamloops	A	—	6799
	Prince George*	A	—	9755
	Prince Rupert	C	—	7029
	Vancouver*	A	—	5515
	Victoria*	A	—	5699
	Victoria	C	—	5579
Man.	Brandon*	A	—	11036
	Churchill	A	—	16728
	The Pas	C	—	12281
	Winnipeg	A	—	10679
N.B.	Fredericton*	A	—	8671
	Moncton	C	—	8727
	St. John	C	—	8219
Nfld.	Argentia	A	—	8440
	Corner Brook	C	—	8978
	Gander	A	—	9254
	Goose*	A	—	11887
	St. John's*	A	—	8991
N.W.T.	Aklavik	C	—	18017
	Fort Norman	C	—	16109
	Resolution Island	C	—	16021
N.S.	Halifax	C	—	7361
	Sydney	A	—	8049
	Yarmouth	A	—	7340
Ont.	Cochrane	C	—	11412
	Fort William	A	—	10405
	Kapuskasing	C	—	11572
	Kitchner	C	—	7566
	London	A	—	7349
	North Bay	C	—	9219
	Ottawa	C	—	8735
	Toronto	C	—	6827
P.E.I.	Charlottertown	C	—	8164
	Summerside	C	—	8488
Que.	Arvida	C	—	10528
	Montreal*	A	—	8203
	Montreal	C	—	7899
	Quebec*	A	—	9372
	Quebec	C	—	8937
Sasks	Prince Albert	A	—	11630
	Regina	A	—	10806
	Saskatoon	C	—	10870
Y.T.	Dawson	C	—	15067
	Mayo Landing	C	—	14454

*The data for these normals were from the full 10-year period 1951-60, adjusted for the standard journal period 1931-1960.

Table 4-9 Equivalent Wind Chill Temperatures

(Table 11, Chapter 8, 1997 *ASHRAE Handbook—Fundamentals*)

Wind Speed, mph	Actual Thermometer Reading, °F											
	50	40	30	20	10	0	−10	−20	−30	−40	−50	−60
	Equivalent Chill Temperature, °F											
0	50	40	30	20	10	0	−10	−20	−30	−40	−50	−60
5	48	37	27	16	6	−5	−15	−26	−36	−47	−57	−68
10	40	28	16	3	−9	−21	−34	−46	−58	−71	−83	−95
15	36	22	9	−5	−18	−32	−45	−59	−72	−86	−99	−113
20	32	18	4	−11	−25	−39	−53	−68	−82	−96	−110	−125
25	30	15	0	−15	−30	−44	−59	−74	−89	−104	−119	−134
30	28	13	−3	−18	−33	−48	−64	−79	−94	−110	−125	−140
35	27	11	−4	−20	−36	−51	−67	−83	−98	−114	−129	−145
40	26	10	−6	−22	−38	−53	−69	−85	−101	−117	−133	−148

Little danger	Increasing danger	Great danger
Little danger: In less than 5 h, with dry skin. Maximum danger from false sense of security. (WCI less than 1400)	**Increasing danger:** Danger of freezing exposed flesh within one minute. (WCI between 1400 and 2000)	**Great danger:** Flesh may freeze within 30 seconds. (WCI greater than 2000)

Notes: Cooling power of environment expressed as an equivalent temperature under calm conditions [Equation (79)].

Winds greater than 43 mph have little added chilling effect.

Source: U.S. Army Research Institute of Environmental Medicine.

4.3 Other Factors Affecting Design

In the interest of energy conservation, new buildings used primarily for human occupancy must meet certain minimum design requirements that enable the efficient use of energy in such new buildings. ASHRAE/IES *Standard* 90.1, "Energy Efficient Design of New Buildings Except New Low-Rise Residential Buildings," has been widely adopted. In fact, the U. S. Energy Policy Act of 1992 requires that each state have energy policies in place that require buildings to conform, on the minimum, to Standard 90.1. Related to design conditions, Standard 90.1 contains such statements as:

"Indoor design temperature and humidity conditions for general comfort applications shall be in accordance with the comfort criteria established in ANSI/ASHRAE *Standard* 55."

"Outdoor design conditions shall be selected from the ASHRAE Handbook... Heating design temperatures shall be no lower than the temperatures listed in the 99% column or statistically similar 0.2% annualized value. Cooling design temperatures shall be no greater than the temperature listed in the 2.5% column or statistically similar 0.5% annualized value."

"If a system is equipped with a means of adding moisture to maintain specific humidity levels in a zone or zones, a humidistat shall be provided. This device shall be capable of being set to prevent the use of fossil fuel or electricity to produce relative humidities in excess of 30% for comfort purposes. Where a humidistat is used for comfort dehumidification, it shall be capable of being set to prevent the use of fossil fuel or electricity to reduce relative humidities below 60%."

Although a heating or cooling system is sized to meet design conditions, it usually functions at only partial capacity. The proper use and application of controls should receive primary consideration at the time the heating or cooling system is being designed. Control devices that produce almost any degree of control required can be used, but it is useless to provide such controls unless the air-conditioning system is capable of properly responding to the demands of the controllers. For example, it is impossible to maintain close control of temperature and humidity by starting and stopping a refrigeration compressor or by opening and closing a refrigerant valve. Instead, refrigeration equipment that permits proportional control, or a chilled-water system with a cooling coil or spray dehumidifier that permits proportional control, must be used. It is neither economical nor good practice to select equipment capable of producing far more precise control than the application requires, or to complicate the system to obtain special sequences or cycles of operation when they are not necessary. Because the system must be adjusted and maintained in operation for many years, the simplest system which produces the necessary results is usually the best.

Another factor at least as important as comfort, first cost, and owning and operating cost, is the application coefficient, which includes such factors as:

- flexibility for change
- suitability for all spaces
- appearance of completed building
- special requirements of project
- income potential
- durability, reliability, and serviceability
- fire and smoke control
- pollution control

Example 4-3: Select appropriate summer and winter, indoor and outdoor, design temperatures and humidities for an office building near the Philadelphia International Airport, Pennsylvania.

Solution:

Based upon *Standard* 90.1 (no lower than 0.2% annualized value winter and no greater than 0.5% annualized value for summer) and the climatic data of Table 4.7, the *outdoor design values* are:

SUMMER: 89°F db and 74°F wb (1% values)
WINTER: 11°F (0.4% value) and 100% rh

Based upon Standard 90.1 and using the limits of the comfort envelope of Standard 55, the selected *indoor design values* are:

SUMMER: 78°F db, 60% rh
WINTER: 72°F db, 30% rh

4.4 Temperatures in Adjacent Unconditioned Spaces

The heat loss or gain between conditioned rooms and unconditioned rooms or spaces must be based on the estimated or assumed temperature in such unconditioned spaces. This temperature normally lies in the range between the indoor and outdoor temperatures. The temperature in the unconditioned space may be estimated by:

$$\begin{aligned} t_u = & [\, t_i(A_1U_1 + A_2U_2 + \ldots + \text{etc.}) \\ & + t_o(KV_o + A_aU_a + A_bU_b + \ldots + \text{etc.})] \\ & \div ([\, (A_1U_1 + A_2U_2 + \ldots + \text{etc.})) \\ & + (KV_o + A_aU_a + A_bU_b + \ldots + \text{etc.})] \end{aligned} \tag{4-6}$$

where

t_u = temperature in unheated space, °F (°C)
t_i = indoor design temperature of heated room, °F (°C)
t_o = outdoor design temperature, °F (°C)
A_1, A_2, etc. = areas of surface of unheated space adjacent to heated space, ft^2 (m^2)
A_a, A_b, etc. = areas of surface of unheated space exposed to outdoors, ft^2 (m^2)
U_1, U_2, etc. = heat transfer coefficients of surfaces of A_1, A_2, etc., Btu/h· ft^2·°F (W/(m^2· °C))
U_a, U_b, etc = heat transfer coefficients of surfaces of A_a, A_b, etc. Btu/h· ft^2· °F (W/(m^2· °C))
V_o = rate of introduction of outside air into the unheated space by infiltration and/or ventilation, cfm (L/s)
K = 1.10 (1200)

Reasonable accuracy for ordinary unconditioned spaces may be attained if the following approximations for adjacent rooms are used:

1. Cooling with adjacent unconditioned room. Select for computation a temperature equal to $t_i + 0.667(t_o - t_i)$ in the unconditioned space.
2. Heating with adjacent room unheated. Select for computation a temperature equal to $t_i - 0.50(t_i - t_o)$ in the unconditioned space.

Temperatures in unconditioned spaces having large glass areas and two or more surfaces exposed to the outdoors (such as sleeping porches or sun parlors) and/or large amounts of infiltration (such as garages with poor fitting doors) are generally assumed to be that of the outdoors.

Example 4-4: Calculate the temperature in an unheated space adjacent to a conditioned room with three common surface areas of 100, 120, and 140 ft^2 and overall heat transfer coefficients of 0.15, 0.20, and 0.25 Btu/h·ft^2·°F, respectively. The surface areas of the unheated space exposed to the outdoors are 100 and 140 ft^2 with corresponding overall heat transfer coefficients are 0.10 and 0.30 Btu/h·ft^2·°F. The sixth surface is on the ground and can be neglected for this example as can be the effect of any outdoor air entering the space. Inside and outside design temperatures are 70°F and −10°F, respectively.

Solution:
Substituting into Eq. 4-6,

$$\begin{aligned} t_u = & [70(100 \times 0.15 + 120 \times 0.20 + 140 \times 0.25) \\ & + (-10)(100 \times 0.10 + 140 \times 0.30)]/ \\ & [100 \times 0.15 + 120 \times 0.20 + 140 \times 0.25 \\ & + 100 \times 0.10 + 140 \times 0.30] \\ = & 4660/126 = 37°\text{F} \end{aligned}$$

4.5 Problems

4.1 Describe the various processes of heat transfer involved in maintaining heat balance between the human body and the surrounding space.

4.2 Solve the following:
(a) What single factor governs most specifications of outdoor air ratio?
(b) How does the fresh air rate vary with the allowable air space per person?
(c) What are typical outdoor air rates for large air spaces? for small (<100 ft^3 per person) air spaces?

4.3 Solve the following:
(a) What factors affect the temperature and humidity required for comfort?
(b) Of what is "effective temperature" (ET*) a function?
(c) What are the criteria on which the values given on the ET* chart are based?

4.4 How must the ASHRAE Comfort Chart Data be altered for (a) women, (b) older people, (c) people in warm climates, and (d) hot or cold radiative walls or windows?

4.5 What are the disadvantages of specifying a high humidity? A low humidity? Answer with respect to both equipment and room occupancy consideration. What are recommended limits of humidity?

4.6 For an office building in St. Louis, Missouri, the inside dry-bulb temperature is maintained at 24°C (75°F) during the summer. What is the maximum allowable humidity ratio consistent with the ASHRAE Comfort Standard?
[Ans: 0.012]

4.7 A person reclining nude would probably consider which of the following interior environments comfortable?

(a) $t = 78°F$; $\phi = 50\%$; 25 fpm; MRT = 78°F
(b) $t = 75°F$; $\phi = 10\%$; 25 fpm; MRT = 75°F
(c) $t = 75°F$; $\phi = 70\%$; 30 fpm; MRT = 82°F
(d) $t = 80°F$; $\phi = 50\%$; 20 fpm; MRT = 80°F

(e) $t = 90°F$; $\phi = 20\%$; 30 fpm; MRT = 80°F
(f) $t = 70°F$; $\phi = 70\%$; 20 fpm; MRT = 70°F

4.8 For the person in Problem 4.7 (5 ft, 5 in., 120 lb), compute the body surface area (ft^2).

4.9 Compute your body surface area based on the DuBois formula and estimate your current rate of dry heat exchange with the surroundings.

4.10 From weather data, estimate the lowest equivalent wind chill temperature which will be exceeded 22 h per year for the following locations:
(a) Barrow, Alaska
(b) Los Angeles, California
(c) Denver, Colorado
(d) New Haven, Connecticut
(e) Rochester, Minnesota
(f) Manhattan, Kansas

4.11 Specify comfortable environments for the following space usage:
(a) senior citizens retirement home in Florida
(b) gymnasium in Missouri
(c) office building in Colorado
(d) residence in Nevada

4.12 The living room in a home is occupied by adults at rest wearing medium clothing. The mean radiant temperature is 18°C (64°F). Determine the air temperature necessary for comfort. [Ans: 30°C (86°F)]

4.13 A room has a net outside wall area of 275 ft^2 with a surface temperature of 54°F, 45 ft^2 of glass with a surface temperature of 20°F, 540 ft^2 of ceiling with a surface temperature of 60°F, 670 ft^2 of partitions with a surface temperature of 70°F, and 540 ft^2 of floor with a surface temperature of 70°F. If the air movement is 20 fpm and light clothing is being worn, determine the air temperature necessary for comfort.

4.14 Workers on an assembly line making electronic equipment dissipate 700 Btu/h, of which 310 Btu/h is latent heat. When the MRT for the area is 69°F, what air temperature must the heating system maintain for comfort of the workers if the air movement is 40 fpm?

4.15 A room has 1000 ft^2 of surface, of which 120 ft^2 is to be heated, and the balance has an average surface temperature of 60°F. The air temperature in the room is 68°F. The room is occupied by light clothed adults at rest. Determine the surface temperature of the heated panel necessary to produce comfort if the air velocity is 20 fpm.
[Ans: 243°F ? unfeasible]

4.16 Assume that in *Problem* 4.15, the maximum allowable panel temperature is 120°F. The average temperature of other surfaces in the room remains at 60°F and the air temperature is still 68°F. What panel area will be required if the room is occupied by adults at rest?

4.17 In an auditorium, 17,150 students are watching slides. The MRT is 80°F and the average room air temperature is 72°F. Air enters the room at 57°F. Assume the lights are out and no heat gain or loss occurs through the walls, floor, and ceiling.
(a) How much air (cfm) should be supplied to remove the sensible heat?
(b) Explain what must be done to remove the latent heat.

4.18 Two hundred people attend a theater matinee. Air is supplied at 60°F. Determine the required flow rate (lb/h) to handle the heat gain from the occupants if the return air temperature is not to exceed 75°F.

4.19 A meeting room designed to accommodate 25 people who smoke heavily is 6 m by 12 m by 2.4 m high. Specify the minimum outdoor air requirement in L/s.

4.20 Determine the increase in humidity ratio due to 80 people in a dance hall if air is circulated at the rate of 0.64 m^3/s (1350 cfm).

4.21 Specify the MRT for comfort in a space where the air temperature is 68°F and the relative velocity is 20 fpm, for medium activity and light clothing. [Ans: 92°F]

4.22 Specify completely a suitable set of indoor and outdoor design conditions for each of the following cases:
(a) winter; apartment building; St. Louis, Missouri
(b) summer; apartment building; St. Louis, Missouri
(c) winter; factory (medium activity); Rochester, Minnesota
(d) summer; $250,000 residence; Chicago, Illinois
(e) winter; $70,000 residence; Chicago, Illinois

4.23 The mean radiant temperature in a bus is 6°C lower in winter than the air temperature. For passengers seated without coats, determine the desired air temperature if the relative air velocity is 0.2 m/s.

4.24 For Atlanta, Georgia, specify the normal indoor design conditions listed below for:

(a) Winter: Dry bulb = _____ °C; W = _______ kg/kg

(b) Summer: Dry bulb = _____ °C; W = _______ kg/kg

4.25 Specify completely indoor and outdoor design conditions for both summer and winter for a clean room in Kansas City, Missouri, having a 1.2 m by 1.2 m radiant panel at 49°C on each of the four walls. The room is 6 m by 4 m by 3 m high and the other surfaces are all at 22°C. Assume very little activity and light clothing.

4.6 Bibliography

ASHRAE. 1995. *Applications Handbook*.

ASHRAE. 1992. Thermal environmental conditions for human occupancy. *Standard* 55-1992.

ASHRAE. 1989. Energy-efficient design of new buildings except low-rise residential buildings. *Standard* 90.1-1989.

ASHRAE. 1992. Energy-efficient design of new low-rise residential buildings. *Standard* 90.2-1992.

SI Tables and Figures

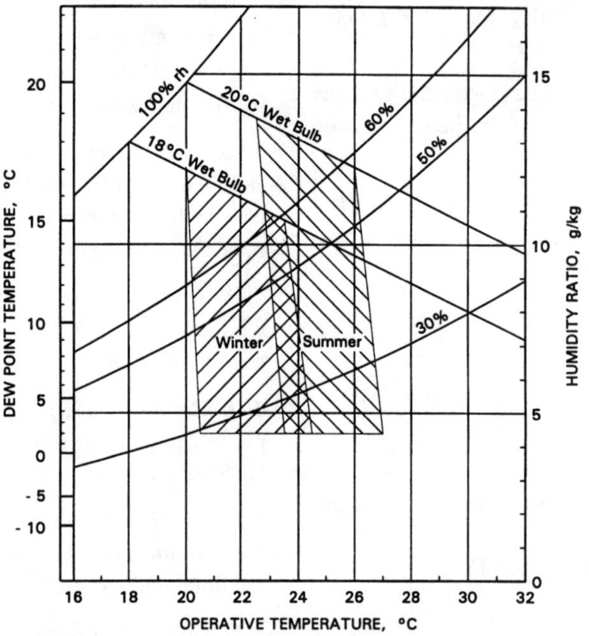

Fig. 4-2 SI ASHRAE Summer and Winter Comfort Zones

(Acceptable ranges of operative temperature and humidity for people in typical summer and winter clothing during primarily sedentary activity.)

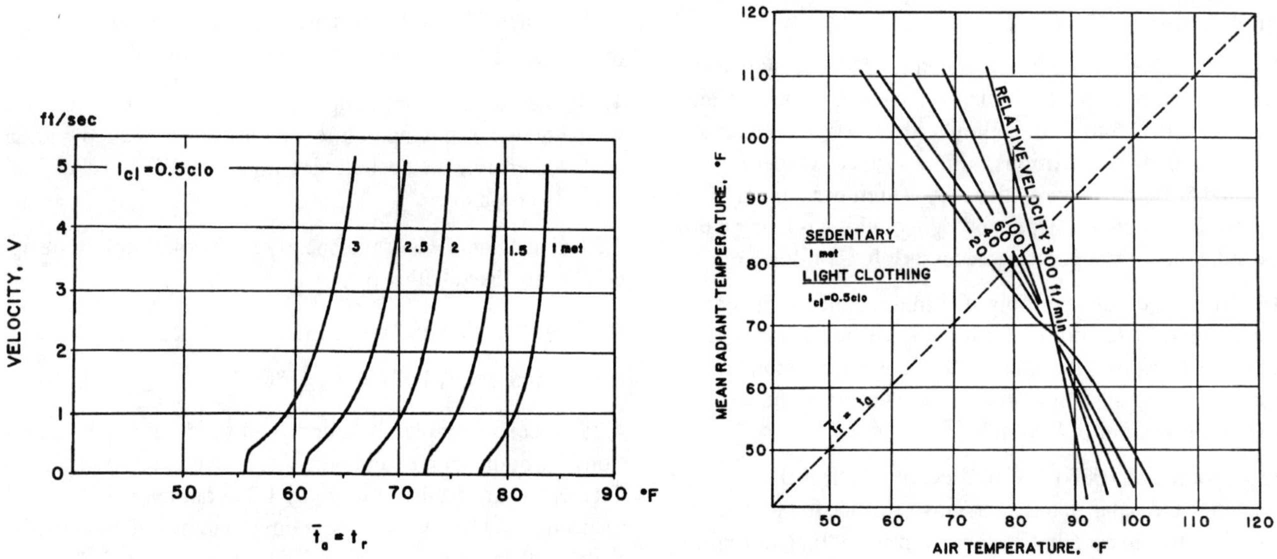

Fig. 4-3 SI Examples of Fanger's Charts

(Figs. 10 & 11, Chapter 8, 1997 ASHRAE Handbook—Fundamentals)

Table 4-1 SI Equations for Prediction Thermal Sensation (Y)[a,b]

Exposure Period, h	Sex	Regression Equations t = dry-bulb temperature, °C p = vapor pressure, kPa
	Male	$Y = 0.220\,t + 0.233\,p - 5.673$
1.0	Female	$Y = 0.272\,t + 0.248\,p - 7.245$
	Combined	$Y = 0.245\,t + 0.248\,p - 6.475$
	Male	$Y = 0.221\,t + 0.270\,p - 6.024$
2.0	Female	$Y = 0.283\,t + 0.210\,p - 7.694$
	Combined	$Y = 0.252\,t + 0.240\,p - 6.859$
	Male	$Y = 0.212\,t + 0.293\,p - 5.949$
3.0	Female	$Y = 0.275\,t + 0.255\,p - 8.622$
	Combined	$Y = 0.243\,t + 0.278\,p - 6.802$

[a] Y values refer to the ASHRAE thermal sensation scale.
[b] For young adult subjects with sedentary activity and wearing clothing with a thermal resistance of approximately 0.5 clo, $\bar{t}_r \approx \bar{t}_a$ and air velocities are < 0.2 m/s.

Table 4-9 SI Equivalent Wind Chill Temperatures[a]

(Table 11, Chapter 8, 1997 *ASHRAE Handbook—Fundamentals*)

Wind Speed, km/h	Actual Thermometer Reading, °C												
	10	5	0	−5	−10	−15	−20	−25	−30	−35	−40	−45	−50
	Equivalent Chill Temperature, °C												
Calm	10	5	0	−5	−10	−15	−20	−25	−30	−35	−40	−45	−50
10	8	2	−3	−9	−14	−20	−25	−31	−37	−42	−48	−53	−59
20	3	−3	−10	−16	−23	−29	−35	−42	−48	−55	−61	−68	−74
30	1	−6	−13	−20	−27	−34	−42	−49	−56	−63	−70	−77	−84
40	−1	−8	−16	−23	−31	−38	−46	−53	−60	−68	−75	−83	−90
50	−2	−10	−18	−25	−33	−41	−48	−56	−64	−71	−79	−87	−94
60	−3	−11	−19	−27	−35	−42	−50	−58	−66	−74	−82	−90	−97
70	−4	−12	−20	−28	−35	−43	−51	−59	−67	−75	−83	−91	−99

Little danger	Increasing danger	Great danger
Little danger: In less than 5 h, with dry skin. Maximum danger from false sense of security. (WCI less than 1400)	**Increasing danger:** Danger of freezing exposed flesh within one minute. (WCI between 1400 and 2000)	**Great danger:** Flesh may freeze within 30 seconds. (WCI greater than 2000)

Note: Cooling power of environment expressed as an equivalent temperature under calm conditions [Equation (79)].

Winds greater than 70 km/h have little added chilling effect.

Source: U.S. Army Research Institute of Environmental Medicine.

Chapter 5

LOAD ESTIMATING FUNDAMENTALS

In this chapter, the fundamental elements that accompany the load calculations for sizing heating and cooling systems are presented. The material includes the estimation of outside air quantities and the evaluation of the overall coefficient of heat transfer for building components. Chapters 22 through 25 of the 1997 *ASHRAE Handbook—Fundamentals* and the *ASHRAE Cooling and Heating Load Calculation Manual* are the major sources of information.

5.1 General Considerations

The basic components of heating and cooling loads are illustrated in Figure 5-1.

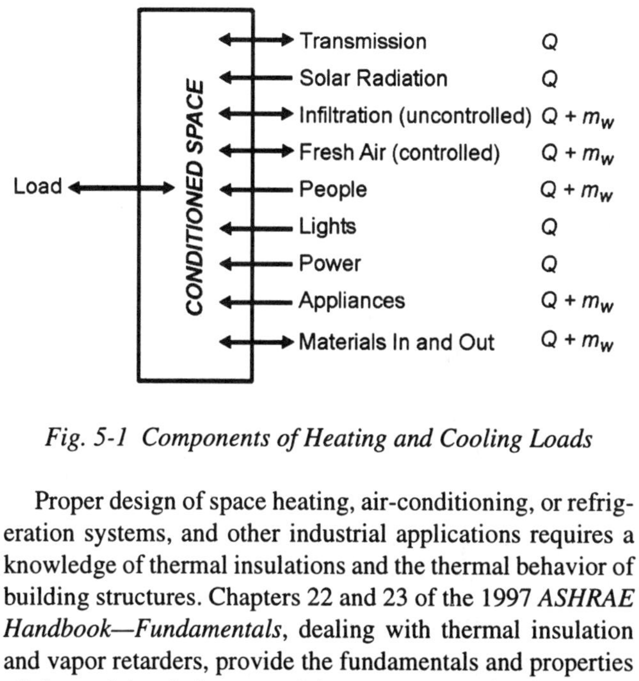

Fig. 5-1 Components of Heating and Cooling Loads

Proper design of space heating, air-conditioning, or refrigeration systems, and other industrial applications requires a knowledge of thermal insulations and the thermal behavior of building structures. Chapters 22 and 23 of the 1997 *ASHRAE Handbook—Fundamentals*, dealing with thermal insulation and vapor retarders, provide the fundamentals and properties of thermal insulating materials, water vapor barriers, economic thickness of insulation, general practices for building and industrial insulation, and the insulating of mobile equipment and environmental spaces.

Flowing fluids such as air, water, and refrigerants are used in heating, ventilating, air-conditioning, and refrigeration systems to carry heat or mass. An understanding of fluid flow and the nature of its mechanisms is vital to engineers working in these fields. Chapter 2, Fluid Flow, of the 1997 *ASHRAE Handbook—Fundamentals* introduces the principles of fluid mechanics relevant to these processes.

Heating or cooling air involves only heat transfer, resulting in a temperature change of the air. However, in a true air-conditioning process, there is a simultaneous transfer of heat and mass (water vapor). Chapter 5 of the 1997 *ASHRAE Handbook—Fundamentals* presents the elementary principles of mass transfer to provide a basic understanding of the air-conditioning processes involving mass transfer.

The humidification or dehumidification load depends primarily on the ventilation rate of the space to be conditioned, but other sources of moisture gain or loss should be considered. Chapter 6, Psychrometrics, of the 1997 *ASHRAE Handbook—Fundamentals* contains equations and examples for determining loads and energy requirements associated with humidification or dehumidification.

5.2 Outdoor Air Load Components

5.2.1 Basic Concepts

Outdoor air that flows through a building is often used to dilute and remove indoor air contaminants. However, the energy required to condition this outdoor air can be a significant portion of the total space-conditioning load. The magnitude of the outdoor airflow into the building must be known for proper sizing of the HVAC equipment and evaluation of energy consumption. For buildings without mechanical cooling and dehumidification, proper ventilation and infiltration airflows are important for providing comfort for occupants.

A conditioned space may be ventilated by natural infiltration, alone or in combination with intentional mechanical ventilation. Natural infiltration varies with indoor-outdoor temperature difference, wind velocity, and the tightness of the construction, as discussed in Chapter 25, Ventilation and Infiltration, of the 1997 *ASHRAE Handbook—Fundamentals*. Related information is presented in Chapter 15, Airflow Around Buildings, of the 1997 *ASHRAE Handbook—Fundamentals*.

Air exchange of outdoor air with the air already in a building can be divided into two broad classifications: ventilation and infiltration. **Ventilation** is the intentional introduction of air from the outside into a building; it is further subdivided into natural ventilation and forced ventilation. **Natural ventilation** is the intentional flow of air through open windows, doors, grilles, and other planned building envelope penetrations, and it is drive by natural and/or artificially produced pressure differentials. **Forced ventilation** is the intentional movement of air into and out of a building using fans and intake and exhaust vents; it is also called **mechanical ventilation**.

Infiltration is the uncontrolled flow of outdoor air into a building through cracks and other unintentional openings and through the normal use of exterior doors for entrance and egress. Infiltration is also known as **air leakage** into a building. **Exfiltration** is the leakage of indoor air out of a building. Like natural ventilation, infiltration and exfiltration are driven by natural and/or artificial pressure differences. *Transfer air* (*ta*) is air that moves from one interior space to another, either intentionally or not.

These modes of air exchange differ significantly in how they affect energy, air quality, and thermal comfort, and they can each vary with weather conditions, building operation, and use. Although one mode may be expected to dominate in a particular building, all must be considered for the proper design and operation of an HVAC system.

Modern commercial and institutional buildings are normally required to have forced ventilation and are usually pressurized somewhat to reduce or eliminate infiltration. Forced ventilation has the greatest potential for control of air exchange when the system is properly designed, installed, and operated; it should provide acceptable indoor air quality when ASHRAE *Standard* 62 requirements are followed. Forced ventilation equipment and systems are described in Chapters 1, 2, and 9 of the 1996 *ASHRAE Handbook—Systems and Equipment*.

In commercial and institutional buildings, uncontrolled natural ventilation, such as through operable windows, may not be desirable from the point of view of energy conservation and comfort. In commercial and institutional buildings with mechanical cooling and forced ventilation, an air- or waterside economizer cycle may be preferable to operable windows for taking advantage of cool outdoor conditions when interior cooling is required. Infiltration may be significant in commercial and institutional buildings, especially in tall, leaky, or underpressurized buildings.

In most of the United States, residential buildings typically rely on infiltration and natural ventilation to meet their ventilation needs. Infiltration is not reliable for ventilation purposes because it depends on weather conditions, building construction, and maintenance. Natural ventilation, usually through operable windows, is dependent on weather and building design but allows occupants to control airborne contaminants and interior air temperature. However, natural ventilation can have a substantial energy cost if used while the residence's heating or cooling equipment is operating.

In place of operable windows, small exhaust fans may be provided for localized venting in residential spaces such as kitchens and bathrooms. Not all local buildings codes require that the exhaust be vented to the outside. Instead, the code may allow the air to be treated and returned to the space or to be discharged to an attic space. Poor maintenance of these treatment devices can make nonducted vents ineffective for ventilation purposes. Condensation in attics should be avoided. In northern Europe and in Canada, some building codes require general forced ventilation in residences, and heat recovery heat exchangers are popular for reducing the energy impact. Residential buildings with low rates of infiltration and natural ventilation require forced ventilation at rates given in ASHRAE *Standard* 62.

Regardless of these complexities and uncertainties, designers and operators need guidance on ventilation and indoor air quality.

ASHRAE *Standard* 62 provides guidance on ventilation and indoor air quality in the form of two alternative procedures. In the **Ventilation Rate Procedure**, indoor air quality is assumed to be acceptable if (1) the concentrations of six pollutants in the incoming outdoor air meet the United States national ambient air quality standards, and (2) the outdoor air supply rates meet or exceed values (which vary depending on the type of space) provided in a table. The minimum outside air supply per person for any type of space is 15 cfm (8 L/s). This minimum rate will maintain an indoor CO_2 concentration below 0.1% (1000 parts per million) assuming a typical CO_2 generation rate per occupant.

The second alternative in ASHRAE *Standard* 62 is the **Indoor Air Quality Procedure**. In this procedure, any outside air supply rate is acceptable if (1) the indoor concentrations of nine pollutants are maintained below specified values, and (2) the air is deemed acceptable via subjective evaluations of order. If users of the IAQ Procedure control pollutant source strengths or use air cleaning of local exhaust ventilation, they may be able to reduce the outside air supply rates to below those specified in the ventilation rate procedure.

As a rough guideline, the minimum infiltration outdoor air allowance may be taken as 0.5 air changes per hour (actually to produce a slight positive pressure within the structure producing exfiltration from the conditioned spaces). The minimum ventilation air allowance based on ASHRAE Standard *62 is 15 cfm (8 L/s) per person. However, local ventilation ordinances must be checked as they may require greater quantities of outdoor air.*

5.2.2 Terminology

Figure 5-2 shows a simple **air-handling unit** (AHU) that conditions air for a building. Air brought back to the air handler from the conditioned space is *return air* (*ra*). The portion of the return air that is discharged to the environment is *exhaust air* (*ea*), and the part of the return air that is reused is *recirculated air* (*ca*). Air brought in intentionally form the environment is *outdoor* or *outside air* (*oa*). Because outside air may need treatment to be acceptable for use in a building, it should not be called "fresh air." The outside air and the recirculated air are combined to form *mixed air* (*ma*), which is then conditioned and delivered to the thermal zone as *supply air* (*sa*). Any portion of the mixed air that intentionally or unintentionally circumvents conditioning is *bypass air* (*ba*). *Ventilation air* is used to provide acceptable indoor air quality. It may be composed of forced or natural ventilation air, infiltration air, suitable treated recirculated air, transfer air, or an appropriate combination. Due to the wide variety of air-

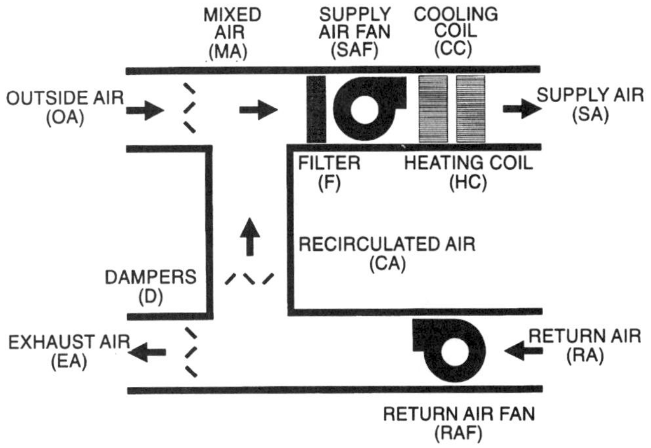

Fig. 5-2 Simple All-Air-Handling Unit with Associated Airflows
(Figure 2, Chapter 25, 1997 *ASHRAE Handbook—Fundamentals*)

handling systems, these airflows may not all be present in a particular system as defined here. Also, more complex systems may have additional airflows.

The outside airflow being introduced to a building or zone by an air-handling unit can also be described by the *outside air fraction* X_{oa}, which is the ratio of the flow rate of outside air brought in by the air handler to the total supply airflow rate. When expressed as a percentage, the outside air fraction is called the *percent outside air*. The design outside airflow rate for a building's ventilation system is found through evaluating the requirements of ASHRAE *Standard* 62. The supply airflow rate is that required to meet the thermal load. The outside air fraction and percent outside air then described the degree of recirculation, where a low value indicates a high rate of recirculation, and a high value shows little recirculation. Conventional all-air-handling systems for commercial and institutional buildings have approximately 10 to 40% outside air. *100% outside air* means no recirculation of return air through the air-handling system. Instead, all the supply air is treated outside air, also known as *makeup air* (*ka*), and all return air is discharged directly to the outside as *relief air* (*la*). An air-handling unit that provides 100% outside air is typically called a **makeup air unit** (MAU).

Outdoor air introduced into a building constitutes a large part of the total space-conditioning (heating, cooling, humidification, and dehumidification) load, which is one reason to limit air exchange rates in buildings to the minimum required. Air exchange typically represents 20 to 40% of a shell-dominated building's thermal load. First, the incoming air must be heated or cooled from the outdoor air temperature to the indoor air temperature. The rate of energy consumption due to this sensible heating or cooling is given by

$$q_s = Q\rho c_p \Delta t \tag{5-1}$$

where

q_s = sensible heat load
Q = airflow rate
ρ = air density
c_p = specific heat of air
Δt = indoor-outdoor temperature difference

Second, air exchange modifies the moisture content of the air in a building. This is particularly important in some locations in the summer when the outdoor air must be dehumidified. In the winter, when the relative humidity of the indoor air is below 30%, humidification may be needed. The rate of energy consumption associated with these latent loads is given by

$$q_l = Q\rho h_{fg} \Delta W \tag{5-2}$$

where

q_l = latent heat load
h_{fg} = latent heat of water
ΔW = humidity ratio of indoor air minus humidity ratio of outdoor air

5.2.3 Infiltration

Infiltration or **exfiltration** is air leakage through cracks and interstices, around windows and doors, and through floors and walls of any type of building. The magnitude of infiltration/exfiltration depends on the type of construction, the workmanship, and the condition of the building.

Outside air infiltration/exfiltration may account for a significant proportion of the heating or cooling requirements for buildings. Thus, it is important to make an adequate estimate of its contribution with respect to both design loads and seasonal energy requirements. Air infiltration is also an important factor in determining the relative humidity that occurs in buildings or, conversely, the amount of humidification or dehumidification required to maintain given humidities.

The rate of airflow into and out of a building due to either infiltration, exfiltration, or natural ventilation depends on the magnitude of the pressure difference between the inside and outside of the structure and on the resistances to airflow offered by openings and interstices in the building. The pressure difference exerted on the building enclosure by the air may be caused either by wind or by a difference in density of the inside and outside air. The effect of the difference in density is often called the **chimney** or **stack effect**, and is often the major factor contributing to air leakage. The pattern of airflow through any part of the structure depends on both the pressure difference and the area of openings.

When the pressure difference is the result of wind pressure, air enters the building through openings in the windward walls and leaves through openings in the leeward walls or, as may be the case in one-story commercial buildings, through ventilating ducts in the roof. When the pressure difference is caused by the indoor-outdoor temperature difference, the flow is along the path of least resistance from inlets at lower levels to outlets at higher levels in a heated building or in the opposite direction for an air-conditioned building, as may be the case in multistory skyscrapers.

In most instances, the pressure difference between inside and outside air results from temperature difference forces. Depending on the design, mechanical ventilation and exhaust systems can affect pressure differences across the building enclosure.

The principles of infiltration calculations are discussed in Chapter 25 of the 1997 *ASHRAE Handbook—Fundamentals*, with emphasis placed on the heating season. For the cooling season, infiltration calculations are usually limited to doors and windows. However, in multistory commercial buildings, a reversed chimney effect may exist.

Heat gain due to infiltration must be included whenever the outdoor air mechanically introduced by the system is unable to maintain a positive pressure within the enclosure to prevent infiltration. Most buildings require input of ventilation air for occupants or processes and by properly balancing or controlling the input air versus exhaust/relief air, a positive pressure can be maintained to minimize infiltration. This excess outdoor air introduced through the air-conditioning equipment will maintain a constant outward escape of air, thereby eliminating the infiltration portion of the gain. The positive pressure maintained must be sufficient to overcome wind pressure through cracks and door openings. When this condition prevails, it is unnecessary to include any infiltration component of heat gain. However, on a typical building, infiltration is usually not eliminated due to the pressure that a 25-30 mph wind can exert and, as buildings age, they develop cracks and leak. When the quantity of outdoor air introduced through the cooling equipment is unable to build up the pressure needed to eliminate infiltration, the entire infiltration load should be included in the space heat gain calculations.

Two methods are used to estimate air infiltration in buildings. In one case, the estimate is based on measured leakage characteristics of the building components and selected pressure differences. This is known as the **crack method**, since cracks around windows and doors are usually the major source of air leakage. The other method is known as the air change method and consists of estimating a certain number of air changes per hour for each room, the number of changes assumed being dependent upon the type, use, and location of the room.

The air change method is used often by engineers and designers both for its simplicity and because either method requires the estimation of at least one appropriate numerical value. The method requires the assumption, based on the performance of similar construction, of the number of air changes per hour (ACH) that a space will experience. The infiltration rate is then obtained as follows:

$$Q = \text{ACH} \times \text{VOL}/60$$

where

Q = infiltration rate, cfm
VOL = gross space volume, ft^3

Table 5-1 presents some values for residential type buildings.

The crack method is more firmly based on scientific principles and is generally regarded as being more accurate, *provided that leakage characteristics and pressure differences can be properly evaluated.* Otherwise, the air change method may be justified. The accuracy of estimating infiltration for design load calculations by the crack or component method is restricted by limitations in information on air leakage characteristics of components and by the difficulty of estimating pressure differences under appropriate design conditions of temperature and wind.

Table 5-1 Change Rates as a Function of Airtightness
(Table 7, Chapter 27, 1997 *ASHRAE Handbook—Fundamentals*)

	Outdoor Design Temperature, °F									
Class	50	40	30	20	10	0	−10	−20	−30	−40
Tight	0.41	0.43	0.45	0.47	0.49	0.51	0.53	0.55	0.57	0.59
Medium	0.69	0.73	0.77	0.81	0.85	0.89	0.93	0.97	1.00	1.05
Loose	1.11	1.15	1.20	1.23	1.27	1.30	1.35	1.40	1.43	1.47

Note: Values are for 15 mph wind and indoor temperature of 68 °F.

A building with only upwind openings is under a *positive pressure* (Figure 5-3). Building pressures are *negative* when there are only downwind openings. A building with internal partitions and openings is under various pressures depending on the relative sizes of the openings and the wind direction. With larger openings on the windward face, the building interior tends to remain under positive pressure; the reverse is also true. Airflow through a wall opening results from positive or negative external and internal pressures. Such differential pressures may exceed 0.5 in. of water during high winds. Supply and exhaust systems, openings, dampers, louvers, doors, and windows make the building flow conditions too complex for most calculations. The opening and closing of doors and windows by building occupants adds further complications.

It is impossible to accurately predict infiltration from theory alone because of the many unknowns. However, it is possible to develop relationships describing the general nature of the problem based on theory and add numerical constants and exponents from experience and experimentation. These semi-

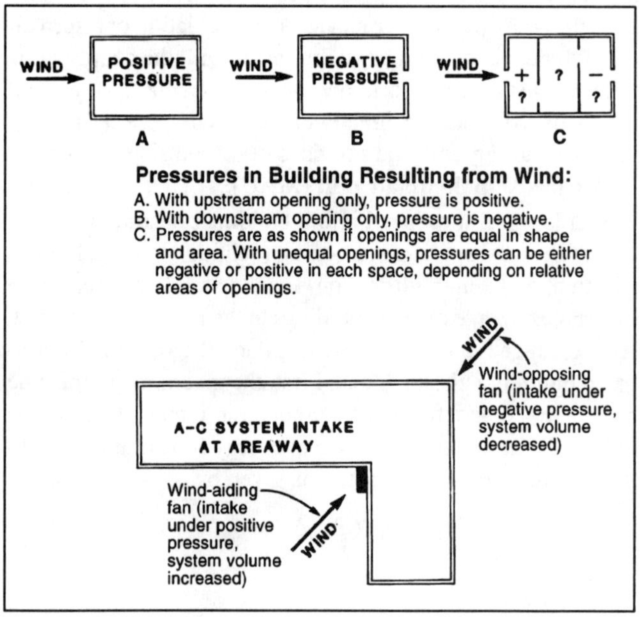

Fig. 5-3 Building Pressure due to Wind Effect
(Figure 11, Chapter 15, 1997 *ASHRAE Handbook—Fundamentals*)

empirical expressions are then useful in estimating infiltration rates.

Infiltration is caused by a greater air pressure on the outside of the building than on the inside. The amount of infiltrated air depends on the pressure difference, the nature of the flow through gaps and cracks (laminar versus turbulent), and the size and shape of the cracks. The relationship between the airflow Q through an opening in the building envelope and the pressure difference Δp across it is called the **leakage function** of the opening. The fundamental equation for the airflow rate through an opening is:

$$Q = C_D A(2\Delta p/\rho)^n \quad (5\text{-}3)$$

where

Q = airflow rate
C_D = discharge coefficient for the opening
A = cross-section area of the opening
ρ = air density
Δp = pressure difference across opening
n = flow exponent (1.0 if laminar; 0.5 if turbulent)

The discharge coefficient C_D is a dimensionless number that depends on the opening geometry and the Reynolds number of the flow.

The above equation is often simplified when evaluating infiltration by combining the discharge coefficient and the crack area into a flow coefficient C yielding

$$Q = C(\Delta p)^n$$

The pressure difference is given by:

$$\Delta p = \Delta p_s + \Delta p_w + \Delta p_p$$

where

Δp_s = pressure difference caused by stack effect
Δp_w = pressure difference caused by wind
Δp_p = pressure difference due to building pressurization

Stack effect occurs when air densities are different on the inside and outside of a building. The air density decreases with increasing temperature and decreases slightly with increasing humidity. Because the pressure of the air is due to the weight of a column of air, on winter days the air pressure at ground level will be less inside the building due to warmer inside air than outside air. As a result of this pressure difference, air will infiltrate at ground level and flow upward inside the building. Under summer conditions when the air is cooler inside, outside air enters the top of the building and flows downward on the inside. With the stack effect there will be a vertical location in the building where the inside pressure equals the outside pressure, called the neutral pressure level of the building. Unless there is detailed information on the vertical distribution of cracks and other openings, it is assumed that the neutral pressure will be at the building mid-height when under the influence of the stack effect alone.

The theoretical pressure difference due to the stack effect can be found from:

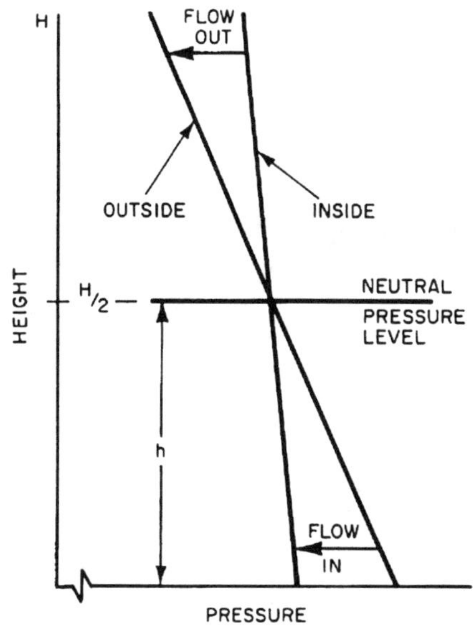

Fig. 5-4 Winter Stack Effect Showing Theoretical Pressure Difference
(Figure 7A, Chapter 25, 1997 *ASHRAE Handbook—Fundamentals*)

$$\Delta p_s = 0.52\, p_b h[(1/T_o) - (1/T_i)] \quad (5\text{-}4)$$

where

Δp_s = theoretical pressure difference, in. water
p_b = outside absolute (barometric) pressure, psi
h = vertical distance from neutral pressure level, ft
T_o = outside absolute temperature, °R
T_i = inside absolute temperature, °R

Figure 5-4 shows the stack effect pressure variations under winter conditions.

The pressure associated with the wind velocity, called velocity pressure, is

$$p_v = \rho V_w^2/2$$

Even on the windward side of a building the wind velocity does not go to zero as the air comes in contact with the building. To account for this, a wind pressure coefficient Cp is used when determining the static pressure obtained from the velocity pressure of the wind:

$$\Delta p_w = 0.5 C_p \rho V_w^2 \quad (5\text{-}5)$$

The pressure coefficient will always have a value less than 1.0 and can be negative when the wind causes outdoor pressures below atmospheric such as on the leeward side of buildings. Figure 5-5 provides average pressure coefficients for tall buildings.

The building pressure and the corresponding pressure difference Δp_p depend on the design and operation of the HVAC system. A building can be operated either at a positive or negative pressure depending upon the relative flow resistances of

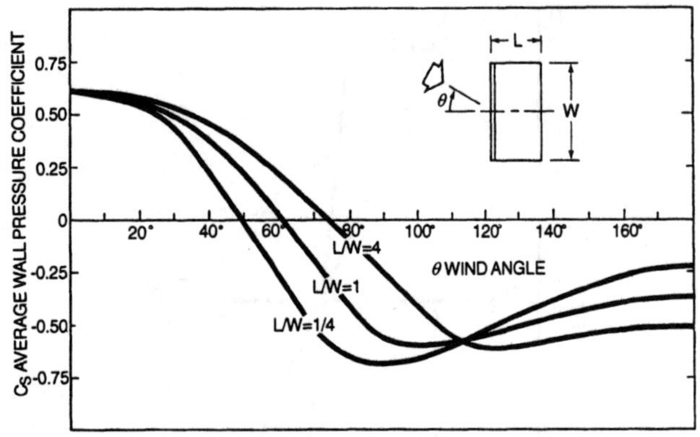

Fig. 5-5 Wind Pressure Coefficients for Tall Buildings
(Figure 7, Chapter 15, 1997 *ASHRAE Handbook—Fundamentals*)

the supply and return duct systems. A positive building pressure results in a negative pressure difference Δp_p and a reduction in infiltration from wind and stack effects. While building pressurization is usually desired and assumed to occur, the air circulation system must be carefully designed and balanced to achieve this effect. Care must be taken to estimate a realistic value that the system can actually achieve.

The flow coefficient C in Equation (5-2) has a particular value for each crack and each window and door perimeter gap. Although values of C are determined experimentally for window and door gaps, this procedure does not work for cracks. Cracks occur at random in fractures of building materials and at the interface of materials. The number and size of cracks depend on the type of construction, the workmanship during construction, and the maintenance of the building after construction. To determine a value of C for each crack is impractical; however, an overall leakage coefficient can used by modifying Equation (5-2) into the following form:

$$Q = KA(\Delta p)^n \tag{5-6}$$

where

A = wall area

K = leakage coefficient

Table 5-2 provides typical values of the leakage coefficient for various types of curtain wall construction. The associated infiltration can be determined from Figure 5-6.

Table 5-2 Curtain Wall Leakage Coefficients
(Table 6.1, *ASHRAE Load Calculation Manual*)

Leakage Coefficient	Description	Curtain Wall Construction
$K = 0.22$	Tight-fitting wall	Constructed under close supervision of workmanship on wall joints. When joints seals appear inadequate they must be redone
$K = 0.66$	Average fitting wall	Conventional construction procedures are used
$K = 1.30$	Loose-fitting wall	Poor construction quality control or an older building having separated joints

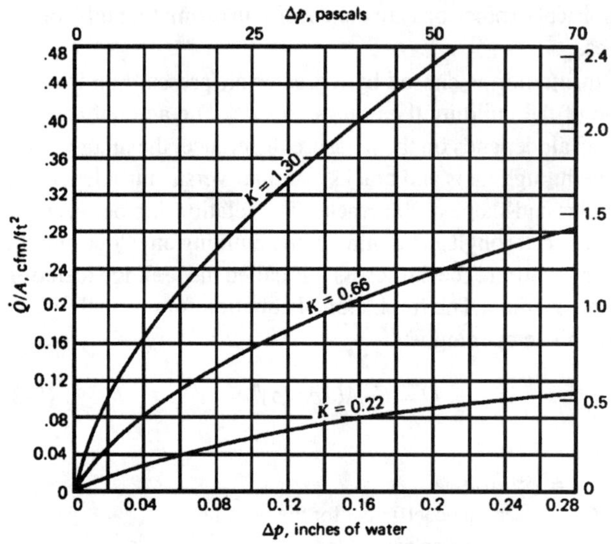

Fig. 5-6 Curtain Wall Infiltration Rates
(Figure 6.7, *ASHRAE Load Calculation Manual*)

Although the terms infiltration and air leakage are sometimes used synonymously, they are different, though related, quantities. Infiltration is the rate of uncontrolled air exchange through unintentional openings that occur under given conditions, while air leakage is a measure of the airtightness of the building shell. The greater the air leakage of a building, the greater its infiltration rate. The infiltration rate of an individual building depends on weather conditions, equipment operation, and occupant activities. The rate can vary by a factor of five from weather effects alone.

Typical infiltration values in housing in North America vary by about a factor of ten, from tight housing with seasonal air change rates of 0.2 per hour (ACH), to housing with infiltration rates as great as 2.0 per hour. Histograms of infiltration rates measured in two different samples of North American housing are shown in Figures 5-7 and 5-8. The average seasonal infiltration of 312 houses located in many different areas in North America is shown in Figure 5-7. The median infiltration value of this sample is 0.50 ACH. Measurements in 266 houses located in 16 cities in the United States are represented in Figure 5-8. The median value of this sample is 0.90 ACH. The group of houses in the Figure 5-7 sample is biased toward new energy-efficient houses, while the group in Figure 5-8 represents older, low-income housing in the United States. While these two samples are not a valid random sample of North American housing, they indicate the distribution expected in an appropriate building sample. Note that infiltration values listed are appropriate for unoccupied structures. Although occupancy influences have not been measured directly, estimates add an average of 0.10 to 0.15 ACH to unoccupied values.

When estimating infiltration rates for a large group of houses to determine gross energy loads, an adequate assumption for infiltration rates is obtained by using Figures 5-7 and 5-8. A combination of the median values in these figures, with an additional 0.10 to 0.15 ACH to account for occupancy

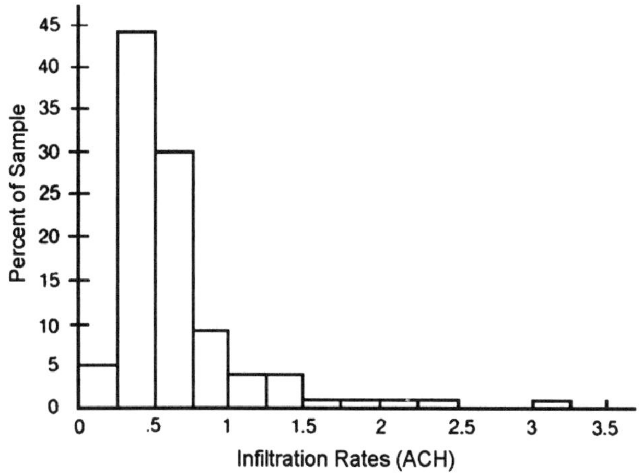

Fig. 5-7 Histogram of Infiltration Values—New Construction
(Fig. 10, Chapter 25, 1997 *ASHRAE Handbook—Fundamentals*)

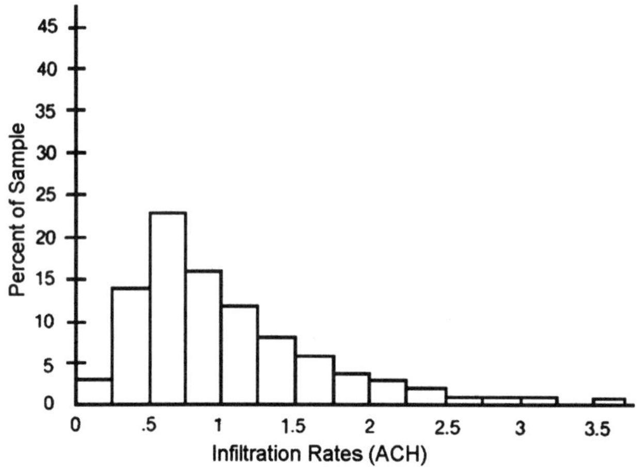

Fig. 5-8 Histogram of Infiltration Values—Low-Income Housing
(Fig. 11, Chapter 25, 1997 *ASHRAE Handbook—Fundamentals*)

effects, represents average infiltration for a large group of houses.

The building envelopes of large commercial buildings are often thought to be nearly airtight. The National Association of Architectural Metal Manufacturers specifies a maximum leakage per unit of exterior wall area of 0.060 cfm/ft^2 at a pressure difference of 0.30 in. of water, exclusive of leakage through operable windows. Recent measurements on eight U.S. office buildings ranged from 0.213 to 1.028 cfm/ft^2 at 0.30 in. of water (0.1 to 0.6 air changes per hour) with no outdoor air intake. Therefore, office building envelopes may leak more than expected. Typical air leakage values per unit wall area at 0.30 in. of water are 0.10, 0.30, and 0.60 for tight, average, and leaky walls, respectively.

Infiltration may also be estimated by statistical analysis of long-term data of infiltration measurements for specific sites. Weather-related pressures that drive infiltration are estimated by finding the regression constants in a function of the form:

$$I = K_1 + K_2\Delta t + K_3 V \tag{5-7}$$

where

I = air change rate, h^{-1}
Δt = indoor-outdoor temperature difference, °F
V = wind speed, mph
K_1, K_2, K_3 = empirical regression constants derived from measurements at the site

The analysis reveals that correlation with weather variables are only moderately successful. Because the regression coefficients reflect structural characteristics, as well as shielding effects and occupants' behavior, the values of K_1, K_2, and K_3 have varied by 20:1 between similar residences, and the model may be inappropriate as a design tool or for inclusion in computer simulations for building energy analysis.

Several procedures have been developed that treat the building as a well-mixed zone. But a study of a large variety of single-cell models found that these models can only be used to calculate air change rates in structures that can be assumed to have a uniform internal pressure.

Multicell models treat the actual complexity of flows in a building by recognizing effects of internal flow restrictions. They require extensive information on flow characteristics and pressure distributions, and, in many cases, are too complex to justify their use to predict flow for simple structures such as single-family residences.

A simple, single-zone approach to calculating air infiltration rates in houses requires an effective leakage area at 0.016 in. of water. The data in Table 5-3 can be used to estimate the leakage area of a building. The values in the table present results in terms of leakage area per component. Per unit component means either per component, per unit surface area, or per unit length of crack, whichever is appropriate. To obtain the buildings' total leakage area, multiply the overall dimensions or number of occurrences of each building component by the appropriate table entry. The sum of the resulting products is the total building leakage area. Using the effective leakage area, the airflow rate due to infiltration is calculated according to the following equation:

$$Q = A_L(C_S\Delta t + C_W V^2)^{0.5} \tag{5-8}$$

where

Q = airflow rate, cfm
A_L = effective leakage area, in^2
C_S = stack coefficient, cfm^2/(in$^4\cdot$°F)
Δt = average indoor-outdoor temp. difference, °F
C_W = wind coefficient, cfm^2/(in$^4\cdot$ mph^2)
V = average wind speed, mph

The infiltration rate of the building is obtained by dividing Q by the building volume. The value of C_W depends on the local shielding class of the building. Five different shielding classes are listed in Table 5-4. Values for C_S for one-, two-, and three-story houses are presented in Table 5-5. Values of C_W for one-, two-, and three-story houses in shielding classes one through five are found in Table 5-6. The heights of

Table 5-3 Effective Leakage Area of Building Components (0.016 in. of water pressure difference)

(Table 3, Chapter 25, 1997 *ASHRAE Handbook—Fundamentals*)

	Units (see note)	Best Estimate	Minimum	Maximum
Ceiling				
General	in^2/ft^2	0.026	0.011	0.04
Drop	in^2/ft^2	0.0027	0.00066	0.003
Ceiling penetrations				
Whole-house fans	in^2 ea	3.1	0.25	3.3
Recessed lights	in^2 ea	1.6	0.23	3.3
Ceiling/Flue vent	in^2 ea	4.8	4.3	4.8
Surface-mounted lights	in^2 ea	0.13		
Chimney	in^2 ea	4.5	3.3	5.6
Crawl space				
General (area for exposed wall)	in^2/ft^2	0.144	0.1	0.24
8 in. by 16 in. vents	in^2 ea	20		
Door frame				
General	in^2 ea	1.9	0.37	3.9
Masonry, not caulked	in^2/ft^2	0.07	0.024	0.07
Masonry, caulked	in^2/ft^2	0.014	0.004	0.014
Wood, not caulked	in^2/ft^2	0.024	0.009	0.024
Wood, caulked	in^2/ft^2	0.004	0.001	0.004
Trim	in^2/lftc	0.05		
Jamb	in^2/lftc	0.4	0.3	0.5
Threshold	in^2/lftc	0.1	0.06	1.1
Doors				
Attic/crawl space, not weatherstripped	in^2 ea	4.6	1.6	5.7
Attic/crawl space, weatherstripped	in^2 ea	2.8	1.2	2.9
Attic fold down, not weatherstripped	in^2 ea	6.8	3.6	13
Attic fold down, weatherstripped	in^2 ea	3.4	2.2	6.7
Attic fold down, with insulated box	in^2 ea	0.6		
Attic from unconditioned garage	in^2 ea	0	0	0
Double, not weatherstripped	in^2/ft^2	0.16	0.1	0.32
Double, weatherstripped	in^2/ft^2	0.12	0.04	0.33
Elevator (passenger)	in^2 ea	0.04	0.022	0.054
General, average	in^2/lftc	0.015	0.011	0.021
Interior (pocket, on top floor)	in^2 ea	2.2		
Interior (stairs)	in^2/lftc	0.04	0.012	0.070
Mail slot	in^2/lftc	0.2		
Sliding exterior glass patio	in^2 ea	3.4	0.46	9.3
Sliding exterior glass patio	in^2/ft^2	0.079	0.009	0.22
Storm (difference between with and without)	in^2 ea	0.9	0.46	0.96
Single, not weatherstripped	in^2 ea	3.3	1.9	8.2
Single, weatherstripped	in^2 ea	1.9	0.6	4.2
Vestibule (subtract per each location)	in^2 ea	1.6		
Electrical outlets/Switches				
No gaskets	in^2 ea	0.38	0.08	0.96
With gaskets	in^2 ea	0.023	0.012	0.54
Furnace				
Sealed (or no) combustion	in^2 ea	0	0	0
Retention head or stack damper	in^2 ea	4.6	3.1	4.6
Retention head and stack damper	in^2 ea	3.7	2.8	4.6
Floors over crawl spaces				
General	in^2/ft^2	0.032	0.006	0.071
Without ductwork in crawl space	in^2/ft^2	0.0285		
With ductwork in crawl space	in^2/ft^2	0.0324		
Fireplace				
With damper closed	in^2/ft^2	0.62	0.14	1.3
With damper open	in^2/ft^2	5.04	2.09	5.47
With glass doors	in^2/ft^2	0.58	0.06	0.58
With insert and damper closed	in^2/ft^2	0.52	0.37	0.66
With insert and damper open	in^2/ft^2	0.94	0.58	1.3
Gas water heater	in^2 ea	3.1	2.3	3.9
Joints				
Ceiling-wall	in^2/lftc	0.070	0.0075	0.12
Sole plate, floor/wall, uncaulked	in^2/lftc	0.2	0.018	0.26
Sole plate, floor/wall, caulked	in^2/lftc	0.04	0.0035	0.056
Top plate, band joist	in^2/lftc	0.005	0.0035	0.018

	Units (see note)	Best Estimate	Minimum	Maximum
Piping/Plumbing/Wiring penetrations				
Uncaulked	in^2 ea	0.9	0.31	3.7
Caulked	in^2 ea	0.3	0.16	0.3
Vents				
Bathroom with damper closed	in^2 ea	1.6	0.39	3.1
Bathroom with damper open	in^2 ea	3.1	0.95	3.4
Dryer with damper	in^2 ea	0.46	0.45	1.1
Dryer without damper	in^2 ea	2.3	1.9	5.3
Kitchen with damper open	in^2 ea	6.2	2.2	11
Kitchen with damper closed	in^2 ea	0.8	0.16	1.1
Kitchen with tight gasket	in^2 ea	0.16		
Walls (exterior)				
Cast-in-place concrete	in^2/ft^2	0.007	0.0007	0.026
Clay brick cavity wall, finished	in^2/ft^2	0.0098	0.0007	0.033
Precast concrete panel	in^2/ft^2	0.017	0.0004	0.024
Lightweight concrete block, unfinished	in^2/ft^2	0.05	0.019	0.058
Lightweight concrete block, painted or stucco	in^2/ft^2	0.016	0.0075	0.016
Heavyweight concrete block, unfinished	in^2/ft^2	0.0036		
Continuous air infiltration barrier	in^2/ft^2	0.0022	0.0008	0.003
Rigid sheathing	in^2/ft^2	0.005	0.0042	0.006
Window framing				
Masonry, uncaulked	in^2/ft^2	0.094	0.082	0.148
Masonry, caulked	in^2/ft^2	0.019	0.016	0.03
Wood, uncaulked	in^2/ft^2	0.025	0.022	0.039
Wood, caulked	in^2/ft^2	0.004	0.004	0.007
Windows				
Awning, not weatherstripped	in^2/ft^2	0.023	0.011	0.035
Awning, weatherstripped	in^2/ft^2	0.012	0.006	0.017
Casement, weatherstripped	in^2/lftc	0.011	0.005	0.14
Casement, not weatherstripped	in^2/lftc	0.013		
Double horizontal slider, not weatherstripped	in^2/lftc	0.052	0.0009	0.16
Double horizontal slider, wood, weatherstripped	in^2/lftc	0.026	0.0070	0.081
Double horizontal slider, aluminum, weatherstripped	in^2/lftc	0.034	0.027	0.038
Double-hung, not weatherstripped	in^2/lftc	0.12	0.040	0.29
Double-hung, weatherstripped	in^2/lftc	0.031	0.009	0.089
Double-hung with storm, not weatherstripped	in^2/lftc	0.046	0.023	0.080
Double-hung with storm, weatherstripped	in^2/lftc	0.037	0.021	0.05
Double-hung with pressurized track, weatherstripped	in^2/lftc	0.023	0.018	0.026
Jalousie	in^2/louver	0.524		
Lumped	in^2/lfts	0.022	0.00042	0.097
Single horizontal slider, weatherstripped	in^2/lfts	0.031	0.009	0.097
Single horizontal slider, aluminum	in^2/lfts	0.04	0.013	0.097
Single horizontal slider, wood	in^2/lfts	0.021	0.013	0.047
Single horizontal slider, wood clad	in^2/lfts	0.030	0.025	0.038
Single-hung, weatherstripped	in^2/lfts	0.041	0.029	0.058
Sill	in^2/lftc	0.0099	0.0065	0.010
Storm inside, heat shrink	in^2/lfts	0.00085	0.00042	0.00085
Storm inside, rigid sheet with magnetic seal	in^2/lfts	0.0056	0.00085	0.011
Storm inside, flexible sheet with mechanical seal	in^2/lfts	0.0072	0.00085	0.039
Storm inside, rigid sheet with mechanical seal	in^2/lfts	0.019	0.0021	0.039
Storm outside, pressurized track	in^2/lftc	0.025		
Storm outside, 2-track	in^2/lftc	0.058		
Storm outside, 3-track	in^2/lftc	0.116		

Note: Air leakage areas are based on values found in the literature. The effective air leakage area (in square inches) is based on a pressure difference of 0.016 in. of water and $C_D = 1$.

Abbreviations: ft^2 = gross area in square feet; ea = each; lftc = linear foot of crack; lfts = linear foot of sash

Table 5-4 Local Shielding Class
(Table 7, Chapter 25, 1997 *ASHRAE Handbook—Fundamentals*)

Class	Description
1	No obstructions or local shielding
2	Light local shielding; few obstructions, few trees, or small shed
3	Moderate local shielding; some obstructions within two house heights, thick hedge, solid fence, or one neighboring house
4	Heavy shielding; obstructions around most of perimeter, buildings or trees within 30 ft in most directions; typical suburban shielding
5	Very heavy shielding; large obstructions surrounding perimeter within two house heights; typical downtown shielding

Table 5-5 Stack Coefficient C_S
(Table 6, Chapter 25, 1997 *ASHRAE Handbook—Fundamentals*)

	House Height (Stories)		
	One	Two	Three
Stack coefficient	0.0150	0.0299	0.0449

Table 5-6 Wind Coefficient C_W
(Table 8, Chapter 25, 1997 *ASHRAE Handbook—Fundamentals*)

Shielding Class	House Height (Stories)		
	One	Two	Three
1	0.0119	0.0157	0.0184
2	0.0092	0.0121	0.0143
3	0.0065	0.0086	0.0101
4	0.0039	0.0051	0.0060
5	0.0012	0.0016	0.0018

the one-, two-, and three-story buildings are 8, 16, and 24 ft, respectively.

Example 5-1 A double-slider, weather-stripped window is mounted in a masonry wall and is caulked. The window is 4 ft by 5 ft and is on the second story of an unshielded building. The design wind velocity is 20 mph; the inside temperature is 75°F while the outside temperature is 0°F. Estimate the cfm of infiltration air.

Solution: The leakage area method is used.

From Table 5-3 for a double-slider, weather-stripped window, the best estimate for infiltration area is 0.37 in^2/ft of crack length. From Table 5-3, for the window frame leakage in the wall, the best estimate is 0.019 in^2/ft^2.

Infiltration
area = 0.37(4 + 4 + 4 + 5 + 5) + (0.019)(4 × 5) = 8.52 in^2

From Equation (5-8):

$$Q = A_L(C_S \Delta t + C_W V^2)^{0.5}$$

From Table 5-4, this window is classed as class 1 shielding. From Table 5-5, C_S = 0.0313 for a two-story window. For a two-story window with class 1 shielding, C_W = 0.0157, from Table 5-6. Substitution yields:

$$Q = 8.52(0.0313 \times 75 + 0.0157 \times 20^2)^{0.5} = 25.0 \text{ cfm}$$

Example 5-2 Estimate the infiltration at design conditions for a two-story house in Lincoln, Nebraska. The house has an effective leakage area of 77 in^2, and is surrounded by a thick hedge.

Solution: The design temperature for Lincoln is −2°F. Design wind speed is 15 mph. Shielding Class 3 due to hedge. From Table 5-5, CS = 0.0313, and from Table 5-6, C_W = 0.0086. The airflow rate due to infiltration is thus:

$$Q = 77[(0.0313 \times 70) + (0.0086 \times 15^2)]^{0.5}$$
$$= 156 \text{ cfm} = 9384 \text{ ft}^3/\text{h}$$

Infiltration rate I equals Q divided by the building volume:

$$I = 9384/12000 = 0.78 \text{ ACH}$$

Commercial-type doors have different infiltration characteristics than those given in Table 5-3 in that they normally have larger cracks and are used more often.

Data for the infiltration through cracks in swinging doors is given in Figure 5-9. Commercial buildings often have a large number of people entering and leaving with associated infiltration. Figures 5-10 and 5-11 provide data for estimating the infiltration due to traffic in and out of the building. The figures are based on a standard sized (3 ft by 7 ft) door. There is no published information on automatically operated doors, but automatic doors stay open two to four times longer than manually operated doors. Thus, doubling of the infiltration obtained for manually operated doors would be a reasonable estimate for automatic doors.

The total infiltration is the infiltration through the cracks when the door is closed added to the infiltration due to traffic.

Figure 5-12 shows the infiltration due to a pressure difference across the seals of a standard sized revolving door. Figure 5-13 and 5-14 provide data for estimating the infiltration caused by the rotation of the standard-sized door. The amount of infiltration depends upon the inside-outside temperature difference and the rotational speed of the door. The total infiltration is the infiltration due to leakage through the door seals and the infiltration due to the mechanical interchange of air due to the rotation of the door.

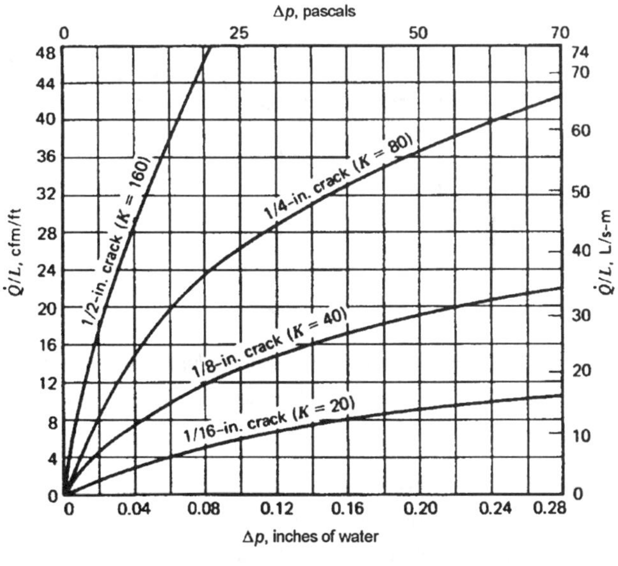

Fig. 5-9 Infiltration through Closed Swinging Door Cracks
(Fig. 6.10, *ASHRAE Load Calculation Manual*)

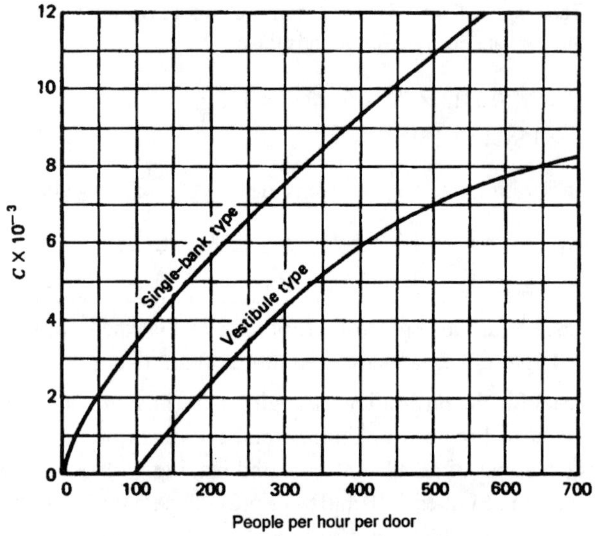

Fig. 5-10 Flow Coefficients for Swinging Doors
(Fig. 6.12, *ASHRAE Load Calculation Manual*)

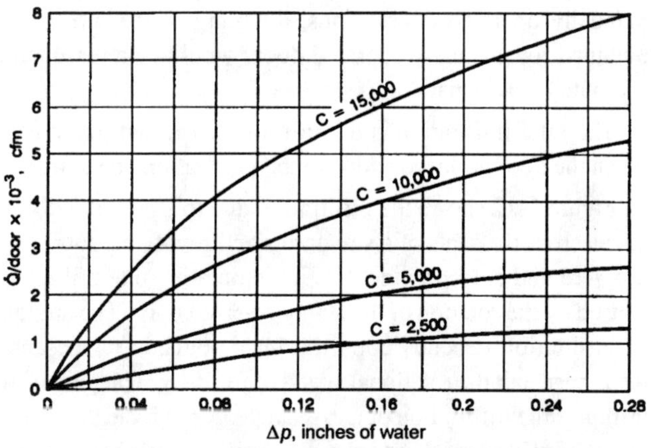

Fig. 5-11 Infiltration for Swinging Doors with Traffic
(Fig. 6.11, ASHRAE Load Calculation Manual)

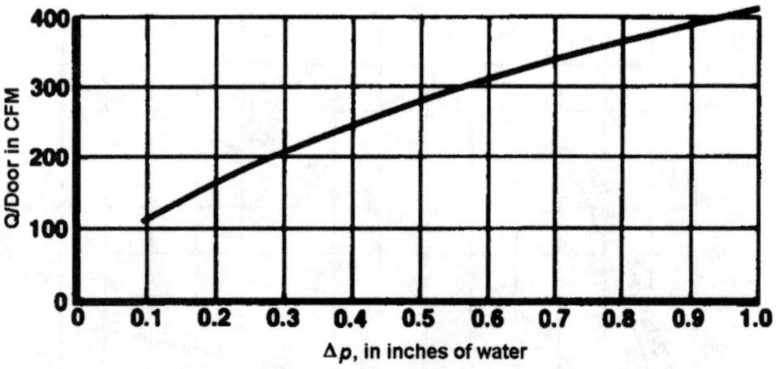

Fig. 5-12 Infiltration Through Revolving Door Seals while Stationary
(Fig. 6.13, ASHRAE Load Calculation Manual)

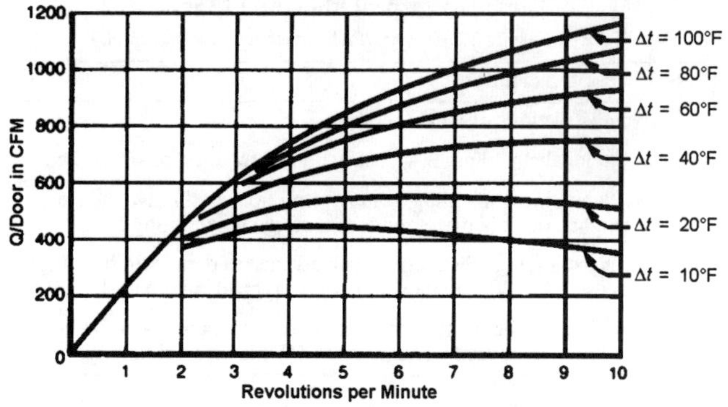

Fig. 5-13 Infiltration for Motor-Operated Revolving Door
(Fig. 6.14, ASHRAE Load Calculation Manual)

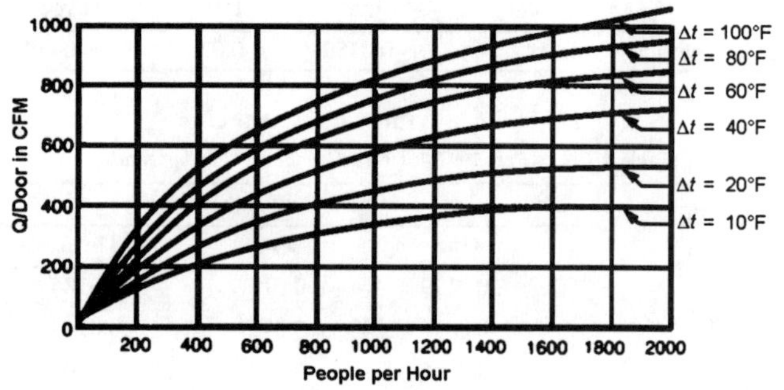

Fig. 5-14 Infiltration for Manual Revolving Door
(Fig. 6.15, ASHRAE Load Calculation Manual)

5.2.4 Ventilation Air

Outdoor air requirements for acceptable indoor air quality (IAQ) have long been debated and different rationales have produced quite different ventilation standards. Historically, the major considerations have included the amount of outdoor air required to control moisture, carbon dioxide, odors, and tobacco smoke generated by occupants. These considerations have led to the minimum rate of outside air supply per occupant. More recently, the maintenance of acceptable indoor concentrations of a variety of additional pollutants that are not generated primarily by occupants has been a major concern. The most common pollutants of concern and their sources are given in Table 5-7.

Regardless of the complexities and uncertainties that exist regarding proper ventilation, building designers and operators require guidance on minimum outside air quantities and indoor air quality. ASHRAE *Standard* 62-1989 provides guidance on ventilation and indoor air quality in the form of two alternative procedures. In the **ventilation rate procedure**, indoor air quality is assumed to be acceptable if the concentrations of pollutants in the incoming outdoor air meet the U.S. national ambient air quality standards (Table 5-8) and the outside air supply rates meet or exceed values provided in Table 5-9. The minimum outside air supply per person for any type of space is 15 cfm. This minimum rate will maintain indoor CO_2 concentrations below 0.1% (1000 parts per million) assuming a typical generation rate per occupant. Table 5-9 lists the required ventilation rates in cfm (L/s) per person or cfm/ft^2 [L/(s·m^2)] for a variety of indoor spaces. In most cases, the contamination produced is presumed to be proportional to the number of persons in the spaces. In other cases, the contamination is presumed to be chiefly due to other factors and the ventilating rates given are based on more appro-

Table 5-7 Indoor Air Pollutants and Sources

Sources	Contaminants
OUTDOOR	
Ambient air	SO_2, NO, NO_2, O_3, hydrocarbons, CO, particulates, bioaerosols
Motor vehicles	CO, Pb, hydrocarbons, particulates
Soil	Radon organics
INDOOR	
Building construction materials	
Concrete, stone	Radon
Particleboard, plywood	Formaldehyde
Insulation	Formaldehyde, fiberglass
Fire retardant	Asbestos
Adhesives	Organics
Paint	Mercury, organics
Building Contents	
Heating and cooking combustion appliances	CO, NO, NO_2, formaldehyde, particulates, organics
Furnishings	Organics
Water service, natural gas	Radon
Human Occupants	
Tobacco smoke	CO, NO_2, organics, particulates, odors
Aerosol sprays	Fluorocarbons, vinyl chloride, organices
Cleaning and cooking products	Organics NH_2, odors
Hobbies and crafts	Organics
Damp orgainic materials, stagnant water	
Coil drain pans	Bioaerosols
Humidifiers	

Table 5-8 United States Ambient Air Quality *Standards*

Contaminant	Averaging Time	Primary Standard Levels	Secondary Standard Levels
Particulate matter	Annual (geometric mean)	75 $\mu g/m^3$	60 $\mu g/m^3$
	24 h	260 $\mu g/m^3$	150 $\mu g/m^3$
Sulfur oxides	Annual (arithmetic mean)	80 $\mu g/m^3$ (0.03 ppm)	—
	24 h	365 $\mu g/m^3$ (0.14 ppm)	—
	3 h	—	1300 $\mu g/m^3$ (0.5 ppm)
Carbon monoxide	8 h	10 mg/m^3 (9 ppm)	10 mg/m^3 (9 ppm)
	1 h	40 mg/m^3 (35 ppm)	40 mg/m^3 (35 ppm)
Nitrogen dioxide	Annual (arithmetic mean)	100 $\mu g/m^3$ (0.05 ppm)	100 $\mu g/m^3$ (0.05 ppm)
Ozone	1 h	240 $\mu g/m^3$ (0.12 ppm)	240 $\mu g/m^3$ (0.12 ppm)
Hydrocarbons (nonmethane)	3 h (6 A.M. to 9 A.M.)	160 $\mu g/m^3$ (0.24 ppm)	160 $\mu g/m^3$ (0.24 ppm)
Lead	3 months	1.5 $\mu g/m^3$	1.5 $\mu g/m^3$

priate parameters. Where appropriate, the table lists the estimated density of people for design purposes. The requirements for ventilation air quantities given in Table 5-9 are for 100% outdoor air when the outdoor air quality meets the national specifications for acceptable outdoor air quality.

Properly cleaned air may be recirculated. Under the ventilation rate procedure, for other than intermittent variable occupancy, outdoor air flow rates may not be reduced below the requirements in Table 5-9. If cleaned, recirculated air is used to reduce the outdoor air flow rate below the values of Table 5-9, the indoor air quality procedure must be used. The ***indoor air quality procedure*** provides an alternative performance method to the ***ventilation rate procedure*** for achieving acceptable air quality. The ventilation rate procedure is deemed to provide acceptable indoor air quality. Nevertheless that procedure, through prescription of required ventilation rates, provides only an indirect solution to the control of indoor contaminants. The indoor air quality procedure provides a direct solution by restricting contaminant concentration concern to acceptable levels.

The amount of outdoor air specified in Table 5-9 may be reduced by recirculating air from which offending contaminants have been removed or converted to less objectionable forms. The amount of outdoor air required depends on the contaminant concentrations in the indoor and outdoor air, the contaminant generation in the space, the filter location, the filter efficiency for the contaminants in question, the ventilation effectiveness, the supply air circulation rate, and the fraction recirculated.

Figure 5-15 shows a representative HVAC ventilation system. A filter may be located in the recirculated airstream (location A) or in the supply (mixed) airstream (location B). Variable-air-volume (VAV) systems reduce the circulation

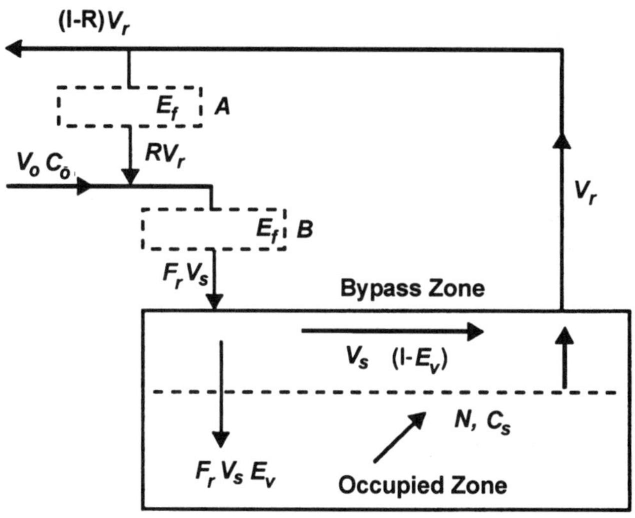

A, B = Filter Location
V = Volumetric Flow
C = Contaminate Concentration
E = Efficiency or Effectiveness
F_r = Flow Reduction Factor
N = Contaminate Generation Rate
R = Recirculation Flow Factor

Subscripts
f = filter
o = outdoor
r = return
s = supply
v = ventilation

Fig. 5-15 HVAC Ventilation System Schematic
(Figure E-1, ASHRAE Standard 62-1989)

Table 5-9 ASHRAE *Standard* 62-1989 Ventilation Rates

OUTDOOR AIR REQUIREMENTS FOR VENTILATION*

2.1 COMMERCIAL FACILITIES (offices, stores, shops, hotels, sports facilities)

Application	Estimated Maximum** Occupancy P/1000 ft² or 100 m²	Outdoor Air Requirements cfm/person	L/s·person	cfm/ft²	L/s·m²	Comments
Dry Cleaners, Laundries						Dry-cleaning processes may require more air.
Commercial laundry	10	25	13			
Commercial dry cleaner	30	30	15			
Storage, pick up	30	35	18			
Coin-operated laundries	20	15	8			
Coin-operated dry cleaner	20	15	8			
Food and Beverage Service						
Dining rooms	70	20	10			
Cafeteria, fast food	100	20	10			
Bars, cocktail lounges	100	30	15			Supplementary smoke-removal equipment may be required.
Kitchens (cooking)	20	15	8			Makeup air for hood exhaust may require more ventilating air. The sum of the outdoor air and transfer air of acceptable quality from adjacent spaces shall be sufficient to provide an exhaust rate of not less than 1.5 cfm/ft² (7.5 L/s·m²).
Garages, Repair, Service Stations						
Enclosed parking garage				1.50	7.5	Distribution among people must consider worker location and concentration of running engines; stands where engines are run must incorporate systems for positive engine exhaust withdrawal. Contaminant sensors may be used to control ventilation.
Auto repair rooms				1.50	7.5	
Hotels, Motels, Resorts, Dormitories						
				cfm/room	L/s·room	Independent of room size.
Bedrooms				30	15	
Living rooms				30	15	
Baths				35	18	Installed capacity for intermittent use.
Lobbies	30	15	8			
Conference rooms	50	20	10			
Assembly rooms	120	15	8			
Dormitory sleeping areas	20	15	8			See also food and beverage services, merchandising, barber and beauty shops, garages.
Gambling casinos	120	30	15			Supplementary smoke-removal equipment may be required.
Offices						
Office space	7	20	10			Some office equipment may require local exhaust.
Reception areas	60	15	8			
Telecommunication centers and data entry areas	60	20	10			
Conference rooms	50	20	10			Supplementary smoke-removal equipment may be required.
Public Spaces				cfm/ft²	L/s·m²	
Corridors and utilities				0.05	0.25	
Public restrooms, cfm/wc or urinal		50	25			Mechanical exhaust with no recirculation is recommended.
Locker and dressing rooms				0.5	2.5	
Smoking lounge	70	60	30			Normally supplied by transfer air, local mechanical exhaust; with no recirculation recommended.
Elevators				1.00	5.0	Normally supplied by transfer air.

* Table 2 prescribes supply rates of acceptable outdoor air required for acceptable indoor air quality. These values have been chosen to control CO_2 and other contaminants with an adequate margin of safety and to account for health variations among people, varied activity levels, and a moderate amount of smoking. Rational of CO_2 control is presented in Appendix D.

**Net occupiable space.

Table 5-9 ASHRAE *Standard* 62-1989 Ventilation Rates (*Continued*)

OUTDOOR AIR REQUIREMENTS FOR VENTILATION* (*Continued*)

2.1 COMMERCIAL FACILITIES (offices, stores, shops, hotels, sports facilities)

Application	Estimated Maximum** Occupancy P/1000 ft² or 100 m²	Outdoor Air Requirements cfm/person	L/s·person	cfm/ft²	L/s·m²	Comments
Retail Stores, Sales Floors, and Show Room Floors						
Basement and street	30			0.30	1.50	
Upper floors	20			0.20	1.00	
Storage rooms	15			0.15	0.75	
Dressing rooms				0.20	1.00	
Malls and arcades	20			0.20	1.00	
Shipping and receiving	10			0.15	0.75	
Warehouses	5			0.05	0.25	
Smoking lounge	70	60	30			Normally supplied by transfer air, local mechanical exhaust; exhaust with no recirculation recommended.
Specialty Shops						
Barber	25	15	8			
Beauty	25	25	13			
Reducing salons	20	15	8			
Florists	8	15	8			Ventilation to optimize plant growth may dictate requirements.
Clothiers, furniture				0.30	1.50	
Hardware, drugs, fabric	8	15	8			
Supermarkets	8	15	8			
Pet shops				1.00	5.00	
Sports and Amusement						
Spectator areas	150	15	8			When internal combustion engines are operated for maintenance of playing surfaces, increased ventilation rates may be required.
Game rooms	70	25	13			
Ice arenas (playing areas)				0.50	2.50	
Swimming pools (pool and deck area)				0.50	2.50	Higher values may be required for humidity control.
Playing floors (gymnasium)	30	20	10			
Ballrooms and discos	100	25	13			
Bowling alleys (seating areas)	70	25	13			
Theaters						Special ventilation will be needed to eliminate special stage effects (e.g., dry ice vapors, mists, etc.)
Ticket booths	60	20	10			
Lobbies	150	20	10			
Auditorium	150	15	8			
Stages, studios	70	15	8			
Transportation						Ventilation within vehicles may require special considerations.
Waiting rooms	100	15	8			
Platforms	100	15	8			
Vehicles	150	15	8			
Workrooms						
Meat processing	10	15	8			Spaces maintained at low temperatures (−10 °F to + 50 °F, or −23 °C to + 10 °C) are not covered by these requirements unless the occupancy is continuous. Ventilation from adjoining spaces is permissible. When the occupancy is intermittent, infiltration will normally exceed the ventilation requirement. (See Ref 18).

* Table 2 prescribes supply rates of acceptable outdoor air required for acceptable indoor air quality. These values have been chosen to control CO_2 and other contaminants with an adequate margin of safety and to account for health variations among people, varied activity levels, and a moderate amount of smoking. Rational of CO_2 control is presented in Appendix D.

**Net occupiable space.

Table 5-9 ASHRAE *Standard* 62-1989 Ventilation Rates (*Continued*)

OUTDOOR AIR REQUIREMENTS FOR VENTILATION* (*Concluded*)

2.1 COMMERCIAL FACILITIES (offices, stores, shops, hotels, sports facilities)

Application	Estimated Maximum** Occupancy P/1000 ft² or 100 m²	Outdoor Air Requirements cfm/person	L/s·person	cfm/ft²	L/s·m²	Comments
Photo studios	10	15	8			
Darkrooms	10			0.50	2.50	
Pharmacy	20	15	8			
Bank vaults	5	15	8			
Duplicating, printing				0.50	2.50	Installed equipment must incorporate positive exhaust and control (as required) of undesirable contaminants (toxic or otherwise).

2.2 INSTITUTIONAL FACILITIES

Application	Estimated Maximum** Occupancy P/1000 ft² or 100 m²	cfm/person	L/s·person	cfm/ft²	L/s·m²	Comments
Education						
Classroom	50	15	8			
Laboratories	30	20	10			Special contaminant control systems may be required for processes or functions including laboratory animal occupancy.
Training shop	30	20	10			
Music rooms	50	15	8			
Libraries	20	15	8			
Locker rooms				0.50	2.50	
Corridors				0.10	0.50	
Auditoriums	150	15	8			
Smoking lounges	70	60	30			Normally supplied by transfer air. Local mechanical exhaust with no recirculation recommended.
Hospitals, Nursing and Convalescent Homes						
Patient rooms	10	25	13			Special requirements or codes and pressure relationships may determine minimum ventilation rates and filter efficiency. Procedures generating contaminants may require higher rates.
Medical procedure	20	15	8			
Operating rooms	20	30	15			
Recovery and ICU	20	15	8			
Autopsy rooms				0.50	2.50	Air shall not be recirculated into other spaces.
Physical Therapy	20	15	8			
Correctional Facilities						
Cells	20	20	10			
Dining halls	100	15	8			
Guard stations	40	15	8			

* Table 2 prescribes supply rates of acceptable outdoor air required for acceptable indoor air quality. These values have been chosen to control CO_2 and other contaminants with an adequate margin of safety and to account for health variations among people, varied activity levels, and a moderate amount of smoking. Rationale, for CO_2 control is presented in Appendix D.

**Net occupiable space.

OUTDOOR AIR REQUIREMENTS FOR VENTILATION OF RESIDENTIAL FACILITIES
(Private Dwellings, Single, Multiple)

Applications	Outdoor Requirements	Comments
Living areas	0.35 air changes per hour but not less than 15 cfm (7.5 L/s) per person	For calculating the air changes per hour, the volume of the living spaces shall include all areas within the conditioned space. The ventilation is normally satisfied by infiltration and natural ventilation. Dwellings with tight enclosures may require supplemental ventilation supply for fuel-burning appliances, including fireplaces and mechanically exhausted appliances. Occupant loading shall be based on the number of bedrooms as follows: first bedroom, two persons; each additional bedroom, one person. Where higher occupant loadings are known, they shall be used.
Kitchens[b]	100 cfm (50 L/s) intermittent or 25 cfm (12 L/s) continuous or openable windows	Installed mechanical exhaust capacity[c] Climatic conditions may affect choice of the ventilation system.
Baths, Toilets[b]	50 cfm (25 L/s) intermittent or 20 cfm (10 L/s) continuous or openable windows	Installed mechanical exhaust capacity[c]
Garages:		
Separate for each dwelling unit	100 cfm (50 L/s) per car	Normally satisfied by infiltration or natural ventilation
Common for several units	1.5 cfm/ft² (7.5 L/s·m²)	See "Enclosed parking garages," Table 2.1

[a] In using this table, the outdoor air is assumed to be acceptable.
[b] Climatic conditions may affect choice of ventilation option chosen.
[c] The air exhausted from kitchens, bath, and toilet rooms may utilize air supplied through adjacent living areas to compensate for the air exhausted. The air supplied shall meet the requirements of exhaust systems as described in 5.8 and be of sufficient quantities to meet the requirements of this table.

Table 5-10 Required Outdoor Air or Space Contaminant Concentration with Recirculation and Filtration
(Table E-1, ASHRAE *Standard* 62-1989)

Class	Required Recirculation Rate				Required Outdoor Air	Space Contaminant Concentration	Required Recirculation Rate
	Filter Location	Flow	Temperature	Outdoor Air			
I	None	VAV	Constant	100%	$V_o = \frac{N}{E_v F_r (C_s - C_o)}$	$C_s = C_o + \frac{N}{E_v F_r V_o}$	Not applicable
II	A	Constant	Variable	Constant	$V_o = \frac{N - E_v RV_r E_f C_s}{E_v (C_s - C_o)}$	$C_s = \frac{N + E_v V_o C_o}{E_v (V_o + RV_r E_f)}$	$RV_r = \frac{N + E_v V_o (C_o - C_s)}{E_v E_f C_s}$
III	A	VAV	Constant	Constant	$V_o = \frac{N - E_v F_r RV_r E_f C_s}{E_v (C_s - C_o)}$	$C_s = \frac{N + E_v V_o C_o}{E_v (V_o + F_r RV_r E_f)}$	$RV_r = \frac{N + E_v V_o (C_o - C_s)}{E_v F_r E_f C_s}$
IV	A	VAV	Constant	Proportional	$V_o = \frac{N - E_v F_r RV_r E_f C_s}{E_v F_r (C_s - C_o)}$	$C_s = \frac{N + E_v F_r V_o C_o}{F_r E_v (V_o + RV_r E_f)}$	$RV_r = \frac{N + E_v F_r V_o (C_o - C_s)}{E_v F_r E_f C_s}$
V	B	Constant	Variable	Constant	$V_o = \frac{N - E_v RV_r E_f C_s}{E_v [C_s - (1 - E_f) C_o]}$	$C_s = \frac{N + E_v V_o (1 - E_f) C_o}{E_v (V_o + RV_r E_f)}$	$RV_r = \frac{N + E_v V_o [(1 - E_f) C_o - C_s]}{E_v E_f C_s}$
VI	B	VAV	Constant	Constant	$V_o = \frac{N - E_v F_r RV_r E_f C_s}{E_v [C_s - (1 - E_f) C_o]}$	$C_s = \frac{N + E_v V_o (1 - E_f) C_o}{E_v (V_o + F_r RV_r E_f)}$	$RV_r = \frac{N + E_v V_o [(1 - E_f) C_o - C_s]}{E_v F_r E_f C_s}$
VII	B	VAV	Constant	Proportional	$V_o = \frac{N - E_v F_r RV_r E_f C_s}{E_v F_r [C_s - (1 - E_f)(C_o)]}$	$C_s = \frac{N + E_v F_r V_o (1 - E_f) C_o}{E_v F_r (V_o + RV_r E_f)}$	$RV_r = \frac{N + E_v F_r V_o [(1 - E_f) C_o - C_s]}{E_v F_r E_f C_s}$

rate when the thermal load is satisfied. This is accounted for by a flow reduction factor F_r. A mass balance for the contaminant may be written to determine the space contaminant concentration for each of the system arrangements. The various permutations for the air-handling and distribution systems are described in Table 5-10. The mass balance equations for computing the space contaminant concentration for each system are included in Table 5-10.

If the allowable space contamination is specified, the equations in Table 5-10 may be solved for the outdoor flow rate. When the outdoor flow rate is specified, the equations may be used to determine the resulting contaminant concentration.

Local codes and ordinances frequently specify outdoor air ventilation requirements for public places and for industrial installations and must be checked and complied with if their requirements are for greater quantities of outdoorair than provided above.

Example 5-3 A small fast-food cafeteria building, 30 × 100 × 9 ft, located in downtown Chicago, IL, has windows and doors on the east and north sides, but none on the south and west. The HVAC system is to include a humidifier. Estimate the winter design heat losses due to ventilation and/or infiltration. Indoor and outdoor design conditions are 72°F, 30% rh and −3°F, respectively.

Based on ASHRAE *Standard* 62-1989, ventilation is to be at the rate of 20 cfm/person with a density of 100 people per 1000 ft^2. Thus,

$$\text{Ventilation} = [(30 \times 100)/1000] \times 100 \times 20 = 6000 \text{ cfm}$$

With the limited number of openings, infiltration is estimated as 1/2 AC/h plus that due to traffic through swinging doors, approximated as 2000 CFM from Figs. 5-10 and 5-11. Thus,

$$\text{Infiltration} = (1/2)(30 \times 100 \times 9)/60 + 2000 = 2225 \text{ cfm}$$

The ventilation airflow of 6000 cfm is considerably larger than the estimated 2225 cfm of infiltration and should be sufficient to pressurize the building, actually producing exfiltration, rather that having infiltration.

The design heat losses due to outside air entering the building due to ventilation are determined as:

$$q_s = 1.10(6000)([72-(-3)] = 495{,}000 \text{ Btu/h}$$

$$q_l = 4840(6000)(0.005 - 0.0007) = 125{,}000 \text{ Btu/h}$$

$$q_{total} = 495{,}000 + 125{,}000 = 620{,}000 \text{ Btu/h}$$

5.3 Heat Transfer Coefficients

5.3.1 Modes of Heat Transfer

The design of a heating, refrigerating, or air-conditioning system, including selection of building insulation or sizing of piping and ducts, or the evaluation of the thermal performance of system parts such as chillers, heat exchangers, and fans, is based on the principles of heat transfer given in Chapter 3, Heat Transfer, of the 1997 *ASHRAE Handbook—Fundamentals*.

Whenever a temperature difference between two areas (indoor-outdoor) exists, heat flows from the warmer area to the cooler area. The flow or transfer of heat takes place by one or more of three modes—conduction, convection, or radiation.

Conduction is the transfer of heat through a solid. When a poker is left in a fire, the handle is also warmed even though it is not in direct contact with the flame. The flow of heat along the poker is by conduction. The rate of flow is influenced by the temperature difference, the area of the material, the distance through the material from warm side to cool side, and the thermal conductivity of the material. Insulating materials have low thermal conductivity, which, combined with their thickness, provide a barrier that slows conductive heat transfer.

Convection transfers heat by movement through liquids or gases. As a gas (e.g., air) is heated, it expands, becomes lighter, and rises. It is then displaced with cooler air which follows the same cycle, carrying heat with it. The continuous cycle of rising warm air and descending cool air is a convection current. By dividing a large space into many small spaces and providing barriers that restrict convection, the flow of heat can be slowed. The mat of random fibers in batt-type insulation, such as mineral wool or wood fiber insulation, provides such barriers.

Radiation is a method of heat transfer whereby a warm object can heat a cool object without the need of a solid, liquid, or gas between them. An example of radiation is heat from the sun passing through the vacuum of space and warming the earth. In another example, standing in front of a campfire results in the warming of those parts of the body that face the fire. For other body parts to be warmed, the body position must be reversed. The body can also be the radiator and radiate heat to cooler objects.

The **U-factor** and the **R-number** or **R-value** are used to indicate the relative insulating value of materials and sections of walls, floors, and ceilings. The U-factor indicates the rate at which heat flows through a specific material or a building section (Figure 5-16). The smaller the U-factor, the better the insulating value of the material or group of materials making up the wall, ceiling, or floor.

The R-number indicates the ability of one specific material, or a group of materials in a building section, to resist heat flow through them. Many insulating materials now have their R-number stamped on the outside of the package, batt, or blanket. The R-number and relative heat-resisting values of several of these materials are listed in Table 5-11. The R-number for batt, blanket, and loose-fill insulation as listed in this figure is for a thickness of 1 in. The R-number for greater thicknesses can be determined by multiplying the thickness desired, in inches, by the R-number listed.

The greater the R-number, the greater the insulating value of the material, and the lower the heat loss. Thus, a high R-number means lower heating and cooling costs and less energy used to maintain a comfortable temperature.

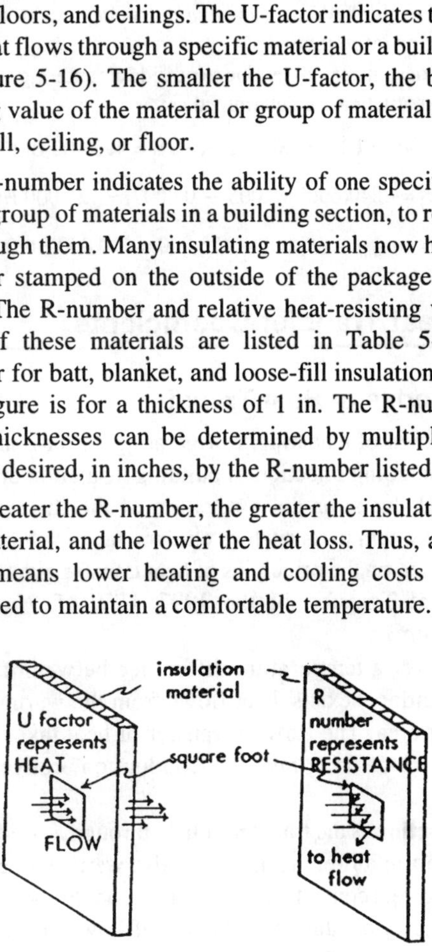

Fig. 5-16 U-Factor and R-Number

Thermal conductivity k is a property of a homogeneous material. Building materials, such as lumber, brick, and stone, are usually considered homogeneous. Most thermal insulation and many other building materials are porous and consist of combinations of solid matter with small voids. For most insulating materials, conduction is not the only mode of heat transfer. Consequently, the term **apparent thermal conductivity** describes the heat flow properties of most materials. Some materials with low thermal conductivities are almost purely conductive (silica opacified aerogel, corkboard, etc.). The apparent thermal conductivity of insulation varies with form and physical structure, environment, and application conditions. Form and physical structure vary with the basic material and manufacturing process. Typical variations include density, cell size, diameter and arrangement of fibers or particles, degree and extent of bonding materials, transparency to thermal radiation, and the type and pressure of gas within the insulation.

The method of calculating an overall coefficient of heat transmission requires knowledge of (1) the apparent thermal conductivity and thickness of homogeneous components, (2) thermal conductance of nonhomogeneous components, (3) surface conductances of both sides of the construction, and (4) conductance of air spaces in the construction.

Surface conductance is the heat transfer to or from the surface by the combined effects of radiation, convection, and conduction. Each of these transport modes can vary independently. Heat transfer by radiation between two surfaces is controlled by the character of the surfaces (emittance and reflectivity), the temperature difference between them, and the solid angle through which they see each other. Heat transfer by convection and conduction is controlled by surface roughness, air movement, and temperature difference between the air and surface.

Heat transfer across an air space is affected by the nature of the boundary surfaces, as well as the intervening air space, the orientation of the air space, the distance between boundary surfaces, and the direction of heat flow. Air space conductance coefficients represent the total conductance from one surface bounding the air space to the other. The total conductance is the sum of a radiation component and a convection and conduction component. In all cases, the spaces are considered airtight with no through air leakage.

The combined effect of the emittances of the boundary surfaces of an air space is expressed by the effective emittance E of the air space. The radiation component is affected only slightly by the thickness of the space, its orientation, the direction of heat flow, or the order of emittance (hot or cold surface). The heat transfer by convection and conduction combined is affected markedly by orientation of the air space and the direction of heat flow, by the temperature difference across the space, and, in some cases, by the thickness of the space. It is also slightly affected by the mean temperature of its surfaces.

The steady-state thermal resistances (R-values) of building components (walls, floors, windows, roof systems, etc.) can be calculated from the thermal properties of the materials in the component; or the heat flow through the assembled com-

Table 5-11 Relative Thermal Resistances of Building Materials

Material Description	Material Density, lb/ft³	Material Thickness, in.	Resistance for Thickness Listed, °F·ft²·h/Btu
Building paper	–	–	0.06
Gypsum plaster, sand aggregate	105	1/2	0.09
Structural glass	–	–	0.10
Air surface, 15 mph wind, outside surface	–	–	0.17
Gypsum or plaster board	50	3/8	0.32
Stone, lime, or sand	–	4	0.32
Concrete, sand-gravel aggregate	140	4	0.32
Built-up roofing	70	3/8	0.33
Brick, face	130	4	0.44
Still air surface, horiz., ordinary materials, heat flow up	–	–	0.61
Aluminum, steel, or vinyl over sheathing, hollow backed	–	–	0.61
Plywood	34	1/2	0.63
Still air surface, vertical, ordinary mtrls, horiz. heat flow	–	–	0.68
Wood siding, bevel, 1/2 in 8 in. lapped	–	–	0.81
Wood shingle siding, 16 in., 7 1/2 in. exposure	–	–	0.87
Oak, maple, and similar hardwoods	45	1	0.91
Air space, vertical, ordinary materials, horiz. heat flow	–	3/4 to 4	0.97
Clay tile, one cell deep	–	4	1.11
Concrete block, 3 core, sand-gravel aggregate	–	8	1.11
Acoustical tile, wood or cane fiber	–	1/2	1.19
Fir, pine, and similar softwoods	32	1	1.25
Insulation board, impregnated	20	1/2	1.32
Concrete, lightweight aggregate	80	4	1.50
Air space, vertical, bounded by reflective material	–	3/4 to 4	1.70
Concrete block, 3 core, cinder aggregate	–	8	1.72
Concrete block, 3 core, lightweight aggregate	–	8	2.00
Vermiculite, expanded	7	1	2.08
Carpet and fibrous pad	–	–	2.08
Cellular glass insulation board	9	1	2.50
Roof insulation, preformed for above deck	–	1	2.78
Mineral wool, loose fill, from slag glass or rock	2–5	1	3.33
Wood fiber, loose fill, hemlock, fir or redwood	2–3.5	1	3.33
Plastic, foamed	1.62	1	3.45
Macerated paper or pulp	2–3.5	1	3.57
Corkboard, without added binder	6.5–8	1	3.70
Batt and Blankets Bounded by Nonreflective Materials			
Mineral wool, fibrous form, rock, slag, or glass	1.5–4	1	3.70
Wood fiber, multilayer, stitched expanded	1.5–2	1	3.70
Cotton fiber	0.8–2	1	3.85
Wood fiber	3.2–3.6	1	4.00

Relative Value of Resistance to Heat flow

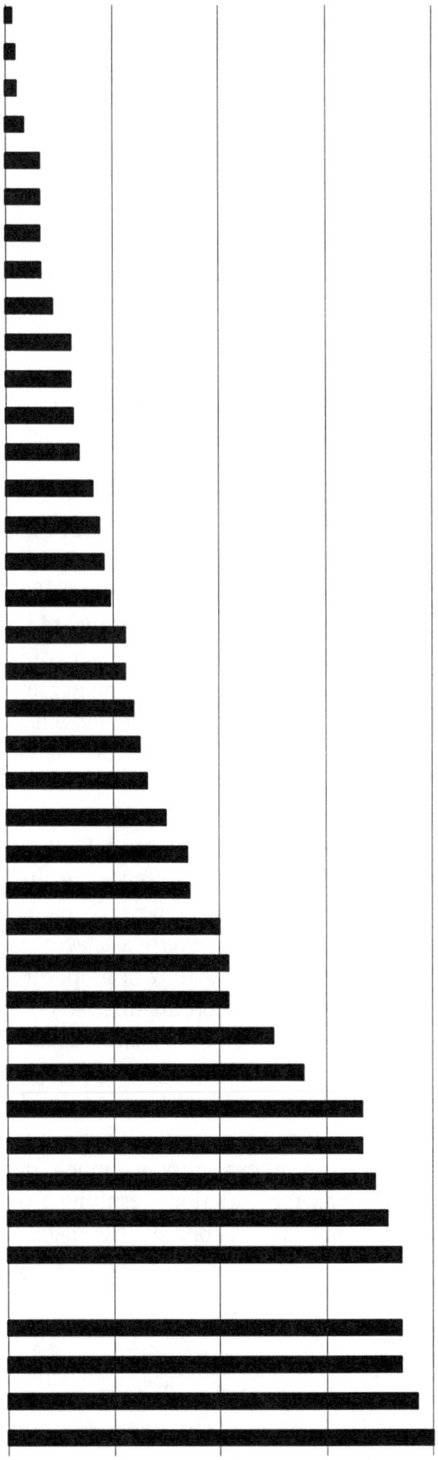

ponent can be measured directly with laboratory equipment such as the guarded hot box (ASTM *Standard* C236) or the calibrated hot box (ASTM *Standard* C976).

Tables 5-12 through 5-15 list thermal values which may be used to calculate thermal resistances of building wall, floors, and ceilings. The values shown in these tables were developed under ideal conditions. In practice, overall thermal performance can be reduced significantly by such factors as improper installation and shrinkage, settling, or compression of the insulation.

The performance of materials fabricated in the field is especially subject to the quality of workmanship during construction and installation. Good workmanship becomes increasingly important as the insulation requirement becomes greater. Therefore, some engineers include additional insulation or other safety factors based on experience in their design.

When installing insulation, irregular areas must be given careful attention. Blanket-type insulation should be sealed by stapling or taping it to the floor, ceiling plates, and studs. Insulating material should be carefully fitted around all plumbing, wiring, and other projections. The proper thickness should be maintained throughout the walls, ceilings, and floors. To get the most value from reflective materials, such as aluminum foil facing on batts or blankets, allow a 0.6-in. (15-mm) airspace between the foil and the wallboard.

In order to obtain the proper density of insulation, competent operators using special equipment blow loose fill insulation (be it for new or remodeled homes) into the walls, floors, and ceilings. Insulation should be blown into each wall cavity at both top and bottom so that all spaces are filled and variations in density are minimized. Variations in insulation density affect the resistance value and the R-number of material. Loose fill insulation tends to settle, resulting in high density insulation below and none above. Therefore, batt or blanket insulation is preferable for vertical spaces in new construction.

Insulation resists heat flow in proportion to its R-number *only* if it is installed according to these general recommendations and the manufacturer's instructions. Wall voids are frequently left open at the top of the stud space, thereby allowing outside air to enter and greatly affect the U-value of the wall.

Common variations in conditions, materials, workmanship, and so forth, can introduce much greater variations in U-values than the variations resulting from assumed mean temperatures and temperature differences. *Therefore, stating a U-value of more than two significant figures may assume more precision than can possibly exist.*

Shading devices, such as venetian blinds, draperies, and roller shades, substantially reduce the U-value for windows and/or glass doors if they fit tightly to the window jambs, head, and sill, and are made of nonporous material. As a rough approximation, tight-fitting shading devices may be considered to reduce the U-value of vertical exterior single glazing by 25% and of vertical exterior double glazing and glass block by 15%. These adjustments should not be considered in choosing heating equipment, but may be used for calculating design cooling loads.

Table 5-12 Surface Conductances and Resistances
(Table 1, Chapter 24, 1997 *ASHRAE Handbook—Fundamentals*)

		Surface Emittance, ε					
		Non-reflective		Reflective			
		ε = 0.90		ε = 0.20		ε = 0.05	
Position of Surface	**Direction of Heat Flow**	h_i	R	h_i	R	h_i	R
STILL AIR							
Horizontal	Upward	1.63	0.61	0.91	1.10	0.76	1.32
Sloping—45°	Upward	1.60	0.62	0.88	1.14	0.73	1.37
Vertical	Horizontal	1.46	0.68	0.74	1.35	0.59	1.70
Sloping—45°	Downward	1.32	0.76	0.60	1.67	0.45	2.22
Horizontal	Downward	1.08	0.92	0.37	2.70	0.22	4.55
MOVING AIR (Any position)		h_o	R				
15-mph Wind (for winter)	Any	6.00	0.17	—	—	—	—
7.5-mph Wind (for summer)	Any	4.00	0.25	—	—	—	—

Notes:
1. Surface conductance h_i and h_o measured in Btu/h·ft²·°F; resistance R in °F·ft²·h/Btu.
2. No surface has both an air space resistance value and a surface resistance value.
3. For ventilated attics or spaces above ceilings under summer conditions (heat flow down), see Table 5.
4. Conductances are for surfaces of the stated emittance facing virtual blackbody surroundings at the same temperature as the ambient air. Values are based on a surface-air temperature difference of 10°F and for surface temperatures of 70°F.
5. See Chapter 3 for more detailed information, especially Tables 5 and 6, and see Figure 1 for additional data.
6. Condensate can have a significant impact on surface emittance (see Table 2).

Table 5-13 Emittance Values of Various Surfaces and Effective Emittances of Airspaces
(Table 2, Chapter 24, 1997 *ASHRAE Handbook—Fundamentals*)

		Effective Emittance ε_{eff} of Air Space	
Surface	**Average Emittance ε**	**One Surface Emittance ε; Other, 0.9**	**Both Surfaces Emittance ε**
Aluminum foil, bright	0.05	0.05	0.03
Aluminum foil, with condensate just visible (> 0.7 gr/ft²)	0.30[b]	0.29	—
Aluminum foil, with condensate clearly visible (> 2.9 gr/ft²)	0.70[b]	0.65	—
Aluminum sheet	0.12	0.12	0.06
Aluminum coated paper, polished	0.20	0.20	0.11
Steel, galvanized, bright	0.25	0.24	0.15
Aluminum paint	0.50	0.47	0.35
Building materials: wood, paper, masonry, nonmetallic paints	0.90	0.82	0.82
Regular glass	0.84	0.77	0.72

[a]These values apply in the 4 to 40 μm range of the electromagnetic spectrum.
[b]Values are based on data presented by Bassett and Trethowen (1984).

5.3.2 Determining U-Factors

The total resistance to heat flow through building construction such as a flat ceiling, floor, or wall (or curved surface if the curvature is small) is the numerical sum of the resistances (R-values) of all parts of the construction in series:

$$R = R_1 + R_2 + R_3 + R_4 + ... + R_n$$

where

$R_1, R_2, ..., R_n$ = individual resistances of the parts
R = resistance of the construction from inside surface to outside surface

Table 5-14 Thermal Resistances of Plane Airspaces
(Table 3, Chapter 24, 1997 *ASHRAE Handbook—Fundamentals*)

Position of Air Space	Direction of Heat Flow	Air Space Mean Temp.[d], °F	Air Space Temp. Diff.[d], °F	0.5-in. Air Space[c] Effective Emittance ε_{eff}[d,e] 0.03	0.05	0.2	0.5	0.82	0.75-in. Air Space[c] Effective Emittance ε_{eff}[d,e] 0.03	0.05	0.2	0.5	0.82
		90	10	2.13	2.03	1.51	0.99	0.73	2.34	2.22	1.61	1.04	0.75
		50	30	1.62	1.57	1.29	0.96	0.75	1.71	1.66	1.35	0.99	0.77
		50	10	2.13	2.05	1.60	1.11	0.84	2.30	2.21	1.70	1.16	0.87
Horiz.	Up ↑	0	20	1.73	1.70	1.45	1.12	0.91	1.83	1.79	1.52	1.16	0.93
		0	10	2.10	2.04	1.70	1.27	1.00	2.23	2.16	1.78	1.31	1.02
		−50	20	1.69	1.66	1.49	1.23	1.04	1.77	1.74	1.55	1.27	1.07
		−50	10	2.04	2.00	1.75	1.40	1.16	2.16	2.11	1.84	1.46	1.20
		90	10	2.44	2.31	1.65	1.06	0.76	2.96	2.78	1.88	1.15	0.81
		50	30	2.06	1.98	1.56	1.10	0.83	1.99	1.92	1.52	1.08	0.82
		50	10	2.55	2.44	1.83	1.22	0.90	2.90	2.75	2.00	1.29	0.94
45° Slope	Up ↗	0	20	2.20	2.14	1.76	1.30	1.02	2.13	2.07	1.72	1.28	1.00
		0	10	2.63	2.54	2.03	1.44	1.10	2.72	2.62	2.08	1.47	1.12
		−50	20	2.08	2.04	1.78	1.42	1.17	2.05	2.01	1.76	1.41	1.16
		−50	10	2.62	2.56	2.17	1.66	1.33	2.53	2.47	2.10	1.62	1.30
		90	10	2.47	2.34	1.67	1.06	0.77	3.50	3.24	2.08	1.22	0.84
		50	30	2.57	2.46	1.84	1.23	0.90	2.91	2.77	2.01	1.30	0.94
		50	10	2.66	2.54	1.88	1.24	0.91	3.70	3.46	2.35	1.43	1.01
Vertical	Horiz. →	0	20	2.82	2.72	2.14	1.50	1.13	3.14	3.02	2.32	1.58	1.18
		0	10	2.93	2.82	2.20	1.53	1.15	3.77	3.59	2.64	1.73	1.26
		−50	20	2.90	2.82	2.35	1.76	1.39	2.90	2.83	2.36	1.77	1.39
		−50	10	3.20	3.10	2.54	1.87	1.46	3.72	3.60	2.87	2.04	1.56
		90	10	2.48	2.34	1.67	1.06	0.77	3.53	3.27	2.10	1.22	0.84
		50	30	2.64	2.52	1.87	1.24	0.91	3.43	3.23	2.24	1.39	0.99
		50	10	2.67	2.55	1.89	1.25	0.92	3.81	3.57	2.40	1.45	1.02
45° Slope	Down ↘	0	20	2.91	2.80	2.19	1.52	1.15	3.75	3.57	2.63	1.72	1.26
		0	10	2.94	2.83	2.21	1.53	1.15	4.12	3.91	2.81	1.80	1.30
		−50	20	3.16	3.07	2.52	1.86	1.45	3.78	3.65	2.90	2.05	1.57
		−50	10	3.26	3.16	2.58	1.89	1.47	4.35	4.18	3.22	2.21	1.66
		90	10	2.48	2.34	1.67	1.06	0.77	3.55	3.29	2.10	1.22	0.85
		50	30	2.66	2.54	1.88	1.24	0.91	3.77	3.52	2.38	1.44	1.02
		50	10	2.67	2.55	1.89	1.25	0.92	3.84	3.59	2.41	1.45	1.02
Horiz.	Down ↓	0	20	2.94	2.83	2.20	1.53	1.15	4.18	3.96	2.83	1.81	1.30
		0	10	2.96	2.85	2.22	1.53	1.16	4.25	4.02	2.87	1.82	1.31
		−50	20	3.25	3.15	2.58	1.89	1.47	4.60	4.41	3.36	2.28	1.69
		−50	10	3.28	3.18	2.60	1.90	1.47	4.71	4.51	3.42	2.30	1.71

Position of Air Space	Direction of Heat Flow	Air Space Mean Temp.[d], °F	Air Space Temp. Diff.[d], °F	1.5-in. Air Space[c] 0.03	0.05	0.2	0.5	0.82	3.5-in. Air Space[c] 0.03	0.05	0.2	0.5	0.82
		90	10	2.55	2.41	1.71	1.08	0.77	2.84	2.66	1.83	1.13	0.80
		50	30	1.87	1.81	1.45	1.04	0.80	2.09	2.01	1.58	1.10	0.84
		50	10	2.50	2.40	1.81	1.21	0.89	2.80	2.66	1.95	1.28	0.93
Horiz.	Up ↑	0	20	2.01	1.95	1.63	1.23	0.97	2.25	2.18	1.79	1.32	1.03
		0	10	2.43	2.35	1.90	1.38	1.06	2.71	2.62	2.07	1.47	1.12
		−50	20	1.94	1.91	1.68	1.36	1.13	2.19	2.14	1.86	1.47	1.20
		−50	10	2.37	2.31	1.99	1.55	1.26	2.65	2.58	2.18	1.67	1.33
		90	10	2.92	2.73	1.86	1.14	0.80	3.18	2.96	1.97	1.18	0.82
		50	30	2.14	2.06	1.61	1.12	0.84	2.26	2.17	1.67	1.15	0.86
		50	10	2.88	2.74	1.99	1.29	0.94	3.12	2.95	2.10	1.34	0.96
45° Slope	Up ↗	0	20	2.30	2.23	1.82	1.34	1.04	2.42	2.35	1.90	1.38	1.06
		0	10	2.79	2.69	2.12	1.49	1.13	2.98	2.87	2.23	1.54	1.16
		−50	20	2.22	2.17	1.88	1.49	1.21	2.34	2.29	1.97	1.54	1.25
		−50	10	2.71	2.64	2.23	1.69	1.35	2.87	2.79	2.33	1.75	1.39
		90	10	3.99	3.66	2.25	1.27	0.87	3.69	3.40	2.15	1.24	0.85
		50	30	2.58	2.46	1.84	1.23	0.90	2.67	2.55	1.89	1.25	0.91
		50	10	3.79	3.55	2.39	1.45	1.02	3.63	3.40	2.32	1.42	1.01
Vertical	Horiz. →	0	20	2.76	2.66	2.10	1.48	1.12	2.88	2.78	2.17	1.51	1.14
		0	10	3.51	3.35	2.51	1.67	1.23	3.49	3.33	2.50	1.67	1.23
		−50	20	2.64	2.58	2.18	1.66	1.33	2.82	2.75	2.30	1.73	1.37
		−50	10	3.31	3.21	2.62	1.91	1.48	3.40	3.30	2.67	1.94	1.50
		90	10	5.07	4.55	2.56	1.36	0.91	4.81	4.33	2.49	1.34	0.90
		50	30	3.58	3.36	2.31	1.42	1.00	3.51	3.30	2.28	1.40	1.00
		50	10	5.10	4.66	2.85	1.60	1.09	4.74	4.36	2.73	1.57	1.08
45° Slope	Down ↘	0	20	3.85	3.66	2.68	1.74	1.27	3.81	3.63	2.66	1.74	1.27
		0	10	4.92	4.62	3.16	1.94	1.37	4.59	4.32	3.02	1.88	1.34
		−50	20	3.62	3.50	2.80	2.01	1.54	3.77	3.64	2.90	2.05	1.57
		−50	10	4.67	4.47	3.40	2.29	1.70	4.50	4.32	3.31	2.25	1.68
		90	10	6.09	5.35	2.79	1.43	0.94	10.07	8.19	3.41	1.57	1.00
		50	30	6.27	5.63	3.18	1.70	1.14	9.60	8.17	3.86	1.88	1.22
		50	10	6.61	5.90	3.27	1.73	1.15	11.15	9.27	4.09	1.93	1.24
Horiz.	Down ↓	0	20	7.03	6.43	3.91	2.19	1.49	10.90	9.52	4.87	2.47	1.62
		0	10	7.31	6.66	4.00	2.22	1.51	11.97	10.32	5.08	2.52	1.64
		−50	20	7.73	7.20	4.77	2.85	1.99	11.64	10.49	6.02	3.25	2.18
		−50	10	8.09	7.52	4.91	2.89	2.01	12.98	11.56	6.36	3.34	2.22

[a]See Chapter 22, section Factors Affecting Heat Transfer across Air Spaces. Thermal resistance values were determined from the relation, $R = 1/C$, where $C = h_c + \varepsilon_{eff} h_r$, h_c is the conduction-convection coefficient, $\varepsilon_{eff} h_r$ is the radiation coefficient $\approx 0.0068\varepsilon_{eff}[(t_m + 460)/100]^3$, and t_m is the mean temperature of the air space. Values for h_c were determined from data developed by Robinson et al. (1954). Equations (5) through (7) in Yarbrough (1983) show the data in this table in analytic form. For extrapolation from this table to air spaces less than 0.5 in. (as in insulating window glass), assume $h_c = 0.159(1 + 0.0016\, t_m)/l$ where l is the air space thickness in inches, and h_c is heat transfer through the air space only.

[b]Values are based on data presented by Robinson et al. (1954). (Also see Chapter 3, Tables 3 and 4, and Chapter 36). Values apply for ideal conditions, i.e., air spaces of uniform thickness bounded by plane, smooth, parallel surfaces with no air leakage to or from the space. When accurate values are required, use overall U-factors determined through calibrated hot box (ASTM C 976) or guarded hot box (ASTM C 236) testing. Thermal resistance values for multiple air spaces must be based on careful estimates of mean temperature differences for each air space.

[c]A single resistance value cannot account for multiple air spaces; each air space requires a separate resistance calculation that applies only for the established boundary conditions. Resistances of horizontal spaces with heat flow downward are substantially independent of temperature difference.

[d]Interpolation is permissible for other values of mean temperature, temperature difference, and effective emittance ε_{eff}. Interpolation and moderate extrapolation for air spaces greater than 3.5 in. are also permissible.

[e]Effective emittance ε_{eff} of the air space is given by $1/\varepsilon_{eff} = 1/\varepsilon_1 + 1/\varepsilon_2 - 1$, where ε_1 and ε_2 are the emittances of the surfaces of the air space (see Table 2).

Table 5-15 Typical Thermal Properties of Common Building and Insulating Materials[a]

(Table 4, Chapter 24, 1997 *ASHRAE Handbook—Fundamentals*)

				Resistance[c] (*R*)		
Description	**Density, lb/ft³**	**Conductivity[b] (*k*), Btu·in / h·ft²·°F**	**Conductance (*C*), Btu / h·ft²·°F**	**Per Inch Thickness (1/*k*), °F·ft²·h / Btu·in**	**For Thickness Listed (1/*C*), °F·ft²·h / Btu**	**Specific Heat, Btu / lb·°F**
BUILDING BOARD						
Asbestos-cement board	120	4.0	—	0.25	—	0.24
Asbestos-cement board 0.125 in.	120	—	33.00	—	0.03	
Asbestos-cement board 0.25 in.	120	—	16.50	—	0.06	
Gypsum or plaster board 0.375 in.	50	—	3.10	—	0.32	0.26
Gypsum or plaster board 0.5 in.	50	—	2.22	—	0.45	
Gypsum or plaster board 0.625 in.	50	—	1.78	—	0.56	
Plywood (Douglas Fir)[d]	34	0.80	—	1.25	—	0.29
Plywood (Douglas Fir) 0.25 in.	34	—	3.20	—	0.31	
Plywood (Douglas Fir) 0.375 in.	34	—	2.13	—	0.47	
Plywood (Douglas Fir) 0.5 in.	34	—	1.60	—	0.62	
Plywood (Douglas Fir) 0.625 in.	34	—	1.29	—	0.77	
Plywood or wood panels 0.75 in.	34	—	1.07	—	0.93	0.29
Vegetable fiber board						
Sheathing, regular density[e] 0.5 in.	18	—	0.76	—	1.32	0.31
0.78125 in.	18	—	0.49	—	2.06	
Sheathing intermediate density[e] 0.5 in.	22	—	0.92	—	1.09	0.31
Nail-base sheathing[e] 0.5 in.	25	—	0.94	—	1.06	0.31
Shingle backer 0.375 in.	18	—	1.06	—	0.94	0.31
Shingle backer 0.3125 in.	18	—	1.28	—	0.78	
Sound deadening board 0.5 in.	15	—	0.74	—	1.35	0.30
Tile and lay-in panels, plain or acoustic	18	0.40	—	2.50	—	0.14
0.5 in.	18	—	0.80	—	1.25	
0.75 in.	18	—	0.53	—	1.89	
Laminated paperboard	30	0.50	—	2.00	—	0.33
Homogeneous board from repulped paper	30	0.50	—	2.00	—	0.28
Hardboard[e]						
Medium density	50	0.73	—	1.37	—	0.31
High density, service-tempered grade and service grade	55	0.82	—	1.22	—	0.32
High density, standard-tempered grade	63	1.00	—	1.00	—	0.32
Particleboard[e]						
Low density	37	0.71	—	1.41	—	0.31
Medium density	50	0.94	—	1.06	—	0.31
High density	62	.5	1.18	—	0.85	—
Underlayment 0.625 in.	40	—	1.22	—	0.82	0.29
Waferboard	37	0.63	—	1.59	—	—
Wood subfloor 0.75 in.	—	—	1.06	—	0.94	0.33
BUILDING MEMBRANE						
Vapor—permeable felt	—	—	16.70	—	0.06	
Vapor—seal, 2 layers of mopped 15-lb felt	—	—	8.35	—	0.12	
Vapor—seal, plastic film	—	—	—	—	Negl.	
FINISH FLOORING MATERIALS						
Carpet and fibrous pad	—	—	0.48	—	2.08	0.34
Carpet and rubber pad	—	—	0.81	—	1.23	0.33
Cork tile 0.125 in.	—	—	3.60	—	0.28	0.48
Terrazzo 1 in.	—	—	12.50	—	0.08	0.19
Tile—asphalt, linoleum, vinyl, rubber	—	—	20.00	—	0.05	0.30
vinyl asbestos						0.24
ceramic						0.19
Wood, hardwood finish 0.75 in.	—	—	1.47	—	0.68	
INSULATING MATERIALS						
Blanket and Batt[f,g]						
Mineral fiber, fibrous form processed from rock, slag, or glass						
approx. 3-4 in.	0.4-2.0	—	0.091	—	11	
approx. 3.5 in.	0.4-2.0	—	0.077	—	13	
approx. 3.5 in.	1.2-1.6	—	0.067	—	15	
approx. 5.5-6.5 in.	0.4-2.0	—	0.053	—	19	
approx. 5.5 in.	0.6-1.0	—	0.048	—	21	
approx. 6-7.5 in.	0.4-2.0	—	0.045	—	22	
approx. 8.25-10 in.	0.4-2.0	—	0.033	—	30	
approx. 10-13 in.	0.4-2.0	—	0.026	—	38	
Board and Slabs						
Cellular glass	8.0	0.33	—	3.03	—	0.18
Glass fiber, organic bonded	4.0-9.0	0.25	—	4.00	—	0.23
Expanded perlite, organic bonded	1.0	0.36	—	2.78	—	0.30
Expanded rubber (rigid)	4.5	0.22	—	4.55	—	0.40

Table 5-15 Typical Thermal Properties of Common Building and Insulating Materials[a] (*Continued*)
(Table 4, Chapter 24, 1997 *ASHRAE Handbook—Fundamentals*)

Description	Density, lb/ft³	Conductivity[b] (*k*), Btu·in/h·ft²·°F	Conductance (*C*), Btu/h·ft²·°F	Resistance[c] (*R*) Per Inch Thickness (1/*k*), °F·ft²·h/Btu·in	Resistance[c] (*R*) For Thickness Listed (1/*C*), °F·ft²·h/Btu	Specific Heat, Btu/lb·°F
Expanded polystyrene, extruded (smooth skin surface) (CFC-12 exp.)	1.8-3.5	0.20	—	5.00	—	0.29
Expanded polystyrene, extruded (smooth skin surface) (HCFC-142b exp.)[h]	1.8-3.5	0.20	—	5.00	—	0.29
Expanded polystyrene, molded beads	1.0	0.26	—	3.85	—	—
	1.25	0.25	—	4.00	—	—
	1.5	0.24	—	4.17	—	—
	1.75	0.24	—	4.17	—	—
	2.0	0.23	—	4.35	—	—
Cellular polyurethane/polyisocyanurate[i,l] (CFC-11 exp.) (unfaced)	1.5	0.16-0.18	—	6.25-5.56	—	0.38
Cellular polyisocyanurate[i] (CFC-11 exp.) (gas-permeable facers)	1.5-2.5	0.16-0.18	—	6.25-5.56	—	0.22
Cellular polyisocyanurate[j] (CFC-11 exp.) (gas-impermeable facers)	2.0	0.14	—	7.04	—	0.22
Cellular phenolic (closed cell) (CFC-11, CFC-113 exp.)[k]	3.0	0.12	—	8.20	—	—
Cellular phenolic (open cell)	1.8-2.2	0.23	—	4.40	—	—
Mineral fiber with resin binder	15.0	0.29	—	3.45	—	0.17
Mineral fiberboard, wet felted						
Core or roof insulation	16-17	0.34	—	2.94	—	—
Acoustical tile	18.0	0.35	—	2.86	—	0.19
Acoustical tile	21.0	0.37	—	2.70	—	—
Mineral fiberboard, wet molded						
Acoustical tile[l]	23.0	0.42	—	2.38	—	0.14
Wood or cane fiberboard						
Acoustical tile[l] 0.5 in.	—	—	0.80	—	1.25	0.31
Acoustical tile[l] 0.75 in.	—	—	0.53	—	1.89	—
Interior finish (plank, tile)	15.0	0.35	—	2.86	—	0.32
Cement fiber slabs (shredded wood with Portland cement binder)	25-27.0	0.50-0.53		2.0-1.89	—	
Cement fiber slabs (shredded wood with magnesia oxysulfide binder)	22.0	0.57	—	1.75	—	0.31
Loose Fill						
Cellulosic insulation (milled paper or wood pulp)	2.3-3.2	0.27-0.32	—	3.70-3.13	—	0.33
Perlite, expanded	2.0-4.1	0.27-0.31	—	3.7-3.3	—	0.26
	4.1-7.4	0.31-0.36	—	3.3-2.8	—	—
	7.4-11.0	0.36-0.42	—	2.8-2.4	—	—
Mineral fiber (rock, slag, or glass)[g]						
approx. 3.75-5 in.	0.6-2.0	—	—	—	11.0	0.17
approx. 6.5-8.75 in.	0.6-2.0	—	—	—	19.0	—
approx. 7.5-10 in.	0.6-2.0	—	—	—	22.0	—
approx. 10.25-13.75 in.	0.6-2.0	—	—	—	30.0	—
Mineral fiber (rock, slag, or glass)[g]						
approx. 3.5 in. (closed sidewall application)	2.0-3.5	—	—	—	12.0-14.0	—
Vermiculite, exfoliated	7.0-8.2	0.47	—	2.13	—	0.32
	4.0-6.0	0.44	—	2.27	—	—
Spray Applied						
Polyurethane foam	1.5-2.5	0.16-0.18	—	6.25-5.56	—	—
Ureaformaldehyde foam	0.7-1.6	0.22-0.28	—	4.55-3.57	—	—
Cellulosic fiber	3.5-6.0	0.29-0.34	—	3.45-2.94	—	—
Glass fiber	3.5-4.5	0.26-0.27	—	3.85-3.70	—	—
Reflective Insulation						
Reflective material ($\varepsilon < 0.5$) in center of 3/4 in. cavity forms two 3/8 in. vertical air spaces[m]	—	—	0.31	—	3.2	—
METALS (See Chapter 36, Table 3)						
ROOFING						
Asbestos-cement shingles	120	—	4.76	—	0.21	0.24
Asphalt roll roofing	70	—	6.50	—	0.15	0.36
Asphalt shingles	70	—	2.27	—	0.44	0.30
Built-up roofing 0.375 in.	70	—	3.00	—	0.33	0.35
Slate 0.5 in.	—	—	20.00	—	0.05	0.30
Wood shingles, plain and plastic film faced	—	—	1.06	—	0.94	0.31

Table 5-15 Typical Thermal Properties of Common Building and Insulating Materials[a] (*Continued*)

(Table 4, Chapter 24, 1997 *ASHRAE Handbook—Fundamentals*)

Description	Density, lb/ft³	Conductivity[b] (*k*), Btu·in / h·ft²·°F	Conductance (*C*), Btu / h·ft²·°F	Resistance[c] (*R*): Per Inch Thickness (1/*k*), °F·ft²·h / Btu·in	Resistance[c] (*R*): For Thickness Listed (1/*C*), °F·ft²·h / Btu	Specific Heat, Btu / lb·°F
PLASTERING MATERIALS						
Cement plaster, sand aggregate	116	5.0	—	0.20	—	0.20
Sand aggregate ... 0.375 in.	—	—	13.3	—	0.08	0.20
Sand aggregate ... 0.75 in.	—	—	6.66	—	0.15	0.20
Gypsum plaster:						
Lightweight aggregate ... 0.5 in.	45	—	3.12	—	0.32	—
Lightweight aggregate ... 0.625 in.	45	—	2.67	—	0.39	—
Lightweight aggregate on metal lath ... 0.75 in.	—	—	2.13	—	0.47	—
Perlite aggregate	45	1.5	—	0.67	—	0.32
Sand aggregate	105	5.6	—	0.18	—	0.20
Sand aggregate ... 0.5 in.	105	—	11.10	—	0.09	—
Sand aggregate ... 0.625 in.	105	—	9.10	—	0.11	—
Sand aggregate on metal lath ... 0.75 in.	—	—	7.70	—	0.13	—
Vermiculite aggregate	45	1.7	—	0.59	—	—
MASONRY MATERIALS						
Masonry Units						
Brick, fired clay	150	8.4-10.2	—	0.12-0.10	—	—
	140	7.4-9.0	—	0.14-0.11	—	—
	130	6.4-7.8	—	0.16-0.12	—	—
	120	5.6-6.8	—	0.18-0.15	—	0.19
	110	4.9-5.9	—	0.20-0.17	—	—
	100	4.2-5.1	—	0.24-0.20	—	—
	90	3.6-4.3	—	0.28-0.24	—	—
	80	3.0-3.7	—	0.33-0.27	—	—
	70	2.5-3.1	—	0.40-0.33	—	—
Clay tile, hollow						
1 cell deep ... 3 in.	—	—	1.25	—	0.80	0.21
1 cell deep ... 4 in.	—	—	0.90	—	1.11	—
2 cells deep ... 6 in.	—	—	0.66	—	1.52	—
2 cells deep ... 8 in.	—	—	0.54	—	1.85	—
2 cells deep ... 10 in.	—	—	0.45	—	2.22	—
3 cells deep ... 12 in.	—	—	0.40	—	2.50	—
Concrete blocks[n, o]						
Limestone aggregate						
8 in., 36 lb, 138 lb/ft³ concrete, 2 cores	—	—	—	—	—	—
Same with perlite filled cores	—	—	0.48	—	2.1	—
12 in., 55 lb, 138 lb/ft³ concrete, 2 cores	—	—	—	—	—	—
Same with perlite filled cores	—	—	0.27	—	3.7	—
Normal weight aggregate (sand and gravel)						
8 in., 33-36 lb, 126-136 lb/ft³ concrete, 2 or 3 cores	—	—	0.90-1.03	—	1.11-0.97	0.22
Same with perlite filled cores	—	—	0.50	—	2.0	—
Same with vermiculite filled cores	—	—	0.52-0.73	—	1.92-1.37	—
12 in., 50 lb, 125 lb/ft³ concrete, 2 cores	—	—	0.81	—	1.23	0.22
Medium weight aggregate (combinations of normal weight and lightweight aggregate)						
8 in., 26-29 lb, 97-112 lb/ft³ concrete, 2 or 3 cores	—	—	0.58-0.78	—	1.71-1.28	—
Same with perlite filled cores	—	—	0.27-0.44	—	3.7-2.3	—
Same with vermiculite filled cores	—	—	0.30	—	3.3	—
Same with molded EPS (beads) filled cores	—	—	0.32	—	3.2	—
Same with molded EPS inserts in cores	—	—	0.37	—	2.7	—
Lightweight aggregate (expanded shale, clay, slate or slag, pumice)						
6 in., 16-17 lb 85-87 lb/ft³ concrete, 2 or 3 cores	—	—	0.52-0.61	—	1.93-1.65	—
Same with perlite filled cores	—	—	0.24	—	4.2	—
Same with vermiculite filled cores	—	—	0.33	—	3.0	—
8 in., 19-22 lb, 72-86 lb/ft³ concrete	—	—	0.32-0.54	—	3.2-1.90	0.21
Same with perlite filled cores	—	—	0.15-0.23	—	6.8-4.4	—
Same with vermiculite filled cores	—	—	0.19-0.26	—	5.3-3.9	—
Same with molded EPS (beads) filled cores	—	—	0.21	—	4.8	—
Same with UF foam filled cores	—	—	0.22	—	4.5	—
Same with molded EPS inserts in cores	—	—	0.29	—	3.5	—
12 in., 32-36 lb, 80-90 lb/ft³ concrete, 2 or 3 cores	—	—	0.38-0.44	—	2.6-2.3	—
Same with perlite filled cores	—	—	0.11-0.16	—	9.2-6.3	—
Same with vermiculite filled cores	—	—	0.17	—	5.8	—
Stone, lime, or sand	180	72	—	0.01	—	—
Quartzitic and sandstone	160	43	—	0.02	—	—
	140	24	—	0.04	—	—

Table 5-15 Typical Thermal Properties of Common Building and Insulating Materials[a] (*Continued*)

(Table 4, Chapter 24, 1997 *ASHRAE Handbook—Fundamentals*)

Description	Density, lb/ft³	Conductivity[b] (*k*), Btu·in / h·ft²·°F	Conductance (*C*), Btu / h·ft²·°F	Resistance[c] (*R*): Per Inch Thickness (1/*k*), °F·ft²·h / Btu·in	Resistance[c] (*R*): For Thickness Listed (1/*C*), °F·ft²·h / Btu	Specific Heat, Btu / lb·°F
	120	13	—	0.08	—	0.19
Calcitic, dolomitic, limestone, marble, and granite	180	30	—	0.03	—	—
	160	22	—	0.05	—	—
	140	16	—	0.06	—	—
	120	11	—	0.09	—	0.19
	100	8	—	0.13	—	—
Gypsum partition tile						
3 by 12 by 30 in., solid	—	—	0.79	—	1.26	0.19
3 by 12 by 30 in., 4 cells	—	—	0.74	—	1.35	—
4 by 12 by 30 in., 3 cells	—	—	0.60	—	1.67	—
Concretes[o]						
Sand and gravel or stone aggregate concretes (concretes	150	10.0-20.0	—	0.10-0.05	—	—
with more than 50% quartz or quartzite sand have	140	9.0-18.0	—	0.11-0.06	—	0.19-0.24
conductivities in the higher end of the range)	130	7.0-13.0	—	0.14-0.08	—	—
Limestone concretes	140	11.1	—	0.09	—	—
	120	7.9	—	0.13	—	—
	100	5.5	—	0.18	—	—
Gypsum-fiber concrete (87.5% gypsum, 12.5% wood chips)	51	1.66	—	0.60	—	0.21
Cement/lime, mortar, and stucco	120	9.7	—	0.10	—	—
	100	6.7	—	0.15	—	—
	80	4.5	—	0.22	—	—
Lightweight aggregate concretes						
Expanded shale, clay, or slate; expanded slags;	120	6.4-9.1	—	0.16-0.11	—	—
cinders; pumice (with density up to 100 lb/ft³); and	100	4.7-6.2	—	0.21-0.16	—	0.20
scoria (sanded concretes have conductivities in the	80	3.3-4.1	—	0.30-0.24	—	0.20
higher end of the range)	60	2.1-2.5	—	0.48-0.40	—	—
	40	1.3	—	0.78	—	—
Perlite, vermiculite, and polystyrene beads	50	1.8-1.9	—	0.55-0.53	—	—
	40	1.4-1.5	—	0.71-0.67	—	0.15-0.23
	30	1.1	—	0.91	—	—
	20	0.8	—	1.25	—	—
Foam concretes	120	5.4	—	0.19	—	—
	100	4.1	—	0.24	—	—
	80	3.0	—	0.33	—	—
	70	2.5	—	0.40	—	—
Foam concretes and cellular concretes	60	2.1	—	0.48	—	—
	40	1.4	—	0.71	—	—
	20	0.8	—	1.25	—	—
SIDING MATERIALS (on flat surface)						
Shingles						
Asbestos-cement	120	—	4.75	—	0.21	—
Wood, 16 in., 7.5 exposure	—	—	1.15	—	0.87	0.31
Wood, double, 16-in., 12-in. exposure	—	—	0.84	—	1.19	0.28
Wood, plus ins. backer board, 0.312 in.	—	—	0.71	—	1.40	0.31
Siding						
Asbestos-cement, 0.25 in., lapped	—	—	4.76	—	0.21	0.24
Asphalt roll siding	—	—	6.50	—	0.15	0.35
Asphalt insulating siding (0.5 in. bed.)	—	—	0.69	—	1.46	0.35
Hardboard siding, 0.4375 in.	—	—	1.49	—	0.67	0.28
Wood, drop, 1 by 8 in.	—	—	1.27	—	0.79	0.28
Wood, bevel, 0.5 by 8 in., lapped	—	—	1.23	—	0.81	0.28
Wood, bevel, 0.75 by 10 in., lapped	—	—	0.95	—	1.05	0.28
Wood, plywood, 0.375 in., lapped	—	—	1.69	—	0.59	0.29
Aluminum, steel, or vinyl[p, q], over sheathing						
Hollow-backed	—	—	1.64	—	0.61	0.29[q]
Insulating-board backed nominal 0.375 in.	—	—	0.55	—	1.82	0.32
Insulating-board backed nominal 0.375 in., foil backed	—	—	0.34	—	2.96	—
Architectural (soda-lime float) glass	158	6.9	—	—	—	0.21
WOODS (12% moisture content)[e,r]						
Hardwoods						0.39[s]
Oak	41.2-46.8	1.12-1.25	—	0.89-0.80	—	
Birch	42.6-45.4	1.16-1.22	—	0.87-0.82	—	
Maple	39.8-44.0	1.09-1.19	—	0.92-0.84	—	
Ash	38.4-41.9	1.06-1.14	—	0.94-0.88	—	

Table 5-15 Typical Thermal Properties of Common Building and Insulating Materials[a] (*Continued*)

(Table 4, Chapter 24, 1997 *ASHRAE Handbook—Fundamentals*)

Description	Density, lb/ft^3	Conductivity[b] (k), Btu·in / h·ft^2·°F	Conductance (C), Btu / h·ft^2·°F	Resistance[c] (R) Per Inch Thickness ($1/k$), °F·ft^2·h / Btu·in	Resistance[c] (R) For Thickness Listed ($1/C$), °F·ft^2·h / Btu	Specific Heat, Btu / lb·°F
Softwoods						0.39[s]
Southern Pine	35.6-41.2	1.00-1.12	—	1.00-0.89	—	
Douglas Fir-Larch	33.5-36.3	0.95-1.01	—	1.06-0.99	—	
Southern Cypress	31.4-32.1	0.90-0.92	—	1.11-1.09	—	
Hem-Fir, Spruce-Pine-Fir	24.5-31.4	0.74-0.90	—	1.35-1.11	—	
West Coast Woods, Cedars	21.7-31.4	0.68-0.90	—	1.48-1.11	—	
California Redwood	24.5-28.0	0.74-0.82	—	1.35-1.22	—	

Notes for Table 5-15

[a]Values are for a mean temperature of 75°F. Representative values for dry materials are intended as design (not specification) values for materials in normal use. Thermal values of insulating materials may differ from design values depending on their in-situ properties (e.g., density and moisture content, orientation, etc.) and variability experienced during manufacture. For properties of a particular product, use the value supplied by the manufacturer or by unbiased tests.

[b]To obtain thermal conductivities in Btu/h·ft·°F, divide the k-factor by 12 in/ft.

[c]Resistance values are the reciprocals of C before rounding off C to two decimal places.

[d]Lewis (1967).

[e]U.S. Department of Agriculture (1974).

[f]Does not include paper backing and facing, if any. Where insulation forms a boundary (reflective or otherwise) of an airspace, see Tables 2 and 3 for the insulating value of an airspace with the appropriate effective emittance and temperature conditions of the space.

[g]Conductivity varies with fiber diameter. (See Chapter 22, Factors Affecting Thermal Performance.) Batt, blanket, and loose-fill mineral fiber insulations are manufactured to achieve specified R-values, the most common of which are listed in the table. Due to differences in manufacturing processes and materials, the product thicknesses, densities, and thermal conductivities vary over considerable ranges for a specified R-value.

[h]This material is relatively new and data are based on limited testing.

[i]For additional information, see Society of Plastics Engineers (SPI) *Bulletin* U108. Values are for aged, unfaced board stock. For change in conductivity with age of expanded polyurethane/polyisocyanurate, see Chapter 22, Factors Affecting Thermal Performance.

[j]Values are for aged products with gas-impermeable facers on the two major surfaces. An aluminum foil facer of 0.001 in. thickness or greater is generally considered impermeable to gases. For change in conductivity with age of expanded polyisocyanurate, see Chapter 22, Factors Affecting Thermal Performance, and SPI *Bulletin* U108.

[k]Cellular phenolic insulation may no longer be manufactured. The thermal conductivity and resistance values do not represent aged insulation, which may have a higher thermal conductivity and lower thermal resistance.

[l]Insulating values of acoustical tile vary, depending on density of the board and on type, size, and depth of perforations.

[m]Cavity is framed with 0.75 in. wood furring strips. Caution should be used in applying this value for other framing materials. The reported value was derived from tests and applies to the reflective path only. The effect of studs or furring strips must be included in determining the overall performance of the wall.

[n]Values for fully grouted block may be approximated using values for concrete with a similar unit weight.

[o]Values for concrete block and concrete are at moisture contents representative of normal use.

[p]Values for metal or vinyl siding applied over flat surfaces vary widely, depending on amount of ventilation of airspace beneath the siding; whether airspace is reflective or nonreflective; and on thickness, type, and application of insulating backing used. Values are averages for use as design guides, and were obtained from several guarded hot box tests (ASTM C 236) or calibrated hot box (ASTM C 976) on hollow-backed types and types made using backing-boards of wood fiber, foamed plastic, and glass fiber. Departures of ±50% or more from these values may occur.

[q]Vinyl specific heat = 0.25 Btu/lb·°F

[r]See Adams (1971), MacLean (1941), and Wilkes (1979). The conductivity values listed are for heat transfer across the grain. The thermal conductivity of wood varies linearly with the density, and the density ranges listed are those normally found for the wood species given. If the density of the wood species is not known, use the mean conductivity value. For extrapolation to other moisture contents, the following empirical equation developed by Wilkes (1979) may be used:

$$k = 0.1791 + \frac{(1.874 \times 10^{-2} + 5.753 \times 10^{-4} M)\rho}{1 + 0.01M}$$

where ρ is density of the moist wood in lb/ft^3, and M is the moisture content in percent.

[s]From Wilkes (1979), an empirical equation for the specific heat of moist wood at 75°F is as follows:

$$c_p = \frac{(0.299 + 0.01M)}{(1 + 0.01M)} + \Delta c_p$$

where Δc_p accounts for the heat of sorption and is denoted by

$$\Delta c_p = M(1.921 \times 10^{-3} - 3.168 \times 10^{-5} M)$$

where M is the moisture content in percent by mass.

However, in buildings, to obtain the overall resistance R_T, the air film resistances R_i and R_o must be added to R.

$$R_T = R_i + R + R_o \tag{5-9}$$

The U-factor (thermal transmittance) is the reciprocal of R_T:

$$U = \frac{1}{R_T}$$

Thus, U is computed by adding up all of the R-values, including those of inside- and outside-air films, the air gap, and all building materials.

With the use of higher values of R_T, the corresponding values of U become very small. This is one reason why it is sometimes preferable to specify resistance rather than transmittance. Also, a whole number is more understandable to an insulation buyer than is a decimal or fraction.

For a wall with air space construction, consisting of two homogeneous materials of conductivities k_1 and k_2 and thickness x_1 and x_2, respectively, and separated by an air space of conductance C, the overall resistance would be determined from

$$R_T = \frac{1}{h_i} + \frac{x_1}{k_1} + \frac{1}{C} + \frac{x_2}{k_2} + \frac{1}{h_0}$$

where h_i and h_0 are the heat transfer film coefficients.

Series and Parallel Heat Flow Paths. In many installations, components are arranged so that heat flows in parallel paths of different conductances. If no heat flows between lateral paths, the U-factor for each path is calculated. The average transmittance is then

$$U_{av} = aU_a + bU_b + ... + nU_n \tag{5-10}$$

where a, b, ..., n are respective fractions of a typical basic area composed of several different paths with transmittances U_a, U_b, ..., U_n.

If heat can flow laterally with little resistance in any continuous layer so that transverse isothermal planes result, total average resistance $R_{T(av)}$ is the sum of the resistance of the layers between such planes. This is a series combination of layers, of which one (or more) provides parallel paths. (See Figure 5-17).

The calculated heat flow, assuming parallel heat flow only, is usually considerably lower than that calculated with the assumption of combined series-parallel heat flow. The actual heat flow is some value between the two calculated values. In the absence of test values for the combination, an intermediate value should be used; examination of the construction usually reveals whether a value closer to the higher or lower calculated value should be used. Generally, if the construction contains any highly conductive layer in which lateral conduction is very high compared to heat flow through the wall, a value closer to the series-parallel calculation should be used. If, however, there is no layer of high lateral conductance, a value closer to the parallel heat flow calculation should be used.

The average overall R-values and U-factors of wood frame walls can be calculated by assuming parallel heat flow paths through areas with different thermal resistances.

The following equation is recommended to correct for the effect of framing members.

$$U_{av} = (S/100)U_s + (1 - S/100)U_i \tag{5-11}$$

where

U_{av} = average U-value for building section
U_i = U-value for area between framing members
U_s = U-value for area backed by framing members
S = percentage of area backed by framing members

The framing factor or fraction of the building component that is framing depends on the specific type of construction, and it may vary based on local construction practices--even for the same type of construction. For stud walls 16 in. on center (OC), the fraction of insulated cavity may be as low as 0.75, where the fraction of studs, plates, and sills is 0.21 and the fraction of headers is 0.04, For studs 24 in. OC, the respective values are 0.78, 0.18, and 0.04. These fractions contain an allowance for multiple studs, plates, sills, extra framing around windows, headers, and band joists.

Unequal Areas. A construction may be made up of two or more layers of unequal area, separated by an airspace, and arranged so that heat flows through the layers in series. The most common such construction is a ceiling and roof combination where the attic space is unheated and unventilated. A combined coefficient based on the most convenient area, say the ceiling area, from air inside to air outside can be calculated from

$$R_{T,c} = R_c + R_r/n \text{ and } U_c = 1/R_{T,c} \tag{5-12}$$

where

U_c = combined coefficient based on ceiling area
n = ratio of roof to ceiling area, A_r/A_c

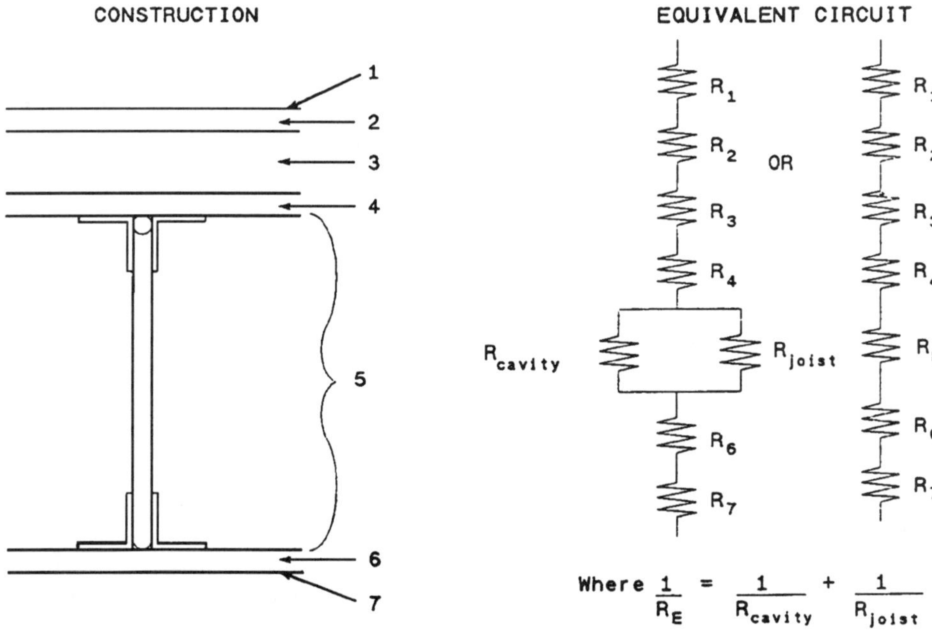

Fig. 5-17 Example of Series/Parallel Unit Flow

Windows and Doors. Table 5-16 lists U-factors for various fenestration products. Table 5-17 provides U-factors for exterior wood and steel doors. All U-factors are approximate, because a significant portion of the resistance of a window or door is contained in the air film resistances, and some parameters that may have important effects are not considered. For example, the listed U-factors assume the surface temperatures of surrounding bodies are equal to the ambient air temperature.

Most fenestration products consist of transparent multipane glazing units and opaque elements comprising the sash and frame (hereafter called frame). The glazing unit's heat transfer paths include a one-dimensional center-of- glass contribution and a two-dimensional edge contribution. The frame contribution is primarily two-dimensional.

Consequently, the total heat transfer can be determined by calculating the separate heat transfer contributions of the center glass, edge glass, and frame. (When present, glazing dividers, such as decorative grilles and muntins, also affect heat transfer, and their contribution must be considered.) The overall U-factor may be estimated by adding the area-weighted U-factors for each contribution.

Table 5-16 lists computed U-factors for a variety of generic fenestration products, *which should only be used as an estimating tool for the early phases of design.* The table is based on ASHRAE-sponsored research involving laboratory testing and computer simulation of various fenestration products. Consequently, computer simulations (with high/low validation by testing) are now accepted as a standard method for determining accurate, product-specific U-factors.

While these U-factors have been determined for winter conditions, they can also be used to estimate heat gain during peak cooling conditions, because conductive gain is usually a small portion of the total heat gain for fenestration in direct sunlight. Glazing designs and framing materials may be compared in choosing a product that needs a specific winter design U-factor.

Table 5-16 lists 48 types of glazing. The multiple glazing categories are appropriate for sealed glass units and the combinations of storm sash and other glazing units. Unless otherwise noted, all multiple-glazed units are filled with dry air.

Six frame types are listed (through not all for any one category), in order of improving thermal performance. The most conservative frame to assume is the aluminum frame **without thermal break** (although some products on the market have higher U-factors). The aluminum frame with thermal break has at least 3/8 in. (10 mm) thermal break between the inside and outside for all members including both the frame and the operable sash, if applicable. (Products are available with significantly wider thermal breaks, which reduce heat flow considerably.)

The **reinforced vinyl/aluminum clad wood** category represents vinyl-frame products, such as sliding glass doors or large windows. These units have extensive metal reinforcing in the frame and wood products with extensive metal, usually on the exterior surface of the frame. The metal, of course, degrades the thermal performance of the frame material.

The **wood/vinyl frame** represents improved thermal performance over reinforced vinyl/aluminum clad wood. **Insulated fiberglass/vinyl frames** do not have metal reinforcing and the frame cavities are filled with insulation.

Shading devices, such as venetian blinds, draperies, and roller shades, substantially reduce the U-value for windows and/or glass doors if they fit tightly to the window jambs, head, and sill, and are made of nonporous material. As a rough approximation, tight-fitting shading devices may be considered to reduce the U-value of vertical exterior single glazing by 25% and of vertical exterior double glazing and glass block by 15%. These adjustments should not be considered in choosing heating equipment, but may be used for calculating design cooling loads.

5.3.3 The Overall Thermal Transmittance

U_o is the combined thermal transmittance of the respective areas of gross exterior wall, roof or ceiling or both, and floor assemblies. The overall thermal transmittance of the building envelope assembly shall be calculated from:

$$\begin{aligned} U_o &= \Sigma U_i A_i / A_o \\ &= (U_1 A_1 + U_2 A_2 + \ldots + U_n A_n)/A_o \end{aligned} \tag{5-13}$$

where

U_o = the area-weighted average thermal transmittance of the gross area of an envelope assembly; i.e., the exterior wall assembly including fenestration and doors, the roof and ceiling assembly, and the floor assembly, Btu/(h·ft²·°F)

A_o = The gross area of the envelope assembly, ft²

U_i = the thermal transmittance of each individual path of the envelope assembly, i.e., the opaque portion or the fenestration, Btu/(h·ft²·°F)

U_i = $1/R_i$ (where R_i is the total resistance to heat flow of an individual path through an envelope assembly).

A_i = the area of each individual element of the envelope assembly, ft²

5.4 Calculating Surface Temperatures

The temperature at any interface can be calculated, since the temperature drop through any component of the wall is proportional to its resistance. Thus, the temperature drop Δt through R_1 is

$$\Delta t_1 = \frac{R_1(t_i - t_0)}{R_T} \tag{5-14}$$

where t_1 and t_0 are the indoor and outdoor temperatures, respectively. Hence, the temperature at the interface between R_1 and R_2 is

$$t_{1\text{-}2} = t_i - \Delta t_1$$

If the resistances of materials in a wall are highly dependent on temperature, the mean temperature must be known to assign the correct value. In such cases, it is perhaps most convenient to use a trial-and-error procedure for the calculation

Table 5-16 Overall Coefficients of Heat Transmission of Various Fenestrations

(Table 5, Page 29.8 only, Chapter 29, 1997 *ASHRAE Handbook—Fundamentals*)

Product Type		Glass Only		Vertical Installation									
				Operable (including sliding and swinging glass doors)					Fixed				
Frame Type		Center of Glass	Edge of Glass	Aluminum without Thermal Break	Aluminum with Thermal Break	Reinforced Vinyl/ Aluminum Clad Wood	Wood/ Vinyl	Insulated Fiberglass/ Vinyl	Aluminum without Thermal Break	Aluminum with Thermal Break	Reinforced Vinyl/ Aluminum Clad Wood	Wood/ Vinyl	Insulated Fiberglass/ Vinyl
ID	Glazing Type												
	Single Glazing												
1	1/8 in. glass	*1.04*	*1.04*	1.27	1.08	0.90	0.89	0.81	1.13	1.07	0.98	0.98	0.94
2	1/4 in. acrylic/polycarb	*0.88*	*0.88*	1.14	0.96	0.79	0.78	0.71	0.99	0.92	0.84	0.84	0.81
3	1/8 in. acrylic/polycarb	*0.96*	*0.96*	1.21	1.02	0.85	0.83	0.76	1.06	1.00	0.91	0.91	0.87
	Double Glazing												
4	1/4 in. airspace	*0.55*	*0.64*	0.87	0.65	0.57	0.55	0.49	0.69	0.63	0.56	0.56	0.53
5	1/2 in. airspace	*0.48*	*0.59*	0.81	0.60	0.53	0.51	0.44	0.64	0.57	0.50	0.50	0.48
6	1/4 in. argon space	*0.51*	*0.61*	0.84	0.62	0.55	0.53	0.46	0.66	0.59	0.53	0.52	0.50
7	1/2 in. argon space	*0.45*	*0.57*	0.79	0.58	0.51	0.49	0.43	0.61	0.54	0.48	0.48	0.45
	Double Glazing, *e* = 0.60 on surface 2 or 3												
8	1/4 in. airspace	*0.52*	*0.62*	0.84	0.63	0.55	0.53	0.47	0.67	0.60	0.54	0.53	0.51
9	1/2 in. airspace	*0.44*	*0.56*	0.78	0.57	0.50	0.48	0.42	0.60	0.53	0.47	0.47	0.45
10	1/4 in. argon space	*0.47*	*0.58*	0.81	0.59	0.52	0.50	0.44	0.63	0.56	0.50	0.49	0.47
11	1/2 in. argon space	*0.41*	*0.54*	0.76	0.55	0.48	0.46	0.40	0.58	0.51	0.45	0.44	0.42
	Double Glazing, *e* = 0.40 on surface 2 or 3												
12	1/4 in. airspace	*0.49*	*0.60*	0.82	0.61	0.53	0.51	0.45	0.64	0.58	0.51	0.51	0.49
13	1/2 in. airspace	*0.40*	*0.54*	0.75	0.54	0.48	0.45	0.40	0.57	0.50	0.44	0.44	0.41
14	1/4 in. argon space	*0.43*	*0.56*	0.78	0.57	0.50	0.47	0.41	0.59	0.53	0.46	0.46	0.44
15	1/2 in. argon space	*0.36*	*0.51*	0.72	0.52	0.45	0.43	0.37	0.53	0.47	0.41	0.40	0.38
	Double Glazing, *e* = 0.20 on surface 2 or 3												
16	1/4 in. airspace	*0.45*	*0.57*	0.79	0.58	0.51	0.49	0.43	0.61	0.54	0.48	0.48	0.45
17	1/2 in. airspace	*0.35*	*0.50*	0.71	0.51	0.44	0.42	0.36	0.53	0.46	0.40	0.39	0.37
18	1/4 in. argon space	*0.38*	*0.52*	0.74	0.53	0.46	0.44	0.38	0.55	0.48	0.42	0.42	0.40
19	1/2 in. argon space	*0.30*	*0.46*	0.67	0.47	0.41	0.39	0.33	0.48	0.41	0.36	0.35	0.33
	Double Glazing, *e* = 0.10 on surface 2 or 3												
20	1/4 in. airspace	*0.42*	*0.55*	0.77	0.56	0.49	0.47	0.41	0.59	0.52	0.46	0.45	0.43
21	1/2 in. airspace	*0.32*	*0.48*	0.69	0.49	0.42	0.40	0.35	0.50	0.43	0.37	0.37	0.35
22	1/4 in. argon space	*0.35*	*0.50*	0.71	0.51	0.44	0.42	0.36	0.53	0.46	0.40	0.39	0.37
23	1/2 in. argon space	*0.27*	*0.44*	0.65	0.45	0.39	0.37	0.31	0.46	0.39	0.33	0.33	0.31
	Double Glazing, *e* = 0.05 on surface 2 or 3												
24	1/4 in. airspace	*0.41*	*0.54*	0.76	0.55	0.48	0.46	0.40	0.58	0.51	0.45	0.44	0.42
25	1/2 in. airspace	*0.30*	*0.46*	0.67	0.47	0.41	0.39	0.33	0.48	0.41	0.36	0.35	0.33
26	1/4 in. argon space	*0.33*	*0.48*	0.70	0.49	0.43	0.41	0.35	0.51	0.44	0.38	0.38	0.36
27	1/2 in. argon space	*0.25*	*0.42*	0.63	0.44	0.38	0.36	0.30	0.44	0.37	0.32	0.31	0.29
	Triple Glazing												
28	1/4 in. airspaces	*0.38*	*0.52*	0.72	0.51	0.44	0.43	0.38	0.55	0.48	0.42	0.41	0.40
29	1/2 in. airspaces	*0.31*	*0.47*	0.67	0.46	0.40	0.39	0.34	0.49	0.42	0.36	0.35	0.34
30	1/4 in. argon spaces	*0.34*	*0.49*	0.69	0.48	0.42	0.41	0.35	0.51	0.45	0.39	0.38	0.36
31	1/2 in. argon spaces	*0.29*	*0.45*	0.65	0.44	0.38	0.37	0.32	0.47	0.40	0.34	0.34	0.32
	Triple Glazing, *e* = 0.20 on surface 2,3,4, or 5												
32	1/4 in. airspaces	*0.33*	*0.48*	0.69	0.47	0.41	0.40	0.35	0.50	0.44	0.38	0.37	0.36
33	1/2 in. airspaces	*0.25*	*0.42*	0.62	0.41	0.36	0.35	0.30	0.43	0.37	0.31	0.30	0.29
34	1/4 in. argon spaces	*0.28*	*0.45*	0.65	0.44	0.38	0.37	0.32	0.46	0.40	0.34	0.33	0.32
35	1/2 in. argon spaces	*0.22*	*0.40*	0.60	0.39	0.34	0.33	0.28	0.41	0.34	0.29	0.28	0.27
	Triple Glazing, *e* = 0.20 on surfaces 2 or 3 and 4 or 5												
36	1/4 in. airspaces	*0.29*	*0.45*	0.65	0.44	0.38	0.37	0.32	0.47	0.40	0.34	0.34	0.32
37	1/2 in. airspaces	*0.20*	*0.39*	0.58	0.38	0.32	0.31	0.27	0.39	0.33	0.27	0.26	0.25
38	1/4 in. argon spaces	*0.23*	*0.41*	0.61	0.40	0.34	0.33	0.29	0.42	0.35	0.30	0.29	0.28
39	1/2 in. argon spaces	*0.17*	*0.36*	0.56	0.36	0.30	0.29	0.25	0.37	0.30	0.25	0.24	0.23
	Triple Glazing, *e* = 0.10 on surfaces 2 or 3 and 4 or 5												
40	1/4 in. airspaces	*0.27*	*0.44*	0.64	0.43	0.37	0.36	0.31	0.45	0.39	0.33	0.32	0.31
41	1/2 in. airspaces	*0.18*	*0.37*	0.57	0.36	0.31	0.30	0.25	0.37	0.31	0.25	0.25	0.23
42	1/4 in. argon spaces	*0.21*	*0.39*	0.59	0.39	0.33	0.32	0.27	0.40	0.34	0.28	0.27	0.26
43	1/2 in. argon spaces	*0.14*	*0.34*	0.54	0.33	0.28	0.27	0.23	0.34	0.28	0.22	0.21	0.20
	Quadruple Glazing, *e* = 0.10 on surfaces 2 or 3 and 4 or 5												
44	1/4 in. airspaces	*0.22*	*0.40*	0.60	0.39	0.34	0.33	0.28	0.41	0.34	0.29	0.28	0.27
45	1/2 in. airspaces	*0.15*	*0.35*	0.54	0.34	0.29	0.28	0.24	0.35	0.28	0.23	0.22	0.21
46	1/4 in. argon spaces	*0.17*	*0.36*	0.56	0.36	0.30	0.29	0.25	0.37	0.30	0.25	0.24	0.23
47	1/2 in. argon spaces	*0.12*	*0.32*	0.52	0.32	0.27	0.26	0.22	0.32	0.26	0.20	0.20	0.19
48	1/4 in. krypton spaces	*0.12*	*0.32*	0.52	0.32	0.27	0.26	0.22	0.32	0.26	0.20	0.20	0.19

Notes:

1. All heat transmission coefficients in this table include film resistances and are based on winter conditions of 0°F outdoor air temperature and 70°F indoor air temperature, with 15 mph outdoor air velocity and zero solar flux. With the exception of single glazing, small changes in the indoor and outdoor temperatures will not significantly affect overall U-factors. The coefficients are for vertical position except skylight and sloped glazing values, which are for 20° from horizontal with heat flow up.

2. Glazing layer surfaces are numbered from the outdor to the indor. Double, triple and quadruple refer to the number of glazing panels. All data are based on 1/8 inch glass, unless otherwise noted. Thermal conductivities are: 0.53 Btu/(h·ft·°F) for glass, and 0.11 Btu/(h·ft·°F) for acrylic and polycarbonate.

3. Standard spacers are metal. Edge-of-glass effects assumed to extend over the 2 1/2 inch band around perimeter of each glazing unit as in Figure 3.

Table 5-17 Transmission Coefficients for Wood and Steel Doors

(Table 6, Chapter 24, 1997 *ASHRAE Handbook—Fundamentals*)

Nominal Door Thickness, in.	Description	No Storm Door	Wood Storm Door[c]	Metal Storm Door[d]
Wood Doors[a,b]				
1-3/8	Panel door with 7/16-in. panels[e]	0.57	0.33	0.37
1-3/8	Hollow core flush door	0.47	0.30	0.32
1-3/8	Solid core flush door	0.39	0.26	0.28
1-3/4	Panel door with 7/16-in. panels[e]	0.54	0.32	0.36
1-3/4	Hollow core flush door	0.46	0.29	0.32
1-3/4	Panel door with 1-1/8-in. panels[e]	0.39	0.26	0.28
1-3/4	Solid core flush door	0.40	—	0.26
2-1/4	Solid core flush door	0.27	0.20	0.21
Steel Doors[b]				
1-3/4	Fiberglass or mineral wool core with steel stiffeners, no thermal break[f]	0.60	—	—
1-3/4	Paper honeycomb core without thermal break[f]	0.56	—	—
1-3/4	Solid urethane foam core without thermal break[a]	0.40	—	—
1-3/4	Solid fire rated mineral fiberboard core without thermal break[f]	0.38	—	—
1-3/4	Polystyrene core without thermal break (18 gage commercial steel)[f]	0.35	—	—
1-3/4	Polyurethane core without thermal break (18 gage commercial steel)[f]	0.29	—	—
1-3/4	Polyurethane core without thermal break (24 gage residential steel)[f]	0.29	—	—
1-3/4	Polyurethane core with thermal break and wood perimeter (24 gage residential steel)[f]	0.20	—	—
1-3/4	Solid urethane foam core with thermal break[a]	0.20	—	0.16

Note: All U-factors for exterior doors in this table are for doors with no glazing, except for the storm doors which are in addition to the main exterior door. Any glazing area in exterior doors should be included with the appropriate glass type and analyzed as a window (see Chapter 29). Interpolation and moderate extrapolation are permitted for door thicknesses other than those specified.

[a]Values are based on a nominal 32 in. by 80 in. door size with no glazing.

[b]Outside air conditions: 15 mph wind speed, 0°F air temperature; inside air conditions: natural convection, 70°F air temperature.

[c]Values for wood storm door are for approximately 50% glass area.

[d]Values for metal storm door are for any percent glass area.

[e]55% panel area.

[f]ASTM C 236 hotbox data on a nominal 3 ft by 7 ft door size with no glazing.

of the total resistance R_T. First the mean operating temperature for each layer is estimated, and R-values for the particular materials are selected. The total resistance R_T is then calculated and the temperature at each interface is calculated.

The mean temperature of each component (arithmetic mean of its surface temperatures) can then be used to obtain second generation R-values. This procedure can then be repeated until the R-values have been correctly selected for the resulting mean temperatures. Generally, this can be done in two or three trial calculations.

Figure 5-18 illustrates the procedure for determining the temperatures throughout the structure.

Example 5-3 Determine the winter U-value for a cavity wall consisting of face brick, 8-in. concrete block (three oval core, lightweight aggregate), a 3/4-in. airspace as the cavity, another layer of the same type of concrete block, 2 in. of rigid organic bonded glass fiber insulation, and 1/2-in. plasterboard.

Solution:

Component	Resistance	
Outside air	0.17	(Table 5-13)
Brick, 4-in. face	0.44	(Table 5-12)
Concrete block, 8 in.	2.00	(Table 5-15)
Airspace, 3/4 in.	1.00	(Table 5-14)
Concrete block, 8 in.	2.00	(Table 5-15)
Glass fiber insulation, 2 in.	8.00	(Table 5-15)
Plasterboard, 1/2 in.	0.45	(Table 5-14)
Inside air	0.68	(Table 5-12)
Total $R =$	14.74	

$$U = 1/R_T = 1/14.74 = 0.068 \text{ Btu/h·ft}^2\text{·°F}$$

	Item	R	R_T	U
①	Outside air film	0.17	0.17	
②	8" concrete block, light aggregate vermiculite filled core	4.6	4.77	
③	3-1/2" mineral fiber insulation	11.0	15.77	
④	1/2" mineral fiber insulation	0.45	16.22	
⑤	Inside air film	0.68	16.9	0.059

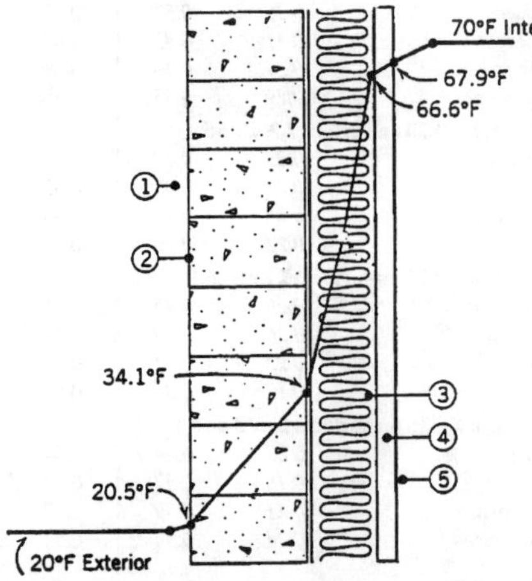

Component	Component Temperature Rise	Temperatures Cold Side	Temperatures Warm Side
① Air film	0.17/16.9 × 50°F = 0.5°	20°F	20.5°F
② 8 in. block	4.6/16.9 × 50°F = 13.6°	20°F	20.5°F
③ 3-1/2 in. insul.	11/16.9 × 50°F = 32.5°	20°F	20.5°F
④ Gypsum board	0.45/16.9 × 50°F = 1.3°	20°F	20.5°F
⑤ Inside air film	0.68/16.9 × 50°F = 2.1°	20°F	20.5°F

Fig. 5-18 Temperatures Throughout Wall

Example 5-4 Determine the overall coefficients (U-values) for winter for (a) a solid wood door, 1 3/4 in. thick, with glass storm door and (b) the flat ceiling/roof of an industrial building, which consists of a painted sheet metal exterior, 1/2-in. nail-base fiberboard sheathing, and wood rafters.

Solution:

(a) Use Table 5-17 to find the U-value.

$$U = 0.26 \text{ Btu/h}\cdot\text{ft}^2\cdot°\text{F}$$

(b) To calculate the U-value of the ceiling, add the resistance values of each element.

Component	Resistance	
Inside Air	0.61	(Table 5-13)
Sheathing	1.14	(Table 5-15)
Outside Air	0.17	(Table 5-13)
Total $R =$	1.92	

$$U = 1/1.92 = 0.52 \text{ Btu/h}\cdot\text{ft}^2\cdot°\text{F} \quad (5\text{-}15)$$

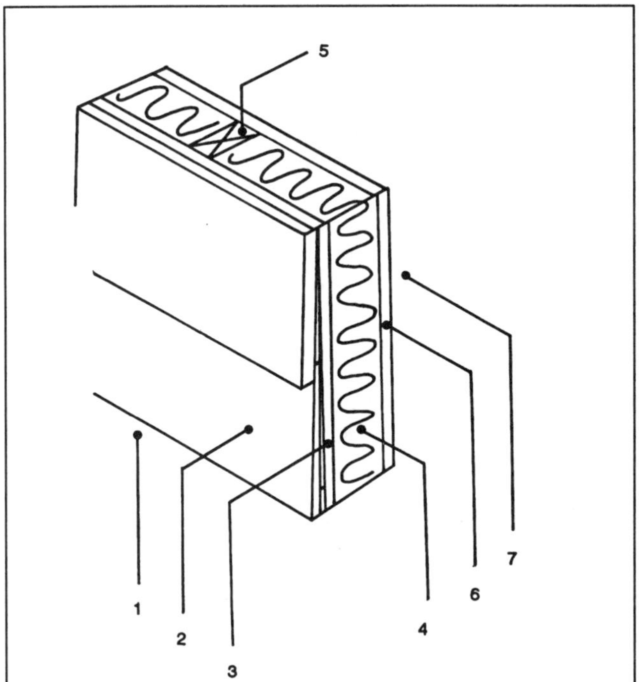

Fig. 5-19 Insulated Wood Frame Wall (Example 5-5)

Example 5-5 Calculate the U-factor of the 2 by 4 stud wall shown in Figure 5-19. The studs are at 16 in. OC. There is 3.5 in. mineral fiber batt insulation (R-13) in the stud space. The inside finish is 0.5 in. gypsum wallboard; the outside is finished with rigid foam insulating sheathing (R-4) and 0.5 in. by 8 in. wood bevel lapped siding. The insulated cavity occupies approximately 75% of the transmission area; the studs, plates, and sills occupy 21%; and the headers occupy 4%.

Solution. Obtain the R-values of the various building elements from Tables 5-12 and 5-15. Assume the $R = 1.25$ per inch for the wood framing. Also, assume the headers are solid wood, in this case, and group them with the studs, plates, and sills.

Element	R (Insulated Cavity)	R (Studs, Plates, and Headers)
1. Outside surface, 15 mphwind	0.17	0.17
2. Wood bevel lapped siding	0.81	0.81
3. Rigid foam insulating sheathing	4.0	4.0
4. Mineral fiber batt insulation, 3.5 in.	13.0	—
5. Wood stud, nominal 2 × 4	—	4.38
6. Gypsum wallboard, 0.5 in.	0.45	0.45
7. Inside surface, still air	0.68	0.68
	$R_1 = 19.11$	$R_2 = 10.49$

Since the U-factor is the reciprocal of R-value, $U_1 = 0.052$ and $U_2 = 0.095$ Btu/h·ft²·°F.

If the wood framing (thermal bridging) is not included, Equation (3) from Chapter 22 may be used to calculate the U-factor of the wall as follows:

$$U_{av} = U_1 = \frac{1}{R_1} = 0.052 \text{ Btu/h}\cdot\text{ft}^2\cdot°\text{F}$$

If the wood framing is accounted for using the parallel-path flow method, the U-factor of the wall is determined using Equation (5) from Chapter 22 as follows:

$$U_{av} = (0.75 \times 0.052) + (0.25 \times 0.095) = 0.063 \text{ Btu/h}\cdot\text{ft}^2\cdot°\text{F}$$

If the wood framing is included using the isothermal planes method, the U-factor of the wall is determined using Equations (2) and (3) from Chapter 22 as follows:

$$R_{T(av)} = 4.98 + 1/[(0.75/13.0) + (0.25/4.38)] + 1.13$$

$$= 14.82°\text{F}\cdot\text{ft}^2\cdot\text{h/Btu}$$

$$U_{av} = 0.067 \text{ Btu/h}\cdot\text{ft}^2\cdot°\text{F}$$

For a frame wall with a 24-in. OC stud space, the average overall R-value is 15.18°F·ft²·h/Btu. Similar calculation procedures may be used to evaluate other wall designs, except those with thermal bridges.

5.5 Problems

5.1 With an 11.2-m/s wind blowing uniformly against one face of a building, what pressure differential would be used to calculate the air leakage into the building?

5.2 Assuming a zero wind velocity, what would be the leakage rate through a nonweather-stripped aluminum 3 ft by 5 ft casement window (reasonably tight) set in a masonry wall (caulked) when the pressure inside the building is 0.2 in. of water?

5.3 A double door has a 1/8-in. crack on all sides except between the two doors, which has a 1/4-in. crack. What would be the leakage rate for the building of *Problem* 5.1?

[Ans: 453 cfm]

5.4 Assuming a 20-mph wind blowing against the window and an inside pressure of 0.05 in. of water, find the infiltration through a wood, double-hung, 3 ft by 2 ft, locked, non-weather-stripped, loosely fit window set in a masonry wall and caulked. There is no temperature difference, no shielding, and it is on the first floor.

5.5 Determine the heat loss due to infiltration of 236 L/s of outdoor air at 9°C when the indoor air is 24°C.

5.6 Give an expression for (a) the sensible load due to infiltration, and (b) the latent load due to infiltration.

5.7 Can wind forces and Δt forces cancel each other when predicting infiltration? Reinforce? How can infiltration be prevented entirely?

5.8 What methods does ASHRAE suggest using to estimate infiltration rate? Which method appears to be most accurate? Which method is most used? How are infiltration rates determined by test?

5.9 A building is 75 ft wide by 100 ft long and 10 ft high. The indoor conditions are 75°F and 24% rh, and the outside conditions are 0°F and saturated. The infiltration rate is estimated to be 0.75 ACH. Calculate the sensible and latent heat loss. [Ans: 77,300 Btu/h; 17,700 Btu/h]

5.10 How can infiltration rates be reduced? Does a reduction in the infiltration rate always result in a reduction of the air-conditioning load? In air-conditioning equipment size? Explain.

5.11 A 3 ft by 3 ft ventilation opening is in a wall facing in the prevalent wind direction. There are adequate openings in the roof for the passage of exhaust air. Estimate the ventilation rate for a 25-mph wind.

5.12 A building 20 ft by 40 ft by 9 ft has an anticipated infiltration rate of 0.75 air changes per hour. Indoor design conditions are 75°F, 30% rh minimum. Outdoor design temperature is 5°F.

(a) Determine sensible, latent, and total heat loads (Btu/h) due to infiltration.

(b) Specify the necessary humidifier size (lb/h).

[Ans: 8890 Btu/h, 1.8 lb/h]

5.13 A small factory with a 10-ft high ceiling is shown. There are 22 employees normally in the shop area and 4 employees in the office area. On a winter day when the outside temperature is 0°F, the office is maintained at 75°F, 25% rh, and the

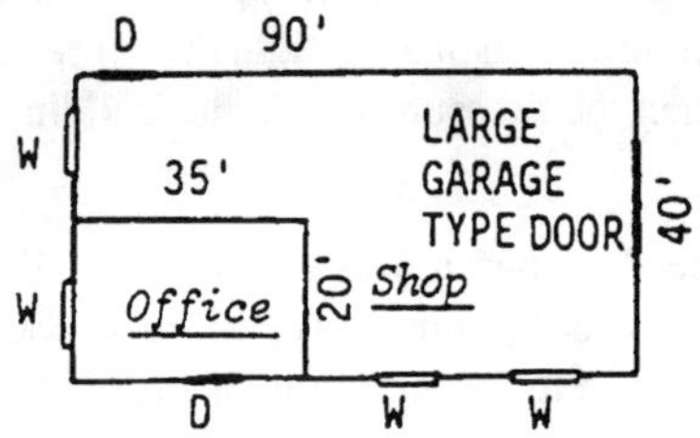

shop is kept at 68°F with no humidity control. Determine for each area:

(a) infiltration, cfm

(b) minimum required outside air, cfm

(c) sensible heat loss due to infiltration, Btu/h

(d) latent heat loss due to infiltration, Btu/h

5.14 Specify the required amount of outside air for ventilation of the following:

(a) 12 ft by 12 ft private office with 8 ft high walls

(b) department store with 20,000 ft2 of floor area

5.15 A wall consists of 4 in. of face brick, 1/2 in. of cement mortar, 8-in. hollow clay tile, an airspace 1 5/8 in. wide, and wood lath and plaster totaling 3/4 in. Find the U-values for both winter and summer.

5.16 The ceiling of a house is 3/4-in. (19-mm) acoustical tile on furring strips with highly reflective aluminum foil across the top of the ceiling joists. Determine the U-value for cooling load calculations.

5.17 Calculate the winter U-value for a wall consisting of 4-in. (100-mm) face brick, 4-in. (100-mm) common brick, and 1/2 in. (13 mm) of gypsum plaster (sand aggregate).

[Ans: 0.459 Btu/h$\cdot$ ft$^2\cdot$°F [2.61 W/(m$^2\cdot$ K)]]

5.18 Find the overall coefficient of heat transmission U for a wall consisting of 4 in. of face brick, 1/2 in. of cement mortar, 8 in. of stone, and 3/4 in. of gypsum plaster. The outside air velocity is 15 mph and the inside air is still.

5.19 A wall has an overall coefficient $U = 1.31$ W/(m$^2\cdot$K). What is the conductance of the wall when its outside surface is exposed to a wind velocity of 6.7 m/s and the inside air is still?

5.20 Compute the U-value for a wall of frame construction consisting of 1/2 by 8 bevel siding, permeable felt building paper, 25/32-in. wood fiber sheathing, 2 by 4 studding on 16-in. centers, and 3/4-in. metal lath and sand plaster. Outside wind velocity is 15 mph. [Ans: 0.206 Btu/ h$\cdot$ ft$^2\cdot$°F]

5.21 For the wall of *Problem* 5.20, determine *U* if the space between the studs is filled with fiberglass blanket insulation. Neglect the effect of the studs.

5.22 Rework *Problem* 5.21 including the effect of the studs.

5.23 A concrete wall 250 mm thick is exposed to outside air at −15°C with a velocity of 6.7 m/s. Inside air temperature is 15.6°C. Determine the heat flow through 14.9 m^2 of this wall. [Ans: 1548 W]

5.24 Find the overall coefficient of heat transfer and the total thermal resistance for the following exterior wall exposed to a 25-mph wind: face brick veneer, 25/32-in. insulating board sheathing, 3-in. fiberglass insulation in stud space, and 1/4-in. walnut veneer plywood panels for the interior.

5.25 What is the thermal resistance of 12.1 cm (4-3/4 in.) thick precast concrete (stone aggregate, oven dried)?

5.26 A composite wall structure experiences a -10°F air temperature on the outside and a 75°F air temperature on the inside. The wall consists of a 4 in. thick outer facebrick, a 2-in. batt of fiberglass insulation, and a 3/8-in. sheet of gypsum board. Determine the U-value and the heat flow rate, per ft^2. Plot the steady-state temperature profile across the wall. [Ans: 0.118 Btu/h· ft2·°F, 10.07 Btu/h· ft^2]

5.27 Find the overall heat transmission coefficient for a floor-ceiling sandwich (heat flow up) having the following construction. [Ans: 0.22 Btu/h· ft·°F]

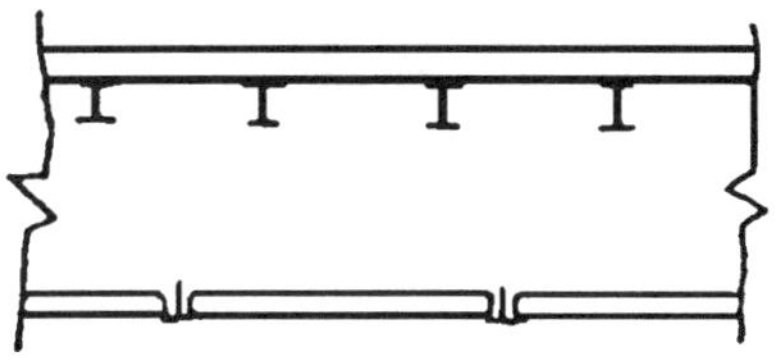

5.28 The exterior windows of a house are of double insulating glass with 1/4-in. airspace and have metal sashes. Determine the design U-value for heating.

5.29 In designing a house, the total heat loss is calculated as 17.9 kW. The heat loss through the outside walls is 28% of this total when the overall coefficient for the outside walls is 1.4 W/(m^2· K). If 50-mm organic bonded fiberglass is added to the wall in the stud space, determine the new total heat loss for the house. [Ans: 14.6 kW]

5.30 The top floor ceiling of a building 30 ft by 36 ft is constructed of 2 in. by 4 in. joists on 18-in. centers. On the underside is metal lath with plaster, 3/4 in. thick. On top of the joists there are only scattered walking planks, but the space between the joists is filled with rock wool. The air temperature at the ceiling in the room is 78°F and the attic temperature is 25°F. Find the coefficient of heat transfer for the ceiling.

5.31 Determine the U-value and the temperature at each point of change of material for the flat roof shown below. The roof has 3/8-in. built-up roofing, 1 1/2-in. roof insulation, 2-in. thick, 80 lb/ft^3 lightweight aggregate concrete on corrugated metal over steel joists, with a metal lath and 3/4-in. (sand) plaster ceiling. Omit correction for framing.

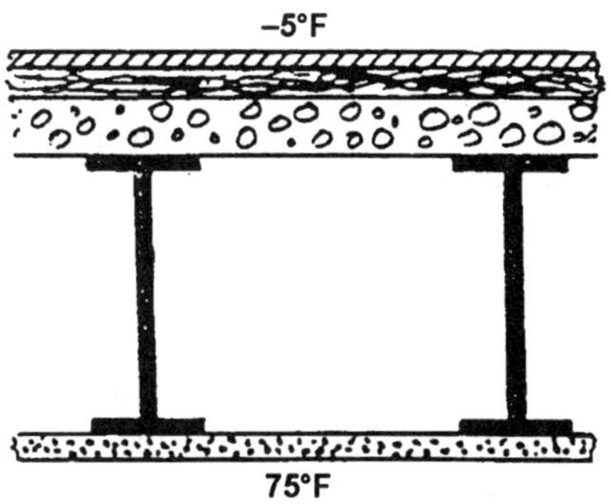

5.32 Calculate the heat loss through a roof of 100 ft^2 area where the inside air temperature is to be 70°F, outside air 10°F, and the composition from outside to inside: 3/8-in. built-up roofing, 1-in. cellular glass insulation, 4-in. concrete slab, and 3/4-in. acoustical tile. [Ans: 1030 Btu/h (0.30 kW)]

5.33 Calculate the heat loss through 100 ft2 (9.29 m2) of 1/4-in. (6.5-mm) plate glass with inside and outside air temperatures of 70°F and 10°F (21.1°C and −12.2°C), respectively.

5.34 A building has single glass windows and an indoor temperature of 75°F. The outside air temperature is 40°F. With a 15-mph outside wind, still air inside, and after sundown, what can the maximum relative humidity of the inside air be without condensation forming on the glass?

5.35 Repeat *Problem* 5.34 for a double glass window with a 1/2-in. airspace. [Ans: 67% rh]

5.36 A wall is constructed of 4-in. face brick, pressed fiber board sheathing (k = 0.44), 3 1/2-in. airspace, and 1/2-in. lightweight gypsum plaster on 1/2-in. plasterboard. When the inside air temperature is 70°F and the outside temperature is −15°F, how thick must the sheathing be to prevent water pipes in the stud space from freezing?

5.37 The roof of a rapid transit car is constructed of 3/8-in. plywood (C = 2.12), a vapor seal having negligible thermal resistance, expanded polystyrene insulation (k = 0.24), 3/4-in. airspace, 1/16-in. steel with welded joints and aluminum paint. If the car is traveling at 60 mph (film coefficient is 20.0 Btu/h· ft^2·°F) when the ambient temperature is −20°F, what thickness of insulation is necessary to prevent condensation when the inside conditions in the car are 72°F dry bulb and 55% rh?

5.38 A roof is constructed of 2-in. wood decking, insulation on top of deck, and 3/8-in. built-up roofing. It has no ceiling. Assuming that the insulation forms a perfect vapor barrier, determine the required resistance of the insulation to prevent condensation from occurring at the deck-insulation interface when indoor conditions are 70°F and 40% rh, and the outside temperature is 20°F. [Ans: 2.48 ft^2·°F· h/Btu]

5.39 Find the surface conductance of:

(a) clear pine when wind velocity = 15 mph (6.7 m/s)
(b) stucco when wind velocity = 0 mph (0 m/s)
(c) stucco when wind velocity = 25 mph (11.2 m/s)

5.40 Determine the summer U-value for each of the following:

(a) building wall consisting of face brick veneer, 3/4-in. plywood sheathing, 2 by 6 studs on 24-in. centers, no insulation, and 5/32-in. plywood paneling
(b) ceiling/roof where the ceiling is composed of 1/2-in. plasterboard nailed to 2 by 6 joists on 16-in. centers and the roof consists of asphalt shingles on 3/4-in. plywood on 2

by 4 rafters on 16-in. centers. The roof area is 2717 ft^2 while the ceiling area is 1980 ft^2.

(c) sliding patio door with insulating glass (double) having a 0.50-in. airspace in a metal frame

(d) a 2-in. solid wood door with a wood storm door

5.41 A residence has an unheated basement. Determine the U-value applicable for heat transfer between the first floor rooms and the basement if the floor joists are 2 by 10; there is a basement ceiling of 1/2-in. plasterboard, and the floor proper has a carpet and rubber pad laid on 5/8-in. particle board underlayment on a 3/4-in. wood subfloor. There is no insulation between the joists. Neglect the effect of the joists. [Ans: 0.140 Btu/h· ft^2·°F [0.795 W/(m^2 · K)]

5.42 Determine the thermal conductivity in both IP and SI units of:

(a) plywood
(b) lightweight concrete (100 lb/ft^3)
(c) oak

5.43 Determine the thermal conductance in both Btu/h· ft^2 and W/m^2 of:

(a) 3/4-in. plywood
(b) 2 in. nominal thickness insulating roof deck
(c) 1/2-in. sand aggregate gypsum plaster

5.44 A prefabricated commercial building has exterior walls constructed of 2-in. expanded polyurethane bonded between 1/8-in. aluminum sheet and 1/4-in. veneer plywood. Design conditions include 105°F outside air temperature, 72°F indoor air, and 7.5-mph wind. Determine:

(a) overall thermal resistance
(b) value of U
(c) heat gain per ft2

[Ans: (a) 13.74 ft^2·°F· h/Btu; (b) 0.073 Btu/h· ft^2·°F; (c) 2.41 Btu/h· ft^2]

5.45 An outside wall consists of 4-in. face brick, 25/32-in. insulating board sheathing 2-in. mineral fiber batt between the 2 by 4 studs, and 1/2-in. plasterboard. Determine the winter U-value.

5.46 Solve the following:

(a) Compute the winter U-value for the wall of *Problem* 5.45 if the wind velocity is 30 mph.
(b) Compute the summer U-value for the wall of *Problem* 5.45.
(c) If full wall insulation is used, compute the summer U-value for the wall of *Problem* 5.45.

5.47 An exterior wall contains a 3 ft by 7 ft solid wood door, 1-3/8 in. thick, and a 6 ft by 7 ft sliding patio door with double insulating glass having a 1/2-in. airspace and metal frame. Determine the summer U-value for each door.

[Ans: 0.39 Btu/h· ft^2·°F; 0.74 Btu/h· ft^2·°F]

5.48 If the doors of *Problem* 5.47 are between the residence and a completely enclosed swimming pool area, determine the U-value for each door.

5.49 Determine the winter U-value in W/(m^2 · K) for the wall of a building which has the following construction: face brick, 4 in.; airspace, 3/4 in.; concrete, 9 in.; cellular glass board insulation, 1 in.; plywood paneling, 1/4 in.

5.50 Determine the summer U-value for the following building components:

(a) Wall: wood drop siding, 1 by 8 in.; 1/2-in. nail-base insulating board sheathing; 2 by 4 studs (16-in. oc) with full wall fiberglass insulation; 1/4-in. paneling
(b) Door: solid wood, 1 1/2 in. thick, with wood and glass storm door

5.51 Determine the combined ceiling and roof winter U-value for the following construction: The ceiling consists of 3/8-in. gypsum board on 2 by 6 in. ceiling joists. Six inches of fiberglass (mineral/glass wool) insulation fills the space between the joists. The pitched roof has asphalt shingles on 25/32-in. solid wood sheathing with no insulation between the rafters. The ratio of roof area to ceiling area is 1:3. The attic is unvented in winter.

5.52 The west wall of a residence is 70 ft long by 8 ft high. The wall contains four 3 ft by 5 ft wood sash 80% glass single pane windows each with a storm window; one double-glazed (1/2-in. airspace) picture window, 5 1/2 ft by 10 ft; and one 1 3/4 in. thick solid wood door, 3 ft by 7 ft, with a glass storm door. The wall itself has the construction of *Problem* 5.24. Specify the U-value and corresponding area for each of the various parts of the wall with normal winter air velocities.

5.53 A wall is 20 m by 3 m, which includes 14% doubleinsulating glass windows with a 6-mm airspace. The wall proper consists of one layer of face brick backed by 250 mm of concrete with 12 mm of gypsum plaster on the inside. For indoor and outdoor design temperatures of 22°C and −15°C, respectively, determine the heat loss through this wall, kW.

5.6 Bibliography

ASHRAE *Standard* 55-1992, Thermal Environmental Conditions for Human Occupancy.

ASHRAE *Standard* 62-1989, Ventilation for Acceptable Indoor Air Quality.

ASHRAE *Standard* 90.1-1989, Energy Efficient Design of New Buildings Except New Low-Rise Residential Buildings.

McQuiston, F.C. and J. D. Spitler. 1992. *Cooling and Heating Load Calculation Manual*, 2nd ed. ASHRAE.

SI Figures and Tables

Example 5-5 Calculate the U-factor of the 38 mm by 90 mm stud wall shown in Figure 5-19. The studs are at 400 mm OC. There is 90 mm mineral fiber batt insulation (R = 2.3 m^2·K/W) in the stud space. The inside finish is 13 mm gypsum wallboard; the outside is finished with rigid foam insulating sheathing (R = 0.7 m^2·K/W) and 13 mm by 200 mm wood bevel lapped siding. The insulated cavity occupies approximately 75% of the transmission area; the studs, plates, and sills occupy 21%; and the headers occupy 4%.

Solution. Obtain the R-values of the various building elements from Tables 5-12 and 5-15. Assume the $R = 7.0$ m^2·K/W for the wood framing. Also, assume the headers are solid wood, in this case, and group them with the studs, plates, and sills.

Element	*R* (Insulated Cavity)	*R* (Studs, Plates, and Headers)
1. Outside surface, 24 km/h wind	0.03	0.03
2. Wood bevel lapped siding	0.14	0.14
3. Rigid foam insulating sheathing	0.70	0.70
4. Mineral fiber batt insulation	2.30	—
5. Wood stud	—	0.63
6. Gypsum wallboard	0.08	0.08
7. Inside surface, still air	0.12	0.12
	3.37	1.70

Since the U-factor is the reciprocal of R-value, U_1 = 0.297 W/(m^2·K) and U_2 = 0.588 W/(m^2·K).

If the wood framing (thermal bridging) is not included, Equation (3) from Chapter 22 may be used to calculate the U-factor of the wall as follows:

$$U_{av} = U_1 = \frac{1}{R_1} = 0.30 \text{ W/(m}^2 \cdot \text{K)}$$

If the wood framing is accounted for using the parallel-path flow method, the U-factor of the wall is determined using Equation (5) from Chapter 22 as follows:

$$U_{av} = (0.75 \times 0.297) + (0.25 \times 0.588) = 0.37 \text{ W/(m}^2 \cdot \text{K)}$$

If the wood framing is included using the isothermal planes method, the U-factor of the wall is determined using Equations (2) and (3) from Chapter 22 as follows:

$$R_{T(av)} = 4.98 + 1/[(0.75/2.30) + (0.25/0.63)] + 0.22$$

$$= 2.47 \text{ K} \cdot \text{m}^2/\text{W}$$

$$U_{av} = 0.40 \text{ W/(m}^2 \cdot \text{K)}$$

For a frame wall with a 600 mm OC stud space, the average overall R-value is 0.25 m^2·K/W. Similar calculation procedures may be used to evaluate other wall designs, except those with thermal bridges.

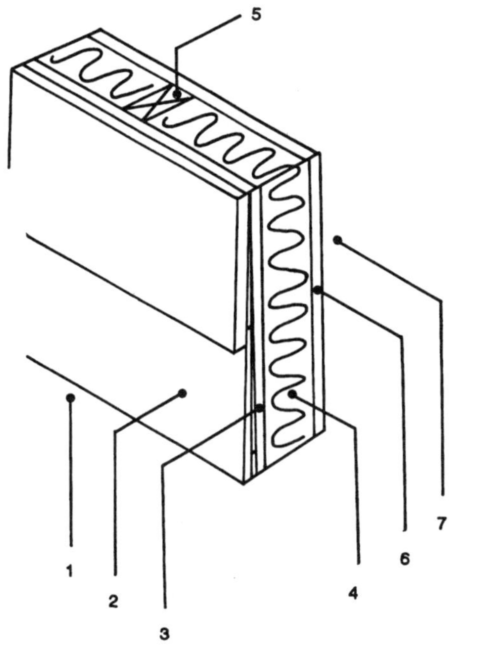

Fig. 5-19 Insulated Wood Frame Wall (Example 5-5)

Table 5-1 SI Change Rates as a Function of Airtightness
(Table 7, Chapter 27, 1997 *ASHRAE Handbook—**Fundamentals***)

	Outdoor Design Temperature, °C									
Class	**10**	**4**	**−1**	**−7**	**−12**	**−18**	**−23**	**−29**	**−34**	**−40**
Tight	0.41	0.43	0.45	0.47	0.49	0.51	0.53	0.55	0.57	0.59
Medium	0.69	0.73	0.77	0.81	0.85	0.89	0.93	0.97	1.00	1.05
Loose	1.11	1.15	1.20	1.23	1.27	1.30	1.35	1.40	1.43	1.47

Note: Values are for 6.7 m/s (24 km/h) wind and indoor temperature of 20°C.

Table 5-3 SI Effective Leakage Area of Building Components

(Table 3, Chapter 25, 1997 *ASHRAE Handbook—Fundamentals*)

	Units (see note)	Best Estimate	Mini-mum	Maxi-mum
Ceiling				
General	cm^2/m^2	1.8	0.79	2.8
Drop	cm^2/m^2	0.19	0.046	0.19
Ceiling penetrations				
Whole-house fans	cm^2 ea	20	1.6	21
Recessed lights	cm^2 ea	10	1.5	21
Ceiling/Flue vent	cm^2 ea	31	28	31
Surface-mounted lights	cm^2 ea	0.82		
Chimney	cm^2 ea	29	21	36
Crawl space				
General (area for exposed wall)	cm^2/m^2	10	8	17
200 mm by 400 mm vents	cm^2 ea	129		
Door frame				
General	cm^2 ea	12	2.4	25
Masonry, not caulked	cm^2/m^2	5	1.7	5
Masonry, caulked	cm^2/m^2	1	0.3	1
Wood, not caulked	cm^2/m^2	1.7	0.6	1.7
Wood, caulked	cm^2/m^2	0.3	0.1	0.3
Trim	cm^2/lmc	1		
Jamb	cm^2/lmc	8	7	10
Threshold	cm^2/lmc	2	1.2	24
Doors				
Attic/crawl space, not weatherstripped	cm^2 ea	30	10	37
Attic/crawl space, weatherstripped	cm^2 ea	18	8	18.5
Attic fold down, not weatherstripped	cm^2 ea	44	23	86
Attic fold down, weatherstripped	cm^2 ea	22	14	43
Attic fold down, with insulated box	cm^2 ea	4		
Attic from unconditioned garage	cm^2 ea	0	0	0
Double, not weatherstripped	cm^2/m^2	11	7	22
Double, weatherstripped	cm^2/m^2	8	3	23
Elevator (passenger)	cm^2 ea	0.26	0.14	0.35
General, average	cm^2/lmc	0.31	0.23	0.45
Interior (pocket, on top floor)	cm^2 ea	14		
Interior (stairs)	cm^2/lmc	0.9	0.25	1.5
Mail slot	cm^2/lmc	4		
Sliding exterior glass patio	cm^2 ea	22	3	60
Sliding exterior glass patio	cm^2/m^2	5.5	0.6	15
Storm (difference between with and without)	cm^2 ea	6	3	6.2
Single, not weatherstripped	cm^2 ea	21	12	53
Single, weatherstripped	cm^2 ea	12	4	27
Vestibule (subtract per each location)	cm^2 ea	10		
Electrical outlets/Switches				
No gaskets	cm^2 ea	2.5	0.5	6.2
With gaskets	cm^2 ea	0.15	0.08	3.5
Furnace				
Sealed (or no) combustion	cm^2 ea	0	0	0
Retention head or stack damper	cm^2 ea	30	20	30
Retention head and stack damper	cm^2 ea	24	18	30
Floors over crawl spaces				
General	cm^2/m^2	2.2	0.4	4.9
Without ductwork in crawl space	cm^2/m^2	1.98		
With ductwork in crawl space	cm^2/m^2	2.25		
Fireplace				
With damper closed	cm^2/m^2	43	10	92
With damper open	cm^2/m^2	350	145	380
With glass doors	cm^2/m^2	40	4	40
With insert and damper closed	cm^2/m^2	36	26	46
With insert and damper open	cm^2/m^2	65	40	90
Gas water heater	cm^2 ea	20	15	25
Joints				
Ceiling-wall	cm^2/lmc	1.5	0.16	2.5
Sole plate, floor/wall, uncaulked	cm^2/lmc	4	0.38	5.6
Sole plate, floor/wall, caulked	cm^2/lmc	0.8	0.075	1.2
Top plate, band joist	cm^2/lmc	0.1	0.075	0.38

	Units (see note)	Best Estimate	Mini-mum	Maxi-mum
Piping/Plumbing/Wiring penetrations				
Uncaulked	cm^2 ea	6	2	24
Caulked	cm^2 ea	2	1	2
Vents				
Bathroom with damper closed	cm^2 ea	10	2.5	20
Bathroom with damper open	cm^2 ea	20	6.1	22
Dryer with damper	cm^2 ea	3	2.9	7
Dryer without damper	cm^2 ea	15	12	34
Kitchen with damper open	cm^2 ea	40	14	72
Kitchen with damper closed	cm^2 ea	5	1	7
Kitchen with tight gasket	cm^2 ea	1		
Walls (exterior)				
Cast-in-place concrete	cm^2/m^2	0.5	0.049	1.8
Clay brick cavity wall, finished	cm^2/m^2	0.68	0.05	2.3
Precast concrete panel	cm^2/m^2	1.2	0.28	1.65
Low-density concrete block, unfinished	cm^2/m^2	3.5	1.3	4
Low-density concrete block, painted or stucco	cm^2/m^2	1.1	0.52	1.1
High-density concrete block, unfinished	cm^2/m^2	0.25		
Continuous air infiltration barrier	cm^2/m^2	0.15	0.055	0.21
Rigid sheathing	cm^2/m^2	0.35	0.29	0.41
Window framing				
Masonry, uncaulked	cm^2/m^2	6.5	5.7	10.3
Masonry, caulked	cm^2/m^2	1.3	1.1	2.1
Wood, uncaulked	cm^2/m^2	1.7	1.5	2.7
Wood, caulked	cm^2/m^2	0.3	0.3	0.5
Windows				
Awning, not weatherstripped	cm^2/m^2	1.6	0.8	2.4
Awning, weatherstripped	cm^2/m^2	0.8	0.4	1.2
Casement, weatherstripped	cm^2/lmc	0.24	0.1	3
Casement, not weatherstripped	cm^2/lmc	0.28		
Double horizontal slider, not weatherstripped	cm^2/lmc	1.1	0.019	3.4
Double horizontal slider, wood, weatherstripped	cm^2/lmc	0.55	0.15	1.72
Double horizontal slider, aluminum, weatherstripped	cm^2/lmc	0.72	0.58	0.8
Double-hung, not weatherstripped	cm^2/lmc	2.5	0.86	6.1
Double-hung, weatherstripped	cm^2/lmc	0.65	0.2	1.9
Double-hung with storm, not weatherstripped	cm^2/lmc	0.97	0.48	1.7
Double-hung with storm, weatherstripped	cm^2/lmc	0.79	0.44	1
Double-hung with pressurized track, weatherstripped	cm^2/lmc	0.48	0.39	0.56
Jalousie	cm^2/louver	3.38		
Lumped	cm^2/lms	0.471	0.009	2.06
Single horizontal slider, weatherstripped	cm^2/lms	0.67	0.2	2.06
Single horizontal slider, aluminum	cm^2/lms	0.8	0.27	2.06
Single horizontal slider, wood	cm^2/lms	0.44	0.27	0.99
Single horizontal slider, wood clad	cm^2/lms	0.64	0.54	0.81
Single-hung, weatherstripped	cm^2/lms	0.87	0.62	1.24
Sill	cm^2/lmc	0.21	0.139	0.212
Storm inside, heat shrink	cm^2/lms	0.018	0.009	0.018
Storm inside, rigid sheet with magnetic seal	cm^2/lms	0.12	0.018	0.24
Storm inside, flexible sheet with mechanical seal	cm^2/lms	0.154	0.018	0.833
Storm inside, rigid sheet with mechanical seal	cm^2/lms	0.4	0.045	0.833
Storm outside, pressurized track	cm^2/lmc	0.528		
Storm outside, 2-track	cm^2/lmc	1.23		
Storm outside, 3-track	cm^2/lmc	2.46		

Note: Air leakage areas are based on values found in the literature. The effective air leakage area (in square centimetres) is based on a pressure difference of 4 Pa and $C_D = 1$.

Abbreviations: m^2 = gross area in square metres; ea = each; lmc = linear metre of crack; lms = linear metre of sash

Table 5-4 SI Stack Coefficient C_S

(Table 6, Chapter 25, 1997 *ASHRAE Handbook—Fundamentals*, SI Version)

	House Height (Stories)		
	One	Two	Three
Stack coefficient	0.000 145	0.000 290	0.000 435

Table 5-5 SI Wind Coefficient C_W

(Table 8, Chapter 25, 1997 *ASHRAE Handbook—Fundamentals*, SI Version)

Shielding Class	House Height (Stories)		
	One	Two	Three
1	0.000 319	0.000 420	0.000 494
2	0.000 246	0.000 325	0.000 382
3	0.000 174	0.000 231	0.000 271
4	0.000 104	0.000 137	0.000 161
5	0.000 032	0.000 042	0.000 049

Table 5-12 SI Surface Conductances and Resistances

(Table 1, Chapter 24, 1997 *ASHRAE Handbook—Fundamentals*, SI Version)

		Surface Emittance, ε					
		Non-reflective ε = 0.90		Reflective ε = 0.20		ε = 0.05	
Position of Surface	Direction of Heat Flow	h_i	R	h_i	R	h_i	R
STILL AIR							
Horizontal	Upward	9.26	0.11	5.17	0.19	4.32	0.23
Sloping—45°	Upward	9.09	0.11	5.00	0.20	4.15	0.24
Vertical	Horizontal	8.29	0.12	4.20	0.24	3.35	0.30
Sloping—45°	Downward	7.50	0.13	3.41	0.29	2.56	0.39
Horizontal	Downward	6.13	0.16	2.10	0.48	1.25	0.80
MOVING AIR (Any position)		h_o	R				
Wind (for winter) 6.7 m/s (24 km/h)	Any	34.0	0.030	—	—	—	—
Wind (for summer) 3.4 m/s (12 km/h)	Any	22.7	0.044	—	—	—	—

Notes:

1. Surface conductance h_i and h_o measured in W/(m^2·K); resistance R in m^2·K/W.
2. No surface has both an air space resistance value and a surface resistance value.
3. For ventilated attics or spaces above ceilings under summer conditions (heat flow down), see Table 5.
4. Conductances are for surfaces of the stated emittance facing virtual blackbody surroundings at the same temperature as the ambient air. Values are based on a surface-air temperature difference of 5.5°C and for surface temperatures of 21°C.
5. See Chapter 3 for more detailed information, especially Tables 5 and 6, and see Figure 1 for additional data.
6. Condensate can have a significant impact on surface emittance (see Table 2).

Table 5-13 SI Emittance Values of Various Surfaces and Effective Emmittances of Airspaces

(Table 2, Chapter 24, 1997 *ASHRAE Handbook—Fundamentals*, SI Version)

		Effective Emittance ε_{eff} of Air Space	
Surface	Average Emittance ε	One Surface Emittance ε; Other, 0.9	Both Surfaces Emittance ε
Aluminum foil, bright	0.05	0.05	0.03
Aluminum foil, with condensate just visible (> 0.5 g/m^2)	0.30[b]	0.29	—
Aluminum foil, with condensate clearly visible (> 2.0 g/m^2)	0.70[b]	0.65	—
Aluminum sheet	0.12	0.12	0.06
Aluminum coated paper, polished	0.20	0.20	0.11
Steel, galvanized, bright	0.25	0.24	0.15
Aluminum paint	0.50	0.47	0.35
Building materials: wood, paper, masonry, nonmetallic paints	0.90	0.82	0.82
Regular glass	0.84	0.77	0.72

[a]These values apply in the 4 to 40 μm range of the electromagnetic spectrum.
[b]Values are based on data presented by Bassett and Trethowen (1984).

Table 5-14 Thermal Resistances of Plane Airspaces

(Table 3, Chapter 24, 1997 *ASHRAE Handbook—Fundamentals*, SI Version)

Position of Air Space	Direction of Heat Flow	Air Space Mean Temp.[d], °C	Air Space Temp. Diff.[d], °C	13 mm Air Space[c] Effective Emittance ε_{eff}[d,e] 0.03	0.05	0.2	0.5	0.82	20 mm Air Space[c] Effective Emittance ε_{eff}[d,e] 0.03	0.05	0.2	0.5	0.82
		32.2	5.6	0.37	0.36	0.27	0.17	0.13	0.41	0.39	0.28	0.18	0.13
		10.0	16.7	0.29	0.28	0.23	0.17	0.13	0.30	0.29	0.24	0.17	0.14
		10.0	5.6	0.37	0.36	0.28	0.20	0.15	0.40	0.39	0.30	0.20	0.15
Horiz.	Up	−17.8	11.1	0.30	0.30	0.26	0.20	0.16	0.32	0.32	0.27	0.20	0.16
		−17.8	5.6	0.37	0.36	0.30	0.22	0.18	0.39	0.38	0.31	0.23	0.18
		−45.6	11.1	0.30	0.29	0.26	0.22	0.18	0.31	0.31	0.27	0.22	0.19
		−45.6	5.6	0.36	0.35	0.31	0.25	0.20	0.38	0.37	0.32	0.26	0.21
		32.2	5.6	0.43	0.41	0.29	0.19	0.13	0.52	0.49	0.33	0.20	0.14
		10.0	16.7	0.36	0.35	0.27	0.19	0.15	0.35	0.34	0.27	0.19	0.14
		10.0	5.6	0.45	0.43	0.32	0.21	0.16	0.51	0.48	0.35	0.23	0.17
45° Slope	Up	−17.8	11.1	0.39	0.38	0.31	0.23	0.18	0.37	0.36	0.30	0.23	0.18
		−17.8	5.6	0.46	0.45	0.36	0.25	0.19	0.48	0.46	0.37	0.26	0.20
		−45.6	11.1	0.37	0.36	0.31	0.25	0.21	0.36	0.35	0.31	0.25	0.20
		−45.6	5.6	0.46	0.45	0.38	0.29	0.23	0.45	0.43	0.37	0.29	0.23
		32.2	5.6	0.43	0.41	0.29	0.19	0.14	0.62	0.57	0.37	0.21	0.15
		10.0	16.7	0.45	0.43	0.32	0.22	0.16	0.51	0.49	0.35	0.23	0.17
		10.0	5.6	0.47	0.45	0.33	0.22	0.16	0.65	0.61	0.41	0.25	0.18
Vertical	Horiz.	−17.8	11.1	0.50	0.48	0.38	0.26	0.20	0.55	0.53	0.41	0.28	0.21
		−17.8	5.6	0.52	0.50	0.39	0.27	0.20	0.66	0.63	0.46	0.30	0.22
		−45.6	11.1	0.51	0.50	0.41	0.31	0.24	0.51	0.50	0.42	0.31	0.24
		−45.6	5.6	0.56	0.55	0.45	0.33	0.26	0.65	0.63	0.51	0.36	0.27
		32.2	5.6	0.44	0.41	0.29	0.19	0.14	0.62	0.58	0.37	0.21	0.15
		10.0	16.7	0.46	0.44	0.33	0.22	0.16	0.60	0.57	0.39	0.24	0.17
		10.0	5.6	0.47	0.45	0.33	0.22	0.16	0.67	0.63	0.42	0.26	0.18
45° Slope	Down	−17.8	11.1	0.51	0.49	0.39	0.27	0.20	0.66	0.63	0.46	0.30	0.22
		−17.8	5.6	0.52	0.50	0.39	0.27	0.20	0.73	0.69	0.49	0.32	0.23
		−45.6	11.1	0.56	0.54	0.44	0.33	0.25	0.67	0.64	0.51	0.36	0.28
		−45.6	5.6	0.57	0.56	0.45	0.33	0.26	0.77	0.74	0.57	0.39	0.29
		32.2	5.6	0.44	0.41	0.29	0.19	0.14	0.62	0.58	0.37	0.21	0.15
		10.0	16.7	0.47	0.45	0.33	0.22	0.16	0.66	0.62	0.42	0.25	0.18
		10.0	5.6	0.47	0.45	0.33	0.22	0.16	0.68	0.63	0.42	0.26	0.18
Horiz.	Down	−17.8	11.1	0.52	0.50	0.39	0.27	0.20	0.74	0.70	0.50	0.32	0.23
		−17.8	5.6	0.52	0.50	0.39	0.27	0.20	0.75	0.71	0.51	0.32	0.23
		−45.6	11.1	0.57	0.55	0.45	0.33	0.26	0.81	0.78	0.59	0.40	0.30
		−45.6	5.6	0.58	0.56	0.46	0.33	0.26	0.83	0.79	0.60	0.40	0.30

Position of Air Space	Direction of Heat Flow	Air Space Mean Temp.[d], °C	Air Space Temp. Diff.[d], °C	40 mm Air Space[c] 0.03	0.05	0.2	0.5	0.82	90 mm Air Space[c] 0.03	0.05	0.2	0.5	0.82
		32.2	5.6	0.45	0.42	0.30	0.19	0.14	0.50	0.47	0.32	0.20	0.14
		10.0	16.7	0.33	0.32	0.26	0.18	0.14	0.27	0.35	0.28	0.19	0.15
		10.0	5.6	0.44	0.42	0.32	0.21	0.16	0.49	0.47	0.34	0.23	0.16
Horiz.	Up	−17.8	11.1	0.35	0.34	0.29	0.22	0.17	0.40	0.38	0.32	0.23	0.18
		−17.8	5.6	0.43	0.41	0.33	0.24	0.19	0.48	0.46	0.36	0.26	0.20
		−45.6	11.1	0.34	0.34	0.30	0.24	0.20	0.39	0.38	0.33	0.26	0.21
		−45.6	5.6	0.42	0.41	0.35	0.27	0.22	0.47	0.45	0.38	0.29	0.23
		32.2	5.6	0.51	0.48	0.33	0.20	0.14	0.56	0.52	0.35	0.21	0.14
		10.0	16.7	0.38	0.36	0.28	0.20	0.15	0.40	0.38	0.29	0.20	0.15
		10.0	5.6	0.51	0.48	0.35	0.23	0.17	0.55	0.52	0.37	0.24	0.17
45° Slope	Up	−17.8	11.1	0.40	0.39	0.32	0.24	0.18	0.43	0.41	0.33	0.24	0.19
		−17.8	5.6	0.49	0.47	0.37	0.26	0.20	0.52	0.51	0.39	0.27	0.20
		−45.6	11.1	0.39	0.38	0.33	0.26	0.21	0.41	0.40	0.35	0.27	0.22
		−45.6	5.6	0.48	0.46	0.39	0.30	0.24	0.51	0.49	0.41	0.31	0.24
		32.2	5.6	0.70	0.64	0.40	0.22	0.15	0.65	0.60	0.38	0.22	0.15
		10.0	16.7	0.45	0.43	0.32	0.22	0.16	0.47	0.45	0.33	0.22	0.16
		10.0	5.6	0.67	0.62	0.42	0.26	0.18	0.64	0.60	0.41	0.25	0.18
Vertical	Horiz.	−17.8	11.1	0.49	0.47	0.37	0.26	0.20	0.51	0.49	0.38	0.27	0.20
		−17.8	5.6	0.62	0.59	0.44	0.29	0.22	0.61	0.59	0.44	0.29	0.22
		−45.6	11.1	0.46	0.45	0.38	0.29	0.23	0.50	0.48	0.40	0.30	0.24
		−45.6	5.6	0.58	0.56	0.46	0.34	0.26	0.60	0.58	0.47	0.34	0.26
		32.2	5.6	0.89	0.80	0.45	0.24	0.16	0.85	0.76	0.44	0.24	0.16
		10.0	16.7	0.63	0.59	0.41	0.25	0.18	0.62	0.58	0.40	0.25	0.18
		10.0	5.6	0.90	0.82	0.50	0.28	0.19	0.83	0.77	0.48	0.28	0.19
45° Slope	Down	−17.8	11.1	0.68	0.64	0.47	0.31	0.22	0.67	0.64	0.47	0.31	0.22
		−17.8	5.6	0.87	0.81	0.56	0.34	0.24	0.81	0.76	0.53	0.33	0.24
		−45.6	11.1	0.64	0.62	0.49	0.35	0.27	0.66	0.64	0.51	0.36	0.28
		−45.6	5.6	0.82	0.79	0.60	0.40	0.30	0.79	0.76	0.58	0.40	0.30
		32.2	5.6	1.07	0.94	0.49	0.25	0.17	1.77	1.44	0.60	0.28	0.18
		10.0	16.7	1.10	0.99	0.56	0.30	0.20	1.69	1.44	0.68	0.33	0.21
		10.0	5.6	1.16	1.04	0.58	0.30	0.20	1.96	1.63	0.72	0.34	0.22
Horiz.	Down	−17.8	11.1	1.24	1.13	0.69	0.39	0.26	1.92	1.68	0.86	0.43	0.29
		−17.8	5.6	1.29	1.17	0.70	0.39	0.27	2.11	1.82	0.89	0.44	0.29
		−45.6	11.1	1.36	1.27	0.84	0.50	0.35	2.05	1.85	1.06	0.57	0.38
		−45.6	5.6	1.42	1.32	0.86	0.51	0.35	2.28	2.03	1.12	0.59	0.39

[a]See Chapter 22, section Factors Affecting Heat Transfer across Air Spaces. Thermal resistance values were determined from the relation, $R = 1/C$, where $C = h_c + \varepsilon_{eff} h_r$, h_c is the conduction-convection coefficient, $\varepsilon_{eff} h_r$ is the radiation coefficient ≈ $0.227\varepsilon_{eff}[(t_m + 273)/100]^3$, and t_m is the mean temperature of the air space. Values for h_c were determined from data developed by Robinson et al. (1954). Equations (5) through (7) in Yarbrough (1983) show the data in this table in analytic form. For extrapolation from this table to air spaces less than 12.5 mm (as in insulating window glass), assume $h_c = 21.8(1 + 0.00274\, t_m)/l$ where l is the air space thickness in mm, and h_c is heat transfer in W/(m²·K) through the air space only.

[b]Values are based on data presented by Robinson et al. (1954). (Also see Chapter 3, Tables 3 and 4, and Chapter 36). Values apply for ideal conditions, i.e., air spaces of uniform thickness bounded by plane, smooth, parallel surfaces with no air leakage to or from the space. When accurate values are required, use overall U-factors determined through calibrated hot box (ASTM C 976) or guarded hot box (ASTM C 236) testing. Thermal resistance values for multiple air spaces must be based on careful estimates of mean temperature differences for each air space.

[c]A single resistance value cannot account for multiple air spaces; each air space requires a separate resistance calculation that applies only for the established boundary conditions. Resistances of horizontal spaces with heat flow downward are substantially independent of temperature difference.

[d]Interpolation is permissible for other values of mean temperature, temperature difference, and effective emittance ε_{eff}. Interpolation and moderate extrapolation for air spaces greater than 90 mm are also permissible.

[e]Effective emittance ε_{eff} of the air space is given by $1/\varepsilon_{eff} = 1/\varepsilon_1 + 1/\varepsilon_2 - 1$, where ε_1 and ε_2 are the emittances of the surfaces of the air space (see Table 2).

Table 5-15 Typical Thermal Properties of Common Building and Insulating Materials[a]
(Table 4, Chapter 24, 1997 *ASHRAE Handbook—Fundamentals*, SI Version)

Description	Density, kg/m³	Conductivity[b] (*k*), W/(m·K)	Conductance (*C*), W/(m²·K)	Resistance[c] (*R*) Per Inch Thickness (1/*k*), K·m/W	Resistance[c] (*R*) For Thickness Listed (1/*C*), K·m²/W	Specific Heat, kJ/(kg·K)
BUILDING BOARD						
Asbestos-cement board	1900	0.58	—	1.73	—	1.00
Asbestos-cement board ... 3.2 mm	1900	—	187.4	—	0.005	—
Asbestos-cement board ... 6.4 mm	1900	—	93.7	—	0.011	—
Gypsum or plaster board ... 9.5 mm	800	—	17.6	—	0.056	1.09
Gypsum or plaster board ... 12.7 mm	800	—	12.6	—	0.079	—
Gypsum or plaster board ... 15.9 mm	800	—	10.1	—	0.099	—
Plywood (Douglas Fir)[d]	540	0.12	—	8.66	—	1.21
Plywood (Douglas Fir) ... 6.4 mm	540	—	18.2	—	0.055	—
Plywood (Douglas Fir) ... 9.5 mm	540	—	12.1	—	0.083	—
Plywood (Douglas Fir) ... 12.7 mm	540	—	9.1	—	0.11	—
Plywood (Douglas Fir) ... 15.9 mm	540	—	7.3	—	0.14	—
Plywood or wood panels ... 19.0 mm	540	—	6.1	—	0.16	1.21
Vegetable fiber board						
Sheathing, regular density[e] ... 12.7 mm	290	—	4.3	—	0.23	1.30
... 19.8 mm	290	—	2.8	—	0.36	—
Sheathing intermediate density[e] ... 12.7 mm	350	—	5.2	—	0.19	1.30
Nail-base sheathing[e] ... 12.7 mm	400	—	5.3	—	0.19	1.30
Shingle backer ... 9.5 mm	290	—	6.0	—	0.17	1.30
Shingle backer ... 7.9 mm	290	—	7.3	—	0.14	—
Sound deadening board ... 12.7 mm	240	—	4.2	—	0.24	1.26
Tile and lay-in panels, plain or acoustic	290	0.058	—	17.	—	0.59
... 12.7 mm	290	—	4.5	—	0.22	—
... 19.0 mm	290	—	3.0	—	0.33	—
Laminated paperboard	480	0.072	—	13.9	—	1.38
Homogeneous board from repulped paper	480	0.072	—	13.9	—	1.17
Hardboard[e]						
Medium density	800	0.105	—	9.50	—	1.30
High density, service-tempered grade and service grade	880	0.82	—	8.46	—	1.34
High density, standard-tempered grade	1010	0.144	—	6.93	—	1.34
Particleboard[e]						
Low density	590	0.102	—	9.77	—	1.30
Medium density	800	0.135	—	7.35	—	1.30
High density	1000	0.170	—	5.90	—	1.30
Underlayment ... 15.9 mm	640	—	6.9	—	0.14	1.21
Waferboard	590	0.01	—	11.0	—	—
Wood subfloor ... 19.0 mm	—	—	6.0	—	0.17	1.38
BUILDING MEMBRANE						
Vapor—permeable felt	—	—	94.9	—	0.011	
Vapor—seal, 2 layers of mopped 0.73 kg/m² felt	—	—	47.4	—	0.21	
Vapor—seal, plastic film	—	—	—	—	Negl.	
FINISH FLOORING MATERIALS						
Carpet and fibrous pad	—	—	2.73	—	0.37	1.42
Carpet and rubber pad	—	—	4.60	—	0.22	1.38
Cork tile ... 3.2 mm	—	—	20.4	—	0.049	2.01
Terrazzo ... 25 mm	—	—	71.0	—	0.014	0.80
Tile—asphalt, linoleum, vinyl, rubber	—	—	113.6	—	0.009	1.26
vinyl asbestos						1.01
ceramic						0.80
Wood, hardwood finish ... 19 mm	—		8.35	—	0.12	
INSULATING MATERIALS						
Blanket and Batt[f,g]						
Mineral fiber, fibrous form processed from rock, slag, or glass						
approx. 75-100 mm	6.4-32	—	0.52	—	1.94	
approx. 90 mm	6.4-32	—	0.44	—	2.29	
approx. 90 mm	19-26	—	0.38	—	2.63	
approx. 140-165 mm	6.4-32	—	0.30	—	3.32	
approx. 140 mm	10-16	—	0.27	—	3.67	
approx. 150-190 mm	6.4-32	—	0.26	—	3.91	
approx. 210-250 mm	6.4-32	—	0.19	—	5.34	
approx. 250-330 mm	6.4-32	—	0.15	—	6.77	
Board and Slabs						
Cellular glass	136	0.050	—	19.8	—	0.75
Glass fiber, organic bonded	64-140	0.036	—	27.7	—	0.96
Expanded perlite, organic bonded	16	0.052	—	19.3	—	1.26
Expanded rubber (rigid)	72	0.032	—	31.6	—	1.68
Expanded polystyrene, extruded (smooth skin surface) (CFC-12 exp.)	29-56					

Table 5-15 Typical Thermal Properties of Common Building and Insulating Materials[a] (*Continued*)

(Table 4, Chapter 24, 1997 *ASHRAE Handbook—Fundamentals*, SI Version)

Description	Density, kg/m³	Conductivity[b] (*k*), W/(m·K)	Conductance (*C*), W/(m²·K)	Resistance[c] (*R*) Per Inch Thickness (1/*k*), K·m/W	Resistance[c] (*R*) For Thickness Listed (1/*C*), K·m²/W	Specific Heat, kJ/(kg·K)
Expanded polystyrene, extruded (smooth skin surface) (HCFC-142b exp.)[h]	29-56	0.029	—	34.7	—	1.21
Expanded polystyrene, molded beads	16	0.037	—	26.7	—	—
	20	0.036	—	27.7	—	—
	24	0.035	—	28.9	—	—
	28	0.035	—	28.9	—	—
	32	0.033	—	30.2	—	—
Cellular polyurethane/polyisocyanurate[i] (CFC-11 exp.) (unfaced)	24	0.023-0.026	—	43.3-38.5	—	1.59
Cellular polyisocyanurate[i] (CFC-11 exp.) (gas-permeable facers)	24-40	0.023-0.026	—	43.3-38.5	—	0.92
Cellular polyisocyanurate[j] (CFC-11 exp.) (gas-impermeable facers)	32	0.020	—	48.8	—	0.92
Cellular phenolic (closed cell) (CFC-11, CFC-113 exp.)[k]	32	0.017	—	56.8	—	—
Cellular phenolic (open cell)	29-35	0.033	—	30.5	—	—
Mineral fiber with resin binder	240	0.042	—	23.9	—	0.71
Mineral fiberboard, wet felted						
Core or roof insulation	260-270	0.049	—	20.4	—	
Acoustical tile	290	0.050	—	19.8	—	0.80
Acoustical tile	340	0.053	—	18.7	—	
Mineral fiberboard, wet molded						
Acoustical tile[l]	370	0.060	—	16.5	—	0.59
Wood or cane fiberboard						
Acoustical tile[l] 12.7 mm	—	—	4.5	—	0.22	1.30
Acoustical tile[l] 19.0 mm	—	—	3.0	—	0.33	
Interior finish (plank, tile)	240	0.050	—	19.8	—	1.34
Cement fiber slabs (shredded wood with Portland cement binder)	400-430	0.072-0.076	—	13.9-13.1	—	—
Cement fiber slabs (shredded wood with magnesia oxysulfide binder)	350	0.082	—	12.1	—	1.30
Loose Fill						
Cellulosic insulation (milled paper or wood pulp)	37-51	0.039-0.046	—	25.6-21.7	—	1.38
Perlite, expanded	32-66	0.039-0.045	—	25.6-22.9	—	1.09
	66-120	0.045-0.052	—	22.9-19.4	—	—
	120-180	0.052-0.060	—	19.4-16.6	—	—
Mineral fiber (rock, slag, or glass)[g]						
approx. 95-130 mm	9.6-32	—	—	—	1.94	0.71
approx. 170-220 mm	9.6-32	—	—	—	3.35	—
approx. 190-250 mm	9.6-32	—	—	—	3.87	—
approx. 260-350 mm	9.6-32	—	—	—	5.28	—
Mineral fiber (rock, slag, or glass)[g]						
approx. 90 mm (closed sidewall application)	32-56	—	—	—	2.1-2.5	
Vermiculite, exfoliated	110-130	0.068	—	14.8	—	1.34
	64-96	0.063	—	15.7	—	—
Spray Applied						
Polyurethane foam	24-40	0.023-0.026	—	43.3-38.5	—	—
Ureaformaldehyde foam	11-26	0.032-0.040	—	31.5-24.7	—	—
Cellulosic fiber	56-96	0.042-0.049	—	23.9-20.4	—	—
Glass fiber	56-72	0.038-0.039	—	26.7-25.6	—	—
Reflective Insulation						
Reflective material ($\varepsilon < 0.5$) in center of 20 mm cavity forms two 10 mm vertical air spaces[m]	—	—	1.76	—	0.57	—
METALS						
(See Chapter 36, Table 3)						
ROOFING						
Asbestos-cement shingles	1900	—	27.0	—	0.037	1.00
Asphalt roll roofing	1100	—	36.9	—	0.026	1.51
Asphalt shingles	1100	—	12.9	—	0.077	1.26
Built-up roofing 10 mm	1100	—	17.0	—	0.058	1.46
Slate 13 mm	—	—	114	—	0.009	1.26
Wood shingles, plain and plastic film faced	—	—	6.0	—	0.166	1.30
PLASTERING MATERIALS						
Cement plaster, sand aggregate	1860	0.72	—	1.39	—	0.84
Sand aggregate 10 mm	—	—	75.5	—	0.013	0.84
Sand aggregate 20 mm	—	—	37.8	—	0.026	0.84

Table 5-15 Typical Thermal Properties of Common Building and Insulating Materials[a] (*Continued*)

(Table 4, Chapter 24, 1997 *ASHRAE Handbook—Fundamentals*, SI Version)

Description	Density, kg/m³	Conductivity[b] (*k*), W/(m·K)	Conductance (*C*), W/(m²·K)	Resistance[c] (*R*) Per Inch Thickness (1/*k*), K·m/W	Resistance[c] (*R*) For Thickness Listed (1/*C*), K·m²/W	Specific Heat, kJ/(kg·K)
Gypsum plaster:						
Lightweight aggregate ... 13 mm	720	—	17.7	—	0.056	—
Lightweight aggregate ... 16 mm	720	—	15.2	—	0.066	—
Lightweight aggregate on metal lath ... 19 mm	—	—	12.1	—	0.083	—
Perlite aggregate ...	720	0.22	—	4.64	—	1.34
Sand aggregate ...	1680	0.81	—	1.25	—	0.84
Sand aggregate ... 13 mm	1680	—	63.0	—	0.016	—
Sand aggregate ... 16 mm	1680	—	51.7	—	0.019	—
Sand aggregate on metal lath ... 19 mm	—	—	43.7	—	0.023	—
Vermiculite aggregate ...	720	0.24	—	4.09	—	—
MASONRY MATERIALS						
Masonry Units						
Brick, fired clay ...	2400	1.21-1.47	—	0.83-0.68	—	—
	2240	1.07-1.30	—	0.94-0.77	—	—
	2080	0.92-1.12	—	1.08-0.89	—	—
	1920	0.81-0.98	—	1.24-1.02	—	0.79
	1760	0.71-0.85	—	1.42-1.18	—	—
	1600	0.61-0.74	—	1.65-1.36	—	—
	1440	—0.52-0.62	—	1.93-1.61	—	—
	1280	0.43-0.53	—	2.31-1.87	—	—
	1120	0.36-0.45	—	2.77-2.23	—	—
Clay tile, hollow						
1 cell deep ... 75 mm	—	—	7.10	—	0.14	0.88
1 cell deep ... 100 mm	—	—	5.11	—	0.20	—
2 cells deep ... 150 mm	—	—	3.75	—	0.27	—
2 cells deep ... 200 mm	—	—	3.07	—	0.33	—
2 cells deep ... 250 mm	—	—	2.56	—	0.39	—
3 cells deep ... 300 mm	—	—	2.27	—	0.44	—
Concrete blocks[n, o]						
Limestone aggregate						
200 mm, 16.3 kg, 2210 kg/m³ concrete, 2 cores ...	—	—	—	—	—	—
Same with perlite filled cores ...	—	—	2.73	—	0.37	—
300 mm, 25 kg, 2210 kg/m³ concrete, 2 cores ...	—	—	—	—	—	—
Same with perlite filled cores ...	—	—	1.53	—	0.65	—
Normal mass aggregate (sand and gravel) 200 mm						
15-16 kg, 2020-2180 kg/m³ concrete, 2 or 3 cores	—	—	5.1-5.8	—	0.20-0.17	0.92
Same with perlite filled cores ...	—	—	2.84	—	0.35	—
Same with vermiculite filled cores ...	—	—	3.0-4.1	—	0.34-0.24	—
300 mm, 22.7 kg, 2000 kg/m³ concrete, 2 cores ...	—	—	4.60	—	0.217	0.92
Medium mass aggregate (combinations of normal and low mass aggregate) 200 mm, 12-13 kg,						
1550-1790 kg/m³ concrete, 2 or 3 cores ...	—	—	3.3-4.4	—	0.30-0.22	—
Same with perlite filled cores ...	—	—	1.5-2.5	—	0.65-0.41	—
Same with vermiculite filled cores ...	—	—	1.70	—	0.58	—
Same with molded EPS (beads) filled cores ...	—	—	1.82	—	0.56	—
Same with molded EPS inserts in cores ...	—	—	2.10	—	0.47	—
Low mass aggregate (expanded shale, clay, slate or slag, pumice) 150 mm						
7.3-7.7 kg, 1360-1390 kg/m³ concrete, 2 or 3 cores	—	—	3.0-3.5	—	0.34-0.29	—
Same with perlite filled cores ...	—	—	1.36	—	0.74	—
Same with vermiculite filled cores ...	—	—	1.87	—	0.53	—
200 mm, 8.6-10.0 mm, 1150-1380 kg/m³ concrete,	—	—	1.8-3.1	—	0.56-0.33	0.88
Same with perlite filled cores ...	—	—	0.9-1.3	—	1.20-0.77	—
Same with vermiculite filled cores ...	—	—	1.1-1.5	—	0.93-0.69	—
Same with molded EPS (beads) filled cores ...	—	—	1.19	—	0.85	—
Same with UF foam filled cores ...	—	—	1.25	—	0.79	—
Same with molded EPS inserts in cores ...	—	—	1.65	—	0.62	—
300 mm, 14.5-16.3 kg, 1280-1440 kg/m³ concrete,						
2 or 3 cores ...	—	—	2.2-2.5	—	0.46-0.40	—
Same with perlite filled cores ...	—	—	0.6-0.9	—	1.6-1.1	—
Same with vermiculite filled cores ...	—	—	0.97	—	1.0	—
Stone, lime, or sand						
Quartzitic and sandstone ...	2880	10.4	—	0.10	—	—
	2560	6.2	—	0.16	—	—
	2240	3.5	—	0.29	—	—
	1920	1.9	—	0.53	—	0.79
Calcitic, dolomitic, limestone, marble, and granite ...	2880	4.3	—	0.23	—	—
	2560	3.2	—	0.32	—	—
	2240	2.3	—	0.43	—	—
	1920	1.6	—	0.63	—	0.79
	1600	1.1	—	0.90	—	—

Table 5-15 Typical Thermal Properties of Common Building and Insulating Materials[a] (*Continued*)

(Table 4, Chapter 24, 1997 *ASHRAE Handbook—Fundamentals*, SI Version)

				Resistance[c] (R)		
Description	**Density, kg/m^3**	**Conductivity[b] (k), W/(m·K)**	**Conductance (C), W/(m^2·K)**	**Per Inch Thickness ($1/k$), K·m/W**	**For Thickness Listed ($1/C$), K·m^2/W**	**Specific Heat, kJ/(kg·K)**
Gypsum partition tile						
75 by 300 by 760 mm, solid	—	—	4.50	—	0.222	0.79
75 by 300 by 760 mm, 4 cells	—	—	4.20	—	0.238	—
100 by 300 by 760 mm, 3 cells	—	—	3.40	—	0.294	—
Concretes[o]						
Sand and gravel or stone aggregate concretes (concretes with more than 50% quartz or quartzite sand have conductivities in the higher end of the range)	2400	1.4-2.9	—	0.69-0.35	—	—
	2240	1.3-2.6	—	0.77-0.39	—	0.8-1.0
	2080	1.0-1.9	—	0.99-053	—	—
Limestone concretes	2240	1.60	—	0.62	—	—
	1920	1.14	—	0.88	—	—
	1600	0.79	—	1.26	—	—
Gypsum-fiber concrete (87.5% gypsum, 12.5% wood chips)	816	0.24	—	4.18	—	0.88
Cement/lime, mortar, and stucco	1920	1.40	—	0.71	—	—
	1600	0.97	—	1.04	—	—
	1280	0.65	—	1.54	—	—
Lightweight aggregate concretes						
Expanded shale, clay, or slate; expanded slags; cinders; pumice (with density up to 1600 kg/m^3); and scoria (sanded concretes have conductivities in the higher end of the range)	1920	0.9-1.3	—	1.08-0.76	—	—
	1600	0.68-0.89	—	1.48-1.12	—	0.84
	1280	0.48-0.59	—	2.10-1.69	—	0.84
	960	0.30-0.36	—	3.30-2.77	—	—
	640	0.18	—	5.40	—	—
Perlite, vermiculite, and polystyrene beads	800	0.26-0.27	—	3.81-3.68	—	
	640	0.20-0.22	—	4.92-4.65	—	0.63-0.96
	480	0.16	—	6.31	—	—
	320	0.12	—	8.67	—	—
Foam concretes	1920	0.75	—	1.32	—	—
	1600	0.60	—	1.66	—	—
	1280	0.44	—	2.29	—	—
	1120	0.36	—	2.77	—	—
Foam concretes and cellular concretes	960	0.30	—	3.33	—	—
	640	0.20	—	4.92	—	—
	320	0.12	—	8.67	—	—
SIDING MATERIALS (on flat surface)						
Shingles						
Asbestos-cement	1900	—	27.0	—	0.037	—
Wood, 400 mm, 190-mm exposure	—	—	6.53	—	0.15	1.30
Wood, double, 400 mm, 300-mm exposure	—	—	4.77	—	0.21	1.17
Wood, plus insul. backer board, 8 mm	—	—	4.03	—	0.25	1.30
Siding						
Asbestos-cement, 6.4 mm, lapped	—	—	27.0	—	0.037	1.01
Asphalt roll siding	—	—	36.9	—	0.026	1.47
Asphalt insulating siding (12.7 mm bed.)	—	—	3.92	—	0.26	1.47
Hardboard siding, 11 mm	—	—	8.46	—	0.12	1.17
Wood, drop, 20 by 200 mm	—	—	7.21	—	0.14	1.17
Wood, bevel, 13 by 200 mm, lapped	—	—	6.98	—	0.14	1.17
Wood, bevel, 19 by 250 mm, lapped	—	—	5.40	—	0.18	1.17
Wood, plywood, 9.5 mm, lapped	—	—	9.60	—	0.10	1.22
Aluminum, steel, or vinyl[p, q], over sheathing						
Hollow-backed	—	—	9.31	—	0.11	1.22[q]
Insulating-board backed						
9.5 mm nominal	—	—	3.12	—	0.32	1.34
9.5 mm nominal, foil backed	—	—	1.93	—	0.52	—
Architectural (soda-lime float) glass	—	—	56.8	—	0.018	0.84
WOODS (12% moisture content)[e,r]						
Hardwoods						1.63[s]
Oak	659-749	0.16-0.18	—	6.2-5.5	—	
Birch	682-726	0.167-0.176	—	6.0-5.7	—	
Maple	637-704	0.157-0.171	—	6.4-5.8	—	
Ash	614-670	0.153-0.164	—	6.5-6.1	—	
Softwoods						1.63[s]
Southern Pine	570-659	0.144-0.161	—	6.9-6.2	—	
Douglas Fir-Larch	536-581	0.137-0.145	—	7.3-6.9	—	
Southern Cypress	502-514	0.130-0.132	—	7.7-7.6	—	
Hem-Fir, Spruce-Pine-Fir	392-502	0.107-0.130	—	9.3-7.7	—	
West Coast Woods, Cedars	347-502	0.098-0.130	—	10.3-7.7	—	
California Redwood	392-448	0.107-0.118	—	9.4-8.5	—	

Notes for Table 5-15 SI

[a] Values are for a mean temperature of 24 °C. Representative values for dry materials are intended as design (not specification) values for materials in normal use. Thermal values of insulating materials may differ from design values depending on their in-situ properties (e.g., density and moisture content, orientation, etc.) and variability experienced during manufacture. For properties of a particular product, use the value supplied by the manufacturer or by unbiased tests.

[b] The symbol λ is also used to represent thermal conductivity.

[c] Resistance values are the reciprocals of *C* before rounding off *C* to two decimal places.

[d] Lewis (1967).

[e] U.S. Department of Agriculture (1974).

[f] Does not include paper backing and facing, if any. Where insulation forms a boundary (reflective or otherwise) of an airspace, see Tables 2 and 3 for the insulating value of an airspace with the appropriate effective emittance and temperature conditions of the space.

[g] Conductivity varies with fiber diameter. (See Chapter 22, Factors Affecting Thermal Performance.) Batt, blanket, and loose-fill mineral fiber insulations are manufactured to achieve specified R-values, the most common of which are listed in the table. Due to differences in manufacturing processes and materials, the product thicknesses, densities, and thermal conductivities vary over considerable ranges for a specified R-value.

[h] This material is relatively new and data are based on limited testing.

[i] For additional information, see Society of Plastics Engineers (SPI) *Bulletin* U108. Values are for aged, unfaced board stock. For change in conductivity with age of expanded polyurethane/polyisocyanurate, see Chapter 22, Factors Affecting Thermal Performance.

[j] Values are for aged products with gas-impermeable facers on the two major surfaces. An aluminum foil facer of 25 μm thickness or greater is generally considered impermeable to gases. For change in conductivity with age of expanded polyisocyanurate, see Chapter 22, Factors Affecting Thermal Performance, and SPI *Bulletin* U108.

[k] Cellular phenolic insulation may no longer be manufactured. The thermal conductivity and resistance values do not represent aged insulation, which may have a higher thermal conductivity and lower thermal resistance.

[l] Insulating values of acoustical tile vary, depending on density of the board and on type, size, and depth of perforations.

[m] Cavity is framed with 20 mm wood furring strips. Caution should be used in applying this value for other framing materials. The reported value was derived from tests and applies to the reflective path only. The effect of studs or furring strips must be included in determining the overall performance of the wall.

[n] Values for fully grouted block may be approximated using values for concrete with a similar unit density.

[o] Values for concrete block and concrete are at moisture contents representative of normal use.

[p] Values for metal or vinyl siding applied over flat surfaces vary widely, depending on amount of ventilation of airspace beneath the siding; whether airspace is reflective or nonreflective; and on thickness, type, and application of insulating backing-board used. Values are averages for use as design guides, and were obtained from several guarded hot box tests (ASTM C 236) or calibrated hot box (ASTM C 976) on hollow-backed types and types made using backing of wood fiber, foamed plastic, and glass fiber. Departures of ±50% or more from these values may occur.

[q] Vinyl specific heat = 1.0 kJ/(kg·K)

[r] See Adams (1971), MacLean (1941), and Wilkes (1979). The conductivity values listed are for heat transfer across the grain. The thermal conductivity of wood varies linearly with the density, and the density ranges listed are those normally found for the wood species given. If the density of the wood species is not known, use the mean conductivity value. For extrapolation to other moisture contents, the following empirical equation developed by Wilkes (1979) may be used:

$$= 0.7494 + \frac{(4.895 \times 10^{-3} + 1.503 \times 10^{-4} M}{1 + 0.01M}$$

where ρ is density of the moist wood in kg/m^3, and *M* is the moisture content in percent.

[s] From Wilkes (1979), an empirical equation for the specific heat of moist wood at 24°C is as follows:

$$= 0.1442\left[\frac{(0.299 + 0.01M)}{(1 + 0.01M)}\right] + \Delta$$

where Δc_p accounts for the heat of sorption and is denoted by

$$c_p = M(0.008037 - 1.325 \times 10^{-4} M$$

where *M* is the moisture content in percent by mass.

Table 5-16 SI Overall Coefficients of Heat Transmission of Various Fenestrations

(Table 5, Page 29.8 only, Chapter 29, 1997 *ASHRAE Handbook—Fundamentals*, SI Version)

Product Type	Glass Only		Vertical Installation									
			Operable (including sliding and swinging glass doors)					Fixed				
Frame Type / **ID Glazing Type**	**Center of Glass**	**Edge of Glass**	**Aluminum without Thermal Break**	**Aluminum with Thermal Break**	**Reinforced Vinyl/ Aluminum Clad Wood**	**Wood/ Vinyl**	**Insulated Fiberglass/ Vinyl**	**Aluminum without Thermal Break**	**Aluminum with Thermal Break**	**Reinforced Vinyl/ Aluminum Clad Wood**	**Wood/ Vinyl**	**Insulated Fiberglass/ Vinyl**
Single Glazing												
1 3.2 mm glass	*5.91*	*5.91*	7.24	6.12	5.14	5.05	4.61	6.42	6.07	5.55	5.55	5.35
2 6.4 mm acrylic/polycarb	*5.00*	*5.00*	6.49	5.43	4.51	4.42	4.01	5.60	5.25	4.75	4.75	4.58
3 3.2 mm acrylic/polycarb	*5.45*	*5.45*	6.87	5.77	4.82	4.73	4.31	6.01	5.66	5.15	5.15	4.97
Double Glazing												
4 6.4 mm airspace	*3.12*	*3.63*	4.93	3.70	3.25	3.13	2.77	3.94	3.56	3.19	3.17	3.04
5 12.7 mm airspace	*2.73*	*3.36*	4.62	3.42	3.00	2.87	2.53	3.61	3.22	2.86	2.84	2.72
6 6.4 mm argon space	*2.90*	*3.48*	4.75	3.54	3.11	2.98	2.63	3.75	3.37	3.00	2.98	2.85
7 12.7 mm argon space	*2.56*	*3.24*	4.49	3.30	2.89	2.76	2.42	3.47	3.08	2.73	2.70	2.58
Double Glazing, *e* = 0.60 on surface 2 or 3												
8 6.4 mm airspace	*2.95*	*3.52*	4.80	3.58	3.14	3.02	2.67	3.80	3.41	3.05	3.03	2.90
9 12.7 mm airspace	*2.50*	*3.20*	4.45	3.26	2.85	2.73	2.39	3.42	3.03	2.68	2.66	2.54
10 6.4 mm argon space	*2.67*	*3.32*	4.58	3.38	2.96	2.84	2.49	3.56	3.17	2.82	2.80	2.67
11 12.7 mm argon space	*2.33*	*3.08*	4.31	3.13	2.74	2.62	2.28	3.28	2.89	2.54	2.52	2.40
Double Glazing, *e* = 0.40 on surface 2 or 3												
12 6.4 mm airspace	*2.78*	*3.40*	4.66	3.46	3.03	2.91	2.56	3.66	3.27	2.91	2.89	2.76
13 12.7 mm airspace	*2.27*	*3.04*	4.27	3.09	2.70	2.58	2.25	3.23	2.84	2.49	2.47	2.35
14 6.4 mm argon space	*2.44*	*3.16*	4.40	3.21	2.81	2.69	2.35	3.37	2.98	2.63	2.61	2.49
15 12.7 mm argon space	*2.04*	*2.88*	4.09	2.93	2.55	2.43	2.10	3.04	2.65	2.31	2.29	2.17
Double Glazing, *e* = 0.20 on surface 2 or 3												
16 6.4 mm airspace	*2.56*	*3.24*	4.49	3.30	2.89	2.76	2.42	3.47	3.08	2.73	2.70	2.58
17 12.7 mm airspace	*1.99*	*2.83*	4.05	2.89	2.52	2.39	2.07	2.99	2.60	2.26	2.24	2.13
18 6.4 mm argon space	*2.16*	*2.96*	4.18	3.01	2.63	2.51	2.17	3.13	2.74	2.40	2.38	2.26
19 12.7 mm argon space	*1.70*	*2.62*	3.83	2.68	2.33	2.21	1.89	2.75	2.36	2.03	2.01	1.90
Double Glazing, *e* = 0.10 on surface 2 or 3												
20 6.4 mm airspace	*2.39*	*3.12*	4.36	3.17	2.78	2.65	2.32	3.32	2.93	2.59	2.56	2.45
21 12.7 mm airspace	*1.82*	*2.71*	3.92	2.77	2.41	2.28	1.96	2.84	2.45	2.12	2.10	1.99
22 6.4 mm argon space	*1.99*	*2.83*	4.05	2.89	2.52	2.39	2.07	2.99	2.60	2.26	2.24	2.13
23 12.7 mm argon space	*1.53*	*2.49*	3.70	2.56	2.22	2.10	1.79	2.60	2.21	1.89	1.86	1.76
Double Glazing, *e* = 0.05 on surface 2 or 3												
24 6.4 mm airspace	*2.33*	*3.08*	4.31	3.13	2.74	2.62	2.28	3.28	2.89	2.54	2.52	2.40
25 12.7 mm airspace	*1.70*	*2.62*	3.83	2.68	2.33	2.21	1.89	2.75	2.36	2.03	2.01	1.90
26 6.4 mm argon space	*1.87*	*2.75*	3.96	2.81	2.44	2.32	2.00	2.89	2.50	2.17	2.15	2.03
27 12.7 mm argon space	*1.42*	*2.41*	3.61	2.48	2.15	2.02	1.71	2.50	2.11	1.79	1.77	1.67
Triple Glazing												
28 6.4 mm airspace	*2.16*	*2.96*	4.11	2.89	2.51	2.45	2.16	3.10	2.73	2.38	2.33	2.25
29 12.7 mm airspace	*1.76*	*2.67*	3.80	2.60	2.25	2.19	1.91	2.76	2.39	2.05	2.01	1.93
30 6.4 mm argon space	*1.93*	*2.79*	3.94	2.73	2.36	2.30	2.01	2.90	2.54	2.19	2.15	2.07
31 12.7 mm argon space	*1.65*	*2.58*	3.71	2.52	2.17	2.12	1.84	2.66	2.30	1.96	1.91	1.84
Triple Glazing, *e* = 0.20 on surface 2,3,4, or 5												
32 6.4 mm airspace	*1.87*	*2.75*	3.89	2.69	2.32	2.27	1.98	2.86	2.49	2.15	2.10	2.03
33 12.7 mm airspace	*1.42*	*2.41*	3.54	2.36	2.02	1.97	1.70	2.47	2.10	1.77	1.73	1.66
34 6.4 mm argon space	*1.59*	*2.54*	3.67	2.48	2.13	2.08	1.80	2.61	2.25	1.91	1.87	1.80
35 12.7 mm argon space	*1.25*	*2.28*	3.40	2.23	1.91	1.86	1.59	2.32	1.96	1.63	1.59	1.52
Triple Glazing, *e* = 0.20 on surfaces 2 or 3 and 4 or 5												
36 6.4 mm airspace	*1.65*	*2.58*	3.71	2.52	2.17	2.12	1.84	2.66	2.30	1.96	1.91	1.84
37 12.7 mm airspace	*1.14*	*2.19*	3.31	2.15	1.84	1.78	1.52	2.23	1.86	1.54	1.49	1.43
38 6.4 mm argon space	*1.31*	*2.32*	3.45	2.27	1.95	1.90	1.62	2.37	2.01	1.68	1.63	1.56
39 12.7 mm argon space	*0.97*	*2.05*	3.18	2.03	1.72	1.67	1.41	2.08	1.71	1.39	1.35	1.29
Triple Glazing, *e* = 0.10 on surfaces 2 or 3 and 4 or 5												
40 6.4 mm airspace	*1.53*	*2.49*	3.63	2.44	2.10	2.05	1.77	2.57	2.20	1.86	1.82	1.75
41 12.7 mm airspace	*1.02*	*2.10*	3.22	2.07	1.76	1.71	1.45	2.13	1.76	1.44	1.40	1.33
42 6.4 mm argon space	*1.19*	*2.23*	3.36	2.19	1.87	1.82	1.55	2.27	1.91	1.58	1.54	1.47
43 12.7 mm argon space	*0.80*	*1.92*	3.05	1.90	1.61	1.56	1.30	1.93	1.57	1.25	1.21	1.15
Quadruple Glazing, *e* = 0.10 on surfaces 2 or 3 and 4 or 5												
44 6.4 mm airspaces	*1.25*	*2.28*	3.40	2.23	1.91	1.86	1.59	2.32	1.96	1.63	1.59	1.52
45 12.7 mm airspaces	*0.85*	*1.96*	3.09	1.94	1.65	1.60	1.34	1.98	1.62	1.30	1.26	1.19
46 6.4 mm argon spaces	*0.97*	*2.05*	3.18	2.03	1.72	1.67	1.41	2.08	1.71	1.39	1.35	1.29
47 12.7 mm argon spaces	*0.68*	*1.83*	2.96	1.82	1.54	1.48	1.23	1.84	1.47	1.16	1.11	1.05
48 6.4 mm krypton spaces	*0.68*	*1.83*	2.96	1.82	1.54	1.48	1.23	1.84	1.47	1.16	1.11	1.05

Notes:

1. All heat transmission coefficients in this table include film resistances and are based on winter conditions of −18°C outdoor air temperature and 21°C indoor air temperature, with 24 km/h outdoor air velocity and zero solar flux. With the exception of single glazing, small changes in the indoor and outdoor temperatures will not significantly affect overall U-factors. The coefficients are for vertical position except skylight values, which are for 20° from horizontal with heat flow up.

2. Glazing layer surfaces are numbered from the outdoor to the indoor. Double, triple and quadruple refer to the number of glazing panels. All data are based on 3 mm glass, unless otherwise noted. Thermal conductivities are: 0.917 W/(m·K) for glass, and 0.19 W/(m·K) for acrylic and polycarbonate.

3. Standard spacers are metal. Edge-of-glass effects assumed to extend over the 65 mm band around perimeter of each glazing unit as in Figure 3.

Table 5-17 SI Transmission Coefficients for Wood and Steel Doors

(Table 6, Chapter 24, 1997 *ASHRAE Handbook—Fundamentals*, SI Version)

Nominal Door Thickness, mm	Description	No Storm Door	Wood Storm Door[c]	Metal Storm Door[d]
Wood Doors[a,b]				
35	Panel door with 11 mm panels[e]	3.24	1.87	2.10
35	Hollow core flush door	2.67	1.70	1.82
35	Solid core flush door	2.21	1.48	1.59
45	Panel door with 11 mm panels[e]	3.07	1.82	2.04
45	Hollow core flush door	2.61	1.65	1.82
45	Panel door with 29 mm panels[e]	2.21	1.48	1.59
45	Solid core flush door	2.27	—	1.48
57	Solid core flush door	1.53	1.14	1.19
Steel Doors[b]				
45	Fiberglass or mineral wool core with steel stiffeners, no thermal break[f]	3.41	—	—
45	Paper honeycomb core without thermal break[f]	3.18	—	—
45	Solid urethane foam core without thermal break[a]	2.27	—	—
45	Solid fire rated mineral fiberboard core without thermal break[f]	2.16	—	—
45	Polystyrene core without thermal break [18 gage (1.31 mm) commercial steel][f]	1.99	—	—
45	Polyurethane core without thermal break (18 gage commercial steel)[f]	1.65	—	—
45	Polyurethane core without thermal break [24 gage (0.70 mm) residential steel][f]	1/65	—	—
45	Polyurethane core with thermal break and wood perimeter (24 gage residential steel)[f]	1.14	—	—
45	Solid urethane foam core with thermal break[a]	1.14	—	0.91

Note: All U-factors for exterior doors in this table are for doors with no glazing, except for the storm doors which are in addition to the main exterior door. Any glazing area in exterior doors should be included with the appropriate glass type and analyzed as a window (see Chapter 29). Interpolation and moderate extrapolation are permitted for door thicknesses other than those specified.

[a]Values are based on a nominal 810 mm by 2030 mm door size with no glazing.

[b]Outside air conditions: 24 km/h wind speed, −18°C air temperature; inside air conditions: natural convection, 21°C air temperature.

[c]Values for wood storm door are for approximately 50% glass area.

[d]Values for metal storm door are for any percent glass area.

[e]55% panel area.

[f]ASTM C 236 hotbox data on a nominal 910 mm by 2130 mm door size with no glazing.

Chapter 6

HEATING LOAD CALCULATION

The procedures described in this chapter are for calculating the design heating loads for both commercial and residential buildings. Additional details can be found in Chapters 27 and 28 of the 1997 *ASHRAE Handbook—Fundamentals*, and *Cooling and Heating Load Calculation Manual*, Second Edition, 1992.

6.1 Heating Load Principles

Techniques for estimating design heating load for commercial, institutional, and industrial applications are essentially the same as for those estimating design cooling loads, except that (1) temperatures outside the conditioned spaces are generally lower than the space temperatures maintained; (2) credit for solar heat gains or for internal heat gains is not included; and (3) the thermal storage effect of building structure or content is ignored. Heat losses (negative heat gains) are thus considered to be instantaneous, heat transfer essentially conductive, and latent heat treated only as a function of replacing space humidity lost to the exterior environment. The actual heat loss problem is transient because outdoor temperature, wind velocity, and sunlight are constantly changing. The Transfer Function Method (discussed in Chapter 7, in connection with the cooling load) may be used under winter conditions to account for changing solar radiation, outdoor temperature, internal gains, and the energy storage capacity of the structure. During the coldest months, however, sustained periods of cold and cloudy weather with relatively small variation in outdoor conditions may occur. In this situation, heat loss from the space will be relative constant, and in the absence of internal gains, will peak during the early morning hours. Therefore, for design purposes the heat loss is usually estimated based on steady-state heat transfer for some reasonable design temperature. Transient analyses are often used to predict the *energy* requirements of the building, where solar and storage effects and internal heat gains are taken into account. Thus, the general methodology is applicable for all types of buildings, including residential.

This simplified approach can be used to estimate a heating load for the "worst case" conditions that can reasonably be anticipated during a heating season. Traditionally this is considered as the load that must be met under design interior and exterior conditions, including infiltration and/or ventilation, but in the absence of solar effect (at night or cloudy winter days) and before the periodic presence of people, lights, and appliances can begin to have an offsetting effect. The primary orientation is thus toward identification of adequately sized heating equipment to handle the normal worst-case condition.

Safety Factors and Load Allowances. Before mechanical cooling of buildings became a usual procedure, buildings included much less insulation, large operable windows, and generally more infiltration-prone assemblies than the energy-efficient and much tighter buildings typical of post-1975 design. Allowances of 10 to 20% of the net calculated heating load for piping losses to unheated spaces, and 10 to 20% more for a warm-up load were common practice, along with occasional other safety factors reflecting the experience and/or concern of the individual designer. Except for possibly including as much as 10% for warm-up with intermittently heated buildings (such as churches), such measures are infrequently used in estimating heating loads for contemporary buildings, with the uncompensated net heating load normally considered as having an adequate margin for error.

Cooling Needs During Noncooling Months. Perimeter spaces exposed to high solar heat gain often justify mechanical cooling during sunlit portions of traditional heating months, as will completely interior spaces with significant internal heat gain. These conditions require special attention by the system designer for proper accommodation as needed, but such spaces can also represent significant heating loads during nonsunlit hours or after periods of nonoccupancy when adjacent spaces have been allowed to cool below interior design temperatures. The loads involved can be estimated conventionally for the purpose of designing the means to offset or to compensate for them and prevent overheating and they have **no direct relationship to design heating loads** for the spaces in question.

Prior to designing a heating system, the engineer must estimate the maximum probable (design) heat loss of each room or space to be heated, based on maintaining a selected indoor air temperature during periods of design outdoor weather conditions. Heat losses may be divided into two groups: (1) transmission losses or heat transmitted through the confining walls, floor, ceiling, glass, or other surfaces and (2) infiltration losses or heat required to warm outdoor air which leaks in through cracks and crevices, around doors and windows, or through open doors and windows, or heat required to warm outdoor air used for ventilation.

The ideal solution is to select a system with a capacity at maximum output just equal to the heating load that develops when the most severe weather conditions for the locality occur. However, where night setback is used, some excess capacity may be needed unless the owner understands that under some conditions of operation, it may be impossible to elevate the set-back temperature.

The heating load is normally estimated for the winter design temperature, which usually occurs at night; therefore, no credit is taken for the heat given off by such internal sources like persons, lights, motors, and equipment. This heat energy supplied by people, lights, motors, and machinery should always be estimated, but any actual allowance for these heat sources requires careful consideration. The full complement of people may not occupy certain spaces in the evenings, on weekends, and during other periods, but generally these spaces must be heated to a reasonably comfortable temperature for the few who may be using the space during these periods as well as prior to occupancy.

In industrial plants, heat sources may be substituted for part of the heating requirement. In fact, there are situations where so much process heat is present that outdoor air must be used to prevent overheating of the space. However, sufficient heating equipment must still be provided to prevent freezing or other damage during periods when a facility or process is shut down.

6.2 Heating Load Methodology

The general procedure for calculating design heating loads using information in the 1997 *ASHRAE Handbook—Fundamentals* and from the *ASHRAE Cooling and Heating Load Calculation Manual, Second Edition,* is summarized in Table 6-1 and described in the following sections.

Table 6-1 Summary of Loads, Equations and References for Calculating Design Heating Loads in Residential and Light Commercial Buildings

(References refer to Table 12, Chapter 27, 1997 *ASHRAE Handbook—Fundamentals*)

Heating Load	Equation	Reference, Table, Description
Roofs, ceilings, walls, glass	$q = U A \Delta t$	U → Chapter 24, Tables 1, 2, and 4 Δt → Temperature difference between inside and outside design dry bulbs, Chapter 26. For temperatures in unheated spaces, see Equation (2); for attic temperatures, see Equation (3). A → Area calculated from plans
Walls below grade	$q = U A \Delta t$	U → See Table 14. Δt → Use Figure 6 to assist in determining Δt.
Floors Above grade	$q = U A \Delta t$	Δt → For crawl space temperatures, see Equation (4).
On grade	$q = F_2 P \Delta t$	F_2 → See Table 16. Δt → See Equation (6). P → Perimeter of slab
Below grade	$q = U A \Delta t$	Δt → Use Figure 6 to assist in determining Δt. A → See Table 15.
Infiltration and ventilation air Sensible	$q_s = 0.018\ Q\ \Delta t$	Q → Volume of outdoor air entering building. See Chapter 25 for estimating methods for infiltration.
Latent	$q_l = 80.7\ Q\ \Delta W$	ΔW → Humidity ratio difference, if humidification is to be added

Note: SI equations for infiltration and ventilation air are $q_s = 1.2Q\Delta t$ and $q_l = 3.0Q\Delta W$

6.2.1 General Procedure

To calculate a design heating load, prepare the following information about building design and weather data at design conditions.

1. Select outdoor design weather conditions: temperature, wind direction, and wind speed.
2. Select the indoor air temperature to be maintained in each space and the humidity level of the return air, if a humidifier is to be installed, during design weather conditions.
3. Estimate temperatures in adjacent unheated spaces and, if there are below grade spaces, determine the ground surface temperature at design winter conditions.
4. Select or compute heat transfer coefficients for outside walls and glass; for inside walls, nonbasement floors, and ceilings, if these are next to unheated spaces; and for the roof if it is next to heated spaces.
5. Determine the net area of outside wall, glass, and roof next to heated spaces, as well as any cold walls, floors, or ceilings next to unheated spaces. These determinations can be made from building plans or from the actual buildings, using inside dimensions.
6. Compute heat transmission losses for each kind of wall, glass, floor, ceiling, and roof in the building by multiplying the overall heat transfer coefficient in each case by the area of the surface and the temperature difference between indoor air and outdoor air, adjacent space air, or ground surface, as appropriate.
7. Compute heat losses from grade-level slab floors using the heat loss rate per unit length of exposed perimeter using the method in this chapter.
8. Compute the energy associated with infiltration of cold air around outside doors, windows, porous building materials, and other openings. These unit values depend on the kind or width of crack, wind speed, and the temperature difference between indoor and outdoor air.
9. When positive ventilation using outdoor air is provided by the conditioning unit, the energy required to warm and humidify the ventilation outdoor air to the space conditions must be provided by the unit. Unless mechanical ventilation is sufficient to maintain the building at a slightly positive pressure at all time (producing exfiltration and preventing infiltration), the heating unit must provide for both ventilation and natural infiltration losses.
10. Sum the coincidental transmission losses or heat transmitted through the confining walls, floor, ceiling, glass, and other surfaces, and the energy associated with cold air entering by infiltration and/or the ventilation air, to obtain the total heating load.
11. Include the pickup loads that may be required in intermittently heated buildings or when using night thermostat setback. Pickup loads frequently require an increase in heating capacity to bring the temperature of structure, air, and material contents to the specified temperature.

With the exception of slab-on-grade heat transfer, the basic formula for the heat loss by conduction and convection heat transfer through any surface is

$$q = AU(t_i - t_o) \tag{6-1}$$

where

q = heat transfer through wall, roof, ceiling, floor, or glass, Btu/h (W)
A = area of wall, glass, roof, ceiling, floor, or other exposed surface, ft^2 (m^2)
U = air-to-air (ground surface) heat transfer coefficient, Btu/h·ft^2·°F (W/m^2·K)
t_i = indoor air temperature near surface involved, °F (°C)
t_o = outdoor air temperature, temperature of adjacent unheated space, or ground surface temperature, °F (°C)

Example 6-1 Calculate the design heat loss q_t for the following wall:

Wall size: 10 ft high by 50 ft long

Wall construction: 4-in. face brick; building paper, vapor seal, 2 layers of mopped 15-lb felt; 4-in. concrete block (cinder aggregate); 1-in. glass fiber, organic bonded; 3/8-in. painted plasterboard.

Design conditions: Indoor, 72°F dry bulb, relative humidity = 30%; Outdoor, 32°F dry bulb

Solution:

	R-Value	
Outside air	0.17	(Table 5-12)
Brick	0.44	(Table 5-15)
Felt	0.12	(Table 5-15)
Block	1.11	(Table 5-15)
Glass fiber	4.00	(Table 5-15)
Plasterboard	0.32	(Table 5-13)
Inside air	0.68	(Table 5-12)
ΣR =	6.84	

$$U = 1/R = 1/6.84 = 0.146 \text{ Btu/h·ft}^2\text{·°F}$$

$$A = 10 \times 50 = 500 \text{ ft}^2$$

$$\Delta t = 72 - 32 = 40\text{°F}$$

$$q_t = UA\Delta t = 0.146 \times 500 \times 40 = 2920 \text{ Btu/h } (0.856 \text{ W})$$

6.2.2 Selecting Heating Design Conditions

The ideal solution to a basic heating system design is a plant with a maximum output capacity equal to the heating load that develops with the most severe local weather conditions. However, this solution is usually uneconomical. Weather records show that severe weather conditions do not repeat annually. If heating systems were designed for maximum weather conditions, excess capacity would exist during most of the system's operating life.

In many cases, an occasional failure of a heating plant to maintain a preselected indoor design temperature during brief periods of severe weather is not critical. However, the successful completion of some industrial or commercial processes may depend on close regulation of indoor temperatures. The specific requirements for each building should be carefully evaluated.

Before selecting an outdoor design temperature from Chapter 26 of the 1997 *ASHRAE Handbook—Fundamentals*, the designer should consider the following:

- Is the type of structure heavy, medium, or light?
- Is the structure insulated?
- Is the structure exposed to high wind?
- Is the load from infiltration or ventilation high?
- Is there more glass area than normal?
- During what part of the day will the structure be used?
- What is the nature of occupancy?
- Will there be long periods of operation at reduced indoor temperature?
- What is the amplitude between local maximum and minimum daily temperatures?
- Are there local conditions that cause significant variation from temperatures reported by the Weather Bureau?
- What auxiliary heating devices will be in the building?

Before selecting an outdoor design temperature, the designer must keep in mind that, if the outdoor to indoor design temperature difference is exceeded, the indoor temperature may fall, depending on the thermal mass of the structure and its contents and whether or not the internal load was included in calculations and the duration of the cold period.

The effect of wind on the heating requirements of any building should be considered because

- Wind movement increases the heat transmission of walls, glass, and roof, affecting poorly insulated walls to a much greater extent than well-insulated walls.
- Wind increases the infiltration of cold air through cracks around doors and windows and even through building materials themselves.

Although 72°F and 75°F are the most commonly selected indoor temperature for comfort heating design; local code requirements must be checked. ASHRAE *Standard* 55, Chapter 8 of the 1997 *ASHRAE Handbook—Fundamentals* and the 1995 *ASHRAE Handbook—Applications* provide additional details on selecting indoor design conditions.

6.2.3 Heat Loss from Crawl Spaces

To prevent ground moisture from evaporating and causing a condensation problem in crawl spaces, sheets of vapor retardant (e.g., polyethylene film) are used to cover the ground surface (see Chapter 23 of the 1997 *ASHRAE Handbook—Fundamentals*). Most codes require crawl spaces to be adequately vented all year round. However, venting the crawl space in the heating season causes substantial heat loss through the floor.

The space may be insulated in several ways; the crawl space ceiling (floor above the crawl space) can be insulated, or the perimeter wall can be insulated either on the outside or on the inside of the wall. If the floor above is insulated, the crawl space vents should be kept open, because the temperature of the crawl space is likely to be below the dew point of the indoor space. If the perimeter wall is insulated, the vents should be kept closed in the heating season and open the remainder of the year.

6.2.4 Heat Loss Through Ceiling and Roof

Transmission heat loss through top floor ceilings, attics and roofs may be estimated by either of two methods:

1. Substitute in Equation (6-1) the ceiling area A, the indoor/outdoor temperature difference $(t_i - t_o)$, and the proper U-factor.
2. For *pitched roofs*, estimate the attic temperature (based on the indoor and outdoor design temperatures) and substitute for t_o in Equation (6-1). Attic temperatures do not need to be calculated for flat roofs, as the ceiling-roof heat loss can be determined using an overall coefficient of heat transfer for the combined ceiling and roof structure.

6.2.5 Heat Loss From Basements

Heat transfer through basement walls and floors to the ground depends on (1) the difference between the air temperature within the room and that of the ground and outside air, (2) the material of the walls or floor, and (3) conductivity of the surrounding earth. Conductivity of the earth is usually unknown. Because of thermal inertia, ground temperature varies with depth, and there is a substantial time lag between changes in outdoor air temperatures and corresponding changes in ground temperature. As a result, ground-coupled heat transfer is less amenable to steady-state representation than is the case for above-grade building elements.

Heat transmission from the below-grade portion of the basement wall to the ambient air cannot be approximated by one-dimensional heat conduction. The heat flux through the basement wall is not uniform with the depth of the wall. Listed in Table 6-2 are heat loss values at different depths for an uninsulated and insulated concrete wall. The conductivity of the soil was assumed to be 9.6 Btu·in/h·ft²·°F (1.4 W/m·K).

The same steady-state design used for the basement wall can be applied to the basement floor, except that the length of the heat flow path is longer. Thus, heat loss through the basement floor is smaller than that from the wall. To find total heat loss from the floor, take an average value for the heat loss and multiply by the floor area. Typical values are estimated and given in Table 6-3. Selecting the appropriate design temperature difference can be a problem with below-grade spaces. Although internal design temperature is given by the basement (or below-grade space) air temperature, none of the usual external design air temperatures are applicable because of the heat capacity of the soil. Ground surface temperature fluctuates about a mean value by an amplitude A, which varies with geographic location and surface cover (Figure 6-1). Suitable external design temperatures can be obtained by subtracting A for the location from the average winter air temperature t_a.

Table 6-2 Below-Grade Wall U-Factors, Btu/h·ft²·°F
(Table 14, Chapter 27 of the 1997 *ASHRAE Handbook—Fundamentals*)

Depth, ft	Path Length Through Soil, ft	Heat Loss Coefficient, Btu/h·ft²·°F[a] Uninsulated		R-4.17		R-8.34		R-12.5	
0 to 1	0.68	0.410	Σ[b]	0.152	Σ[b]	0.093	Σ[b]	0.067	Σ[b]
1 to 2	2.27	0.222	0.632	0.116	0.268	0.079	0.172	0.059	0.126
2 to 3	3.88	0.155	0.787	0.094	0.362	0.068	0.240	0.053	0.179
3 to 4	5.52	0.119	0.906	0.079	0.441	0.060	0.300	0.048	0.227
4 to 5	7.05	0.096	1.002	0.069	0.510	0.053	0.353	0.044	0.271
5 to 6	8.65	0.079	1.081	0.060	0.570	0.048	0.401	0.040	0.311
6 to 7	10.28	0.069	1.150	0.054	0.624	0.044	0.445	0.037	0.348

Source: Latta and Boileau (1969).
[a]Soil conductivity was assumed to be 9.6 Btu·in/h·ft²·°F.
[b]Σ = heat loss to current depth.
Note: The second column under each level of insulation is a summation of the first column.

Table 6-3 Below-Grade Floor U-Factors, Btu/h·ft²·°F
(Table 15, Chapter 27 of the 1997 *ASHRAE Handbook—Fundamentals*)

Depth of Foundation Wall below Grade, ft	Heat Loss Coefficient, Btu/h·ft²·°F — Shortest Width of House, ft: 20	24	28	32
5	0.032	0.029	0.026	0.023
6	0.030	0.027	0.025	0.022
7	0.029	0.026	0.023	0.021

Note: $\Delta t = (t_a - A)$

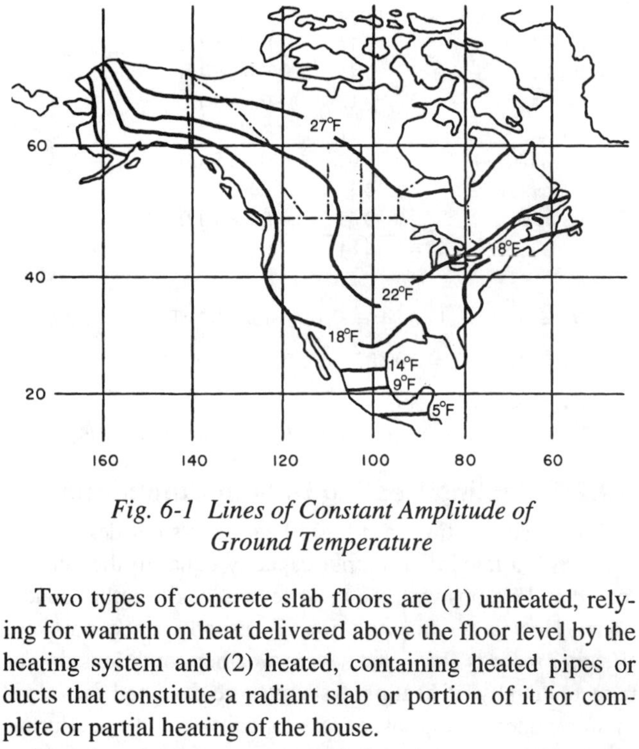

Fig. 6-1 Lines of Constant Amplitude of Ground Temperature

Two types of concrete slab floors are (1) unheated, relying for warmth on heat delivered above the floor level by the heating system and (2) heated, containing heated pipes or ducts that constitute a radiant slab or portion of it for complete or partial heating of the house.

Heat loss from a concrete slab floor is mostly through the perimeter rather than through the floor and into the ground. Total heat loss is more nearly proportional to the length of the perimeter than to the area of the floor. It can be estimated by the following equation for both unheated and heated slab floors:

$$q = F_2 P(t_i - t_o) \tag{6-2}$$

where

q = heat loss through the perimeter, Btu/h (W)
F_2 = heat loss coefficient, Btu/h·°F·ft of perimeter (W/m·K)
P = perimeter of exposed edge of floor, ft (m)
t_i = indoor temperature, °F (°C)
t_o = outdoor temperature, °F (°C)

Four basic slab-on-grade constructions have been analyzed with a finite element computer program and are shown in Figure 6-2. Figure 6-2(a) through (c) represent unheated slabs; Figure 6-2(d) can be considered a heated slab. Each was investigated with and without insulation of $R = 5.4$ h·ft^2·°F/Btu ($R = 0.95$ m^2·K/W) under three climatic conditions [7433, 5350 and 2950 degree Rankine days (4130, 2970, and 1640 degree Kelvin days)]. The results in terms of heat loss coefficient F_2, based on degree-days, are listed in Table 6-4.

Table 6-4 can be used to estimate F_2 under different degree-days of heating season weather. It is accurate enough to assign F_2 values between 0.8 and 0.93 for an uninsulated, unheated slab floor. The coefficient is reduced to between 0.47 and 0.54 when insulation of $R = 5.4$ h·ft^2·°F/Btu ($R = 0.95$ m^2·K/W) is applied to the slab edge and extended below grade to the frost line.

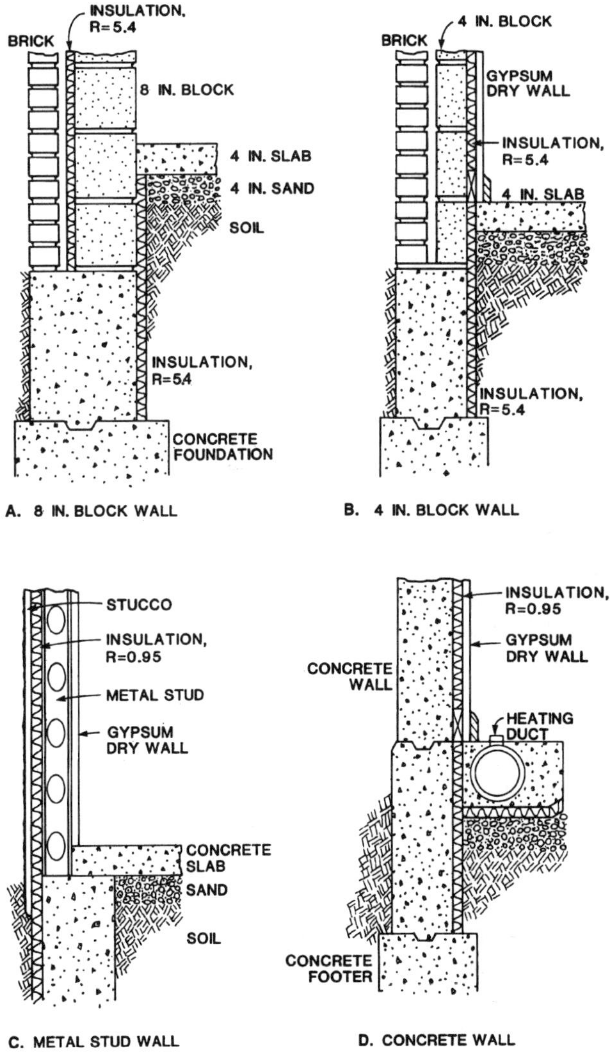

Fig. 6-2 Slab-on-Grade Configurations

Table 6-4 Heat Loss Coefficients F_2 for Slab Floors (Btu/h·°F·ft)

(Table 16, Chapter 27 of the 1997 *ASHRAE Handbook—Fundamentals*)

		Degree-Days (65°F Base)		
Construction	**Insulation**	**2950**	**5350**	**7433**
8 in. block wall, brick facing	Uninsulated	0.62	0.68	0.72
	R-5.4 from edge to footer	0.48	0.50	0.56
4 in. block wall, brick facing	Uninsulated	0.80	0.84	0.93
	R-5.4 from edge to footer	0.47	0.49	0.54
Metal stud wall, stucco	Uninsulated	1.15	1.20	1.34
	R-5.4 from edge to footer	0.51	0.53	0.58
Poured concrete wall with duct near perimeter[a]	Uninsulated	1.84	2.12	2.73
	R-5.4 from edge to footer, 3 ft under floor	0.64	0.72	0.90

[a]Weighted average temperature of the heating duct was assumed at 110°F during the heating season (outdoor air temperature less than 65°F).

For the heated slab floor, F_2 is estimated at between 1.2 and 1.8 for severe winters and 1.3 and 2.7 for mild winters, when no insulation is provided at the perimeter. When insulation of $R = 5.4$ ($R = 0.95$) is applied down to the frost line, the coefficient is reduced to between 0.5 and 0.64 in severe climates and between 0.58 and 0.9 in mild climates.

Example 6-2 Determine the heat loss for a basement in St. Louis, Missouri, which is 60 ft by 40 ft by 8 ft high, of standard concrete construction, and entirely below grade. Average winter temperature in St. Louis is 44°F.

Solution:

$$\text{Design } \Delta t = t_i - (t_a - A) = 70 - (44 - 22) = 48 \qquad \text{(Figure 6-1)}$$

Wall U-factors (Table 6-2)

1st ft	0.41
2nd ft	0.222
3rd ft	0.155
4th ft	0.119
5th ft	0.096
6th ft	0.079
7th ft	0.069
8th ft	0.069 (conservative)
	1.219 Btu/h·ft^2·°F

$$\text{Wall loss} = \Sigma U(P \times 1 \text{ ft})\Delta t = 1.219(200)(48) = 11{,}700 \text{ Btu/h}$$

Floor heat loss (Table 6-3)

$$U_{floor} = 0.021 \text{ Btu/h·ft}^2\text{·°F}$$

$$A = 60 \times 40 = 2400 \text{ ft}^2$$

$$\text{Floor heat loss} = 0.021(2400)(48) = 2420 \text{ Btu/h}$$

$$q_{total} = 11{,}700 + 2420 = 14{,}100 \text{ Btu/h (4.13 kW)}$$

6.2.6 Infiltration Heat Loss

Heat loss due to infiltration of outside air can be divided into sensible and latent components. The energy quantity that raises the temperature of outdoor infiltrating air up to indoor air temperature is the sensible component. The energy quantity associated with net loss of moisture from the space is the latent component. These calculations are discussed in Chapter 5.

Example 6-3 The west brick wall of a residence in Louisville, Kentucky, has a net area (excluding windows and doors) of 506 ft^2 and a U-factor of 0.067 Btu/h·ft^2·°F. Determine the heating load for the wall, Btu/h.

Solution:

$$q_s = UA\Delta t = 0.067(506)(72-10)$$
$$= 2101 \text{ Btu/h}$$

Example 6-4 A large window, essentially all glass, 10 ft by 5 ft, is located in the west wall of a residence in Kansas City, Missouri, where the indoor and outdoor winter design conditions have been selected as 72 and 6°F, respectively. To reduce energy requirements, the window is heat absorbing double glass ($e = 0.40$), 1/2-in. air space, wood framing, and has inside draperies which are closed at peak conditions. Determine the heating load for the window, Btu/h.

Solution:

From the Chapter 5 table for fenestration U-factors,

$$U_{window\ w/o\ draperies} = 0.45 \text{ Btu/h·ft}^2\text{·°F}$$

The major effect of the draperies will be to create an air space that will add approximately 1 °F·ft^2·F/Btu of thermal resistance. Thus,

$$R_{with\ drapes} = 1/U_{w/o} = 1/0.45 + 1 = 3.22$$
$$U_{with\ drapes} = 1/3.22 = 0.31 \text{ Btu/h·ft}^2\text{·°F}$$
$$q_s = UA\Delta t = 0.31(50)(72-6) = 1023 \text{ Btu/h}$$

Example 6-5 For the commercial building located in St. Louis, Missouri, and described below, determine the design heating load. The outside winter design temperature is 6°F and inside winter design conditions are 72°F, 30% rh. The 8-in. concrete floor is a slab-on-grade with $R = 5.4$ insulation, properly installed. There are 4900 (base 65°F) degree-days.

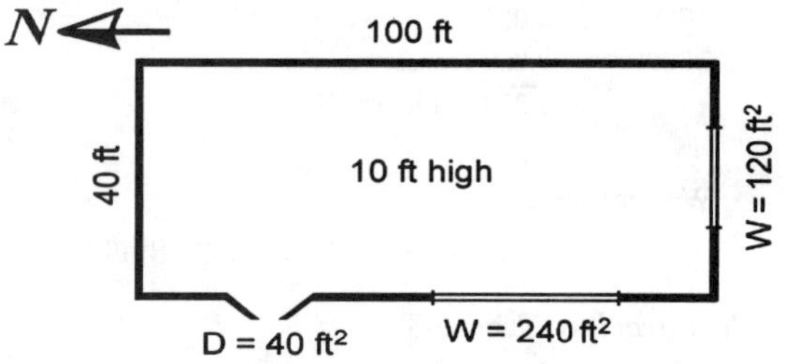

People: 35 at moderate office activity
Lights: 5600 W, fluorescent
Infiltration: 0.5 air changes per hour (ACH)
Wall: 1 in. dark stucco on 4 in. regular concrete, $U = 0.350$ Btu/h·ft^2·°F
Roof: 8 in. lightweight concrete, $U = 0.12$ Btu/h·ft^2·°F
Door: 2 in. solid wood, $U = 0.42$ Btu/h·ft^2·°F, $A = 40$ ft^2
Windows:
South: 1/8 in. regular sheet, $A = 120$ ft^2, $U = 1.30$ Btu/h·ft^2·°F
West: Insulating glass, regular sheet out/regular sheet in, 1/4 in. air space, 1/4 in. thick glass; $A = 240$ ft^2, $U = 0.69$ Btu/h·ft^2·°F

Solution:

Construction Element	U	A	Δt	q
East wall	0.35	1000	66	23,100
North wall	0.35	400	66	9,240
West wall	0.35	720	66	16,632
South wall	0.35	280	66	6,468
Door	0.43	40	66	1,135
South glass	1.30	120	66	10,296
West glass	0.69	240	66	10,930
Roof	0.12	4000	66	31,680
Floor	$F_2 = 0.485$	$P = 280$	66	8,963
			Subtotal =	118,444

Infiltration:

$$q_s = 1.10Q(t_i - t_o)$$
$$q_l = 4840Q(W_i - W_o)$$

where, at 0.5 ACH,

$$Q = 0.5(40 \times 100 \times 10)/60 = 333$$

Thus,

$$q_s = 1.10 \times 333 \times 66 = 24{,}200 \text{ Btu/h}$$

$$q_l = 4840 \times 333 \times (0.005 - 0.001) = 6447 \text{ Btu/h}$$

Total design heating load =

$$118{,}444 + 24{,}200 + 6447 = 149{,}100 \text{ Btu/h}$$

Note: Ventilation air requirements will produce additional load, but may eliminate infiltration load if sufficient to pressurize the building.

Example 6.6 Redo the design heating load for the building of Example 6.5 if, instead of a slab floor, the building is constructed over a full, conditioned basement that has a height of 8 ft, all below grade.

Solution:

All values are the same as for the previous problem except that the previously calculated floor loss must be replaced with losses for below grade walls and floor.

$$\text{Below-grade wall loss} = \Sigma U(P \times 1 \text{ ft})[t_i - (t_a - A)]$$
$$\text{Below-grade floor loss} = UA[t_i - (t_a - A)]$$

The average winter air temperature t_a (Chapter 4) is found to be 43.1°F, and the ground temperature amplitude from Fig. 6-1 is 22°F.

For the wall, $\Sigma U = 1.219$ (Table 6-2).

$$q_{wall} = 1.219(280 \times 1 \text{ ft})[72 - (43.1 - 22)] = 17{,}373 \text{ Btu/h}$$

For the floor, U ≅ 0.021.

$$q_{floor} = 0.021 \times 4000 \times 50.9 = 4276 \text{ Btu/h}$$

Thus, total load =

$$149{,}100 - 8963 + 17{,}373 + 4276 = 161{,}700 \text{ Btu/h}$$

Example 6.7 Redo the design heating load for the building of Example 6.5 if, instead of a slab floor on grade, the 8-in. concrete floor is above an open parking garage.

Solution:

All values are the same as for Example 6-5 except that the previously calculated floor loss must be replaced with one appropriately calculated for air-to-air heat transfer.

The air beneath the floor in the garage may be considered to be at outside air temperature and with the normal winter wind velocity. Thus, the U-factor for the floor can be determined as

$$U = \frac{1}{0.92 + 0.075 \times 8 + 0.17} = 0.59 \text{ Btu/h}\cdot\text{ft}^2\cdot{}^\circ\text{F}$$

The design heat loss becomes

$$q = 0.59 \times 4000 \times 66 = 156{,}213 \text{ Btu/h}$$

Total design heating load =

$$149{,}100 - 8963 + 156{,}213 = 296{,}300 \text{ Btu/h}$$

Note: Floor needs several inches of insulation.

6.2.7 Heating Load Summary Form

When preparing a set of design heating loads for a multi-space building, either a computer spreadsheet software program or a summary sheet such as provided as Figure 6-3 (adapted from Fig. 7.1, ASHRAE *Cooling and Heating Load Calculation Manual)* might prove useful.

HEAT LOSS CALCULATION SHEET

	Design Conditions		
Job Name ______	t_o = ______	t_i = ______	Δt = ______
Location ______	rh_o = ______	rh_i = ______	
Date ______	W_o = ______	W_i = ______	ΔW = ______

Room Number or Name												
Length of Exposed Slab Perim., ft												
Room Dimension, Height, Length, Width, ft												
Component	**No.**	***U* or *U'***	**Δt or ΔW**	**Area**	**Btu/h Sens.**	**Btu/h Lat.**	**Area**	**Btu/h Sens.**	**Btu/h Lat.**	**Area**	**Btu/h Sens.**	**Btu/h Lat.**
Gross Exposed Walls and Partitions												
Windows and Doors												
Net Exposed Walls and Partitions												
Ceilings and Roofs												
Floors												
Infiltration												
Heat Loss, Subtotal												
Duct Heat Loss												
Total Heat Loss												
Air Quantity, cfm												

Fig. 6-3 Heat Loss Calculation Sheet

6.3 Problems

6.1 Determine which of the following walls of 150 ft^2 gross area will have the greatest heat loss:

(a) Wall of 25% single glass and the remainder brick veneer ($U = 0.25$ Btu/h·ft^2·°F)

(b) Wall of 50% double-glazed windows with the remainder of the wall brick veneer ($U = 0.25$ Btu/h·ft^2·°F)

(c) Wall of 10% single pane glass and 90% of 6-in. poured concrete with $h_o = 6.0$ and $h_i = 1.6$ Btu/h·ft^2

6.2 In calculating heating estimates, the solar load on a building

(a) Is neglected because there is not much data on winter solar conditions

(b) Is neglected because the solar load is not large enough to worry about

(c) Is included because it gives a better estimate

(d) Is neglected because furnaces are so large that the heating estimate is not really necessary

(e) None of the above

6.3 A house has a pitched roof with an area of 159 m^2 and a U of 1.6 W/(m^2·K). The ceiling beneath the roof has an area of 133 m^2 and a U of 0.42 W/(m^2·K). The attic is unvented in winter for which the design conditions are −19°C outside and 22°C inside. Determine the heat loss through the ceiling. [Ans: 1.88 kW (6400 Btu/h)]

6.4 Determine the design winter heat loss through each of the following components of a building located in Minneapolis, Minnesota:

(a) Wall having 648 ft^2 of area and construction of 4-in. face brick; 3/4-in. plywood sheathing; 2-1/2-in. glass fiber insulation in 2 by 4 stud space (16-in. on centers); 1/2-in. plasterboard interior wall.

(b) A 2185 ft^2 ceiling topped by a 2622 ft^2 hip roof. The ceiling consists of 1/2-in. acoustical tile with R-19 insulation between the 2 by 6 (16-in. on centers) ceiling joists. The roof has asphalt shingles on 3/4-in. plywood sheathing on the roof rafters. The attic is unvented in winter.

(c) Two 4 ft by 6 ft single pane glass windows with storm windows.

6.5 If the building of *Problem* 6.4 is a residence having a volume of 17,480 ft^3 and is equipped with a humidifier set for 25% rh, determine

(a) Sensible heat load due to infiltration

(b) Latent heat load due to infiltration

6.6 For a building with design conditions of 72°F indoor and 12°F outdoor, determine the heat loss through each of the following components:

(a) Slab floor, 56 ft by 28 ft, on grade without perimeter insulation [Ans: 8165 Btu/h]

(b) Single glass double-hung window, 3 ft by 5 ft, with storm window in common metal frame [Ans: 730 Btu/h]

(c) 1-3/8-in. thick solid wood door, 3 ft by 7 ft, with wood storm door [Ans: 328 Btu/h]

(d) Sliding patio door, 6 ft by 7 ft, metal frame with double insulating glass having 1/4-in. air space [Ans: 2192 Btu/h]

6.7 Determine the heat loss for a basement in Chicago, Illinois, which is 8 m by 12 m by 2.1 m high, of standard concrete construction, and entirely below grade.

6.8 A residence located in Chicago, Illinois, has a total ceiling area of 1960 ft^2 and consists of 3/8-in. gypsum board on 2 by 6 ceiling joists. Six inches of fiberglass (mineral/glass wool) insulation fills the space between the joists. The pitched roof has asphalt shingles on 25/32-in. solid wood sheathing with no insulation between the rafters. The ratio of roof area to ceiling area is 1.3. The attic is unvented in winter. For winter design conditions, including a 72°F inside dry bulb at the 5-ft line, determine

(a) Outside design temperature, °F

(b) Appropriate temperature difference, °F

(c) Appropriate overall coefficient U, Btu/h·ft^2·°F

(d) Ceiling heat loss q, Btu/h

6.9 What will be the heat loss per hour due to infiltration through four windows that are double-hung metal sash with no weather strip and locked? The windows are 3 ft wide by 3 ft high and wind velocity is 30 mph outside at a temperature of 0°F. Inside temperature is 72°F. [Ans: 360 Btu/h]

6.10 A building has 8-in. concrete block walls, no insulating fill, 8 ft high walls, 1 window on each side and at the back end. Each window is 4 ft wide by 6 ft high. The building is 20 ft wide by 40 ft long with plaster ceiling, 2 by 12 wood joists, 1-in. plywood deck, 1-in. rigid roof insulation, and a built-up roof. The floor is concrete and there is a 3 ft wide by 7 ft high glass door in the front. There are 1500 W of incandescent lighting and eight 1/2-hp electric motors. On the average there will be 10 moderately active people in the building. There is no direct ventilation. Calculate the heating load for this structure.

6.11 Determine the heating load and specify the furnace for the following residence (located in St. Louis, Missouri) with

(a) 1-in. fiberglass wall insulation and 2-in. fiberglass ceiling insulation

(b) Full wall fiberglass insulation and 4-in. fiberglass ceiling insulation

Basic Plan

Wall Construction: Face brick, 25/32-in. insulating board sheathing, 2 by 4 studs on 16-in. centers, 3/8-in. gypsum board interior

Ceiling: 2 by 6 ceiling joists, 16-in. on center, no flooring above, 3/8-in. gypsum board ceiling

Roof: Asphalt shingles on solid wood sheathing, 2 by 6 rafters, no insulation between rafters, no ceiling applied

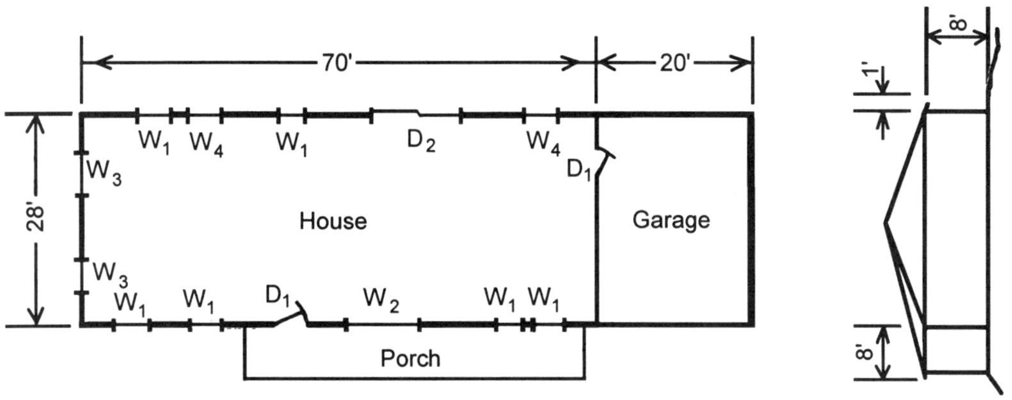

Diagram for Problem 6.11

to rafters, 1:4 pitch, 1-ft overhang on eaves, no overhang on gables

Full basement: Heated, 10-in. concrete walls, all below grade, 4-in. concrete floor over 4-in. gravel

Fireplaces: One in living room on first floor

Garage: Attached but unheated

Windows:

W1: 3 ft by 5 ft singles glazed, double-hung wood sash, weather stripped with storm window

W2: 10 ft by 5 1/2 ft picture window, double glazed, 1/2-in. airspace

W3: 5 ft by 3 ft wood sash casement, double glazed, 1/2-in. airspace

W4: 3 ft by 3 ft wood sash casement, double glazed, 1/2-in. airspace

Doors:

D1: 3 ft by 6 ft-8 in, 1 3/4-in. solid with glass storm door

D2: Sliding glass door, two section, each 3 ft by 6 ft, 8 in. double glazed, 1/2-in. airspace, aluminum frame

[Ans: (b) 50,000 Btu/h (14.6 kW)]

6.12 Determine the total conductance loss through the wall panel as shown below. The window has a wooden sill and the plate glass ($U = 1.06$) covers 85% of the window area.

[Ans: 9640 Btu/h (2.77 kW)]

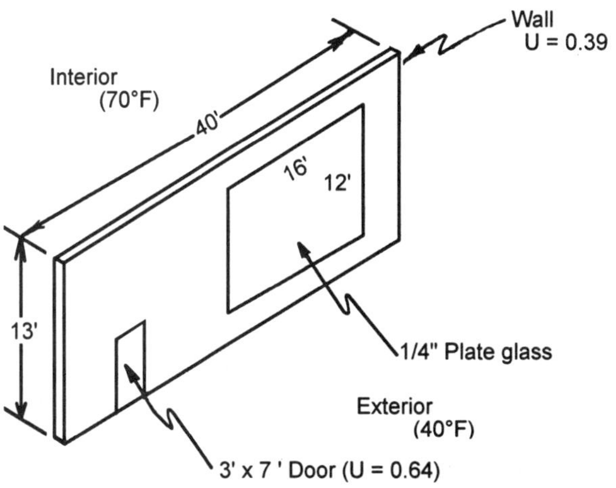

6.13 A building used as a meeting hall is 50 ft wide by 90 ft long. The walls are 10 ft high with a pitched roof rising to 20 ft at the center. Walls are lightweight concrete blocks faced with brick. Floor is a 4-in. concrete slag on 4 in. of gravel with 2-in. edge insulation. It has no ceiling. The roof has light asphalt shingles and building paper on 25/32-in. wood sheathing with 2-in. fiberglass insulation. Three windows on each of the two sides of double insulation glass with 1/4-in. airspace in metal sashes. Each window is 4 ft by 3 ft, horizontally pivoted. The doors are solid wood, 2 in. thick and each is 7 ft by 3 ft. There are double doors on front and a single door in the rear. The building is located in St. Louis, Missouri. Determine the necessary furnace size. (Prepare a table showing each heat loss separately.)

6.14 Make a dimensional takeoff for heat loss calculations of the structure shown in the diagram. Report the results in SI units.

6.15 Calculate, for design purposes, the heat losses from a room of a building as shown in the diagram, if the outside ambient is 0 °F.

[Ans: 62,820 Btu/h (18.4 kW)]

6.16 A room has three 760 mm by 1520 mm well-fitted double hung windows. For design conditions of -1°C and 21°C, calculate (a) heating load from air leakage and (b) heating load from transmission through the windows.

6.17 A residence has a total ceiling area of 1960 ft^2 and consists of 3/8-in. gypsum board on 2 in. by 6 in. ceiling joists. Six inches of fiberglass (mineral/glass wool) insulation fills the space between the joists. The effect of the joists themselves can be neglected. The pitched roof has asphalt shingles on 5/8-in. plywood with no insulation between the rafters. The ratio of roof area to ceiling area is 1:3. The attic contains louvers which remain open all year. The residence is located in Louisville, Kentucky. For winter design conditions, determine: (a) appropriate temperature difference Δt; (b) overall coefficient U; and (c) ceiling heat loss.

6.18 Estimate the heat loss from the uninsulated slab floor of a frame house having dimensions of 18 m by 38 m. The house

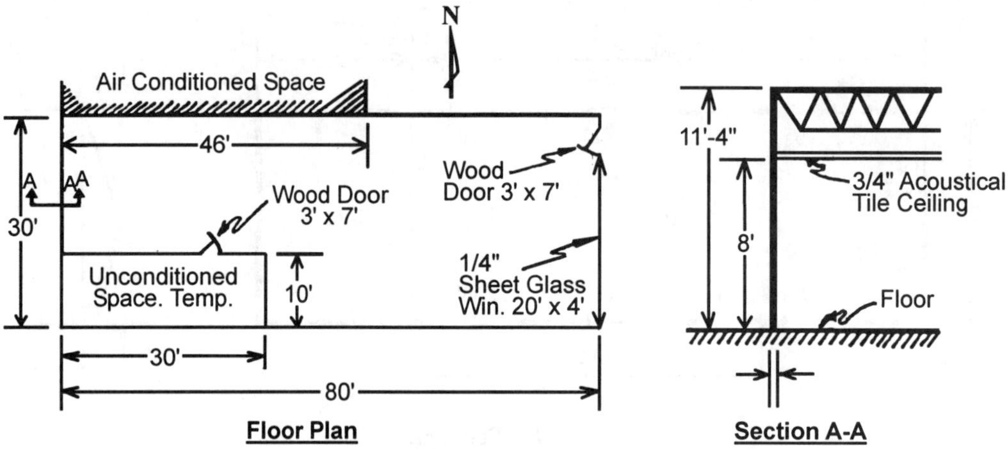

Diagram for Problem 6.14

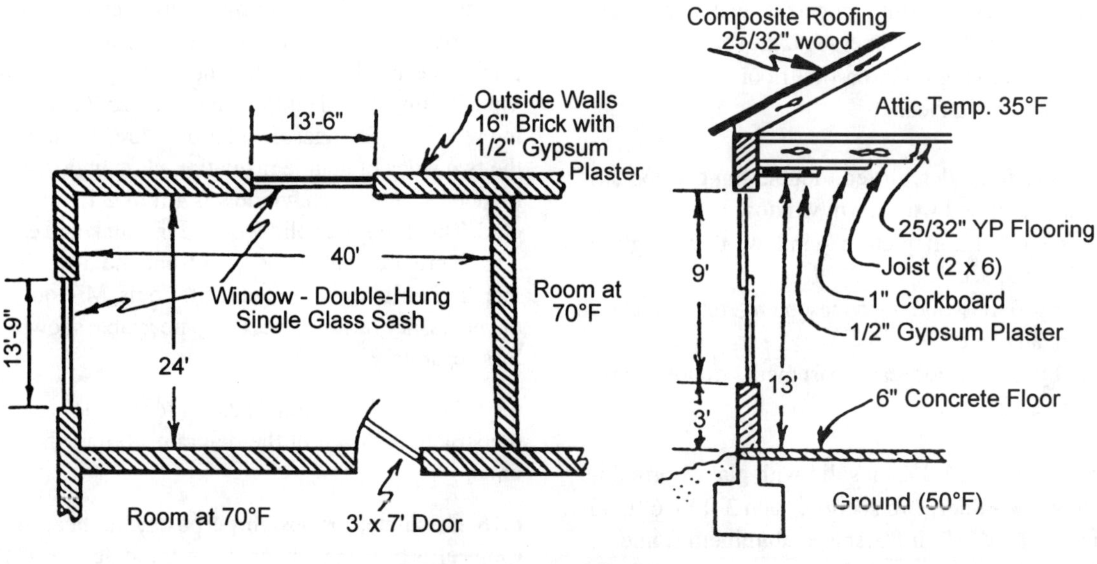

Diagram for Problem 6.15

is maintained at 22°C. Outdoor design temperature is -15°C in a region with 5400 kelvin days.

[Ans: 8.6 kW]

6.19 Repeat *Problem* 6.18 for the case where insulation (R = 0.9 $m^2 \cdot K/W$) is applied to the slab edge and extended below grade to the frost line.

6.20 To preclude attic condensation, an attic ventilation rate of 59 L/s is provided with outside air at -13°C. The roof area is 244 m^2 and U_{roof} = 2.7 $W/m^2 \cdot K$. The ceiling area is 203 m^2 and U_{clg} = 0.30 $W/m^2 \cdot K$. Inside design temperature is 22°C. Determine the ceiling heat loss W with ventilation and compare to the loss if there had been no ventilation.

6.21 Determine the design heating load for the office portion of the building described below if the factory area is 65°F in winter. Indoor and outdoor design temperatures are 70°F and 2°F, respectively. [Ans: 195,000 Btu/h]

Location: Indianapolis, Indiana
Occupancy: 20 people
East and south walls: 8-in. concrete block
U = 0.3 Btu/h·ft^2·°F
North and west walls: Concrete block
U = 0.5 Btu/h·ft^2·°F
Floor: Concrete slab
Ceiling: U = 0.5 Btu/h·ft^2·°F
Lights: 5 W/ft^2
Windows: Insulating glass, 0.25-in. gray plate outside, regular plate inside

6.22 For a residence in Roanoke, Virginia, the hip roof consisting of asphalt shingles on 1/2-in. plywood has an area of 2950 ft^2. The 2300 ft^2 ceiling consists of 3/8-in. plasterboard on 2 by 6 joists on 24-in. centers. The attic has forced ventilation at the rate of 325 cfm. Determine the attic air temperature at winter design conditions.

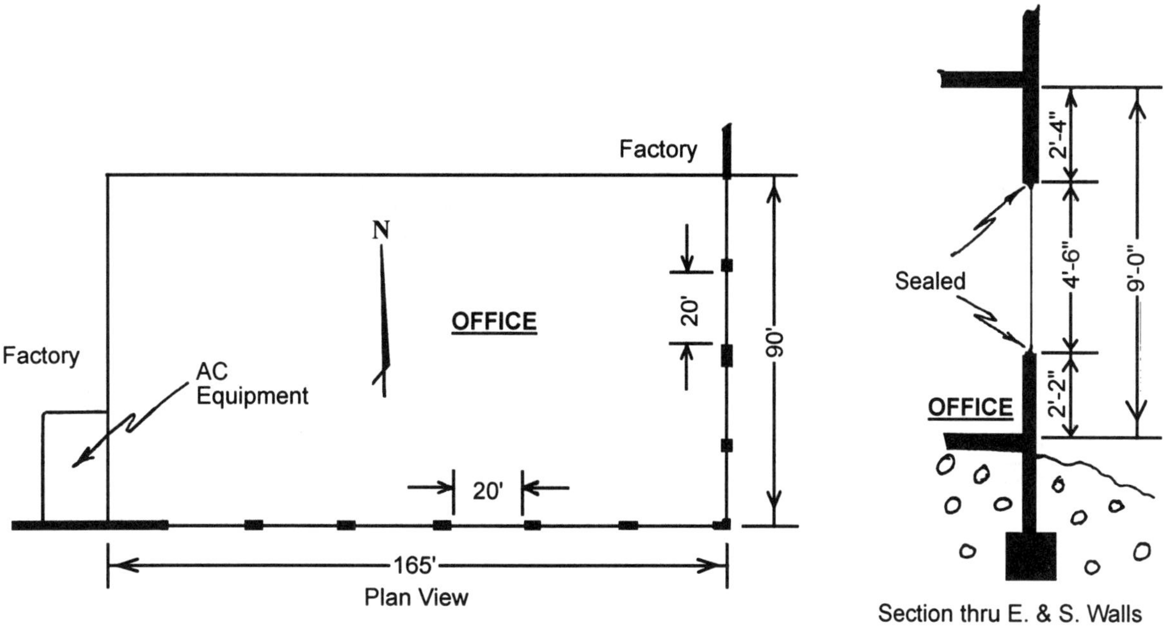

Diagram for Problem 6.21

6.23 Solve the following:

(a) A 115 ft by 10 ft high wall in Minneapolis, Minnesota, consists of face brick, a 3/4-in. air gap, 8-in. cinder aggregate concrete blocks, 1-in. organic bonded glass fiber insulation, and 4-in. clay tile interior. Determine the design heat loss through the wall in winter, Btu/h.

(b) If the wall of Part (a) is converted to 60% single glazed glass, what is the winter design heat loss through the total wall, Btu/h?

6.24 A small commercial building, 30 ft by 100 ft, located in Des Moines, Iowa, has a conditioned space which extends 9 ft below grade level. Determine the design heat loss from the uninsulated below grade concrete walls and floor.

6.25 A new gambling casino is being designed for Jefferson City, Missouri. The building is to be 150 ft by 200 ft by 10 ft. The long sides of the building face east and west and the building has glass only on the west side where there are 900 ft^2 of double glazed (1/4 in. thick glass, 1/4 in. space) windows. There are eight 1-3/4 in. thick solid wood doors on both the east and west sides, 21 ft^2 each. The exterior walls are all constructed of face brick, 2 in. of rigid organic bonded glass fiber insulation, and another of face brick on the interior. The roof is 6 in. thick lightweight aggregate concrete (120 lb/ft^3 density) with 3/8 in. built-up roofing on top and 6 in. of glass fiber insulation immediately underneath. There is a suspended ceiling of 3/4 in. acoustical tile and the floor is a 4 in. thick uninsulated concrete slab. No humidifier is planned. Determine the design heating load.

6.26 Determine the design heating load for a small commercial office building, 30 ft by 100 ft by 10 ft, to be located in Windsor Locks, Connecticut, which has an uninsulated slab on grade concrete floor. The construction consists of

Walls: 4 in. face brick, 3/4 in. plywood sheathing, 4 in. cellular glass insulation, and 1/2 in. plasterboard

Ceiling/roof: 3 in. lightweight concrete deck, built-up roofing, 2 in. of rigid, expanded rubber insulation, and a drop ceiling of 1/2 in. acoustical tiles, some 18 in. below the roof.

Windows: 45% of each wall is double pane, nonoperable, metal-framed glass (1/4 in. air gap).

Doors: Two 3 ft by 7 ft, 1.75 in. thick, solid wood doors are located in each wall.

6.4 Bibliography

Kusuda, T. and J.W. Bean. 1984. Simplified methods for determining seasonal heat loss from uninsulated slab-on-grade floors. *ASHRAE Transactions* 89(2A).

McQuiston, F.C. and J.D. Spitler. 1992. *Cooling and Heating Load Calculation Manual*, Second Edition, ASHRAE, Atlanta, GA.

Mitalas, G.P. 1983. Calculation of basement heat loss. *ASHRAE Transactions* 89(1B).

SI Tables and Figures

Table 6-2 SI Below-Grade Wall U-Factors, W/m²·K

Depth, m	Path Length Through Soil, m	Heat Loss Coefficient, W/(m²·K)[a] Un-insulated		R = 0.73 m²·K/W		R = 1.47 m²·K/W		R = 2.20 m²·K/W	
0 to 0.3	0.2	2.33	Σ[b]	0.86	3.53	0.53	Σ[b]	0.38	Σ[b]
0.3 to 0.6	0.69	1.26	3.59	0.66	1.52	0.45	0.98	0.36	0.74
0.6 to 0.9	1.18	0.88	4.47	0.53	2.05	0.38	1.36	0.30	1.04
0.9 to 1.2	1.68	0.67	5.14	0.45	2.50	0.34	1.70	0.27	1.31
1.2 to 1.5	2.15	0.54	5.68	0.39	2.89	0.30	2.00	0.25	1.56
1.5 to 1.8	2.64	0.45	6.13	0.34	3.23	0.27	2.27	0.23	1.79
1.8 to 2.1	3.13	0.39	6.52	0.30	3.53	0.25	2.52	0.21	2.00

Source: Latta and Boileau (1969).
[a]Soil conductivity was assumed to be 1.38 W/(m·K).
[b]Σ = heat loss to current depth.

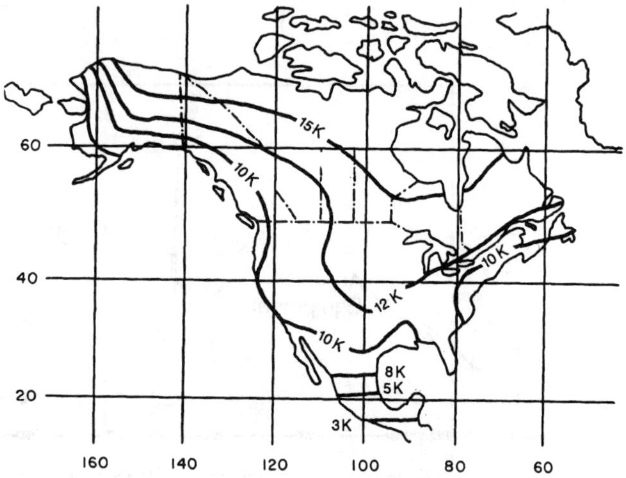

Fig. 6-1 SI Lines of Constant Amplitude of Ground Temperature

Table 6-3 SI Below-Grade Floor U-Factors, W/m²·K

Depth of Foundation Wall below Grade, m	Heat Loss Coefficient, W/(m²·K) Shortest Width of House, m 6	7.3	8.5	9.7
1.5	0.18	0.16	0.15	0.13
1.8	0.17	0.15	0.14	0.12
2.1	0.16	0.15	0.13	0.12

Note: $\Delta t = (t_a - A)$

Table 7 Heat Loss Coefficients F_2 for Slab Floors (W/K per metre of perimeter)

Construction	Insulation	Kelvin Days (18 °C Base) 4130 K·d/yr	2970 K·d/yr	1640 K·d/yr
200 mm block wall, brick facing	Uninsulated	1.07	1.17	1.24
	R = 0.95 K·m²/W from edge to footer	0.83	0.86	0.97
100 mm block wall, brick facing	Uninsulated	1.38	1.45	1.61
	R = 0.95 from edge to footer	0.81	0.85	0.93
Metal stud wall, stucco	Uninsulated	1.99	2.07	2.32
	R = 0.95 from edge to footer	0.88	0.92	1.00
Poured concrete wall with duct near perimeter[a]	Uninsulated	3.18	3.67	4.72
	R = 0.95 from edge to footer, 910 mm under floor	1.11	1.24	1.56

[a]Weighted average temperature of the heating duct was assumed at 43 °C during the heating season (outdoor air temperature less than 18 °C).

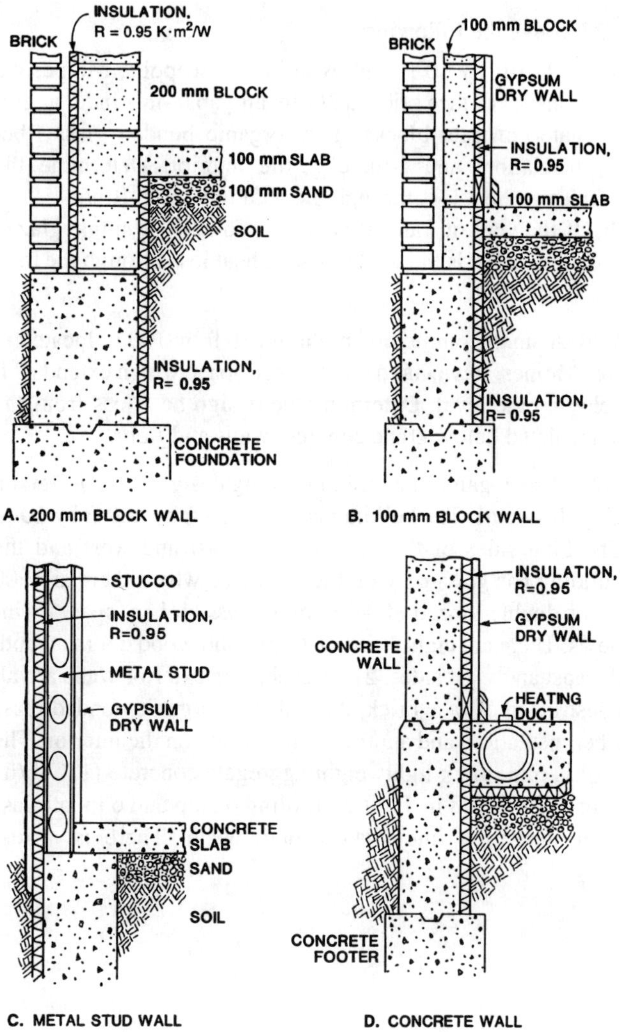

Fig. 6-2 SI Slab-on-Grade Configurations

Chapter 7

COOLING LOAD CALCULATION

This chapter discusses three methods of calculating the air-conditioning cooling load which is used for sizing cooling equipment. For residential applications, a simplified method is also presented here. A more detailed discussion of the cooling loads for buildings is given in Chapters 27 and 28 of the 1997 *ASHRAE Handbook—Fundamentals*.

7.1 Principles

The heat balance approach is a fundamental concept in calculating cooling loads. While generally cumbersome for wide-spread or routine use, this underlying concept is the basis for each of the three simplified procedures outlined for varying purposes.

The cooling calculation procedure most closely approximating the heat balance concept is the transfer function method (TFM), which was first introduced in the 1972 *ASHRAE Handbook—Fundamentals*. This computer-based procedure takes place in two steps, first establishing the heat gain from all sources and then determining the conversion of such heat gain into cooling load. Developed as an hour-by-hour calculation procedure oriented to simulate annual energy use, its normalizing characteristics make it particularly appropriate for that application.

A simplified version of the TFM, which apply to certain types of buildings for which application data are available, was presented in the 1977 *ASHRAE Handbook—Fundamentals*. This one-step procedure uses cooling load temperature differences (CLTD), solar cooling load factors (SCL), and internal cooling load factors (CLF), to calculate cooling loads as an approximation of the TFM. Where applicable, this method may be suitable for hand calculations.

An alternative simplification of the heat balance technique uses total equivalent temperature differential values and a system of time-averaging (TETD/TA) to calculate cooling loads. Also a computer-based, two-step procedure (heat gain, then cooling load), first introduced in the 1967 *ASHRAE Handbook—Fundamentals*, gives valid broad-range results to experienced users.

The variables affecting cooling load calculations are numerous, often difficult to define precisely, and always intricately interrelated. Many cooling load components vary in magnitude over a wide range during a 24-h period. Since these cyclic changes in load components are often not in phase with each other, each must be analyzed to establish the resultant maximum cooling load for a building or zone. A zoned system (a system of conditioning equipment serving several independent areas, each with its own temperature control) needs no greater total cooling load capacity than the largest hourly summary of simultaneous zone loads throughout a design day; however, it must handle the peak cooling load for each zone at its individual peak hour. At certain times of the day during the heating or intermediate seasons, some zones may need heating while others need cooling.

Calculation Accuracy. The concept of determining the cooling load for a given building must be kept in perspective. A proper cooling load calculation gives values adequate for proper performance. Variation in the heat transmission coefficient of typical building materials and composite assemblies, the differing motivations and skills of those who physically construct the building, and the manner in which the building is actually operated are some of the variables that make a numerically precise calculation impossible. While the designer uses reasonable procedures to account for these factors, the calculation can never be more than a good estimate of the actual cooling load.

Heat Flow Rates. In air-conditioning design, four related heat flow rates, each of which varies with time, must be differentiated: (1) space heat gain, (2) space cooling load, (3) space heat extraction rate, and (4) cooling coil load.

Space Heat Gain. This instantaneous rate of heat gain is the rate heat enters into and/or is generated within a space at a given instant. Heat gain is classified by (1) the mode in which it enters the space and (2) whether it is a sensible or latent gain.

Mode of Entry. The modes of heat gain may be (1) solar radiation through transparent surfaces; (2) heat conduction through exterior walls and roofs; (3) heat conduction through interior partitions, ceilings, and floors; (4) heat generated within the space by occupants, lights, and appliances; (5) energy transfer as a result of ventilation and infiltration of outdoor air; or (6) miscellaneous heat gains.

Sensible or Latent Heat. Sensible heat gain is directly added to the conditioned space by conduction, convection, and/or radiation. Latent heat gain occurs when moisture is added to the space (e.g., from vapor emitted by occupants and equipment). To maintain a constant humidity ratio, water vapor must condense on the cooling apparatus at a rate equal to its rate of addition into the space. The amount of energy required to offset the latent heat gain essentially equals the product of the rate of condensation and the latent heat of condensation. In selecting cooling apparatus, it is necessary to distinguish between sensible and latent heat gain. Every cooling apparatus has a maximum latent heat removal capacity for particular operating conditions.

Space Cooling Load. This is the rate at which heat must be removed from the space to maintain a constant space air temperature. The sum of all space instantaneous heat gains at any given time does not necessarily (or even frequently) equal the cooling load for the space at that same time.

Radiant Heat Gain. Space heat gain by radiation is not immediately converted into cooling load. Radiant energy must first be absorbed by the surfaces that enclose the space (walls, floor, and ceiling) and the objects in the space (furniture, etc.). As soon as these surfaces and objects become warmer than the space air, some of their heat is transferred in the air space by convection. The composite heat storage capacity of these surfaces and objects determines the rate at which their respective surface temperatures increase for a given radiant input, and thus governs the relationship between the radiant portion of heat gain and its corresponding part of the space cooling load (Figure 7-1). The thermal storage effect is critically important in differentiating between instantaneous heat gain for a given space and its cooling load for that moment. Predicting the nature and magnitude of this elusive phenomenon in order to estimate a realistic cooling load for a particular combination of circumstances has long been a subject of major interest to design engineers.

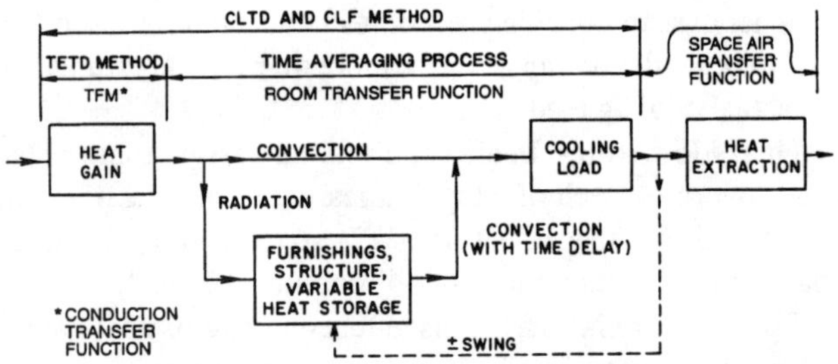

Fig. 7-1 Origin of Difference Between Magnitude of Instantaneous Heat Gain and Instantaneous Cooling Load

Space Heat Extraction Rate. The rate at which heat is removed from the conditioned space equals the space cooling load only to the degree that room air temperature is held constant. In conjunction with intermittent operation of the cooling equipment, the control system characteristics usually permit a minor cyclic variation or swing in room temperature. Therefore, a proper simulation of the control system gives a more realistic value of energy removal over a fixed period than using the values of the space cooling load. This concept is primarily important for estimating energy use over time; however, it is not needed to calculate design peak cooling load for equipment selection.

Cooling Coil Load. The rate at which energy is removed at the cooling coil that serves one or more conditioned spaces equals the sum of the instantaneous space cooling loads (or space heat extraction rate if it is assumed that the space temperature does not vary) for all the spaces served by the coil, plus any external loads. Such external loads include heat gain by the distribution system between the individual spaces and the cooling equipment, and outdoor air heat and moisture introduced into the distribution system through the cooling equipment.

7.1.1 Heat Balance Fundamentals

The calculation of cooling load for a space involves calculating a surface-by-surface conductive, convective, and radiative heat balance for each room surface and a convective heat balance for the room air. Sometimes called "the exact solution," these principles form the foundation for all other methods described in this chapter.

To calculate space cooling load directly by heat balance procedures requires a laborious solution of energy balance equations involving the space air, surrounding walls and windows, infiltration and ventilation air, and internal energy sources. To demonstrate the calculation principle, consider a sample room enclosed by four walls, a ceiling, and a floor, with infiltration air and normal internal energy sources. The energy exchange at each inside surface at a given time can be calculated from the following equation:

$$q_{i,\theta} = \left[h_{ci}(t_{a,\theta} - t_{i,\theta}) + \sum_{j=1 \neq i}^{m} g_{ij}(t_{j,\theta} - t_{i,\theta}) \right] A_i + RS_{i,\theta} + RL_{i,\theta} + RE_{i,\theta} \qquad (7\text{-}1)$$

$$\text{for } i = 1, 2, 3, 4, 5, 6$$

where

m = number of surfaces in room (6 in this case)

$q_{i,\theta}$ = rate of heat conducted into surface i at inside surface at time θ

A_i = area of surface i

h_{ci} = convective heat transfer coefficient at interior surface i

g_{ij} = a radiation heat transfer factor between interior surface i and interior surface j

$t_{a,\theta}$ = inside air temperature at time θ

$t_{i,\theta}$ = average temperature of interior surface i at time θ

$RS_{i,\theta}$ = rate of solar energy coming through windows and absorbed by surface i at time θ

$RL_{i,\theta}$ = rate of heat radiated from lights and absorbed by surface i at time θ

$RE_{i,\theta}$ = rate of heat radiated from equipment and occupants and absorbed by surface i at time θ

Conduction Transfer Functions. The equations governing conduction within the six surfaces cannot be solved independently of Equation (7-1), since the energy exchanges occurring within the room affect the inside surface conditions, in turn affecting the internal conduction. Consequently, the six formulations of Equation (7-1) must be solved simultaneously with the governing equations of conduction within the six surfaces in order to calculate the space cooling load. Typically, these equations are formulated as conduction transfer functions in the form

$$q_{in,\theta} = \sum_{m=1}^{M} Y_{k,m} t_{o,\theta-m+1} - \sum_{m=1}^{M} Z_{k,m} t_{o,\theta-m+1} + \sum_{m=1}^{M} F_m q_{in,\theta-m} \quad (7\text{-}2)$$

where

- q = rate of heat conducted into a specific surface at a specific hour
- in = inside surface subscript
- k = order of CTF
- m = time index variable
- M = number of nonzero CTF values
- o = outside surface subscript
- t = temperature
- θ = time
- Y = cross CTF values
- Z = interior CTF values
- F_m = flux history coefficients

Space Air Energy Balance. Note that the interior surface temperature, $t_{i,\theta}$ in Equation (7-1) and $t_{in,\theta}$ in Equation (7-2), requires simultaneous solution. In addition, Equation (7-3), which represents an energy balance on the space air must also be solved simultaneously.

$$Q_{L,\theta} = \left[\sum_{i=1}^{6} h_{ci}(t_{i,\theta} - t_{a,\theta})\right] A_i + \rho C V_{L,\theta}(t_{o,\theta} - t_{a,\theta}) + \rho C V_{v,\theta}(t_{v,\theta} - t_{a,\theta}) + RS_{a,\theta} + RL_{a,\theta} + RE_{a,\theta} \quad (7\text{-}3)$$

where

- ρ = air density
- C = air specific heat
- $V_{L,\theta}$ = volume flow rate of outdoor air infiltrating into room at time θ
- $t_{o,\theta}$ = outdoor air temperature at time θ
- $V_{v,\theta}$ = volume rate of flow of ventilation air at time θ
- $t_{v,\theta}$ = ventilation air temperature at time θ
- $RS_{a,\theta}$ = rate of solar heat coming through windows and convected into room air at time θ
- $RL_{a,\theta}$ = rate of heat from lights convected into room air at time θ
- $RE_{a,\theta}$ = rate of heat from equipment and occupants and convected into room air at time θ

Note that the space air temperature is allowed to float. By fixing the space air temperature, the cooling load need not be determined simultaneously.

This rigorous approach to calculating space cooling load is impractical without the speed at which some computations can be done by modern digital computers. Computer programs that calculate instantaneous space cooling loads in this exact manner are primarily oriented to energy use calculations over extended periods (Mitalas and Stephenson 1967, Buchberg 1958).

The transfer function concept is a simplification to the strict heat balance calculation procedure. In the transfer function concept, Mitalas and Stephenson (1967) used room thermal response factors. In their procedure, room surface temperatures and cooling load were first calculated by the rigorous method just described, for several typical constructions representing offices, schools, and dwellings of heavy, medium, and light construction. In these calculations, components such as solar heat gain, conduction heat gain, or heat gain from the lighting, equipment, and occupants were simulated by pulses of unit strength. The transfer functions were then calculated as numerical constants representing the cooling load corresponding to the input excitation pulses. Once these transfer functions were determined for typical constructions they were assumed independent of input pulses, thus permitting cooling loads to be determined without the more rigorous calculation. Instead, the calculation requires simple multiplication of the transfer functions by a time-series representation of heat gain and subsequent summation of these products, which can be carried out on a small computer. The same transfer function concept can be applied to calculating heat gain components themselves, as explained later.

7.1.2 Total Equivalent Temperature Differential Method

In the total equivalent temperature differential (TETD) method, the response factor technique was used with a number of representative wall and roof assemblies from which data were derived to calculate TETD values as functions of sol-air temperature and maintained room temperature. Various components of space heat gain are calculated using associated TETD values, and the results are added to internal heat gain elements to get an instantaneous total rate of space heat gain. This gain is converted to an instantaneous space cooling load by the time-averaging (TA) technique of averaging the radiant portions of the heat gain load components for the current hour with related values from an appropriate period of immediately preceding hours. This technique provides a rational means to deal quantitatively with the thermal storage phenomenon, but it is best solved by computer because of its complexity.

7.1.3 Transfer Function Method

Although similar in principle to TETD/TA, the transfer function method (TFM) (Mitalas 1972) applies a series of weighting factors, or conduction transfer function (CTF) coefficients to the various exterior opaque surfaces and to differences between sol-air temperature and inside space temperature to determine heat gain with appropriate reflection of thermal inertia of such surfaces. Solar heat gain through glass and various forms of internal heat gain are calculated directly for the load hour of interest. The TFM next applies a second series of weighting factors, or coefficients of room transfer functions (RTF), to heat gain and cooling load values from all load elements having radiant components, to account for the thermal storage effect in converting heat gain to cooling load. Both evaluation series consider data from several previous hours as well as the current hour. RTF coefficients relate specifically to the spatial geometry, configuration, mass, and other characteristics of the space so as to reflect weighted variations in thermal storage effect on a time basis rather than a straight-line average.

Transfer Functions. These coefficients relate an output function at a given time to the value of one or more driving functions at a given time and at a set period immediately preceding. The CTF described in this chapter is no different from the thermal response factor used for calculating wall or roof heat conduction, while the RTF is the weighting factor for obtaining cooling load components (ASHRAE 1975). Chapter 28 of the 1997 *ASHRAE Handbook—Fundamentals* lists reports of various experimental work that has validated the predictive accuracy of the TFM. While the TFM is scientifically appropriate and technically sound for a specific cooling load analysis, its computational complexity requires computer use for effective application in a commercial design environment.

7.1.4 CLTD/SCL/CLF Method

ASHRAE has sponsored research to compare the TETD/TA and the TFM (Rudoy and Duran 1975). As part of this work, data obtained by using the TFM on a group of applications considered representative were then used to generate cooling load temperature differential (CLTD) data, for direct one-step calculation of cooling load from conduction heat gain through sunlit walls and roofs and conduction through glass exposures. Cooling load factors (CLF) for similar one-step calculation of solar load through glass and for loads from internal sources were also developed. More recent research (McQuiston 1992) developed an improved factor for solar load through glass, the solar cooling load (SCL) factor, which allows additional influencing parameters to be considered for greater accuracy. CLTDs, SCLs, and CLFs all include the effect of (1) time lag in conductive heat gain through opaque exterior surfaces and (2) time delay by thermal storage in converting radiant heat gain to cooling load. This simplification allows cooling loads to be calculated manually; thus, when data are available and are appropriately used, the results are consistent with those from the TFM, thus making the method popular for instruction.

7.1.5 Application Experience

The CLTD and CLF tables published in previous editions of the Fundamentals volume and in the original Cooling and Heating Load Calculation Manual (ASHRAE 1979) are normalized data, based on applications of the original TFM data presented in the 1972 Fundamentals volume. Subsequent studies investigating the effects of 1981 to 1985 RTF data indicated results generally less conservative than those computed with the 1972 data. More recent research, however, suggests otherwise (McQuiston 1992), and the revised values for 1993, including the new SCLs, are currently considered realistic for design load purposes.

CLTD Data. The originally developed CLTD data were so voluminous that they were first limited to 13 representative flat roof assemblies (with and without ceilings, for 26 total cases) and 7 wall groups (into which 41 different wall assemblies can be categorized). Twenty-four hourly CLTD values were tabulated for each of the 26 roof cases and each of the 7 wall groups, broken down for walls into 8 primary orientations. Adjustments were then required for specific north latitude and month of calculation. Reliability of adjustments was reasonably consistent during summer months but became much less realistic for early and late hours during traditionally noncooling load months.

Solar Heat Gain Data. Solar heat gain through glass required similar data compression to present a corresponding range of conditions. Tables of maximum solar heat gain factors (SHGF) were listed for every 4° of north latitude between 0 and 64°, for each month and by 16 compass directions and horizontal. Cooling load factors (CLF), decimal multipliers for SHGF data, were tabulated for unshaded glass in spaces having carpeted or uncarpeted floors and for inside-shaded glass with any room construction. Unshaded CLFs were presented for each of 24 h by 8 compass directions plus horizontal, further categorized by light, medium, or heavy room construction. Inside-shaded CLFs disregarded construction mass but included 16 orientations plus horizontal. The product of the selected CLTD and CLF values represented cooling load per unit area as a single process. CLF values published in the Chapter 28 of the 1997 *ASHRAE Handbook—Fundamentals* were derived for the period May through September as normally the hottest months for load calculation purposes. As with CLTDs, the reliability of CLF data deteriorated rapidly for applications during early and late hours of months considered "noncooling load" periods.

ASHRAE Research. For some space geometries and building constructions, the tabulated CLTD and CLF data published through 1989 were found also to be too restrictive or limited. The weighting factors used to generate these data, based on representative spaces in schools, offices, and dwellings at the time of the original research, did not reflect current design and construction practices. ASHRAE research investigated the sensitivity of the weighting factors to variations in space construction, size, exposure, and related conditions to update the tabular data. However, the investigators discovered that the range and amplitude of this sensitivity was much broader than previously thought, rendering even more impractical the generation of enough tabular material to cover the majority of normal applications. Accordingly, two significant changes in direction have occurred:

1. The section describing the CLTD/CLF in the 1985 and 1989 *ASHRAE Handbook—Fundamentals* recommended caution in application of this procedure for general practice, and this cautionary notice was also added as an insert to the Cooling and Heating Load Calculation Manual (McQuiston and Spitler 1992).
2. The system itself was modified for more specific tabulation of data, abandoning the maximum SHGF concept and incorporating solar cooling load (SCL) factors for estimating cooling load from glass.

Recent research supported by ASHRAE has been used to update the *Cooling and Heating Load Calculation Manual.* Information from earlier research was used to revise the original factors by incorporating additional parameters, including separating solar load through glass from the CLF category and creating more appropriate SCL factors for that component. Still faced with too much tabular data, information was tabulated only for limited use and representative examples, but it was accompanied by instructions for customizing similar data for specific application; a microcomputer database was also provided to facilitate such calculations. Certain limitations resulting from normalization of data remain, for which anticipated error ranges are listed to aid in evaluating results. The section in this chapter describing the CLTD/SCL/CLF method has incorporated this latest research, but it does not provide the microcomputer program.

TETD/TA Method. Prior to introduction of the CLTD/CLF, most users had turned to computer-based versions of the time-averaging technique, proven successful and practical in ten years of heavy use. Most users, however, recognized the subjectivity of determining the relative percentages of radiant heat in the various heat gain components and selecting the number of hours over which to average such loads-both of which must rely on the individual experience of the user rather than on research or support in the scientific literature. Harris and McQuiston (1988) developed decrement factors and time lag values. In this chapter, these factors have been keyed to typical walls and roofs. All other tabular data pertaining to this method has been deleted, so that since 1989, information has been confined to basic algorithms intended for continued computer applications.

Primary Emphasis of Future Research. Because of the increasing availability and power of microcomputers, emphasis has refocused on the more specific and flexible transfer function method as the fundamental computational technique. Future research will concentrate on refining the weighting factors and broadening the range of circumstances to which the TFM can be applied.

Alternative Procedures. The CLTD/SCL/CLF and TETD/TA procedures, tables, and related data will continue to be appropriate and dependable when applied within the limitations identified. Users will likely incorporate newer relationships developed for TFM usage in the development of specific CLTD/SCL/CLF or TETD/TA tabular data, customized for their specialized projects.

The CLTD/SCL/CLF method is the only method presented in detail in this chapter. If the reader is interested in details of using the other cooling/heating methods, Chapter 28 of the 1997 *ASHRAE Handbook—Fundamentals* should be consulted.

7.2 Initial Design Considerations

To calculate a space cooling load, detailed building design information and weather data at selected design conditions are required. Generally, the following steps should be followed:

Building Characteristics. Characteristics of the building, such as building materials, component size, external surface colors, and shape, can usually be obtained from building plans and specifications.

Configuration. Determine building location, orientation, and external shading from plans and specifications. Shading from adjacent buildings can be determined by a site plan or by visiting the proposed site. The probable permanence of shading should be evaluated before it is included in the calculations. Possible high ground-reflected solar radiation from adjacent water, sand, parking lots, or solar load from adjacent reflective buildings should not be overlooked.

Outdoor Design Conditions. Obtain appropriate weather data and select outdoor design conditions. Weather data can be obtained from local weather stations or (in the United States) from the National Climatic Data Center (NCDC), Asheville, North Carolina 28801. (See Chapter 4 for outdoor design conditions for a large number of weather stations.) The designer should exercise judgment to ensure that results are consistent with expectations. Prevailing wind velocity and the relationship of a project site to a selected weather station should also be considered.

Indoor Design Conditions. Select indoor design conditions such as indoor dry-bulb temperature, indoor wet-bulb temperature, and ventilation rate. Include permissible variations and control limits.

Operating Schedules. Obtain a proposed schedule of lighting, occupants, internal equipment, appliances, and processes that contribute to the internal thermal load. Determine the probability that the cooling equipment will be operated continuously or shut off during unoccupied periods (e.g., nights and/or weekends).

Date and Time. Select the time of day and month to do the cooling load calculation. Frequently, several times of day and several months are required. The particular day and month are often dictated by peak solar conditions. For southern exposures in latitudes north of 32°, the peak space cooling load usually occurs in December or January. To calculate a space cooling load under these conditions, the warmest temperature for the winter months must be known. These data can be found in the NCDC's *Climatic Atlas of the United States.*

Additional Considerations. The proper design and sizing of all-air or air-and-water central air-conditioning systems require more than calculation of the cooling load in the space to be conditioned. The type of air-conditioning system, fan energy, fan location, duct heat loss and gain, duct leakage, heat-extraction lighting systems, and type of return air system all affect system load and component sizing. Adequate system design and component sizing require that system performance be analyzed as a series of psychrometric processes.

7.3 Heat Gain Calculation Concepts

The primary weather-related variable influencing a building's cooling load is solar radiation. The effect of solar radiation is more pronounced and immediate on exposed, nonopaque surfaces. The calculation of solar heat gain and conductive heat transfer through various glazing materials and associated mounting frames is discussed in Chapter 29 of the 1997 *ASHRAE Handbook—Fundamentals.*

7.3.1 Heat Gain Through Exterior Walls and Roofs

Heat gain through exterior opaque surfaces is derived in the same way as for fenestration areas. It differs primarily as a function of the mass and nature of wall or roof construction, since those elements affect the rate of conductive transfer through the composite assembly to the interior surface.

Sol-Air Temperature. This temperature of the outdoor air that, in the absence of all radiation changes, gives the same rate of heat entry into the surface as would the combination of incident solar radiation, radiant energy exchange with the sky and other outdoor surroundings, and convective heat exchange with outdoor air.

Heat Gain Through Exterior Surfaces. The heat balance at a sunlit surface gives the heat flux into the surface q/A in Btu/h·ft^2 (W/m^2), as

$$q/A = \alpha I_t + h_o(t_o - t_s) - \varepsilon\Delta R \tag{7-4}$$

where

α = absorptance of surface for solar radiation

I_t = total solar radiation incident on surface, Btu/h·ft^2 (W/m^2)

h_o = coefficient of heat transfer by long-wave radiation and convection at outer surface, Btu/h·ft^2·°F (W/m^2·K)

t_o = outdoor air temperature, °F (°C)

t_s = surface temperature, °F (°C)

ε = hemispherical emittance of surface

ΔR = difference between long-wave radiation incident on surface from sky and surroundings and radiation emitted by blackbody at outdoor air temperature, Btu/h·ft^2 (W/m^2)

Assuming the rate of heat transfer can be expressed in terms of the sol-air temperature t_e:

$$q/A = h_o(t_e - t_s) \tag{7-5}$$

From Equations (7-4) and (7-5):

$$t_e = t_o + \alpha I_t/h_o - \varepsilon\Delta R/h_o \tag{7-6}$$

For horizontal surfaces that receive long-wave radiation from the sky only, an appropriate value of ΔR is about 20 Btu/h·ft^2, so if $\varepsilon = 1$ and $h_o = 3.0$ Btu/h·ft^2·°F, the long-wave correction term is about −7°F.

Because vertical surfaces receive long-wave radiation from the ground and surrounding buildings, as well as from the sky, accurate ΔR values are difficult to determine. When solar radiation intensity is high, surfaces of terrestrial objects usually have a higher temperature than the outdoor air; thus, their long-wave radiation compensates to some extent for the sky's low emittance. Therefore, it is assumed that $\Delta R = 0$ for vertical surfaces.

The sol-air temperatures in Table 7-1 are calculated based on $\varepsilon\Delta R/h_o = -7$°F for horizontal surfaces and 0°F for vertical surfaces; total solar intensity values for the calculation were the same as those used to evaluate the solar heat gain factors (SHGF) for July 21 at 40°N latitude (Chapter 29 of the 1997 *ASHRAE Handbook—Fundamentals*). These values of I_t incorporate diffuse radiation from a clear sky and ground reflection, but make no allowance for reflection from adjacent walls.

Surface Colors. Sol-air temperature values are given for two values of the parameter α/h_o (Table 7-1); 0.15 is appropriate for a light-colored surface, while 0.30 is the usual maximum value for this parameter (i.e., for a darkcolored surface, or any surface for which the permanent lightness cannot be reliably anticipated).

Air Temperature Cycle. The air temperature cycle used to calculate sol-air temperatures is given in Column 2, Table 7-1. Sol-air temperatures can be adjusted to any other air temperature cycle by adding or subtracting the difference between the desired air temperature and the air temperature value given in Column 2.

Adjustments. Sol-air temperature cycles can be estimated for other dates and latitudes by using the data in Tables 15 through 21, Chapter 29 of the 1997 *ASHRAE Handbook—Fundamentals*. For any of the times, dates, and wall orientations listed in these tables, the value of It is approximately 1.15. However, the 1.15 factor only accounts for the solar energy excluded by a single sheet of ordinary window glass. For surfaces with other orientations or with slope angles above 50° (particularly critical for southern exposures), the solar intensity can be found by the method outlined in Chapter 29 of the 1997 *ASHRAE Handbook—Fundamentals*.

Average Sol-Air Temperature. Average daily sol-air temperature tea can be calculated for any situation covered by Tables 15 through 21, Chapter 29 in the 1997 *ASHRAE Handbook—Fundamentals*:

$$t_{ea} = t_{oa} + \frac{\alpha}{h_o}\left(\frac{I_{DT}}{24}\right) - \frac{\varepsilon\Delta R}{h_o} \tag{7-7}$$

where I_{DT} is the sum of two appropriate half-day totals of solar heat gain in Btu/h·ft^2. For example, the average sol-air temperature for a wall facing southeast at 40°N latitude on August 21 would be

$$t_{ea} = t_{oa} + \frac{\alpha}{h_o}\left[\frac{1.15(205 + 956)}{24}\right] \tag{7-8}$$

The daily solar heat gain of double-strength sheet glass is (205 + 956) Btu/ft^2 in a southeast facade at this latitude and date (Table 18, Chapter 29 of the 1997 *ASHRAE Handbook—Fundamentals*), and $\varepsilon\Delta R/h_o$ is assumed to be zero for this vertical surface.

Table 7-1 Sol-Air Temperature (t_e) for July 21, 40 °N Latitude

$$t_e = t_o + \alpha I_t/h_o - \varepsilon \Delta R/h_o$$

Time	Air Temp. t_o, °F	Light Colored Surface, $\alpha/h_o = 0.15$ N	NE	E	SE	S	SW	W	NW	HOR
1	76	76	76	76	76	76	76	76	76	69
2	76	76	76	76	76	76	76	76	76	69
3	75	75	75	75	75	75	75	75	75	68
4	74	74	74	74	74	74	74	74	74	67
5	74	74	74	74	74	74	74	74	74	67
6	74	80	93	95	84	76	76	76	76	72
7	75	80	99	106	94	78	78	78	78	81
8	77	81	99	109	101	82	81	81	81	92
9	80	85	96	109	106	88	85	85	85	102
10	83	88	91	105	107	95	88	88	88	111
11	87	93	93	99	106	102	93	93	93	118
12	90	96	96	96	102	106	102	96	96	122
13	93	99	99	99	99	108	112	105	99	124
14	94	99	99	99	99	106	118	116	102	122
15	95	100	100	100	100	103	121	124	111	117
16	94	98	98	98	98	99	118	126	116	109
17	93	98	96	96	96	96	112	124	117	99
18	91	97	93	93	93	93	101	112	110	89
19	87	87	87	87	87	87	87	87	87	80
20	85	85	85	85	85	85	85	85	85	78
21	83	83	83	83	83	83	83	83	83	76
22	81	81	81	81	81	81	81	81	81	74
23	79	79	79	79	79	79	79	79	79	72
24	77	77	77	77	77	77	77	77	77	70
Avg.	**83**	**86**	**88**	**90**	**90**	**87**	**90**	**90**	**88**	**90**

Time	Air Temp. t_o, °F	Dark Colored Surface, $\alpha/h_o = 0.30$ N	NE	E	SE	S	SW	W	NW	HOR
1	76	76	76	76	76	76	76	76	76	69
2	76	76	76	76	76	76	76	76	76	69
3	75	75	75	75	75	75	75	75	75	68
4	74	74	74	74	74	74	74	74	74	67
5	74	74	75	75	74	74	74	74	74	67
6	74	85	112	115	94	77	77	77	77	77
7	75	84	124	136	113	81	81	81	81	94
8	77	85	121	142	125	86	85	85	85	114
9	80	90	112	138	131	96	89	89	89	131
10	83	94	100	127	131	107	94	94	94	145
11	87	98	99	111	125	118	100	98	98	156
12	90	101	101	102	114	123	114	102	101	162
13	93	104	104	104	106	124	131	117	105	162
14	94	105	105	105	105	118	142	138	111	156
15	95	105	104	104	104	111	146	153	127	146
16	94	102	102	102	102	103	142	159	138	131
17	93	102	99	99	99	99	131	154	142	112
18	91	102	94	94	94	94	111	132	129	94
19	87	87	87	87	87	87	87	88	88	80
20	85	85	85	85	85	85	85	85	85	78
21	83	83	83	83	83	83	83	83	83	76
22	81	81	81	81	81	81	81	81	81	74
23	79	79	79	79	79	79	79	79	79	72
24	77	77	77	77	77	77	77	77	77	70
Avg.	**83**	**89**	**94**	**99**	**97**	**93**	**97**	**99**	**94**	**104**

Note: Sol-air temperatures are calculated based on $\varepsilon \Delta R/h_o$ = 7°F for horizontal surfaces and 0°F for vertical surfaces.

Table 7-2 Percentage of Daily Range

Time, h	%	Time, h	%	Time, h	%
1	87	9	71	17	10
2	92	10	56	18	21
3	96	11	39	19	34
4	99	12	23	20	47
5	100	13	11	21	58
6	98	14	3	22	68
7	93	15	0	23	76
8	84	16	3	24	82

Hourly Air Temperatures. The hourly air temperatures in Column 2, Table 7-1 are for a location with a design temperature of 95 °F and a range of 21 °F. To compute corresponding temperatures for other locations, select a suitable design temperature and note the outdoor daily range.

For each hour, take the percentage of the daily range indicated in Table 7-2 and subtract from the design temperature.

7.3.2 Heat Gain Through Fenestration

Fenestration is the term used here to designate any light-transmitting opening in a building wall or roof. The opening may be glazed with single or multiple sheet, plate or float glass, pattern glass, plastic panels, or glass block. Interior or exterior shading devices are usually employed, and some glazing systems incorporate integral sun control devices.

Calculating heat transfer through fenestration is explained in detail in Chapter 29 of the 1997 *ASHRAE Handbook—Fundamentals* while Chapter 28 presents only the portion of this operation required in the calculation of space cooling load due to heat transfer through fenestration.

Heat admission or loss through fenestration areas is affected by many factors, including

1. Solar radiation intensity and incident angle
2. Outdoor-indoor temperature difference
3. Velocity and direction of airflow across the exterior and interior fenestration surfaces
4. Low-temperature radiation exchange between the surfaces of the fenestration and the surroundings
5. Exterior and/or interior shading

When solar radiation strikes an unshaded window (Figure 7-2), part of the radiant energy (8% for uncoated clear glass) is reflected back outdoors, part is absorbed within the glass (from 5 to 50%, depending upon the composition and thickness of the glass), and the remainder is transmitted directly indoors to become part of the cooling load. The solar heat gain is the sum of the transmitted radiation and the portion of the absorbed radiation that flows inward.

The total instantaneous rate of heat gain through a glazing material can be obtained from the heat balance between a unit area of fenestration and its thermal environment:

[Total heat transmission through glass] = [Heat flow due to outdoor-indoor temp. difference] + [Inward flow of absorbed solar radiation] + [Radiation transmiitted through glass]

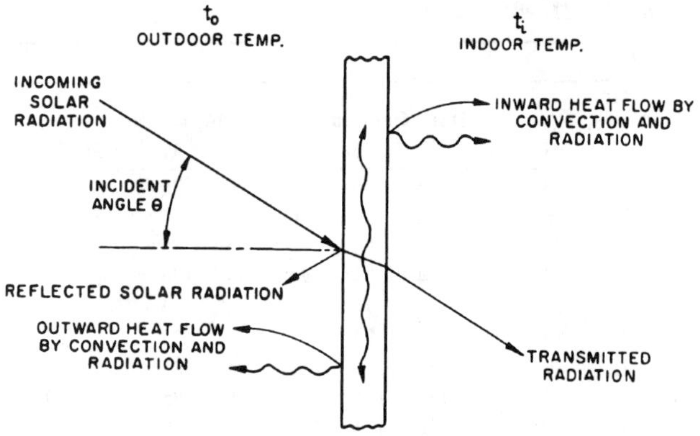

Fig. 7-2 Instantaneous Heat Balance for Sunlit Glazing Material

In this equation, the last two terms on the right are present only when the fenestration is irradiated and are therefore related to the incident radiation. The first term occurs whether or not the sun is shining, since it represents the heat flow through fenestration by thermal conduction.

Combining the last two terms:

Total heat transmission through glass	=	Conduction heat gain	+	Solar heat gain

In this way, heat gain is divided into two components: (1) the conduction heat gain (or loss), due to differences in outdoor and indoor air temperature, and (2) the solar heat gain (SHG), due to transmitted and absorbed solar energy. The total load through fenestration is the sum of the load due to conductive heat gain and the load due to solar heat gain.

Whether or not sunlight is present, heat flows through fenestration by thermal conduction, as expressed by:

Conduction heat flow	=	Overall coefficient of heat transfer	×	Outdoor-indoor temperature difference

or

$$q/A = U(t_o - t_i) \tag{7-9}$$

where

q/A = instantaneous rate of heat transfer through fenestration
U = overall coefficient of heat transfer for the glazing
t_o = outside air temperature
ti = inside air temperature

Values of the overall coefficient of heat transfer for a number of widely used fenestrations are in Chapter 29 of the 1997 *ASHRAE Handbook—Fundamentals* (see Chapter 5).

Heat gain due to transmitted and absorbed solar energy or solar heat gain (SHG) is present in cooling load calculations only when fenestration is irradiated. The SHG factor values used to estimate solar heat gain are given in Tables 15 through 21 in Chapter 29 of the 1997 *ASHRAE Handbook—Fundamentals* for double-strength glass with transmittance of 0.87, reflectance of 0.08, and 0.05 absorptance.

Table 7-3 presents SHG factors (SHGF) for 40°N latitude.

The *instantaneous rate* of heat gain through fenestrations is given by

$$q/A = [\text{SHGF} + u(t_o - t_i)]$$

However this "instantaneous" heat rate will not be the cooling requirement at that instant due to thermal storage in the space.

The solar heat gain factor for each exposure is determined by the latitude, date, and time of day. The outdoor air temperature is a matter of local climatology (Table 7-2).

To account for the different types of fenestration and shading devices used, the shading coefficient SC, which relates the solar heat gain through a glazing system under a specific set of conditions to the solar heat gain through the reference glazing material under the same conditions, is defined as follows:

$$\text{SC} = \frac{\text{Solar heat gain of actual fenestration}}{\text{Solar heat gain of standard double-strength glass}}$$

Most fenestration has some type of internal shading to provide privacy and aesthetic effects, as well as to give varying degrees of sun control. The SC values applicable to typical internal shading devices are given in Tables 7-4 through 7-11 for various fenestrations and shading device combinations.

The instantaneous heat rate through the fenestration with shading then becomes

$$q/A = [\text{SHGF(SC)} + u(t_o - t_i)]$$

The selection of the value for SC is based on the *combination* of the fenestration and the shading device. Only a single value is used for SC in the above equation when shading is present.

The effectiveness of any internal shading device depends on its ability to reflect incoming solar radiation back through the fenestration before it can be absorbed and converted into heat within the building.

In general, external shading devices that eliminate all direct radiation and still permit free air movement at the outer fenestration surface reduce solar heat gain by as much as 80%. Such devices include overhangs, wings, screen walls, horizontal and vertical louvers, and vented awnings.

During certain seasons of the year and for some exposures, horizontal projections can result in considerable reductions in solar heat gain by providing shade. This is particularly applicable to south, southeast, and southwest exposures during the late spring, summer, and early fall. On east and west exposures during the entire year, and on southerly exposures during the winter, the solar altitude is generally so low that horizontal projections, in order to be effective, would have to be excessively long.

Table 7-3 Solar Intensity and Solar Heat Gain Factors for 40°N Latitude

Date	Solar Time	Direct Normal Btu/(h·ft²)	N	NNE	NE	ENE	E	ESE	SE	SSE	S	SSW	SW	WSW	W	WNW	NW	NNW	Hor.	Solar Time
			Solar Heat Gain Factors, Btu/(h·ft²)																	
Jan	0800	142	5	5	17	71	111	132	133	114	75	22	6	5	5	5	5	5	14	1600
	0900	239	12	12	13	74	154	205	224	209	160	82	13	12	12	12	12	12	55	1500
	1000	274	16	16	16	31	124	199	241	246	213	146	51	17	16	16	16	16	96	1400
	1100	289	19	19	19	20	61	156	222	252	244	198	118	28	19	19	19	19	124	1300
	1200	294	20	20	20	20	21	90	179	234	254	234	179	90	21	20	20	20	133	1200
HALF DAY TOTALS			61	61	73	199	452	734	904	932	813	561	273	101	62	61	61	61	354	
Feb	0700	55	2	3	23	40	51	53	47	34	14	2	2	2	2	2	2	2	4	1700
	0800	219	10	11	50	129	183	206	199	160	94	18	10	10	10	10	10	10	43	1600
	0900	271	16	16	22	107	186	234	245	218	157	66	17	16	16	16	16	16	98	1500
	1000	294	21	21	21	49	143	211	246	243	203	129	38	21	21	21	21	21	143	1400
	1100	304	23	23	23	24	71	160	219	244	231	184	103	27	23	23	23	23	171	1300
	1200	307	24	24	24	24	25	86	170	222	241	222	170	86	25	24	24	24	180	1200
HALF DAY TOTALS			84	86	152	361	648	916	1049	1015	821	508	250	114	85	84	84	84	548	
Mar	0700	171	9	29	93	140	163	161	135	86	22	8	8	8	8	8	8	8	26	1700
	0800	250	16	18	91	169	218	232	211	157	74	17	16	16	16	16	16	16	85	1600
	0900	282	21	22	47	136	203	238	236	198	128	40	22	21	21	21	21	21	143	1500
	1000	297	25	25	27	72	153	207	229	216	171	95	29	25	25	25	25	25	186	1400
	1100	305	28	28	28	30	78	151	198	213	197	150	77	30	28	28	28	28	213	1300
	1200	307	29	29	29	29	31	75	145	191	206	191	145	75	31	29	29	29	223	1200
HALF DAY TOTALS			114	139	302	563	832	1035	1087	968	694	403	220	132	114	113	113	113	764	
Apr	0600	89	11	46	72	87	88	76	52	18	5	5	5	5	5	5	5	5	11	1800
	0700	206	16	71	140	185	201	186	143	75	16	14	14	14	14	14	14	14	61	1700
	0800	252	22	44	128	190	224	223	188	124	41	22	21	21	21	21	21	21	123	1600
	0900	274	27	29	80	155	202	219	203	156	83	29	27	27	27	27	27	27	177	1500
	1000	286	31	31	37	92	152	187	193	170	121	56	32	31	31	31	31	41	217	1400
	1100	292	33	33	34	39	81	130	160	166	146	102	52	35	33	33	33	33	243	1300
	1200	293	34	34	34	34	36	62	108	142	154	142	108	62	36	34	34	34	252	1200
HALF DAY TOTALS			154	265	501	758	957	1051	994	782	488	296	199	157	148	147	147	147	957	
May	0500	1	0	1	1	1	1	1	0	0	0	0	0	0	0	0	0	0	0	1900
	0600	144	36	90	128	145	141	115	71	18	10	10	10	10	10	10	10	11	31	1800
	0700	216	28	102	165	202	209	184	131	54	20	19	19	19	19	19	19	19	87	1700
	0800	250	27	73	149	199	220	208	164	93	29	25	25	25	25	25	25	25	146	1600
	0900	267	31	42	105	164	197	200	175	121	53	32	30	30	30	30	30	30	195	1500
	1000	277	34	36	54	105	148	168	163	133	83	40	35	34	34	34	34	34	234	1400
	1100	283	36	36	38	48	81	113	130	127	105	70	42	38	36	36	36	36	257	1300
	1200	284	37	37	37	38	40	54	82	104	113	104	82	54	40	38	37	37	265	1200
HALF DAY TOTALS			215	404	666	893	1024	1025	881	601	358	247	200	180	176	175	174	175	1083	
Jun	0500	22	10	17	21	22	20	14	6	2	1	1	1	1	1	1	1	2	3	1900
	0600	155	48	104	143	159	151	121	70	17	13	13	13	13	13	13	13	14	40	1800
	0700	216	37	113	172	205	207	178	122	46	22	21	21	21	21	21	21	21	97	1700
	0800	246	30	85	156	201	216	199	152	80	29	27	27	27	27	27	27	27	153	1600
	0900	263	33	51	114	166	192	190	161	105	45	33	32	32	32	32	32	32	201	1500
	1000	272	35	38	63	109	145	158	148	116	69	39	36	35	35	35	35	35	238	1400
	1100	277	38	39	40	52	81	105	116	110	88	60	41	39	38	38	38	38	260	1300
	1200	279	38	38	38	40	41	52	72	89	95	89	72	52	41	40	38	38	267	1200
HALF DAY TOTALS			253	470	734	941	1038	999	818	523	315	236	204	191	188	187	186	188	1126	
Jul	0500	2	1	2	2	2	2	1	1	0	0	0	0	0	0	0	0	0	0	1900
	0600	138	37	89	125	142	137	112	68	18	11	11	11	11	11	11	11	12	32	1800
	0700	208	30	102	163	198	204	179	127	53	21	20	20	20	20	20	20	20	88	1700
	0800	241	28	75	148	196	216	203	160	90	30	26	26	26	26	26	26	26	145	1600
	0900	259	32	44	106	163	193	196	170	118	52	33	31	31	31	31	31	31	194	1500
	1000	269	35	37	56	106	146	165	159	129	81	41	36	35	35	35	35	35	231	1400
	1100	275	37	38	40	50	81	111	127	123	102	69	43	39	37	37	37	37	254	1300
	1200	276	38	38	38	40	41	55	80	101	109	101	80	55	41	40	38	38	262	1200
HALF DAY TOTALS			223	411	666	885	1008	1003	858	584	352	248	204	186	181	180	180	181	1076	
Aug	0600	81	12	44	68	81	82	71	48	17	6	5	5	5	5	5	5	5	12	1800
	0700	191	17	71	135	177	191	177	135	70	17	16	16	16	16	16	16	16	62	1700
	0800	237	24	47	126	185	216	214	180	118	41	23	23	23	23	23	23	23	122	1600
	0900	260	28	31	82	153	197	212	196	151	80	31	28	28	28	28	28	28	174	1500
	1000	272	32	33	40	93	150	182	187	165	116	56	34	32	32	32	32	32	214	1400
	1100	278	35	35	36	41	81	128	156	160	141	99	52	37	35	35	35	35	239	1300
	1200	280	35	35	35	36	38	63	106	138	149	138	106	63	38	36	35	35	247	1200
HALF DAY TOTALS			164	273	498	741	928	1013	956	751	474	296	205	166	157	156	156	156	946	
Sep	0700	149	9	27	84	125	146	144	121	77	21	9	9	9	9	9	9	9	25	1700
	0800	230	17	19	87	160	205	218	199	148	71	18	17	17	17	17	17	17	82	1600
	0900	263	22	23	47	131	194	227	226	190	124	41	23	22	22	22	22	22	138	1500
	1000	280	27	27	28	71	148	200	221	209	165	93	30	27	27	27	27	27	180	1400
	1100	287	29	29	29	31	78	147	192	207	191	146	77	31	29	29	29	29	206	1300
	1200	290	30	30	30	30	32	75	142	185	200	185	142	75	32	30	30	30	215	1200
HALF DAY TOTALS			119	142	291	534	787	980	1033	925	672	396	222	137	119	118	118	118	738	
Oct	0700	48	2	3	20	36	45	47	42	30	12	2	2	2	2	2	2	2	4	1700
	0800	204	11	12	49	123	173	195	188	151	89	18	11	11	11	11	11	11	43	1600
	0900	257	17	17	23	104	180	225	235	209	151	64	18	17	17	17	17	17	97	1500
	1000	280	21	21	22	50	139	205	238	235	196	125	38	22	21	21	21	21	140	1400
	1100	291	24	24	24	25	71	156	212	236	224	178	101	28	24	24	24	24	168	1300
	1200	294	25	25	25	25	27	85	165	216	234	216	165	85	27	25	25	25	177	1200
HALF DAY TOTALS			88	89	152	351	623	878	1006	974	791	493	247	117	89	88	88	88	540	
Nov	0800	136	5	5	18	69	108	128	129	110	72	21	6	5	5	5	5	5	14	1600
	0900	232	12	12	13	73	151	201	219	204	156	80	13	12	12	12	12	12	55	1500
	1000	268	16	16	16	31	122	196	237	242	209	143	50	17	16	16	16	16	96	1400
	1100	283	19	19	19	20	61	154	218	248	240	194	116	28	19	19	19	19	123	1300
	1200	288	20	20	20	20	21	89	176	231	250	231	176	89	21	20	20	20	132	1200
HALF DAY TOTALS			63	63	75	198	445	721	887	914	798	551	269	101	63	63	63	63	354	
Dec	0800	89	3	3	8	41	67	82	84	73	50	17	3	3	3	3	3	3	6	1600
	0900	217	10	10	11	60	135	185	205	194	151	83	13	10	10	10	10	10	39	1500
	1000	261	14	14	14	25	113	188	232	239	210	146	55	15	14	14	14	14	77	1400
	1100	280	17	17	17	17	56	151	217	249	242	198	120	28	17	17	17	17	104	1300
	1200	285	18	18	18	18	19	89	178	233	253	233	178	89	19	18	18	18	113	1200
HALF DAY TOTALS			52	52	56	146	374	649	822	867	775	557	276	94	53	52	52	52	282	
			N	NNW	NW	WNW	W	WSW	SW	SSW	S	SSE	SE	ESE	E	ENE	NE	NNE	Hor.	PM

Notes: 1. Clearness number = 1.00; Ground reflectance = 0.20. 2. Figures shown are for 21st day of each month.

Table 7-4 Visible Transmission (VT), Shading Coefficients (SC), and Solar Heat Gain Coefficient (SHGC) at Normal Incidence for Single Pane Glass and Insulating Glass

Glazing System		Center Glazing	Center Glazing	Glazing SHGC at Specified Incidence Angles						Total Window SHGC at Normal Incidence				Total Window VT at Normal Incidence	
				Normal						Aluminum		Other Frames		All Frames	
ID	Glass Thick, in.	VT	SC	0°	40°	50°	60°	70°	Hemis. (Diffuse)	Operable	Fixed	Operable	Fixed	Operable	Fixed
Uncoated Single Glazing															
1a	1/8 Clear	0.90	1.00	0.86	0.85	0.83	0.78	0.67	0.78	0.75	0.78	0.63	0.75	0.65	0.78
1b	1/4 Clear	0.89	0.94	0.81	0.80	0.77	0.73	0.62	0.73	0.71	0.74	0.60	0.71	0.65	0.78
1c	1/8 Bronze	0.68	0.85	0.73	0.71	0.69	0.64	0.55	0.65	0.64	0.67	0.54	0.64	0.49	0.59
1d	1/4 Bronze	0.55	0.73	0.62	0.60	0.58	0.54	0.46	0.55	0.55	0.57	0.46	0.54	0.40	0.48
1e	1/8 Green	0.82	0.82	0.71	0.68	0.66	0.62	0.53	0.63	0.62	0.65	0.53	0.62	0.60	0.71
1f	1/4 Green	0.74	0.68	0.58	0.56	0.54	0.51	0.44	0.52	0.51	0.53	0.43	0.51	0.54	0.64
1g	1/8 Gray	0.62	0.82	0.70	0.68	0.66	0.61	0.53	0.63	0.61	0.64	0.52	0.61	0.45	0.54
1h	1/4 Gray	0.43	0.65	0.56	0.53	0.51	0.48	0.41	0.49	0.50	0.51	0.42	0.49	0.31	0.37
1i	1/4 Bluegreen	0.75	0.72	0.62	0.59	0.57	0.54	0.46	0.55	0.55	0.57	0.46	0.54	0.54	0.65
Reflective Single Glazing															
1j	1/4 SS on CLR 8%	0.08	0.22	0.19	0.19	0.18	0.17	0.15	0.17	0.18	0.18	0.15	0.17	0.06	0.07
1k	1/4 SS on CLR 14%	0.14	0.29	0.25	0.25	0.24	0.23	0.20	0.23	0.23	0.24	0.19	0.22	0.10	0.12
1l	1/4 SS on CLR 20%	0.20	0.36	0.31	0.30	0.30	0.28	0.24	0.28	0.28	0.29	0.24	0.27	0.15	0.17
1m	1/4 SS on GRN 14%	0.12	0.29	0.25	0.25	0.24	0.23	0.20	0.23	0.23	0.24	0.19	0.22	0.09	0.10
1n	1/4 TI on CLR 20%	0.20	0.34	0.29	0.29	0.28	0.26	0.23	0.27	0.27	0.27	0.22	0.26	0.15	0.17
1o	1/4 TI on CLR 30%	0.30	0.45	0.39	0.38	0.37	0.35	0.30	0.35	0.35	0.36	0.29	0.34	0.22	0.26
Uncoated Double Glazing															
5a	1/8 CLR CLR	0.81	0.87	0.75	0.73	0.70	0.63	0.49	0.65	0.66	0.68	0.55	0.66	0.59	0.71
5b	1/4 CLR CLR	0.78	0.81	0.70	0.68	0.65	0.58	0.45	0.60	0.61	0.64	0.52	0.61	0.57	0.68
5c	1/8 BRZ CLR	0.62	0.72	0.62	0.59	0.57	0.51	0.39	0.53	0.55	0.57	0.46	0.54	0.45	0.54
5d	1/4 BRZ CLR	0.48	0.59	0.50	0.47	0.45	0.40	0.31	0.42	0.45	0.46	0.37	0.44	0.35	0.42
5e	1/8 GRN CLR	0.74	0.70	0.60	0.57	0.55	0.49	0.38	0.51	0.53	0.55	0.45	0.53	0.54	0.64
5f	1/4 GRN CLR	0.66	0.54	0.47	0.44	0.42	0.38	0.30	0.40	0.42	0.43	0.35	0.41	0.48	0.57
5g	1/8 GRY CLR	0.56	0.69	0.59	0.57	0.54	0.48	0.37	0.50	0.52	0.54	0.44	0.52	0.41	0.49
5h	1/4 GRY CLR	0.40	0.51	0.44	0.42	0.40	0.35	0.28	0.38	0.39	0.41	0.33	0.39	0.29	0.35
5i	1/4 BLUGRN CLR	0.67	0.58	0.50	0.47	0.45	0.40	0.32	0.43	0.45	0.46	0.37	0.44	0.49	0.58
5j	1/4 HI-P GRN CLR	0.59	0.46	0.39	0.37	0.35	0.31	0.25	0.33	0.35	0.36	0.29	0.34	0.43	0.51
Reflective Double Glazing															
5k	1/4 SS on CLR 8%,CLR	0.07	0.15	0.13	0.13	0.12	0.12	0.10	0.12	0.13	0.13	0.10	0.12	0.05	0.06
5l	1/4 SS on CLR 14%, CLR	0.13	0.20	0.17	0.17	0.16	0.15	0.12	0.15	0.17	0.16	0.13	0.15	0.09	0.11
5m	1/4 SS on CLR 20%, CLR	0.18	0.26	0.22	0.21	0.21	0.19	0.16	0.19	0.21	0.21	0.17	0.20	0.13	0.16
5n	1/4 SS on GRN 14%, CLR	0.11	0.18	0.16	0.16	0.15	0.14	0.12	0.14	0.16	0.16	0.13	0.14	0.08	0.10
5o	1/4 TI on CLR 20%, CLR	0.18	0.24	0.21	0.20	0.20	0.18	0.15	0.19	0.20	0.20	0.16	0.19	0.13	0.16
5p	1/4 TI on CLR 30%, CLR	0.27	0.33	0.29	0.28	0.27	0.25	0.20	0.25	0.27	0.27	0.22	0.26	0.20	0.24
Low-e Double Glazing, e = 0.2 on Surface 2															
17a	1/8 LE CLR	0.76	0.76	0.65	0.63	0.61	0.55	0.43	0.57	0.57	0.59	0.48	0.57	0.55	0.66
17b	1/4 LE CLR	0.73	0.70	0.60	0.58	0.56	0.51	0.40	0.52	0.53	0.55	0.45	0.53	0.53	0.64
Low-e Double Glazing, e = 0.2 on Surface 3															
17c	1/8 CLR LE	0.76	0.81	0.70	0.68	0.65	0.59	0.46	0.61	0.61	0.64	0.52	0.61	0.55	0.66
17d	1/4 CLR LE	0.73	0.75	0.65	0.63	0.60	0.54	0.42	0.56	0.57	0.59	0.48	0.57	0.53	0.64
17e	1/8 BRZ LE	0.58	0.66	0.57	0.54	0.52	0.46	0.36	0.48	0.50	0.52	0.42	0.50	0.42	0.51
17f	1/4 BRZ LE	0.45	0.52	0.45	0.42	0.40	0.35	0.27	0.37	0.40	0.41	0.34	0.40	0.33	0.39
17g	1/8 GRN LE	0.70	0.63	0.55	0.52	0.50	0.44	0.34	0.46	0.49	0.50	0.41	0.48	0.51	0.61
17h	1/4 GRN LE	0.61	0.48	0.42	0.39	0.37	0.33	0.25	0.35	0.38	0.39	0.32	0.37	0.44	0.53
17i	1/8 GRY LE	0.53	0.63	0.54	0.51	0.49	0.43	0.33	0.46	0.48	0.50	0.40	0.47	0.38	0.46
17j	1/4 GRY LE	0.37	0.46	0.39	0.36	0.34	0.31	0.24	0.33	0.35	0.36	0.29	0.34	0.27	0.32
17k	1/4 BLUGRN LE	0.62	0.52	0.45	0.42	0.40	0.35	0.27	0.37	0.40	0.41	0.34	0.40	0.45	0.54
17l	1/4 HI-P GRN LE	0.55	0.40	0.34	0.31	0.29	0.26	0.20	0.28	0.31	0.32	0.26	0.30	0.40	0.48
Low-e Double Glazing, e = 0.1 on Surface 2															
21a	1/8 LE CLR	0.75	0.62	0.54	0.52	0.49	0.44	0.34	0.46	0.48	0.50	0.40	0.47	0.54	0.65
21b	1/4 LE CLR	0.72	0.59	0.51	0.49	0.47	0.42	0.32	0.44	0.45	0.47	0.38	0.45	0.52	0.63
21l	1/4 HI-P GRN W/LE CLR	0.57	0.36	0.31	0.30	0.29	0.26	0.21	0.27	0.28	0.29	0.24	0.27	0.41	0.50
Low-e Double Glazing, e = 0.1 on Surface 3															
21c	1/8 CLR LE	0.75	0.69	0.60	0.58	0.56	0.51	0.41	0.53	0.53	0.55	0.45	0.53	0.54	0.65
21d	1/4 CLR LE	0.72	0.66	0.56	0.54	0.52	0.47	0.38	0.49	0.50	0.51	0.42	0.49	0.52	0.63
21e	1/8 BRZ LE	0.57	0.56	0.48	0.46	0.43	0.39	0.31	0.41	0.43	0.44	0.36	0.42	0.41	0.50
21f	1/4 BRZ LE	0.45	0.45	0.39	0.37	0.34	0.31	0.24	0.33	0.35	0.36	0.29	0.34	0.33	0.39
21g	1/8 GRN LE	0.68	0.57	0.49	0.47	0.44	0.40	0.31	0.42	0.44	0.45	0.37	0.43	0.49	0.59
21h	1/4 GRN LE	0.61	0.45	0.39	0.36	0.34	0.30	0.24	0.33	0.35	0.36	0.29	0.34	0.44	0.53
21i	1/8 GRY LE	0.52	0.53	0.46	0.44	0.41	0.37	0.29	0.39	0.41	0.42	0.34	0.41	0.38	0.45
21j	1/4 GRY LE	0.37	0.40	0.35	0.33	0.31	0.28	0.22	0.29	0.32	0.33	0.26	0.31	0.27	0.32
21k	1/4 BLUGRN LE	0.62	0.48	0.42	0.39	0.37	0.33	0.26	0.35	0.38	0.39	0.32	0.37	0.45	0.54

Table 7-4 Visible Transmission (VT), Shading Coefficients (SC), and Solar Heat Gain Coefficient (SHGC) at Normal Incidence for Single Pane Glass and Insulating Glass (*Continued*)

Glazing System					Glazing SHGC at Specified Incidence Angles						Total Window SHGC at Normal Incidence				Total Window VT at Normal Incidence	
					Normal						Aluminum		Other Frames		All Frames	
ID	Glass Thick, in.		Center Glazing VT	Center Glazing SC	0°	40°	50°	60°	70°	Hemis. (Diffuse)	Operable	Fixed	Operable	Fixed	Operable	Fixed
Low-e Double Glazing, e = 0.05 on Surface 2																
25a	1/8	LE CLR	0.72	0.48	0.41	0.38	0.34	0.26	0.14	0.35	0.37	0.38	0.31	0.36	0.52	0.63
25b	1/4	LE CLR	0.70	0.43	0.37	0.34	0.31	0.24	0.13	0.32	0.33	0.34	0.28	0.33	0.51	0.61
25c	1/4	BRZ W/LE CLR	0.42	0.30	0.26	0.24	0.22	0.18	0.10	0.23	0.24	0.24	0.20	0.23	0.31	0.37
25d	1/4	GRN W/LE CLR	0.60	0.35	0.30	0.28	0.25	0.20	0.11	0.26	0.28	0.28	0.23	0.27	0.44	0.52
25e	1/4	GRY W/LE CLR	0.35	0.27	0.24	0.22	0.20	0.16	0.10	0.20	0.22	0.23	0.18	0.21	0.25	0.30
25f	1/4	BLUE W/LE CLR	0.45	0.32	0.27	0.25	0.23	0.18	0.10	0.23	0.25	0.25	0.21	0.24	0.33	0.39
25g	1/4	HI-P GRN W/LE CLR	0.53	0.31	0.27	0.26	0.25	0.23	0.18	0.24	0.25	0.25	0.22	0.25	0.38	0.46
Triple Glazing																
29a	1/8	CLR CLR CLR	0.74	0.78	0.67	0.65	0.61	0.53	0.39	0.57	0.59	0.61	0.50	0.59	0.54	0.64
29b	1/4	CLR CLR CLR	0.70	0.71	0.61	0.58	0.55	0.48	0.35	0.51	0.54	0.56	0.45	0.54	0.51	0.61
29c	1/4	HI-P GRN CLR CLR	0.53	0.39	0.34	0.31	0.29	0.25	0.19	0.27	0.31	0.32	0.26	0.30	0.38	0.46
Triple Glazing, e = 0.2 on Surface 2																
32a	1/8	LE CLR CLR	0.68	0.69	0.60	0.58	0.55	0.48	0.35	0.51	0.53	0.55	0.45	0.53	0.49	0.59
32b	1/4	LE CLR CLR	0.64	0.62	0.53	0.50	0.47	0.41	0.30	0.44	0.47	0.49	0.39	0.47	0.46	0.56
Triple Glazing, e = 0.2 on Surface 5														0.00	0.00	
32c	1/8	CLR CLR LE	0.68	0.72	0.62	0.60	0.56	0.49	0.36	0.52	0.55	0.57	0.46	0.54	0.49	0.59
32d	1/4	CLR CLR LE	0.64	0.65	0.56	0.53	0.50	0.44	0.32	0.47	0.50	0.51	0.42	0.49	0.46	0.56
Triple Glazing, e = 0.1 on Surface 2 and 5																
40a	1/8	LE CLR LE	0.62	0.52	0.45	0.43	0.40	0.36	0.26	0.38	0.40	0.41	0.34	0.40	0.45	0.54
40b	1/4	LE CLR LE	0.59	0.47	0.41	0.39	0.37	0.32	0.24	0.34	0.37	0.38	0.31	0.36	0.43	0.51
Triple Glazing, e = 0.05 on Surface 2 and 4								0.00	0.00							
40c	1/8	LE LE CLR	0.58	0.37	0.32	0.30	0.29	0.26	0.19	0.27	0.29	0.30	0.24	0.28	0.42	0.51
40d	1/4	LE LE CLR	0.55	0.36	0.31	0.29	0.28	0.25	0.19	0.26	0.28	0.29	0.24	0.27	0.40	0.48

KEY:

CLR = clear, GRN = green, GRY = gray, SS = stainless steel reflective coating, TI = titanium reflective coating

Reflective coating decsriptors include percent visible transmittance as x%.

Hi-P GRN = high performance green tinted glass, LE = glass with a low-emissivity coating with an emittance of *e* = 0.xx

Low-e coating with an emittance of 0.2 is a pyrolytic coating. Other low-e coatings are sputtered coatings.

VT is Visible Transmittance, SC is Shading Coefficient, SHGC, is Solar Heat Gain Coefficient, and HEMIS is the hemispherical SHGC

ID numberss refer to U-factors in Table 5

SHGC at 90° is 0.

Table 7-5 Shading Coefficients for Domed Horizontal Skylights

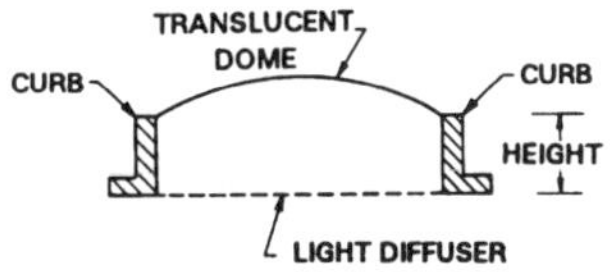

Dome	Light Diffuser (Translucent)	Curb Height, in.	Curb Width to Height Ratio	Shading Coefficient
Clear	Yes	0	∞	0.61
τ = 0.86	τ = 0.58	9	5	0.58
		18	2.5	0.50
Clear		0	∞	0.99
τ = 0.86	None	9	5	0.88
		18	2.5	0.80
Translucent	None	0	∞	0.57
τ = 0.52		18	2.5	0.46
Translucent	None	0	∞	0.34
τ = 0.27		9	5	0.30
		18	2.5	0.28

Table 7-6 Shading Coefficients and U-Factors for Standard Hollow Glass Block Wall Panels

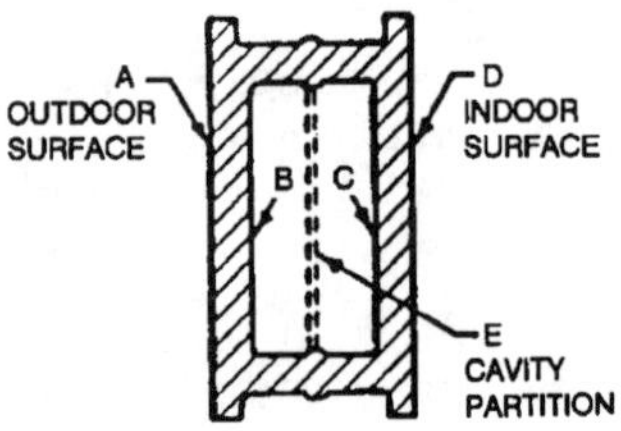

Type of Glass Block[a]	Description of Glass Block	Shading Coefficient[b]: Panels[c] in Sun	Shading Coefficient[b]: Panels[d] in Shade (N, NW, W, SW)	U-Factor,[e] Btu/h·ft²·°F
Type I	Glass colorless or aqua A, D: Smooth B, C: Smooth or wide ribs, or flutes horizontal or vertical, or shallow configuration E: None	0.65	0.40	0.51
Type IA	Same as Type I except ceramic enamel on A	0.27	0.20	0.51
Type II	Same as Type I except glass fiber screen partition E	0.44	0.34	0.48
Type III	Glass colorless or aqua A, D: Narrow vertical ribs or flutes. B, C: Horizontal light-diffusing prisms, or horizontal light-directing prisms E: Glass fiber screen	0.33	0.27	0.48
Type IIIA	Same as Type III except E: Glass fiber screen with green ceramic spray coating or glass fiber screen and gray glass or glass fiber screen with light-selecting prisms	0.25	0.18	0.48
Type IV	Same as Type I except reflective oxide coating on A	0.16	0.12	0.51

[a]All values are for 7 3/4 by 7 3/4 by 3 7/8 in. block, set in light-colored mortar. For 11 3/4 by 11 3/4 by 3 7/8 in. block, increase coefficients by 15%, and for 5 3/4 by 5 3/4 by 3 7/8 in. block reduce coefficents by 15%.
[b]Shading coefficients are applied to heat gain factors for one hour earlier than the load calculation time to allow for heat storage in the panel.
[c]Shading coefficients are for peak load condition, but provide a close approximation for other conditions.
[d]For NE, E, and SE panels in shade, add 50% to the values listed for panels in the shade.
[e]Values shown are the same for all size block.

Table 7-7 Shading Coefficients for Louvered Sun Screens

Profile Angle	Group 1 Transmittance	Group 1 SC	Group 2 Transmittance	Group 2 SC	Group 3 Transmittance	Group 3 SC	Group 4 Transmittance	Group 4 SC	Group 5 Transmittance	Group 5 SC	Group 6 Transmittance	Group 6 SC
10°	0.23	0.35	0.25	0.33	0.40	0.51	0.48	0.59	0.15	0.27	0.26	0.45
20°	0.06	0.17	0.14	0.23	0.32	0.42	0.39	0.50	0.04	0.11	0.20	0.35
30°	0.04	0.15	0.12	0.21	0.21	0.31	0.28	0.38	0.03	0.10	0.13	0.26
≥ 40°	0.04	0.15	0.11	0.20	0.07	0.18	0.20	0.30	0.03	0.10	0.04	0.13

Group 1. Black, width over spacing ratio 1.15/1; 23 louvers/in. Group 2. Light color; high reflectance, otherwise same as Group 1. Group 3. Black or dark color; w/s ratio 0.85/1; 17 louvers/in. Group 4. Light color or unpainted aluminum; high reflectance; otherwise same as Group 3. Group 5. Same as Group 1, except two lights of 0.25 in. clear glass with 0.5 in. air space. Group 6. Same as Group 3, except two lights of 0.25 in. clear glass with 0.5 in. air space. U-value = 0.85 Btu/h·ft²·°F for all groups when used with single glazing.

Table 7-8 Shading Coefficients for Single Glass with Indoor Shading by Venetian Blinds or Roller Shades

Type of Glass	Nominal Thickness,[a] in.	Solar Transmittance[b]	Venetian Blinds: Medium	Venetian Blinds: Light	Roller Shade, Opaque: Dark	Roller Shade, Opaque: White	Roller Shade, Translucent: Light
Clear	3/32[c]	0.87 to 0.80	0.74[d] (0.63)[e]	0.67[d] (0.58)[e]	0.81	0.39	0.44
Clear	1/4 to 1/2	0.80 to 0.71					
Clear pattern	1/8 to 1/2	0.87 to 0.79					
Heat-absorbing pattern	1/8	—					
Tinted	3/16, 7/32	0.74, 0.71					
Heat-absorbing[f]	3/16, 1/4	0.46					
Heat-absorbing pattern	3/16, 1/4	—	0.57	0.53	0.45	0.30	0.36
Tinted	1/8, 7/32	0.59, 0.45					
Heat-absorbing or pattern	—	0.44 to 0.30	0.54	0.52	0.40	0.28	0.32
Heat-absorbing[f]	3/8	0.34					
Heat-absorbing or pattern		0.29 to 0.15					
	—	0.24	0.42	0.40	0.36	0.28	0.31
Reflective coated glass	S.C. = 0.30[g]		0.25	0.23			
	= 0.40		0.33	0.29			
	= 0.50		0.42	0.38			
	= 0.60		0.50	0.44			

[a]Refer to manufacturers' literature for values.
[b]For vertical blinds with opaque white and beige louvers in the tightly closed position, SC is 0.25 and 0.29 when used with glass of 0.71 to 0.80 transmittance.
[c]Typical residential glass thickness.
[d]From Van Dyck and Konen (1982), for 45° open venetian blinds, 35° solar incidence, and 35° profile angle.
[e]Values for closed venetian blinds. Use these values only when operation is automated for solar gain reduction (as opposed to daylight use).
[f]Refers to gray, bronze, and green tinted heat-absorbing glass.
[g]SC for glass with no shading device.

Table 7-9 Shading Coefficients for Double Glazing with Indoor Shading by Venetian Blinds or Roller Shades

				Type of Shading				
						Roller Shade		
	Nominal Thickness,	Solar Transmittance[a]		Venetian Blinds[b]		Opaque		Translucent
Type of Glass	Each Light	Outer Pane	Inner Pane	Medium	Light	Dark	White	Light
Clear out	3/32, 1/8 in.	0.87	0.87	0.62[c]	0.58[c]	0.71	0.35	0.40
Clear in				(0.63)[d]	(0.58)[d]			
Clear in	1/4 in.	0.80	0.80					
Heat-absorbing[e] out	1/4 in.	0.46	0.80	0.39	0.36	0.40	0.22	0.30
Clear in								
Reflective coated glass	SC = 0.20[f]			0.19	0.18			
	= 0.30			0.27	0.26			
	= 0.40			0.34	0.33			

Table refers to factory-fabricated units with 3/16, 1/4, or 1/2 in. air space, or to prime windows plus storm windows.

[a]Refer to manufacturers' literature for exact values.
[b]For vertical blinds with opaque white or beige louvers, tightly closed, SC is approximately the same as for opaque white roller shades.
[c]From Van Dyck and Konen (1982), for 45° open venetian blinds, 35° solar incidence, and 35° profile angle.
[d]Values for closed venetian blinds. Use these values only when operation is automated for solar gain reduction (as opposed to daylight use).
[e]Refers to bronze, or green tinted, heat-absorbing glass.
[f]SC for glass with no shading device.

Table 7-10 Shading Coefficients for Double Glazing with Between-Glass Shading

					Type of Shading		
	Nominal Thickness,	Solar Transmittance[a]			Venetian Blinds		Louvered
Type of Glass	Each Pane	Outer Pane	Inner Pane	Description of Air Space	Light	Medium	Sun Screen
Clear out, Clear in	3/32, 1/8 in.	0.87	0.87	Shade in contact with glass or shade separated from glass by air space.	0.33	0.36	0.43
Clear out, Clear in	1/4 in.	0.80	0.80	Shade in contact with glass-voids filled with plastic.	—	—	0.49
Heat-absorbing[b] out, Clear in				Shade in contact with glass or shade separated from glass by air space.	0.28	0.30	0.37
	1/4 in.	0.46	0.80	Shade in contact with glass-voids filled with plastic.	—	—	0.41

[a]Refer to manufacturers' literature for exact values.
[b]Refers to grey, bronze and green tinted heat-absorbing glass.

A vertical fin or projection P_v required to produce a given shadow width S_W on a window or wall for any given time of day and year is related to the vertical surface-solar azimuth (see Table 7-12) by

$$P_V = S_W/|\tan\gamma| \tag{7-10}$$

The horizontal projection P_H required to produce a given shadow height S_H on a window or wall for any time of day or year is related to the profile angle Ω (Table 7-13) by

$$P_H = S_H/\tan\Omega \tag{7-11}$$

The profile angle, also called the vertical shadow line angle, is the angle between a line perpendicular to the plane of the window and the projection of the earth-sun line in a vertical plane that is also normal to the window and is given by

$$\tan\Omega = \tan\beta/\cos\gamma$$

The use of an overhang to shade glass is an excellent way of reducing the solar heat gain. Use the values for north glass when reducing solar heat gain for a shaded window. North glass does not have sun shining directly on it, so the SHGFs listed for it are based on only diffuse solar radiation (as on shaded glass). If a window is partially shaded, use the north value of SHGF for the shaded portion and the regular (east, west, south, etc.) SHGF for the rest of the window.

A window with a significant depth of reveal generally has part of its glass area shaded by the mullions and the transom. The area that is shaded varies throughout the day, but it can be estimated by treating mullions and transoms as vertical and horizontal projections.

The width S_W of the shadow from a mullion which projects a distance P_V beyond the plane of the glass is

$$S_W = P_V|\tan\gamma| \tag{7-12}$$

where γ is the wall-solar azimuth. When γ is greater than 90°, the entire window is in the shade.

Similarly, the height of the shadow cast by a transom that projects PH beyond the plane of the glass is

$$S_H = P_H\tan\beta/\cos\gamma \tag{7-13}$$

where β is the solar altitude. The solar angles are shown in Figure 7-3.

Table 7-11 Shading Coefficients for Single and Double Glazing with Draperies

Glazing	Glass Trans- mission	Glass Alone SC (No Drapes)	A	B	C	D	E	F	G	H	I	J
Single glass												
1/8 in. Clear	0.86	1.00	0.87	0.82	0.74	0.69	0.64	0.59	0.53	0.48	0.42	0.37
1/4 in. Clear	0.80	0.95	0.80	0.75	0.70	0.65	0.60	0.55	0.50	0.45	0.40	0.35
1/2 in. Clear	0.71	0.88	0.74	0.70	0.66	0.61	0.56	0.52	0.48	0.43	0.39	0.35
1/4 in. Heat absorbing	0.46	0.67	0.57	0.54	0.52	0.49	0.46	0.44	0.41	0.38	0.36	0.33
1/2 in. Heat absorbing	0.24	0.50	0.43	0.42	0.40	0.39	0.38	0.36	0.34	0.33	0.32	0.30
Reflective coated	—	0.60	0.57	0.54	0.51	0.49	0.46	0.43	0.41	0.38	0.36	0.33
(see manufacturers' literature for exact values)	—	0.50	0.46	0.44	0.42	0.41	0.39	0.38	0.36	0.34	0.33	0.31
	—	0.40	0.36	0.35	0.34	0.33	0.32	0.30	0.29	0.28	0.27	0.26
	—	0.30	0.25	0.24	0.24	0.23	0.23	0.23	0.22	0.21	0.21	0.20
Insulating glass, 1/4-in. air space												
(1/8 in. out and 1/8 in. in)	0.76	0.89	0.75	0.71	0.65	0.63	0.57	0.53	0.48	0.45	0.38	0.36
Insulating glass 1/2-in. air space												
clear out and clear in	0.64	0.83	0.66	0.62	0.58	0.56	0.52	0.48	0.45	0.42	0.37	0.35
Heat absorbing out and clear in	0.37	0.55	0.49	0.47	0.45	0.43	0.41	0.39	0.37	0.35	0.33	0.32
Reflective coated	—	0.40	0.38	0.37	0.37	0.36	0.34	0.32	0.31	0.29	0.28	0.28
(see manufacturers' literature for exact values)	—	0.30	0.29	0.28	0.27	0.27	0.26	0.26	0.25	0.25	0.24	0.24
	—	0.20	0.19	0.19	0.18	0.18	0.17	0.17	0.16	0.16	0.15	0.15

Shading Coefficient Index Letter

Notes:

1. Shading coefficients are for draped fabrics.
2. Other properties are for fabrics in flat orientation.
3. Use fabric reflectance and transmittance to obtain accurate shading coefficients.
4. Use openness and yarn reflectance or openness and fabric reflectance to obtain the various environmental characteristics, or to obtain approximate shading coefficients.

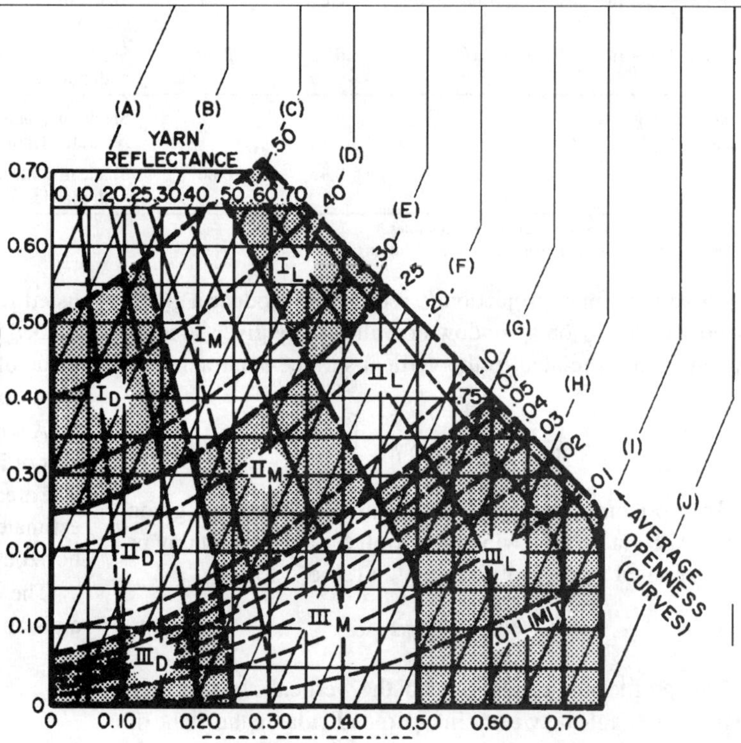

Classification of Fabrics

I = Open weave

II = Semiopen weave

III = Closed weave

D = Dark color

M = Medium color

L = Light color

To obtain fabric designator (III_L, I_M, etc.). Using either (1) Fabric Transmittance and Fabric Reflectance coordinates, or (2) Openness and Yarn Reflectance coordinates, find a point on the chart and note the designator for that area. If properties are not known, the classification may be approximated by eye as described in the note in Figure 34. Table 31 lists appropriate classifications for various applications.

To obtain shading coefficient (SC). (1) Locate drapery fabric as a point using its known properties, or approximate using its fabric classification designator. For accuracy, use fabric transmittance and fabric reflectance; (2) follow diagonal SC lines to lettered columns in the table. Find SC on line with glazing used. For example, SC is 0.45 for 0.25-in. clear single glass with III_L drapery (Column H).

Note: Shading coefficients are for 45° incident angle. For 30° or less, add 5% to the number found in the table.

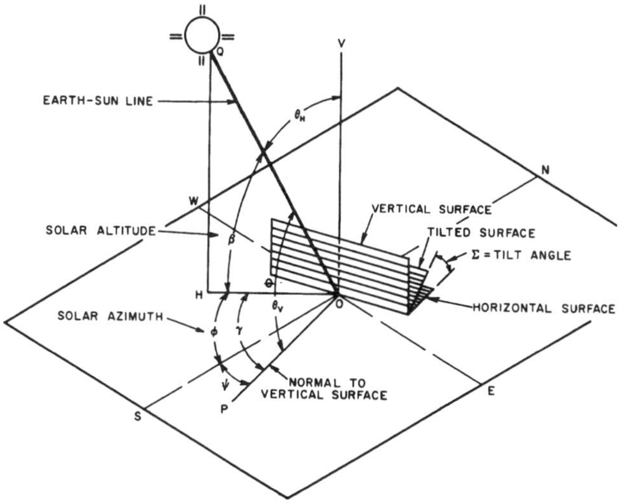

Fig. 7-3 Solar Angles

Table 7-12 Surface Orientations and Azimuths, Measured from South

	N	NE	E	SE	S	SW	W	NW
Surface azimuth, ψ	180°	−135°	−90°	−45°	0°	45°	90°	135°

Thus, the sunlit area of the window is

$$\text{Area in Sun} = (\text{Width} - S_W)(\text{Height} - S_H) \tag{7-14}$$

7.3.3 Heat Gain Through Interior Surfaces

Whenever a conditioned space is adjacent to a space with a different temperature, heat transfer through the separating physical section must be considered. The heat transfer rate q, in Btu/h, is given by

$$q = UA(t_b - t_i) \tag{7-15}$$

where

U = coefficient of overall heat transfer between the adjacent and the conditioned space, Btu/h·ft^2·F

A = area of separating section concerned, ft^2

t_b = average air temperature in adjacent space, °F

t_i = air temperature in conditioned space, °F

Temperature t_b may have any value over a considerable range according to conditions in the adjacent space. The temperature in a kitchen or boiler room may be as much as 15 to 50°F above the outdoor air temperature. The actual temperatures in adjoining spaces should be measured wherever practicable; where nothing is known except that the adjacent space is of conventional construction and contains no heat sources, $t_b - t_i$ may be considered to be the difference between the outdoor air and conditioned-space design dry-bulb temperatures minus 5°F (2.8°C). In some cases, the air temperature in the adjacent space corresponds to the outdoor air temperature or higher.

Table 7-13 Solar Position and Profile Angles for 40°N Latitude

	Solar Time	Solar Time		Profile (Shadow Line) Angles												Angles of Incidence Vertical Surfaces													Solar Time
DATE		ALT	AZ	N	NNE	NE	ENE	E	ESE	SE	SSE	S	SSW	SW	WSW	N	NNE	NE	ENE	E	ESE	SE	SSE	S	SSW	SW	WSW	HOR	
DEC	0800	5	53			35	11	7	6	6	6	9	21					82	60	37	16	10	31	53	76			85	1600
	0900	14	42				37	20	15	14	15	18	30	78					71	50	29	14	24	44	65	87		76	1500
	1000	21	29				72	38	26	21	21	23	31	54					84	63	43	26	22	35	55	75		69	1400
	1100	25	15					61	37	28	25	26	31	43	75					76	56	38	26	29	44	63	83	65	1300
	1200	27	0					90	53	35	28	27	28	35	53					90	70	51	34	27	34	51	70	63	1200
JAN	0800	8	55			38	15	10	8	8	10	14	34					80	58	36	15	13	34	56	78			82	1600
+	0900	17	44				40	24	18	17	18	23	37	87					70	48	29	17	27	46	68	89		73	1500
NOV	1000	24	31				72	41	29	24	24	27	36	61					82	62	43	27	25	38	57	77		66	1400
	1100	28	16					63	41	32	29	29	35	48	78					76	57	40	29	32	47	65	84	62	1300
	1200	30	0					90	56	39	32	30	32	39	56					90	71	52	37	30	37	52	71	60	1200
FEB	0700	4	72		43	9	6	4	4	5	7	14					85	63	41	18	6	27	50	72				86	1700
+	0800	15	62			43	23	17	15	15	19	29	69					74	52	32	16	22	41	63	84			75	1600
OCT	0900	24	50			80	45	31	25	24	27	35	56					86	65	46	30	25	36	54	74			66	1500
	1000	32	35				70	47	36	32	33	38	50	75					79	61	44	33	34	46	63	82		58	1400
	1100	37	19					67	49	40	37	39	45	60	85					75	58	45	37	41	53	69	87	53	1300
	1200	39	0					90	65	49	41	39	41	49	65					90	73	57	44	39	44	57	73	51	1200
MAR	0700	11	80		43	13	13	12	12	14	21	50					78	56	34	15	17	37	58	80				79	1700
+	0800	23	70		85	45	29	24	23	25	31	50					88	67	47	30	23	33	51	71				67	1600
SEP	0900	33	57			72	48	37	33	33	38	50	75					80	61	45	34	35	46	63	81			57	1500
	1000	42	42				69	53	45	42	43	50	64	87					76	60	48	42	45	56	71	88		48	1400
	1100	48	23				90	71	57	50	48	50	57	71					90	75	62	52	48	52	62	75		42	1300
	1200	50	0					90	72	59	52	50	52	59	72					90	76	63	54	50	54	63	76	40	1200
APR	0600	7	99	40	14	9	8	8	9	12	29					81	59	37	15	12	32	54	77					83	1800
+	0700	19	89		42	26	20	19	20	26	41	88					69	48	29	19	29	48	68	89				71	1700
AUG	0800	30	79		71	46	35	31	31	35	47	72					80	61	44	32	32	44	62	81				60	1600
	0900	41	67			67	51	44	41	43	51	66	90					74	58	46	41	46	58	73	90			49	1500
	1000	51	51			85	69	58	52	51	55	63	77					86	72	61	53	51	57	67	80			39	1400
	1100	59	29				86	73	64	60	59	62	69	81					87	75	66	60	59	63	71	82		31	1300
	1200	62	0					90	78	69	63	62	63	69	78					90	80	70	64	62	64	70	80	28	1200
MAY	0500	2	115	5	3	2	2	2	3	6						65	43	20	3	25	47	70						88	1900
+	0600	13	106	40	20	15	13	13	16	25	62					75	53	32	14	20	40	61	83					77	1800
JUL	0700	24	97	75	42	30	25	24	27	36	58					84	64	44	28	25	37	55	76					66	1700
	0800	35	87		65	47	38	35	37	44	59	86					74	57	43	36	40	53	70	88				55	1600
	0900	47	76		82	64	53	48	47	51	61	77					84	69	57	48	47	54	66	80				43	1500
	1000	57	61			80	68	61	58	58	63	73	86					82	70	62	58	59	65	75	86			33	1400
	1100	66	37				84	75	69	66	67	71	77	87					84	76	70	66	67	71	78	87		24	1300
	1200	70	0					90	82	76	71	70	71	76	82					90	82	76	72	70	72	76	82	20	1200
JUN	0500	4	117	9	6	4	4	5	7	14						63	40	18	6	28	50	72						86	1900
	0600	15	108	40	22	16	15	16	19	31	75					72	51	30	15	23	43	64	86					75	1800
	0700	26	100	71	42	31	27	26	30	40	66					81	61	43	29	28	40	59	79					64	1700
	0800	37	91	89	63	47	39	37	40	48	64					89	72	55	42	37	43	56	73					53	1600
	0900	49	80		79	63	54	49	50	54	65	82					82	68	56	50	50	57	69	84				41	1500
	1000	60	66			78	68	62	60	61	67	77	89					80	70	63	60	62	69	78	89			30	1400
	1100	69	42				83	76	71	69	70	74	81	89					83	76	71	69	70	75	81	89		21	1300
	1200	73	0					90	84	78	75	73	75	78	84					90	84	78	75	73	75	78	84	17	1200
				N	NNW	NW	WNW	W	WSW	SW	SSW	S	SSE	SE	ESE	N	NNW	NW	WNW	W	WSW	SW	SSW	S	SSE	SE	ESE	HOR	

Dates vary year to year within plus or minus two days of the twenty-first day of the month.

For floors in direct contact with the ground, or over an underground basement that is neither ventilated nor conditioned, heat transfer may be neglected for cooling load estimates.

7.3.4 Heat Sources in Conditioned Spaces

People. Representative rates at which heat and moisture are given off by human beings in different states of activity are listed in Table 7-14. Often, these sensible and latent heat gains constitute a large fraction of the total load. For short occupancy, the extra heat and moisture brought in by people may be significant.

The conversion of sensible heat gain from people to space cooling load is affected by the thermal storage characteristics of that space, and it is thus subject to application of appropriate room transfer functions (RTF). Latent heat gains are instantaneous.

Lighting. Since lighting is often the major component of space load, an accurate estimate of the space heat gain it imposes is needed. The rate of heat gain at any moment can be different from the heat equivalent of power supplied instantaneously to those lights.

Only part of the energy from lights is in the form of convective heat, which is immediately picked up by the air-conditioning apparatus. The remaining portion is in the form of radiation that affects the conditioned space once it has been absorbed and re-released by the walls, floors, furniture, etc. This absorbed energy contributes to space cooling load only after a time lag, so part of this energy is reradiating after the lights have been turned off (Figure 7-4).

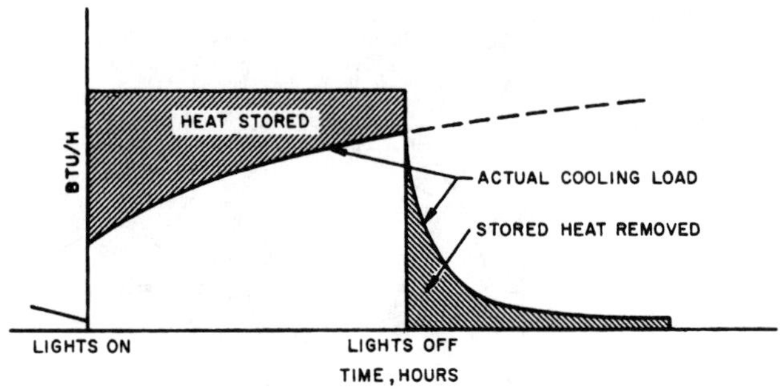

Fig. 7-4 Thermal Storage Effect in Cooling Load from Lights

Time lag effect should always be considered when calculating cooling load, since load felt by the space can be lower than the instantaneous heat gain generated, and peak load for the space may be affected.

The primary source of heat from lighting comes from the light-emitting elements (lamps), although additional heat may be generated from associated components in the light fixtures housing such lamps. Generally, the instantaneous rate of heat gain from electric lighting may be calculated from

$$q_{el} = 3.41 W F_{ul} F_{sa} \quad (7\text{-}16)$$

where

q_{el} = heat gain, Btu/h
W = total light wattage
F_{ul} = lighting use factor
F_{sa} = lighting special allowance factor

Table 7-14 Rates of Heat Gain from Occupants

		Total Heat, Btu/h		Sensible	Latent	% Sensible Heat that is Radiant[b]	
Degree of Activity		**Adult Male**	**Adjusted, M/F[a]**	**Heat, Btu/h**	**Heat, Btu/h**	**Low *V***	**High *V***
Seated at theater	Theater, matinee	390	330	225	105		
Seated at theater, night	Theater, night	390	350	245	105	60	27
Seated, very light work	Offices, hotels, apartments	450	400	245	155		
Moderately active office work	Offices, hotels, apartments	475	450	250	200		
Standing, light work; walking	Department store; retail store	550	450	250	200	58	38
Walking, standing	Drug store, bank	550	500	250	250		
Sedentary work	Restaurant[c]	490	550	275	275		
Light bench work	Factory	800	750	275	475		
Moderate dancing	Dance hall	900	850	305	545	49	35
Walking 3 mph; light machine work	Factory	1000	1000	375	625		
Bowling[d]	Bowling alley	1500	1450	580	870		
Heavy work	Factory	1500	1450	580	870	54	19
Heavy machine work; lifting	Factory	1600	1600	635	965		
Athletics	Gymnasium	2000	1800	710	1090		

Notes:
1. Tabulated values are based on 75°F room dry-bulb temperature. For 80°F room dry bulb, the total heat remains the same, but the sensible heat values should be decreased by approximately 20%, and the latent heat values increased accordingly.
2. Also refer to Table 4, Chapter 8, for additional rates of metabolic heat generation.
3. All values are rounded to nearest 5 Btu/h.

[a]Adjusted heat gain is based on normal percentage of men, women, and children for the application listed, with the postulate that the gain from an adult female is 85% of that for an adult male, and that the gain from a child is 75% of that for an adult male.

[b]Values approximated from data in Table 6, Chapter 8, where is air velocity with limits shown in that table.

[c]Adjusted heat gain includes 60 Btu/h for food per individual (30 Btu/h sensible and 30 Btu/h latent).

[d]Figure one person per alley actually bowling, and all others as sitting (400 Btu/h) or standing or walking slowly (550 Btu/h).

Total light wattage is obtained from the ratings of all lamps installed, both for general illumination and for display use.

The **use factor** is the ratio of the wattage in use for the conditions under which the load estimate is being made to the total installed wattage. For commercial applications, such as stores, the use factor generally is unity.

The **special allowance factor** is for fluorescent fixtures or for fixtures that are ventilated or installed so that only part of their heat goes to the conditioned space. For fluorescent fixtures, the special allowance factor accounts primarily for the ballast losses and can be as high as 2.19 for 32-W single-lamp, high-output fixtures on 277-V circuits. Rapid start, 40-W lamp fixtures have special allowance factors varying from a low of 1.18 for two lamps at 277 V, to a high of 1.30 for one lamp at 118 V, with a recommended value of 1.20 for general applications. Industrial fixtures, such as sodium lamps, may have special allowance factors varying from 1.04 to 1.37, depending on the manufacturer, and should be dealt with individually.

For ventilated or recessed fixtures, manufacturers' or other data must be sought to establish the fraction of the total wattage expected to enter the conditioned space directly (and subject to time lag effect) versus that which must be picked up by return air or in some other appropriate manner.

Cooling load caused by lights recessed into ceiling cavities is made up of two components: one part comes from the light heat directly contributing to the space heat gain; the other is the light heat released into the above-ceiling cavity, which (if used as a return air plenum) is mostly picked up by the return air passing over or through the light fixtures. In such a ceiling return air plenum, the second part of the load (sometimes referred to as **heat-to-return**), never enters the conditioned space. It does, however, add to the overall load and significantly influences the load calculation.

Even though the total cooling load imposed by these two components remains the same, the larger the fraction of heat picked up by the return air, the more the space cooling load is reduced. The minimum required airflow rate for the conditioned space is decreased if the space cooling load is reduced. Supply fan power is reduced accordingly, which ultimately results in reduced energy consumption for the system and, possibly, reduced equipment size.

For ordinary design load estimation, the heat gain for each component may be calculated as a fraction of the total lighting load by using judgment to estimate heat-to-space and heat-to-return percentages.

Two generic types of light fixtures are those that allow and those that do not allow return air to flow through the lamp chamber. The first type is sometimes called a **heat-of-light fixture**. The percent of light heat released through the plenum side of various ventilated fixtures can be obtained from lighting fixture manufacturers. Even unventilated fixtures lose some heat to plenum spacc; however, most of the heat ultimately enters the conditioned space from a dead-air plenum or is picked up by return air via ceiling return air openings. The percentage of heat from fixtures ranges from 40 to 60% heat-to-return for ventilated fixtures or 15 to 25% for unventilated fixtures.

Plenum Temperatures. As heat from lighting is picked up by the return air, the temperature differential between the ceiling space and the conditioned space causes part of that heat to flow from the ceiling back to the conditioned space. Return air from the conditioned space can be ducted to capture light heat without passing through a ceiling plenum as such, or the ceiling space can be used as a return air plenum, causing the distribution of light heat to be handled in distinctly different ways. Most plenum temperatures do not rise more than 1 to 3 °F above space temperature, thus generating only a relatively small thermal gradient for heat transfer through plenum surfaces but a relatively large percentage reduction in space cooling load.

Energy Balance. Where the ceiling space is used as a return air plenum, an energy balance requires that the heat picked up from the lights into the return air do one or more of the following:

1. Become a part of the cooling load to the return air (represented by a temperature rise of the return air as it passes through the ceiling space)
2. Be partially transferred back into the conditioned space through the ceiling material below
3. Be partially lost (from the space) through the floor surfaces above the plenum

In a multistory building, the conditioned space frequently gains heat through its floor from a similar plenum below, offsetting the loss just mentioned. The radiant component of heat leaving the ceiling or floor surface of a plenum is normally so small that all such heat transfer is considered convective in calculations.

Figure 7-5 shows a schematic diagram of a typical return air plenum. Equations (7-17) through (7-21), using the sign convention as shown in Figure 7-5, represent the heat balance of a return air plenum design for a typical interior room in a multifloor building:

$$q_1 = U_c A_c (t_p - t_r) \tag{7-17}$$

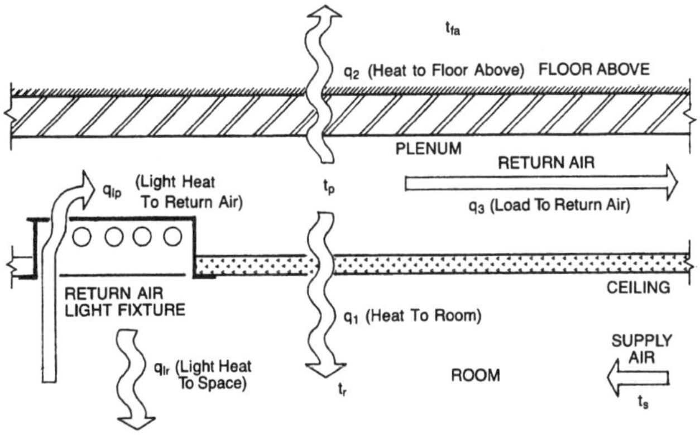

Fig. 7-5 Heat Balance of Typical Ceiling Return Plenum

$$q_2 = U_f A_f (t_p - t_{fa}) \tag{7-18}$$

$$q_3 = 1.1Q(t_p - t_r) \tag{7-19}$$

$$q_{lp} - q_2 - q_1 - q_3 = 0 \tag{7-20}$$

$$Q = \frac{q_r + q_1}{1.1(t_r - t_s)} \tag{7-21}$$

where

q_1 = heat gain to space from plenum through ceiling, Btu/h
q_2 = heat loss from plenum through floor above, Btu/h
q_3 = heat gain "pickup" by return air, Btu/h
Q = return airflow, cfm
q_{lp} = light heat gain to plenum via return air, Btu/h
q_{lr} = light heat gain to space, Btu/h
q_f = heat gain from plenum below, through floor, Btu/h
q_w = heat gain from exterior wall, Btu/h
q_r = space cooling load, Btu/h, including appropriate treatment of q_{lr}, q_f, and/or q_w
t_p = plenum temperature, °F
t_r = space temperature, °F
t_{fa} = space temperature of floor above, °F
t_s = supply air temperature, °F

By substituting Equations (7-17), (7-18), (7-19), and (7-21) into heat balance equation (7-20), t_p can be found as the resultant return air temperature or plenum temperature, by means of a quadratic equation derived from such relationships. The results, although rigorous and best solved by computer, are important in determining the cooling load, which affects equipment size selection, future energy consumption and other factors.

Equations (7-17) through (7-21) are simplified to illustrate the heat balance relationship. Heat gain into a return air plenum is not limited to the heat of lights alone. Exterior walls directly exposed to the ceiling space will transfer heat directly to or from the return air. For single-story buildings or the top floor of a multistory building, the roof heat gain or loss enters or leaves the ceiling plenum rather than entering or leaving the conditioned space directly. The supply air quantity calculated by Equation (7-21) is for the conditioned space under consideration only, and it is assumed equal to the return air quantity.

The amount of airflow through a return plenum above a conditioned space may not be limited to that supplied into the space under consideration; it will, however, have no noticeable effect on plenum temperature if the surplus comes from an adjacent plenum operating under similar conditions. Where special conditions exist, heat balance Equations (7-17) through (7-21) must be modified appropriately. Finally, even though the building's thermal storage has some effect, the amount of heat entering the return air is small and may be considered as convective for calculation purposes.

Power. When equipment is operated by electric motors within a conditioned space, the heat equivalent is calculated as follows:

$$q_{em} = 2545(P/E_M)F_{LM}F_{UM} \tag{7-22}$$

where

q_{em} = heat equivalent of equipment operation, Btu/h
P = motor horsepower rating
E_M = motor efficiency, as decimal fraction
F_{LM} = motor load factor
F_{UM} = motor use factor

The motor use factor may be applied when motor use is known to be intermittent with significant nonuse during all hours of operation (i.e., overhead door operator, and so forth). For conventional applications, its value is 1.0.

The motor load factor is the fraction of the rated load delivered under the conditions of the cooling load estimate. In Equation (7-22), both the motor and the driven equipment are assumed to be within the conditioned space. If the motor is outside the space or airstream, Equation (7-23) is used:

$$q_{em} = 2545PF_{LM}F_{UM} \tag{7-23}$$

When the motor is inside the conditioned space or airstream but the driven machine is outside, Equation (7-24) is used:

$$q_{em} = 2545P[(1 - E_M)/E_M]F_{LM}F_{UM} \tag{7-24}$$

Equation (7-24) also applies to a fan or pump in the conditioned space that exhausts air or pumps fluid outside that space.

Heat gains, average efficiencies, and related data representative of typical electric motors, generally derived from the lower efficiencies reported by several manufacturers of open, drip-proof motors, are given in Table 7-15. Unless the manufacturers' technical literature indicates otherwise, the heat gain may be divided equally between radiant and convective components for subsequent cooling load calculations.

Appliances. In a cooling load estimate, heat gain from all appliances—electrical, gas, or steam—should be considered. Food preparation equipment is among the most common types of heat-producing appliances found in conditioned areas. Appliance surfaces contribute most of the heat to commercial kitchens. When installed under an effective hood, cooling load is independent of the fuel or energy used for similar equipment performing the same operations. Because the heat is primarily radiant energy from the appliance surfaces and cooking utensils, convected and latent heat are negligible.

To establish a heat gain value, actual input values and various factors, efficiencies, or other judgmental modifiers are preferred. Where specific rating data are unavailable (nameplate missing, equipment not yet purchased, and so forth), recommended heat gains tabulated in this chapter may be used. In estimating the appliance load, probabilities of simultaneous use and operation for different appliances located in the same space must be considered.

Radiation contributes up to 32% of the hourly heat input to hooded appliances (for a conservative radiation factor F_{RA} = 0.32). Radiant heat temperature rises can be substantially

Table 7-15 Heat Gain from Typical Electric Motors

Motor Nameplate or Rated Horsepower	Motor Type	Nominal rpm	Full Load Motor Efficiency, %	Location of Motor and Driven Equipment with Respect to Conditioned Space or Airstream: A — Motor in, Driven Equipment in, Btu/h	B — Motor out, Driven Equipment in, Btu/h	C — Motor in, Driven Equipment out, Btu/h
0.05	Shaded pole	1500	35	360	130	240
0.08	Shaded pole	1500	35	580	200	380
0.125	Shaded pole	1500	35	900	320	590
0.16	Shaded pole	1500	35	1160	400	760
0.25	Split phase	1750	54	1180	640	540
0.33	Split phase	1750	56	1500	840	660
0.50	Split phase	1750	60	2120	1270	850
0.75	3-Phase	1750	72	2650	1900	740
1	3-Phase	1750	75	3390	2550	850
1.5	3-Phase	1750	77	4960	3820	1140
2	3-Phase	1750	79	6440	5090	1350
3	3-Phase	1750	81	9430	7640	1790
5	3-Phase	1750	82	15,500	12,700	2790
7.5	3-Phase	1750	84	22,700	19,100	3640
10	3-Phase	1750	85	29,900	24,500	4490
15	3-Phase	1750	86	44,400	38,200	6210
20	3-Phase	1750	87	58,500	50,900	7610
25	3-Phase	1750	88	72,300	63,600	8680
30	3-Phase	1750	89	85,700	76,300	9440
40	3-Phase	1750	89	114,000	102,000	12,600
50	3-Phase	1750	89	143,000	127,000	15,700
60	3-Phase	1750	89	172,000	153,000	18,900
75	3-Phase	1750	90	212,000	191,000	21,200
100	3-Phase	1750	90	283,000	255,000	28,300
125	3-Phase	1750	90	353,000	318,000	35,300
150	3-Phase	1750	91	420,000	382,000	37,800
200	3-Phase	1750	91	569,000	509,000	50,300
250	3-Phase	1750	91	699,000	636,000	62,900

reduced by shielding the fronts of cooking appliances. These reductions amount to 61% with glass panels and 78% with polished aluminum shielding. A floor-slot air curtain in front of appliances reduces the radiant temperature rise by 15%.

For each meal served, the heat transferred to the dining space is approximately 50 Btu/h, 75% of which is sensible and 25% is latent.

The maximum hourly input can be estimated as 50% of the total nameplate or catalog input q_i ratings because of the diversity of appliance use and the effect of thermostatic controls, giving a usage factor $F_{UA} = 0.50$. Therefore, the maximum hourly heat gain q_m for generic types of **electric and steam appliances** installed under a hood can be estimated from the following equations:

$$q_a = q_i F_{UA} F_{RA} \tag{7-25}$$

or

$$q_a = 0.16 q_i \tag{7-26}$$

Direct fuel-fired cooling appliances require more heat input than electric or steam equipment of the same type and size. In the case of gas fuel, the American Gas Association established an overall figure of approximately 60% more. Where appliances are installed under an effective hood, only radiant heat adds to the cooling load; convected and latent heat from the cooking process and combustion products are exhausted and do not enter the kitchen. To compensate for 60% higher input ratings, Equation (7-27) must be used with **fuel-fired appliances**, since the appliance surface temperatures are the same and the extra heat input combustion products are exhausted to outdoors. This correction is made by introducing a flue loss factor (F_{FL}) of 1.60 as follows:

$$q_a = (q_i F_{UA} F_{RA})/F_{FL} \tag{7-27}$$

or

$$q_a = 0.10 q_i \tag{7-28}$$

Factors for seven typical electrical and steam appliances are found in Table 7-16. Recommended rates of heat gain from selected restaurant equipment are listed in Table 7-17.

Table 7-16 Heat Gain Factors of Typical Appliances under Hoods

Appliance	Usage Factor F_U	Radiation Factor F_R	Load Factor $F_L = F_U F_R$ Elec/Steam
Griddle	0.16	0.45	0.07
Fryer	0.06	0.43	0.03
Convection oven	0.42	0.17	0.07
Charbroiler	0.83	0.29	0.24
Open-top range without oven	0.34	0.46	0.16
Hot-top range			
without oven	0.79	0.47	0.37
with oven	0.59	0.48	0.28
Steam cooker	0.13	0.30	0.04

Hospital and Laboratory Equipment. As with large kitchen installations, hospital and laboratory equipment is a major source of heat gain in conditioned spaces. Care must be taken in evaluating the probability and duration of simultaneous usage when many components are concentrated in one area, such as in a laboratory, operating room, and so forth. Commonly, heat gain from such equipment in a laboratory ranges from 15 to 70 Btu/h·ft^2 or, in laboratories with outdoor exposure, as much as four times the heat gain from all of the sources combined. Heat gain values for hospital and laboratory equipment are listed in Table 1 in Chapter 13 of the 1995 *ASHRAE Handbook—Applications*.

Office Appliances. Electric typewriters, calculators, checkwriters, teletype units, posting machines, and the like can generate 3 to 4 Btu/h·ft^2 for general offices and 6 to 7 Btu/h·ft^2 for purchasing and accounting departments. However, in offices with computer display terminals at most desks, heat gains range up to 15 Btu/h·ft^2 (Table 7-18).

Computer rooms housing mainframe or minicomputer equipment must be considered individually. Computer manufacturers have data pertaining to various individual

Table 7-17 Heat Gain from Selected Restaurant Equipment[a]

		Energy Rate, Btu/h		Recommended Rate of Heat Gain,[a] Btu/h			
				Without Hood			With Hood
Appliance	**Size**	**Rated**	**Standby**	**Sensible**	**Latent**	**Total**	**Sensible**
Electric, No Hood Required							
Barbeque (pit), per pound of food capacity	80 to 300 lb	136	—	86	50	136	42
Barbeque (pressurized), per pound of food capacity	44 lb	327	—	109	54	163	50
Blender, per quart of capacity	1 to 4 qt	1550	—	1000	520	1520	480
Braising pan, per quart of capacity	108 to 140 qt	360	—	180	95	275	132
Cabinet (large hot holding)	16.2 to 17.3 ft^3	7100	—	610	340	960	290
Cabinet (large hot serving)	37.4 to 406 ft^3	6820	—	610	310	920	280
Cabinet (large proofing)	16 to 17 ft^3	693	—	610	310	920	280
Cabinet (small hot holding)	3.2 to 6.4 ft^3	3070	—	270	140	410	130
Cabinet (very hot holding)	17.3 ft^3	21000	—	1880	960	2830	850
Can opener		580	—	580	—	580	0
Coffee brewer	12 cup/2 brnrs	5660	—	3750	1910	5660	1810
Coffee heater, per boiling burner	1 to 2 brnrs	2290	—	1500	790	2290	720
Coffee heater, per warming burner	1 to 2 brnrs	340	—	230	110	340	110
Coffee/hot water boiling urn, per quart of capacity	11.6 qt	390	—	256	132	388	123
Coffee brewing urn (large), per quart of capacity	23 to 40 qt	2130	—	1420	710	2130	680
Coffee brewing urn (small), per quart of capacity	10.6 qt	1350	—	908	445	1353	416
Cutter (large)	18 in. bowl	2560	—	2560	—	2560	0
Cutter (small)	14 in. bowl	1260	—	1260	—	1260	0
Cutter and mixer (large)	30 to 48 qt	12730	—	12730	—	12730	0
Dishwasher (hood type, chemical sanitizing), per 100 dishes/h	950 to 2000 dishes/h	1300	—	170	370	540	170
Dishwasher (hood type, water sanitizing), per 100 dishes/h	950 to 2000 dishes/h	1300	—	190	420	610	190
Dishwasher (conveyor type, chemical sanitizing), per 100 dishes/h	5000 to 9000 dishes/h	1160	—	140	330	470	150
Dishwasher (conveyor type, water sanitizing), per 100 dishes/h	5000 to 9000 dishes/h	1160	—	150	370	520	170
Display case (refrigerated), per 10 ft^3 of interior	6 to 67 ft^3	1540	—	617	0	617	0
Dough roller (large)	2 rollers	5490	—	5490	—	5490	0
Dough roller (small)	1 roller	1570	—	140	—	140	0
Egg cooker	12 eggs	6140	—	2900	1940	4850	1570
Food processor	2.4 qt	1770	—	1770	—	1770	0
Food warmer (infrared bulb), per lamp	1 to 6 bulbs	850	—	850	—	850	850
Food warmer (shelf type), per square foot of surface	3 to 9 ft^2	930	—	740	190	930	260
Food warmer (infrared tube), per foot of length	39 to 53 in.	990	—	990	—	990	990
Food warmer (well type), per cubic foot of well	0.7 to 2.5 ft^3	3620	—	1200	610	1810	580
Freezer (large)	73	4570	—	1840	—	1840	0
Freezer (small)	18	2760	—	1090	—	1090	0
Griddle/grill (large), per square foot of cooking surface	4.6 to 11.8 ft^2	9200	—	615	343	958	343
Griddle/grill (small), per square foot of cooking surface	2.2 to 4.5 ft^2	8300	—	545	308	853	298
Hot dog broiler	48 to 56 hot dogs	3960	—	340	170	510	160
Hot plate (double burner, high speed)		16720	—	7810	5430	13240	6240
Hot plate (double burner, stockpot)		13650	—	6380	4440	10820	5080
Hot plate (single burner, high speed)		9550	—	4470	3110	7580	3550
Hot water urn (large), per quart of capacity	56 qt	416	—	161	52	213	68
Hot water urn (small), per quart of capacity	8 qt	738	—	285	95	380	123
Ice maker (large)	220 lb/day	3720	—	9320	—	9320	0
Ice maker (small)	110 lb/day	2560	—	6410	—	6410	0
Microwave oven (heavy duty, commercial)	0.7 ft^3	8970	—	8970	—	8970	0
Microwave oven (residential type)	1 ft^3	2050 to 4780	—	2050 to 4780	—	2050 to 4780	0
Mixer (large), per quart of capacity	81 qt	94	—	94	—	94	0
Mixer (small), per quart of capacity	12 to 76 qt	48	—	48	—	48	0
Press cooker (hamburger)	300 patties/h	7510	—	4950	2560	7510	2390
Refrigerator (large), per 10 ft^3 of interior space	25 to 74 ft^3	753	—	300	—	300	0
Refrigerator (small), per 10 ft^3 of interior space	6 to 25 ft^3	1670	—	665	—	665	0
Rotisserie	300 hamburgers/h	10920	—	7200	3720	10920	3480
Serving cart (hot), per cubic foot of well	1.8 to 3.2 ft^3	2050	—	680	340	1020	328
Serving drawer (large)	252 to 336 dinner rolls	3750	—	480	34	510	150
Serving drawer (small)	84 to 168 dinner rolls	2730	—	340	34	380	110
Skillet (tilting), per quart of capacity	48 to 132 qt	580	—	293	161	454	218
Slicer, per square foot of slicing carriage	0.65 to 0.97 ft^2	680	—	682	—	682	216
Soup cooker, per quart of well	7.4 to 11.6 qt	416	—	142	78	220	68
Steam cooker, per cubic foot of compartment	32 to 64 qt	20700	—	1640	1050	2690	784
Steam kettle (large), per quart of capacity	80 to 320 qt	300	—	23	16	39	13
Steam kettle (small), per quart of capacity	24 to 48 qt	840	—	68	45	113	32
Syrup warmer, per quart of capacity	11.6 qt	284	—	94	52	146	45

Table 7-17 Heat Gain from Selected Restaurant Equipment[a] *(Continued)*

		Energy Rate, Btu/h		Recommended Rate of Heat Gain,[a] Btu/h			
				Without Hood			With Hood
Appliance	**Size**	**Rated**	**Standby**	**Sensible**	**Latent**	**Total**	**Sensible**
Toaster (bun toasts on one side only)	1400 buns/h	5120	—	2730	2420	5150	1640
Toaster (large conveyor)	720 slices/h	10920	—	2900	2560	5460	1740
Toaster (small conveyor)	360 slices/h	7170	—	1910	1670	3580	1160
Toaster (large pop-up)	10 slice	18080	—	9590	8500	18080	5800
Toaster (small pop-up)	4 slice	8430	—	4470	3960	8430	2700
Waffle iron	75 in^2	5600	—	2390	3210	5600	1770
Electric, Exhaust Hood Required							
Broiler (conveyor infrared), per square foot of cooking area/minute	2 to 102 ft^2	19230	—	—	—	—	3840
Broiler (single deck infrared), per square foot of broiling area	2.6 to 9.8 ft^2	10870	—	—	—	—	2150
Charbroiler, per linear foot of cooking surface	2 to 8 linear ft	11,000	9300	—	—	—	2800
Fryer (deep fat)	35 - 50 lb oil	48,000	2900	—	—	—	1200
Fryer (pressurized), per pound of fat capacity	13 to 33 lb	1565	—	—	—	—	59
Oven (full-size convection)		41,000	4600	—	—	—	2900
Oven (large deck baking with 537 ft^3 decks), per cubic foot of oven space	15 to 46 ft^3	1670	—	—	—	—	69
Oven (roasting), per cubic foot of oven space	7.8 to 23 ft^3	27350	—	—	—	—	113
Oven (small convection), per cubic foot of oven space	1.4 to 5.3 ft^3	10340	—	—	—	—	147
Oven (small deck baking with 272 ft^3 decks), per cubic foot of oven space	7.8 to 23 ft^3	2760	—	—	—	—	113
Open range top, per 2 element section	2 to 6 elements	14,000	4600	—	—	—	2100
Range (hot top/fry top), per square foot of cooking surface	4 to 8 ft^2	7260	—	—	—	—	2690
Range (oven section), per cubic foot of oven space	4.2 to 11.3 ft^3	3940	—	—	—	—	160
Griddle, per linear foot of cooking surface	2 to 8 linear feet	19,500	3100	—	—	—	1400
Gas, No Hood Required							
Broiler, per square foot of broiling area	2.7 ft^2	14800	660[b]	5310	2860	8170	1220
Cheese melter, per square foot of cooking surface	2.5 to 5.1 ft^2	10300	660[b]	3690	1980	5670	850
Dishwasher (hood type, chemical sanitizing), per 100 dishes/h	950 to 2000 dishes/h	1740	660[b]	510	200	710	230
Dishwasher (hood type, water sanitizing), per 100 dishes/h	950 to 2000 dishes/h	1740	660[b]	570	220	790	250
Dishwasher (conveyor type, chemical sanitizing), per 100 dishes/h	5000 to 9000 dishes/h	1370	660[b]	330	70	400	130
Dishwasher (conveyor type, water sanitizing), per 100 dishes/h	5000 to 9000 dishes/h	1370	660[b]	370	80	450	140
Griddle/grill (large), per square foot of cooking surface	4.6 to 11.8 ft^2	17000	330	1140	610	1750	460
Griddle/grill (small), per square foot of cooking surface	2.5 to 4.5 ft^2	14400	330	970	510	1480	400
Hot plate	2 burners	19200	1325[b]	11700	3470	15200	3410
Oven (pizza), per square foot of hearth	6.4 to 12.9 ft^2	4740	660[b]	623	220	843	85
Gas, Exhaust Hood Required							
Braising pan, per quart of capacity	105 to 140 qt	9840	660[b]	—	—	—	2430
Broiler, per square foot of broiling area	3.7 to 3.9 ft^2	21800	530	—	—	—	1800
Broiler (large conveyor, infrared), per square foot of cooking area/minute	2 to 102 ft^2	51300	1990	—	—	—	5340
Broiler (standard infrared), per square foot of broiling area	2.4 to 9.4 ft^2	1940	530	—	—	—	1600
Charbroiler (large), per linear foot of cooking area	2 to 8 linear feet	36,000	22,000	—	—	—	3800
Fryer (deep fat)	35 to 50 oil cap.	80,000	5600	—	—	—	1900
Oven (bake deck), per cubic foot of oven space	5.3 to 16.2 ft^3	7670	660[b]	—	—	—	140
Oven (convection), full size		70,000	29,400	—	—	—	5700
Oven (pizza), per square foot of oven hearth	9.3 to 25.8 ft^2	7240	660[b]	—	—	—	130
Oven (roasting), per cubic foot of oven space	9 to 28 ft^3	4300	660[b]	—	—	—	77
Oven (twin bake deck), per cubic foot of oven space	11 to 22 ft^3	4390	660[b]	—	—	—	78
Range (burners), per 2 burner section	2 to 10 brnrs	33600	1325	—	—	—	6590
Range (hot top or fry top), per square foot of cooking surface	3 to 8 ft^2	11800	330	—	—	—	3390
Range (large stock pot)	3 burners	100000	1990	—	—	—	19600
Range (small stock pot)	2 burners	40000	1330	—	—	—	7830
Griddle, per linear foot of cooking surface	2 to 8 linear feet	25,000	6300				1600
Range top, open burner (per 2 burner section)	2 to 6 elements	40,000	13,600				2200
Steam							
Compartment steamer, per pound of food capacity/h	46 to 450 lb	280	—	22	14	36	11
Dishwasher (hood type, chemical sanitizing), per 100 dishes/h	950 to 2000 dishes/h	3150	—	880	380	1260	410
Dishwasher (hood type, water sanitizing), per 100 dishes/h	950 to 2000 dishes/h	3150	—	980	420	1400	450
Dishwasher (conveyor, chemical sanitizing), per 100 dishes/h	5000 to 9000 dishes/h	1180	—	140	330	470	150
Dishwasher (conveyor, water sanitizing), per 100 dishes/h	5000 to 9000 dishes/h	1180	—	150	370	520	170
Steam kettle, per quart of capacity	13 to 32 qt	500	—	39	25	64	19

[a]In some cases, heat gain data are given per unit of capacity. In those cases, the heat gain is calculated by: q = (recommended heat gain per unit of capacity) * (capacity)

[b]Standby input rating is given for entire appliance regardless of size.

Table 7-18 Heat Gain from Selected Office and Hospital Equipment

Appliance	Size	Maximum Input Rating, Btu/h	Standby Input Rating, Btu/h	Recommended Rate of Heat Gain, Btu/h
Check processing workstation	12 pockets	16400	8410	8410
Computer devices				
Card puncher	—	2730 to 6140	2200 to 4800	2200 to 4800
Card reader	—	7510	5200	5200
Communication/transmission	—	6140 to 15700	5600 to 9600	5600 to 9600
Disk drives/mass storage	—	3410 to 34100	3412 to 22420	3412 to 22420
Magnetic ink reader	—	3280 to 16000	2600 to 14400	2600 to 14400
Microcomputer	16 to 640 Kbyte[a]	340 to 2050	300 to 1800	300 to 1800
Minicomputer	—	7500 to 15000	7500 to 15000	7500 to 15000
Optical reader	—	10240 to 20470	8000 to 17000	8000 to 17000
Plotters	—	256	128	214
Printers				
Letter quality	30 to 45 char/min	1200	600	1000
Line, high speed	5000 or more lines/min	4300 to 18100	2160 to 9040	2500 to 13000
Line, low speed	300 to 600 lines/min	1540	770	1280
Tape drives	—	4090 to 22200	3500 to 15000	3500 to 15000
Terminal	—	310 to 680	270 to 600	270 to 600
Copiers/Duplicators				
Blue print	—	3930 to 42700	1710 to 17100	3930 to 42700
Copiers (large)	30 to 67[a] copies/min	5800 to 22500	3070	5800 to 22500
Copiers (small)	6 to 30[a] copies/min	1570 to 5800	1020 to 3070	1570 to 5800
Feeder	—	100	—	100
Microfilm printer	—	1540	—	1540
Sorter/collator	—	200 to 2050	—	200 to 2050
Electronic equipment				
Cassette recorders/players	—	200	—	200
Receiver/tuner	—	340	—	340
Signal analyzer	—	90 to 2220	—	90 to 2220
Mailprocessing				
Folding machine	—	430	—	270
Inserting machine	3600 to 6800 pieces/h	2050 to 11300	—	1330 to 7340
Labeling machine	1500 to 30000 pieces/h	2050 to 22500	—	1330 to 14700
Postage meter	—	780	—	510
Wordprocessors/Typewriters				
Letter quality printer	30 to 45 char/min	1200	600	1000
Phototypesetter	—	5890	—	5180
Typewriter	—	270	—	230
Wordprocessor	—	340 to 2050	—	300 to 1800
Vending machines				
Cigarette	—	250	51 to 85	250
Cold food/beverage	—	3920 to 6550	—	1960 to 3280
Hot beverage	—	5890	—	2940
Snack	—	820 to 940	—	820 to 940
Miscellaneous				
Barcode printer	—	1500	—	1260
Cash registers	—	200	—	160
Coffee maker	10 cups	5120	—	3580 sens., 1540 latent
Microfiche reader	—	290	—	290
Microfilm reader	—	1770	—	1770
Microfilm reader/printer	—	3920	—	3920
Microwave oven	1 ft^3	2050	—	1360
Paper shredder	—	850 to 10240	—	680 to 8250
Water cooler	32 qt/h	2390	—	5970

[a]Input is not proportional to capacity.

Table 7-18 Heat Gain from Selected Office and Hospital Equipment (*Concluded*)

Appliance Type	Size	Maximum Input Rating, Btu/h	Recommended Rate of Heat Gain, Btu/h[a]
Autoclave (bench)	0.7 ft^3	4270	480
Bath, hot or cold circulating, small	1.0 to 9.7 gal, −22 to 212°F	2560 to 6140	40 to 1060 (sensible) 850 to 2010 (latent)
Blood analyzer	120 samples/h	2510	2510
Blood analyzer with CRT screen	115 samples/h	5120	5120
Centrifuge (large)	8 to 24 places	3750	3580
Centrifuge (small)	4 to 12 places	510	480
Chromatograph	—	6820	6820
Cytometer (cell sorter/analyzer)	1000 cells/s	73,230	73,230
Electrophoresis power supply	—	1360	850
Freezer, blood plasma, medium	13 ft^3, down to −40°F	340[b]	136[b]
Hot plate, concentric ring	4 holes, 212°F	3750	2970
Incubator, CO_2	5 to 10 ft^3, up to 130°F	9660	4810
Incubator, forced draft	10 ft^3, 80 to 140°F	2460	1230
Incubator, general application	1.4 to 11 ft^3, up to 160°F	160 to 220[b]	80 to 110[b]
Magnetic stirrer	—	2050	2050
Microcomputer	16 to 256 kbytes[c]	341 to 2047	300 to 1800
Minicomputer	—	7500 to 15,000	7500 to 15,000
Oven, general purpose, small	1.4 to 2.8 ft^3, 460°F	2120[b]	290[b]
Refrigerator, laboratory	22 to 106 ft^3, 39°F	80[d]	34[d]
Refrigerator, blood, small	7 to 20 ft^3, 39°F	260[b]	102[b]
Spectrophotometer	—	1710	1710
Sterilizer, freestanding	3.9 ft^3, 212 to 270°F	71,400	8100
Ultrasonic cleaner, small	1.4 ft^3	410	410
Washer, glassware	7.8 ft^3 load area	15,220	10,000
Water still	5 to 15 gal	14,500[e]	320[e]

Source: Alereza and Breen (1984).
[a]For hospital equipment installed under a hood, the heat gain is assumed to be zero.
[b]Heat gain per cubic foot of interior space.
[c]Input is not proportional to memory size.
[d]Heat gain per 10 ft^3 of interior space.
[e]Heat gain per gallon of capacity.

components. In addition, such things as computer schedules and near-term future planning should be considered. Heat gains from digital computer equipment range from 75 to 175 Btu/h·ft^2. While the trend in hardware development is toward less heat release on a component basis, the associated miniaturization tends to offset such unitary reduction by a higher concentration of equipment.

7.3.5 Ventilation and Infiltration Air

Wind and pressure differences cause outdoor air to infiltrate into the cracks around doors and windows, resulting in localized sensible and latent heat gains. Also, some outdoor ventilation air is needed to eliminate any odors. This outdoor air imposes a cooling and dehumidifying load on the cooling coil because heat and/or moisture must be removed from the air. Heat gains due to infiltration and ventilation can be computed using equations in Chapter 5.

These equations are valid for calculating the cooling load due to infiltration of outside air and also due to the positive introduction of air for ventilation, provided it is introduced directly into the space.

7.3.6 Moisture Transfer Through Permeable Building Materials

In the usual comfort air-conditioning application, moisture transfer through walls is often neglected, since the actual rate is small and the corresponding latent heat gain is insignificant. On the other hand, industrial applications frequently call for a low moisture content in a conditioned space. Here, moisture transfer cannot be neglected, as the latent heat gain accompanying this transfer may be of greater magnitude than any other latent heat gain. Under these conditions, proper calculation of the moisture transfer due to both air infiltration and diffusion through building materials is important.

7.3.7 Miscellaneous Sources of Heat

Fans that circulate air through HVAC systems add energy to the system by one or all of the following processes:

Temperature rise in the airstream from fan inefficiency. Depending on the equipment, fan efficiencies generally range between 50 and 70%, with an average value of 65%. Thus, some 35% of the energy required by the fan appears as instantaneous heat gain to the air being transported.

Temperature rise in the airstream as a consequence of air static and velocity pressure. The fan energy that creates pressure to move air spreads throughout the entire air transport system in the process of conversion into sensible heat. Designers commonly assume that the temperature change equivalent of this heat occurs in one point in the system, depending on fan location.

Temperature rise from heat generated by motor and drive inefficiencies. The relatively small gains from fan motors and drives are normally disregarded unless the motor and/or drive are physically located within the conditioned airstream. Equations (7-22), (7-23), and (7-24) may be used to estimate heat gains from typical motors. Belt drive losses are often estimated as 3% of the rated motor power.

The location of each fan relative to other elements (primarily the cooling coil), the type of system (single zone, multizone, double-duct, terminal reheat, VAV, etc.), and the type of equipment control (space temperature alone, space temperature and relative humidity, and so forth) must be known before the analysis can be completed. A fan located upstream of the cooling coil (blow-through supply fan, return air fan, outside air fan) adds the heat equivalent to its inefficiency to the airstream temperature at that point; the cooling coil sees this as elevated entering dry-bulb temperature. Afan located downstream of the cooling coil raises the dry-bulb temperature of air leaving the cooling coil. This rise can be offset by reducing the cooling coil temperature, or alternatively, by increasing airflow across the cooling coil.

Unless return air duct systems are extensive or subjected to rigorous conditions, only the heat gained or lost by supply duct systems is significant. It is estimated as a percentage of space sensible cooling load (normally about 1%) and applied to the air dry-bulb temperature of the air leaving the coil in the form of an equivalent temperature reduction.

Losses from air leakage out of (or into) ductwork or equipment can be greater than conventional duct heat gain or loss, but is normally about the same or less. Outward duct leakage is a direct loss of cooling and/or dehumidifying capacity and must be offset by increased airflow (sometimes reduced supply air temperature) unless it enters the conditioned space directly. Inward duct leakage causes temperature and/or humidity variations, but it is often ignored under ordinary circumstances due to the low temperature and pressure differentials involved.

A well-designed and properly installed duct system should not leak more than 1 to 3% of the total system airflow. HVAC equipment and volume control units connected into a duct system should be delivered from manufacturers with allowable leakage rates not exceeding 1 or 2% of maximum airflow. Where duct systems are specified to be sealed and leak-tested, both low- and high-pressure types can be constructed and be required to fall in this range. Latent heat considerations are frequently ignored.

Poorly designed or installed duct systems can have leakage rates of 10 to 30%. Leakage from low-pressure lighting troffer connections lacking proper taping and sealing runs up to 35% or more of the terminal air supply. Such extremes can ruin the validity of any load calculation. As such, they may not affect overall system loads enough to cause problems; they will, however, always adversely impact required supply air quantities for most air-conditioning systems. Also, using uninsulated supply ductwork running through return air plenums results in high thermal leakage, loss of space cooling capability by the supply air, and condensation difficulties during a warm start-up.

7.4 Transfer Function Method

The **transfer function method** (TFM) applies a series of weighting factors, or coefficients of *room transfer functions*, to heat gain and cooling load values from previous hours as well as the current hour. These factors account for the thermal storage effect in converting heat gain to cooling load. Such weighting factors relate to spatial geometry, configuration, mass, and other characteristics of the space, and reflect weighted variations in thermal storage effect on a time basis, rather than a straight-line average.

Transfer functions relate an output function to the value of one or more driving functions at a given time and at a set period immediately preceding. While the TFM is preferable to other methods and technically sound for a specific cooling load analysis, its computational complexity requires computer use.

A transfer function is a set of coefficients that relates an output function at some specific time to the value of one or more driving functions at that time and to previous values of both the input and output functions. For example, a component of cooling load at time θ, Q_θ can be related to the corresponding component of the heat gain q_θ by an expression of the form:

$$Q_\theta = v_o q_\theta + v_1 q_{\theta-\Delta} + v_2 q_{\theta-2\Delta} + \cdots - w_1 Q_{\theta-\Delta} - w_2 Q_{\theta-2\Delta} - w_3 Q_{\theta-3\Delta} - \cdots \quad (7\text{-}29)$$

Values of the v_o, v_1, ... and the w_1, w_2, ... coefficients depend on heat storage characteristics of the building and on the nature of the particular heat gain component.

The main advantage of the TFM is that it takes the calculation a step beyond the determination of cooling load and evaluates both the rate at which heat is removed from a space and the temperature of the space when a specific size and type of cooling unit is used. This phase of the analysis also allows the designer to evaluate the effects of different schedules of operation. By evaluating the deviations of room air temperature from the nominal design value, the entire width of the comfort zone can be used and equipment can be selected that can maintain conditions within this zone.

Calculation of heat gains due to (1) solar radiation, (2) heat sources within the conditioned space, and (3) ventilation and infiltration air are identical to those given for space cooling load in prior sections.

Specific details of using this method are given in Chapter 28 of the 1997 *ASHRAE Handbook—Fundamentals*.

7.5 CLTD/SCL/CLF Calculation Procedure

The CLTD/SCL/CLF method is a one-step, hand calculation procedure, based on the transfer function method (TFM) which is applicable to commercial and institutional buildings. It may be used to approximate the cooling load corresponding

Table 7-19 Procedure for Calculating Space Design Cooling Load by CLTD/SCL/CLF Method

External Cooling Load

Roofs, walls, and conduction through glass

$$q = UA(\text{CLTD})$$

U = design heat transfer coefficient for roof or wall from Chapter 5

A = area of roof, wall, or glass, calculated from building plans

CLTD = cooling load temperature difference, roof, wall, or glass, Tables 7-20, 7-22, and 7-25.

Solar load through glass

$$q = A(\text{SC})(\text{SCL})$$

SC = shading coefficient, Tables 7-4 through 7-11

SCL = solar cooling load factor with no interior shade or with shade, Table 7-27.

Cooling load from partitions, ceilings, floors

$$q = UA(t_o - t_{rc})$$

U = design heat transfer coefficient for partition, ceiling, or floor, from Chapter 5

A = area of partition, ceiling, or floor, calculated from building plans

t_b = temperature in adjacent space

t_{rc} = inside design temperature (constant) in conditioned space

Internal Cooling Load

People

$$q_{sensible} = N(\text{Sensible heat gain})\text{CLF}$$

$$q_{latent} = N(\text{Latent heat gain})$$

N = number of people in space, from best available source. Sensible and latent heat gain from occupancy—Table 7-14

CLF = cooling load factor, by hour of occupancy, Table 7-28

Note: CLF 1.0 with high density or 24-h occupancy and/or if cooling off at night or during weekends.

Lights

$$q_{el} = 3.41 W F_{ul} F_{sa}\,(\text{CLF})$$

W = watts input from electrical plans or lighting fixture data

F_{ul} = lighting use factor, as appropriate

F_{sa} = special allowance factor, as appropriate

CLF = cooling load factor, by hour of occupancy, Table 7-29

Note: CLF = 1.0 with 24-h light usage and/or if cooling off at night or during weekends.

Power

$$q_p = 2545\, P E_F\, \text{CLF}$$

P = horsepower rating from electrical plans or manufacturer's data

E_F = efficiency factors and arrangements to suit circumstances

CLF = cooling load factor, by hour of occupancy, Table 7-28

Note: CLF = 1.0 with 24-h power operation and/or if cooling off at night or during weekends.

Appliances

$$q_{sensible} = q_{input} F_U F_R (\text{CLF})$$

or

$$q_{sensible} = q_{input} F_L (\text{CLF})$$

q_{input} = rated energy input from appliances—Tables 7-17 and 7-18

F_U, F_R, F_L = usage factors, radiation factors,and load factors from the General Principles section

CLF = cooling load factor, by scheduled hours and hooded or not; Tables 7-28 and 7-30

Note 1: CLF = 1.0 with 24-h appliance operation and/or if cooling off at night or during weekends.

Note 2: Set latent load = 0 if appliance under exhaust hood.

Ventilation and Infiltration Air

$$q_{sensible} = 1.10\, Q\, (t_o - t_i)$$

$$q_{latent} = 4840\, Q\, (W_o - W_i)$$

$$q_{total} = 4.5\, Q\, (h_o - h_i)$$

Q = ventilation cfm from ASHRAE *Standard* 62; infiltration from Chapter 5

t_o, t_i = outside, inside air temperature, °F

W_o, W_i = outside, inside air humidity ratio, lb (water)/lb (dry air)

h_o, h_i = outside, inside air enthalpy, Btu/lb (dry air)

to the first three modes of heat gain (conductive heat gain through surfaces such as windows, walls, and roofs; solar heat gain through fenestrations; and internal heat gain from lights, people, and equipment) and the cooling load from infiltration and ventilation. The acronyms are defined as follows:

CLTD—Cooling Load Temperature Difference

SCL—Solar Cooling Load

CLF—Cooling Load Factor

The following sections give details of how the CLTD/SCL/CLF technique relates to and differs from the TFM. The sources of the space cooling load, forms of equations to use in the calculations, and appropriate references and tables are summarized in Table 7-19.

This method was developed by using the TFM to compute one-dimensional transient heat flow through various sunlit roofs and walls. Heat gain was converted to cooling load using the room transfer function for rooms with light, medium, and heavy thermal characteristics. **All calculations for data tabulated were based on the sol-air temperatures in Table 7-1. The inside air temperature was assumed to be constant at 78°F (cooling system in operation 24 h/day, seven days a week) and the outside mean daily temperature was assumed to be 85°F.**

7.5.1 Basic CLTD Cooling Load for Exterior Surfaces

The results were generalized to some extent by dividing the cooling load by the U-factor for each roof or wall and are in units of total equivalent CLTD. This establishes the basic cooling load equation for exterior surfaces as

$$q = UA(\text{CLTD}) \tag{7-30}$$

where

q = cooling load, Btu/h
U = coefficient of heat transfer, Btu/h·ft²·°F
A = area of surface, ft²
CLTD = cooling load temperature difference, °F

In developing the method, it was assumed that the heat flow through a similar roof or wall (similar in thermal mass as well as U-factor) can be obtained by multiplying the total CLTDs listed in Tables 7-20 or 7-22 by the U-factor of the roof or wall at hand, respectively. The errors introduced by this approach depend on the extent of the differences between the construction in question (components, size, configuration, and general mass of building and contents) and the one used for calculating the CLTDs. The code numbers and thermal properties for the roofs and walls are listed in Table 7-23.

The sol-air temperature value depends on outdoor air temperature as well as the intensity of solar radiation. Consequently, a change in either outdoor air temperature or geographic location changes the sol-air temperature. The CLTD values in the tables were computed for an indoor air temperature of 78°F, an outdoor maximum temperature of 95°F, and an outdoor mean temperature of 85°F, with an outdoor daily range of 21°F and a solar radiation variation typical of 40°N latitude on July 21.

The notes associated with Table 7-20 and 7-22 provide descriptions of the conditions under which the CLTD values were calculated. While variations in exterior color and/or outside and inside surface film resistances do have some effect, their impact on roofs or walls of contemporary construction is relatively minor and can be ignored with data that is already normalized for convenience. Variations in inside space temperature or the mean outdoor temperature are of much more significance, and the means of appropriate adjustment are thus outlined. Additional guidance for specific application may be found along with tables for a broad range of latitudes and months in the *Cooling and Heating Load Calculation Manual* (McQuiston and Spitler 1992).

7.5.2 Space Cooling Load from Fenestration

The principles of calculating heat gain for fenestration consists of two components, conduction and solar heat gain.

CLTD Cooling Load from Conduction. For conduction heat gain, the overall heat transfer coefficient accounts for the heat transfer processes of (1) convection and long-wave radiation exchange outside and inside the conditioned space and (2) conduction through the fenestration material. To calculate cooling load for this component, the conduction heat gain is treated in similar to that through walls and roofs. The coefficients used to convert the heat gain to cooling load are the same as those for walls and roofs. The resulting CLTDs are given in Table 7-25, again presenting only a single set of factors for all room construction types, neglecting the effects of mass and latitude due to the generally low density and the small magnitude of these components.

The CLTDs from Table 7-25 can also be used for doors with reasonable accuracy. The cooling load from conduction and convection heat gain is calculated by

$$q_{cond} = UA(\text{CLTD}) \tag{7-31}$$

where A is the net glass area of the fenestration in square feet. [Note that this equation is identical to Equation (7-30).]

Solar Heat Gain. The basic principles of evaluating heat gain from transmitted and absorbed solar energy through fenestration, including the primary terms solar heat gain factor (SHGF) and shading coefficient (SC), are the same for the CLTD/CLF procedure as previously described.

Previous *ASHRAE Handbooks* tabulated values of maximum SHGFs for sunlit or externally shaded double-strength sheet glass, used as the heat gain input for calculating CLFs, using appropriate coefficients. This process, however, introduced new variables into the calculations: (1) the presence or absence of interior shading devices, which is pivotal, and (2) the construction, furnishings, floor coverings, and relative amounts of fenestration, which are critical when interior shading is absent. Results obtained with this method do not recognize the significant variation of solar cooling load profiles (SCL) due to different latitudes, months, and other factors. The term SCL is introduced to more closely approximate cooling loads due to solar radiation transmitted through fenestration.

Cooling load caused by solar radiation through fenestration is calculated by

$$q_{rad} = A(\text{SC})(\text{SCL}) \tag{7-32}$$

where

q_{rad} = cooling load caused by solar radiation, Btu/h
A = net glass area of fenestration, ft²
SC = shading coefficient, for combination of fenestration and shading device
SCL = solar cooling load, Btu/h·ft²

Total Cooling Load from Fenestration. The total cooling load due to fenestration is the sum of the conductive and radiant components q_{cond} and q_{rad}.

Zone Influencing Parameters. For purposes of estimating a cooling load, a zone is a particular combination of conditions defining the space under consideration. The SCL for a particular zone depends on latitude, direction, nature, and quantity of enclosing surfaces, as well as various internal parameters that influence the SHGF for each glass exposure in that zone.

To determine the most appropriate zone for finding the SCL, refer to Tables 7-26A through 7-26E, where zone types

Table 7-20-J24 July Cooling Load Temperature Differences for Calculating Cooling Load from Flat Roofs at 24° North Latitude

Roof No.	Solar time, hr 1	2	3	4	5	6	7	8	9	10	11	12	13	14	15	16	17	18	19	20	21	22	23	24
1	0	-2	-4	-5	-6	-6	-3	9	26	44	62	76	87	92	92	86	74	58	39	23	14	8	4	2
2	2	0	-2	-4	-5	-6	-5	1	14	30	48	64	77	86	90	89	82	70	53	36	23	14	8	5
3	12	8	5	2	0	-2	-2	3	11	22	35	47	59	68	74	77	74	68	58	47	37	29	22	16
4	16	11	6	3	0	-2	-3	-4	-1	5	15	27	41	55	67	75	80	80	76	67	55	43	32	23
5	21	16	12	8	5	3	1	1	4	10	19	30	42	52	61	68	71	70	66	59	50	41	33	27
8	28	24	20	17	14	11	9	9	10	14	20	27	35	43	49	54	58	58	56	52	47	42	37	32
9	31	25	20	16	12	9	6	4	3	5	10	17	26	36	46	54	61	65	66	63	58	51	44	37
10	36	31	27	22	19	15	12	9	8	8	11	16	22	30	37	45	52	56	59	59	56	52	47	41
13	34	31	28	25	22	20	17	16	15	16	19	23	28	33	38	43	47	49	50	49	46	43	40	37
14	34	32	30	27	25	23	21	19	19	19	21	24	27	32	36	40	43	45	46	45	44	42	39	37

Table 7-20-J32 July Cooling Load Temperature Differences for Calculating Cooling Load from Flat Roofs at 32° North Latitude

Roof No.	Solar time, hr 1	2	3	4	5	6	7	8	9	10	11	12	13	14	15	16	17	18	19	20	21	22	23	24
1	0	-2	-4	-5	-6	-6	-1	11	27	45	62	76	86	91	91	85	75	59	41	25	15	9	5	2
2	2	0	-2	-4	-5	-6	-4	3	16	32	48	64	76	85	89	88	82	70	55	38	24	15	9	5
3	12	8	5	2	0	-2	-1	4	12	23	35	48	59	68	74	76	74	68	59	48	38	29	22	17
4	17	11	7	3	1	-1	-3	-3	0	6	16	28	42	55	66	75	79	80	76	67	56	44	33	24
5	21	16	12	8	5	3	1	1	5	12	21	31	42	52	61	67	71	70	66	59	51	42	34	27
8	29	25	21	17	14	12	10	9	11	15	21	28	35	43	49	54	57	58	57	53	48	43	38	33
9	32	26	21	16	12	9	6	4	4	6	11	18	27	37	46	54	61	65	66	64	59	52	45	38
10	37	32	27	23	19	15	12	10	9	9	12	16	23	30	38	45	52	56	59	59	56	52	47	42
13	34	31	28	25	23	20	18	16	16	17	20	24	28	33	39	43	47	49	50	49	47	44	41	38
14	35	32	30	28	25	23	21	20	19	20	22	24	28	32	36	40	43	45	46	46	44	42	40	37

Table 7-20-J40 July Cooling Load Temperature Differences for Calculating Cooling Load from Flat Roofs at 40° North Latitude

Roof No.	Solar time, hr 1	2	3	4	5	6	7	8	9	10	11	12	13	14	15	16	17	18	19	20	21	22	23	24
1	0	-2	-4	-5	-6	-6	0	13	29	45	60	73	83	88	88	83	73	60	43	26	15	9	5	2
2	2	0	-2	-4	-5	-6	-4	4	17	32	48	62	74	82	86	85	80	70	56	39	25	15	9	5
3	12	8	5	2	0	-2	0	5	13	24	35	47	57	66	72	74	73	67	59	48	38	30	23	17
4	17	11	7	3	1	-1	-3	-3	0	7	17	29	42	54	65	73	77	78	74	67	56	45	34	24
5	21	16	12	8	5	3	1	2	6	12	21	31	41	51	60	66	69	69	65	59	51	42	34	27
8	28	24	21	17	14	12	10	10	12	16	21	28	35	42	48	53	56	57	56	52	48	43	38	33
9	32	26	21	16	13	9	6	4	4	7	12	19	27	36	45	53	59	63	64	63	58	52	45	38
10	37	32	27	23	19	15	12	10	9	10	12	17	23	30	37	44	50	55	57	58	56	52	47	42
13	34	31	28	25	22	20	18	16	16	17	20	24	28	33	38	42	46	48	49	48	46	44	40	37
14	35	32	30	27	25	23	21	20	19	20	22	24	28	32	36	39	42	44	45	45	44	42	40	37

Table 7-20-J48 July Cooling Load Temperature Differences for Calculating Cooling Load from Flat Roofs at 48° North Latitude

Roof No.	Solar time, hr 1	2	3	4	5	6	7	8	9	10	11	12	13	14	15	16	17	18	19	20	21	22	23	24
1	0	-2	-4	-5	-6	-5	3	15	29	44	58	69	78	83	83	79	71	59	44	29	17	9	5	2
2	2	0	-2	-4	-5	-5	-2	6	19	32	47	60	70	78	82	81	76	68	55	41	27	16	10	5
3	12	8	5	2	0	-1	1	6	14	24	35	45	55	63	68	71	70	65	58	48	38	30	23	17
4	17	12	7	3	1	-1	-3	-2	2	8	18	29	40	52	62	69	73	74	71	65	55	45	34	25
5	21	16	12	8	5	3	2	3	7	13	21	31	40	49	57	63	66	66	63	58	50	42	34	27
8	28	24	20	17	14	11	10	10	12	16	21	27	34	40	46	51	54	55	54	51	47	42	37	32
9	31	26	21	16	12	9	6	5	5	8	12	19	27	35	43	51	57	60	62	61	57	51	44	38
10	36	31	27	22	19	15	12	10	9	10	13	17	23	29	36	43	48	53	55	56	54	51	46	41
13	33	30	27	25	22	20	17	16	16	18	20	24	28	32	37	41	44	47	48	47	45	43	40	37
14	34	32	29	27	25	23	21	20	19	20	22	24	27	31	35	38	41	43	44	44	43	41	39	36

1. Direct Application of Data,
   - Dark surface
   - Indoor temperature of 78°F
   - Outdoor maximum temperature of 95°F with mean temperature of 85°F and daily range of 21°F
   - Solar radiation typical of clear day on 21st day of month
   - Outside surface film resistance of 0.333 (h·ft²·°F)/Btu
   - With or without suspended ceiling but no ceiling plenum air return systems
   - Inside surface film resistance of 0.685 (h·ft²·°F)/Btu

2. Adjustments to Table Data
   Design temperatures:

$$\text{Corr. CLTD} = \text{CLTD} + (78 - T_r) + (T_m - 85)$$

   where T_r = inside temperature and
   T_m = mean outdoor temperature,
   T_m = maximum outdoor temperature − (daily range)/2
   - No adjustment recommended for color
   - No adjustment recommended for ventilation of air space above a ceiling

Table 7-20-A24 August Cooling Load Temperature Differences for Calculating Cooling Load from Flat Roofs at 24° North Latitude

Roof No.	1	2	3	4	5	6	7	8	9	10	11	12	13	14	15	16	17	18	19	20	21	22	23	24
	Solar time, hr																							
1	-1	-2	-4	-5	-6	-7	-5	5	22	41	59	75	86	91	91	84	72	55	35	21	13	8	4	1
2	1	-1	-2	-4	-5	-6	-6	-1	11	27	45	62	76	85	89	88	80	67	50	33	21	13	8	4
3	11	7	4	2	-1	-2	-3	1	9	20	33	46	57	67	73	75	73	66	55	44	35	27	21	15
4	15	10	6	3	0	-2	-3	-4	-3	3	13	25	39	53	65	74	79	79	74	64	53	41	30	22
5	20	15	11	7	5	2	0	0	2	8	17	28	40	51	60	66	69	69	64	56	47	39	32	25
8	27	23	19	16	13	11	8	7	9	13	18	25	33	41	48	53	56	56	54	50	45	40	35	31
9	29	24	19	15	11	8	6	3	2	4	8	16	24	34	44	53	60	63	64	61	56	49	42	35
10	34	30	25	21	18	14	11	9	7	7	9	14	20	28	36	43	50	55	57	57	54	50	45	39
13	32	29	26	24	21	19	16	15	14	15	17	21	26	32	37	42	45	47	48	47	44	42	38	35
14	33	31	28	26	24	22	20	18	17	18	19	22	26	30	34	38	41	43	44	43	42	40	38	35

Table 7-20-A32 August Cooling Load Temperature Differences for Calculating Cooling Load from Flat Roofs at 32° North Latitude

Roof No.	1	2	3	4	5	6	7	8	9	10	11	12	13	14	15	16	17	18	19	20	21	22	23	24
	Solar time, hr																							
1	-1	-2	-4	-5	-6	-7	-4	6	23	41	58	72	82	88	88	82	70	54	36	21	13	8	4	1
2	1	-1	-2	-4	-5	-6	-6	-1	11	27	44	60	73	82	86	85	78	66	50	33	21	13	8	4
3	11	7	4	1	-1	-2	-2	1	9	20	32	44	56	65	71	73	70	64	54	44	35	27	20	15
4	15	10	6	3	0	-2	-3	-4	-2	3	13	25	38	51	63	71	76	76	72	63	52	40	30	22
5	19	15	11	7	4	2	0	0	3	9	17	28	39	49	58	64	67	67	62	55	47	39	31	25
8	26	23	19	16	13	10	8	8	9	13	18	25	32	40	46	51	54	55	53	49	44	39	35	30
9	29	24	19	15	11	8	5	3	3	4	9	15	24	33	43	51	58	61	62	60	55	48	41	35
10	34	29	25	21	17	14	11	9	7	7	10	14	20	27	35	42	48	53	55	55	53	49	44	39
13	32	29	26	23	21	18	16	14	14	15	17	21	26	31	36	40	44	46	47	46	43	41	38	35
14	32	30	28	25	23	21	19	18	17	17	19	22	25	29	33	37	40	42	43	42	41	39	37	35

Table 7-20-A40 August Cooling Load Temperature Differences for Calculating Cooling Load from Flat Roofs at 40° North Latitude

Roof No.	1	2	3	4	5	6	7	8	9	10	11	12	13	14	15	16	17	18	19	20	21	22	23	24
	Solar time, hr																							
1	-1	-2	-4	-5	-6	-7	-3	7	22	39	55	68	78	83	83	77	67	53	36	22	13	7	4	1
2	1	-1	-3	-4	-5	-6	-5	0	11	26	42	57	69	77	81	80	74	63	48	33	21	13	8	4
3	10	7	4	1	-1	-2	-2	2	9	19	30	42	53	61	67	69	67	61	52	43	34	26	20	15
4	15	10	6	2	0	-2	-4	-4	-2	4	13	24	36	49	59	67	72	72	68	61	50	39	29	21
5	19	14	10	7	4	2	0	0	3	9	17	26	37	46	55	61	64	63	60	53	45	37	30	24
8	25	22	18	15	12	10	8	7	9	12	17	24	31	38	44	49	51	52	51	47	43	38	34	29
9	28	23	18	14	11	8	5	3	3	4	8	15	23	32	41	48	55	58	59	57	52	46	40	34
10	33	28	24	20	17	13	10	8	7	7	9	13	19	26	33	40	46	50	53	53	50	47	42	37
13	30	28	25	22	20	17	15	14	13	14	17	20	24	29	34	38	42	44	45	44	42	39	36	33
14	31	29	26	24	22	20	18	17	16	17	18	21	24	28	32	35	38	40	41	41	39	37	35	33

Table 7-20-A48 August Cooling Load Temperature Differences for Calculating Cooling Load from Flat Roofs at 48° North Latitude

Roof No.	1	2	3	4	5	6	7	8	9	10	11	12	13	14	15	16	17	18	19	20	21	22	23	24
	Solar time, hr																							
1	-1	-3	-4	-5	-6	-7	-3	7	21	36	50	62	71	76	76	72	63	50	35	21	13	7	4	1
2	1	-1	-3	-4	-5	-6	-5	1	11	25	39	52	63	71	75	74	69	59	46	32	21	13	7	4
3	10	6	3	1	-1	-3	-2	2	9	18	28	39	48	56	61	64	62	57	50	40	32	25	19	14
4	14	9	5	2	0	-2	-4	-4	-2	4	12	22	34	45	55	62	66	67	64	57	48	37	28	20
5	18	13	10	6	4	1	0	0	3	8	16	25	34	43	50	56	59	59	56	50	43	35	29	23
8	24	20	17	14	11	9	7	7	8	12	16	22	28	35	40	45	48	48	47	44	40	36	32	28
9	26	22	17	13	10	7	4	3	2	4	8	14	21	29	37	45	50	54	55	53	49	44	38	32
10	31	26	22	19	15	12	10	7	6	7	9	13	18	24	31	37	42	46	49	49	47	44	40	35
13	28	26	23	21	18	16	14	13	12	13	16	19	23	27	31	35	39	41	41	41	39	37	34	31
14	29	27	25	23	21	19	17	16	15	16	17	20	23	26	29	33	35	37	38	38	37	35	33	31

1. Direct Application of Data,
   - Dark surface
   - Indoor temperature of 78°F
   - Outdoor maximum temperature of 95°F with mean temperature of 85°F and daily range of 21°F
   - Solar radiation typical of clear day on 21st day of month
   - Outside surface film resistance of 0.333 (h·ft²·°F)/Btu
   - With or without suspended ceiling but no ceiling plenum air return systems
   - Inside surface film resistance of 0.685 (h·ft²·°F)/Btu

2. Adjustments to Table Data
   Design temperatures:

$$\text{Corr. CLTD} = \text{CLTD} + (78 - T_r) + (T_m - 85)$$

where T_r = inside temperature and

T_m = mean outdoor temperature,

T_m = maximum outdoor temperature − (daily range)/2

   - No adjustment recommended for color
   - No adjustment recommended for ventilation of air space above a ceiling

Table 7-21 Roof Numbers Used In Table 7-20

Mass Location**	Suspended Ceiling	R-Value, h·ft²·°F/Btu	B7, Wood 1 in.	C12, HW Concrete 2 in.	A3, Steel Deck	Attic-Ceiling Combination
Mass inside the insulation	Without	0 to 5	*	2	*	*
		5 to 10	*	2	*	*
		10 to 15	*	4	*	*
		15 to 20	*	4	*	*
		20 to 25	*	5	*	*
		25 to 30	*	*	*	*
	With	0 to 5	*	5	*	*
		5 to 10	*	8	*	*
		10 to 15	*	13	*	*
		15 to 20	*	13	*	*
		20 to 25	*	14	*	*
		25 to 30	*	*	*	*
Mass evenly placed	Without	0 to 5	1	2	1	1
		5 to 10	2	*	1	2
		10 to 15	2	*	1	2
		15 to 20	4	*	2	2
		20 to 25	4	*	2	4
		25 to 30	*	*	*	*
	With	0 to 5	*	3	1	*
		5 to 10	4	*	1	*
		10 to 15	5	*	2	*
		15 to 20	9	*	2	*
		20 to 25	10	*	4	*
		25 to 30	10	*	*	*
Mass outside the insulation	Without	0 to 5	*	2	*	*
		5 to 10	*	3	*	*
		10 to 15	*	4	*	*
		15 to 20	*	5	*	*
		20 to 25	*	5	*	*
		25 to 30	*	*	*	*
	With	0 to 5	*	3	*	*
		5 to 10	*	3	*	*
		10 to 15	*	4	*	*
		15 to 20	*	5	*	*
		20 to 25	*	*	*	*
		25 to 30	*	*	*	*

*Denotes a roof that is not possible with the chosen parameters.

**The 2 in. concrete is considered massive and the others nonmassive.

Table 7-22-J24 July Cooling Load Temperature Differences for Calculating Cooling Load from Sunlit Walls 24° North Latitude

Wall No. 1 — Solar time, hr

Wall Facing	1	2	3	4	5	6	7	8	9	10	11	12	13	14	15	16	17	18	19	20	21	22	23	24
N	1	0	-1	-2	-3	-2	5	13	17	18	19	22	26	28	30	32	34	34	27	17	11	7	5	3
NE	1	0	-1	-2	-3	0	17	39	51	53	48	39	32	30	30	30	28	24	18	13	10	7	5	3
E	1	0	-1	-2	-3	0	18	44	59	63	59	48	36	32	31	30	28	24	19	13	10	7	5	3
SE	1	0	-1	-2	-3	-2	8	25	38	44	45	42	35	32	31	30	27	24	18	13	10	7	5	3
S	1	0	-1	-2	-3	-3	-1	3	8	12	18	24	29	31	31	30	27	23	18	13	9	7	4	3
SW	1	0	-1	-2	-3	-3	-1	3	8	13	17	22	29	40	51	58	59	52	36	20	12	8	5	3
W	2	0	-1	-2	-2	-3	-1	3	8	13	17	22	27	42	59	73	80	75	52	27	14	9	5	3
NW	2	0	-1	-2	-2	-3	-1	3	8	13	17	22	27	37	50	62	69	67	48	25	13	8	5	3

Wall No. 2 — Solar time, hr

Wall Facing	1	2	3	4	5	6	7	8	9	10	11	12	13	14	15	16	17	18	19	20	21	22	23	24
N	5	3	2	0	-1	-2	-1	2	7	12	15	18	20	23	25	28	30	32	32	29	23	17	12	8
NE	5	3	2	0	-1	-2	0	9	23	36	44	46	43	38	34	32	31	29	26	22	18	14	10	7
E	5	3	2	0	-1	-2	0	10	26	42	52	55	52	44	38	35	32	30	27	23	18	14	10	8
SE	5	3	2	0	-1	-2	-1	4	14	26	35	40	41	38	35	33	31	29	26	22	18	14	10	7
S	5	3	1	0	-1	-2	-2	-1	1	4	8	13	19	24	27	29	29	28	26	22	17	13	10	7
SW	6	4	2	1	-1	-2	-2	-1	1	5	9	13	18	24	32	42	50	54	52	44	33	22	15	10
W	8	5	2	1	0	-1	-2	-1	1	5	9	13	17	23	33	46	59	69	71	61	45	30	19	12
NW	7	4	2	1	-1	-1	-2	-1	1	5	9	13	17	22	30	40	51	60	62	55	41	28	18	12

Wall No. 3 — Solar time, hr

Wall Facing	1	2	3	4	5	6	7	8	9	10	11	12	13	14	15	16	17	18	19	20	21	22	23	24
N	8	5	4	2	1	0	1	5	8	11	14	16	19	21	24	26	29	30	30	26	21	17	13	10
NE	7	5	3	2	1	0	4	14	25	34	38	38	36	35	33	32	31	29	26	22	19	15	12	9
E	7	5	3	2	1	0	5	16	29	39	45	46	43	40	37	35	33	30	27	23	19	16	12	10
SE	7	5	3	2	0	0	2	8	17	25	31	34	35	34	33	32	31	29	26	22	18	15	12	9
S	7	5	3	1	0	-1	-1	0	2	5	9	13	18	22	25	26	26	26	23	20	17	14	11	9
SW	10	7	5	3	1	0	0	1	3	6	9	13	17	24	32	40	46	48	45	37	30	23	18	14
W	13	9	6	4	2	1	0	1	3	6	9	13	17	24	34	46	56	62	59	50	39	30	23	17
NW	12	8	6	4	2	1	0	1	3	6	9	13	17	22	30	39	48	54	53	45	35	27	21	16

Wall No. 4 — Solar time, hr

Wall Facing	1	2	3	4	5	6	7	8	9	10	11	12	13	14	15	16	17	18	19	20	21	22	23	24
N	12	8	6	4	2	1	0	0	3	6	10	13	15	18	21	23	26	28	30	30	28	24	20	15
NE	10	7	5	3	2	0	0	3	10	20	29	36	39	39	37	35	34	32	30	27	24	20	16	13
E	10	8	5	3	2	1	0	3	11	22	34	43	47	46	43	40	37	34	32	28	25	21	17	13
SE	10	7	5	3	2	0	0	1	5	13	21	28	33	35	35	35	33	32	30	27	24	20	16	13
S	10	7	5	3	2	0	-1	-1	-1	1	4	7	11	16	20	24	26	27	27	25	22	19	16	12
SW	15	11	7	5	3	1	0	-1	0	1	4	7	11	15	21	29	37	43	47	47	42	35	27	21
W	20	14	9	6	4	2	0	0	0	2	4	7	11	15	21	30	41	52	60	61	56	46	36	27
NW	18	13	9	6	3	1	0	0	0	2	4	7	11	15	20	27	36	45	52	54	50	42	33	25

Wall No. 5 — Solar time, hr

Wall Facing	1	2	3	4	5	6	7	8	9	10	11	12	13	14	15	16	17	18	19	20	21	22	23	24
N	13	11	9	7	5	3	2	3	5	7	10	12	14	16	19	21	23	25	27	27	25	22	19	16
NE	13	11	8	7	5	3	3	6	12	20	26	31	33	33	32	32	31	31	29	27	24	21	18	16
E	14	11	9	7	5	4	3	6	13	22	31	36	39	39	37	36	35	33	31	29	26	22	19	16
SE	13	10	8	6	5	3	2	4	8	14	20	25	28	30	30	30	30	30	28	26	24	21	18	15
S	11	9	7	6	4	3	2	1	1	3	5	7	11	14	18	20	22	23	23	22	20	18	16	14
SW	18	15	12	9	7	5	3	3	3	4	5	8	11	14	20	26	32	38	41	40	36	31	27	22
W	23	19	15	12	9	7	5	4	4	4	6	8	11	15	20	28	37	45	51	51	47	41	34	28
NW	21	17	14	11	8	6	4	3	3	4	6	8	11	14	19	25	32	40	45	46	42	37	31	26

Wall No. 6 — Solar time, hr

Wall Facing	1	2	3	4	5	6	7	8	9	10	11	12	13	14	15	16	17	18	19	20	21	22	23	24
N	14	12	10	8	7	5	4	5	6	8	10	11	13	15	17	20	22	24	25	25	23	21	19	16
NE	14	12	10	8	7	5	5	8	14	20	25	28	29	30	30	30	30	29	28	26	24	22	19	17
E	15	13	11	9	7	6	6	9	15	22	29	33	35	35	34	34	33	32	30	28	26	23	20	18
SE	14	12	10	8	7	5	4	6	10	14	19	23	26	27	28	28	28	28	27	25	23	21	19	16
S	12	10	8	7	5	4	3	3	3	4	5	8	11	14	16	19	20	21	21	21	19	17	16	14
SW	19	16	14	11	9	7	6	5	5	6	7	9	11	15	19	25	30	34	36	36	33	29	26	22
W	24	21	17	14	12	9	8	7	6	7	8	10	12	15	20	27	35	42	46	46	42	37	33	28
NW	22	19	16	13	11	8	7	6	6	6	7	9	11	14	18	24	31	37	41	41	38	34	29	25

Wall No. 7 — Solar time, hr

Wall Facing	1	2	3	4	5	6	7	8	9	10	11	12	13	14	15	16	17	18	19	20	21	22	23	24
N	14	12	11	9	8	7	7	7	9	10	11	12	14	15	17	19	20	22	23	22	21	19	17	16
NE	16	14	12	11	9	8	9	12	17	21	24	26	26	27	27	28	28	27	26	25	23	21	19	17
E	17	15	13	11	10	9	9	13	19	24	28	30	31	31	31	31	30	30	28	27	25	23	21	19
SE	15	13	12	10	9	7	7	9	13	16	20	22	24	25	25	26	26	26	25	23	22	20	18	17
S	12	10	9	8	7	6	5	5	5	6	7	9	11	14	16	17	18	19	19	18	17	16	15	13
SW	19	17	15	13	11	10	8	8	8	8	9	11	13	16	20	24	28	31	32	30	28	26	23	21
W	24	21	19	16	14	12	11	10	10	10	11	12	14	17	22	28	34	39	40	39	36	32	29	26
NW	21	19	17	15	13	11	10	9	9	9	10	11	13	16	20	24	30	34	36	35	32	29	26	24

Wall No. 9 — Solar time, hr

Wall Facing	1	2	3	4	5	6	7	8	9	10	11	12	13	14	15	16	17	18	19	20	21	22	23	24
N	19	16	14	11	9	7	5	4	4	5	6	8	10	12	14	16	18	21	23	25	26	25	23	21
NE	18	16	13	11	9	7	5	4	6	9	15	20	25	29	30	31	31	31	31	30	28	26	24	21
E	19	17	14	12	9	7	6	5	6	10	17	24	30	34	36	36	36	35	34	32	30	28	25	22
SE	18	15	13	11	9	7	5	4	4	6	10	15	20	24	27	28	29	29	29	29	27	25	23	21
S	15	13	11	9	8	6	4	3	2	2	3	4	6	8	11	14	17	20	21	22	22	21	19	18
SW	26	22	18	15	12	10	8	6	4	4	4	5	7	9	12	16	21	27	32	36	37	36	33	30
W	33	28	23	19	16	13	10	8	6	5	5	6	7	9	12	16	22	30	37	44	47	46	43	38
NW	30	25	21	18	14	11	9	7	5	5	5	6	7	9	12	15	20	26	33	38	41	41	38	34

Table 7-22-J24 July Cooling Load Temperature Differences for Calculating Cooling Load from Sunlit Walls 24° North Latitude (*Concluded*)

Wall No. 10

Wall Facing	1	2	3	4	5	6	7	8	9	10	11	12	13	14	15	16	17	18	19	20	21	22	23	24
N	18	16	14	12	10	8	6	5	5	6	7	8	10	12	14	16	18	20	22	24	24	24	22	21
NE	19	16	14	12	9	8	6	6	7	11	16	20	24	27	29	30	30	30	30	29	28	26	24	21
E	20	17	15	12	10	8	6	6	8	12	18	24	29	32	34	34	35	34	33	32	30	28	25	23
SE	18	16	13	11	9	7	6	5	6	8	11	16	20	23	25	27	28	29	29	28	27	25	23	21
S	15	14	12	10	8	6	5	4	3	3	3	4	6	9	11	14	17	19	20	21	21	20	19	17
SW	26	22	19	16	13	11	8	7	5	5	5	6	7	9	12	16	21	26	31	34	35	34	32	29
W	32	28	24	20	17	14	11	9	7	6	6	7	8	10	13	17	23	30	37	42	44	43	40	37
NW	29	25	22	18	15	12	10	8	6	6	6	6	8	10	12	16	21	27	32	37	39	38	36	33

Wall No. 11

Wall Facing	1	2	3	4	5	6	7	8	9	10	11	12	13	14	15	16	17	18	19	20	21	22	23	24
N	17	16	14	13	11	10	8	8	8	8	9	10	11	12	14	15	17	18	20	21	22	21	20	19
NE	19	17	16	14	12	11	10	9	11	14	17	21	23	25	26	26	27	27	27	26	26	24	23	21
E	21	19	17	15	13	12	10	10	12	15	19	24	27	29	30	30	30	30	30	29	28	26	25	23
SE	18	17	15	13	12	10	9	8	9	11	14	17	19	21	23	24	25	25	25	25	24	23	22	20
S	14	13	12	11	9	8	7	6	5	5	6	6	8	10	12	14	15	17	18	18	18	18	17	16
SW	23	21	19	17	15	13	12	10	9	9	9	9	10	11	14	17	20	24	28	30	30	29	27	25
W	29	26	24	21	19	17	15	13	12	11	11	11	12	13	15	18	23	28	33	36	37	36	34	32
NW	26	24	21	19	17	15	13	12	10	10	10	10	11	12	14	17	20	25	29	32	33	33	31	29

Wall No. 12

Wall Facing	1	2	3	4	5	6	7	8	9	10	11	12	13	14	15	16	17	18	19	20	21	22	23	24
N	17	16	14	13	12	10	9	8	8	9	9	10	11	12	14	15	16	18	19	20	21	20	19	18
NE	20	18	16	15	13	12	11	10	12	14	17	20	22	24	25	25	26	26	26	26	25	24	23	21
E	21	19	18	16	14	13	12	11	13	16	19	23	26	28	29	29	29	29	29	28	27	26	25	23
SE	19	17	16	14	13	11	10	9	10	11	14	16	19	21	22	23	24	24	25	24	24	23	21	20
S	14	13	12	11	10	9	8	7	6	6	6	7	8	10	11	13	15	16	17	17	17	17	16	15
SW	23	21	19	17	16	14	12	11	10	10	9	10	11	12	14	17	20	23	26	28	28	28	26	25
W	29	26	24	22	20	18	16	14	13	12	12	12	12	13	15	18	22	27	31	35	35	35	33	31
NW	26	24	22	20	18	16	14	13	11	11	11	11	12	13	14	17	20	24	28	31	32	31	30	28

Wall No. 13

Wall Facing	1	2	3	4	5	6	7	8	9	10	11	12	13	14	15	16	17	18	19	20	21	22	23	24
N	16	15	14	13	12	11	10	9	9	10	10	11	12	13	14	15	16	17	19	19	20	19	18	17
NE	19	18	17	16	14	13	12	12	13	16	18	20	22	23	24	24	25	25	25	25	24	23	22	21
E	21	20	18	17	15	14	13	13	15	17	20	23	25	27	27	28	28	28	28	27	26	25	24	23
SE	18	17	16	15	13	12	11	11	11	13	15	17	19	20	21	22	23	23	23	23	23	22	21	20
S	14	13	12	11	10	9	8	7	7	7	7	8	9	10	12	13	14	15	16	16	16	16	15	15
SW	22	20	19	17	16	15	13	12	11	11	11	11	12	13	15	17	20	23	25	26	26	26	25	23
W	27	25	23	22	20	18	17	15	14	14	13	13	14	15	16	19	23	27	30	33	33	32	31	29
NW	24	23	21	20	18	16	15	14	13	12	12	12	13	14	15	17	20	24	27	29	29	29	28	26

Wall No. 14

Wall Facing	1	2	3	4	5	6	7	8	9	10	11	12	13	14	15	16	17	18	19	20	21	22	23	24
N	17	16	15	14	13	12	11	11	10	10	11	11	12	12	13	14	15	16	17	18	18	18	18	17
NE	20	19	18	17	16	15	14	13	14	15	17	19	21	22	22	23	24	24	24	24	24	23	22	21
E	22	21	20	19	17	16	15	15	15	17	19	21	23	25	26	26	27	27	27	27	26	25	24	23
SE	19	18	17	16	15	14	13	12	12	13	14	16	18	19	20	21	21	22	22	22	22	22	21	20
S	14	13	12	12	11	10	9	9	8	8	8	8	9	10	11	12	13	14	15	15	15	15	15	15
SW	22	21	20	18	17	16	15	14	13	12	12	12	13	13	14	16	18	20	22	24	25	24	24	23
W	27	26	24	23	21	20	19	17	16	16	15	15	15	15	16	18	21	24	27	29	30	30	30	29
NW	24	23	22	21	19	18	17	16	15	14	14	14	14	14	15	17	19	21	24	26	27	27	27	26

Wall No. 15

Wall Facing	1	2	3	4	5	6	7	8	9	10	11	12	13	14	15	16	17	18	19	20	21	22	23	24
N	21	19	17	15	13	11	9	8	7	6	6	7	8	9	11	13	15	17	19	21	22	23	23	22
NE	22	20	18	16	14	11	10	8	7	8	11	14	18	22	24	26	28	29	29	29	29	28	26	24
E	24	22	19	17	14	12	10	9	8	9	12	16	21	25	29	31	32	33	33	33	32	30	29	26
SE	22	20	17	15	13	11	9	8	7	7	8	11	14	17	20	23	25	26	27	27	27	26	25	24
S	17	16	14	13	11	9	8	6	5	4	4	4	5	6	8	10	13	15	17	19	19	20	20	19
SW	29	26	24	21	18	15	13	11	9	7	6	6	6	7	9	11	15	19	23	27	31	32	32	31
W	37	33	30	26	23	20	16	14	11	9	8	8	8	9	10	12	16	21	26	32	37	40	40	39
NW	33	30	27	24	21	18	15	12	10	8	7	7	7	8	9	12	15	19	23	28	33	35	36	35

Wall No. 16

Wall Facing	1	2	3	4	5	6	7	8	9	10	11	12	13	14	15	16	17	18	19	20	21	22	23	24
N	20	18	17	15	14	12	11	9	8	8	8	8	9	10	11	13	14	16	17	19	20	21	21	21
NE	22	21	19	17	15	13	12	10	10	10	12	15	18	21	23	24	26	27	27	27	27	26	25	24
E	24	22	20	18	16	14	12	11	10	11	13	17	20	24	26	28	30	30	31	31	30	29	28	26
SE	21	20	18	16	14	13	11	10	9	9	10	12	14	17	19	21	23	24	25	25	25	25	24	23
S	17	16	14	13	12	10	9	8	6	6	5	5	6	7	8	10	12	14	16	17	18	18	18	17
SW	27	25	23	21	19	17	15	13	11	10	9	8	8	9	10	12	15	18	22	25	28	29	29	28
W	34	32	29	26	24	21	18	16	14	12	11	10	10	11	11	13	16	20	25	30	33	36	36	35
NW	30	28	26	24	21	19	17	14	12	11	10	9	9	10	11	12	15	18	22	26	30	32	32	32

1. Direct Application of Data,
   - Dark surface
   - Indoor temperature of 78°F
   - Outdoor maximum temperature of 95°F with mean temperature of 85°F and daily range of 21°F
   - Solar radiation typical of clear day on 21st day of month
   - Outside surface film resistance of 0.333 (h·ft^2·°F)/Btu
   - Inside surface film resistance of 0.685 (h·ft^2·°F)/Btu

2. Adjustments to Table Data
   Design temperatures:

$$\text{Corr. CLTD} = \text{CLTD} + (78 - T_r) + (T_m - 85)$$

where T_r = inside temperature and
T_m = mean outdoor temperature,
T_m = maximum outdoor temperature − (daily range)/2

- No adjustment recommended for color

Table 7-22-J32 July Cooling Load Temperature Differences for Calculating Cooling Load from Sunlit Walls 32° North Latitude

Wall No. 1 — Solar time, hr

Wall Facing	1	2	3	4	5	6	7	8	9	10	11	12	13	14	15	16	17	18	19	20	21	22	23	24
N	1	0	-1	-2	-3	-2	6	12	14	15	18	22	25	28	29	29	30	31	27	17	11	7	5	3
NE	1	0	-1	-2	-3	1	21	41	49	48	41	33	29	29	30	29	28	24	19	14	10	7	5	3
E	1	0	-1	-2	-3	1	23	48	61	64	59	48	36	32	31	30	28	24	19	14	10	7	5	3
SE	1	0	-1	-2	-3	-1	12	29	42	50	52	49	42	35	32	30	28	24	19	14	10	7	5	3
S	1	0	-1	-2	-3	-3	0	4	8	16	25	34	40	42	41	36	30	25	19	13	10	7	5	3
SW	2	0	-1	-2	-2	-2	0	4	8	13	17	23	34	47	58	65	64	57	41	22	13	8	5	3
W	2	1	-1	-2	-2	-2	0	4	8	13	17	22	27	42	59	73	80	77	58	30	15	9	6	3
NW	2	0	-1	-2	-2	-2	0	4	8	13	17	21	26	32	43	56	65	66	52	27	14	8	5	3

Wall No. 2 — Solar time, hr

Wall Facing	1	2	3	4	5	6	7	8	9	10	11	12	13	14	15	16	17	18	19	20	21	22	23	24
N	5	3	2	0	-1	-2	-1	3	7	10	13	15	18	22	25	27	28	29	30	28	23	17	12	8
NE	5	3	2	0	-1	-2	1	11	25	37	42	42	38	34	32	31	30	29	26	23	18	14	10	7
E	5	3	2	0	-1	-2	1	13	30	45	54	56	52	45	38	35	32	30	27	23	18	14	11	8
SE	5	3	2	0	-1	-2	0	6	17	29	39	45	47	44	40	36	33	30	27	23	18	14	10	8
S	5	3	2	0	-1	-2	-2	-1	1	5	11	18	26	33	37	39	37	34	29	24	19	14	10	7
SW	7	4	2	1	-1	-2	-2	-1	2	5	9	13	18	26	37	47	56	60	58	49	36	25	16	11
W	8	5	3	1	0	-1	-2	-1	2	5	9	13	17	23	33	46	59	69	72	64	48	32	20	13
NW	7	4	2	1	-1	-2	-2	-1	2	5	9	13	17	22	27	36	46	55	60	55	42	29	19	12

Wall No. 3 — Solar time, hr

Wall Facing	1	2	3	4	5	6	7	8	9	10	11	12	13	14	15	16	17	18	19	20	21	22	23	24
N	8	5	3	2	1	0	2	5	7	9	12	15	18	21	23	25	26	28	28	25	21	17	13	10
NE	7	5	3	2	1	0	6	16	26	33	35	35	33	32	31	31	30	28	26	22	18	15	12	9
E	7	5	4	2	1	0	7	19	31	41	46	47	44	40	37	35	33	31	27	23	19	16	13	10
SE	7	5	3	2	1	0	3	10	20	29	35	39	40	39	36	35	33	30	27	23	19	16	13	10
S	7	5	3	2	0	0	-1	1	3	6	12	18	25	30	33	34	33	30	27	23	19	16	12	10
SW	11	8	5	3	2	0	0	1	3	6	9	13	19	27	36	44	50	53	49	41	33	25	20	15
W	13	10	7	4	2	1	1	2	4	6	9	13	17	24	34	45	56	62	62	52	41	32	24	18
NW	12	9	6	4	2	1	0	1	3	6	9	13	16	21	27	35	44	51	52	45	35	28	21	16

Wall No. 4 — Solar time, hr

Wall Facing	1	2	3	4	5	6	7	8	9	10	11	12	13	14	15	16	17	18	19	20	21	22	23	24
N	11	8	6	4	2	0	0	0	3	6	8	11	14	17	20	22	25	26	28	28	27	23	19	15
NE	10	7	5	3	2	0	0	3	11	21	29	34	36	35	34	33	32	31	29	27	24	20	16	13
E	10	8	5	4	2	1	0	4	13	25	36	44	48	47	44	40	37	34	32	29	25	21	17	13
SE	10	8	5	3	2	0	0	2	7	15	24	32	38	41	41	39	37	34	32	29	25	21	17	13
S	10	8	5	3	2	0	-1	-1	0	2	5	9	15	22	28	32	34	34	33	30	26	21	17	14
SW	17	12	8	5	3	1	0	0	0	2	4	7	11	17	24	32	41	48	53	52	47	38	30	23
W	21	15	10	6	4	2	0	0	0	2	4	8	11	15	21	30	41	52	60	63	58	49	38	28
NW	18	13	9	6	3	1	0	0	0	2	4	7	11	15	19	25	32	41	48	52	49	42	33	25

Wall No. 5 — Solar time, hr

Wall Facing	1	2	3	4	5	6	7	8	9	10	11	12	13	14	15	16	17	18	19	20	21	22	23	24
N	13	11	8	6	5	3	2	3	5	7	8	10	12	15	18	20	22	24	25	25	24	21	18	16
NE	13	10	8	6	5	3	3	7	13	20	26	29	30	30	30	30	30	29	28	26	24	21	18	15
E	14	11	9	7	5	4	3	7	15	24	32	38	40	39	38	37	35	34	32	29	26	23	20	17
SE	13	11	9	7	5	3	3	5	9	16	23	28	33	35	35	34	33	32	31	28	25	22	19	16
S	13	10	8	6	5	3	2	2	2	3	6	10	14	20	24	27	29	29	28	27	24	21	18	15
SW	20	16	13	10	8	6	4	3	3	4	6	8	11	16	22	29	36	42	45	44	40	35	29	24
W	24	20	16	12	9	7	5	4	4	5	6	9	11	15	20	28	37	46	52	53	49	42	36	29
NW	21	17	14	11	8	6	4	3	3	4	6	8	11	14	18	23	29	37	42	44	41	36	31	25

Wall No. 6 — Solar time, hr

Wall Facing	1	2	3	4	5	6	7	8	9	10	11	12	13	14	15	16	17	18	19	20	21	22	23	24
N	14	12	10	8	6	5	4	5	6	7	9	10	12	14	17	19	20	22	23	23	22	20	18	16
NE	14	12	10	8	7	5	6	9	15	20	24	26	27	28	28	28	28	28	27	26	24	21	19	16
E	16	13	11	9	7	6	6	10	17	24	30	34	36	36	35	34	34	32	31	29	26	23	21	18
SE	15	13	11	9	7	6	5	7	11	16	22	26	30	31	32	32	31	31	29	27	25	22	20	17
S	14	12	10	8	6	5	4	3	4	5	7	10	14	18	22	25	26	27	26	25	23	20	18	16
SW	21	18	15	12	10	8	7	6	6	6	7	9	12	16	22	28	34	38	40	39	36	32	28	25
W	25	21	18	15	12	10	8	7	7	7	8	10	12	15	20	27	35	42	47	47	44	39	34	29
NW	22	18	15	13	10	8	7	6	6	6	8	9	11	14	17	22	28	34	39	39	37	33	29	25

Wall No. 7 — Solar time, hr

Wall Facing	1	2	3	4	5	6	7	8	9	10	11	12	13	14	15	16	17	18	19	20	21	22	23	24
N	13	12	10	9	8	7	7	7	8	9	10	11	13	14	16	18	19	20	21	21	20	18	17	15
NE	15	13	12	10	9	8	9	13	17	21	23	24	25	25	26	26	26	26	25	24	22	21	19	17
E	17	15	13	12	10	9	10	15	20	25	29	31	32	32	32	31	31	30	29	27	25	23	21	19
SE	16	14	12	11	9	8	8	11	14	19	22	25	27	28	28	29	28	28	27	25	24	22	20	18
S	14	12	11	9	8	7	6	6	6	7	9	12	15	18	21	23	23	23	23	22	20	19	17	16
SW	21	18	16	14	12	11	9	9	9	9	10	11	14	18	22	27	32	35	35	34	31	28	26	23
W	24	22	19	17	15	13	11	10	10	10	11	12	14	17	22	28	34	39	41	40	37	34	30	27
NW	21	19	16	14	12	11	9	9	9	9	10	11	13	15	18	23	28	32	35	34	31	29	26	23

Wall No. 9 — Solar time, hr

Wall Facing	1	2	3	4	5	6	7	8	9	10	11	12	13	14	15	16	17	18	19	20	21	22	23	24
N	18	15	13	11	9	7	5	4	4	4	6	7	9	11	13	15	17	20	21	23	24	24	22	20
NE	18	16	13	11	9	7	5	5	6	10	15	21	25	27	28	29	29	29	29	29	27	25	23	21
E	20	17	14	12	10	8	6	5	7	11	18	25	31	35	37	37	36	36	34	33	31	28	26	23
SE	19	16	14	11	9	7	6	5	5	8	12	17	23	27	31	32	33	33	32	31	30	27	25	22
S	18	15	13	11	9	7	5	4	3	3	3	5	7	11	15	20	23	26	27	28	27	25	23	20
SW	28	24	20	17	14	11	9	7	5	5	5	6	7	9	13	18	23	30	35	40	41	40	37	33
W	34	29	24	20	16	13	10	8	6	6	6	6	8	10	12	17	22	30	37	44	48	48	44	39
NW	29	25	21	17	14	11	9	7	5	5	5	6	7	9	12	15	19	24	30	36	39	40	37	34

Table 7-22-J32 July Cooling Load Temperature Differences for Calculating Cooling Load from Sunlit Walls 32° North Latitude (*Concluded*)

Wall Facing	Wall No. 10												Solar time, hr											
	1	2	3	4	5	6	7	8	9	10	11	12	13	14	15	16	17	18	19	20	21	22	23	24
N	18	15	13	11	9	7	6	5	5	5	6	7	9	11	13	15	17	19	21	22	23	23	21	20
NE	18	16	14	11	9	7	6	6	8	12	16	20	23	26	27	28	28	29	29	28	27	25	23	21
E	20	17	15	12	10	8	7	6	9	13	19	25	30	33	35	35	35	35	34	32	31	28	26	23
SE	19	17	14	12	10	8	6	6	6	9	13	18	22	26	29	31	32	32	31	31	29	27	25	22
S	18	16	13	11	9	7	6	4	4	3	4	6	8	12	15	19	22	25	26	26	26	24	22	20
SW	28	24	21	18	15	12	9	7	6	5	6	6	8	10	14	18	24	29	34	38	39	38	35	32
W	34	29	25	21	18	14	11	9	7	7	6	7	8	10	13	17	23	30	37	42	45	44	42	38
NW	29	25	21	18	15	12	10	8	6	6	6	6	8	10	12	15	19	25	30	35	37	37	35	32

Wall Facing	Wall No. 11												Solar time, hr											
	1	2	3	4	5	6	7	8	9	10	11	12	13	14	15	16	17	18	19	20	21	22	23	24
N	16	15	13	12	11	9	8	7	7	8	8	9	10	11	13	14	16	17	19	20	20	20	19	18
NE	19	17	15	14	12	11	9	9	11	14	17	20	22	23	24	25	25	26	26	25	25	23	22	20
E	21	19	17	15	14	12	11	11	13	16	21	25	28	30	31	31	31	31	30	30	28	27	25	23
SE	20	18	16	14	13	11	10	9	10	12	15	19	22	25	26	27	28	28	28	27	26	25	23	22
S	17	16	14	13	11	10	8	7	7	6	7	8	10	12	15	18	20	22	22	23	22	21	20	19
SW	25	23	21	19	17	15	13	11	10	10	10	10	11	12	15	19	23	27	30	33	33	32	30	28
W	30	27	24	22	19	17	15	13	12	11	11	11	12	13	15	18	23	28	33	37	38	38	35	33
NW	26	23	21	19	17	15	13	11	10	10	10	10	11	12	14	16	19	23	27	31	32	32	30	28

Wall Facing	Wall No. 12												Solar time, hr											
	1	2	3	4	5	6	7	8	9	10	11	12	13	14	15	16	17	18	19	20	21	22	23	24
N	16	15	14	12	11	10	9	8	8	8	9	9	10	11	13	14	15	17	18	19	20	19	18	17
NE	19	17	16	14	13	12	10	10	12	14	17	20	22	23	23	24	25	25	25	25	24	23	22	21
E	22	20	18	16	15	13	12	12	14	17	21	24	27	29	29	30	30	30	30	29	28	27	25	23
SE	20	18	17	15	14	12	11	10	11	13	16	19	21	24	25	26	27	27	27	27	26	25	23	22
S	17	16	14	13	12	10	9	8	7	7	8	9	10	12	15	17	19	21	21	22	21	21	20	18
SW	25	23	21	19	17	15	14	12	11	11	11	11	12	13	15	18	22	26	29	31	31	31	29	27
W	29	27	25	22	20	18	16	15	13	13	12	12	13	14	16	19	23	27	32	35	36	36	34	32
NW	25	23	21	19	17	15	14	12	11	11	11	11	11	12	14	16	19	22	26	29	30	30	29	27

Wall Facing	Wall No. 13												Solar time, hr											
	1	2	3	4	5	6	7	8	9	10	11	12	13	14	15	16	17	18	19	20	21	22	23	24
N	16	15	14	12	11	10	9	9	9	9	10	10	11	12	13	14	15	16	17	18	18	18	17	17
NE	19	18	16	15	14	13	12	12	13	16	18	20	21	22	23	23	24	24	24	24	23	22	21	20
E	22	20	19	17	16	14	13	14	15	18	21	24	26	28	28	28	29	29	28	28	27	26	25	23
SE	20	19	17	16	15	13	12	12	13	14	17	19	21	23	24	25	25	26	26	25	25	24	23	21
S	17	15	14	13	12	11	10	9	9	8	9	10	11	13	15	17	19	20	20	20	20	19	19	18
SW	24	22	21	19	18	16	15	14	13	12	12	12	13	14	16	19	22	25	28	29	29	29	27	26
W	28	26	24	22	21	19	17	16	15	14	14	14	14	15	17	19	23	27	31	33	34	33	32	30
NW	24	22	21	19	17	16	15	13	13	12	12	12	13	14	15	17	19	22	25	28	28	28	27	25

Wall Facing	Wall No. 14												Solar time, hr											
	1	2	3	4	5	6	7	8	9	10	11	12	13	14	15	16	17	18	19	20	21	22	23	24
N	16	15	14	13	12	12	11	10	10	10	10	10	11	12	12	13	14	15	16	17	17	17	17	16
NE	20	19	18	17	15	14	13	13	14	15	17	19	20	21	21	22	22	23	23	23	23	22	22	21
E	23	22	20	19	18	17	16	15	16	18	20	22	24	26	26	27	27	27	27	27	27	26	25	24
SE	21	20	19	17	16	15	14	13	14	14	16	18	20	21	23	23	24	24	25	25	24	24	23	22
S	17	16	15	14	13	12	11	11	10	10	10	10	11	12	14	15	17	18	19	19	19	19	18	18
SW	24	23	22	20	19	18	17	15	15	14	14	13	14	14	16	18	20	23	25	27	27	27	26	25
W	28	27	25	24	22	21	19	18	17	16	16	15	16	16	17	19	21	24	27	30	31	31	31	29
NW	24	23	21	20	19	17	16	15	14	14	13	13	14	14	15	16	18	20	23	25	26	26	26	25

Wall Facing	Wall No. 15												Solar time, hr											
	1	2	3	4	5	6	7	8	9	10	11	12	13	14	15	16	17	18	19	20	21	22	23	24
N	20	18	16	14	13	11	9	7	6	6	6	6	7	9	10	12	14	16	17	19	21	22	22	21
NE	22	20	17	15	13	11	9	8	7	9	11	14	18	21	23	25	26	27	28	28	27	27	25	24
E	24	22	19	17	15	12	10	9	8	10	13	17	22	26	30	32	33	34	34	33	32	31	29	27
SE	23	21	19	16	14	12	10	8	7	8	9	12	16	20	23	26	28	30	30	30	30	29	27	25
S	21	19	17	15	13	11	9	7	6	5	5	5	6	8	10	14	17	20	22	24	25	25	24	22
SW	32	29	26	23	20	17	14	12	10	8	7	7	7	8	10	13	16	21	26	30	34	36	36	34
W	38	35	31	27	24	20	17	14	12	10	9	8	8	9	10	12	16	21	26	32	37	40	41	40
NW	32	29	26	23	20	17	15	12	10	8	7	7	7	8	9	11	14	17	22	27	31	34	34	34

Wall Facing	Wall No. 16												Solar time, hr											
	1	2	3	4	5	6	7	8	9	10	11	12	13	14	15	16	17	18	19	20	21	22	23	24
N	19	18	16	15	13	12	10	9	8	7	7	8	8	9	10	12	13	15	16	18	19	20	20	20
NE	22	20	18	17	15	13	11	10	10	10	12	15	18	20	22	23	24	25	26	26	26	25	25	23
E	25	23	21	19	16	15	13	11	11	12	14	18	22	25	27	29	30	31	31	31	31	30	28	27
SE	23	21	19	18	16	14	12	10	10	10	11	13	16	19	22	24	26	27	28	28	28	27	26	25
S	20	19	17	15	14	12	11	9	8	7	6	6	7	9	11	13	16	18	20	22	22	22	22	21
SW	30	28	26	23	21	18	16	14	12	11	10	9	9	10	11	13	16	20	24	28	31	32	32	31
W	35	33	30	27	24	22	19	17	14	13	12	11	11	11	12	14	16	20	25	30	34	36	37	36
NW	29	28	26	23	21	19	16	14	12	11	10	9	9	10	11	12	14	17	21	25	28	30	31	31

1. Direct Application of Data,
   - Dark surface
   - Indoor temperature of 78°F
   - Outdoor maximum temperature of 95°F with mean temperature of 85°F and daily range of 21°F
   - Solar radiation typical of clear day on 21st day of month
   - Outside surface film resistance of 0.333 (h·ft²·°F)/Btu
   - Inside surface film resistance of 0.685 (h·ft²·°F)/Btu

2. Adjustments to Table Data
   Design temperatures:

$$\text{Corr. CLTD} = \text{CLTD} + (78 - T_r) + (T_m - 85)$$

where T_r = inside temperature and
T_m = mean outdoor temperature,
T_m = maximum outdoor temperature − (daily range)/2
   - No adjustment recommended for color

Table 7-22-J40 July Cooling Load Temperature Differences for Calculating Cooling Load from Sunlit Walls 40° North Latitude

Wall No. 1

Wall Facing	1	2	3	4	5	6	7	8	9	10	11	12	13	14	15	16	17	18	19	20	21	22	23	24
N	1	0	-1	-2	-3	-1	7	11	11	13	17	21	25	27	29	29	28	29	27	17	11	7	5	3
NE	1	0	-1	-2	-3	2	24	42	47	43	35	28	27	28	29	29	27	24	20	14	10	7	5	3
E	1	0	-1	-2	-2	2	28	51	62	64	59	48	36	31	30	30	28	25	20	14	10	7	5	3
SE	1	0	-1	-2	-3	0	15	32	46	55	58	56	49	39	33	31	28	25	20	14	10	7	5	3
S	1	0	-1	-2	-3	-2	0	4	11	21	33	43	50	52	50	44	34	27	20	14	10	7	5	3
SW	2	0	-1	-2	-2	-2	0	4	8	13	17	25	39	53	64	70	69	61	45	24	13	8	5	3
W	2	1	-1	-2	-2	-2	1	4	8	13	17	21	27	42	59	73	80	79	62	32	16	9	6	3
NW	2	0	-1	-2	-2	-2	0	4	8	13	17	21	25	29	38	50	61	64	55	29	15	9	5	3

Wall No. 2

Wall Facing	1	2	3	4	5	6	7	8	9	10	11	12	13	14	15	16	17	18	19	20	21	22	23	24
N	5	3	2	0	-1	-2	-1	3	7	9	11	14	18	21	24	26	27	28	28	27	22	17	12	8
NE	5	3	2	0	-1	-2	2	13	26	36	39	37	33	31	29	29	29	28	26	23	18	14	10	7
E	5	3	2	0	-1	-1	2	15	32	47	55	57	52	44	38	34	32	30	27	23	19	14	11	8
SE	5	3	2	0	-1	-2	0	8	20	33	43	50	53	51	45	39	35	31	28	24	19	14	11	8
S	5	3	2	0	-1	-2	-2	-1	2	7	14	24	33	42	47	48	46	40	33	27	21	15	11	8
SW	7	4	2	1	0	-1	-2	0	2	5	9	13	20	30	41	53	61	65	62	53	39	27	17	11
W	8	5	3	1	0	-1	-2	0	2	5	9	13	17	23	33	46	59	69	73	66	50	34	22	14
NW	8	4	2	1	-1	-2	-2	-1	2	5	9	13	17	21	25	32	41	51	57	54	42	29	19	12

Wall No. 3

Wall Facing	1	2	3	4	5	6	7	8	9	10	11	12	13	14	15	16	17	18	19	20	21	22	23	24
N	7	5	3	2	1	0	2	5	7	8	11	14	17	20	23	24	25	26	27	24	20	16	13	10
NE	7	5	3	2	0	0	7	17	26	31	33	31	30	29	29	29	29	28	25	22	18	15	12	9
E	7	5	4	2	1	1	8	21	33	42	47	47	44	40	37	35	33	31	28	24	20	16	13	10
SE	8	5	4	2	1	0	4	12	22	32	39	44	46	44	41	38	35	32	29	24	20	16	13	10
S	8	6	4	2	1	0	0	1	4	9	16	24	31	38	41	42	40	36	31	26	22	17	14	11
SW	12	9	6	4	2	1	1	2	4	6	9	14	21	30	40	49	55	57	54	45	36	28	21	16
W	14	10	7	5	3	1	1	2	4	6	9	13	17	24	34	45	56	63	63	54	43	33	25	19
NW	12	8	6	4	2	1	0	2	3	6	9	13	16	20	25	32	40	48	50	44	35	27	21	16

Wall No. 4

Wall Facing	1	2	3	4	5	6	7	8	9	10	11	12	13	14	15	16	17	18	19	20	21	22	23	24
N	11	8	6	4	2	0	0	1	3	5	7	10	13	16	19	22	24	26	27	27	26	22	19	15
NE	10	7	5	3	2	0	0	4	12	21	29	32	33	32	31	30	30	29	28	26	23	20	16	13
E	10	8	5	4	2	1	1	5	15	27	38	45	49	47	44	40	37	34	32	29	25	21	17	14
SE	11	8	6	4	2	1	0	2	8	17	27	36	43	46	46	44	41	37	34	30	26	22	18	14
S	11	8	6	4	2	1	0	-1	0	2	6	13	20	28	35	41	43	42	39	35	30	24	19	15
SW	18	13	9	6	3	2	0	0	0	2	5	8	12	18	27	36	46	53	57	57	51	42	33	25
W	21	15	10	7	4	2	1	0	1	2	5	8	11	15	21	30	40	51	60	64	60	50	40	30
NW	18	13	9	6	3	1	0	0	0	2	4	8	11	15	19	23	30	37	45	49	48	41	33	25

Wall No. 5

Wall Facing	1	2	3	4	5	6	7	8	9	10	11	12	13	14	15	16	17	18	19	20	21	22	23	24
N	13	10	8	6	5	3	2	3	5	6	8	9	12	14	17	19	21	23	24	24	23	21	18	15
NE	13	10	8	6	5	3	3	7	14	20	25	27	28	28	28	28	28	28	27	26	23	21	18	15
E	14	11	9	7	5	4	4	8	17	26	33	39	40	40	38	37	35	34	32	29	26	23	20	17
SE	14	12	9	7	5	4	3	6	11	18	25	32	37	39	39	38	37	35	33	30	27	24	20	17
S	15	12	9	7	5	4	3	2	3	4	8	13	19	25	31	35	36	36	34	32	28	24	21	18
SW	22	18	14	11	8	6	5	4	4	5	6	9	12	17	25	33	40	46	49	48	44	38	32	26
W	25	20	16	13	10	7	5	4	4	5	7	9	11	15	20	28	37	45	52	54	50	44	37	30
NW	21	17	13	10	8	6	4	3	4	4	6	8	11	14	17	21	27	34	40	42	40	35	30	25

Wall No. 6

Wall Facing	1	2	3	4	5	6	7	8	9	10	11	12	13	14	15	16	17	18	19	20	21	22	23	24
N	13	11	9	8	6	5	4	5	6	7	8	10	12	14	16	18	20	21	22	23	21	20	17	15
NE	14	12	10	8	6	5	6	10	15	20	23	25	25	26	26	27	27	27	26	25	23	21	18	16
E	16	13	11	9	7	6	7	11	18	25	31	35	36	36	35	35	34	33	31	29	26	24	21	18
SE	16	14	11	9	8	6	6	8	13	18	24	29	33	35	36	35	34	33	32	29	27	24	21	18
S	16	13	11	9	7	6	5	4	4	6	9	13	18	24	28	31	33	33	31	29	27	24	21	18
SW	23	19	16	14	11	9	7	6	6	7	8	10	13	18	24	31	37	42	44	43	40	35	31	27
W	26	22	18	15	13	10	8	7	7	7	8	10	12	15	20	27	35	42	47	48	45	40	35	30
NW	21	18	15	12	10	8	7	6	6	6	8	9	11	14	16	21	26	32	36	38	36	32	28	25

Wall No. 7

Wall Facing	1	2	3	4	5	6	7	8	9	10	11	12	13	14	15	16	17	18	19	20	21	22	23	24
N	13	12	10	9	7	6	6	7	8	8	9	11	12	14	16	17	18	19	20	20	19	18	16	15
NE	15	13	11	10	9	8	9	13	17	20	22	23	23	24	24	25	25	25	24	23	22	20	18	16
E	17	15	13	12	10	9	11	16	21	26	30	32	32	32	32	32	31	30	29	27	25	23	21	19
SE	17	15	13	12	10	9	9	12	16	21	25	28	31	32	32	32	31	30	29	27	25	23	21	19
S	16	14	13	11	10	8	7	7	7	9	12	15	19	23	26	28	29	29	28	26	24	22	20	18
SW	23	20	18	16	13	12	10	10	10	10	11	12	15	20	25	30	35	38	39	37	34	31	28	25
W	25	22	20	17	15	13	12	11	11	11	12	13	14	17	22	28	34	39	42	41	38	34	31	28
NW	20	18	16	14	12	10	9	9	9	9	10	11	13	15	17	21	26	30	33	33	30	28	25	23

Wall No. 9

Wall Facing	1	2	3	4	5	6	7	8	9	10	11	12	13	14	15	16	17	18	19	20	21	22	23	24
N	17	15	13	11	9	7	5	4	4	4	5	7	8	10	12	15	17	19	21	22	23	23	22	20
NE	18	15	13	11	9	7	5	5	6	10	16	20	23	25	26	27	27	28	28	27	26	25	23	20
E	20	17	14	12	10	8	6	5	7	12	19	26	32	36	37	37	37	36	34	33	31	29	26	23
SE	20	17	15	12	10	8	6	5	6	9	13	19	25	31	34	36	37	36	35	34	32	29	26	23
S	21	18	15	12	10	8	6	5	4	3	4	6	10	14	20	25	29	33	34	34	32	30	27	24
SW	31	26	22	18	15	12	9	7	6	5	5	6	8	10	14	19	26	33	39	43	45	44	40	36
W	35	30	25	21	17	14	11	8	7	6	6	7	8	10	12	16	22	30	37	44	48	48	45	41
NW	29	25	21	17	14	11	9	7	5	5	5	6	7	9	11	14	18	22	28	34	37	38	36	33

Column headings 1–24: Solar time, hr

Table 7-22-J40 July Cooling Load Temperature Differences for Calculating Cooling Load from Sunlit Walls 40° North Latitude (*Concluded*)

Wall No. 10 — Solar time, hr

Wall Facing	1	2	3	4	5	6	7	8	9	10	11	12	13	14	15	16	17	18	19	20	21	22	23	24
N	17	15	13	11	9	7	6	5	5	5	6	7	8	10	12	14	17	18	20	22	22	22	21	19
NE	18	16	13	11	9	7	6	6	8	12	16	20	22	24	25	26	27	27	27	27	26	24	22	20
E	20	17	15	12	10	8	7	7	10	14	20	26	31	34	35	36	36	35	34	33	31	28	26	23
SE	21	18	15	13	10	8	7	6	7	10	15	20	25	30	33	34	35	35	34	33	31	29	26	23
S	21	18	15	13	11	9	7	5	4	4	5	7	11	15	20	24	28	31	32	32	31	29	26	24
SW	31	27	23	19	16	13	10	8	7	6	6	7	8	11	15	20	26	32	38	41	42	41	38	35
W	34	30	26	22	18	15	12	9	8	7	7	7	8	10	13	17	23	30	37	42	45	45	42	39
NW	28	24	21	18	15	12	10	8	6	6	6	6	8	10	12	14	18	23	28	33	35	36	34	31

Wall No. 11 — Solar time, hr

Wall Facing	1	2	3	4	5	6	7	8	9	10	11	12	13	14	15	16	17	18	19	20	21	22	23	24
N	16	14	13	12	10	9	8	7	7	7	8	9	10	11	12	14	15	17	18	19	20	19	18	17
NE	18	17	15	13	12	10	9	9	11	14	17	20	21	22	23	23	24	24	25	25	24	23	21	20
E	21	19	17	16	14	12	11	11	13	17	22	26	29	30	31	31	31	31	31	30	29	27	25	23
SE	21	19	17	16	14	12	11	10	11	14	17	21	24	27	29	30	31	31	30	30	29	27	25	23
S	20	18	16	15	13	11	10	9	8	8	8	10	13	16	19	23	25	27	28	28	27	25	24	22
SW	28	25	23	20	18	16	14	12	11	11	10	11	12	14	17	21	25	30	33	36	36	35	33	30
W	31	28	25	22	20	18	16	14	12	12	11	12	12	13	15	19	23	28	33	37	39	38	36	33
NW	25	23	20	18	16	14	12	11	10	9	9	10	11	12	13	15	18	22	26	29	31	31	29	27

Wall No. 12 — Solar time, hr

Wall Facing	1	2	3	4	5	6	7	8	9	10	11	12	13	14	15	16	17	18	19	20	21	22	23	24
N	16	14	13	12	11	10	8	8	8	8	8	9	10	11	12	14	15	16	17	18	19	19	18	17
NE	18	17	15	14	13	11	10	10	12	14	17	19	21	21	22	23	23	24	24	24	23	22	21	20
E	22	20	18	17	15	13	12	12	14	17	21	25	28	29	30	30	30	30	30	29	28	27	25	24
SE	22	20	18	16	15	13	12	11	12	14	17	21	24	26	28	29	30	30	30	29	28	27	25	23
S	20	19	17	15	14	12	11	10	9	9	9	11	13	16	19	22	24	26	26	26	26	25	23	22
SW	27	25	23	21	19	17	15	14	12	12	12	12	12	14	17	20	24	28	32	34	34	34	32	30
W	30	28	25	23	21	19	17	15	14	13	13	13	13	14	16	19	23	27	32	35	37	36	35	33
NW	24	22	20	19	17	15	13	12	11	10	10	11	11	12	13	15	18	21	25	28	29	29	28	26

Wall No. 13 — Solar time, hr

Wall Facing	1	2	3	4	5	6	7	8	9	10	11	12	13	14	15	16	17	18	19	20	21	22	23	24
N	15	14	13	12	11	10	9	9	9	9	9	10	10	11	12	14	15	16	17	18	18	18	17	16
NE	18	17	16	15	13	12	11	12	13	16	18	19	20	21	21	22	23	23	23	23	23	22	21	20
E	22	20	19	17	16	15	14	14	16	19	22	25	27	28	29	29	29	29	29	28	27	26	25	23
SE	22	20	19	17	16	14	13	13	14	16	18	21	24	26	27	28	28	28	28	28	27	26	24	23
S	20	18	17	16	14	13	12	11	10	10	11	12	14	16	19	21	23	24	25	25	24	23	22	21
SW	26	25	23	21	19	18	16	15	14	13	13	13	14	15	18	21	24	28	30	32	32	31	30	28
W	29	27	25	23	21	19	18	16	15	15	14	14	15	15	17	20	23	27	31	34	34	34	32	31
NW	23	22	20	18	17	15	14	13	12	12	12	12	12	13	14	16	18	21	24	26	27	27	26	25

Wall No. 14 — Solar time, hr

Wall Facing	1	2	3	4	5	6	7	8	9	10	11	12	13	14	15	16	17	18	19	20	21	22	23	24
N	15	15	14	13	12	11	10	10	10	10	10	10	10	11	12	13	14	15	15	16	17	17	16	16
NE	19	18	17	16	15	14	13	13	14	15	17	18	19	20	20	21	21	22	22	22	22	22	21	20
E	23	22	21	19	18	17	16	15	16	18	21	23	25	26	27	27	28	28	28	28	27	26	25	24
SE	23	21	20	19	18	16	15	15	15	16	18	20	22	24	25	26	27	27	27	27	26	26	25	24
S	20	19	18	17	16	15	14	13	12	12	12	12	14	15	17	19	21	22	23	23	23	23	22	21
SW	26	25	24	22	21	19	18	17	16	15	15	15	15	16	17	19	22	25	27	29	30	30	29	28
W	29	27	26	24	23	21	20	18	17	16	16	16	16	16	17	19	21	24	27	30	32	32	31	30
NW	23	22	21	19	18	17	16	15	14	13	13	13	13	14	14	15	17	19	21	24	25	25	25	24

Wall No. 15 — Solar time, hr

Wall Facing	1	2	3	4	5	6	7	8	9	10	11	12	13	14	15	16	17	18	19	20	21	22	23	24
N	19	18	16	14	12	10	9	7	6	6	6	6	7	8	9	11	13	15	17	19	20	21	21	20
NE	21	19	17	15	13	11	9	8	7	9	11	14	18	20	22	23	25	25	26	26	26	26	25	23
E	25	22	20	17	15	12	10	9	9	10	14	18	23	27	30	32	34	34	34	33	32	31	29	27
SE	25	22	20	17	15	13	11	9	8	8	10	14	18	22	26	30	32	33	34	33	33	31	30	27
S	25	22	20	17	15	13	11	9	7	6	6	6	7	10	13	17	21	25	28	30	30	30	29	27
SW	35	32	28	25	22	18	16	13	11	9	8	8	8	9	11	14	18	23	28	33	37	39	39	37
W	39	35	32	28	24	21	18	15	12	10	9	8	8	9	10	13	16	21	26	32	38	41	42	41
NW	31	28	26	23	20	17	14	12	10	8	7	7	7	8	9	11	13	16	20	25	29	32	33	33

Wall No. 16 — Solar time, hr

Wall Facing	1	2	3	4	5	6	7	8	9	10	11	12	13	14	15	16	17	18	19	20	21	22	23	24
N	18	17	16	14	13	11	10	9	8	7	7	7	8	9	10	11	13	14	16	17	18	19	19	19
NE	21	20	18	16	14	13	11	10	10	11	13	15	17	19	21	22	23	24	24	25	25	24	24	23
E	25	23	21	19	17	15	13	11	11	12	15	19	22	26	28	30	31	31	32	32	31	30	29	27
SE	25	23	21	19	17	15	13	11	10	11	12	15	18	21	25	27	29	30	31	31	31	30	29	27
S	24	22	20	18	16	14	12	11	9	8	8	8	9	11	14	17	20	23	25	27	27	27	27	25
SW	33	30	28	25	23	20	18	15	13	12	11	10	10	11	12	15	18	22	27	30	33	35	35	34
W	36	33	31	28	25	22	20	17	15	13	12	11	11	11	12	14	17	20	25	30	34	37	38	37
NW	29	27	25	23	20	18	16	14	12	11	10	9	9	10	11	12	14	16	19	23	27	29	30	30

1. Direct Application of Data,
   - Dark surface
   - Indoor temperature of 78°F
   - Outdoor maximum temperature of 95°F with mean temperature of 85°F and daily range of 21°F
   - Solar radiation typical of clear day on 21st day of month
   - Outside surface film resistance of 0.333 (h·ft²·°F)/Btu
   - Inside surface film resistance of 0.685 (h·ft²·°F)/Btu

2. Adjustments to Table Data
   Design temperatures:

$$\text{Corr. CLTD} = \text{CLTD} + (78 - T_r) + (T_m - 85)$$

where T_r = inside temperature and
T_m = mean outdoor temperature,
T_m = maximum outdoor temperature − (daily range)/2
   - No adjustment recommended for color

Table 7-22-J48 July Cooling Load Temperature Differences for Calculating Cooling Load from Sunlit Walls 48° North Latitude

Wall No. 1 — Solar time, hr

Wall Facing	1	2	3	4	5	6	7	8	9	10	11	12	13	14	15	16	17	18	19	20	21	22	23	24
N	1	0	-1	-2	-2	3	9	10	10	13	17	21	24	27	28	28	27	27	27	21	13	8	5	3
NE	1	0	-1	-2	-1	10	30	42	44	38	30	26	26	28	29	29	27	24	20	15	10	7	5	3
E	1	0	-1	-2	-1	10	34	54	63	64	58	47	35	31	30	29	28	25	20	15	10	7	5	3
SE	2	0	-1	-2	-2	4	19	36	50	59	63	61	55	45	36	31	28	25	20	15	10	7	5	3
S	2	0	-1	-2	-2	-2	1	5	15	28	41	52	59	62	59	51	40	29	22	15	11	7	5	3
SW	2	1	-1	-2	-2	-1	1	5	8	12	18	29	45	59	70	75	74	65	49	29	16	9	6	3
W	2	1	-1	-2	-2	-1	1	5	9	13	17	21	26	41	58	72	80	80	67	41	20	11	6	4
NW	2	0	-1	-2	-2	-2	1	5	8	12	17	21	24	27	33	45	56	62	57	37	19	10	6	3

Wall No. 2 — Solar time, hr

Wall Facing	1	2	3	4	5	6	7	8	9	10	11	12	13	14	15	16	17	18	19	20	21	22	23	24
N	6	3	2	0	-1	-1	1	5	7	9	11	14	17	21	24	26	27	27	27	27	24	18	13	9
NE	5	3	2	0	-1	0	6	18	29	36	37	34	30	28	28	28	28	28	26	23	19	14	11	8
E	5	3	2	0	-1	0	6	20	36	49	56	57	52	44	38	34	31	29	27	23	19	15	11	8
SE	5	3	2	0	-1	-1	2	11	23	36	48	55	58	56	51	43	37	33	29	24	20	15	11	8
S	6	4	2	0	-1	-1	-1	0	3	9	19	30	41	50	55	57	54	47	38	30	23	17	12	8
SW	8	5	3	1	0	-1	-1	0	2	6	9	14	22	33	46	58	66	69	67	57	44	30	20	13
W	9	6	3	1	0	-1	-1	0	3	6	9	13	17	22	32	45	58	69	73	69	55	38	25	15
NW	8	5	3	1	0	-1	-1	0	2	5	9	13	17	20	24	29	37	46	54	54	46	33	22	14

Wall No. 3 — Solar time, hr

Wall Facing	1	2	3	4	5	6	7	8	9	10	11	12	13	14	15	16	17	18	19	20	21	22	23	24
N	8	6	4	2	1	1	3	5	7	8	11	14	17	20	22	24	25	25	26	25	21	17	14	10
NE	7	5	3	2	1	3	11	20	27	31	30	29	28	28	28	28	28	27	25	22	19	15	12	9
E	8	5	4	2	1	3	12	24	36	44	48	48	44	40	37	35	33	31	28	24	20	16	13	10
SE	8	6	4	2	1	1	6	15	25	35	43	49	51	49	45	41	37	34	30	26	21	17	14	11
S	9	6	4	3	1	0	0	2	5	12	20	29	38	45	49	50	47	42	36	30	24	19	15	12
SW	13	9	7	4	2	1	1	2	4	6	10	15	24	34	45	54	60	61	58	50	39	31	23	18
W	15	11	8	5	3	2	2	2	4	7	9	13	16	23	33	45	55	62	64	58	46	36	27	20
NW	12	9	6	4	2	1	1	2	4	6	9	13	16	19	23	29	37	44	49	46	38	29	22	17

Wall No. 4 — Solar time, hr

Wall Facing	1	2	3	4	5	6	7	8	9	10	11	12	13	14	15	16	17	18	19	20	21	22	23	24
N	12	9	6	4	2	1	1	2	4	6	8	10	13	16	19	21	24	25	26	26	26	23	19	16
NE	10	8	5	3	2	1	2	7	15	23	29	31	31	30	29	29	29	28	28	26	23	20	17	13
E	11	8	6	4	2	1	2	8	18	30	40	47	49	48	44	40	37	34	31	29	25	21	18	14
SE	11	8	6	4	2	1	1	4	11	20	30	40	47	51	51	49	45	40	36	32	27	23	18	14
S	12	9	6	4	2	1	0	0	1	3	9	16	25	34	43	48	51	50	46	40	34	27	22	17
SW	20	14	10	6	4	2	1	0	1	3	5	8	13	20	30	40	50	58	62	61	55	46	36	27
W	24	17	11	7	5	2	1	0	1	3	5	8	11	15	21	29	40	51	60	64	62	54	43	32
NW	20	14	10	6	4	2	0	0	1	2	5	8	11	14	18	22	27	34	42	47	47	43	35	27

Wall No. 5 — Solar time, hr

Wall Facing	1	2	3	4	5	6	7	8	9	10	11	12	13	14	15	16	17	18	19	20	21	22	23	24
N	13	11	9	7	5	3	3	4	5	6	8	10	12	14	17	19	21	22	23	24	23	21	19	16
NE	13	10	8	6	5	4	5	10	16	22	25	26	26	26	27	27	27	27	27	25	23	21	18	15
E	14	12	9	7	5	4	6	11	20	28	35	40	41	40	39	37	35	34	32	29	27	23	20	17
SE	15	12	10	8	6	4	4	7	13	20	28	35	40	43	44	42	40	38	35	32	29	25	21	18
S	16	13	11	8	6	5	3	3	3	6	10	16	23	31	37	41	43	43	40	37	32	28	24	20
SW	24	19	15	12	9	7	5	4	4	5	7	9	13	19	27	36	44	50	53	52	48	41	35	29
W	27	21	17	14	10	8	6	5	5	6	7	9	11	15	20	27	36	45	52	55	52	46	39	32
NW	21	17	14	11	8	6	5	4	4	5	6	8	11	14	16	20	25	31	37	41	40	36	31	26

Wall No. 6 — Solar time, hr

Wall Facing	1	2	3	4	5	6	7	8	9	10	11	12	13	14	15	16	17	18	19	20	21	22	23	24
N	14	12	10	8	6	5	5	6	6	7	8	10	12	14	16	18	19	21	22	22	22	20	18	16
NE	14	12	10	8	6	6	7	12	17	21	23	24	24	25	25	26	26	26	26	25	23	21	18	16
E	16	14	11	9	8	7	9	14	20	27	33	36	37	37	36	35	34	33	31	29	27	24	21	19
SE	17	14	12	10	8	7	7	10	15	21	27	33	37	39	40	39	38	36	34	32	29	26	23	20
S	18	15	13	11	9	7	6	5	6	8	12	17	23	29	34	37	39	39	37	34	31	28	24	21
SW	25	21	18	15	12	10	8	7	7	7	9	11	14	20	27	34	40	45	48	47	43	39	34	29
W	27	23	19	16	13	11	9	8	8	8	9	10	12	15	20	27	34	42	47	49	47	42	37	32
NW	22	18	15	13	10	8	7	6	6	7	8	9	11	14	16	19	24	29	34	37	36	33	29	25

Wall No. 7 — Solar time, hr

Wall Facing	1	2	3	4	5	6	7	8	9	10	11	12	13	14	15	16	17	18	19	20	21	22	23	24
N	13	12	10	9	8	7	7	8	8	8	9	11	12	14	16	17	18	19	20	20	19	18	16	15
NE	15	13	11	10	9	9	11	15	18	21	22	22	22	23	24	24	25	25	24	23	21	20	18	16
E	17	16	14	12	10	10	13	18	23	28	31	33	33	33	32	32	32	31	30	28	26	24	22	20
SE	18	16	14	13	11	10	11	14	18	23	27	31	34	35	35	35	34	33	32	30	27	25	23	21
S	19	17	15	13	11	10	9	8	9	11	15	19	23	28	31	34	34	34	32	30	28	26	23	21
SW	25	22	19	17	15	13	12	11	11	11	12	14	17	22	28	33	38	41	42	40	37	34	31	28
W	26	23	21	18	16	14	12	12	11	11	12	13	14	17	22	28	34	39	42	42	40	36	33	29
NW	21	18	16	14	12	11	10	9	9	9	10	11	13	14	17	20	24	28	32	33	31	28	26	23

Wall No. 9 — Solar time, hr

Wall Facing	1	2	3	4	5	6	7	8	9	10	11	12	13	14	15	16	17	18	19	20	21	22	23	24
N	18	15	13	11	9	7	5	5	5	5	6	7	8	10	12	14	17	19	20	22	23	23	22	20
NE	18	15	13	11	9	7	6	6	8	12	17	21	23	25	25	26	26	27	27	27	26	24	22	20
E	20	17	15	12	10	8	6	6	9	15	22	28	34	37	38	38	37	36	35	33	31	29	26	23
SE	21	18	15	13	10	8	7	6	7	10	16	22	28	34	38	41	41	40	39	37	34	31	28	25
S	24	20	17	14	11	9	7	5	4	4	5	8	12	18	24	30	35	39	40	40	38	35	31	27
SW	34	29	24	20	16	13	10	8	7	6	6	7	8	11	15	22	29	36	43	47	49	48	44	39
W	37	32	27	22	18	15	12	9	7	7	6	7	8	10	12	16	22	29	37	44	49	50	47	43
NW	29	25	21	18	14	12	9	7	6	5	5	6	7	9	11	14	17	21	26	31	36	38	36	33

Table 7-22-J48 July Cooling Load Temperature Differences for Calculating Cooling Load from Sunlit Walls 48° North Latitude (*Concluded*)

Wall No. 10

Wall Facing	1	2	3	4	5	6	7	8	9	10	11	12	13	14	15	16	17	18	19	20	21	22	23	24
N	17	15	13	11	9	7	6	5	5	6	6	7	9	10	12	14	16	18	20	21	22	22	21	19
NE	18	15	13	11	9	7	6	7	10	13	17	20	22	23	24	25	26	26	26	26	25	24	22	20
E	20	18	15	13	10	8	7	8	11	16	22	28	32	35	36	36	36	35	34	33	31	29	26	23
SE	22	19	16	14	11	9	7	7	9	12	17	22	28	33	36	38	39	39	38	36	34	31	28	25
S	24	21	18	15	12	10	8	6	5	5	7	9	14	19	24	30	34	37	38	38	36	34	31	27
SW	34	29	25	21	17	14	11	9	8	7	7	7	9	12	17	22	29	36	41	45	46	45	42	38
W	36	32	27	23	19	16	13	10	9	8	7	8	9	10	13	17	23	30	37	42	46	46	44	41
NW	29	25	22	18	15	12	10	8	7	6	6	7	8	10	12	14	17	21	26	31	34	35	34	32

Wall No. 11

Wall Facing	1	2	3	4	5	6	7	8	9	10	11	12	13	14	15	16	17	18	19	20	21	22	23	24
N	16	15	13	12	10	9	8	8	8	8	8	9	10	11	12	14	15	17	18	19	19	19	19	18
NE	18	16	15	13	12	10	10	10	12	15	18	20	21	22	22	23	23	24	24	24	23	22	21	20
E	22	20	18	16	14	12	12	12	15	19	23	27	30	32	32	32	32	32	31	30	29	28	26	24
SE	23	21	19	17	15	13	12	12	13	15	19	23	27	30	33	34	34	34	33	32	31	29	27	25
S	23	21	19	17	15	13	12	10	10	9	10	12	16	19	23	27	30	32	33	33	31	30	28	26
SW	30	28	25	22	20	18	15	14	13	12	12	12	13	15	18	23	28	32	36	39	39	38	36	33
W	32	29	26	23	21	19	16	15	13	12	12	12	13	14	16	19	23	28	33	38	40	40	38	35
NW	25	23	21	18	16	14	13	11	10	10	10	10	11	12	13	15	17	20	24	28	30	30	29	27

Wall No. 12

Wall Facing	1	2	3	4	5	6	7	8	9	10	11	12	13	14	15	16	17	18	19	20	21	22	23	24
N	16	15	13	12	11	10	9	8	8	8	9	9	10	11	12	14	15	16	17	18	19	19	18	17
NE	18	17	15	14	12	11	11	11	13	15	18	19	20	21	22	22	23	23	24	23	23	22	21	20
E	22	20	19	17	15	14	13	13	16	19	23	26	29	30	31	31	31	31	30	30	29	27	26	24
SE	23	21	20	18	16	14	13	13	14	16	19	23	26	29	31	33	33	33	32	32	30	29	27	25
S	23	22	20	18	16	14	13	12	11	11	11	13	16	19	23	26	29	31	31	31	30	29	27	25
SW	30	28	25	23	21	19	17	15	14	13	13	13	14	16	19	22	27	31	35	37	38	37	35	33
W	32	29	26	24	22	19	17	16	15	14	13	13	14	14	16	19	23	27	32	36	38	38	36	34
NW	25	23	21	19	17	15	14	12	11	11	11	11	11	12	13	15	17	20	23	26	29	29	28	27

Wall No. 13

Wall Facing	1	2	3	4	5	6	7	8	9	10	11	12	13	14	15	16	17	18	19	20	21	22	23	24
N	15	14	13	12	11	10	10	9	9	9	9	10	11	11	13	14	15	16	17	17	18	18	17	16
NE	18	17	16	14	13	12	12	13	14	16	18	19	20	20	21	22	22	22	23	23	22	21	20	19
E	22	21	19	18	16	15	14	15	17	20	24	26	28	29	29	30	30	30	29	29	28	27	25	24
SE	23	22	20	19	17	16	15	15	16	18	20	23	26	29	30	31	31	31	31	30	29	28	27	25
S	23	21	20	18	17	15	14	13	12	12	13	15	17	20	23	26	28	29	30	29	29	27	26	25
SW	29	27	25	23	21	19	18	16	15	15	14	15	15	17	20	23	27	30	33	35	35	34	33	31
W	30	28	26	24	22	20	18	17	16	15	15	15	15	16	17	20	23	27	31	34	35	35	34	32
NW	23	22	20	19	17	16	14	13	12	12	12	12	13	13	14	16	17	20	23	25	27	27	26	25

Wall No. 14

Wall Facing	1	2	3	4	5	6	7	8	9	10	11	12	13	14	15	16	17	18	19	20	21	22	23	24
N	16	15	14	13	12	11	11	10	10	10	10	10	11	11	12	13	14	15	15	16	17	17	17	16
NE	19	18	17	16	15	14	13	13	14	16	17	18	19	20	20	21	21	21	22	22	22	21	21	20
E	24	22	21	20	18	17	16	16	18	20	22	24	26	27	28	28	28	28	28	28	28	27	26	25
SE	24	23	22	20	19	18	17	16	17	18	20	22	24	26	28	29	29	30	30	29	29	28	27	26
S	24	22	21	20	18	17	16	15	14	14	14	15	16	18	21	23	25	27	27	28	27	27	26	25
SW	29	27	26	24	23	21	20	19	18	17	16	16	16	17	19	21	24	27	30	32	33	32	32	30
W	30	28	27	25	23	22	20	19	18	17	17	16	16	17	18	19	22	24	28	30	32	33	32	31
NW	23	22	21	20	18	17	16	15	14	13	13	13	13	14	14	15	17	18	21	23	24	25	25	24

Wall No. 15

Wall Facing	1	2	3	4	5	6	7	8	9	10	11	12	13	14	15	16	17	18	19	20	21	22	23	24
N	19	18	16	14	13	11	9	8	7	6	6	7	7	8	10	11	13	15	17	18	20	21	21	20
NE	21	19	17	15	13	11	9	8	8	10	13	16	18	20	22	23	24	25	25	26	26	25	24	23
E	25	22	20	17	15	13	11	9	10	12	15	20	25	29	32	34	34	35	34	34	33	31	30	27
SE	27	24	21	18	16	14	11	10	9	10	12	16	20	25	29	33	35	37	37	37	36	34	32	29
S	29	26	23	20	17	15	12	10	8	7	7	7	9	12	17	21	26	30	33	35	36	35	33	31
SW	38	35	31	27	24	20	17	14	12	10	9	8	9	10	12	15	20	25	31	36	40	42	42	41
W	40	37	33	29	26	22	19	16	13	11	10	9	9	10	11	13	16	21	26	32	38	41	43	42
NW	31	29	26	23	20	17	15	12	10	9	8	7	8	8	9	11	13	16	19	23	28	31	32	32

Wall No. 16

Wall Facing	1	2	3	4	5	6	7	8	9	10	11	12	13	14	15	16	17	18	19	20	21	22	23	24
N	18	17	16	15	13	12	10	9	8	8	8	8	8	9	10	11	13	14	16	17	18	19	19	19
NE	21	19	18	16	14	13	11	10	10	12	14	16	18	19	20	22	22	23	24	24	24	24	23	22
E	25	23	21	19	17	15	13	12	12	14	17	20	24	27	29	31	32	32	32	32	31	30	29	27
SE	27	25	22	20	18	16	14	12	12	12	14	17	20	24	27	30	32	34	34	34	33	32	31	29
S	28	26	23	21	19	16	14	12	11	10	9	10	11	14	17	21	24	28	30	32	33	32	31	30
SW	36	33	31	28	25	22	19	17	15	13	12	11	11	12	13	16	20	24	29	33	36	38	38	38
W	37	35	32	29	26	23	21	18	16	14	13	12	12	12	12	14	17	20	25	30	34	37	39	38
NW	29	27	25	23	21	18	16	14	12	11	10	9	9	10	11	12	13	16	19	22	25	28	29	29

Column headings 1–24: Solar time, hr.

1. Direct Application of Data,
   - Dark surface
   - Indoor temperature of 78°F
   - Outdoor maximum temperature of 95°F with mean temperature of 85°F and daily range of 21°F
   - Solar radiation typical of clear day on 21st day of month
   - Outside surface film resistance of 0.333 (h·ft²·°F)/Btu
   - Inside surface film resistance of 0.685 (h·ft²·°F)/Btu

2. Adjustments to Table Data
   Design temperatures:

$$\text{Corr. CLTD} = \text{CLTD} + (78 - T_r) + (T_m - 85)$$

where T_r = inside temperature and
T_m = mean outdoor temperature,
T_m = maximum outdoor temperature − (daily range)/2

   - No adjustment recommended for color

Table 7-22-A24 August Cooling Load Temperature Differences for Calculating Cooling Load from Sunlit Walls 24° North Latitude

Wall No. 1 — Solar time, hr

Wall Facing	1	2	3	4	5	6	7	8	9	10	11	12	13	14	15	16	17	18	19	20	21	22	23	24
N	1	0	-1	-2	-3	-3	0	6	9	12	17	21	25	28	29	29	27	26	20	13	9	7	4	3
NE	1	0	-1	-2	-3	-2	8	31	44	46	41	33	29	29	30	29	27	23	17	13	9	7	5	3
E	1	0	-1	-2	-3	-2	10	39	59	65	60	49	36	32	31	30	27	23	18	13	10	7	5	3
SE	1	0	-1	-2	-3	-2	5	26	43	52	54	51	43	35	32	30	27	23	17	13	9	7	5	3
S	1	0	-1	-2	-3	-3	-2	2	8	17	26	35	41	43	42	37	30	24	18	13	9	7	4	3
SW	2	0	-1	-2	-2	-3	-2	2	7	12	17	23	34	48	60	67	68	57	35	19	12	8	5	3
W	2	0	-1	-2	-2	-3	-1	3	7	12	17	21	27	43	61	75	82	73	45	23	13	8	5	3
NW	1	0	-1	-2	-3	-3	-2	2	7	12	17	21	25	32	44	56	63	60	38	20	12	8	5	3

Wall No. 2 — Solar time, hr

Wall Facing	1	2	3	4	5	6	7	8	9	10	11	12	13	14	15	16	17	18	19	20	21	22	23	24
N	5	3	1	0	-1	-2	-2	-1	2	5	9	13	17	21	24	27	27	27	26	23	18	14	10	7
NE	5	3	2	0	-1	-2	-1	5	17	30	38	39	36	33	31	30	30	28	25	21	17	13	10	7
E	5	3	2	0	-1	-2	-1	6	22	40	52	56	52	45	39	35	32	29	26	22	17	13	10	7
SE	5	3	2	0	-1	-2	-2	3	15	29	40	47	49	46	41	36	33	30	26	22	17	13	10	7
S	5	3	1	0	-1	-2	-2	-2	0	4	11	19	27	34	38	40	38	34	29	23	18	14	10	7
SW	6	4	2	1	-1	-2	-2	-2	1	4	8	13	18	26	37	49	58	62	59	47	34	23	15	10
W	7	4	2	1	0	-1	-2	-2	1	4	8	13	17	23	33	47	61	70	70	58	41	27	18	11
NW	6	4	2	1	-1	-2	-2	-2	0	4	8	12	17	21	27	36	45	54	55	47	34	23	15	10

Wall No. 3 — Solar time, hr

Wall Facing	1	2	3	4	5	6	7	8	9	10	11	12	13	14	15	16	17	18	19	20	21	22	23	24
N	7	5	3	2	0	-1	-1	1	3	6	9	13	16	20	22	24	25	25	24	21	17	14	11	9
NE	7	5	3	2	0	0	2	10	20	28	32	32	31	30	30	30	29	27	25	21	18	14	12	9
E	7	5	3	2	1	0	2	13	27	38	45	46	43	40	37	35	33	30	26	23	19	15	12	10
SE	7	5	3	2	1	0	1	8	18	29	36	41	41	39	37	35	33	30	26	22	19	15	12	9
S	7	5	3	2	0	-1	-1	0	2	6	12	19	25	30	34	35	34	31	27	23	19	15	12	9
SW	11	8	5	3	2	0	0	0	2	5	9	13	19	27	37	46	52	54	49	40	31	25	19	14
W	12	9	6	4	2	1	0	1	3	5	9	12	16	24	34	46	57	62	57	47	37	28	22	16
NW	10	7	5	3	1	0	0	0	2	5	9	12	16	20	27	35	44	49	46	38	30	24	18	14

Wall No. 4 — Solar time, hr

Wall Facing	1	2	3	4	5	6	7	8	9	10	11	12	13	14	15	16	17	18	19	20	21	22	23	24
N	10	7	5	3	2	0	-1	-1	0	2	4	8	11	15	18	21	24	25	26	25	23	19	16	13
NE	10	7	5	3	2	0	0	1	6	15	24	30	33	33	32	32	31	30	28	26	23	19	16	13
E	10	7	5	3	2	0	0	1	8	20	32	42	46	46	44	40	37	34	31	28	24	20	16	13
SE	10	7	5	3	2	0	0	0	5	13	23	32	39	42	42	40	37	35	32	28	24	20	16	13
S	10	7	5	3	2	0	-1	-1	-1	1	4	9	16	22	28	33	35	35	33	30	25	21	17	13
SW	16	11	8	5	3	1	0	-1	-1	1	3	7	11	16	24	33	42	50	54	52	46	37	29	22
W	18	13	9	6	3	2	0	-1	0	1	4	7	11	15	21	30	42	53	60	61	54	44	34	25
NW	16	11	8	5	3	1	0	-1	-1	1	3	7	10	14	19	25	32	40	47	48	43	36	28	21

Wall No. 5 — Solar time, hr

Wall Facing	1	2	3	4	5	6	7	8	9	10	11	12	13	14	15	16	17	18	19	20	21	22	23	24
N	11	9	7	6	4	3	2	1	2	3	5	8	10	13	16	19	21	22	23	22	20	18	16	14
NE	12	10	8	6	4	3	2	4	9	16	22	26	27	28	28	28	29	28	27	25	23	20	17	15
E	13	11	9	7	5	3	3	4	11	20	29	36	39	38	37	36	35	33	31	28	25	22	19	16
SE	13	11	9	7	5	3	2	3	8	15	22	29	33	35	35	35	34	32	30	28	25	22	19	16
S	13	10	8	6	5	3	2	1	1	3	6	10	15	20	25	28	30	30	29	27	24	21	18	15
SW	19	16	13	10	7	5	4	3	3	4	5	8	11	15	22	30	37	43	46	44	39	34	28	24
W	22	18	14	11	9	6	5	3	3	4	6	8	11	14	20	28	37	46	51	50	45	39	33	27
NW	18	15	12	9	7	5	3	2	2	3	5	7	10	13	17	23	29	36	40	40	37	32	27	22

Wall No. 6 — Solar time, hr

Wall Facing	1	2	3	4	5	6	7	8	9	10	11	12	13	14	15	16	17	18	19	20	21	22	23	24
N	12	10	8	7	5	4	3	3	3	4	6	8	10	13	15	17	19	20	21	20	19	17	16	14
NE	14	11	10	8	6	5	4	6	11	16	21	23	25	25	26	27	27	27	26	24	22	20	18	16
E	15	13	11	9	7	6	5	7	13	21	28	32	34	35	34	34	33	32	30	28	25	23	20	18
SE	15	13	11	9	7	5	4	6	10	16	22	27	30	32	32	32	32	31	29	27	25	22	20	17
S	14	12	10	8	6	5	4	3	3	4	7	10	15	19	23	26	27	27	26	25	23	20	18	16
SW	21	18	15	12	10	8	6	5	5	6	7	9	11	16	22	28	34	39	41	39	36	32	28	24
W	23	20	17	14	11	9	7	6	6	6	7	9	11	15	20	27	35	42	46	44	41	36	31	27
NW	19	16	14	11	9	7	6	5	5	5	7	8	11	13	17	22	28	33	36	36	33	29	26	22

Wall No. 7 — Solar time, hr

Wall Facing	1	2	3	4	5	6	7	8	9	10	11	12	13	14	15	16	17	18	19	20	21	22	23	24
N	12	10	9	8	7	5	5	5	5	6	7	9	11	13	15	16	17	18	19	18	17	16	14	13
NE	14	13	11	10	8	7	7	10	14	18	20	22	22	23	24	25	25	25	24	22	21	19	18	16
E	16	15	13	11	10	8	8	12	17	23	27	30	31	31	30	30	30	29	28	26	24	22	20	18
SE	16	14	12	11	9	8	7	10	14	18	22	26	28	28	29	29	29	28	27	25	23	21	20	18
S	14	12	11	9	8	7	6	5	6	7	9	12	15	19	21	23	24	24	23	22	20	19	17	16
SW	20	18	16	14	12	10	9	8	8	9	10	11	14	18	22	28	32	35	35	33	31	28	25	23
W	23	20	18	16	14	12	10	9	9	10	10	12	13	17	22	28	34	39	39	37	34	31	28	26
NW	19	17	15	13	11	9	8	8	7	8	9	10	12	14	18	22	27	31	32	30	28	26	23	21

Wall No. 9 — Solar time, hr

Wall Facing	1	2	3	4	5	6	7	8	9	10	11	12	13	14	15	16	17	18	19	20	21	22	23	24
N	15	13	11	9	8	6	4	3	2	2	3	4	6	8	11	13	16	18	20	21	21	21	19	17
NE	17	15	13	10	8	7	5	4	4	7	11	17	21	24	26	27	27	28	28	27	26	24	22	20
E	19	16	14	11	9	7	6	4	5	9	15	22	29	33	35	36	36	35	34	32	30	28	25	22
SE	19	16	14	11	9	7	5	4	4	6	11	17	23	28	31	33	33	33	33	31	29	27	24	22
S	18	15	13	11	9	7	5	4	3	2	3	4	7	11	16	20	24	27	28	28	27	25	23	20
SW	28	24	20	16	13	11	8	6	5	4	4	5	6	9	12	17	24	30	36	41	42	40	36	32
W	32	27	23	19	15	12	10	7	6	5	5	5	7	9	12	16	22	30	38	44	46	45	41	37
NW	26	22	19	15	13	10	8	6	4	4	4	5	6	8	11	14	18	24	30	35	37	36	33	30

Table 7-22-A24 August Cooling Load Temperature Differences for Calculating Cooling Load from Sunlit Walls 24° North Latitude (*Concluded*)

Wall No. 10

Wall Facing	1	2	3	4	5	6	7	8	9	10	11	12	13	14	15	16	17	18	19	20	21	22	23	24
N	15	13	12	10	8	6	5	4	3	3	4	5	6	9	11	13	16	18	19	20	20	20	19	17
NE	17	15	13	11	9	7	6	5	6	9	13	17	20	23	24	26	27	27	27	27	25	24	22	20
E	19	17	14	12	10	8	6	5	7	11	16	22	28	31	33	34	34	34	33	32	30	27	25	22
SE	19	17	14	12	10	8	6	5	6	8	12	17	22	26	29	31	32	32	32	31	29	27	24	22
S	18	16	13	11	9	7	6	4	3	3	4	5	8	12	16	20	23	25	27	27	26	24	23	20
SW	28	24	21	17	14	12	9	7	6	5	5	6	7	10	13	18	24	30	35	38	39	37	35	31
W	31	27	23	20	16	13	10	8	7	6	6	6	8	9	12	17	23	30	37	42	43	42	39	35
NW	26	22	19	16	13	11	8	7	5	5	5	5	7	9	11	15	19	24	29	33	34	34	32	29

Wall No. 11

Wall Facing	1	2	3	4	5	6	7	8	9	10	11	12	13	14	15	16	17	18	19	20	21	22	23	24
N	14	13	12	10	9	8	7	6	6	6	6	7	8	9	11	13	14	16	17	18	18	17	16	15
NE	18	16	14	13	11	10	9	8	9	11	14	17	20	21	22	23	24	24	24	24	23	22	21	19
E	20	18	17	15	13	12	10	9	11	14	18	23	26	28	29	30	30	30	29	29	27	26	24	22
SE	20	18	16	14	13	11	10	9	9	11	15	18	22	25	26	27	28	28	28	27	26	25	23	21
S	17	16	14	13	11	10	8	7	6	6	7	8	10	13	16	18	21	22	23	23	22	21	20	19
SW	25	23	21	18	16	14	13	11	10	9	9	9	10	12	15	18	23	27	31	33	33	32	30	27
W	28	25	23	20	18	16	14	12	11	10	10	10	11	12	14	18	23	28	33	36	37	35	33	31
NW	23	21	19	17	15	13	11	10	9	8	8	9	10	11	13	15	18	22	26	29	29	29	27	25

Wall No. 12

Wall Facing	1	2	3	4	5	6	7	8	9	10	11	12	13	14	15	16	17	18	19	20	21	22	23	24
N	14	13	12	11	10	8	7	7	6	6	6	7	8	9	11	12	14	15	16	17	17	17	16	15
NE	18	16	15	14	12	11	10	9	10	12	14	17	19	20	21	22	23	23	24	23	23	22	21	19
E	21	19	17	16	14	13	11	11	12	14	18	22	25	27	28	29	29	29	29	28	27	26	24	22
SE	20	18	17	15	14	12	11	10	10	12	15	18	21	24	25	26	27	27	27	27	26	24	23	21
S	17	16	14	13	12	10	9	8	7	7	7	8	10	13	15	18	20	21	22	22	22	21	20	18
SW	25	23	21	19	17	15	14	12	11	10	10	10	11	13	15	18	22	26	30	31	31	30	29	27
W	28	25	23	21	19	17	15	14	12	11	11	11	12	13	15	18	22	27	31	34	35	34	32	30
NW	23	21	19	17	15	14	12	11	10	9	9	10	10	11	13	15	18	22	25	27	28	27	26	24

Wall No. 13

Wall Facing	1	2	3	4	5	6	7	8	9	10	11	12	13	14	15	16	17	18	19	20	21	22	23	24
N	14	13	12	11	10	9	8	7	7	7	7	8	9	10	11	12	14	15	16	16	16	16	15	14
NE	18	17	15	14	13	12	11	10	11	13	15	17	19	20	21	21	22	22	22	22	22	21	20	19
E	21	19	18	17	15	14	13	12	13	16	19	22	25	26	27	27	28	28	27	27	26	25	24	22
SE	20	18	17	16	14	13	12	11	12	14	16	19	21	23	24	25	26	26	26	25	25	24	22	21
S	17	16	14	13	12	11	10	9	8	8	9	10	11	13	15	17	19	20	21	21	20	20	19	18
SW	24	22	21	19	17	16	15	13	12	12	12	12	12	14	16	19	22	26	28	29	29	28	27	25
W	26	25	23	21	19	18	16	15	14	13	13	13	13	14	16	19	23	27	30	32	32	31	30	28
NW	22	20	19	17	16	14	13	12	11	11	11	11	11	12	14	16	18	21	24	26	26	25	24	23

Wall No. 14

Wall Facing	1	2	3	4	5	6	7	8	9	10	11	12	13	14	15	16	17	18	19	20	21	22	23	24
N	14	13	12	12	11	10	9	9	8	8	8	8	9	9	10	11	12	13	14	15	15	15	15	14
NE	18	17	16	15	14	13	12	12	12	13	15	16	18	19	19	20	21	21	21	21	21	21	20	19
E	22	21	19	18	17	16	15	14	14	16	18	21	23	24	25	26	26	26	26	26	26	25	24	23
SE	21	19	18	17	16	15	14	13	13	14	16	18	20	21	23	23	24	24	25	24	24	23	23	22
S	17	16	15	14	13	12	11	11	10	9	9	10	11	12	14	16	17	18	19	19	19	19	18	18
SW	24	23	21	20	19	18	16	15	14	14	13	13	13	14	15	17	20	23	25	27	27	27	26	25
W	26	25	24	22	21	19	18	17	16	15	15	14	15	15	16	18	20	24	27	29	30	30	29	28
NW	22	20	19	18	17	16	15	14	13	12	12	12	12	13	14	15	17	19	21	23	24	24	23	23

Wall No. 15

Wall Facing	1	2	3	4	5	6	7	8	9	10	11	12	13	14	15	16	17	18	19	20	21	22	23	24
N	17	16	14	13	11	9	8	6	5	4	4	4	5	6	8	10	12	14	16	18	19	19	19	18
NE	21	19	17	15	13	11	9	7	6	7	9	12	15	18	20	22	24	25	26	26	26	25	24	22
E	24	21	19	16	14	12	10	8	7	8	11	15	20	24	28	30	32	32	33	32	31	30	28	26
SE	23	21	18	16	14	12	10	8	7	7	8	11	15	20	23	26	28	30	30	31	30	29	27	25
S	21	19	17	15	13	11	9	7	6	5	4	4	6	8	10	14	17	20	23	24	25	25	24	23
SW	32	29	26	23	20	17	14	12	9	8	7	6	7	8	9	12	16	21	26	31	34	36	36	34
W	35	32	29	25	22	19	16	13	11	9	8	7	7	8	9	12	15	20	26	32	37	39	39	38
NW	29	26	24	21	18	15	13	11	9	7	6	6	6	7	9	11	13	17	21	26	29	31	32	31

Wall No. 16

Wall Facing	1	2	3	4	5	6	7	8	9	10	11	12	13	14	15	16	17	18	19	20	21	22	23	24
N	16	15	14	13	12	10	9	8	6	6	5	6	6	7	8	10	11	13	15	16	17	18	18	17
NE	21	19	17	16	14	12	11	9	8	9	10	12	15	17	19	21	22	23	24	24	24	24	23	22
E	24	22	20	18	16	14	12	11	10	10	12	16	19	23	26	28	29	30	30	30	30	29	27	26
SE	23	21	19	17	15	14	12	10	9	9	10	13	16	19	22	24	26	27	28	28	28	27	26	25
S	20	19	17	15	14	12	11	9	8	7	6	6	7	9	11	13	16	19	21	22	23	23	22	21
SW	30	28	25	23	20	18	16	14	12	10	9	9	9	9	11	13	16	20	24	28	31	32	32	31
W	33	31	28	26	23	20	18	15	13	12	10	10	10	10	11	13	16	20	25	30	33	35	35	35
NW	27	25	23	21	19	17	15	13	11	9	8	8	8	9	10	11	13	16	20	24	26	28	28	28

1. Direct Application of Data,
   - Dark surface
   - Indoor temperature of 78°F
   - Outdoor maximum temperature of 95°F with mean temperature of 85°F and daily range of 21°F
   - Solar radiation typical of clear day on 21st day of month
   - Outside surface film resistance of 0.333 (h·ft^2·°F)/Btu
   - Inside surface film resistance of 0.685 (h·ft^2·°F)/Btu

2. Adjustments to Table Data

   Design temperatures:

$$\text{Corr. CLTD} = \text{CLTD} + (78 - T_r) + (T_m - 85)$$

where T_r = inside temperature and

T_m = mean outdoor temperature,

T_m = maximum outdoor temperature − (daily range)/2

- No adjustment recommended for color

Table 7-22-A32 August Cooling Load Temperature Differences for Calculating Cooling Load from Sunlit Walls 32° North Latitude

Wall No. 1 — Solar time, hr

Wall Facing	1	2	3	4	5	6	7	8	9	10	11	12	13	14	15	16	17	18	19	20	21	22	23	24
N	1	0	-1	-2	-3	-3	1	5	8	12	17	21	25	27	29	28	27	24	20	14	9	7	4	3
NE	1	0	-1	-2	-3	-1	11	32	42	42	35	28	27	28	29	29	27	23	18	13	9	7	5	3
E	1	0	-1	-2	-3	-1	15	42	60	65	60	49	36	31	30	29	27	23	18	13	10	7	5	3
SE	1	0	-1	-2	-3	-2	8	29	47	57	60	57	50	39	33	30	27	23	18	13	10	7	5	3
S	1	0	-1	-2	-3	-3	-1	3	12	23	35	44	51	54	52	45	36	27	19	13	10	7	5	3
SW	2	0	-1	-2	-2	-3	-1	3	7	12	17	25	39	55	67	73	72	61	39	21	12	8	5	3
W	2	0	-1	-2	-2	-3	-1	3	7	12	17	21	27	42	60	75	81	75	49	25	14	8	5	3
NW	1	0	-1	-2	-3	-3	-1	3	7	12	17	21	25	29	38	50	59	58	41	22	12	8	5	3

Wall No. 2 — Solar time, hr

Wall Facing	1	2	3	4	5	6	7	8	9	10	11	12	13	14	15	16	17	18	19	20	21	22	23	24
N	5	3	1	0	-1	-2	-2	-1	2	5	9	13	17	21	24	26	27	27	25	23	18	14	10	7
NE	5	3	1	0	-1	-2	-1	6	18	29	35	35	32	30	29	29	29	28	25	21	17	13	10	7
E	5	3	2	0	-1	-2	0	8	25	41	52	56	52	45	38	34	32	29	26	22	18	14	10	7
SE	5	3	2	0	-1	-2	-1	5	17	31	44	52	54	52	46	40	35	31	27	22	18	14	10	7
S	5	3	2	0	-1	-2	-2	-2	1	7	15	25	35	43	48	49	47	42	34	27	20	15	11	8
SW	7	4	2	1	0	-1	-2	-1	1	4	8	13	20	30	42	54	63	67	63	51	37	25	16	11
W	7	5	2	1	0	-1	-2	-1	1	4	8	12	17	23	33	46	60	70	71	60	43	29	19	12
NW	7	4	2	1	-1	-2	-2	-1	1	4	8	12	17	21	25	32	41	49	52	46	35	24	16	10

Wall No. 3 — Solar time, hr

Wall Facing	1	2	3	4	5	6	7	8	9	10	11	12	13	14	15	16	17	18	19	20	21	22	23	24
N	7	5	3	1	0	-1	0	1	3	6	9	12	16	19	22	24	25	25	23	21	17	14	11	9
NE	7	5	3	2	0	0	3	11	20	27	29	29	28	28	28	29	28	27	24	21	17	14	12	9
E	7	5	3	2	1	0	4	15	28	39	45	47	43	40	37	35	33	30	27	23	19	15	12	10
SE	7	5	4	2	1	0	2	10	21	31	40	45	47	44	41	38	35	32	28	23	19	16	13	10
S	8	6	4	2	1	0	-1	0	3	9	16	25	32	39	42	43	41	37	32	26	22	17	14	11
SW	11	8	6	4	2	1	0	1	3	5	9	13	21	30	41	50	57	58	53	43	34	26	20	15
W	13	9	6	4	2	1	0	1	3	5	9	12	16	24	34	46	56	62	59	49	38	29	22	17
NW	10	7	5	3	1	0	0	1	2	5	8	12	16	19	25	32	40	46	45	38	30	24	18	14

Wall No. 4 — Solar time, hr

Wall Facing	1	2	3	4	5	6	7	8	9	10	11	12	13	14	15	16	17	18	19	20	21	22	23	24
N	10	7	5	3	2	0	-1	-1	0	2	4	7	11	14	18	21	24	25	25	24	22	19	16	13
NE	10	7	5	3	2	0	0	1	7	15	23	28	30	30	30	29	29	29	27	25	22	19	16	12
E	10	7	5	3	2	0	0	2	10	21	33	42	47	47	44	40	37	34	31	28	24	20	16	13
SE	10	8	5	3	2	1	0	1	6	15	26	36	43	47	47	45	41	37	34	30	25	21	17	13
S	11	8	6	4	2	1	-1	-1	0	2	6	13	21	29	36	42	44	44	41	35	30	24	19	15
SW	17	12	8	5	3	1	0	-1	0	1	4	7	11	18	26	37	47	55	59	57	50	40	31	23
W	19	14	9	6	4	2	0	0	0	1	4	7	10	15	21	30	41	52	60	61	55	46	35	26
NW	16	11	8	5	3	1	0	-1	0	1	4	7	10	14	18	23	29	37	43	45	42	35	28	21

Wall No. 5 — Solar time, hr

Wall Facing	1	2	3	4	5	6	7	8	9	10	11	12	13	14	15	16	17	18	19	20	21	22	23	24
N	11	9	7	6	4	3	2	1	2	3	5	7	10	13	16	18	20	22	22	22	20	18	16	13
NE	12	10	8	6	4	3	2	4	9	16	21	24	25	25	26	27	27	27	26	24	22	20	17	14
E	13	11	9	7	5	3	3	5	13	22	30	36	39	39	37	36	35	33	31	28	25	22	19	16
SE	14	11	9	7	5	4	3	4	9	16	24	32	37	40	40	39	37	35	33	30	26	23	20	17
S	15	12	9	7	5	4	2	2	2	4	8	13	19	26	31	35	38	37	35	32	28	25	21	18
SW	21	17	14	11	8	6	4	3	3	4	6	8	11	17	25	33	41	47	50	48	43	37	31	26
W	23	18	15	12	9	7	5	4	3	4	6	8	11	14	20	28	37	46	51	51	46	40	34	28
NW	18	15	12	9	7	5	3	2	2	3	5	7	10	13	16	21	27	33	38	38	35	31	26	22

Wall No. 6 — Solar time, hr

Wall Facing	1	2	3	4	5	6	7	8	9	10	11	12	13	14	15	16	17	18	19	20	21	22	23	24
N	12	10	8	7	5	4	3	3	3	4	6	8	10	12	15	17	19	20	20	20	19	17	15	14
NE	13	11	9	8	6	5	4	7	11	16	20	22	23	24	24	25	26	26	25	24	22	20	17	15
E	15	13	11	9	7	6	5	8	15	22	29	33	35	35	34	34	33	32	30	28	25	23	20	18
SE	16	13	11	9	7	6	5	7	11	17	24	29	33	36	36	35	34	33	31	29	26	23	21	18
S	16	14	11	9	8	6	5	4	4	6	9	14	19	24	29	32	34	34	32	30	27	24	21	19
SW	22	19	16	13	11	9	7	6	6	6	7	9	12	17	24	31	38	43	44	43	39	34	30	26
W	24	20	17	14	12	9	7	6	6	6	8	9	11	15	20	27	35	42	46	45	41	37	32	28
NW	19	16	13	11	9	7	6	5	5	5	7	8	11	13	16	20	25	31	34	34	32	29	25	22

Wall No. 7 — Solar time, hr

Wall Facing	1	2	3	4	5	6	7	8	9	10	11	12	13	14	15	16	17	18	19	20	21	22	23	24
N	12	10	9	8	7	5	5	5	5	6	7	9	11	13	14	16	17	18	18	18	17	16	14	13
NE	14	12	11	9	8	7	7	10	14	17	19	20	21	22	23	23	24	24	23	22	20	19	17	15
E	17	15	13	11	10	8	9	13	18	24	28	30	31	31	31	31	30	29	28	26	24	22	20	18
SE	17	15	13	11	10	9	8	11	15	20	25	28	31	32	32	32	31	30	29	27	25	23	21	19
S	17	15	13	11	10	8	7	7	7	9	12	16	20	24	27	29	30	29	28	26	24	22	20	18
SW	22	20	17	15	13	11	10	9	9	9	10	12	15	20	25	30	35	38	38	36	33	30	28	25
W	23	21	18	16	14	12	11	10	9	10	11	12	13	17	22	28	34	39	40	38	35	32	29	26
NW	18	16	14	12	11	9	8	7	7	8	9	10	12	14	16	20	25	29	30	29	27	25	23	20

Wall No. 9 — Solar time, hr

Wall Facing	1	2	3	4	5	6	7	8	9	10	11	12	13	14	15	16	17	18	19	20	21	22	23	24
N	15	13	11	9	8	6	4	3	2	2	3	4	6	8	11	13	16	18	20	21	21	20	19	17
NE	17	14	12	10	8	6	5	4	4	7	12	16	20	22	24	25	25	26	26	26	25	23	21	19
E	19	16	14	11	9	7	6	5	6	9	16	23	29	34	36	36	36	35	34	32	30	28	25	22
SE	20	17	14	12	10	8	6	5	5	7	12	18	25	31	35	37	37	37	36	34	32	29	26	23
S	21	18	15	12	10	8	6	4	3	3	4	6	10	15	20	26	30	33	35	35	33	30	27	24
SW	30	26	21	18	14	12	9	7	5	5	5	5	7	9	14	19	26	33	40	44	45	43	40	35
W	32	28	23	19	16	12	10	8	6	5	5	6	7	9	12	16	22	30	37	44	47	46	42	38
NW	25	22	18	15	12	10	8	6	4	4	4	5	6	8	11	14	17	22	27	32	35	35	32	29

Table 7-22-A32 August Cooling Load Temperature Differences for Calculating Cooling Load from Sunlit Walls 32° North Latitude (*Concluded*)

Wall No. 10 — Solar time, hr

Wall Facing	1	2	3	4	5	6	7	8	9	10	11	12	13	14	15	16	17	18	19	20	21	22	23	24
N	15	13	11	10	8	6	5	4	3	3	4	5	6	8	11	13	15	17	19	20	20	20	18	17
NE	17	15	13	11	9	7	5	5	6	9	13	16	19	21	23	24	25	26	26	25	25	23	21	19
E	20	17	14	12	10	8	6	6	7	12	17	23	28	32	34	34	34	34	33	32	30	28	25	22
SE	20	17	15	12	10	8	6	5	6	9	14	19	25	29	33	35	35	35	35	33	31	29	26	23
S	21	18	16	13	11	9	7	5	4	4	5	7	11	15	20	25	29	32	33	33	32	29	27	24
SW	30	26	22	19	15	13	10	8	6	5	5	6	8	10	15	20	26	33	38	42	42	41	38	34
W	32	28	24	20	17	14	11	9	7	6	6	6	8	10	12	17	23	30	37	42	43	43	40	36
NW	25	22	19	16	13	10	8	6	5	5	5	5	7	9	11	14	18	22	27	31	33	32	30	28

Wall No. 11 — Solar time, hr

Wall Facing	1	2	3	4	5	6	7	8	9	10	11	12	13	14	15	16	17	18	19	20	21	22	23	24
N	14	13	12	10	9	8	7	6	5	5	6	7	8	9	11	12	14	16	17	17	17	17	16	15
NE	17	16	14	13	11	10	8	8	9	11	14	17	18	20	21	21	22	23	23	23	22	21	20	19
E	21	19	17	15	13	12	10	10	11	15	19	23	27	29	30	30	30	30	30	29	28	26	24	22
SE	21	19	17	15	14	12	10	10	10	13	16	20	24	27	29	30	31	31	30	30	28	27	25	23
S	20	18	17	15	13	12	10	9	8	8	8	10	13	16	20	23	26	28	28	28	27	26	24	22
SW	27	25	22	20	18	16	14	12	11	10	10	10	11	13	16	20	25	30	34	36	36	35	32	30
W	29	26	23	21	19	16	14	13	11	11	10	11	11	12	15	18	23	28	33	36	37	36	34	31
NW	22	20	18	16	14	13	11	10	9	8	8	9	9	11	12	14	17	21	24	27	28	28	26	24

Wall No. 12 — Solar time, hr

Wall Facing	1	2	3	4	5	6	7	8	9	10	11	12	13	14	15	16	17	18	19	20	21	22	23	24
N	14	13	12	11	9	8	7	7	6	6	6	7	8	9	11	12	14	15	16	17	17	16	16	15
NE	17	16	14	13	12	10	9	9	10	12	14	16	18	19	20	21	22	22	22	22	22	21	20	19
E	21	19	18	16	14	13	11	11	12	15	19	23	26	28	29	29	29	29	29	28	27	26	24	23
SE	21	20	18	16	15	13	12	11	11	13	16	20	23	26	28	29	30	30	29	29	28	26	25	23
S	20	19	17	15	14	12	11	10	9	9	9	11	13	16	19	22	25	26	27	27	26	25	24	22
SW	27	25	23	20	18	17	15	13	12	11	11	11	12	14	16	20	24	29	32	34	34	33	31	29
W	28	26	24	21	19	17	15	14	13	12	11	12	12	13	15	18	22	27	31	34	35	34	33	31
NW	22	20	18	17	15	13	12	11	10	9	9	9	10	11	12	14	17	20	23	26	27	26	25	24

Wall No. 13 — Solar time, hr

Wall Facing	1	2	3	4	5	6	7	8	9	10	11	12	13	14	15	16	17	18	19	20	21	22	23	24
N	13	13	12	11	10	9	8	7	7	7	7	8	9	10	11	12	13	14	15	16	16	15	15	14
NE	17	16	15	14	12	11	10	10	11	13	15	17	18	19	19	20	21	21	21	21	21	20	19	18
E	21	20	18	17	15	14	13	13	14	17	20	23	25	27	27	28	28	28	28	27	26	25	24	22
SE	21	20	18	17	16	14	13	12	13	15	18	21	23	26	27	28	28	28	28	27	27	25	24	23
S	20	19	17	16	15	13	12	11	10	10	11	12	14	17	19	22	24	25	25	25	25	24	23	21
SW	26	24	22	21	19	17	16	14	13	13	13	13	13	15	18	21	24	28	31	32	32	31	29	28
W	27	25	23	21	20	18	16	15	14	13	13	13	14	14	16	19	23	27	30	32	33	32	30	29
NW	21	19	18	17	15	14	13	12	11	10	10	11	11	12	13	15	17	20	23	24	25	24	23	22

Wall No. 14 — Solar time, hr

Wall Facing	1	2	3	4	5	6	7	8	9	10	11	12	13	14	15	16	17	18	19	20	21	22	23	24
N	14	13	12	11	11	10	9	8	8	8	8	8	9	9	10	11	12	13	14	15	15	15	15	14
NE	18	17	16	15	14	13	12	11	12	13	14	16	17	18	18	19	20	20	20	21	20	20	19	19
E	22	21	20	18	17	16	15	14	15	16	19	21	23	25	26	26	26	27	27	26	26	25	24	23
SE	22	21	20	19	17	16	15	14	14	15	17	19	22	24	25	26	27	27	27	27	26	25	24	23
S	20	19	18	17	16	15	14	13	12	12	12	12	14	16	18	20	22	23	24	24	24	23	22	21
SW	26	25	23	22	20	19	18	17	16	15	14	14	14	15	17	19	22	25	27	29	30	29	28	27
W	27	26	24	23	21	20	18	17	16	15	15	15	15	15	16	18	20	24	27	29	30	30	29	28
NW	21	20	19	18	16	15	14	13	12	12	12	12	12	12	13	14	16	18	20	22	23	23	23	22

Wall No. 15 — Solar time, hr

Wall Facing	1	2	3	4	5	6	7	8	9	10	11	12	13	14	15	16	17	18	19	20	21	22	23	24
N	17	16	14	13	11	9	8	6	5	4	4	4	5	6	8	10	12	14	16	17	18	19	19	18
NE	20	18	16	14	12	10	9	7	6	7	9	12	14	17	19	21	22	23	24	25	25	24	23	22
E	24	21	19	16	14	12	10	8	8	8	11	16	20	25	28	31	32	33	33	32	31	30	28	26
SE	25	22	19	17	15	12	10	9	7	8	9	13	17	22	26	29	32	33	34	33	33	31	29	27
S	25	22	20	17	15	13	11	9	7	6	5	6	7	10	14	18	22	26	29	30	31	30	29	27
SW	34	31	28	24	21	18	15	13	10	9	7	7	7	8	10	13	18	23	29	34	37	39	39	37
W	36	33	30	26	23	19	16	14	11	9	8	7	7	8	10	12	15	20	26	32	37	39	40	39
NW	28	25	23	20	18	15	13	10	9	7	6	6	6	7	8	10	13	16	20	24	27	30	30	29

Wall No. 16 — Solar time, hr

Wall Facing	1	2	3	4	5	6	7	8	9	10	11	12	13	14	15	16	17	18	19	20	21	22	23	24
N	16	15	14	13	11	10	9	7	6	6	5	5	6	7	8	10	11	13	14	16	17	17	17	17
NE	20	18	17	15	13	12	10	9	8	9	10	12	14	16	18	19	21	22	23	23	23	23	22	21
E	24	22	20	18	16	14	12	11	10	11	13	16	20	24	26	28	29	30	30	30	30	29	28	26
SE	25	23	21	18	16	14	13	11	10	10	11	14	17	21	24	27	29	30	31	31	31	30	28	27
S	24	22	20	18	16	14	13	11	9	8	8	8	9	11	14	17	21	24	26	27	28	28	27	26
SW	32	30	27	25	22	20	17	15	13	11	10	10	9	10	12	14	18	22	27	31	34	35	35	34
W	33	31	29	26	23	21	18	16	14	12	11	10	10	10	11	13	16	20	25	29	33	35	36	35
NW	26	24	22	20	18	16	14	12	11	9	8	8	8	9	9	11	13	15	19	22	25	27	27	27

1. Direct Application of Data,
   - Dark surface
   - Indoor temperature of 78 °F
   - Outdoor maximum temperature of 95 °F with mean temperature of 85°F and daily range of 21°F
   - Solar radiation typical of clear day on 21st day of month
   - Outside surface film resistance of 0.333 (h·ft^2·°F)/Btu
   - Inside surface film resistance of 0.685 (h·ft^2·°F)/Btu

2. Adjustments to Table Data
   Design temperatures:

$$\text{Corr. CLTD} = \text{CLTD} + (78 - T_r) + (T_m - 85)$$

where T_r = inside temperature and
T_m = mean outdoor temperature,
T_m = maximum outdoor temperature − (daily range)/2

- No adjustment recommended for color

Table 7-22-A40 August Cooling Load Temperature Differences for Calculating Cooling Load from Sunlit Walls 40° North Latitude

Wall No. 1

Wall Facing	1	2	3	4	5	6	7	8	9	10	11	12	13	14	15	16	17	18	19	20	21	22	23	24
N	1	0	-1	-2	-3	-2	1	4	7	12	16	20	24	27	28	28	26	23	20	14	10	7	4	3
NE	1	0	-1	-2	-3	-1	14	32	39	37	29	25	26	27	28	28	26	23	18	13	9	7	4	3
E	1	0	-1	-2	-3	0	18	44	60	64	59	48	35	31	30	29	27	23	18	13	10	7	5	3
SE	1	0	-1	-2	-3	-1	11	32	50	61	65	63	56	45	35	31	28	24	18	13	10	7	5	3
S	1	0	-1	-2	-3	-3	-1	4	15	29	42	53	60	63	60	53	42	29	20	14	10	7	5	3
SW	2	0	-1	-2	-2	-3	-1	3	7	12	17	29	45	61	72	77	75	64	42	23	13	8	5	3
W	2	0	-1	-2	-2	-3	-1	3	7	12	16	20	26	41	59	73	80	75	53	27	14	9	5	3
NW	1	0	-1	-2	-3	-3	-1	3	7	12	16	20	24	27	34	45	54	56	43	23	13	8	5	3

Wall No. 2

Wall Facing	1	2	3	4	5	6	7	8	9	10	11	12	13	14	15	16	17	18	19	20	21	22	23	24
N	5	3	1	0	-1	-2	-2	0	2	5	8	12	16	20	23	26	27	26	25	22	18	14	10	7
NE	5	3	1	0	-1	-2	0	7	19	28	32	31	29	27	27	28	28	27	25	21	17	13	10	7
E	5	3	2	0	-1	-2	0	10	27	43	53	56	52	44	38	34	31	29	26	22	18	14	10	7
SE	5	3	2	0	-1	-2	-1	6	19	34	47	56	59	57	51	44	37	32	28	23	18	14	10	8
S	5	3	2	0	-1	-2	-2	-1	2	9	19	30	42	51	57	58	55	48	39	30	22	16	11	8
SW	7	4	2	1	0	-1	-2	-1	1	4	8	13	22	34	47	59	68	71	67	54	39	26	17	11
W	8	5	2	1	0	-1	-2	-1	1	4	8	12	16	22	32	46	59	69	71	61	45	30	19	12
NW	7	4	2	0	-1	-2	-2	-1	1	4	8	12	16	20	24	29	37	45	50	45	35	24	16	10

Wall No. 3

Wall Facing	1	2	3	4	5	6	7	8	9	10	11	12	13	14	15	16	17	18	19	20	21	22	23	24
N	6	5	3	1	0	-1	0	1	3	5	8	12	15	19	21	23	24	24	23	20	17	14	11	9
NE	7	5	3	2	0	0	4	12	20	25	26	26	26	26	27	27	27	26	24	21	17	14	11	9
E	7	5	3	2	1	0	5	16	29	40	46	46	43	39	36	34	32	30	26	23	19	15	12	10
SE	8	6	4	2	1	0	3	11	23	34	43	49	51	49	45	41	37	33	29	24	20	16	13	10
S	9	6	4	2	1	0	0	1	5	12	20	30	39	46	50	51	48	43	36	30	24	19	15	12
SW	12	9	6	4	2	1	0	1	3	5	9	14	23	34	45	55	61	62	57	46	36	28	22	16
W	13	9	6	4	2	1	0	1	3	5	9	12	16	23	33	45	56	62	60	50	39	30	23	17
NW	10	7	5	3	1	0	0	1	3	5	8	12	15	19	23	29	36	43	43	37	30	23	18	14

Wall No. 4

Wall Facing	1	2	3	4	5	6	7	8	9	10	11	12	13	14	15	16	17	18	19	20	21	22	23	24
N	10	7	5	3	2	0	-1	-1	0	2	4	7	10	14	17	21	23	24	25	24	22	19	16	13
NE	10	7	5	3	2	0	0	2	8	16	22	26	27	27	27	27	28	27	27	25	22	19	16	12
E	10	7	5	3	2	0	0	3	11	23	34	43	47	46	43	40	36	34	31	28	24	20	16	13
SE	11	8	5	4	2	1	0	2	7	17	28	39	47	51	52	49	45	40	36	31	26	22	17	14
S	12	9	6	4	2	1	0	-1	0	3	8	16	26	35	43	49	52	51	47	41	34	27	21	16
SW	18	13	9	6	3	2	0	0	0	1	4	7	12	20	29	41	51	59	63	61	53	43	33	25
W	20	14	9	6	4	2	0	0	0	1	4	7	10	14	21	29	40	51	60	61	56	47	36	27
NW	16	11	8	5	3	1	0	-1	0	1	4	7	10	14	18	22	27	34	40	43	41	35	28	21

Wall No. 5

Wall Facing	1	2	3	4	5	6	7	8	9	10	11	12	13	14	15	16	17	18	19	20	21	22	23	24
N	11	9	7	5	4	3	2	1	2	3	5	7	10	13	15	18	20	21	22	21	20	18	16	13
NE	12	10	8	6	4	3	2	5	10	16	20	22	23	23	24	25	26	26	25	24	22	19	17	14
E	13	11	9	7	5	3	3	6	14	23	31	37	39	39	37	36	34	33	31	28	25	22	19	16
SE	14	12	9	7	5	4	3	5	10	18	26	34	40	43	44	42	40	38	35	31	28	24	21	17
S	16	13	11	8	6	4	3	2	3	5	10	16	24	31	37	42	44	44	41	37	32	28	24	20
SW	22	18	15	11	9	6	5	4	3	4	6	8	12	19	27	36	45	51	53	51	46	39	33	27
W	23	19	15	12	9	7	5	4	4	4	6	8	10	14	19	27	37	45	51	52	47	41	34	28
NW	18	14	11	9	7	5	3	2	2	3	5	7	10	13	16	19	25	30	35	37	34	30	26	21

Wall No. 6

Wall Facing	1	2	3	4	5	6	7	8	9	10	11	12	13	14	15	16	17	18	19	20	21	22	23	24
N	12	10	8	7	5	4	3	3	3	4	5	7	10	12	14	17	18	19	20	20	18	17	15	13
NE	13	11	9	7	6	5	4	7	11	16	19	20	21	22	23	24	24	24	24	23	21	19	17	15
E	15	13	11	9	7	6	6	9	15	23	29	33	35	35	34	33	33	32	30	28	25	23	20	18
SE	16	14	12	10	8	6	6	8	12	19	26	32	36	39	40	39	37	36	33	31	28	25	22	19
S	18	15	13	11	9	7	5	5	5	7	11	17	23	29	34	38	40	40	37	34	31	27	24	21
SW	24	20	17	14	12	9	8	6	6	6	8	10	14	19	26	34	41	46	48	46	42	37	32	28
W	24	21	17	14	12	9	8	6	6	7	8	9	11	14	20	27	34	42	46	46	42	37	33	28
NW	18	15	13	11	9	7	5	5	5	5	6	8	10	13	15	19	23	28	32	33	31	28	24	21

Wall No. 7

Wall Facing	1	2	3	4	5	6	7	8	9	10	11	12	13	14	15	16	17	18	19	20	21	22	23	24
N	11	10	9	8	6	5	5	5	5	6	7	8	10	12	14	16	17	17	18	17	16	15	14	13
NE	13	12	10	9	8	7	7	10	14	16	18	19	19	20	21	22	23	23	22	21	20	18	17	15
E	16	15	13	11	10	8	9	13	19	24	28	31	31	31	31	30	30	29	28	26	24	22	20	18
SE	18	16	14	12	11	9	9	12	16	21	26	31	34	35	35	34	34	32	31	29	27	24	22	20
S	19	17	15	13	11	10	8	8	9	11	14	19	24	28	32	34	35	34	33	30	28	26	23	21
SW	24	21	19	16	14	12	11	10	10	10	11	13	16	22	27	33	38	41	41	39	36	33	30	27
W	24	21	18	16	14	12	11	10	10	10	11	12	13	16	21	27	34	38	40	38	35	32	29	26
NW	18	16	14	12	10	9	8	7	7	8	9	10	12	13	16	19	23	27	29	28	26	24	22	20

Wall No. 9

Wall Facing	1	2	3	4	5	6	7	8	9	10	11	12	13	14	15	16	17	18	19	20	21	22	23	24
N	15	13	11	9	7	6	4	3	2	2	3	4	6	8	10	13	15	17	19	20	20	20	19	17
NE	16	14	12	10	8	6	5	4	5	8	12	16	19	21	22	23	24	25	25	25	24	23	21	19
E	19	16	14	11	9	7	6	5	6	10	17	24	30	34	36	36	35	35	33	32	30	28	25	22
SE	21	18	15	12	10	8	6	5	5	8	13	20	27	33	38	40	41	40	38	36	34	31	27	24
S	24	20	17	14	11	9	7	5	4	4	5	8	12	18	25	31	36	40	41	41	38	35	31	27
SW	32	27	23	19	15	12	10	8	6	5	5	6	7	10	15	21	29	36	43	48	49	47	42	37
W	33	28	23	19	16	13	10	8	6	5	5	6	7	9	12	16	22	29	37	43	47	46	43	38
NW	25	21	18	15	12	10	7	6	4	4	4	5	6	8	11	13	16	20	25	30	33	33	31	28

Columns 1–24: Solar time, hr

Table 7-22-A40 August Cooling Load Temperature Differences for Calculating Cooling Load from Sunlit Walls 40° North Latitude (*Concluded*)

Wall No. 10

Wall Facing	1	2	3	4	5	6	7	8	9	10	11	12	13	14	15	16	17	18	19	20	21	22	23	24
N	15	13	11	9	8	6	5	4	3	3	3	4	6	8	10	13	15	17	18	19	20	19	18	17
NE	17	14	12	10	9	7	5	5	6	9	12	15	18	20	21	22	23	24	25	24	24	22	21	19
E	19	17	14	12	10	8	6	6	8	12	18	24	29	32	34	34	34	34	33	32	30	27	25	22
SE	21	18	16	13	11	9	7	6	7	10	15	21	27	32	36	38	39	38	37	36	33	30	27	24
S	24	21	18	15	12	10	8	6	5	5	6	9	13	19	25	30	35	38	39	38	37	34	31	27
SW	32	28	24	20	16	13	11	8	7	6	6	6	8	11	16	22	29	36	41	45	45	44	40	36
W	32	28	24	20	17	14	11	9	7	6	6	6	8	9	12	17	23	30	36	41	44	43	40	37
NW	24	21	18	15	13	10	8	6	5	4	5	5	7	9	11	13	17	21	25	29	31	31	29	27

Wall No. 11

Wall Facing	1	2	3	4	5	6	7	8	9	10	11	12	13	14	15	16	17	18	19	20	21	22	23	24
N	14	13	11	10	9	8	7	6	5	5	6	6	7	9	10	12	14	15	16	17	17	17	16	15
NE	17	15	14	12	11	9	8	8	9	11	14	16	17	18	19	20	21	22	22	22	21	21	19	18
E	20	19	17	15	13	12	10	10	12	15	20	24	27	29	30	30	30	30	29	29	27	26	24	22
SE	22	20	18	16	14	13	11	10	11	14	17	22	26	30	32	33	34	33	33	32	30	28	26	24
S	23	21	19	17	15	13	12	10	9	9	10	12	16	19	24	28	31	33	33	33	32	30	28	26
SW	29	26	24	21	19	17	15	13	12	11	11	11	12	14	18	22	27	32	36	39	39	37	35	32
W	29	26	24	21	19	17	15	13	12	11	10	11	11	12	14	18	22	28	33	36	37	36	34	32
NW	21	20	18	16	14	12	11	9	8	8	8	8	9	10	12	14	16	19	23	26	27	26	25	23

Wall No. 12

Wall Facing	1	2	3	4	5	6	7	8	9	10	11	12	13	14	15	16	17	18	19	20	21	22	23	24
N	14	13	12	10	9	8	7	6	6	6	6	7	8	9	10	12	13	15	16	16	16	16	15	15
NE	17	15	14	13	11	10	9	9	10	12	14	16	17	18	19	20	20	21	21	21	21	20	19	18
E	21	19	17	16	14	13	11	11	13	16	19	23	26	28	29	29	29	29	29	28	27	26	24	23
SE	23	21	19	17	15	14	12	12	12	14	18	22	25	29	31	32	32	32	32	31	30	28	26	25
S	23	21	20	18	16	14	13	11	10	10	11	13	16	19	23	27	29	31	32	32	31	29	27	25
SW	29	27	24	22	20	18	16	14	13	12	12	12	13	15	18	22	27	31	35	37	37	36	34	31
W	28	26	24	22	19	17	16	14	13	12	12	12	12	13	15	18	22	27	31	34	35	35	33	31
NW	21	19	18	16	14	13	11	10	9	9	9	9	10	11	12	14	16	19	22	24	25	25	24	23

Wall No. 13

Wall Facing	1	2	3	4	5	6	7	8	9	10	11	12	13	14	15	16	17	18	19	20	21	22	23	24
N	13	12	11	10	10	9	8	7	7	7	7	7	8	9	11	12	13	14	15	15	15	15	15	14
NE	17	15	14	13	12	11	10	10	11	13	15	16	17	17	18	19	20	20	21	20	20	19	19	18
E	21	20	18	17	15	14	13	13	14	17	20	23	25	27	27	28	28	28	28	27	26	25	24	22
SE	23	21	20	18	17	15	14	13	14	16	19	22	25	28	30	30	31	31	30	29	28	27	26	24
S	23	21	20	18	17	15	14	13	12	12	13	14	17	20	23	26	28	29	30	30	29	27	26	25
SW	28	26	24	22	20	19	17	16	15	14	14	14	14	16	19	23	27	30	33	34	34	33	32	30
W	27	25	23	22	20	18	17	15	14	14	13	13	14	14	16	19	22	26	30	32	33	32	31	29
NW	20	19	17	16	15	13	12	11	10	10	10	10	11	12	13	14	16	19	21	23	24	23	23	21

Wall No. 14

Wall Facing	1	2	3	4	5	6	7	8	9	10	11	12	13	14	15	16	17	18	19	20	21	22	23	24
N	13	13	12	11	10	10	9	8	8	8	8	8	8	9	10	11	12	13	14	14	14	14	14	14
NE	17	16	15	14	13	12	12	11	12	13	14	15	16	17	17	18	19	19	20	20	20	19	19	18
E	22	21	20	18	17	16	15	14	15	17	19	21	23	25	26	26	26	27	27	26	26	25	24	23
SE	24	22	21	20	19	17	16	15	15	16	18	21	23	25	27	28	29	29	29	29	28	27	26	25
S	24	22	21	20	18	17	16	15	14	14	14	15	16	19	21	23	25	27	28	28	28	27	26	25
SW	28	27	25	24	22	21	19	18	17	16	15	15	15	16	18	21	24	27	30	31	32	32	31	29
W	27	26	24	23	21	20	19	17	16	15	15	15	15	15	16	18	20	23	27	29	30	30	30	28
NW	20	19	18	17	16	15	14	13	12	11	11	11	11	12	13	14	15	17	19	21	22	22	22	21

Wall No. 15

Wall Facing	1	2	3	4	5	6	7	8	9	10	11	12	13	14	15	16	17	18	19	20	21	22	23	24
N	17	15	14	12	11	9	8	6	5	4	4	4	5	6	7	9	11	13	15	17	18	18	18	18
NE	19	18	16	14	12	10	8	7	6	7	9	11	14	16	18	19	21	22	23	23	24	23	22	21
E	24	21	19	16	14	12	10	8	8	9	12	16	21	25	29	31	32	33	33	32	31	30	28	26
SE	26	23	21	18	15	13	11	9	8	8	10	14	19	24	28	32	35	36	37	36	35	33	31	29
S	29	26	23	20	17	15	12	10	8	7	6	7	9	12	17	21	26	31	34	36	36	35	34	31
SW	37	33	30	26	23	19	16	14	11	9	8	7	8	9	11	15	19	25	31	37	40	42	42	40
W	36	33	30	26	23	20	16	14	11	9	8	8	8	8	10	12	15	20	26	32	37	39	40	39
NW	27	25	22	20	17	15	12	10	8	7	6	6	6	7	8	10	12	15	18	22	26	28	29	28

Wall No. 16

Wall Facing	1	2	3	4	5	6	7	8	9	10	11	12	13	14	15	16	17	18	19	20	21	22	23	24
N	16	15	14	12	11	10	9	7	6	6	5	5	6	7	8	9	11	12	14	15	16	17	17	17
NE	19	18	16	15	13	12	10	9	8	9	10	12	14	16	17	18	19	21	21	22	22	22	21	20
E	24	22	20	18	16	14	12	11	10	11	13	17	21	24	26	28	29	30	30	30	30	29	27	26
SE	26	24	22	20	17	15	13	12	11	11	12	15	19	23	27	30	32	33	34	34	33	32	30	28
S	28	26	23	21	19	16	14	12	11	9	9	9	11	13	17	21	25	28	31	32	33	33	31	30
SW	35	32	29	27	24	21	18	16	14	12	11	10	10	11	13	15	19	24	29	33	36	38	38	36
W	34	32	29	26	24	21	18	16	14	12	11	10	10	10	11	13	16	20	24	29	33	35	36	35
NW	25	23	22	20	18	16	14	12	10	9	8	8	8	8	9	11	12	15	18	21	24	25	26	26

Column headings 1–24: Solar time, hr.

1. Direct Application of Data,
   - Dark surface
   - Indoor temperature of 78°F
   - Outdoor maximum temperature of 95°F with mean temperature of 85°F and daily range of 21°F
   - Solar radiation typical of clear day on 21st day of month
   - Outside surface film resistance of 0.333 (h·ft²·°F)/Btu
   - Inside surface film resistance of 0.685 (h·ft²·°F)/Btu

2. Adjustments to Table Data
   Design temperatures:

$$\text{Corr. CLTD} = \text{CLTD} + (78 - T_r) + (T_m - 85)$$

where T_r = inside temperature and
T_m = mean outdoor temperature,
T_m = maximum outdoor temperature − (daily range)/2

- No adjustment recommended for color

Table 7-22-A48 August Cooling Load Temperature Differences for Calculating Cooling Load from Sunlit Walls 48° North Latitude

Wall No. 1

Wall Facing	1	2	3	4	5	6	7	8	9	10	11	12	13	14	15	16	17	18	19	20	21	22	23	24
N	1	0	-1	-2	-3	-2	2	4	7	11	15	20	23	26	27	27	26	23	20	14	10	7	4	2
NE	1	0	-1	-2	-3	0	16	32	36	32	24	22	24	26	28	28	26	23	18	13	9	7	4	3
E	1	0	-1	-2	-3	1	21	45	60	63	58	47	34	30	29	28	26	23	18	13	10	7	5	3
SE	2	0	-1	-2	-3	-1	13	34	52	64	69	68	61	50	37	31	27	24	19	14	10	7	5	3
S	2	0	-1	-2	-2	-3	0	6	19	34	49	60	68	71	67	59	47	33	22	15	10	7	5	3
SW	2	1	-1	-2	-2	-2	0	3	7	11	17	32	50	65	76	81	78	66	45	24	13	8	5	3
W	2	0	-1	-2	-2	-2	0	3	7	11	16	20	25	40	58	72	79	75	55	28	15	9	5	3
NW	1	0	-1	-2	-3	-3	-1	3	7	11	15	20	23	26	29	39	50	54	44	24	13	8	5	3

Wall No. 2

Wall Facing	1	2	3	4	5	6	7	8	9	10	11	12	13	14	15	16	17	18	19	20	21	22	23	24
N	5	3	1	0	-1	-2	-2	0	2	5	8	12	16	19	23	25	26	26	24	22	18	14	10	7
NE	5	3	1	0	-1	-2	0	8	19	27	29	27	25	25	25	26	27	26	24	21	17	13	10	7
E	5	3	2	0	-1	-2	1	12	28	43	52	55	51	43	37	33	30	28	26	22	18	14	10	7
SE	5	3	2	0	-1	-2	0	7	21	36	50	59	63	62	56	47	39	33	28	23	18	14	11	8
S	6	4	2	1	-1	-1	-2	-1	3	11	23	36	48	58	64	65	62	54	43	33	24	17	12	8
SW	7	5	2	1	0	-1	-2	-1	1	4	8	13	23	37	51	63	72	74	70	57	41	28	18	12
W	8	5	3	1	0	-1	-2	-1	1	4	8	12	16	21	31	45	58	68	70	62	46	31	20	13
NW	7	4	2	0	-1	-2	-2	-1	1	4	8	12	16	19	23	27	33	41	46	44	34	24	16	10

Wall No. 3

Wall Facing	1	2	3	4	5	6	7	8	9	10	11	12	13	14	15	16	17	18	19	20	21	22	23	24
N	6	5	3	1	0	-1	0	1	3	5	8	11	15	18	21	23	24	23	23	20	17	14	11	9
NE	7	5	3	2	0	0	4	12	20	23	23	23	23	24	25	26	26	25	23	20	17	14	11	9
E	7	5	3	2	1	0	6	17	30	40	45	46	42	38	36	34	32	29	26	22	19	15	12	10
SE	8	6	4	2	1	0	4	12	24	36	45	52	55	54	49	43	39	34	30	25	21	17	13	10
S	9	7	5	3	1	0	0	2	6	14	24	35	45	52	57	58	55	48	40	33	26	21	16	12
SW	13	9	6	4	2	1	0	1	3	5	9	15	25	37	49	58	64	65	59	49	38	30	23	17
W	13	9	7	4	2	1	0	1	3	5	8	12	15	22	33	44	54	61	60	50	40	31	23	18
NW	10	7	5	3	1	0	0	1	2	5	8	11	15	18	21	26	33	39	41	36	29	23	18	13

Wall No. 4

Wall Facing	1	2	3	4	5	6	7	8	9	10	11	12	13	14	15	16	17	18	19	20	21	22	23	24
N	10	7	5	3	2	0	-1	-1	0	2	4	7	10	13	17	20	22	24	24	24	22	19	16	13
NE	9	7	5	3	2	0	0	2	8	15	21	24	24	24	25	25	26	26	26	24	22	19	15	12
E	10	7	5	3	2	0	0	3	12	23	35	43	46	46	42	39	36	33	30	27	24	20	16	13
SE	11	8	6	4	2	1	0	2	8	18	30	41	50	55	56	53	48	42	37	32	27	22	18	14
S	13	9	7	4	2	1	0	-1	0	4	10	19	30	40	50	56	59	58	53	46	37	30	23	17
SW	19	13	9	6	4	2	0	0	0	1	4	7	12	21	32	44	54	63	66	64	56	45	35	26
W	20	14	10	6	4	2	0	0	0	1	4	7	10	14	20	29	39	50	59	61	56	47	37	28
NW	15	11	8	5	3	1	0	-1	0	1	3	6	10	13	17	20	25	31	37	40	39	34	27	21

Wall No. 5

Wall Facing	1	2	3	4	5	6	7	8	9	10	11	12	13	14	15	16	17	18	19	20	21	22	23	24
N	11	9	7	5	4	2	2	1	2	3	5	7	9	12	15	17	19	21	21	21	20	18	15	13
NE	12	9	7	6	4	3	2	5	10	15	19	20	20	21	22	23	24	25	24	23	21	19	16	14
E	13	11	9	7	5	3	3	7	14	23	31	36	39	38	37	35	34	32	30	28	25	22	19	16
SE	15	12	10	8	6	4	3	5	11	19	28	36	43	46	47	45	43	40	36	33	29	25	21	18
S	18	15	12	9	7	5	3	3	4	7	12	19	28	36	43	48	50	49	46	41	36	31	26	22
SW	24	19	15	12	9	7	5	4	4	4	6	8	13	20	29	39	47	54	56	54	48	41	35	29
W	23	19	15	12	9	7	5	4	4	4	6	8	10	13	19	27	36	44	50	51	47	41	34	28
NW	17	14	11	9	6	5	3	2	2	3	5	7	10	12	15	18	22	28	33	35	33	29	25	21

Wall No. 6

Wall Facing	1	2	3	4	5	6	7	8	9	10	11	12	13	14	15	16	17	18	19	20	21	22	23	24
N	11	10	8	7	5	4	3	3	3	4	5	7	9	12	14	16	18	19	19	19	18	17	15	13
NE	12	11	9	7	6	4	5	7	11	15	17	18	19	20	21	22	23	23	23	22	20	18	16	14
E	15	13	11	9	7	6	6	10	16	23	29	33	35	34	34	33	32	31	30	28	25	23	20	17
SE	17	15	12	10	8	6	6	8	13	20	27	34	39	42	43	41	40	38	35	32	29	26	23	20
S	20	17	14	12	10	8	6	5	6	9	14	20	27	33	39	43	45	45	42	39	35	31	27	23
SW	25	21	18	15	12	10	8	7	6	7	8	10	14	21	28	36	43	48	50	48	44	39	34	29
W	24	21	17	14	12	10	8	7	6	7	8	9	11	14	19	26	34	41	45	45	42	37	33	28
NW	18	15	12	10	8	7	5	4	4	5	6	8	10	12	14	17	21	26	30	31	29	27	23	20

Wall No. 7

Wall Facing	1	2	3	4	5	6	7	8	9	10	11	12	13	14	15	16	17	18	19	20	21	22	23	24
N	11	10	9	7	6	5	5	5	5	6	7	8	10	12	14	15	16	17	17	17	16	15	14	13
NE	13	11	10	9	7	6	7	10	13	16	16	17	18	19	20	21	21	21	21	20	19	18	16	14
E	16	15	13	11	10	8	10	14	19	24	28	30	31	30	30	30	30	29	28	26	24	22	20	18
SE	19	17	15	13	11	10	10	13	17	23	28	33	36	37	37	37	35	34	32	30	28	26	23	21
S	21	19	16	14	12	11	9	9	10	13	17	22	27	32	36	39	40	39	37	34	32	29	26	23
SW	25	22	20	17	15	13	11	11	10	10	11	13	18	23	29	35	40	43	43	41	38	34	31	28
W	24	21	18	16	14	12	11	10	10	10	10	12	13	16	21	27	33	38	40	38	35	32	29	26
NW	17	15	13	11	10	8	7	7	7	7	8	10	11	13	15	17	21	25	27	27	25	23	21	19

Wall No. 9

Wall Facing	1	2	3	4	5	6	7	8	9	10	11	12	13	14	15	16	17	18	19	20	21	22	23	24
N	15	13	11	9	7	6	4	3	2	2	3	4	5	8	10	12	15	17	19	20	20	20	18	17
NE	16	14	12	10	8	6	5	4	5	8	12	15	17	19	20	21	22	23	24	24	23	22	20	18
E	19	16	14	11	9	7	6	5	6	11	17	24	30	34	36	36	35	34	33	31	30	27	25	22
SE	22	18	16	13	10	8	6	5	6	9	14	21	29	35	40	43	44	43	41	38	35	32	28	25
S	26	22	19	15	13	10	8	6	5	4	6	9	15	21	28	35	41	45	47	46	43	39	35	30
SW	34	29	24	20	16	13	10	8	6	5	5	6	7	11	16	23	31	39	46	50	51	49	45	39
W	33	28	24	20	16	13	10	8	6	5	5	6	7	9	11	15	21	28	36	43	46	46	43	38
NW	24	20	17	14	12	9	7	5	4	4	4	4	6	8	10	13	15	19	23	28	31	31	30	27

Column headings 1–24: Solar time, hr

Table 7-22-A48 August Cooling Load Temperature Differences for Calculating Cooling Load from Sunlit Walls 48° North Latitude (*Concluded*)

Wall No. 10 — Solar time, hr

Wall Facing	1	2	3	4	5	6	7	8	9	10	11	12	13	14	15	16	17	18	19	20	21	22	23	24
N	15	13	11	9	8	6	5	4	3	3	3	4	6	8	10	12	14	16	18	19	19	19	18	16
NE	16	14	12	10	8	7	5	5	6	9	12	15	16	18	19	20	22	23	23	23	23	21	20	18
E	19	17	14	12	10	8	6	6	8	13	18	24	29	32	33	34	34	33	32	31	29	27	25	22
SE	22	19	16	14	11	9	7	6	8	11	16	22	29	34	38	41	41	41	40	37	35	32	29	25
S	27	23	19	16	13	11	9	7	6	6	7	11	16	22	28	34	39	43	44	43	41	38	34	31
SW	34	29	25	21	17	14	11	9	7	6	6	7	8	12	17	24	31	38	44	47	48	46	43	38
W	33	28	24	20	17	14	11	9	7	6	6	6	8	9	12	16	22	29	36	41	43	43	40	37
NW	23	20	17	15	12	10	8	6	5	4	4	5	6	8	10	13	15	19	23	27	29	29	28	26

Wall No. 11 — Solar time, hr

Wall Facing	1	2	3	4	5	6	7	8	9	10	11	12	13	14	15	16	17	18	19	20	21	22	23	24
N	14	12	11	10	9	8	7	6	5	5	6	6	7	9	10	12	13	15	16	17	17	16	16	15
NE	16	15	13	12	10	9	8	8	9	11	13	15	16	17	18	19	20	20	21	21	20	20	19	17
E	20	18	17	15	13	12	10	10	12	15	20	24	27	29	30	30	30	30	29	28	27	26	24	22
SE	23	21	19	17	15	13	12	11	12	15	19	23	28	32	34	36	36	36	35	33	32	30	28	25
S	26	24	21	19	17	15	13	12	11	10	12	14	18	23	27	32	35	37	38	37	36	33	31	29
SW	31	28	25	22	20	18	16	14	12	11	11	11	12	15	19	24	29	34	39	41	41	39	37	34
W	29	26	24	21	19	17	15	13	12	11	10	11	11	12	14	17	22	27	32	36	37	36	34	32
NW	21	19	17	15	13	12	10	9	8	8	8	8	9	10	11	13	15	18	21	24	25	25	24	22

Wall No. 12 — Solar time, hr

Wall Facing	1	2	3	4	5	6	7	8	9	10	11	12	13	14	15	16	17	18	19	20	21	22	23	24
N	13	12	11	10	9	8	7	6	6	6	6	7	8	9	10	12	13	14	15	16	16	16	15	14
NE	16	15	13	12	11	10	9	9	10	11	13	15	16	16	17	18	19	20	20	20	20	19	18	17
E	21	19	17	16	14	13	11	11	13	16	20	23	26	28	28	29	29	29	28	28	27	26	24	22
SE	24	22	20	18	16	14	13	12	13	15	19	23	27	30	33	34	35	35	34	33	31	30	28	26
S	26	24	22	20	18	16	14	13	12	12	13	15	18	22	26	30	33	35	36	36	34	33	31	28
SW	31	28	26	23	21	19	17	15	14	13	12	12	13	16	19	24	28	33	37	39	39	38	36	33
W	28	26	24	22	19	17	16	14	13	12	12	12	12	13	15	18	21	26	31	34	35	35	33	31
NW	20	19	17	15	14	12	11	10	9	8	8	9	9	10	12	13	15	17	20	23	24	24	23	22

Wall No. 13 — Solar time, hr

Wall Facing	1	2	3	4	5	6	7	8	9	10	11	12	13	14	15	16	17	18	19	20	21	22	23	24
N	13	12	11	10	9	8	8	7	7	7	7	7	8	9	10	12	13	14	14	15	15	15	14	14
NE	16	15	14	13	12	10	10	10	11	12	14	15	16	16	17	18	18	19	19	19	19	19	18	17
E	21	19	18	17	15	14	13	13	15	17	21	23	25	27	27	27	27	27	27	27	26	25	24	22
SE	24	22	21	19	17	16	15	14	15	17	20	24	27	30	31	32	33	32	32	31	30	29	27	25
S	26	24	22	20	19	17	16	14	14	14	15	17	20	23	26	29	32	33	34	33	32	31	29	28
SW	29	27	25	23	21	20	18	17	15	15	14	14	15	17	20	24	28	32	35	36	36	35	33	31
W	27	25	23	22	20	18	17	15	14	14	13	13	14	14	16	18	22	26	30	32	33	32	31	29
NW	19	18	17	15	14	13	12	11	10	10	10	10	10	11	12	13	15	17	20	22	23	22	22	20

Wall No. 14 — Solar time, hr

Wall Facing	1	2	3	4	5	6	7	8	9	10	11	12	13	14	15	16	17	18	19	20	21	22	23	24
N	13	12	12	11	10	9	9	8	8	8	8	8	8	9	10	11	12	13	13	14	14	14	14	14
NE	16	16	15	14	13	12	11	11	11	12	13	14	15	16	16	17	17	18	18	19	19	18	18	17
E	22	21	19	18	17	16	15	14	15	17	19	21	23	25	25	26	26	26	26	26	26	25	24	23
SE	25	24	22	21	20	18	17	16	16	17	19	22	25	27	29	30	31	31	31	30	30	29	28	26
S	26	25	24	22	21	19	18	17	16	15	16	17	19	21	24	27	29	31	32	32	31	30	29	28
SW	30	28	26	25	23	22	20	19	18	17	16	16	16	17	19	22	25	28	31	33	34	33	32	31
W	27	26	24	23	21	20	18	17	16	15	15	15	15	15	16	18	20	23	26	29	30	30	29	28
NW	19	18	17	16	15	14	13	12	11	11	11	11	11	11	12	13	14	16	18	20	21	21	21	20

Wall No. 15 — Solar time, hr

Wall Facing	1	2	3	4	5	6	7	8	9	10	11	12	13	14	15	16	17	18	19	20	21	22	23	24
N	16	15	14	12	11	9	7	6	5	4	4	4	5	6	7	9	11	13	15	16	17	18	18	17
NE	19	17	15	13	12	10	8	7	6	7	9	11	13	15	17	18	19	20	21	22	22	22	21	20
E	23	21	19	16	14	12	10	8	8	9	12	16	21	25	29	31	32	32	32	32	31	30	28	26
SE	27	24	21	19	16	14	11	9	8	9	11	15	20	25	30	34	37	39	39	38	37	35	33	30
S	32	29	25	22	19	16	14	11	9	8	7	8	11	14	19	25	30	35	39	41	41	40	38	35
SW	39	35	31	28	24	20	17	14	12	10	9	8	8	9	12	16	21	27	33	39	43	44	44	42
W	36	33	30	26	23	20	17	14	11	10	8	8	8	8	9	11	15	20	25	31	36	39	40	39
NW	26	24	21	19	16	14	12	10	8	7	6	6	6	7	8	10	12	14	17	21	24	26	27	27

Wall No. 16 — Solar time, hr

Wall Facing	1	2	3	4	5	6	7	8	9	10	11	12	13	14	15	16	17	18	19	20	21	22	23	24
N	16	15	14	12	11	10	8	7	6	6	5	5	6	6	8	9	11	12	14	15	16	17	17	16
NE	18	17	16	14	13	11	10	8	8	9	10	12	13	15	16	17	18	19	20	21	21	21	20	19
E	24	22	20	18	16	14	12	11	10	11	14	17	21	24	26	28	29	30	30	30	29	28	27	26
SE	28	25	23	20	18	16	14	12	11	12	13	16	20	24	28	32	34	35	36	36	35	34	32	30
S	31	29	26	23	21	18	16	14	12	11	10	11	13	16	19	24	28	32	35	37	37	37	35	33
SW	36	34	31	28	25	22	19	17	15	13	12	11	11	11	13	16	21	26	31	35	38	40	40	39
W	34	32	29	26	24	21	18	16	14	12	11	10	10	10	11	13	15	19	24	29	33	35	36	35
NW	24	22	21	19	17	15	13	11	10	9	8	7	7	8	9	10	12	14	16	19	22	24	25	24

1. Direct Application of Data,
   - Dark surface
   - Indoor temperature of 78°F
   - Outdoor maximum temperature of 95°F with mean temperature of 85°F and daily range of 21°F
   - Solar radiation typical of clear day on 21st day of month
   - Outside surface film resistance of 0.333 (h·ft²·°F)/Btu
   - Inside surface film resistance of 0.685 (h·ft²·°F)/Btu

2. Adjustments to Table Data

   Design temperatures:

$$\text{Corr. CLTD} = \text{CLTD} + (78 - T_r) + (T_m - 85)$$

where T_r = inside temperature and

T_m = mean outdoor temperature,

T_m = maximum outdoor temperature − (daily range)/2

   - No adjustment recommended for color

Table 7-23 Thermal Properties and Code Numbers of Layers Used in Wall and Roof Descriptions

Code Number	Description	Thickness and Thermal Properties					
		L	k	ρ	c_p	R	Mass
A0	Outside surface resistance	0.0	0.0	0.0	0.0	0.33	0.0
A1	1 in. Stucco	0.0833	0.4	116.0	0.20	0.21	9.7
A2	4 in. Face brick	0.333	0.77	125.0	0.22	0.43	41.7
A3	Steel siding	0.005	26.0	480.0	0.10	0.00	2.4
A4	1/2 in. Slag	0.0417	0.11	70.0	0.40	0.38	2.2
A5	Outside surface resistance	0.0	0.0	0.0	0.0	0.33	0.0
A6	Finish	0.0417	0.24	78.0	0.26	0.17	3.3
A7	4 in. Face brick	0.333	0.77	125.0	0.22	0.43	41.7
B1	Air space resistance	0.0	0.0	0.0	0.0	0.91	0.0
B2	1 in. Insulation	0.083	0.025	2.0	0.2	3.33	0.2
B3	2 in. Insulation	0.167	0.025	2.0	0.2	6.67	0.3
B4	3 in. Insulation	0.25	0.025	2.0	0.2	1.19	0.5
B5	1 in. Insulation	0.0833	0.025	5.7	0.2	3.33	0.5
B6	2 in. Insulation	0.167	0.025	5.7	0.2	6.67	1.0
B7	1 in. Wood	0.0833	0.07	37.0	0.6	1.19	3.1
B8	2.5 in. Wood	0.2083	0.07	37.0	0.6	2.98	7.7
B9	4 in. Wood	0.333	0.07	37.0	0.6	4.76	12.3
B10	2 in. Wood	0.167	0.07	37.0	0.6	2.39	6.2
B11	3 in. Wood	0.25	0.07	37.0	0.6	3.57	9.3
B12	3 in. Insulation	0.25	0.025	5.7	0.2	10.00	1.4
B13	4 in. Insulation	0.333	0.025	5.7	0.2	13.33	1.9
B14	5 in. Insulation	0.417	0.025	5.7	0.2	16.67	2.4
B15	6 in. Insulation	0.500	0.025	5.7	0.2	20.00	2.9
B16	0.15 in. Insulation	0.0126	0.025	5.7	0.2	0.50	0.1
B17	0.3 in. Insulation	0.0252	0.025	5.7	0.2	1.00	0.1
B18	0.45 in. Insulation	0.0379	0.025	5.7	0.2	1.50	0.2
B19	0.61 in. Insulation	0.0505	0.025	5.7	0.2	2.00	0.3
B20	0.76 in. Insulation	0.0631	0.025	5.7	0.2	2.50	0.4
B21	1.36 in. Insulation	0.1136	0.025	5.7	0.2	4.50	0.6
B22	1.67 in. Insulation	0.1388	0.025	5.7	0.2	5.50	0.8
B23	2.42 in. Insulation	0.2019	0.025	5.7	0.2	8.00	1.2
B24	2.73 in. Insulation	0.2272	0.025	5.7	0.2	9.00	1.3
B25	3.33 in. Insulation	0.2777	0.025	5.7	0.2	11.00	1.6
B26	3.64 in. Insulation	0.3029	0.025	5.7	0.2	12.00	1.7
B27	4.54 in. Insulation	0.3786	0.025	5.7	0.2	15.00	2.2
C1	4 in. Clay tile	0.333	0.33	70.0	0.2	1.01	23.3
C2	4 in. Lightweight concrete block	0.333	0.22	38.0	0.2	1.51	12.7
C3	4 in. Heavyweight concrete block	0.333	0.47	61.0	0.2	0.71	20.3
C4	4 in. Common brick	0.333	0.42	120.0	0.2	0.79	40.0
C5	4 in. Heavyweight concrete	0.333	1.0	140.0	0.2	0.33	46.7
C6	8 in. Clay tile	0.667	0.33	70.0	0.2	2.00	46.7
C7	8 in. Lightweight concrete block	0.667	0.33	38.0	0.2	2.00	25.3
C8	8 in. Heavyweight concrete block	0.667	0.6	61.0	0.2	1.11	40.7
C9	8 in. Common brick	0.667	0.42	120.0	0.2	1.59	80.0
C10	8 in. Heavyweight concrete	0.667	1.0	140.0	0.2	0.67	93.4
C11	12 in. Heavyweight concrete	1.0	1.0	140.0	0.2	1.00	140.0
C12	2 in. Heavyweight concrete	0.167	1.0	140.0	0.2	0.17	23.3
C13	6 in. Heavyweight concrete	0.5	1.0	140.0	0.2	0.50	70.0
C14	4 in. Lightweight concrete	0.333	0.1	40.0	0.2	3.33	13.3
C15	6 in. Lightweight concrete	0.5	0.1	40.0	0.2	5.00	20.0
C16	8 in. Lightweight concrete	0.667	0.1	40.0	0.2	6.67	26.7
C17	8 in. Lightweight concrete block (filled)	0.667	0.08	18.0	0.2	8.34	12.0
C18	8 in. Heavyweight concrete block (filled)	0.667	0.34	53.0	0.2	1.96	35.4
C19	12 in. Lightweight concrete block (filled)	1.000	0.08	19.0	0.2	12.50	19.0
C20	12 in. Heavyweight concrete block (filled)	1.000	0.39	56.0	0.2	2.56	56.0
E0	Inside surface resistance	0.0	0.0	0.0	0.0	0.69	0.0
E1	3/4 in. Plaster or gypsum	0.0625	0.42	100.0	0.2	0.15	6.3
E2	1/2 in. Slag or stone	0.0417	0.83	55.0	0.40	0.05	2.3
E3	3/8 in. Felt and membrane	0.0313	0.11	70.0	0.40	0.29	2.2
E4	Ceiling air space	0.0	0.0	0.0	0.0	1.00	0.0
E5	Acoustic tile	0.0625	0.035	30.0	0.2	1.79	1.9

L = thickness, ft
k = thermal conductivity, Btu/h·ft·°F
ρ = density, lb/ft^3
c_p = specific heat, Btu/lb·°F
R = thermal resistance, °F·ft^2·h/Btu
Mass = unit mass, lb/ft^2

Table 7-24A Wall Types, Mass Located Inside Insulation, for Use with Table 7-22

Secondary Material	R-Value, ft²·°F·h/Btu	Principal Wall Material**														
		A1	A2	B7	B10	B9	C1	C2	C3	C4	C5	C6	C7	C8	C17	C18
Stucco and/or plaster	0.0 to 2.0	*	*	*	*	*	*	*	*	*	*	*	*	*	*	*
	2.0 to 2.5	*	5	*	*	*	*	*	*	*	5	*	*	*	*	*
	2.5 to 3.0	*	5	*	*	*	3	*	2	5	6	*	*	5	*	*
	3.0 to 3.5	*	5	*	*	*	4	2	2	5	6	*	*	6	*	*
	3.5 to 4.0	*	5	*	*	*	4	2	3	6	6	10	4	6	*	5
	4.0 to 4.75	*	6	*	*	*	5	2	4	6	6	11	5	10	*	10
	4.75 to 5.5	*	6	*	*	*	5	2	4	6	6	11	5	10	*	10
	5.5 to 6.5	*	6	*	*	*	5	2	5	10	7	12	5	11	*	10
	6.5 to 7.75	*	6	*	*	*	5	4	5	11	7	16	10	11	*	11
	7.75 to 9.0	*	6	*	*	*	5	4	5	11	7	*	10	11	*	11
	9.0 to 10.75	*	6	*	*	*	5	4	5	11	7	*	10	11	4	11
	10.75 to 12.75	*	6	*	*	*	5	4	5	11	11	*	10	11	4	11
	12.75 to 15.0	*	10	*	*	*	10	4	5	11	11	*	10	11	9	12
	15.0 to 17.5	*	10	*	*	*	10	5	5	11	11	*	11	12	10	16
	17.5 to 20.0	*	11	*	*	*	10	5	9	11	11	*	15	16	10	16
	20.0 to 23.0	*	11	*	*	*	10	9	9	16	11	*	15	16	10	16
	23.0 to 27.0	*	*	*	*	*	*	*	*	*	*	*	16	*	15	*
Steel or other light-weight siding	0.0 to 2.0	*	*	*	*	*	*	*	*	*	*	*	*	*	*	*
	2.0 to 2.5	*	3	*	*	*	*	*	2	3	5	*	*	*	*	*
	2.5 to 3.0	*	5	*	*	*	2	*	2	5	3	*	*	5	*	*
	3.0 to 3.5	*	5	*	*	*	3	1	2	5	5	*	*	5	*	*
	3.5 to 4.0	*	5	*	*	*	3	2	2	5	5	6	3	5	*	5
	4.0 to 4.75	*	6	*	*	*	4	2	2	5	5	10	4	6	*	5
	4.75 to 5.5	*	6	*	*	*	5	2	2	6	6	11	5	6	*	6
	5.5 to 6.5	*	6	*	*	*	5	2	3	6	6	11	5	6	*	6
	6.5 to 7.75	*	6	*	*	*	5	2	3	6	6	11	5	6	*	10
	7.75 to 9.0	*	6	*	*	*	5	2	3	6	6	12	5	6	*	11
	9.0 to 10.75	*	6	*	*	*	5	2	3	6	6	12	5	6	4	11
	10.75 to 12.75	*	6	*	*	*	5	2	3	6	7	12	6	11	4	11
	12.75 to 15.0	*	6	*	*	*	5	2	4	6	7	12	10	11	5	11
	15.0 to 17.5	*	10	*	*	*	6	4	4	10	7	*	10	11	9	11
	17.5 to 20.0	*	10	*	*	*	10	4	4	10	11	*	10	11	10	11
	20.0 to 23.0	*	11	*	*	*	10	4	5	11	11	*	10	11	10	16
	23.0 to 27.0	*	*	*	*	*	*	*	*	*	*	*	10	*	11	16
Face brick	0.0 to 2.0	*	*	*	*	*	*	*	*	*	*	*	*	*	*	*
	2.0 to 2.5	3	*	*	*	*	*	*	*	*	11	*	*	*	*	*
	2.5 to 3.0	5	11	*	*	*	*	*	6	11	12	*	*	*	*	*
	3.0 to 3.5	5	12	5	*	*	11	*	11	12	12	*	*	12	*	*
	3.5 to 4.0	5	12	6	*	*	12	6	12	12	13	*	*	12	*	*
	4.0 to 4.75	6	13	6	10	*	13	10	12	12	13	*	11	*	*	16
	4.75 to 5.5	6	13	6	11	*	*	11	12	13	13	*	16	*	*	*
	5.5 to 6.5	6	13	6	11	*	*	11	12	13	13	*	*	*	*	*
	6.5 to 7.75	6	13	6	11	*	*	11	13	*	13	*	*	*	*	*
	7.75 to 9.0	6	13	10	16	*	*	11	13	*	13	*	*	*	*	*
	9.0 to 10.75	6	14	10	16	*	*	11	13	*	14	*	*	*	16	*
	10.75 to 12.75	6	14	10	16	*	*	11	13	*	14	*	*	*	16	*
	12.75 to 15.0	6	*	11	16	*	*	12	13	*	*	*	*	*	*	*
	15.0 to 17.5	10	*	11	*	*	*	12	13	*	*	*	*	*	*	*
	17.5 to 20.0	10	*	11	*	*	*	16	*	*	*	*	*	*	*	*
	20.0 to 23.0	11	*	15	*	*	*	16	*	*	*	*	*	*	*	*
	23.0 to 27.0	*	*	*	*	*	*	16	*	*	*	*	*	*	*	*

*Denotes a wall that is not possible with the chosen set of parameters.
**See Table 11 for definition of Code letters

Table 7-24B Wall Types, Mass Evenly Distributed, for Use with Table 7-22

Secondary Material	R-Value, $ft^2 \cdot °F \cdot h/Btu$	Principal Wall Material**														
		A1	A2	B7	B10	B9	C1	C2	C3	C4	C5	C6	C7	C8	C17	C18
Stucco and/or plaster	0.0 to 2.0	1	3	*	*	*	*	*	1	3	3	*	*	*	*	*
	2.0 to 2.5	1	3	1	*	*	2	*	2	4	4	*	*	5	*	*
	2.5 to 3.0	1	4	1	*	*	2	2	2	4	4	*	*	5	*	*
	3.0 to 3.5	1	*	1	*	*	2	2	*	*	*	10	4	5	*	4
	3.5 to 4.0	1	*	1	2	*	*	4	*	*	*	10	4	*	*	4
	4.0 to 4.75	1	*	1	2	*	*	*	*	*	*	10	4	*	*	4
	4.75 to 5.5	1	*	1	2	*	*	*	*	*	*	*	*	*	*	*
	5.5 to 6.5	1	*	2	4	10	*	*	*	*	*	*	*	*	*	*
	6.5 to 7.75	1	*	2	4	11	*	*	*	*	*	*	*	*	*	*
	7.75 to 9.0	1	*	2	4	16	*	*	*	*	*	*	*	*	*	*
	9.0 to 10.75	1	*	2	4	16	*	*	*	*	*	*	*	*	4	*
	10.75 to 12.75	1	*	2	5	*	*	*	*	*	*	*	*	*	4	*
	12.75 to 15.0	2	*	2	5	*	*	*	*	*	*	*	*	*	*	*
	15.0 to 17.5	2	*	2	5	*	*	*	*	*	*	*	*	*	*	*
	17.5 to 20.0	2	*	2	9	*	*	*	*	*	*	*	*	*	*	*
	20.0 to 23.0	2	*	4	9	*	*	*	*	*	*	*	*	*	*	*
	23.0 to 27.0	*	*	*	9	*	*	*	*	*	*	*	*	*	*	*
Steel or other light-weight siding	0.0 to 2.0	1	3	*	*	*	*	*	1	3	2	*	*	*	*	*
	2.0 to 2.5	1	3	1	*	*	2	*	1	3	2	*	*	3	*	*
	2.5 to 3.0	1	4	1	*	*	2	1	2	4	4	*	*	3	*	*
	3.0 to 3.5	1	*	1	*	*	4	1	*	*	*	5	2	4	*	4
	3.5 to 4.0	1	*	1	2	*	*	2	*	*	*	5	2	*	*	4
	4.0 to 4.75	1	*	1	2	*	*	*	*	*	*	10	4	*	*	4
	4.75 to 5.5	1	*	1	2	*	*	*	*	*	*	*	*	*	*	*
	5.5 to 6.5	1	*	1	2	10	*	*	*	*	*	*	*	*	*	*
	6.5 to 7.75	1	*	1	4	11	*	*	*	*	*	*	*	*	*	*
	7.75 to 9.0	1	*	2	4	16	*	*	*	*	*	*	*	*	*	*
	9.0 to 10.75	1	*	2	4	16	*	*	*	*	*	*	*	*	2	*
	10.75 to 12.75	1	*	2	4	*	*	*	*	*	*	*	*	*	4	*
	12.75 to 15.0	1	*	2	5	*	*	*	*	*	*	*	*	*	*	*
	15.0 to 17.5	1	*	2	5	*	*	*	*	*	*	*	*	*	*	*
	17.5 to 20.0	1	*	2	5	*	*	*	*	*	*	*	*	*	*	*
	20.0 to 23.0	2	*	4	9	*	*	*	*	*	*	*	*	*	*	*
	23.0 to 27.0	*	*	*	9	*	*	*	*	*	*	*	*	*	*	*
Face brick	0.0 to 2.0	3	6	*	*	*	*	*	*	*	6	*	*	*	*	*
	2.0 to 2.5	3	10	*	*	*	*	*	5	10	10	*	*	*	*	*
	2.5 to 3.0	4	10	5	*	*	5	*	5	10	11	*	*	10	*	*
	3.0 to 3.5	*	11	5	*	*	10	5	5	11	11	15	10	10	*	10
	3.5 to 4.0	*	11	5	10	*	10	5	5	11	11	16	10	16	*	10
	4.0 to 4.75	*	11	*	11	*	10	5	5	16	11	*	10	16	*	16
	4.75 to 5.5	*	11	*	11	*	10	5	10	16	16	*	10	16	*	16
	5.5 to 6.5	*	16	*	*	*	10	9	10	16	11	*	11	16	*	16
	6.5 to 7.75	*	16	*	*	*	11	9	10	16	16	*	16	16	*	*
	7.75 to 9.0	*	16	*	*	*	15	9	10	16	*	*	15	16	*	*
	9.0 to 10.75	*	16	*	*	*	15	10	10	*	16	*	16	*	10	*
	10.75 to 12.75	*	16	*	*	*	16	10	10	*	*	*	16	*	15	*
	12.75 to 15.0	*	16	*	*	*	16	10	10	*	16	*	*	*	15	*
	15.0 to 17.5	*	*	*	*	*	16	10	15	*	*	*	*	*	16	*
	17.5 to 20.0	*	*	*	*	*	16	15	15	*	*	*	*	*	16	*
	20.0 to 23.0	*	*	*	*	*	*	15	16	*	*	*	*	*	*	*
	23.0 to 27.0	*	*	*	*	*	*	15	*	*	*	*	*	*	*	*

*Denotes a wall that is not possible with the chosen set of parameters.

**See Table 11 for definition of Code letters

Table 7-24C Wall Types, Mass Located Outside Insulation, for Use with Table 7-22

Secondary Material	R-Value, $ft^2 \cdot °F \cdot h/Btu$	Principal Wall Material**														
		A1	A2	B7	B10	B9	C1	C2	C3	C4	C5	C6	C7	C8	C17	C18
Stucco and/or plaster	0.0 to 2.0	1	3	*	*	*	*	*	1	3	3	*	*	*	*	*
	2.0 to 2.5	1	3	1	*	*	2	*	2	4	4	*	*	5	*	*
	2.5 to 3.0	1	4	1	*	*	2	2	2	4	4	*	*	5	*	*
	3.0 to 3.5	1	*	1	*	*	2	2	*	*	*	10	4	5	*	4
	3.5 to 4.0	1	*	1	2	*	*	4	*	*	*	10	4	*	*	4
	4.0 to 4.75	1	*	1	2	*	*	*	*	*	*	10	4	*	*	4
	4.75 to 5.5	1	*	1	2	*	*	*	*	*	*	*	*	*	*	*
	5.5 to 6.5	1	*	2	4	10	*	*	*	*	*	*	*	*	*	*
	6.5 to 7.75	1	*	2	4	11	*	*	*	*	*	*	*	*	*	*
	7.75 to 9.0	1	*	2	4	16	*	*	*	*	*	*	*	*	*	*
	9.0 to 10.75	1	*	2	4	16	*	*	*	*	*	*	*	*	4	*
	10.75 to 12.75	1	*	2	5	*	*	*	*	*	*	*	*	*	4	*
	12.75 to 15.0	2	*	2	5	*	*	*	*	*	*	*	*	*	*	*
	15.0 to 17.5	2	*	2	5	*	*	*	*	*	*	*	*	*	*	*
	17.5 to 20.0	2	*	2	9	*	*	*	*	*	*	*	*	*	*	*
	20.0 to 23.0	2	*	4	9	*	*	*	*	*	*	*	*	*	*	*
	23.0 to 27.0	*	*	*	9	*	*	*	*	*	*	*	*	*	*	*
Steel or other light-weight siding	0.0 to 2.0	1	3	*	*	*	*	*	1	3	2	*	*	*	*	*
	2.0 to 2.5	1	3	1	*	*	2	*	1	3	2	*	*	3	*	*
	2.5 to 3.0	1	4	1	*	*	2	1	2	4	4	*	*	3	*	*
	3.0 to 3.5	1	*	1	*	*	4	1	*	*	*	5	2	4	*	4
	3.5 to 4.0	1	*	1	2	*	*	2	*	*	*	5	2	*	*	4
	4.0 to 4.75	1	*	1	2	*	*	*	*	*	*	10	4	*	*	4
	4.75 to 5.5	1	*	1	2	*	*	*	*	*	*	*	*	*	*	*
	5.5 to 6.5	1	*	1	2	10	*	*	*	*	*	*	*	*	*	*
	6.5 to 7.75	1	*	1	4	11	*	*	*	*	*	*	*	*	*	*
	7.75 to 9.0	1	*	2	4	16	*	*	*	*	*	*	*	*	*	*
	9.0 to 10.75	1	*	2	4	16	*	*	*	*	*	*	*	*	2	*
	10.75 to 12.75	1	*	2	4	*	*	*	*	*	*	*	*	*	4	*
	12.75 to 15.0	1	*	2	5	*	*	*	*	*	*	*	*	*	*	*
	15.0 to 17.5	1	*	2	5	*	*	*	*	*	*	*	*	*	*	*
	17.5 to 20.0	1	*	2	5	*	*	*	*	*	*	*	*	*	*	*
	20.0 to 23.0	2	*	4	9	*	*	*	*	*	*	*	*	*	*	*
	23.0 to 27.0	*	*	*	9	*	*	*	*	*	*	*	*	*	*	*
Face brick	0.0 to 2.0	3	6	*	*	*	*	*	*	*	6	*	*	*	*	*
	2.0 to 2.5	3	10	*	*	*	*	*	5	10	10	*	*	*	*	*
	2.5 to 3.0	4	10	5	*	*	5	*	5	10	11	*	*	10	*	*
	3.0 to 3.5	*	11	5	*	*	10	5	5	11	11	15	10	10	*	10
	3.5 to 4.0	*	11	5	10	*	10	5	5	11	11	16	10	16	*	10
	4.0 to 4.75	*	11	*	11	*	10	5	5	16	11	*	10	16	*	16
	4.75 to 5.5	*	11	*	11	*	10	5	10	16	16	*	10	16	*	16
	5.5 to 6.5	*	16	*	*	*	10	9	10	16	11	*	11	16	*	16
	6.5 to 7.75	*	16	*	*	*	11	9	10	16	16	*	16	16	*	*
	7.75 to 9.0	*	16	*	*	*	15	9	10	16	*	*	15	16	*	*
	9.0 to 10.75	*	16	*	*	*	15	10	10	*	16	*	16	*	10	*
	10.75 to 12.75	*	16	*	*	*	16	10	10	*	*	*	16	*	15	*
	12.75 to 15.0	*	16	*	*	*	16	10	10	*	16	*	*	*	15	*
	15.0 to 17.5	*	*	*	*	*	16	10	15	*	*	*	*	*	16	*
	17.5 to 20.0	*	*	*	*	*	16	15	15	*	*	*	*	*	16	*
	20.0 to 23.0	*	*	*	*	*	*	15	16	*	*	*	*	*	*	*
	23.0 to 27.0	*	*	*	*	*	*	15	*	*	*	*	*	*	*	*

*Denotes a wall that is not possible with the chosen set of parameters.

**See Table 11 for definition of Code letters

A, B, C, or D are given as functions of some of the more common building configurations. The SCLs for sunlit glass are tabulated in Table 7-27 for each zone type. SCLs for externally shaded glass may be taken from these tables as those for North exposure, although with some loss of accuracy at latitudes lower than 24°N. Interpolation between latitudes can be performed with some loss of accuracy. The *Cooling and Heating Load Calculation Manual* (McQuiston and Spitler 1992) includes additional data for multistory buildings and for other latitudes, months, and zone types.

Interior Shading. The cooling load from solar radiation must be analyzed for one of two cases: (1) presence of interior shading or (2) absence of interior shading. Blinds (venetian or roller shades) or drapes absorb the solar energy before it can strike the floor or other interior surfaces of the space, which leads to a rapid response in the cooling load due to the low mass of the shading device.

Table 7-25 Cooling Load Temperature Differences (CLTD) for Conduction Through Glass

Solar Time, h	CLTD, °F	Solar Time, h	CLTD, °F
0100	1	1300	12
0200	0	1400	13
0300	−1	1500	14
0400	−2	1600	14
0500	−2	1700	13
0600	−2	1800	12
0700	−2	1900	10
0800	0	2000	8
0900	2	2100	6
1000	4	2200	4
1100	7	2300	3
1200	9	2400	2

Corrections: The values in the table were calculated for an inside temperature of 78°F and an outdoor maximum temperature of 95°F with an outdoor daily range of 21°F. The table remains nearly correct for other outdoor maximums from 93 to 102°F and other outdoor daily ranges 16 to 34°F, provided the outdoor daily average temperature remains about 85°F. If the room air temperature is different from 78°F and/or the outdoor daily average temperature is different from 85°F, see note 2, Table 7-18.

When interior shading is absent, the solar energy is absorbed by the more massive elements of the space, which results in increased delay in such heat gain being converted to cooling load. Many variables affect this phenomenom, The more important being the presence or absence of carpet on the floor, the mass of the floor and other surfaces, the mass of the contents of the space, the amount of glass in the exposed surfaces, the presence or absence of a ceiling, and the relative size of the space.

The composite effect of the various forms of interior shading on solar radiation from glass, relative to unshaded clear double-strength glass, is represented by a shading coefficient (SC) or decimal multiplier given in Tables 7-4 through 7-11.

Exterior Shading. Where glass is shaded by exterior means of a permanent nature, the hourly mitigating effect of such shading may be estimated by separate evaluations of shaded areas relative to unshaded areas for each situation as previously noted.

Table 7-26A Zone Types for Use With CLF Tables, Interior Rooms

Zone Parameters[a]				Zone Type	
Room Location	Middle Floor	Ceiling Type	Floor Covering	People and Equipment	Lights
Single story	N/A	N/A	Carpet	C	B
	N/A	N/A	Vinyl	D	C
Top floor	2.5 in. Concrete	With	Carpet	D	C
	2.5 in. Concrete	With	Vinyl	D	D
	2.5 in. Concrete	Without	b	D	B
	1 in. Wood	b	b	D	B
Bottom floor	2.5 in. Concrete	With	Carpet	D	C
	2.5 in. Concrete	b	Vinyl	D	D
	2.5 in. Concrete	Without	Carpet	D	D
	1 in. Wood	b	Carpet	D	C
	1 in. Wood	b	Vinyl	D	D
Mid-floor	2.5 in. Concrete	N/A	Carpet	D	C
	2.5 in. Concrete	N/A	Vinyl	D	D
	1 in. Wood	N/A	b	C	B

[a] Fourteen zone parameters are defined in Chapter 26, 1997 *ASHRAE Handbook—Fundamentals*.

[b] The effect of inside shade is negligible in this case.

7.5.3 Heat Sources Within Conditioned Space

People. The heat gain due to people consists of two components, sensible and latent. Latent heat gains are considered instantaneous. The total sensible heat gain from people is not converted directly to cooling load. The radiant portion is first absorbed by the surroundings (floor, ceiling, partitions, furniture) and then convected to the space at a later time, depending on the thermal characteristics of the room. The radiant portion of the sensible heat gain from people varies widely depending on the circumstances. A 70% value was used to generate CLFs for Table 7-28 which considers the storage effect on this radiant load in its results, plus the 30% convective portion. The instantaneous sensible cooling load is thus

$$q_s = N(\mathrm{SHG}_p)(\mathrm{CLF}_p) \tag{7-33}$$

and the latent cooling load is

$$q_l = N(\mathrm{LHG}_p) \tag{7-34}$$

where

q_s = sensible cooling load due to people
N = number of people
SHG_p = sensible heat gain per person (Table 7-14)
CLF_p = cooling load factor for people (Table 7-28)
q_l = latent cooling load due to people
LHG_p = latent heat gain per person (Table 7-14)

The CLF for people load is a function of the time such people spend in the conditioned space and the time elapsed since first entering. As defined for estimating cooling load from fenestration, the space is categorized as a zone, identified in Table

Table 7-26B Zone Types for Use With SCL and CLF Tables, Single-Story Building

Zone Parameters[a]				Zone Type			Error Band	
No. Walls	Floor Covering	Partition Type	Inside Shade	Glass Solar	People and Equipment	Lights	Plus	Minus
1 or 2	Carpet	Gypsum	b	A	B	B	9	2
1 or 2	Carpet	Concrete block	b	B	C	C	9	0
1 or 2	Vinyl	Gypsum	Full	B	C	C	9	0
1 or 2	Vinyl	Gypsum	Half to None	C	C	C	16	0
1 or 2	Vinyl	Concrete block	Full	C	D	D	8	0
1 or 2	Vinyl	Concrete block	Half to None	D	D	D	10	6
3	Carpet	Gypsum	b	A	B	B	9	2
3	Carpet	Concrete block	Full	A	B	B	9	2
3	Carpet	Concrete block	Half to None	B	B	B	9	0
3	Vinyl	Gypsum	Full	B	C	C	9	0
3	Vinyl	Gypsum	Half to None	C	C	C	16	0
3	Vinyl	Concrete block	Full	B	C	C	9	0
3	Vinyl	Concrete block	Half to None	C	C	C	16	0
4	Carpet	Gypsum	b	A	B	B	6	3
4	Vinyl	Gypsum	Full	B	C	C	11	6
4	Vinyl	Gypsum	Half to None	C	C	C	19	−1

Table 7-26C Zone Types for Use With SCL and CLF Tables, First Floor of Multistory Building

Zone Parameters*						Zone Type			Error Band	
No. Walls	Mid-Floor Type	Ceiling Type	Floor Covering	Partition Type	Inside Shade	Glass Solar	People and Equipment	Lights	Plus	Minus
1 or 2	2.5 in. Concrete	With	Carpet	Gypsum	Full	A	C	B	7	1
	2.5 in. Concrete	With	Carpet	Gypsum	Half to None	B	C	B	9	2
	2.5 in. Concrete	With	Carpet	Concrete block	Full	B	D	C	9	2
	2.5 in. Concrete	With	Carpet	Concrete block	Half to None	C	D	C	0	0
	2.5 in. Concrete	With	Vinyl	Gypsum	Full	C	D	D	19	0
	2.5 in. Concrete	With	Vinyl	Gypsum	Half to None	C	D	D	26	0
	2.5 in. Concrete	With	Vinyl	Concrete block	Full	D	D	D	6	3
	2.5 in. Concrete	With	Vinyl	Concrete block	Half to None	D	D	D	16	3
	2.5 in. Concrete	Without	Carpet	Gypsum	**	B	C	B	9	2
	2.5 in. Concrete	Without	Carpet	Concrete block	Full	C	D	C	19	0
	2.5 in. Concrete	Without	Carpet	Concrete block	Half to None	C	D	C	16	0
	2.5 in. Concrete	Without	Vinyl	Gypsum	Full	C	D	D	19	6
	2.5 in. Concrete	Without	Vinyl	Gypsum	Half to None	D	D	D	6	6
	2.5 in. Concrete	Without	Vinyl	Concrete block	Full	C	D	D	16	0
	2.5 in. Concrete	Without	Vinyl	Concrete block	Half to None	D	D	D	6	3
	1 in. Wood	**	Carpet	Gypsum	Full	A	A	B	2	−2
	1 in. Wood	**	Carpet	Gypsum	Half to None	B	A	B	6	6
	1 in. Wood	**	Carpet	Concrete block	Full	B	B	C	6	6
	1 in. Wood	**	Carpet	Concrete block	Half to None	C	B	C	7	3
	1 in. Wood	**	Vinyl	Gypsum	Full	B	B	B	18	6
	1 in. Wood	**	Vinyl	Gypsum	Half to None	C	B	B	14	3
	1 in. Wood	**	Vinyl	Concrete block	Full	C	C	D	14	3
	1 in. Wood	**	Vinyl	Concrete block	Half to None	D	C	D	2	4
3	2.5 in. Concrete	With	Carpet	Gypsum	Full	A	C	B	7	1
	2.5 in. Concrete	With	Carpet	Gypsum	Half to None	B	C	B	9	2
	2.5 in. Concrete	With	Carpet	Concrete block	**	B	C	B	9	2
	2.5 in. Concrete	With	Vinyl	Gypsum	Full	C	D	C	19	0
	2.5 in. Concrete	With	Vinyl	**	Half to None	C	D	C	26	0
	2.5 in. Concrete	With	Vinyl	Concrete block	Full	C	D	C	19	0
	2.5 in. Concrete	Without	Carpet	Gypsum	**	B	C	B	9	2
	2.5 in. Concrete	Without	Carpet	Concrete block	Full	B	C	B	9	2
	2.5 in. Concrete	Without	Carpet	Concrete block	Half to None	C	C	B	0	0
	2.5 in. Concrete	Without	Vinyl	Gypsum	Full	C	D	C	19	6
	2.5 in. Concrete	Without	Vinyl	**	Half to None	C	D	C	26	0
	2.5 in. Concrete	Without	Vinyl	Concrete block	Full	C	D	C	19	0
	1 in. Wood	**	Carpet	Gypsum	Full	A	A	B	2	−2
	1 in. Wood	**	Carpet	Gypsum	Half to None	B	A	B	6	6
	1 in. Wood	**	Carpet	Concrete block	**	B	B	B	6	6
	1 in. Wood	**	Vinyl	Gypsum	Full	B	B	C	18	6
	1 in. Wood	**	Vinyl	Gypsum	Half to None	C	B	C	14	3
	1 in. Wood	**	Vinyl	Concrete block	Full	C	B	C	7	3
	1 in. Wood	**	Vinyl	Concrete block	Half to None	C	B	C	14	3
4	2.5 in. Concrete	With	Carpet	Gypsum	Full	A	B	B	4	−4
	2.5 in. Concrete	With	Carpet	Gypsum	Half to None	B	B	B	18	6
	2.5 in. Concrete	With	Vinyl	Gypsum	**	C	C	C	19	3
	2.5 in. Concrete	Without	Carpet	Gypsum	**	B	C	C	7	6
	2.5 in. Concrete	Without	Vinyl	Gypsum	**	B	C	C	31	6
	1 in. Wood	**	Carpet	Gypsum	Full	A	B	A	0	0
	1 in. Wood	**	Carpet	Gypsum	Half to None	A	B	A	12	0
	1 in. Wood	**	Vinyl	Gypsum	Full	B	B	B	16	8
	1 in. Wood	**	Vinyl	Gypsum	Half to None	C	B	B	20	6

[a]Fourteen zone parameters are defined in Chapter 26, 1997 *ASHRAE Handbook—Fundamentals*.

[b]The effect of inside shade is negligible in this case.

Table 7-26D Zone Types for Use With SCL and CLF Tables, Middle Floor of Multistory Building

	Zone Parameters*					Zone Type			Error Band	
No. Walls	Mid-Floor Type	Ceiling Type	Floor Covering	Partition Type	Inside Shade	Glass Solar	People and Equipment	Lights	Plus	Minus
1 or 2	2.5 in. Concrete	With	Carpet	Gypsum	**	B	B	C	6	6
	2.5 in. Concrete	With	Carpet	Concrete Block	Full	C	C	C	1	4
	2.5 in. Concrete	With	Carpet	Concrete Block	Half to None	C	C	C	10	4
	2.5 in. Concrete	With	Vinyl	Gypsum	Full	C	D	D	10	4
	2.5 in. Concrete	With	Vinyl	Gypsum	Half to None	D	D	D	6	12
	2.5 in. Concrete	With	Vinyl	Concrete Block	**	D	D	D	3	7
	2.5 in. Concrete	Without	Carpet	Gypsum	**	B	B	D	6	6
	2.5 in. Concrete	Without	Carpet	Concrete Block	**	C	C	D	10	4
	2.5 in. Concrete	Without	Vinyl	Gypsum	Full	B	C	C	11	6
	2.5 in. Concrete	Without	Vinyl	Gypsum	Half to None	C	C	C	9	7
	2.5 in. Concrete	Without	Vinyl	Concrete Block	**	C	C	D	9	−1
	1 in. Wood	**	**	Gypsum	**	A	A	A	0	0
	1 in. Wood	**	**	Concrete Block	**	B	A	B	6	8
3	2.5 in. Concrete	With	Carpet	Gypsum	**	B	B	C	6	6
	2.5 in. Concrete	With	Carpet	Concrete Block	Full	B	C	C	6	6
	2.5 in. Concrete	With	Carpet	Concrete Block	Half to None	C	C	C	1	4
	2.5 in. Concrete	With	Vinyl	Gypsum	Full	C	D	D	10	4
	2.5 in. Concrete	With	Vinyl	Gypsum	Half to None	D	D	D	7	12
	2.5 in. Concrete	With	Vinyl	Concrete Block	Full	C	D	D	10	−1
	2.5 in. Concrete	With	Vinyl	Concrete Block	Half to None	D	D	D	7	12
	2.5 in. Concrete	Without	Carpet	Gypsum	**	B	B	C	6	6
	2.5 in. Concrete	Without	Carpet	Concrete Block	Full	C	C	C	1	4
	2.5 in. Concrete	Without	Carpet	Concrete Block	Half to None	B	C	C	6	6
	2.5 in. Concrete	Without	Vinyl	Gypsum	Full	B	C	C	11	6
	2.5 in. Concrete	Without	Vinyl	Gypsum	Half to None	C	C	C	9	7
	2.5 in. Concrete	Without	Vinyl	Concrete Block	Full	B	C	C	11	−2
	2.5 in. Concrete	Without	Vinyl	Concrete Block	Half to None	C	C	C	9	−1
	1 in. Wood	**	**	Gypsum	**	A	A	A	0	0
	1 in. Wood	**	**	Concrete Block	**	A	A	B	10	0
4	2.5 in. Concrete	With	Carpet	Gypsum	**	B	C	C	6	6
	2.5 in. Concrete	With	Vinyl	Gypsum	Full	C	C	C	14	6
	2.5 in. Concrete	With	Vinyl	Gypsum	Half to None	C	C	C	26	6
	2.5 in. Concrete	Without	Carpet	Gypsum	**	B	A	C	6	6
	2.5 in. Concrete	Without	Vinyl	Gypsum	Full	B	A	C	7	6
	2.5 in. Concrete	Without	Vinyl	Gypsum	Half to None	B	A	C	20	6
	1 in. Wood	**	**	**	**	A	A	B	−2	2

[a] Fourteen zone parameters are defined in Chapter 26, 1997 *ASHRAE Handbook—Fundamentals*.
[b] The effect of inside shade is negligible in this case.

7-26. The appropriate CLF is selected from Table 7-28 by zone type, occupancy period, and number of hours after entry.

CLF Usage Exceptions. If the space temperature is not maintained constant during the 24-h period, for example, if the cooling system is shut down during the night (night shutdown), a "pulldown load" results because a major part of the stored sensible heat in the structure has not been removed, thus reappearing as cooling load when the system is started the next day. In this case, a CLF of 1.0 should be used.

When there is a **high occupant density**, as in theaters and auditoriums, the quantity of radiation to the walls and room furnishings is proportionately reduced. In these situations, a CLF of 1.0 should also be used.

Lighting. As previously mentioned, the cooling load from lighting does not immediately reflect the full energy output of the lights. Kimura and Stephenson (1968), Mitalas and Kimura (1971), and Mitalas (1973) indicated the effect on cooling load of light fixture type, type of air supply and return, space furnishings, and the thermal characteristics of the space. The effect of these influencing parameters has been incorporated in the CLF values for lighting listed in Table 7-29; selection zones are identified as appropriate by Table 7-26. At any time, the space cooling load from lighting can be estimated from the following equation:

$$q_{el} = HG_{el}(CLF_{el}) \tag{7-35}$$

where

q_{el} = cooling load from lighting, Btu/h
HG_{el} = heat gain from lighting, Btu/h, as $WF_{ul}F_{sa}$
W = total lamp watts
F_{ul} = lighting use factor
F_{sa} = lighting special allowance factor
CLF_{el} = lighting cooling load factor (Table 7-29)

CLF_{el} data in Table 7-29 are based on the assumptions that (1) the conditioned space temperature is continuously maintained at a constant value, and (2) the cooling load and power input to the lights eventually become equal if the lights are on for long enough.

Operational Exceptions. If the cooling system operates only during occupied hours, the CLF_{el} should be considered 1.0 in lieu of the Table 7-29 values. Where one portion of the

Table 7-26E Zone Types for Use With SCL and CLF Tables, Top Floor of Multistory Building

	Zone Parameters*					Zone Type			Error Band	
No. Walls	**Mid-Floor Type**	**Ceiling Type**	**Floor Covering**	**Partition Type**	**Inside Shade**	**Glass Solar**	**People and Equipment**	**Lights**	**Plus**	**Minus**
1 or 2	2.5 in. Concrete	With	Carpet	Gypsum	Full	A	A	B	2	4
	2.5 in. Concrete	With	Carpet	Gypsum	Half to None	A	A	B	7	−2
	2.5 in. Concrete	With	Carpet	Concrete block	Full	B	A	C	9	6
	2.5 in. Concrete	With	Carpet	Concrete block	Half to None	B	A	C	14	2
	2.5 in. Concrete	With	Vinyl	Gypsum	Full	B	A	C	8	6
	2.5 in. Concrete	With	Vinyl	Gypsum	Half to None	C	A	C	12	10
	2.5 in. Concrete	With	Vinyl	Concrete block	Full	C	B	D	7	7
	2.5 in. Concrete	With	Vinyl	Concrete block	Half to None	C	B	D	19	0
	2.5 in. Concrete	Without	Carpet	Gypsum	**	A	A	B	−4	4
	2.5 in. Concrete	Without	Carpet	Concrete block	**	A	A	C	7	4
	2.5 in. Concrete	Without	Vinyl	Gypsum	**	A	A	B	7	4
	2.5 in. Concrete	Without	Vinyl	Concrete block	Full	B	A	C	8	6
	2.5 in. Concrete	Without	Vinyl	Concrete block	Half to None	B	A	C	10	6
	1 in. Wood	**	**	Gypsum	**	A	A	B	−3	3
	1 in. Wood	**	**	Concrete block	**	A	B	C	13	3
3	2.5 in. Concrete	With	Carpet	Gypsum	Full	A	B	B	2	4
	2.5 in. Concrete	With	Carpet	Gypsum	Half to None	A	A	B	7	−2
	2.5 in. Concrete	With	Carpet	Concrete block	Full	A	A	C	7	−2
	2.5 in. Concrete	With	Carpet	Concrete block	Half to None	B	A	C	9	6
	2.5 in. Concrete	With	Vinyl	Gypsum	Full	B	A	C	8	6
	2.5 in. Concrete	With	Vinyl	Gypsum	Half to None	C	A	C	12	10
	2.5 in. Concrete	With	Vinyl	Concrete block	Full	B	A	C	9	2
	2.5 in. Concrete	With	Vinyl	Concrete block	Half to None	C	A	C	12	7
	2.5 in. Concrete	Without	Carpet	**	**	A	A	B	2	4
	2.5 in. Concrete	Without	Vinyl	Gypsum	Full	A	A	B	7	4
	2.5 in. Concrete	Without	Vinyl	Gypsum	Half to None	A	A	B	4	4
	2.5 in. Concrete	Without	Vinyl	Concrete block	Full	A	A	B	7	4
	2.5 in. Concrete	Without	Vinyl	Concrete block	Half to None	B	A	B	2	6
	1 in. Wood	**	**	Gypsum	**	A	A	B	−3	3
	1 in. Wood	**	**	Concrete block	**	A	A	B	6	3
4	2.5 in. Concrete	With	Carpet	Gypsum	Full	A	A	B	9	6
	2.5 in. Concrete	With	Carpet	Gypsum	Half to None	B	A	B	6	4
	2.5 in. Concrete	With	Vinyl	Gypsum	Full	B	C	C	7	14
	2.5 in. Concrete	With	Vinyl	Gypsum	Half to None	B	B	C	24	4
	2.5 in. Concrete	Without	Carpet	Gypsum	Full	A	A	B	4	6
	2.5 in. Concrete	Without	Carpet	Gypsum	Half to None	A	A	B	−6	6
	2.5 in. Concrete	Without	Vinyl	Gypsum	Full	A	A	B	4	6
	2.5 in. Concrete	Without	Vinyl	Gypsum	Half to None	A	A	B	7	0
	1 in. Wood	**	**	**	**	A	B	B	0	8

[a] Fourteen zone parameters are defined in Chapter 26, 1997 *ASHRAE Handbook—Fundamentals*.

[b] The effect of inside shade is negligible in this case.

lights serving the space is on one schedule of operation and another portion is on a different schedule, each should be treated separately. Where lights are left on for 24 h a day, the CLF_{el} is 1.0.

Power and Appliances. Heat gain of power-driven equipment can be estimated from Equation (7-22), (7-23), or (7-24) as applicable, or taken directly from Table 7-15.

Equations (7-16) through (7-18) can be used to estimate heat gain values under various circumstances, and Tables 7-16 through 7-18 provide representative data for direct use or as input to the equations. Latent heat gain from appliances is considered instantaneous cooling load and is calculated by Equation (7-37), which is in Table 7-19.

The radiant component of sensible heat gain from power-driven equipment or appliances is delayed in becoming cooling load in the same manner as that of other load categories already discussed. For power-driven equipment the CLF values tabulated for unhooded equipment (Table 7-28) are considered appropriate. Tables 7-28 and 7-30 tabulate cooling load factors (CLF_a) for appliances. Multiplying the sensible portion of heat gain by the appropriate CLF_a will produce the following approximate cooling load values:

$$q = SHG(CLF) \qquad (7\text{-}36)$$

7.5.4 Total Space Cooling Load

The estimated total space cooling load for a given application is determined by summing the individual components for each hour of interest. See Table 7-19 for the summary of this procedure.

7.6 Limitations of CLTD/SCL/CLF Method

The results obtained from using CLTD/SCL/CLF data depend on the characteristics of the space and how they vary from those used to generate the weighting factors. Variations can appear in the amplitude and when radiant heat gain

Table 7-27-J24 July Solar Cooling Load for Sunlit Glass 24° North Latitude

Zone type A — Solar time, hr

Glass Facing	1	2	3	4	5	6	7	8	9	10	11	12	13	14	15	16	17	18	19	20	21	22	23	24
N	0	0	0	0	0	19	35	36	36	38	40	42	42	40	38	39	43	32	11	6	3	1	1	0
NE	0	0	0	0	0	54	124	150	144	115	78	58	49	44	38	32	25	14	6	3	1	1	0	0
E	0	0	0	0	0	57	139	177	180	154	107	68	54	46	40	33	25	14	6	3	1	1	0	0
SE	0	0	0	0	0	26	74	104	114	106	83	59	50	44	38	32	25	14	6	3	1	1	0	0
S	0	0	0	0	0	5	15	23	30	35	40	43	43	40	37	32	24	14	6	3	1	1	0	0
SW	0	0	0	0	0	5	15	23	30	35	39	42	61	88	110	118	105	62	24	12	6	3	1	1
W	1	0	0	0	0	5	15	23	30	35	39	41	67	116	160	186	184	118	44	21	11	5	3	1
NW	1	0	0	0	0	5	15	23	30	35	39	41	51	83	122	151	158	106	39	19	9	5	2	1
hor	0	0	0	0	0	10	55	113	170	218	253	271	273	258	225	176	115	54	24	12	6	3	1	1

Zone type B — Solar time, hr

Glass Facing	1	2	3	4	5	6	7	8	9	10	11	12	13	14	15	16	17	18	19	20	21	22	23	24
N	2	2	1	1	1	16	30	32	32	35	37	39	40	39	37	39	42	33	16	10	7	5	4	3
NE	2	1	1	1	1	47	105	128	126	106	78	62	55	50	44	38	31	20	12	9	6	5	3	3
E	2	2	1	1	1	49	118	151	158	141	105	74	63	55	48	41	33	22	13	10	7	5	4	3
SE	2	1	1	1	1	23	63	89	100	95	78	60	53	48	43	37	30	20	12	8	6	4	3	2
S	1	1	1	1	0	5	13	20	26	31	36	39	40	38	36	32	26	17	10	7	5	4	3	2
SW	5	3	3	2	1	5	13	20	26	31	35	38	55	79	98	106	98	63	33	22	15	11	8	6
W	7	6	4	3	2	6	14	21	27	32	35	38	61	102	141	165	167	115	56	37	26	18	13	10
NW	6	5	4	3	2	6	14	21	27	32	35	38	47	75	108	134	142	102	48	32	22	16	11	8
hor	8	6	4	3	3	11	48	97	146	190	224	244	251	243	219	181	130	78	50	35	25	19	14	10

Zone type C — Solar time, hr

Glass Facing	1	2	3	4	5	6	7	8	9	10	11	12	13	14	15	16	17	18	19	20	21	22	23	24
N	5	5	4	4	4	19	31	31	30	32	35	36	36	35	34	36	39	31	14	11	9	8	7	6
NE	8	7	6	6	5	50	104	120	114	92	65	53	50	47	43	38	32	23	16	14	12	11	10	9
E	9	8	7	7	6	53	117	143	143	123	88	62	56	51	47	42	35	26	19	16	14	13	11	10
SE	7	6	6	5	4	26	64	85	92	85	68	51	47	44	40	36	30	21	15	12	11	10	9	8
S	4	4	3	3	3	7	14	20	25	29	33	36	36	34	32	29	24	15	10	8	7	6	5	5
SW	10	9	8	7	7	10	17	23	28	32	34	37	53	75	92	97	87	53	26	20	17	14	13	11
W	15	14	12	11	10	13	20	25	30	34	36	38	60	99	132	152	150	97	43	31	26	22	19	17
NW	13	12	10	9	8	12	19	24	29	33	35	37	45	72	103	125	129	87	36	27	22	19	16	14
hor	24	21	19	17	15	22	57	102	145	181	208	223	226	217	194	160	115	71	51	43	38	33	30	27

Zone type D — Solar time, hr

Glass Facing	1	2	3	4	5	6	7	8	9	10	11	12	13	14	15	16	17	18	19	20	21	22	23	24
N	8	8	7	6	6	17	27	27	27	29	31	33	33	33	33	34	37	30	17	15	13	12	10	9
NE	12	11	10	9	8	43	86	100	97	82	63	54	52	49	46	42	37	29	23	21	18	16	15	13
E	14	13	11	10	9	46	97	118	121	108	83	64	59	56	52	47	41	33	27	24	21	19	17	16
SE	11	10	9	8	7	24	53	71	77	74	62	50	47	45	42	38	33	26	21	18	16	15	13	12
S	6	6	5	5	4	7	13	18	22	25	29	32	32	31	30	28	24	18	13	11	10	9	8	7
SW	15	14	12	11	10	12	18	22	26	29	31	34	47	64	79	84	78	53	32	27	24	21	19	17
W	23	21	19	17	15	17	22	26	29	32	34	36	53	84	112	130	130	91	50	42	36	32	29	26
NW	20	18	16	14	13	15	20	24	28	31	33	34	41	63	88	106	111	80	43	35	30	27	24	22
hor	36	33	30	27	24	29	55	90	124	154	178	193	199	196	181	156	122	88	71	62	56	50	45	40

Table 7-27-J32 July Solar Cooling Load for Sunlit Glass 32° North Latitude

Zone type A — Solar time, hr

Glass Facing	1	2	3	4	5	6	7	8	9	10	11	12	13	14	15	16	17	18	19	20	21	22	23	24
N	0	0	0	0	0	23	31	30	33	36	39	41	41	39	36	33	36	35	12	6	3	1	1	0
NE	0	0	0	0	0	73	128	143	128	94	62	52	46	42	38	32	26	16	6	3	1	1	0	0
E	0	0	0	0	0	78	149	182	182	155	107	68	54	46	40	33	26	16	6	3	2	1	0	0
SE	0	0	0	0	0	37	85	118	133	129	107	75	55	46	40	33	26	16	6	3	2	1	0	0
S	0	0	0	0	0	7	16	24	32	44	56	64	63	55	43	35	27	17	7	3	2	1	0	0
SW	0	0	0	0	0	7	16	24	30	35	39	50	80	111	131	135	120	78	29	14	7	3	2	1
W	1	0	0	0	0	7	16	24	30	35	39	41	67	115	160	188	189	140	50	24	12	6	3	1
NW	1	0	0	0	0	7	16	24	30	35	39	41	42	64	103	137	152	121	42	20	10	5	2	1
hor	0	0	0	0	0	17	62	118	172	217	250	267	269	254	223	178	121	63	27	13	6	3	2	1

Zone type B — Solar time, hr

Glass Facing	1	2	3	4	5	6	7	8	9	10	11	12	13	14	15	16	17	18	19	20	21	22	23	24
N	2	2	1	1	1	20	26	26	29	33	36	38	39	38	36	33	36	35	15	10	7	5	4	3
NE	2	1	1	1	1	62	109	123	114	89	65	57	52	47	42	37	30	22	12	9	6	5	3	3
E	2	2	1	1	1	66	127	156	160	142	106	75	63	55	48	41	34	24	14	10	7	5	4	3
SE	2	2	1	1	1	32	72	101	116	116	100	76	60	53	46	40	32	23	13	9	7	5	4	3
S	2	1	1	1	1	6	14	21	28	39	50	57	58	52	43	36	30	21	12	8	6	4	3	2
SW	5	4	3	2	2	7	15	21	27	32	35	46	71	98	117	123	112	79	39	27	19	13	10	7
W	8	6	5	3	3	8	15	21	27	32	35	37	60	102	140	166	171	133	61	40	28	20	14	11
NW	6	5	4	3	2	7	15	21	27	32	35	37	39	59	92	121	136	113	49	32	22	16	11	8
hor	8	6	5	3	3	16	54	102	148	189	221	241	248	240	218	182	135	85	52	36	26	19	14	11

Zone type C — Solar time, hr

Glass Facing	1	2	3	4	5	6	7	8	9	10	11	12	13	14	15	16	17	18	19	20	21	22	23	24
N	5	5	4	4	3	23	27	25	28	31	34	35	36	35	33	30	34	33	14	10	9	7	7	6
NE	7	7	6	5	5	65	106	115	102	76	54	50	47	45	42	37	32	24	16	13	12	10	9	8
E	9	8	7	7	6	70	125	146	145	124	89	62	56	52	47	42	36	28	20	17	15	13	12	10
SE	8	7	6	6	5	36	73	97	107	104	87	64	52	47	43	39	33	25	17	14	13	11	10	9
S	5	5	4	4	3	9	16	21	27	37	47	53	52	46	38	32	27	20	12	10	8	7	7	6
SW	12	11	10	9	8	13	19	24	29	32	35	44	69	93	108	111	99	67	31	24	20	17	15	13
W	16	14	13	12	10	15	21	26	31	34	36	38	59	99	133	153	154	115	46	33	27	23	20	18
NW	13	11	10	9	8	13	19	25	29	32	35	36	38	57	88	114	124	99	37	26	21	18	16	14
hor	24	22	19	17	16	28	64	106	146	180	205	220	223	215	194	162	121	78	53	44	38	34	30	27

Zone type D — Solar time, hr

Glass Facing	1	2	3	4	5	6	7	8	9	10	11	12	13	14	15	16	17	18	19	20	21	22	23	24
N	8	7	6	6	5	20	24	22	25	28	30	32	33	32	31	30	32	32	17	14	12	11	10	9
NE	11	10	9	8	8	55	87	95	88	69	54	51	49	47	44	40	36	29	22	20	18	16	14	13
E	14	13	12	11	10	60	103	121	123	110	84	65	60	56	53	48	43	35	28	25	22	20	18	16
SE	12	11	10	9	8	32	61	81	90	90	79	62	53	50	46	42	38	31	24	21	19	17	15	14
S	8	7	7	6	5	9	15	19	24	32	40	45	46	42	36	32	28	22	16	14	12	11	10	9
SW	18	16	15	13	12	15	20	24	27	30	32	40	60	79	93	97	89	66	38	32	28	25	22	20
W	24	22	20	18	16	19	23	27	30	33	35	36	53	85	112	131	133	106	53	44	38	34	30	27
NW	19	17	15	14	12	16	20	24	28	30	33	34	35	51	75	97	107	89	42	34	30	26	23	21
hor	37	33	30	27	24	33	60	93	125	154	177	191	197	194	180	158	127	93	72	63	57	51	46	41

Data applies directly to standard, double-strength glass with no inside shade that is exposed to clear sky on the 21st day of the month.

For other types of glass and internal shade, multiply values by shading coefficient (see text). For extremely shaded glass, use north orientation (see text).

Table 7-27-J40 July Solar Cooling Load For Sunlit Glass 40° North Latitude

Zone type A — Solar time, hr

Glass Facing	1	2	3	4	5	6	7	8	9	10	11	12	13	14	15	16	17	18	19	20	21	22	23	24
N	0	0	0	0	1	25	27	28	32	35	38	40	40	39	36	31	31	36	12	6	3	1	1	0
NE	0	0	0	0	2	85	129	134	112	75	55	48	44	40	37	32	26	18	7	3	2	1	0	0
E	0	0	0	0	2	93	157	185	183	154	106	67	53	45	39	33	26	18	7	3	2	1	0	0
SE	0	0	0	0	1	47	95	131	150	150	131	97	63	49	41	34	27	18	7	3	2	1	0	0
S	0	0	0	0	0	9	17	25	41	64	85	97	96	84	63	42	31	20	8	4	2	1	0	0
SW	0	0	0	0	0	9	17	24	30	35	39	64	101	133	151	152	133	93	35	17	8	4	2	1
W	1	0	0	0	0	9	17	24	30	35	38	40	65	114	158	187	192	156	57	27	13	6	3	2
NW	1	0	0	0	0	9	17	24	30	35	38	40	40	50	84	121	143	130	46	22	11	5	3	1
hor	0	0	0	0	0	24	69	120	169	211	241	257	259	245	217	176	125	70	29	14	7	3	2	1

Zone type B — Solar time, hr

Glass Facing	1	2	3	4	5	6	7	8	9	10	11	12	13	14	15	16	17	18	19	20	21	22	23	24
N	2	2	1	1	1	22	23	24	28	32	35	37	38	37	35	32	31	35	16	10	7	5	4	3
NE	2	1	1	1	2	73	109	116	101	73	58	52	48	45	41	36	30	23	13	9	6	5	3	3
E	2	2	1	1	2	80	133	159	162	143	105	74	63	55	48	41	34	25	15	10	7	5	4	3
SE	2	2	1	1	1	40	81	112	131	134	122	96	69	58	49	42	35	26	15	10	8	6	4	3
S	2	2	1	1	1	8	15	21	36	56	74	86	87	79	63	46	37	27	16	11	8	6	4	3
SW	6	5	4	3	2	9	16	22	27	31	36	58	89	117	135	138	126	94	46	31	21	15	11	8
W	8	6	5	4	3	9	16	22	27	31	35	37	59	101	139	166	173	147	66	43	30	21	15	11
NW	6	5	4	3	2	9	16	22	27	31	34	37	37	46	76	108	128	119	51	33	22	16	11	8
hor	8	6	5	4	3	22	60	104	147	185	214	233	239	232	212	180	137	90	53	37	27	19	14	11

Zone type C — Solar time, hr

Glass Facing	1	2	3	4	5	6	7	8	9	10	11	12	13	14	15	16	17	18	19	20	21	22	23	24
N	5	5	4	4	4	24	23	24	27	30	33	34	35	34	32	29	29	34	14	10	8	7	6	6
NE	7	6	6	5	6	75	106	107	88	61	49	47	45	43	40	36	31	25	16	13	11	10	9	8
E	9	8	8	7	8	83	130	148	145	124	89	62	56	52	47	43	37	30	20	17	15	13	12	11
SE	9	8	7	6	6	45	82	107	121	121	107	82	59	51	47	42	36	29	19	16	14	13	11	10
S	7	7	6	5	5	12	18	23	36	54	70	79	79	70	54	40	33	26	16	13	12	10	9	8
SW	14	12	11	10	9	15	21	26	29	33	36	57	86	110	124	125	111	80	37	28	23	20	17	15
W	17	15	13	12	11	17	22	27	31	34	36	37	59	98	132	153	156	128	50	35	28	24	21	19
NW	12	11	10	9	8	14	20	25	29	32	34	36	36	44	73	102	118	107	39	26	21	17	15	13
hor	24	21	19	17	16	34	68	107	144	175	199	212	215	207	189	160	123	83	53	44	38	34	30	27

Zone type D — Solar time, hr

Glass Facing	1	2	3	4	5	6	7	8	9	10	11	12	13	14	15	16	17	18	19	20	21	22	23	24
N	8	7	6	6	6	21	21	21	24	27	29	31	32	31	30	28	29	32	17	14	12	11	10	9
NE	11	10	9	8	9	63	87	90	77	58	49	48	46	44	42	39	35	29	22	19	17	15	14	12
E	15	13	12	11	11	70	107	123	124	110	85	65	60	57	53	48	43	37	29	25	22	20	18	16
SE	14	13	11	10	10	39	68	90	102	104	95	78	60	55	51	47	42	35	27	24	21	19	17	16
S	11	10	9	8	7	12	17	21	32	46	59	67	69	63	52	41	36	30	22	19	17	15	14	12
SW	21	19	17	15	14	18	22	25	28	31	34	51	74	94	106	109	100	78	45	37	33	29	26	23
W	25	23	20	18	17	21	24	28	30	33	34	35	53	84	112	130	135	116	57	46	39	35	31	28
NW	18	16	15	13	12	17	21	24	27	30	32	33	34	41	64	87	101	94	42	33	29	25	22	20
hor	37	33	30	27	24	38	64	95	124	150	171	185	191	188	176	156	128	96	72	63	56	50	45	41

Table 7-27-J48 July Solar Cooling Load For Sunlit Glass 48° North Latitude

Zone type A — Solar time, hr

Glass Facing	1	2	3	4	5	6	7	8	9	10	11	12	13	14	15	16	17	18	19	20	21	22	23	24
N	0	0	0	0	14	28	24	27	31	34	37	38	38	37	35	31	27	34	25	9	4	2	1	1
NE	0	0	0	0	32	101	130	126	95	61	49	44	41	38	35	31	26	19	10	4	2	1	0	0
E	0	0	0	0	31	112	165	188	182	153	104	65	51	43	38	32	27	19	10	4	2	1	0	0
SE	0	0	0	0	11	58	106	143	164	168	152	119	77	54	43	35	28	20	10	4	2	1	1	0
S	0	0	0	0	3	11	18	30	58	90	116	130	130	116	88	56	37	24	12	5	3	1	1	0
SW	1	0	0	0	3	11	18	24	30	34	46	82	122	152	168	166	146	106	50	22	11	5	3	1
W	1	1	0	0	3	11	18	24	30	34	36	38	64	112	156	186	193	167	89	36	17	9	4	2
NW	1	0	0	0	3	11	18	24	30	34	36	38	38	40	67	106	134	134	76	30	14	7	3	2
hor	0	0	0	0	5	32	73	120	163	200	226	241	242	230	205	170	125	76	35	16	8	4	2	1

Zone type B — Solar time, hr

Glass Facing	1	2	3	4	5	6	7	8	9	10	11	12	13	14	15	16	17	18	19	20	21	22	23	24
N	2	2	1	1	13	25	21	24	28	32	34	36	36	36	34	31	28	34	26	12	8	6	4	3
NE	2	1	1	1	28	86	111	110	88	62	53	49	45	42	39	35	30	23	15	9	6	5	3	3
E	2	2	1	1	27	95	141	163	163	143	105	74	62	54	47	41	34	27	17	11	8	6	4	3
SE	3	2	2	1	10	50	91	123	144	151	141	116	83	64	53	45	37	29	19	12	9	6	5	4
S	3	2	2	1	3	10	16	26	50	78	101	115	118	109	88	62	45	34	22	15	11	8	6	4
SW	7	6	4	3	5	11	17	22	27	31	41	72	107	134	150	152	138	107	61	37	26	18	13	10
W	10	7	5	4	5	11	17	22	27	31	34	35	58	99	137	164	174	156	93	51	34	24	17	13
NW	7	5	4	3	4	11	17	22	27	30	33	35	36	38	61	95	119	121	75	38	25	18	13	9
hor	8	6	5	4	7	29	64	104	142	176	202	219	224	218	201	173	136	94	57	38	27	20	15	11

Zone type C — Solar time, hr

Glass Facing	1	2	3	4	5	6	7	8	9	10	11	12	13	14	15	16	17	18	19	20	21	22	23	24
N	5	5	4	4	15	26	21	24	27	30	32	33	34	33	31	29	26	33	25	12	9	8	7	6
NE	7	6	6	5	31	86	106	100	76	51	46	44	43	41	39	35	31	25	18	13	11	10	9	8
E	10	9	8	7	32	97	136	151	146	124	89	62	56	51	47	43	38	31	23	18	16	14	12	11
SE	10	9	8	7	16	54	90	118	133	136	125	101	71	56	50	45	39	33	24	19	16	14	13	11
S	10	9	8	7	9	14	20	29	51	75	95	106	106	96	76	53	40	32	23	18	16	14	12	11
SW	16	14	13	11	13	18	23	27	30	33	42	71	103	126	138	137	122	92	51	33	27	23	20	18
W	18	16	14	13	14	19	24	28	31	33	35	36	58	96	130	152	158	138	77	41	31	26	23	20
NW	12	11	10	9	10	16	21	25	28	31	33	34	35	36	59	90	111	110	63	30	22	18	16	14
hor	23	21	19	17	19	40	72	106	139	167	187	200	202	196	179	154	122	86	57	44	37	33	29	26

Zone type D — Solar time, hr

Glass Facing	1	2	3	4	5	6	7	8	9	10	11	12	13	14	15	16	17	18	19	20	21	22	23	24
N	8	7	7	6	15	23	20	22	24	27	29	30	31	31	30	28	26	31	25	15	13	11	10	9
NE	11	10	9	8	28	71	88	85	68	50	47	45	44	43	41	38	34	29	23	19	17	15	13	12
E	15	14	12	11	30	81	112	126	126	111	85	66	61	57	53	49	44	38	31	26	23	21	19	17
SE	16	14	13	12	18	47	76	99	113	117	111	94	72	61	56	51	46	40	32	27	24	22	20	18
S	15	14	12	11	12	16	20	27	44	64	80	90	93	86	72	55	45	39	31	26	23	21	19	17
SW	24	22	20	18	18	21	24	27	30	32	39	63	88	107	119	120	111	89	57	43	38	33	30	27
W	27	24	22	20	20	23	26	29	31	33	34	35	52	83	110	130	136	123	78	50	43	38	33	30
NW	19	17	15	14	14	18	21	24	27	29	31	32	33	34	53	78	95	96	60	36	30	26	23	21
hor	36	32	29	26	27	42	66	94	120	144	162	175	180	178	167	150	126	98	74	62	55	49	44	40

Data applies directly to standard, double-strength glass with no inside shade that is exposed to clear sky on the 21st day of the month. For other types of glass and internal shade, multiply values by shading coefficient (see text). For extremely shaded glass, use north orientation (see text).

Table 7-27-A24 August Solar Cooling Load For Sunlit Glass 24° North Latitude

Glass Facing	Zone type A					Solar time, hr																		
	1	2	3	4	5	6	7	8	9	10	11	12	13	14	15	16	17	18	19	20	21	22	23	24
N	0	0	0	0	0	5	16	23	29	35	39	41	41	39	36	30	26	14	6	3	1	1	0	0
NE	0	0	0	0	0	23	102	129	122	91	61	51	46	42	37	31	23	10	5	2	1	1	0	0
E	0	0	0	0	0	27	129	177	184	160	110	69	55	46	39	32	23	11	5	2	1	1	0	0
SE	0	0	0	0	0	15	83	125	143	138	113	78	56	47	39	32	24	11	5	2	1	1	0	0
S	0	0	0	0	0	2	13	21	32	46	59	66	66	58	46	34	25	11	5	2	1	1	0	0
SW	0	0	0	0	0	2	13	21	29	34	38	51	83	118	141	147	127	59	25	12	6	3	1	1
W	1	0	0	0	0	2	13	21	29	34	38	41	69	121	166	193	184	88	37	18	9	4	2	1
NW	0	0	0	0	0	2	13	21	29	34	38	41	42	65	102	132	137	68	27	13	7	3	2	1
hor	0	0	0	0	0	4	43	103	162	212	249	269	271	254	219	167	103	44	20	10	5	2	1	1

Glass Facing	Zone type B					Solar time, hr																		
	1	2	3	4	5	6	7	8	9	10	11	12	13	14	15	16	17	18	19	20	21	22	23	24
N	1	1	1	1	0	4	14	19	25	31	35	37	38	37	35	31	27	17	10	7	5	3	3	2
NE	2	1	1	1	1	20	86	110	107	84	62	55	50	46	41	35	28	16	11	8	5	4	3	2
E	2	2	1	1	1	23	110	151	160	144	107	75	63	55	47	40	31	19	13	9	7	5	4	3
SE	2	1	1	1	1	13	71	106	123	123	105	78	62	53	46	39	30	18	12	9	6	5	3	3
S	2	1	1	1	1	2	11	18	28	40	52	59	60	55	45	36	28	17	11	7	5	4	3	2
SW	5	4	3	2	2	3	12	19	25	31	35	46	74	104	125	133	119	64	37	25	18	13	9	7
W	7	5	4	3	2	3	12	19	25	31	35	37	62	106	146	171	167	90	50	34	23	17	12	9
NW	5	4	3	2	2	3	12	19	25	31	34	37	39	59	91	118	123	67	36	24	17	12	9	7
hor	7	6	4	3	2	5	38	88	139	184	219	241	248	239	213	173	119	68	46	32	24	17	13	10

Glass Facing	Zone type C					Solar time, hr																		
	1	2	3	4	5	6	7	8	9	10	11	12	13	14	15	16	17	18	19	20	21	22	23	24
N	4	4	3	3	3	6	15	20	25	29	32	34	34	33	31	27	24	15	9	8	7	6	5	5
NE	7	6	5	5	4	23	87	104	96	72	51	47	45	43	39	35	28	18	14	12	10	9	8	7
E	9	8	7	6	6	28	111	144	146	127	90	62	55	51	46	41	34	23	18	16	14	12	11	10
SE	8	7	6	6	5	17	73	103	114	110	92	66	53	48	43	38	31	21	16	14	12	11	10	9
S	5	5	4	4	3	5	13	20	28	39	48	54	54	48	40	32	25	15	11	9	8	7	6	6
SW	12	11	10	9	8	9	17	23	28	32	34	45	71	98	116	120	105	51	29	23	19	17	15	13
W	15	13	12	11	9	10	18	24	29	33	35	37	61	102	137	157	149	72	38	29	24	21	18	16
NW	10	9	8	8	7	8	16	22	27	31	34	36	37	56	86	110	112	55	28	21	17	15	13	12
hor	23	20	18	16	15	16	48	94	138	176	204	220	223	213	188	152	105	62	48	41	36	32	28	25

Glass Facing	Zone type D					Solar time, hr																		
	1	2	3	4	5	6	7	8	9	10	11	12	13	14	15	16	17	18	19	20	21	22	23	24
N	6	6	5	5	4	7	14	17	21	25	28	30	31	30	29	27	24	17	12	11	10	9	8	7
NE	10	9	8	7	7	21	72	86	81	65	50	47	46	44	41	37	32	24	20	17	16	14	13	11
E	14	12	11	10	9	26	91	118	122	110	84	63	59	55	51	46	40	31	26	23	21	19	17	15
SE	12	11	10	9	8	17	61	85	96	94	82	64	54	50	47	42	36	28	23	21	19	17	15	14
S	8	7	6	6	5	6	12	17	24	33	41	46	47	44	38	32	27	19	15	13	12	11	10	9
SW	18	16	15	13	12	12	18	22	26	29	32	40	62	83	99	104	94	53	37	32	28	25	22	20
W	22	20	18	16	15	15	20	24	28	31	33	35	54	87	116	133	129	72	47	39	34	31	27	25
NW	16	14	13	12	10	11	17	21	25	28	31	33	34	50	74	93	97	54	34	28	25	22	20	18
hor	35	31	28	25	23	23	47	83	118	149	174	190	196	191	175	149	113	80	67	59	53	48	43	39

Table 7-27-A32 August Solar Cooling Load For Sunlit Glass 32° North Latitude

Glass Facing	Zone type A					Solar time, hr																		
	1	2	3	4	5	6	7	8	9	10	11	12	13	14	15	16	17	18	19	20	21	22	23	24
N	0	0	0	0	0	7	15	22	29	34	38	39	40	38	35	30	24	16	6	3	1	1	0	0
NE	0	0	0	0	0	37	103	121	106	72	53	47	43	40	36	30	23	12	5	2	1	1	0	0
E	0	0	0	0	0	44	136	179	184	159	109	68	53	45	38	31	24	12	5	2	1	1	0	0
SE	0	0	0	0	0	25	91	136	157	158	137	100	64	50	41	33	24	12	5	3	1	1	0	0
S	0	0	0	0	0	3	13	24	44	68	88	99	100	88	67	45	29	15	6	3	2	1	0	0
SW	0	0	0	0	0	3	13	22	28	34	39	65	105	139	160	161	138	73	30	14	7	3	2	1
W	1	0	0	0	0	3	13	22	28	34	37	39	68	119	165	192	186	106	41	20	10	5	2	1
NW	0	0	0	0	0	3	13	22	28	34	37	39	40	50	84	117	129	79	30	14	7	3	2	1
hor	0	0	0	0	0	7	46	102	157	205	240	258	260	244	211	163	103	47	21	10	5	3	1	1

Glass Facing	Zone type B					Solar time, hr																		
	1	2	3	4	5	6	7	8	9	10	11	12	13	14	15	16	17	18	19	20	21	22	23	24
N	1	1	1	1	0	7	13	19	25	30	34	36	37	36	34	30	25	18	10	7	5	3	3	2
NE	2	1	1	1	1	32	87	104	93	68	55	50	47	43	39	34	27	17	10	7	5	4	3	2
E	2	2	1	1	1	38	115	153	161	144	107	74	63	54	47	40	31	20	13	9	7	5	4	3
SE	2	2	1	1	1	22	78	116	137	140	127	99	70	58	49	41	32	21	13	10	7	5	4	3
S	2	2	1	1	1	4	12	21	38	59	77	88	90	83	67	49	36	23	15	10	7	6	4	3
SW	6	5	3	3	2	4	12	19	25	30	35	58	92	123	142	147	130	78	43	29	20	15	11	8
W	7	5	4	3	2	5	13	19	25	30	34	36	61	105	145	170	168	105	54	36	25	18	13	10
NW	5	4	3	2	2	4	12	19	25	30	34	36	37	46	75	104	116	75	36	24	17	12	9	6
hor	7	5	4	3	2	7	40	88	135	178	211	232	239	230	206	168	118	70	45	32	23	17	13	10

Glass Facing	Zone type C					Solar time, hr																		
	1	2	3	4	5	6	7	8	9	10	11	12	13	14	15	16	17	18	19	20	21	22	23	24
N	4	4	3	3	3	8	14	19	24	28	31	33	33	33	31	27	23	17	9	8	7	6	5	5
NE	6	6	5	4	4	35	87	97	83	58	46	44	43	41	38	33	28	19	13	11	10	9	8	7
E	9	8	7	6	6	42	115	145	146	126	90	61	55	50	46	41	34	24	18	16	14	12	11	10
SE	9	8	7	6	6	26	79	112	127	126	111	84	59	52	46	41	34	24	18	16	14	12	11	10
S	7	7	6	5	5	7	15	23	39	57	72	81	81	73	58	42	32	21	16	13	12	10	9	8
SW	14	12	11	10	9	11	18	23	28	32	35	57	89	115	131	132	114	64	34	26	22	19	17	15
W	15	14	12	11	10	12	19	24	29	32	35	36	60	101	136	156	151	86	41	31	25	22	19	17
NW	10	9	8	7	6	9	16	22	27	30	33	35	35	44	72	98	106	64	28	20	17	14	13	11
hor	22	20	18	16	14	18	50	93	134	170	196	211	214	205	182	148	104	63	47	40	35	31	28	25

Glass Facing	Zone type D					Solar time, hr																		
	1	2	3	4	5	6	7	8	9	10	11	12	13	14	15	16	17	18	19	20	21	22	23	24
N	6	6	5	5	4	9	13	17	21	25	27	29	30	30	29	26	23	18	12	11	10	9	8	7
NE	10	9	8	7	6	30	71	81	71	53	45	44	43	41	39	35	31	23	19	17	15	13	12	11
E	14	12	11	10	9	37	95	119	123	110	84	63	59	55	51	46	40	32	26	23	21	19	17	15
SE	14	12	11	10	9	25	67	92	106	108	99	79	61	55	51	46	40	32	26	23	21	19	17	15
S	11	10	9	8	7	9	15	21	34	48	61	69	71	65	55	43	35	27	22	19	17	15	14	12
SW	21	19	17	15	14	15	20	24	27	30	33	51	76	98	112	115	103	65	43	36	32	28	26	23
W	23	21	19	17	15	16	21	25	28	31	33	34	53	86	115	133	131	83	49	41	36	32	28	25
NW	15	14	12	11	10	11	17	21	25	28	30	32	32	40	62	84	91	60	33	27	24	21	19	17
hor	34	31	28	25	22	25	48	82	115	144	168	183	189	184	170	145	112	80	66	58	52	46	42	38

Data applies directly to standard, double-strength glass with no inside shade that is exposed to clear sky on the 21st day of the month.

For other types of glass and internal shade, multiply values by shading coefficient (see text). For extremely shaded glass, use north orientation (see text).

Table 7-27-A40 August Solar Cooling Load For Sunlit Glass 40° North Latitude

Glass Facing	Zone type A 1	2	3	4	5	Solar time, hr 6	7	8	9	10	11	12	13	14	15	16	17	18	19	20	21	22	23	24
N	0	0	0	0	0	9	15	22	28	33	36	38	38	37	34	29	23	17	6	3	1	1	0	0
NE	0	0	0	0	0	48	102	112	89	58	47	43	41	38	34	29	23	13	5	3	1	1	0	0
E	0	0	0	0	0	58	140	179	183	157	107	66	52	43	37	31	23	13	5	3	1	1	0	0
SE	0	0	0	0	0	35	99	145	170	174	158	122	78	54	42	33	25	14	6	3	1	1	0	0
S	0	0	0	0	0	5	14	31	61	93	119	133	134	120	93	60	35	19	8	4	2	1	0	0
SW	0	0	0	0	0	5	14	21	28	33	45	83	125	158	176	174	147	86	34	16	8	4	2	1
W	1	0	0	0	0	5	14	21	28	33	36	38	66	117	162	189	185	120	45	22	11	5	3	1
NW	0	0	0	0	0	5	14	21	28	33	36	38	38	40	67	103	121	87	31	15	7	4	2	1
hor	0	0	0	0	0	10	48	99	150	192	224	241	243	228	198	155	101	48	21	10	5	3	1	1

Glass Facing	Zone type B 1	2	3	4	5	Solar time, hr 6	7	8	9	10	11	12	13	14	15	16	17	18	19	20	21	22	23	24
N	1	1	1	1	0	8	13	19	24	29	32	35	35	35	33	29	24	19	10	7	5	3	3	2
NE	2	1	1	1	1	41	87	96	80	56	49	46	43	41	37	32	26	17	10	7	5	4	3	2
E	2	2	1	1	1	50	119	153	160	143	105	73	61	53	46	39	31	21	13	9	7	5	4	3
SE	2	2	1	1	1	30	84	124	148	155	145	119	84	64	53	44	34	23	15	11	8	6	4	3
S	3	2	2	1	1	5	12	27	53	81	104	118	121	112	92	66	45	30	19	14	10	7	5	4
SW	7	5	4	3	2	6	13	19	25	29	40	73	110	139	157	159	140	90	48	32	23	16	12	9
W	8	6	4	3	2	6	13	19	25	29	33	35	59	103	142	167	168	116	56	38	26	19	14	10
NW	5	4	3	2	2	5	12	19	24	29	32	35	35	37	61	92	108	81	36	24	16	12	8	6
hor	7	5	4	3	2	10	42	85	129	168	198	217	223	215	193	159	114	69	44	31	22	16	12	9

Glass Facing	Zone type C 1	2	3	4	5	Solar time, hr 6	7	8	9	10	11	12	13	14	15	16	17	18	19	20	21	22	23	24
N	4	4	3	3	3	10	14	19	24	27	30	32	32	31	29	26	22	18	9	8	6	6	5	4
NE	6	5	5	4	4	44	85	89	70	47	42	41	40	38	36	32	27	19	13	11	9	8	7	7
E	9	8	7	6	6	54	118	145	145	125	88	60	54	49	45	40	34	25	18	16	14	12	11	10
SE	10	9	8	7	6	35	85	119	137	140	128	102	71	56	49	43	36	27	20	18	16	14	12	11
S	10	9	8	7	6	10	16	30	53	78	98	108	109	99	80	56	39	28	21	18	15	14	12	11
SW	15	14	12	11	10	13	19	24	28	31	41	72	105	130	144	142	122	75	39	30	25	22	19	17
W	15	14	12	11	10	13	19	24	28	31	34	35	58	99	134	154	151	98	43	31	26	22	19	17
NW	9	8	8	7	6	9	16	21	26	29	32	33	33	35	58	87	100	71	28	20	16	14	12	11
hor	21	19	17	15	14	20	50	90	127	160	184	198	201	192	171	141	101	63	45	38	33	29	26	23

Glass Facing	Zone type D 1	2	3	4	5	Solar time, hr 6	7	8	9	10	11	12	13	14	15	16	17	18	19	20	21	22	23	24
N	6	5	5	4	4	10	13	17	21	24	26	28	29	29	28	25	22	19	12	11	9	8	8	7
NE	9	8	7	7	6	37	70	74	61	44	41	41	40	39	37	34	29	23	18	16	14	12	11	10
E	14	12	11	10	9	47	97	119	122	110	83	62	58	54	50	46	40	33	26	23	21	19	17	15
SE	15	14	12	11	10	32	72	99	115	120	113	95	72	60	55	50	44	36	29	26	23	21	19	17
S	15	14	12	11	10	12	17	27	46	66	82	92	95	89	75	58	45	36	29	26	23	21	19	17
SW	23	21	19	17	15	17	21	25	28	30	38	63	89	110	123	124	111	76	48	41	36	32	29	26
W	23	21	19	17	15	17	21	25	28	30	32	33	52	85	113	131	130	92	50	42	36	32	29	26
NW	14	13	12	10	9	12	16	20	24	27	29	30	31	33	51	74	85	64	32	26	22	20	18	16
hor	32	29	26	24	21	26	48	79	109	136	157	171	177	173	160	138	108	78	63	55	49	44	40	36

Table 7-27-A48 August Solar Cooling Load For Sunlit Glass 48° North Latitude

Glass Facing	Zone type A 1	2	3	4	5	Solar time, hr 6	7	8	9	10	11	12	13	14	15	16	17	18	19	20	21	22	23	24
N	0	0	0	0	0	10	15	21	27	31	34	36	36	34	32	28	22	18	6	3	1	1	0	0
NE	0	0	0	0	0	57	100	101	74	49	43	40	38	36	32	28	22	14	5	3	1	1	0	0
E	0	0	0	0	0	70	143	178	179	153	104	63	49	41	35	29	23	14	6	3	1	1	0	0
SE	0	0	0	0	0	43	104	152	180	187	175	142	95	58	43	33	25	15	6	3	1	1	0	0
S	0	0	0	0	0	6	15	40	78	116	146	162	163	147	117	77	42	23	10	5	2	1	1	0
SW	1	0	0	0	0	6	14	21	26	31	55	99	143	174	189	183	154	96	37	18	9	4	2	1
W	1	0	0	0	0	6	14	21	26	31	34	36	63	113	157	185	183	131	47	23	11	6	3	1
NW	1	0	0	0	0	6	14	21	26	31	34	36	36	34	53	89	111	92	32	15	7	4	2	1
hor	0	0	0	0	0	13	48	93	138	176	203	218	220	207	181	143	95	49	21	10	5	2	1	1

Glass Facing	Zone type B 1	2	3	4	5	Solar time, hr 6	7	8	9	10	11	12	13	14	15	16	17	18	19	20	21	22	23	24
N	1	1	1	1	0	9	13	18	23	28	31	33	33	33	31	28	23	19	10	7	5	3	2	2
NE	2	1	1	1	0	49	85	87	67	48	44	42	40	38	35	31	25	18	10	7	5	4	3	2
E	2	2	1	1	1	60	121	152	158	140	103	70	59	51	44	37	30	21	13	9	7	5	4	3
SE	3	2	1	1	1	37	89	130	156	167	160	136	99	69	56	45	36	26	16	11	8	6	5	3
S	4	3	2	2	1	6	13	34	67	100	127	144	148	138	115	83	54	37	24	17	12	9	7	5
SW	7	5	4	3	2	7	13	19	24	28	49	87	124	153	169	168	147	101	52	35	25	18	13	10
W	8	6	4	3	2	7	13	19	24	28	31	33	57	99	138	164	166	125	58	39	27	19	14	10
NW	4	3	3	2	1	6	13	18	23	28	31	33	33	33	49	79	99	84	36	23	16	11	8	6
hor	6	5	4	3	2	12	42	80	119	153	180	197	202	195	176	146	107	67	41	29	21	15	11	9

Glass Facing	Zone type C 1	2	3	4	5	Solar time, hr 6	7	8	9	10	11	12	13	14	15	16	17	18	19	20	21	22	23	24
N	4	3	3	3	2	10	14	19	23	26	28	30	30	30	28	25	21	18	9	7	6	5	5	4
NE	6	5	4	4	4	51	83	81	58	40	39	38	37	36	33	30	25	19	12	10	9	8	7	6
E	9	8	7	6	6	64	119	143	143	122	86	58	52	48	43	39	33	26	18	16	14	12	11	10
SE	11	10	9	8	7	42	90	125	145	151	142	118	84	59	51	45	38	30	22	19	17	15	13	12
S	12	11	10	9	8	12	18	38	68	97	119	131	133	122	100	71	47	35	25	22	19	17	15	14
SW	17	15	13	12	11	14	20	24	28	31	50	86	119	143	154	150	129	85	42	32	27	24	21	19
W	15	14	12	11	10	14	19	24	27	30	32	33	56	96	130	151	149	107	44	32	26	22	19	17
NW	9	8	7	6	6	10	16	21	25	28	30	31	32	31	47	76	93	75	27	19	15	13	11	10
hor	19	17	16	14	13	22	49	84	117	146	167	180	182	174	157	130	95	62	42	35	31	27	24	22

Glass Facing	Zone type D 1	2	3	4	5	Solar time, hr 6	7	8	9	10	11	12	13	14	15	16	17	18	19	20	21	22	23	24
N	6	5	5	4	4	10	12	16	20	23	25	26	27	27	26	24	21	19	12	10	9	8	7	7
NE	9	8	7	6	6	43	68	67	51	39	38	38	37	36	34	31	28	22	17	15	13	12	11	9
E	14	12	11	10	9	54	98	118	121	108	82	61	56	53	49	45	39	33	26	23	21	19	17	15
SE	17	15	14	12	11	38	76	104	122	129	125	109	84	65	59	53	47	39	32	28	25	23	21	19
S	19	17	15	14	12	15	19	35	58	82	101	112	115	109	94	73	54	44	36	32	28	25	23	21
SW	25	23	20	18	17	19	22	25	28	30	45	74	101	121	132	132	118	85	52	44	39	35	31	28
W	23	21	19	17	15	18	21	24	27	29	31	32	50	82	110	128	129	99	51	42	36	32	29	26
NW	13	12	11	10	9	12	16	20	23	25	27	29	29	29	42	65	79	67	30	25	21	19	17	15
hor	30	27	24	22	20	26	47	74	101	125	144	156	161	157	146	127	101	74	58	51	45	41	37	33

Data applies directly to standard, double-strength glass with no inside shade that is exposed to clear sky on the 21st day of the month.

For other types of glass and internal shade, multiply values by shading coefficient (see text). For extremely shaded glass, use north orientation (see text).

Table 7-28 Cooling Load Factors for People and Unhooded Equipment

Hours in Space	Number of Hours after Entry into Space or Equipment Turned On																							
	1	2	3	4	5	6	7	8	9	10	11	12	13	14	15	16	17	18	19	20	21	22	23	24
Zone Type A																								
2	0.75	0.88	0.18	0.08	0.04	0.02	0.01	0.01	0.01	0.01	0.00	0.00	0.00	0.00	0.00	0.00	0.00	0.00	0.00	0.00	0.00	0.00	0.00	0.00
4	0.75	0.88	0.93	0.95	0.22	0.10	0.05	0.03	0.02	0.02	0.01	0.01	0.01	0.01	0.00	0.00	0.00	0.00	0.00	0.00	0.00	0.00	0.00	0.00
6	0.75	0.88	0.93	0.95	0.97	0.97	0.23	0.11	0.06	0.04	0.03	0.02	0.02	0.01	0.01	0.01	0.01	0.00	0.00	0.00	0.00	0.00	0.00	0.00
8	0.75	0.88	0.93	0.95	0.97	0.97	0.98	0.98	0.24	0.11	0.06	0.04	0.03	0.02	0.02	0.01	0.01	0.01	0.01	0.01	0.00	0.00	0.00	0.00
10	0.75	0.88	0.93	0.95	0.97	0.97	0.98	0.98	0.99	0.99	0.24	0.12	0.07	0.04	0.03	0.02	0.02	0.01	0.01	0.01	0.01	0.01	0.00	0.00
12	0.75	0.88	0.93	0.96	0.97	0.98	0.98	0.98	0.99	0.99	0.99	0.99	0.25	0.12	0.07	0.04	0.03	0.02	0.02	0.02	0.01	0.01	0.01	0.01
14	0.76	0.88	0.93	0.96	0.97	0.98	0.98	0.99	0.99	0.99	0.99	0.99	1.00	1.00	0.25	0.12	0.07	0.05	0.03	0.03	0.02	0.02	0.01	0.01
16	0.76	0.89	0.94	0.96	0.97	0.98	0.98	0.99	0.99	0.99	0.99	0.99	1.00	1.00	1.00	1.00	0.25	0.12	0.07	0.05	0.03	0.03	0.02	0.02
18	0.77	0.89	0.94	0.96	0.97	0.98	0.98	0.99	0.99	0.99	0.99	1.00	1.00	1.00	1.00	1.00	1.00	1.00	0.25	0.12	0.07	0.05	0.03	0.03
Zone Type B																								
2	0.65	0.74	0.16	0.11	0.08	0.06	0.05	0.04	0.03	0.02	0.02	0.01	0.01	0.01	0.01	0.00	0.00	0.00	0.00	0.00	0.00	0.00	0.00	0.00
4	0.65	0.75	0.81	0.85	0.24	0.17	0.13	0.10	0.07	0.06	0.04	0.03	0.03	0.02	0.02	0.01	0.01	0.01	0.01	0.00	0.00	0.00	0.00	0.00
6	0.65	0.75	0.81	0.85	0.89	0.91	0.29	0.20	0.15	0.12	0.09	0.07	0.05	0.04	0.03	0.02	0.02	0.01	0.01	0.01	0.01	0.01	0.00	0.00
8	0.65	0.75	0.81	0.85	0.89	0.91	0.93	0.95	0.31	0.22	0.17	0.13	0.10	0.08	0.06	0.05	0.04	0.03	0.02	0.02	0.01	0.01	0.01	0.01
10	0.65	0.75	0.81	0.85	0.89	0.91	0.93	0.95	0.96	0.97	0.33	0.24	0.18	0.14	0.11	0.08	0.06	0.05	0.04	0.03	0.02	0.02	0.01	0.01
12	0.66	0.76	0.81	0.86	0.89	0.92	0.94	0.95	0.96	0.97	0.98	0.98	0.34	0.24	0.19	0.14	0.11	0.08	0.06	0.05	0.04	0.03	0.02	0.02
14	0.67	0.76	0.82	0.86	0.89	0.92	0.94	0.95	0.96	0.97	0.98	0.98	0.99	0.99	0.35	0.25	0.19	0.15	0.11	0.09	0.07	0.05	0.04	0.03
16	0.69	0.78	0.83	0.87	0.90	0.92	0.94	0.95	0.96	0.97	0.98	0.98	0.99	0.99	0.99	0.99	0.35	0.25	0.19	0.15	0.11	0.09	0.07	0.05
18	0.71	0.80	0.85	0.88	0.91	0.93	0.95	0.96	0.97	0.98	0.98	0.99	0.99	0.99	0.99	0.99	1.00	1.00	0.35	0.25	0.19	0.15	0.11	0.09
Zone Type C																								
2	0.60	0.68	0.14	0.11	0.09	0.07	0.06	0.05	0.04	0.03	0.03	0.02	0.02	0.01	0.01	0.01	0.01	0.01	0.01	0.00	0.00	0.00	0.00	0.00
4	0.60	0.68	0.74	0.79	0.23	0.18	0.14	0.12	0.10	0.08	0.06	0.05	0.04	0.04	0.03	0.02	0.02	0.02	0.01	0.01	0.01	0.01	0.01	0.01
6	0.61	0.69	0.74	0.79	0.83	0.86	0.28	0.22	0.18	0.15	0.12	0.10	0.08	0.07	0.06	0.05	0.04	0.03	0.03	0.02	0.02	0.01	0.01	0.01
8	0.61	0.69	0.75	0.79	0.83	0.86	0.89	0.91	0.32	0.26	0.21	0.17	0.14	0.11	0.09	0.08	0.06	0.05	0.04	0.04	0.03	0.02	0.02	0.02
10	0.62	0.70	0.75	0.80	0.83	0.86	0.89	0.91	0.92	0.94	0.35	0.28	0.23	0.18	0.15	0.12	0.10	0.08	0.07	0.06	0.05	0.04	0.03	0.03
12	0.63	0.71	0.76	0.81	0.84	0.87	0.89	0.91	0.93	0.94	0.95	0.96	0.37	0.29	0.24	0.19	0.16	0.13	0.11	0.09	0.07	0.06	0.05	0.04
14	0.65	0.72	0.77	0.82	0.85	0.88	0.90	0.92	0.93	0.94	0.95	0.96	0.97	0.97	0.38	0.30	0.25	0.20	0.17	0.14	0.11	0.09	0.08	0.06
16	0.68	0.74	0.79	0.83	0.86	0.89	0.91	0.92	0.94	0.95	0.96	0.96	0.97	0.98	0.98	0.98	0.39	0.31	0.25	0.21	0.17	0.14	0.11	0.09
18	0.72	0.78	0.82	0.85	0.88	0.90	0.92	0.93	0.94	0.95	0.96	0.97	0.97	0.98	0.98	0.99	0.99	0.99	0.39	0.31	0.26	0.21	0.17	0.14
Zone Type D																								
2	0.59	0.67	0.13	0.09	0.08	0.06	0.05	0.05	0.04	0.04	0.03	0.03	0.02	0.02	0.02	0.01	0.01	0.01	0.01	0.01	0.01	0.01	0.01	0.00
4	0.60	0.67	0.72	0.76	0.20	0.16	0.13	0.11	0.10	0.08	0.07	0.06	0.05	0.05	0.04	0.03	0.03	0.03	0.02	0.02	0.02	0.01	0.01	0.01
6	0.61	0.68	0.73	0.77	0.80	0.83	0.26	0.20	0.17	0.15	0.13	0.11	0.09	0.08	0.07	0.06	0.05	0.05	0.04	0.03	0.03	0.03	0.02	0.02
8	0.62	0.69	0.74	0.77	0.80	0.83	0.85	0.87	0.30	0.24	0.20	0.17	0.15	0.13	0.11	0.10	0.08	0.07	0.06	0.05	0.05	0.04	0.04	0.03
10	0.63	0.70	0.75	0.78	0.81	0.84	0.86	0.88	0.89	0.91	0.33	0.27	0.22	0.19	0.17	0.14	0.12	0.11	0.09	0.08	0.07	0.06	0.05	0.05
12	0.65	0.71	0.76	0.79	0.82	0.84	0.87	0.88	0.90	0.91	0.92	0.93	0.35	0.29	0.24	0.21	0.18	0.16	0.13	0.12	0.10	0.09	0.08	0.07
14	0.67	0.73	0.78	0.81	0.83	0.86	0.88	0.89	0.91	0.92	0.93	0.94	0.95	0.95	0.37	0.30	0.25	0.22	0.19	0.16	0.14	0.12	0.11	0.09
16	0.70	0.76	0.80	0.83	0.85	0.87	0.89	0.90	0.92	0.93	0.94	0.95	0.95	0.96	0.96	0.97	0.38	0.31	0.26	0.23	0.20	0.17	0.15	0.13
18	0.74	0.80	0.83	0.85	0.87	0.89	0.91	0.92	0.93	0.94	0.95	0.95	0.96	0.97	0.97	0.97	0.98	0.98	0.39	0.32	0.27	0.23	0.20	0.17

Note: See Table 7-26 for zone type. Data based on a radiative/convective fraction of 0.70/0.30.

components are felt as cooling loads, which affect the hourly cooling loads for the space. Two types of errors are possible:

1. The computer software that generated CLTD/SCL/CLF tables uses the TFM to determine cooling loads based on various types of heat gain. The cooling loads for each type of heat gain are normalized appropriately to obtain CLTDs, SCLs or CLFs. Except, as discussed next, use of the CLTD/SCL/CLF method in conjunction with these tables will yield the same results as the TFM, but only when the same 14 zone parameters are specified.

   Three inherent errors in the TFM are carried through to the CLTD/SCL/CLF data:

   a. Each set of weighting factors or conduction transfer function coefficients is used for a group of walls, roofs, or zones with similar thermal response characteristics. Groups were chosen so that error would be minimal and conservative (Harris and McQuiston 1988, Sowell 1988).

   b. The scheme used for calculating weighting factors is based on 14 discrete parameters applied to a rectangular room. Rarely does a room fit exactly into these parameters. Therefore, engineering judgement must be used to choose the values of the 14 parameters that most closely represent the room for which load calculations are being performed. Deviations of the room from the available levels of the 14 parameters may result in errors that are not easily quantifiable.

   c. A fundamental presupposition of the TFM is that total cooling load for a zone can be calculated by simple addition of the individual componenets. For example, radiation heat transfer from individual walls and roofs is assumed to be independent of the other surfaces.

2. The printed tables for CLTDs, SCLs, and CLFs have undergone a further grouping procedure. The maximum potential errors due to the second grouping procedure are tabulated in Tables 7-26 and 7-31. These errors are in addi-

Table 7-29 Cooling Load Factors for Lights

Lights On For	Number of Hours after Lights Turned On																							
	1	2	3	4	5	6	7	8	9	10	11	12	13	14	15	16	17	18	19	20	21	22	23	24
Zone Type A																								
8	0.85	0.92	0.95	0.96	0.97	0.97	0.97	0.98	0.13	0.06	0.04	0.03	0.02	0.02	0.02	0.01	0.01	0.01	0.01	0.01	0.01	0.01	0.01	0.01
10	0.85	0.93	0.95	0.97	0.97	0.97	0.98	0.98	0.98	0.98	0.14	0.07	0.04	0.03	0.02	0.02	0.02	0.02	0.02	0.02	0.01	0.01	0.01	0.01
12	0.86	0.93	0.96	0.97	0.97	0.98	0.98	0.98	0.98	0.98	0.98	0.98	0.14	0.07	0.04	0.03	0.03	0.02	0.02	0.02	0.02	0.02	0.02	0.02
14	0.86	0.93	0.96	0.97	0.98	0.98	0.98	0.98	0.98	0.98	0.99	0.99	0.99	0.99	0.15	0.07	0.05	0.03	0.03	0.03	0.02	0.02	0.02	0.02
16	0.87	0.94	0.96	0.97	0.98	0.98	0.98	0.99	0.99	0.99	0.99	0.99	0.99	0.99	0.99	0.99	0.15	0.08	0.05	0.04	0.03	0.03	0.03	0.02
Zone Type B																								
8	0.75	0.85	0.90	0.93	0.94	0.95	0.95	0.96	0.23	0.12	0.08	0.05	0.04	0.04	0.03	0.03	0.03	0.02	0.02	0.02	0.02	0.02	0.02	0.01
10	0.75	0.86	0.91	0.93	0.94	0.95	0.95	0.96	0.96	0.97	0.24	0.13	0.08	0.06	0.05	0.04	0.04	0.03	0.03	0.03	0.03	0.02	0.02	0.02
12	0.76	0.86	0.91	0.93	0.95	0.95	0.96	0.96	0.97	0.97	0.97	0.97	0.24	0.14	0.09	0.07	0.05	0.05	0.04	0.04	0.03	0.03	0.03	0.03
14	0.76	0.87	0.92	0.94	0.95	0.96	0.96	0.97	0.97	0.97	0.97	0.98	0.98	0.98	0.25	0.14	0.09	0.07	0.06	0.05	0.05	0.04	0.04	0.03
16	0.77	0.88	0.92	0.95	0.96	0.96	0.97	0.97	0.97	0.98	0.98	0.98	0.98	0.98	0.98	0.99	0.25	0.15	0.10	0.07	0.06	0.05	0.05	0.04
Zone Type C																								
8	0.72	0.80	0.84	0.87	0.88	0.89	0.90	0.91	0.23	0.15	0.11	0.09	0.08	0.07	0.07	0.06	0.05	0.05	0.05	0.04	0.04	0.03	0.03	0.03
10	0.73	0.81	0.85	0.87	0.89	0.90	0.91	0.92	0.92	0.93	0.25	0.16	0.13	0.11	0.09	0.08	0.08	0.07	0.06	0.06	0.05	0.05	0.04	0.04
12	0.74	0.82	0.86	0.88	0.90	0.91	0.92	0.92	0.93	0.94	0.94	0.95	0.26	0.18	0.14	0.12	0.10	0.09	0.08	0.08	0.07	0.06	0.06	0.05
14	0.75	0.84	0.87	0.89	0.91	0.92	0.92	0.93	0.94	0.94	0.95	0.95	0.96	0.96	0.27	0.19	0.15	0.13	0.11	0.10	0.09	0.08	0.08	0.07
16	0.77	0.85	0.89	0.91	0.92	0.93	0.93	0.94	0.95	0.95	0.95	0.96	0.96	0.97	0.97	0.97	0.28	0.20	0.16	0.13	0.12	0.11	0.10	0.09
Zone Type D																								
8	0.66	0.72	0.76	0.79	0.81	0.83	0.85	0.86	0.25	0.20	0.17	0.15	0.13	0.12	0.11	0.10	0.09	0.08	0.07	0.06	0.06	0.05	0.04	0.04
10	0.68	0.74	0.77	0.80	0.82	0.84	0.86	0.87	0.88	0.90	0.28	0.23	0.19	0.17	0.15	0.14	0.12	0.11	0.10	0.09	0.08	0.07	0.06	0.06
12	0.70	0.75	0.79	0.81	0.83	0.85	0.87	0.88	0.89	0.90	0.91	0.92	0.30	0.25	0.21	0.19	0.17	0.15	0.13	0.12	0.11	0.10	0.09	0.08
14	0.72	0.77	0.81	0.83	0.85	0.86	0.88	0.89	0.90	0.91	0.92	0.93	0.94	0.94	0.32	0.26	0.23	0.20	0.18	0.16	0.14	0.13	0.12	0.10
16	0.75	0.80	0.83	0.85	0.87	0.88	0.89	0.90	0.91	0.92	0.93	0.94	0.94	0.95	0.96	0.96	0.34	0.28	0.24	0.21	0.19	0.17	0.15	0.14

Note: See Table 7-26 for zone type. Data based on a radiative/convective fraction of 0.59/0.41.

tion to those inherent in the TFM. However, for usual construction, these errors are modest.

In summary, the CLTD/SCL/CLF method, as with any method, requires engineering judgement in its application. When the method is used in conjunction with custom tables generated by appropriate computer software (McQuiston and Spitler 1992) and for buildings where external shading is not significant, it can be expected to produce results very close to those produced by the TFM. When the printed tables are used, some additional error is introduced. In many cases, the accuracy should be sufficient.

7.7 RESIDENTIAL COOLING LOAD PROCEDURE

The CLTD/SCL/CLF method described in the previous sections of this chapter apply for commercial and institutional buildings. For residential structures there are unique features which allow simplified techniques to be used for cooling load calculations.

The unique features distinguishing residences from other types of buildings, with respect to cooling load calculation and quipment sizing, are

1. Unlike many other structures, residences are usually occupied and conditioned, for 24 h a day, every day of the cooling season.
2. Residential cooling system loads are primarily imposed by heat gain through structural components and by air leakage or ventilation. Internal loads, particularly those from occupants and lights, are small in comparison with those in commercial or industrial installations.
3. Most residences are cooled as a single zone. Cooling unit capacity cannot be redistributed from one area to another as loads change from hour to hour; however, exceptions do occur.
4. Most residential systems use units of relatively small capacity (about 5 to 18 kW or 18,000 to 60,000 Btu/h). Since cooling load is largely affected by outside conditions, and few days each season are design days, only a partial load exists during most of the season; thus, an oversized unit is detrimental to good system performance.
5. Dehumidification occurs only during cooling unit operation, and space condition control is usually restricted to use of room thermostats (sensible heat-actuated devices).
6. Multifamily living units are similar to single-family, detached houses, but each living unit may not have surfaces exposed in all directions. This affects load calculation.

7.7.1 Residential Building Categories

Single-Family Detached. A house in this category usually has exposed walls in four directions, often more than one story, and a roof. The cooling system is a single-zone, unitary system with a single thermostat. Two-story houses may have separate cooling systems for each floor. The rooms are reasonably open with a centralized air return. In this configuration, air and load for all rooms are mixed, and a load leveling effect, which requires a different distribution of air to each room than does a pure commercial system, results. Since the

Table 7-30 Cooling Load Factors for Hooded Equipment

Hours in Operation	Number of Hours after Equipment Turned On																							
	1	2	3	4	5	6	7	8	9	10	11	12	13	14	15	16	17	18	19	20	21	22	23	24
Zone Type A																								
2	0.64	0.83	0.26	0.11	0.06	0.03	0.01	0.01	0.01	0.01	0.00	0.00	0.00	0.00	0.00	0.00	0.00	0.00	0.00	0.00	0.00	0.00	0.00	0.00
4	0.64	0.83	0.90	0.93	0.31	0.14	0.07	0.04	0.03	0.03	0.01	0.01	0.01	0.01	0.00	0.00	0.00	0.00	0.00	0.00	0.00	0.00	0.00	0.00
6	0.64	0.83	0.90	0.93	0.96	0.96	0.33	0.16	0.09	0.06	0.04	0.03	0.03	0.01	0.01	0.01	0.01	0.00	0.00	0.00	0.00	0.00	0.00	0.00
8	0.64	0.83	0.90	0.93	0.96	0.96	0.97	0.97	0.34	0.16	0.09	0.06	0.04	0.03	0.03	0.01	0.01	0.01	0.01	0.01	0.00	0.00	0.00	0.00
10	0.64	0.83	0.90	0.93	0.96	0.96	0.97	0.97	0.99	0.99	0.34	0.17	0.10	0.06	0.04	0.03	0.03	0.01	0.01	0.01	0.01	0.01	0.01	0.00
12	0.64	0.83	0.90	0.94	0.96	0.97	0.97	0.97	0.99	0.99	0.99	0.99	0.36	0.17	0.10	0.06	0.04	0.03	0.03	0.03	0.01	0.01	0.01	0.01
14	0.66	0.83	0.90	0.94	0.96	0.97	0.97	0.99	0.99	0.99	0.99	0.99	1.00	1.00	0.36	0.17	0.10	0.07	0.04	0.04	0.03	0.03	0.03	0.01
16	0.66	0.84	0.91	0.94	0.96	0.97	0.97	0.99	0.99	0.99	0.99	0.99	1.00	1.00	1.00	1.00	0.36	0.17	0.10	0.07	0.04	0.04	0.04	0.03
18	0.67	0.84	0.91	0.94	0.96	0.97	0.97	0.99	0.99	0.99	0.99	1.00	1.00	1.00	1.00	1.00	1.00	1.00	0.36	0.17	0.10	0.08	0.07	0.04
Zone Type B																								
2	0.50	0.63	0.23	0.16	0.11	0.09	0.07	0.06	0.04	0.03	0.03	0.01	0.01	0.01	0.01	0.00	0.00	0.00	0.00	0.00	0.00	0.00	0.00	0.00
4	0.50	0.64	0.73	0.79	0.34	0.24	0.19	0.14	0.10	0.09	0.06	0.04	0.04	0.03	0.03	0.01	0.01	0.01	0.01	0.00	0.00	0.00	0.00	0.00
6	0.50	0.64	0.73	0.79	0.84	0.87	0.41	0.29	0.21	0.17	0.13	0.10	0.07	0.06	0.04	0.03	0.03	0.01	0.01	0.01	0.01	0.01	0.01	0.00
8	0.50	0.64	0.73	0.79	0.84	0.87	0.90	0.93	0.44	0.31	0.24	0.19	0.14	0.11	0.09	0.07	0.06	0.04	0.03	0.03	0.01	0.01	0.01	0.01
10	0.50	0.64	0.73	0.79	0.84	0.87	0.90	0.93	0.94	0.96	0.47	0.34	0.26	0.20	0.16	0.11	0.09	0.07	0.06	0.04	0.03	0.03	0.03	0.01
12	0.51	0.66	0.73	0.80	0.84	0.89	0.91	0.93	0.94	0.96	0.97	0.97	0.49	0.34	0.27	0.20	0.16	0.11	0.09	0.07	0.06	0.05	0.04	0.03
14	0.53	0.66	0.74	0.80	0.84	0.89	0.91	0.93	0.94	0.96	0.97	0.97	0.99	0.99	0.50	0.36	0.27	0.21	0.16	0.13	0.10	0.08	0.07	0.06
16	0.56	0.69	0.76	0.81	0.86	0.89	0.91	0.93	0.94	0.96	0.97	0.97	0.99	0.99	0.99	0.99	0.50	0.36	0.27	0.21	0.16	0.14	0.13	0.10
18	0.59	0.71	0.79	0.83	0.87	0.90	0.93	0.94	0.96	0.97	0.97	0.99	0.99	0.99	0.99	0.99	1.00	1.00	0.50	0.36	0.27	0.23	0.21	0.16
Zone Type C																								
2	0.43	0.54	0.20	0.16	0.13	0.10	0.09	0.07	0.06	0.04	0.04	0.03	0.03	0.01	0.01	0.01	0.01	0.01	0.01	0.00	0.00	0.00	0.00	0.00
4	0.43	0.54	0.63	0.70	0.33	0.26	0.20	0.17	0.14	0.11	0.09	0.07	0.06	0.06	0.04	0.03	0.03	0.03	0.01	0.01	0.01	0.01	0.01	0.01
6	0.44	0.56	0.63	0.70	0.76	0.80	0.40	0.31	0.26	0.21	0.17	0.14	0.11	0.10	0.09	0.07	0.06	0.04	0.04	0.03	0.03	0.02	0.01	0.01
8	0.44	0.56	0.64	0.70	0.76	0.80	0.84	0.87	0.46	0.37	0.30	0.24	0.20	0.16	0.13	0.11	0.09	0.07	0.06	0.06	0.04	0.03	0.03	0.03
10	0.46	0.57	0.64	0.71	0.76	0.80	0.84	0.87	0.89	0.91	0.50	0.40	0.33	0.26	0.21	0.17	0.14	0.11	0.10	0.09	0.07	0.06	0.06	0.04
12	0.47	0.59	0.66	0.73	0.77	0.81	0.84	0.87	0.90	0.91	0.93	0.94	0.53	0.41	0.34	0.27	0.23	0.19	0.16	0.13	0.10	0.09	0.09	0.07
14	0.50	0.60	0.67	0.74	0.79	0.83	0.86	0.89	0.90	0.91	0.93	0.94	0.96	0.96	0.54	0.43	0.36	0.29	0.24	0.20	0.16	0.14	0.13	0.11
16	0.54	0.63	0.70	0.76	0.80	0.84	0.87	0.89	0.91	0.93	0.94	0.94	0.96	0.97	0.97	0.97	0.56	0.44	0.36	0.30	0.24	0.22	0.20	0.16
18	0.60	0.69	0.74	0.79	0.83	0.86	0.89	0.90	0.91	0.93	0.94	0.96	0.96	0.97	0.97	0.99	0.99	0.99	0.56	0.44	0.37	0.33	0.30	0.24
Zone Type D																								
2	0.41	0.53	0.19	0.13	0.11	0.09	0.07	0.07	0.06	0.06	0.04	0.04	0.03	0.03	0.03	0.01	0.01	0.01	0.01	0.01	0.01	0.01	0.01	0.01
4	0.43	0.53	0.60	0.66	0.29	0.23	0.19	0.16	0.14	0.11	0.10	0.09	0.07	0.07	0.06	0.04	0.04	0.04	0.03	0.03	0.03	0.02	0.01	0.01
6	0.44	0.54	0.61	0.67	0.71	0.76	0.37	0.29	0.24	0.21	0.19	0.16	0.13	0.11	0.10	0.09	0.07	0.07	0.06	0.04	0.04	0.04	0.04	0.03
8	0.46	0.56	0.63	0.67	0.71	0.76	0.79	0.81	0.43	0.34	0.29	0.24	0.21	0.19	0.16	0.14	0.11	0.10	0.09	0.07	0.07	0.06	0.06	0.06
10	0.47	0.57	0.64	0.69	0.73	0.77	0.80	0.83	0.84	0.87	0.47	0.39	0.31	0.27	0.24	0.20	0.17	0.16	0.13	0.11	0.10	0.09	0.09	0.07
12	0.50	0.59	0.66	0.70	0.74	0.77	0.81	0.83	0.86	0.87	0.89	0.90	0.50	0.41	0.34	0.30	0.26	0.23	0.19	0.17	0.14	0.13	0.13	0.11
14	0.53	0.61	0.69	0.73	0.76	0.80	0.83	0.84	0.87	0.89	0.90	0.91	0.93	0.93	0.53	0.43	0.36	0.31	0.27	0.23	0.20	0.18	0.17	0.16
16	0.57	0.66	0.71	0.76	0.79	0.81	0.84	0.86	0.89	0.90	0.91	0.93	0.93	0.94	0.94	0.96	0.54	0.44	0.37	0.33	0.29	0.26	0.24	0.21
18	0.63	0.71	0.76	0.79	0.81	0.84	0.87	0.89	0.90	0.91	0.93	0.93	0.94	0.96	0.96	0.96	0.97	0.97	0.56	0.46	0.39	0.35	0.33	0.29

Note: See Table 35 for zone type. Data based on a radiative/convective fraction of 1.0/0.

Table 7-31 Potential Errors for Roof and Wall CLTDs in Tables 7-20 and 7-22

Roof No.	Error, %		Wall No.	Error, %	
	Plus	Minus		Plus	Minus
1	13	5	1	18	7
2	13	5	2	17	8
3	12	5	3	17	7
4	13	5	4	16	7
5	11	4	5	13	8
6	—	—	6	14	6
7	—	—	7	12	6
8	10	4	—	—	—
9	10	4	9	13	6
10	9	3	10	10	6
11	—	—	11	8	3
12	—	—	12	4	7
13	7	4	13	4	4
14	5	4	14	5	8
15	—	—	15	11	6
16	—	—	16	8	7

Note: Percent error = [(Table Value – TFM Value)/TFM Value] × 100

amount of air supplied to each room is based on the load for that room, proper load calculation procedures must be used.

Multifamily Buildings. Unlike single-family detached units, multifamily units do not have exposed surfaces facing in all directions. Rather, each unit has only one or two exposed surfaces and possibly a roof. Two exposed walls will be at right angles, that is, both east and west walls will not be exposed in a given living unit. Each living unit has a single unitary cooling system or a single fan coil unit, and the rooms are relatively open to one another. This configuration does not have the same load leveling effect as the single-family detached house, and it is not a commercial building. Therefore, a specific load calculation procedure is required.

Other Categories. Many buildings do not fall into either of the above categories. Critical to the designation of a single-family detached building is the presence of both east and west walls. Therefore, some multifamily-type structures should be treated as single-family detached when the exposed surfaces are oriented in a particular way. Examples include duplexes or apartments with exposed (1) east, west and south, or (2) east, west, and north walls with or without a roof; and apartments, town houses, or condominiums with only east and west or north and south exposed walls.

Light Commercial Buildings. Many light commercial buildings with single-zone, unitary cooling equipment and three or more exposed walls should be treated as single-family detached, except for their internal loads. Any residential structure that does not have both east and west exposed surfaces should be treated as a multifamily structure. Examples include duplexes and apartments with (1) north, south, and east or (2) north, south, west walls; single-family detached houses zoned so that east and west exposures are not in the same zone; and light commercial buildings with a limited number of zones separating east and west rooms.

7.7.2 Cooling Load Determination

A cooling load calculation determines total sensible cooling load due to heat gain (1) through structural components (walls, floors, and ceilings); (2) through windows; (3) caused by infiltration and ventilation; and (4) due to occupancy. The latent portion of the cooling load is evaluated separately.

While the entire structure may be considered a single zone, equipment selection and system design should be based on a room-by-room calculation. To properly design the distribution system, the amount of conditioned air required by each room must be known.

The tables in this section are based on an assumed indoor temperature swing of not more than 30°F (1.50°C) on a design day when the residence is conditioned for 24 h a day and the thermostat is set at 750°F (240°C).

7.7.3 Cooling Load Due to Heat Gain Through the Structure

The sensible cooling load due to heat gains through walls, floors, and ceilings of each room is calculated using appropriate cooling load temperature differences and U-factors for summer condtions (Table 7-32 and 7-33). For ceilings under naturally vented attics or vented flat roofs, use the combined U-factor for the roof, vented space, and ceiling. The mass of the walls is a variable in Table 7-33, but is not used in Table 7-32 because of the averaging techniques required to develop the CLTDs. A dark color is assumed for values in Table 7-32 and 7-33 because color is an unpredictable variation in any residence.Daily range (outdoor temperature swing on a design day) significantly affects the equivalent temperature difference. Listed in Tables 7-32 and 7-33 are daily temperature ranges classified as high, medium, and low. Daily range may be obtained from the weather data in Chapter 4.

Table 7-32 CLTD Values for Single Family Residences[a]

Daily Temperature Range[b]	Design Temperature, °F											
	85		90			95			100		105	110
	L	M	L	M	H	L	M	H	M	H	M	H
All walls and doors												
North	8	3	13	8	3	18	13	8	18	13	18	23
NE and NW	14	9	19	14	9	24	19	14	24	19	24	29
East and West	18	13	23	18	13	28	23	18	28	23	28	33
SE and SW	16	11	21	16	11	26	21	16	26	21	26	31
South	11	6	16	11	6	21	16	11	21	16	21	26
Roofs and ceilings												
Attic or flat built-up	42	37	47	42	37	51	47	42	51	47	51	56
Floors and ceilings												
Under conditioned space, over unconditioned room, over crawl space	9	4	12	9	4	14	12	9	14	12	14	19
Partitions												
Inside or shaded	9	4	12	9	4	14	12	9	14	12	14	19

[a]Cooling load temperature differences (CLTDs) for single-family detached houses, duplexes, or multifamily, with both east and west exposed walls or only north and south exposed walls, °F.

[b]L denotes low daily range, less than 16°F; M denotes medium daily range, 16 to 25°F; and H denotes high daily range, greater than 25°F.

Table 7-33 CLTD Values for Multifamily Residences[a]

Daily Temperature Range[b]		Design Temperature, °F											
		85		90			95			100		105	110
		L	M	L	M	H	L	M	H	M	H	M	H
Walls and doors[c]													
N	Light	14	11	19	16	12	24	21	17	26	22	27	32
	Medium	13	10	18	15	11	23	20	16	25	21	26	31
	Heavy	9	6	15	11	7	20	16	12	21	17	22	27
NE	Light	23	17	28	22	17	33	27	22	32	26	31	36
	Medium	20	15	25	20	16	30	25	21	29	25	29	34
	Heavy	16	12	21	17	13	26	22	18	26	22	26	31
E	Light	32	27	37	32	27	43	38	32	42	37	42	47
	Medium	30	24	34	29	24	40	34	29	39	33	39	44
	Heavy	23	18	28	23	18	34	29	23	33	28	33	38
SE	Light	31	27	35	31	26	41	37	31	42	37	42	47
	Medium	28	22	32	27	22	37	32	27	37	33	38	43
	Heavy	21	16	26	22	17	32	27	22	31	27	32	37
S	Light	25	22	29	26	22	35	31	26	36	32	37	43
	Medium	22	18	26	22	18	31	26	22	31	27	32	38
	Heavy	16	11	20	16	12	26	21	17	26	21	27	33
SW	Light	39	36	44	40	35	50	46	40	51	47	52	58
	Medium	33	29	37	34	29	44	40	35	45	40	46	52
	Heavy	23	18	28	24	19	36	31	25	35	30	36	42
W	Light	44	41	48	45	40	54	51	46	56	52	57	63
	Medium	37	33	41	38	33	46	42	38	48	43	49	55
	Heavy	26	22	31	27	23	37	32	27	37	32	38	44
NW	Light	33	30	37	34	30	43	39	34	44	40	45	50
	Medium	28	25	32	29	24	37	33	29	39	35	40	45
	Heavy	20	16	25	20	16	31	26	21	31	26	32	37
Roof and ceiling													
Attic or flat built-up	Light	58	53	65	60	55	70	65	60	70	65	72	77
Flat built-up	Medium or heavy	21	18	23	21	18	25	23	21	25	23	25	28
Floors and ceiling													
Under or over unconditioned space, crawl space		9	4	12	9	4	14	12	9	14	12	14	19
Partitions													
Inside or shaded		9	4	12	9	4	14	12	9	14	12	14	19

[a]Cooling load temperature differences (CLTDs) for multifamily low-rise or single-family detached if zoned with separate temperature control for each zone, °F.

[b]L denotes low daily range, less than 16°F; M denotes medium daily range, 16 to 25°F; and H denotes high daily range, greater than 25°F.

[c]Light denotes lightweight; medium denotes medium-weight; and heavy denotes heavy-weight construction.

7.7.4 Cooling Load Due to Heat Gain Through Windows

Window glass load factors (GLF) modified for single- and multifamily residential cooling load calculations and including solar heat load plus air-to-air conduction are given in Tables 7-34 and 7-35. The shading coefficients and U-factors used to compile these tables are listed in Table 7-36.

In application, the area of each window is multiplied by the appropriate GLF. The effects of permanent outside shading devices should be considered separately in determing cooling load. Shaded glass is considered the same as north-facing glass.

The shade line factor (SLF) is the ratio of the distance a shadow falls beneath the edge of an overhang to the width of the overhang (Table 7-37). Therefore, assuming the overhang is at the top of the window, the shade line equals the SLF times the overhang width. The shaded and sunlit glass areas may then be computed separately. The tabulated values are the average of the shade line values for 5 h of maximum solar intensity on each wall orientation shown. Northeast- and northwest-facing windows are not effectively protected by roof overhangs and, in most cases, should not be considered as shaded.

7.7.5 Infiltration

Natural air leakage in residential structures occurs less in summer than in winter, largely because wind velocities are lower in most localities. The data in Table 7-38 applies to both single- and multifamily housing, although most of the raw data is for single-family structures.

Construction may be defined as follows:

Tight. Good multifamily construction with close-fitting doors, windows, and framing is considered tight. New houses with full vapor retardant, no fireplace, well-fitted windows, weather-stripped doors, one story, and less than 1500 ft^2 floor area fall into this category.

Medium. Medium structures include new, two-story frame houses or one-story houses more than 10 years old with average maintenance, a floor area greater than 1500 ft^2, average fit windows and doors, and a fireplace with damper and glass closure. Below-average multifamily construction falls in this category.

Loose. Loose structures are poorly fitted single-family or multifamily residences, with poorly fitted windows and doors. Examples include houses more than 20 years old, of average maintenance, a fireplace without damper or glass closure, and more than an average number of vented appliances. Average mobile homes are in this category.

7.7.6 Ventilation

Residential air-conditioning systems may introduce outdoor air, although it is not a code requirement in most localities. Positive ventilation should be considered, however, if the anticipated infiltration is less than about 0.5 air changes per hour. When positive means of introducing outdoor air are used, controls, either manual or automatic, should be provided and an energy recovery device should be considered.

7.7.7 Occupancy

Even though occupant density is low, occupancy loads should be estimated. Sensible heat gain per sedentary occupant is assumed to be 230 Btu/h. The number of occupants

Table 7-34 Window Glass Load Factors (GLFs) for Single-Family Residences[a]

Design	Regular Single Glass						Regular Double Glass						Heat-Absorbing Double Glass						Clear Triple Glass		
Temperature, °F	85	90	95	100	105	110	85	90	95	100	105	110	85	90	95	100	105	110	85	90	95
No inside shading																					
North	34	36	41	47	48	50	30	30	34	37	38	41	20	20	23	25	26	28	27	27	30
NE and NW	63	65	70	75	77	83	55	56	59	62	63	66	36	37	39	42	44	44	50	50	53
East and West	88	90	95	100	102	107	77	78	81	84	85	88	51	51	54	56	59	59	70	70	73
SE and SW[b]	79	81	86	91	92	98	69	70	73	76	77	80	45	46	49	51	54	54	62	63	65
South[b]	53	55	60	65	67	72	46	47	50	53	54	57	31	31	34	36	39	39	42	42	45
Horizontal skylight	156	156	161	166	167	171	137	138	140	143	144	147	90	91	93	95	96	98	124	125	127
Draperies, venetian blinds, translucent roller shades, fully drawn																					
North	18	19	23	27	29	33	16	16	19	22	23	26	13	14	16	18	19	21	15	16	18
NE and NW	32	33	38	42	43	47	29	30	32	35	36	39	24	24	27	29	29	32	28	28	30
East and West	45	46	50	54	55	59	40	41	44	46	47	50	33	33	36	38	38	41	39	39	41
SE and SW[b]	40	41	46	49	51	55	36	37	39	42	43	46	29	30	32	34	35	37	35	36	38
South[b]	27	28	33	37	38	42	24	25	28	31	31	34	20	21	23	25	26	28	23	24	26
Horizontal skylight	78	79	83	86	87	90	71	71	74	76	77	79	58	59	61	63	63	65	69	69	71
Opaque roller shades, fully drawn																					
North	14	15	20	23	25	29	13	14	17	19	20	23	12	12	15	17	17	20	13	13	15
NE and NW	25	26	31	34	36	40	23	24	27	30	30	33	21	22	24	26	27	29	23	23	26
East and West	34	36	40	44	45	49	32	33	36	38	39	42	29	30	32	34	35	37	32	32	35
SE and SW[b]	31	32	36	40	42	46	29	30	33	35	36	39	26	27	29	31	32	34	29	29	31
South[b]	21	22	27	30	32	36	20	20	23	26	27	30	18	19	21	23	24	26	19	20	22
Horizontal skylight	60	61	64	68	69	72	57	57	60	62	63	65	52	52	55	57	57	59	56	57	59

[a]Glass load factors (GLFs) for single-family detached houses, duplexes, or multifamily residences, with both east and west exposed walls or only north and south exposed walls, Btu/h·ft^2.

[b]Correct by +30% for latitude of 48° and by −30% for latitude of 32°. Use linear interpolation for latitude from 40 to 48 and from 40 to 32°.

To obtain GLF for other combinations of glass and/or inside shading: $GLF_a = (SC_a/SC_t)(GLF_t - U_tD_t) + U_aD_t$, where the subscripts a and t refer to the alternate and table values, respectively. SC_t and U_t are given in Table 5. $D_t = (t_a - 75)$, where $t_a = t_o - (DR/2)$; t_o is the outdoor design temperature and DR is the daily range.

Table 7-35 Window Glass Load Factors (GLFs) for Multifamily Residences[a]

Design Temperature, °F	Regular Single Glass 85	90	95	100	105	110	Regular Double Glass 85	90	95	100	105	110	Heat-Absorbing Double Glass 85	90	95	100	105	110	Clear Triple Glass 85	90	95
No inside shading																					
North	40	44	49	54	58	64	34	36	39	42	44	47	23	24	26	29	30	33	30	32	34
NE	88	89	91	95	97	100	78	79	80	83	84	85	52	52	53	55	55	57	71	71	73
East	136	137	139	142	144	147	120	121	122	125	126	127	79	79	81	83	83	84	109	109	111
SE	129	130	134	139	141	144	109	113	116	119	120	122	72	75	77	79	79	81	99	103	105
South[b]	88	91	96	101	105	110	76	78	81	84	86	89	50	52	54	56	58	60	68	70	72
SW	154	159	164	169	174	179	134	137	140	143	145	148	89	91	93	95	97	99	121	123	125
West	174	178	183	188	192	197	151	154	157	160	162	165	100	102	104	106	108	110	137	139	141
NW	123	127	132	137	141	147	107	109	112	115	117	121	71	72	75	77	79	81	96	98	100
Horizontal	249	252	256	261	264	268	218	220	223	226	228	230	144	146	148	150	152	154	198	200	202
Draperies, venetian blinds, translucent roller shades, fully drawn																					
North	21	25	29	33	36	40	18	21	23	26	28	31	15	17	19	21	23	25	17	19	21
NE	43	44	46	50	51	52	39	40	41	44	45	46	33	33	34	36	36	37	39	39	40
East	67	68	70	74	75	76	61	62	63	65	66	67	50	50	51	54	54	55	60	60	61
SE	64	65	69	73	74	77	58	59	61	63	64	66	48	48	50	52	52	54	57	57	59
South[b]	45	48	52	56	59	63	40	42	44	47	49	52	33	34	36	39	40	42	38	40	42
SW	79	83	87	91	94	98	70	72	75	78	80	83	57	59	62	64	66	68	68	69	71
West	89	92	96	100	103	107	79	81	84	86	88	91	65	66	69	71	72	75	76	78	80
NW	63	66	70	74	77	81	56	58	61	63	66	68	46	48	50	52	54	56	54	55	57
Horizontal	126	128	132	135	137	141	113	115	117	120	121	124	93	94	96	98	100	102	110	111	113
Opaque roller shades, fully drawn																					
North	17	21	25	29	32	36	15	17	20	23	25	28	14	15	18	20	22	24	15	16	18
NE	33	34	35	39	40	42	31	32	33	36	35	37	29	28	30	32	32	34	32	31	33
East	51	52	53	57	61	65	48	49	50	53	52	55	45	45	46	48	48	49	49	49	50
SE	49	50	53	57	58	61	46	47	49	52	52	55	42	43	45	47	47	49	46	46	48
South[b]	35	38	42	46	49	53	32	34	37	40	42	42	29	31	33	35	37	39	32	33	35
SW	61	65	69	73	77	81	57	59	62	65	67	70	52	54	56	58	60	62	56	58	60
West	68	71	75	80	83	87	64	66	68	71	73	76	58	60	62	64	66	68	63	64	66
NW	49	52	56	60	63	67	45	47	50	53	55	58	41	43	45	47	49	51	45	46	48
Horizontal	97	99	102	106	108	111	91	93	95	97	99	102	83	85	87	89	90	92	90	92	93

[a]Glass load factors (GLFs) for multifamily low-rise or single-family detached residences if zoned with separate temperature control for each zone, Btu/h·ft².
[b]Correct by +30% for latitude of 48° and by −30% for latitude of 32°. Use linear interpolation for latitude from 40 to 48 and from 40 to 32°.

To obtain GLF for other combinations of glass and/or inside shading: $GLF_a = (SC_a/SC_t)(GLF_t - U_tD_t) + U_aD_t$, where the subscripts a and t refer to the alternate and table values, respectively. SC_t and U_t are given in Table 5. $D_t = (t_a - 75)$, where $t_a = t_o - (DR/2)$; t_o is the outdoor design temperature and DR is the daily range.

Table 7-36 Shading Coefficients and U-Factors for Residential Windows

Glass Type	None SC	None U	Drapery, Venetian Blind, or Translucent Roller Shade SC	Drapery, Venetian Blind, or Translucent Roller Shade U	Opaque Roller Shade SC	Opaque Roller Shade U
Single	1.00	1.04	0.50	0.81	0.38	0.81
Double	0.88	0.61	0.45	0.55	0.36	0.55
Heat-absorbing	0.58	0.45	0.37	0.44	0.33	0.44
Triple	0.80	0.44	0.44	0.40	0.36	0.40

Note: U is in Btu/h·ft²·°F.

Table 7-37 Shade Line Factors (SLFs)

Direction Window Faces	Latitude, Degrees N 24	32	36	40	44	48	52
East	0.8	0.8	0.8	0.8	0.8	0.8	0.8
SE	1.8	1.6	1.4	1.3	1.1	1.0	0.9
South	9.2	5.0	3.4	2.6	2.1	1.8	1.5
SW	1.8	1.6	1.4	1.3	1.1	1.0	0.9
West	0.8	0.8	0.8	0.8	0.8	0.8	0.8

Note: Shadow length below the overhang equals the shade line factor times the overhang width. Values are averages for the 5 h of greatest solar intensity on August 1.

Table 7-38 Summer Air Exchange Rates (ACH) as Function of Airtightness

Class	Outdoor Design Temperature, °F 85	90	95	100	105	110
Tight	0.33	0.34	0.35	0.36	0.37	0.38
Medium	0.46	0.48	0.50	0.52	0.54	0.56
Loose	0.68	0.70	0.72	0.74	0.76	0.78

Note: Values are for 7.5 mph wind and indoor temperature of 75°F.

should not be overestimated to avoid gross oversizing. Census studies recommend that the toal number of occupants be based on two persons for the first bedroom, plus one person for each additional bedroom. The occupancy load should then be distributed equally among the living areas, because the maximum load occurs when most of the residents occupy these areas.

7.7.8 Household Appliances

Appliance loads are concentrated mainly in the kitchen and laundry areas. Based on contemporary living conditions in single-family houses, a sensible load of 1600 Btu/h (470 W) should be divided between the kitchen, laundry, and the adjoining room or rooms. For multifamily units, the sensible heat gain values should be about 1200 Btu/h (350 W).

These values assume that the cooking range and clothes dryer are vented. Further allowances should be considered when unusual lighting intensities, computers, or other heat-generating equipment are present.

7.7.9 Air Distribution System

Whenever the air distribution system is outside the conditioned space—in attics, crawl spaces, or other unconditioned spaces—heat gains to the ducts or pipes must be included in equipment load and should be considered in equipment selection.

7.7.10 Latent Heat Sources

The latent cooling load has three main sources: outdoor air; occupants; and miscellaneous sources, such as cooking, laundry and bathing. The miscellaneous category is largely covered by outdoor air, because most units have exhaust fans or clothes dryers that vent most of the moisture from these sources. This vent air is accounted for in the infiltration calculation. A latent factor (LF) of 1.3 or a SHF of 0.77 matches the performance of typical residential vapor compression cooling systems. Homes in almost all regions of North America have cooling loads with SHF greater than 0.77 and latent factors less than 1.3. Figure 7-6 may be used to estimate the total cooling load by reading LF as a function of the design humidity ratio and airtightness. Then,

$$q_{total} = \text{LF}q_{sens}$$

If the humidity ratio is less than 0.01, set LF = 1.0.

7.7.11 Selection of Cooling Equipment

Residential cooling equipment that is flexible in application helps match the space SHF to the system. Usually equipment is designed for a standard operating condition of 800°F dry-bulb and 670°F wet-bulb (26.70°C dry-bulb, 19.40°C

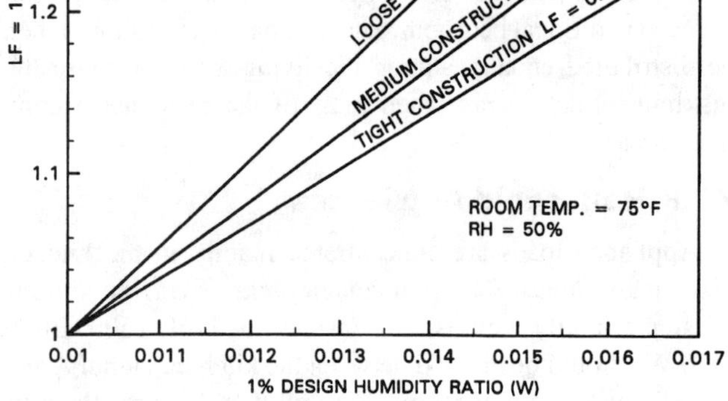

Fig. 7-6 Effect of Infiltration on Latent Load Factor

wet-bulb) air entering the coil, and airflow of 400 ft^3/min per ton of refrigeration (54 L/s per kW), and SHF of 0.77 (LF = 1.3). Most regions require a coil SHF greater than 0.77; therefore a mismatch often occurs. A coil designed with a given latent capacity generally transfers more sensible heat in the absence of moistrue in the air, but not in the same amount as the design latent heat transfer capacity.

Cooling equipment should be sized on the basis of the estimated sensible cooling load, taking into account the effect of outdoor ambient conditions on the unit performance. The unit should not be oversized more than 25% of the estimated sensible load or the next available size. After selecting a unit, its latent capacity should be checked to ensure that it is equal to or greater than the calculated latent cooling load. The latent capacity of the unit generally is ample, except in very wet climates with excessive infiltration. If the latent cooling capacity is less than the calculated latent load, the unit size must be increased.

The residential cooling load method is summarized in Table 7-39.

Example 7.1 Determine the cooling load caused by glass on the south and west walls of a building at 1200, 1400, and 1600 h in July. The building is located at 40°N latitude with outside design conditions of 90°F dry-bulb temperature and a 20°F daily range. The inside design dry-bulb temperature is 78°F. Assume that the room configuration includes two exposed walls, vinyl floor covering, and gypsum partitions, and that the building is a single story. The south glass is insulating type (0.25-in. air space) with an area of 100 ft^2 and no interior shading. The west glass is 7/32-in. single grey-tinted glass with an area of 100 ft^2 and has light-colored venetian blinds.

Solution:

By the room configuration described and with inside shading for half the exposed glass area, Table 7-26B indicates the SCL factors should be selected for a Zone C condition.

Data required for the calculation are as follows:

Variable	Time	South Glass	West Glass
U, Btu/h·ft^2·F		0.61	0.81
Area A, ft^2		100	100
SC		0.82	0.53
SCL	1200	79	37
	1400	70	98
	1600	40	153

The conduction heat gain component of cooling load by Equation (7-31) is

Time	CLTD (Table 7-21)	CLTD Corrected	South Glass, Btu/h	West Glass, Btu/h
1200	9	4	244	324
1400	13	8	488	648
1600	14	9	549	729

The correction factor applied to the above CLTDs was −5°F, computed from the notes of Table 7-25. Heat gain values are rounded.

Table 7-39 Summary of Procedures for Residential Cooling Load Calculations

Load Source	Equation	Tables and Notes
Glass and window areas	$q = (\text{GLF})A$	Glass load factors may be found in Tables 7-34 and 7-35 according to window orientation, type of glass, type of interior shading, and outdoor design temperature. The GLF includes effects of both transmission and solar radiation. Glass shaded by overhangs is treated as north glass. Table 7-37 gives shade line factors.
Doors	$q = U_dA(\text{CLTD})$	Door CLTD values are in Tables 7-32 and 7-33 according to orientation, outdoor design temperature, and design daily temperature range.
Above-grade exterior walls	$q = U_wA(\text{CLTD})$	Wall CLTD values are in Tables 7-32 and 7-33 based on the outdoor design temperature, daily range, and orientation.
Partitions to unconditioned space	$q = U_pA\Delta t$	Where Δt is the temperature difference across the partition.
Ceilings and roofs	$q = U_rA(\text{CLTD})$	Tables 7-32 and 7-33 for CLTD, based on outdoor design temperature and daily range.
Exposed floors	$q = U_fA(\text{CLTD})$	Tables 7-32 and 7-33 for CLTD, based on outdoor design temperature and daily range.
Infiltration	$q = 1.1Q\Delta t$ $Q = \text{ACH} \times (\text{room volume})/60$	Air exchange rates are given in Table 7-38.
Internal loads— People, appliances, lights	Plan 230 Btu/h per person.	Divide occupants evenly among rooms not used as bedrooms. If number of occupants is not known, assume two people for first bedroom and one person for each additional bedroom. The appliance and light load of 1600 Btu/h is divided between the kitchen and adjoining room and the laundry and adjoining room. Use 1200 Btu/h for multifamily units.
Total loads	Total cooling load = LF × (Sum of individual sensible cooling load components)	Load factors are from Figure 7-6 according to outdoor design humidity ratio and airtightness classification.

q = sensible cooling load, Btu/h
Δt = design temperature difference between outside and inside air, °F
A = area of applicable surface, ft^2
U = U-factors for appropriate construction, Btu/h·ft^2·°F
Q = volumetric airflow rate, cfm
ACH = air changes per hour, 1/h
GLF = glass load factor, Btu/h·ft^2
CLTD = cooling load temperature difference, °F
LF = latent load multiplier

The solar heat gaincomponent of cooling load by Equation (7-32) is

Time	South Glass SC	South Glass SCL	SHG, Btu/h	West Glass SC	West Glass SCL	SHG, Btu/h
1200	0.82	79	6478	0.53	37	1961
1400	0.82	70	5740	0.53	98	5194
1600	0.82	40	3280	0.53	153	8109

The total cooling load due to heat gain through the glass is, therefore,

Time	South Glass, Btu/h	West Glass, Btu/h
1200	6722	2285
1400	6198	5842
1600	3829	8838

Example 7.2 Estimate the cooling load in a building at 1200, 1400, and 1600 h from four moderately active people occupying an office from 0900 to 1700 h. The office temperature is 78°F, and the cooling system operates continuously. Assume the conditions of the space define it as zone Type D.

Solution:

The sensible cooling load is calculated by Equation (7-33), and the latent cooling load is calculated by Equation (7-34). The period of occupancy is 8 h.

Time	No. of People	Hours in Space	Hours after Entry	Heat, each (Table 7-14) Sens., Btu	Heat, each (Table 7-14) Latent, Btu	CLF_p (Table 7-28) Zone D	Cooling Load Sens., Btu/h	Cooling Load Latent, Btu/h
1200	4	8	3	250	200	0.74	740	800
1400	4	8	5	250	200	0.80	800	800
1600	4	8	7	250	200	0.85	850	800

Example 7.3 Estimate the cooling load in a building at 1200, 1400, and 1600 h from recessed fluorescent lights, turned on at 0800 h and turned off at 1800 h. Lamp wattage is 800 W. The use factor is 1.0 and the special allowance factor is 1.25. The interior room is in a one-story building, has tile flooring over a 3-in concrete floor, and has a suspended ceiling. The cooling system runs 24 h per day, including weekends.

Solution:

From Table 7-26, the room is categorized as Type C for lighting load purposes. Therefore,

Time	Hours Lights on	Hours after on	Lamp Watts	Heat Gain, Btu/h [Eq. (7-20)]	CLF_{el} (Table 7-29) Zone C	Cooling Load, Btu/h [Eq. (7-35)]
1200	10	4	800	3410	0.87	2698
1400	10	6	800	3410	0.90	3069
1600	10	8	800	3410	0.92	3137

Example 7.4 Determine the cooling load in a building at 1200, 1400, and 1600 h caused by an electric coffee brewer with one brewer and one warmer. The brewer operates continuously from 0900 to 1500 h and does not have an exhaust hood. The midfloor room is in a multistory building, has carpet over a 3-in. concrete floor,

and has a suspended ceiling. The cooling system runs 24 h/day, including weekends.

Solution:

From Table 7-17, q_s and q_l for an unhooded, two-burner coffee brewer are 3750 and 1910 Btu/h, respectively (thus 1875 and 955 each burner), and for a coffee heater (per warming burner) are 230 and 110 Btu/h, respectively. The brewer is on for 6 h, and 1200 h is 3 h after the brewer is turned on. From Table 7-26B, the room is categorized as zone Type D for equipment load purposes. Therefore,

Time	q, Btu/h	Hours in Use	Hours after Start	CLF_a (Table 7-24)	Cooling Load Sensible, Btu/h	Latent, Btu/h	Total, Btu/h
1200	2105	6	3	0.73	1537	1065	2602
1400	2105	6	5	0.80	1684	1065	2749
1600	2105	6	7	0.26	547	0	547

Example 7.5 For the commercial building described below, determine the sensible, latent, and total cooling load at 4:00 P.M. on July 21 for an inside design temperature of 75 °F and 55% rh.

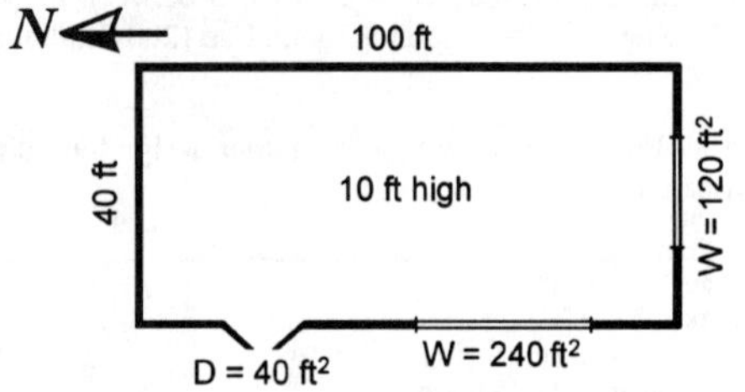

People: 35 at moderate office activity
Lights: 5600 W, fluorescent
Infiltration: 0.5 air changes per hour
Wall: 1 in. dark stucco on 4 in. regular concrete, U = 0.340 Btu/h·ft²·°F
Roof: 8 in. lightweight concrete, U = 0.11 Btu/h·ft²·°F
Door: 2 in. solid wood, U = 0.42 Btu/h·ft²·°F, A = 40 ft²
Windows:

South: 1/8 in. regular sheet glass with white roller shades drawn half-way, A = 120 ft²

West: Insulating glass, regular sheet out/regular sheet in, no internal shading, 1/4 in. air space, 1/4 in. thick glass; A = 240 ft²

Solution:

Outside Design: 94/75, 21 °F range, 83.5 °F average, correction = −1.5 °F
Inside Design: 75 °F, correction = +3.0 °F
Latitude: ≈ 40 °N

Walls/Roof/Door	U	A	CLTD	$Q_{cooling}$
East wall (type 5)	0.34	1000	38.5	13,090
North wall (5)	0.34	400	20.5	2,788
West wall (5)	0.34	720	29.5	7,222
South wall (5)	0.34	280	36.5	3,475
Door (west) (2)	0.42	40	47.5	798
Roof (type 3)	0.11	4000	75.5	33,220
			Subtotal =	60,593

Lighting: 5600 × 3.41 × 1.2 × 0.92 = 21,082 Btu/h
Zone C

Glass Exposure

	South (Shade)	South	West
A	60	60	240
U	1.17	1.17	0.69
CLTD	15.5	15.5	15.5
Q_c	1088	1088	2418
Zone	B	B	B
SCL	32	46	153
SC	0.35	1.0	0.81
Q_s	672	2760	29,743
Q_{cool}	1760	3848	32,161
		Subtotal = ΣQ_{cool} =	37,770 Btu/h

On at 8 A.M. for 10 h
People: Enter at 8 A.M. for 8 h
Sensible: 35 × 250 × 0.91 = 7962 Btu/h
Latent: 35 × 200 = 7000 Btu/h
Infiltration:
Sensible: 1/2(4000 × 10)(1/60)(1.10)(94 × 75) = 6970 Btu/h
Latent: 1/2(4000 × 10)(1/60)(4840)(0.0144 − 0.0102) = 6780 Btu/h

Sensible Total = 134,380 Btu/h
Latent Total = 13,780 Btu/h
Grand Total = 148,160 Btu/h

Example 7.6 A one-story small commercial building is located in the eastern United States near 40 °N latitude. The adjoining buildings on the north and west are not conditioned, and the air temperature within them is approximately equal to the outdoor air temperature at any time of day.

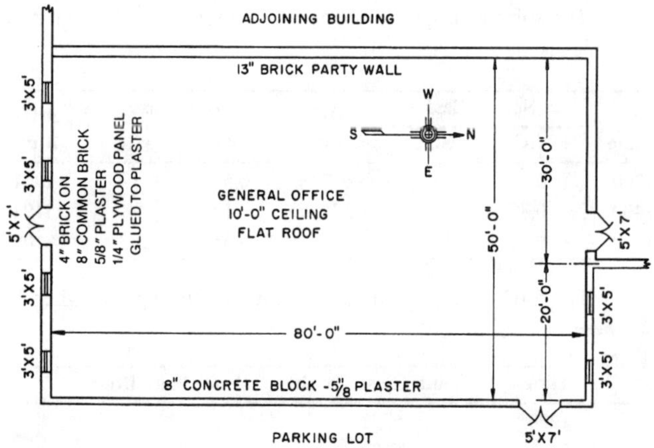

Building Data:

South wall construction. 4-in. light-colored face brick, 8-in. common brick, 0.625-in. plaster, 0.25-in. plywood panel glued on plaster (Summer U = 0.24 Btu/h·ft²·°F, or R = 4.14).

East wall and outside north wall construction. 8-in. light-colored heavy concrete block, 5/8-in. plaster on walls (Summer U = 0.48 Btu/h·ft²·°F, or R = 2.083).

West wall and adjoining north party wall construction. 13-in. solid brick (color N/A), no plaster: with U for a 12-in. brick interior wall = 0.26, R for that wall = 1/0.26 = 3.846; subtracting 2 still air film coefficients with R_{fc} = 0.68 each leaves R_b = 2.486. Thus, for this wall,

$$R_w = 0.68 + (2.486 \times 13/12) + 0.68 = 4.053$$

and

$$U_w = 1/4.053 = 0.25 \text{ Btu/h·ft}^2\text{·°F}$$

Roof construction. 4-1/2-in. (nominal) flat roof of 2-in gypsum slab on metal roof deck, 2-in. rigid roof insulation, surfaced with two layers of mopped 15-lb felt vapor-seal built-up roofing having dark-colored gravel surface, and with no false ceiling below underside of roof deck (Summer U = 0.09 Btu/h·ft^2·°F, or R = 11.11).

Floor construction. 4-in concrete on ground.

Fenestration. 3 ft by 5 ft nonoperable windows of regular plate glass with light colored venetian blinds (Summer U = 0.81 Btu/h·ft^2·°F).

Door construction. Light-colored 1.75-in. steel door with solid urethane core and thermal break (Summer U = 0.19 Btu/h·ft^2·°F, or R = 5.26 for exterior doors, and U = 0.18 Btu/h·ft^2·°F, or R = 5.56 for interior doors).

Front doors: Two 30 in. by 7 ft

Side doors: Two 30 in. by 7 ft

Rear doors: Two 30 in. by 7 ft (interior)

Note: U-factors for all exterior surfaces assume a summer wind velocity of 7.5 mph. Those for party walls and other interior surfaces assume still air.

Summer outdoor design conditions. Dry bulb 94°F, daily range 20°F, wet bulb 77°F: W_o = 0.0161 lb vapor/lb dry air, h_o = 40.3 Btu/lb dry air.

Winter outdoor design conditions. Dry bulb 10°F.

Summer indoor design conditions. Dry bulb 75°F, wet bulb 62.5°F; W_i = 0.0092 lb vapor/lb dry air; h_i = 28.07 Btu/lb dry air.

Winter indoor design conditions. Dry bulb 75°F

Occupancy. 85 office workers from 0800 to 1700 h.

Lights. 17,500 W, fluorescent, operating from 0800 to 1700 hours daily; along with 4000 W, tungsten, operated continuously. Lighting fixtures are nonventilated type.

Power equipment and appliances. For this example, none are assumed.

Ventilation. From ASHRAE *Standard* 62, a ventilation rate of 15 cfm/person is selected as representative of a drugstore or hardware store. With 85 people, the total ventilation air quantity is thus 1275 cfm. Floor area of 4000 ft^2 with 10 ft ceiling height gives a space volume of 40,000 ft^3, corresponding to (1275 cfm × 60)/40,000 = 1.91 air changes per hour.

In practice, ventilation air is normally conditioned to some extent by the air-conditioning equipment before being admitted to the conditioned space. However, the variety of such arrangements and the varying impact felt by the load calculation process are not covered by this chapter and should be evaluated as part of a system analysis procedure. For this example, assume the ventilation air is introduced directly into the space and included as part of the space cooling load, but only during scheduled operating hours of the cooling equipment.

Infiltration. Window infiltration is considered zero, since the windows are sealed. Infiltration through wall surfaces is also neglected as insignificant, particularly with plastered interior surfaces. Calculation of door infiltration however, requires some judgement. The pressure of 1.91 air changes per hour in the form of positive ventilation could be sufficient to prevent door infiltration, depending on the degree of simultaneous door openings and the wind direction and velocity.

For this example, assume that outside and inside doors are frequently opened simultaneously, and that door infiltration should be included as part of the cooling load, estimating 100 ft^3 per person per door passage. Further estimating outside door use at 10 persons/h, and inside doors (to unconditioned space, previously estimated to be at ambient temperature and humidity) at 30 persons/h, generates the following infiltration rate:

$$Q_{inf} = 40 \times 100/60 = 67 \text{ cfm}$$

Thermal responsiveness of building and contents. For this example, mass of building construction and contents is medium.

Conditioning equipment location. Conditioning equipment is in an adjoining structure to the north, thus having no direct impact on heat gain.

Find (for stated design conditions):

1. Sensible cooling load
2. Latent cooling load
3. Total cooling load

Solution:

By inspection, the cooling load from the roof can be expected to be the variable making the greatest contribution to the overall cooling load for the building. Therefore, the time of cooling load occurrence will probably be close to the time of maximum CLTD for the roof. The maximum cooling load for the building as a whole can be expected to occur in one of the summer months-June, July, or August. From Table 7-21, a "mass inside" roof with no ceiling and an R-value of 11.1 is classified as Type 4. From Table 7-20C, the CLTD for Roof No. 4 at 40°N latitude has a maximum tabulated value of 78°F at 1800 h, but is only somewhat less (73°F) at 1600 h.

South-facing glass can also be expected to wield considerable influence on the cooling load for this particular building. From Table 7-26B, a one-story building with three exposed walls, uncarpeted floor, masonry partitions, and fully inside-shaded windows is classified B for solar loads, and C for loads from people, equipment, or lights. Cross-checking the variation of SCLs for glass facing south, in Table 7-24C, the maximum cooling load from these windows would be only slightly more at noon or 1300 h than at 1400 for 40°N latitude. Sometime in the early afternoon seems obvious, but it is necessary to make a quick estimate to establish the peak load hour:

Roof [Equation (7-30)]:

U = 0.098 Btu/h·ft^2·°F, Area = 4000 ft^2

Time	1300	1400	1500	1600	1700
CLTD	42	54	65	73	77
C_1	3	3	3	3	3
C_2	−1	−1	−1	−1	−1
Corr. CLTD	44	56	67	75	79
Btu/h	15,840	20,160	24,120	27,000	28,440

C_1 = (78 − 75) = indoor design temperature correction

C_2 = (94 + 74)/2 − 85 = daily average temperature correction

South Glass, Solar [Equation (7-32)]:

SC = 0.55, Area = 60 ft^2

Time	1300	1400	1500	1600	1700
SCL at 40°,	87	79	63	46	37
Btu/h	2871	2607	2079	1518	1221
Roof and south glass, Btu/h	18,711	22,767	26,199	28,518	29,661

Evaluation of the foregoing indicates that 1600 h will be the probable hour of maximum cooling load for this building, considering that although the roof and south glass loads increase another 1143 Btu/h for 1700 h, the trend has slowed and most other load components of significance can be expected to be leveling off or moving toward lower values at that time. In some cases there would be no such clear cut indication, and it would be necessary to estimate the total load for a number of hours, including the potential impact of other significant variables that could exert a determining influence at a different time (such as a major load from appliances known to occur only in the morning, etc.), before selecting the peak load hour for the overall calculation.

Cooling Load from Heat Gain Through Roof, Exposed Walls, and Doors. Such loads are estimated using Equation (7-30), where the CLTDs are taken from Table 7-20C after determining appropriate type numbers from Table 7-21, with insulation placement, U-factors, and general construction are as close to the actual components as possible. Corrections to CLTD values are made according to footnote instructions to Table 7-20C, similar to the preliminary evaluation. (Note that there are no corrections to CLTD values for building mass variations because they have little effect on the overall results. Tabulated data for roofs, walls and doors assume room transfer functions for "light to medium" construction.)

Cooling Load from Heat Gain Through Fenestration Areas. The load component from conduction heat gain is calculated using Equation (7-31), where the CLTD value is taken from Table 7-25, corrected by −1°F because of a 1°F lower average daily temperature than that for which the table was generated, and +3°F to recognize the 75°F design space temperature. The U-factor of the glass is taken as 0.81 Btu/h·ft^2·°F for single sheet plate glass, during summer.

The load component from solar heat gain is calculated using Equation (7-32) as indicated above. A shading coefficient (SC) of 0.55 is used for clear glass with light-colored venetian blinds. SCL values are taken from Table 7-27C, after first identifying the appropriate zone type as B for solar load from Table 7-26B. Results are in the next column.

Cooling Load from Heat Gain Through Party Walls. For the north and west party walls, cooling load is calculated using appropriate U-factors and the temperature differential existing at 1600 h, 18.4°F. The results are tabulated in the next column.

Solar Cooling Load for Windows

Section	Net ft^2	SC	CLF (Table 7-27)	Cooling Load, Btu/h
South Windows	60	0.55	46	1518
North windows	30	0.55	32	528

Cooling Load from Internal Heat Sources. For the cooling load component from lights, Equation (7-16) is used to obtain the heat gain. Assuming a use factor of 1.0, and a special allowance factor of 1.0 for tungsten lamps and 1.20 for fluorescent lamps, these gains are

$$q_{tung} = 4000 \times 1.0 \times 1.0 \times 3.41 = 13{,}640 \text{ Btu/h}$$

$$q_{fluor} = 17{,}500 \times 1.0 \times 1.2 \times 3.41 = 71{,}610 \text{ Btu/h}$$

Since the tungsten lamps are operated continuously, the previously stored radiant heat from this source currently being

Conduction Cooling Load Summary for Enclosing Surfaces

Section	Net ft^2	U-Factor, $\frac{\text{Btu}}{\text{h}\cdot\text{ft}^2\cdot°\text{F}}$	Δt, °F	CLTD, °F	Ref. for CLTD	1600 h Cooling Load, Btu/h
Roof	4000	0.09		73	Table 7-22C Roof 4	27,000
South wall	405	0.24		19	Table 7-22C Wall 16	1,847
East wall	765	0.48		38	Table 7-22C Wall 10	13,954
North exposed wall	170	0.48		16	Table 7-22C Wall 10	1,306
W. and N. party wall	1065	0.25	18.4			4,899
Doors in S. wall	35	0.19		50	Table 7-22C Wall 2	333
Doors in N. wall	35	0.18	18.4			116
Doors in E. wall	60	0.19		36	Table 7-22C Wall 2	239
South windows	60	0.81		16	Table 7-25	778
North windows	30	0.81		16	Table 7-25	389

reconvected to the space equals the rate of new radiant heat from this source being stored; thus the cooling load from this source equals heat gain. The fluorescent lamps, however, are operated only 9 h per day, 0800 through hour 1700, and thus contribute radiant heat to cooling load in a cyclic and somewhat delayed manner. From Table 7-26B, the zone type is identified as C for lighting loads, and from Table 7-29 a CLF value of 0.92 is obtained for lights that are operated for 10 hours, for a calculation hour 9 h after the lights have been turned on. The cooling load from fluorescent lights for this estimate is

$$q_{cl\ fluor} = 71{,}610 \times 0.92 = 65{,}881 \text{ Btu/h}$$

For people, Table 7-14 is used to select heat gains for seated occupants doing light office work, as 250 Btu/h per person, sensible, and 200 Btu/h, latent, for 75°F space temperature. The CLF for the sensible component is taken from Table 7-28 as 0.92, for a condition of 10 total hours in a type C space and a load calculation taken 9 h after entry. Cooling load from people is thus estimated as

$$q_{ps} = 85 \text{ people} \times 250 \times 0.92 = 19{,}550 \text{ Btu/h}$$

$$q_{pl} = 85 \text{ people} \times 200 = 17{,}000 \text{ Btu/h}$$

Cooling Load from Power Equipment and Appliances. For this example, none are assumed.

Cooling Load from Infiltration and Ventilation Air. Ventilation for this building is established at 15 cfm/person, or 1275 cfm, and infiltration (through doors) at 67 cfm. For this example, ventilation is assumed to enter directly into the space (as opposed to first passing through the cooling equipment), so it is included as part of the space pcooling load.

The sensible and latent portions of each load component are calculated using Equations (7-38) and (7-39), given in Table 7-19, where at 1600 h, t_o = 93.4°F, t_i = 75°F, W_o = 0.0161, and W_i = 0.0093.

For ventilation,

cfm	Factor	$t_o - t_i$	$W_o - W_i$	Load, Btu/h
1275	1.1	18.4		25,806 sensible
1275	4840		0.0068	41,963 latent

For infiltration,

cfm	Factor	$t_o - t_i$	$W_o - W_i$	Load, Btu/h
67	1.1	18.4		1356 sensible
67	4840		0.0068	2205 latent

Summary of Calculations

	Dry Bulb, °F	Wet Bulb, °F	Humidity Ratio
Outdoor conditions	93.4	76.8	0.0161
Indoor conditions	75	62.5	0.0093
Difference	19		0.0068

Sensible cooling load at 1600 h	**Btu/h**
Roof and Exposed Walls	
Roof	27,000
South wall	1,847
East wall	13,954
North wall	1,306
South wall doors	333
East wall doors	239
Fenestration Areas	
South windows	2,296
North Windows	917
Party Walls	
West and North walls	4,899
North wall doors	116
Internal Sources	
People	19,550
Tungsten lights	13,640
Fluorescent lights	65,881
Outside Air	
Infiltration	1,356
Ventilation	25,806
Total	179,140
Latent Cooling Load at 1600 h	**Btu/h**
People	17,000
Infiltration	2,205
Ventilation	41,963
Total	63,208
Grand Total Load	**242,348**

Example 7.7 The west brick wall of a residence in Louisville, Kentucky, has a net area (excluding windows and doors) of 506 ft^2 and a U-factor of 0.067 Btu/h·ft^2·°F for both winter and summer. Determine

(a) The heating load for the wall, Btu/h
(b) The cooling load for the wall, Btu/h

Solution:

$$\text{(a) } q_s = UA\Delta t = 0.067(506)(72-10) = 2101 \text{ Btu/h}$$

$$\text{(b) } q_s = UA(\text{CLTD}) = 0.067(506)(21) = 712 \text{ Btu/h}$$

Example 7.8 A large window, essentially all glass, 10 ft by 5 ft, is located in the west wall of a residnece in Kansas City, Missouri. To reduce energy requirements, the window is heat absorbing double glass, 1/2-in. air space, coating emissivity of 0.15, and has inside draperies which are closed at peak conditions. Determine

(a) The heating load for the window, Btu/h
(b) The cooling load for the window, Btu/h

Solution:

$$\text{(a) } q_s = UA\Delta t = 0.039(50)(72-6) = 1287 \text{ Btu/h}$$

$$\text{(b) } q_s = (\text{GLF})A = 36.9 \text{ Btu/h}\cdot\text{ft}^2 \times 50 \text{ ft}^2 = 1820 \text{ Btu/h}$$

7.8 Problems

7.1 The exterior windows are of double insulating glass with 0.25-in. (6-mm) airspace and have metal sashes. Determine the design U-factor for cooling for the window.

7.2 Find the heat gain through a 10 ft by 5 ft heat-absorbing 0.25-in. plate glass in a window fully exposed to the sun, with light-colored inside venetian blind set at an angle where no direct sunlight can enter the space at 4:00 P.M. solar time, July 21st, for the west-facing wall of a building located at 40°N latitude. Assume outside and inside dry-bulb temperature to be 92°F and 75°F. [Ans: 6574 Btu/h (1.92 kW)]

7.3 Calculate the solar radiation entering through the glass having a SC = 1.0 as shown to the left. [Ans 59.2 Btu/h]

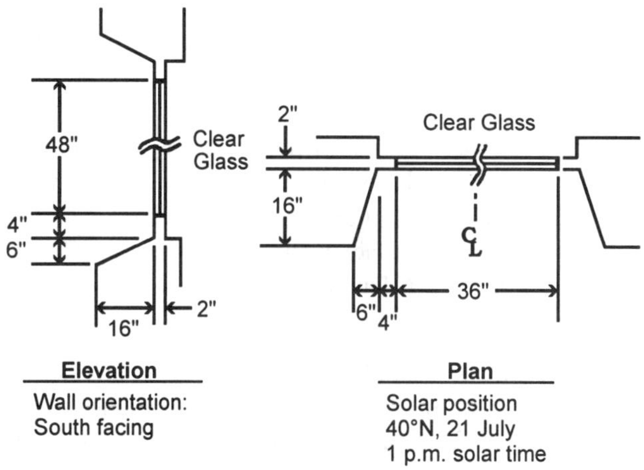

7.4 Calculate the instantaneous rate of heat flow (to the inside) through a west facing vertical window of common window glass that measures 6 ft high by 30 ft wide. The location is Dallas, Texas, latitude 32°47′N, at 4:00 p.m. solar time on August 1. The solar altitude angle is 34°38′; the solar azimuth angle is 89°37′; and the incident angle for the west facing vertical surface is 34°38′. Outdoor air and space temperatures are 101°F (38.3°C) and 80°F (26.7°C), respectively, and the window is set back 6 in. (152 mm).

7.5 Find the total heat gain through a 3-mm (0.125-in.) double-strength (DS) glass window as shown at solar noon for the south facing wall of a building located at 40°N latitude on August 21. Outdoor air temperature is 92°F (33.3°C). Room temperature is 75°F (23.9°C). [Ans: 1335 Btu/h (0.39 kW)]

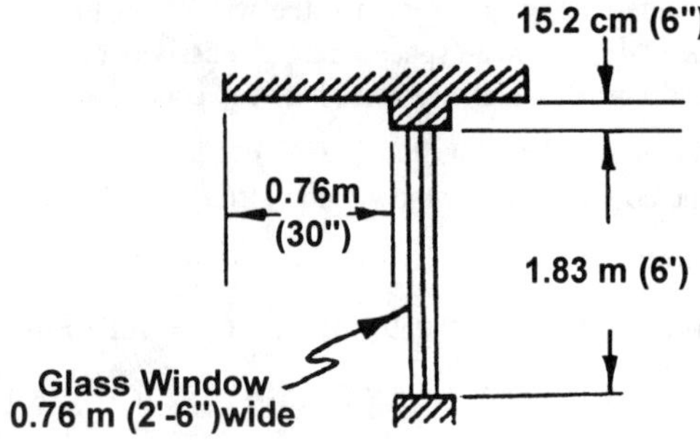

7.6 A store in Lafayette, Indiana, is on the northeast corner of an intersection with one street running due north. The bottom of the show windows are 2 ft 6 in. above the sidewalk; the show windows are 7 ft high. An aluminum awning with a 3-in. rise per horizontal foot is to be hung with the bottom strut at the window header. Both south and west awnings are to have the same dimensions.

(a) What minimum distance should the strut extend from the building to keep the shade line on the windows at 3 p.m. sun time?
(b) Which face of the building governs the awning dimensions?
(c) Where will the shade line be at 3 p.m. on the other face of the building?
(d) What is the elevation of the top of the awnings above the sidewalk?

7.7 Solve the following problems.

(a) Determine the solar angle of incidence for a vertical wall facing 15° west of south when the sun has an azimuth of 79.2° west of south and an altitude of 75.7°. [Ans: 83.8°]
(b) Find the solar incident angle (for direct solar radiation) for a vertical surface facing southeast at 8:30 a.m. CST on October 22 at 32°N latitude and 95°W longitude. [Ans: 28.4°]

7.8 The southwest wall of a school building in Fort Collins, Colorado, is 76 m by 2.7 m overall. It has 30 windows, each 1.8 m by 1.2 m. The wall is 200-mm heavyweight concrete with 25.4-mm (R = 0.53 $K \cdot m^2/W$) insulation. The windows are insulating glass (clear-out, clear-in, 6.4-mm glass, 13-mm airspace) with translucent roller shades. Determine the design cooling load for the complete wall, assuming this wall determines the design time for the building.

7.9 What environmental factors affect the solar intensity reaching the earth's surface?

7.10 Solve the following problems.

(a) List at least three principles of luminaire design and installation which determine how heat is dissipated to the building interior.
(b) What procedure would be followed to determine wattage values of luminaires when calculating the heat gain of a structure?
(c) What factors determine the input wattage to a fluorescent type luminaire?

7.11 Determine the heat being dissipated by 50 pendant mounted fluorescent luminaires with four 40 W lamps in each luminaire.

7.12 How much sensible, latent, and total heat is contributed by 50 customers shopping in a drugstore?

7.13 A 1-hp motor driving a pump is located in a space to be air conditioned. Determine heat dissipated to the space from the motor and pump. [Ans: 3390 Btu/h]

7.14 Calculate the heat gain to a room from a 21-lb deep fat fryer (8-kW input rating) if (a) hooded and (b) nonhooded.

7.15 A 20 ft by 20 ft by 8 ft room has a sensible heat gain of 3700 Btu/h and latent gain due to infiltration of 1270 Btu/h. The room also has a lighting load of 5 W/ft^2, six 0.5-hp electric motors, and 12 adult males performing light bench work. Find the total cooling load.

7.16 Calculate the maximum heat gain through the floor for a room directly over a boiler room. The air temperature at the underside of the floor is 100°F, and the room air temperature desired close to the floor is 70°F. The floor is 4-in. concrete with vinyl tile finish.
[Ans: 18.87 $Btu/h \cdot ft^2$ (18.9 W/m^2)]

7.17 An air-conditioning unit serves an office having the following areas:

Description	Size	Occupancy
General office	25 ft by 50 ft	75 ft^2 per person
Director's room	25 ft by 25 ft	16 people
Conference room	10 ft by 25 ft	Plush furnishings
5 private offices	10 ft by 10 ft	Smoking permitted

What quantity of outdoor air must be brought into the air-conditioning unit for ventilation?

7.18 Suppose the fan of the air-conditioning unit in Problem 7.17 supplies 3200 cfm to the ductwork.

(a) How many air changes per hour are being used? (Assume a ceiling height of 9 ft.)
(b) What is the percentage of outdoor air?
(c) Suppose the minimum recommended quantities of total air and outside air are used, what will be the percentage of outdoor air?
[Ans: 8.1, 32%, 43%]

7.19 A small parts assembly area in a factory has a working force of 25 men and occupies a space 27.4 m by 9.1 m with a 3-m ceiling. Smoking is not allowed. Determine

(a) Sensible heat load from the occupants
(b) Latent heat load from the occupants

(c) Moisture added from the occupants
(d) The minimum volume of outdoor air for ventilation
(e) Suitable summer design inside dry-bulb temperature

7.20 The west wall of a school building in Abilene, Texas, is 250 ft by 9 ft overall and includes 10 windows, each 6 ft by 4 ft. The 12-in. wall concrete (k = 12 Btu·in/h·ft^2·°F) is followed by 8-in. cinder aggregate concrete block. The windows are single pane, 0.25-in. regular plate glass, with light venetian blinds. For design conditions in late July at 6 P.M., determine the cooling load for the complete wall.

7.21 The southwest wall of a school building in Jefferson City, Missouri, is 250 ft by 9 ft overall and includes 30 windows, each 6 ft by 4 ft. The wall is 12-in. concrete (k = 12 Btu·in/h·ft^2·°F) followed by 8-in. cinder aggregate concrete block. The windows are single pane, 0.25-in. regular plate glass, with light venetian blinds.

Determine the design cooling load for the complete wall assuming this wall determines the design time for the building. [Ans: 62,400 Btu/h]

7.22 A bowling alley located in Cincinnati, Ohio, has total space cooling loads of 140 kW sensible and 49 kW latent. Estimate accurately:

(a) Number of people present
(b) Outdoor air requirements, L/s
(c) Space design temperature for comfort, °C

7.23 The office portion of a multistory commercial building, located at 40°N latitude, is shown in the sketch below. Neglecting any outside air load, for August 21 determine the cooling load at 4 P.M. if it is located at 40°N.

Inside design: 75°F, W = 0.0102

Outside design: 95°F, 22°F daily range, W = 0.0168

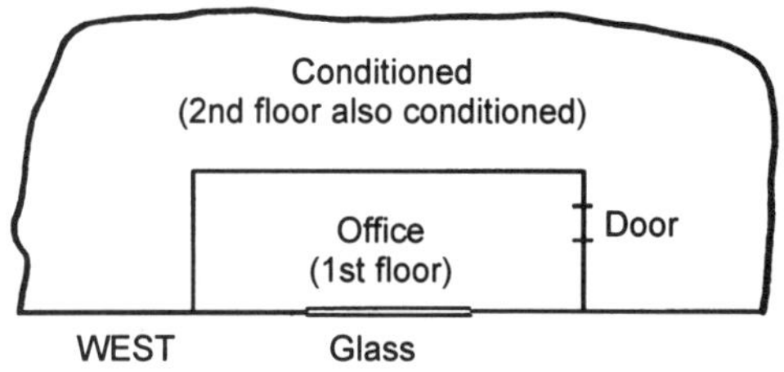

For Office Portion:

West wall: Net area = 230 ft^2, U = 0.333
4-in. red face brick, 4-in. low weight concrete block, and 0.75-in. plaster
Window: Area = 90 ft^2, U = 0.59
double pane, regular sheet, insulating glass
People: 4, moderately active office work
Lights: 800 W fluorescent, on continuously

7.24 Calculate the cooling load for the office shown in the diagram below.

Location: Indianapolis, Indiana
Occupancy: 180 people
Factory temperature: Assume 5°F below outside ambient
Equipment: 35 business machines, each 110 V at 4.0 A
East and south walls: 8-in. concrete block, U = 0.3 Btu/h·ft^2·°F
North and west walls: Concrete block, U = 0.5 Btu/h·ft^2·°F
Floor transmission: Neglect
Ceiling: U = 0.5 Btu/h·ft^2·°F
Lights: 6 W/ft^2
Windows: Insulating glass, 0.25-in. gray plate outside, regular plate inside

Direct-expansion packaged air-conditioning unit will be used.

Locate equipment in factory west of office.

Calculate the heat gain for this office.

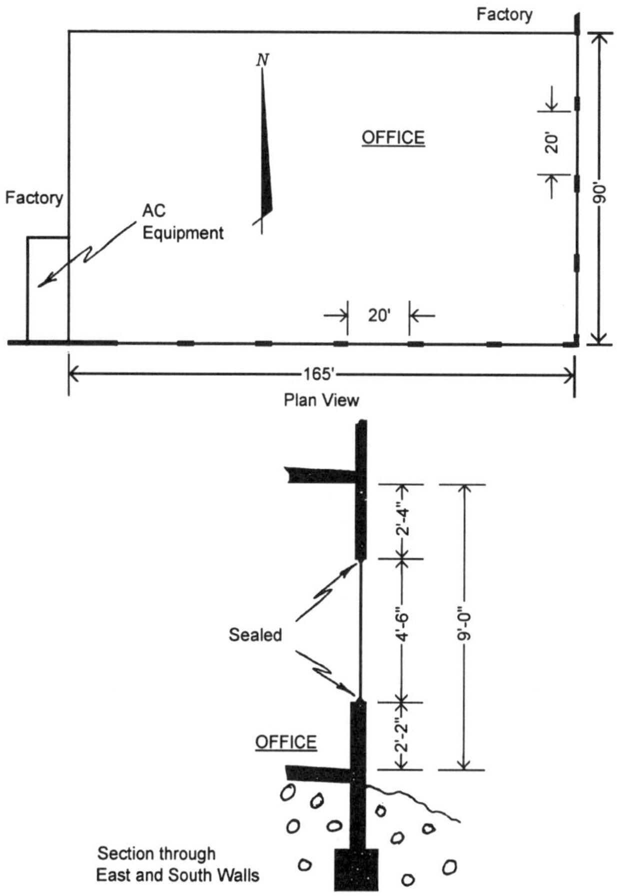

Diagram for Problem 7.24

7.25 An architect provides the following data for a new cafeteria in Tampa, Florida:

Size: 80 ft wide by 100 ft deep; 30-ft deep area in rear is for kitchen and storage. Wall separating this area from main dining area is made of concrete block.

Walls: 4-in. concrete block with an outside facing of 1/2-in. cement mortar; 3/8-in. air space filled with fiberglass insulation, backed by 1-mil aluminum foil; 3/8-in. gypsum wallboard; 2 coats light green paint; front wall has a canopy projection of 4 ft (located 12 ft above ground level).

Windows: On front wall: 80% of front wall is composed of 1/4-in. gray plate glass, backed by fiberglass draperies of a medium-colored yarn of a close weave; windows are well sealed. On side walls: No windows. On back walls: No windows.

Roof: Flat, stone aggregation on tar base outside; 3/8-in. roofing board; 1/2-in. roof insulation; metal decking; 2-ft air space between steel beams (for lighting fixtures and ductwork); suspended acoustical ceiling.

Floor: 8-in. concrete slab with 1/4-in. floor tile: 1-in. edge insulation.

Doors: Two sets of double swinging doors on opposite sides of front wall; single bank; 7 ft wide (total of 2 doors); 7 ft high; peak traffic expected is 300 people per hour. There are two service entrance doors on rear, normally closed, 3 ft by 7 ft, with slight cracks all around.

Occupancy: Maximum expected occupancy is 300 between the hours of 5:00 P.M. and 7:00 P.M.

Internal equipment: Usual cooking, washing, and food service-storage trays for a cafeteria; a refrigerated food locker is in the rear.

Lighting: Indirect neon lights on ceiling.

Location: Front faces southwest; located in Tampa, Florida.

Calculate the sensible cooling load (using your best judgment as to the number of people present at off-hours) for 10 A.M.; 2 P.M.; and 6 P.M. Consider the cafeteria as a single zone and plan to air condition the kitchen also.

7.26 Size the cooling system by determining the design cooling loads for the following pharmacy building to be built in Tulsa, Oklahoma.

Overall size: 60 ft by 130 ft by 12 ft high [long sides on east and west]

Walls: 8 inch concrete block with normal weight sand and gravel aggregazte with 1-in. stucco on the outside and 3/4-in. cement plaster with sand aggregate on the inside

Doors: Double 2-1/4-in. solid core doors (6 ft by 7 ft) on north and south

Window: One 6 ft by 90 ft double glass with thermal break frames, 1/8-in. thick glass with 3/8-in. air gap, with translucent roller shades, on west side

Roof/Ceiling: 4-in. lightweight concrete with 3/8-in. built-up roofing on the exterior and 3/4-in. cement plaster with sand aggregate on the inside

Carefully state all assumptions.

7.27 Solve the following:

(a) A 115 ft by 10 ft high wall in Minneapolis, Minnesota consists of face brick, a 3/4-in. air gap, 8-in. cinder aggregate concrete blocks, 1-in. organic bonded glass fiber insulation, and 4-in. clay tile interior. Determine the design heat loss through the wall in winter in Btu/h.

(b) If the wall of *Part* (a) is converted to 60% single glazed glass, what is the winter design heat loss through the total wall in Btu/h?

7.28 The living room in a home in Lafayette, Indiana, has a 4-ft 2-in. by 15-ft window facing south and a 4-ft 2-in. by 11-ft window facing west. What width soffit should be put on the house to keep the shade line on the windows at 3 p.m. sun time? (Assume soffit will always be 8 in. above the window.) [Ans: 6.4 ft]

7.29 A naturally vented attic of a residence has a roof with U = 0.23 Btu/h·ft^2·°F [1.30 W/(m^2·K)]. Beneath the roof, the attic has an area of 1960 ft^2 (182 m^2) and U = 0.048 (0.27). The ratio of roof to ceiling area is 1.2. For a dark roof, medium daily temperature range, and outdoor design temperature of 90°F (32.2°C), determine the heat gain to the residence through the ceiling.

7.30 For a design outside temperature of 100°F, compute the heat gain through a 10-ft by 15-ft ceiling if the naturally vented attic has a dark roof. The ceiling is constructed of 3/8-in. gypsum board on 2 by 6 ceiling joists with 2-in. fibrous insulation in the space between joists.

7.31 Estimate the total (sensible and latent) cooling load due to infiltration for a single-story house, which is 21 m long by 8.5 m deep and is in Houston, Texas.

7.32 For the house in *Problem* 7.31 and an occupancy of six people, determine the occupancy load. [Ans: 2700 Btu/h]

7.33 The south wall of a residence located in Manhattan, Kansas, has one 3-ft by 5-ft double glass, 0.25-in. airspace, window with wood sash. The remainder of the 30 ft by 8 ft high wall is constructed as follows: face brick; 3/4-in. air space, 25/32-in. insulating board siding; full wall glass fiber insulation in the stud space; and 1/4-in. wood paneling. Neglecting the effect of the studs, determine the cooling load through the wall and window if there are closed draperies at the window.

7.34 A 6 ft high by 4 ft wide west window of single pane glass is immediately below the 4-ft overhang of the roof. There are draperies inside the window. Design outdoor temperature is 105°F. Determine the sensible heat gain through the window.

7.35 As a move to conserve energy, a three-bedroom underground house is being designed to be built in Jefferson City, Missouri. It will have 10-in. thick concrete walls, floor, and roof/ceiling. The roof is covered with 6 in. of dirt having a thermal conductivity of 9.0 Btu·in/h·ft^2·°F. The overall interior dimensions of the house are 70 ft by 28 ft by 8 ft. One air change per hour is provided. Continuous lighting of a minimum of 1120 watts is required. Determine the size air conditioner required. [Ans: 58,000 Btu/h (17 kW)]

7.36 An underground house in Rolla, Missouri, has 250 mm thick concrete walls, floor, and roof/ceiling. The walls and roof/ceiling are insulated (R = 0.7 m^2·K/W). The roof is covered with 150 mm of dirt having a thermal conductivity of

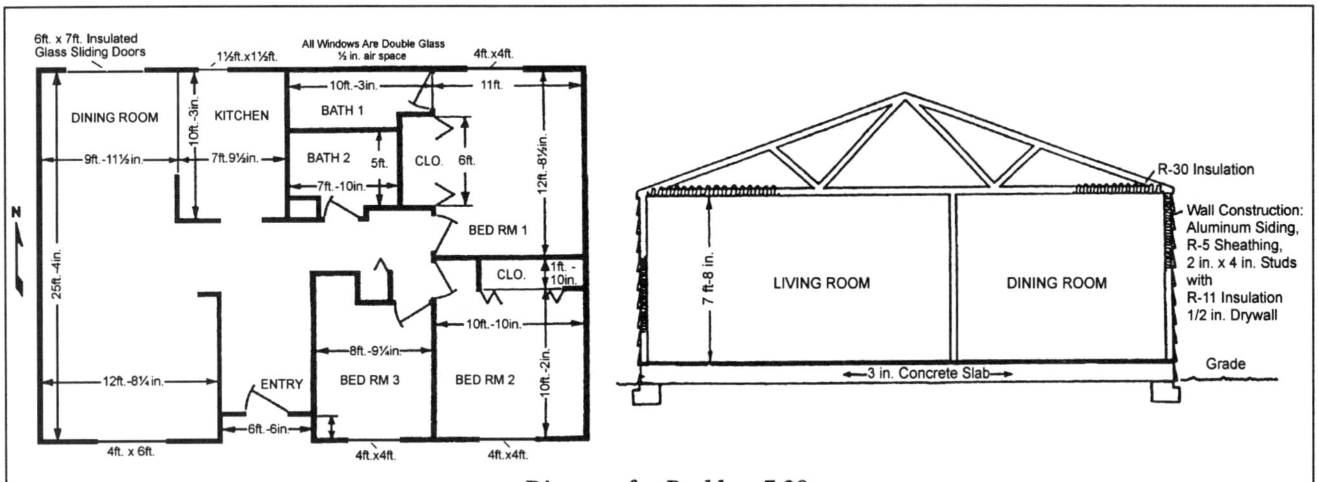

Diagram for Problem 7.38

15.6 W/(m·K). The three-bedroom house overall interior dimensions are 21.3 m by 8.5 m by 2.4 m. One-half air change per hour is provided. Continuous lighting of a minimum of 1120 watts is used. Determine the size air conditioner required.

7.37 As an attempt to minimize energy requirements, a new residence has been constructed in Dallas, Texas (100°F dry bulb; 20°F daily range; $W = 0.0156$). Size the air-conditioning unit (Btu/h) for this residence with the following features:

- No windows
- Inside design conditions: 75°F, 60% rh ($W = 0.0112$)
- One 3-ft by 7-ft, 2 in. thick wood door with storm door on south side, $U = 0.26$ Btu/h ft2 °F, one 3-ft by 7-ft, 2-in. thick wood door with storm door on east side, $U = 0.26$ Btu/h·ft^2·°F
- Overall size: 70 ft by 28 ft by 8 ft high
- Walls are frame construction with 2 by 6 studs and full insulation for $U = 0.043$
- Attic has natural ventilation, 12-in. fiberglass insulation, and overall U of roof and ceiling of 0.021 based on ceiling area, light-colored roof
- Infiltration is so small that outside air must be brought in at a rate of 9 cfm/person
- Estimated occupancy at design condition is 15 people
- Fluorescent tights rated at 320 W will be on all the time
- Floor is concrete slab on ground.

7.38 Determine design heating and cooling loads for the residence shown in the figure and located in Manhattan, Kansas.

7.39 Determine the cooling load and specify the central air-conditioning system for the following residence in St. Louis, Missouri, having

(a) black asphalt shingles, full-wall fiberglass insulation, 4in. fiberglass ceiling insulation, no drapes, no attic fan

(b) same as (a) except silver-white asphalt shingles

(c) same as (a) except lined drapes at all windows

(d) same as (a) except large attic vent fan

Basic Plan

Wall construction: Face brick, 25/32-in. insulating board sheathing, 2 by 4 studs on 16-in. centers, 3/8-in. gypsum board interior

Ceiling: 2 by 6 ceiling joists, 16-in. on-center, no flooring above, 3/8-in. gypsum board ceiling

Roof: Asphalt shingles on solid wood sheathing, 2 by 6 rafters, no insulation between rafters, no ceiling applied to rafters, 1:4 pitch, 1-ft overhang on eaves, no overhang on gables

Full basement: Heated, 10-in. concrete watts, all below grade, 4-in. concrete floor over 4-in. gravel

Fireplace: One in living room of first floor

Garage: Attached but unheated

Windows:

W1: 3 ft by 5 ft single-glazed, double-hung wood sash, weather stripped with storm window

W2: 10 ft by 5.5 ft picture window, double-glazed, 1/2 in. airspace

W3: 5 ft by 3 ft wood-sash casement, double-glazed, 1/2-in. airspace

W4: 3 ft by 3 ft wood-sash casement, double-glazed, 1/2-in. airspace

Doors:

D1: 3 ft by 6 ft 8 in., 1 3/4 in. solid with glass storm door

D2: Sliding glass door, two 3 ft by 6 ft 8 in sections, double-glazed, 1/2-in. airspace, aluminum frame

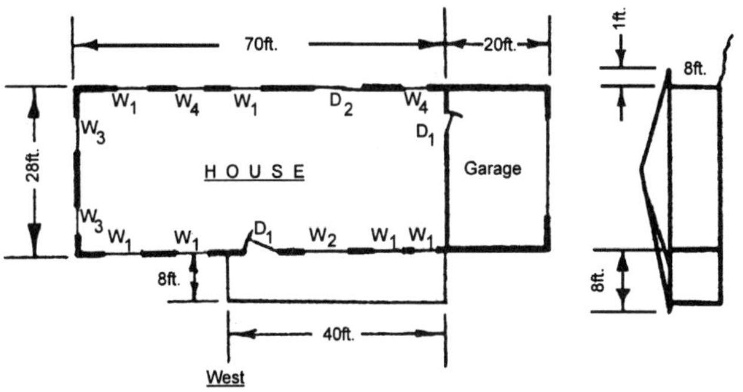

7.40 Write a computer program for calculating the cooling load for a residence.

7.41 Apply the computer program to the residence of *Problem* 7.39.

7.9 References

ASHRAE. 1975. Procedure for determining heating and cooling loads for computerized energy calculations, algorithms for building heat transfer subroutines.

ASHRAE. 1979. *Cooling and Heating Load Calculation Manual.*

Buchberg, H. 1958. Cooling load from thermal network solutions *ASHAE Transactions* 64:111.

Harris, S.M. and F.C. McQuiston. 1988. A study to categorize walls and roofs on the basis of thermal response. *ASHRAE Transactions* 94(2):688-715.

Kimura and Stephenson. 1968. Theoretical study of cooling loads caused by lights. *ASHRAE Transactions* 74(2):189-97.

McQuiston, F.C. and J.D. Spitler. 1992. *Cooling and Heating Load Calculation Manual*, 2nd ed. ASHRAE.

Mitalas, G.P. 1972. Transfer function method of calculating cooling loads, heat extraction rate, and space temperature. *ASHRAE Journal* 14(12):52.

Mitalas, G.P. 1973. Calculating cooling load caused by lights. *ASHRAE Journal* 15(6):7.

Mitalas, G.P. and K. Kimura, 1971. A calorimeter to determine cooling load caused lights. *ASHRAE Transactions* 77(2):65.

Mitalas, G.P. and D.G. Stephenson. 1967. Room thermal response factors. *ASHRAE Transactions* 73(2):III.2.1.

Rudoy, W. and F. Duran. 1975. Development of an improved cooling load calculation method. *ASHRAE Transactions* 81(2):1969

Sowell, E.F. 1988a. Classification of 200,640 parametric zones for cooling load calculations. *ASHRAE Transactions* 94(2):754-77.

Sowell, E.F. 1988b. Cross-check and modification of the DOE program for calculation of zone weighting factors. *ASHRAE Transactions* 94(2):737-53.

Sowell, E.F. 1988c. Load calculations for 200,640 zones. *ASHRAE Transactions* 94(2):716-36.

SI Tables and Figures

Table 7-1 SI Sol-Air Temperatures (t_e) for July 21, 40°N Latitude

$$t_e = t_o + \alpha I_t/h_o - \varepsilon\Delta R/h_o$$

Time	Air Temp. t_o, °C	Light Colored Surface, $\alpha/h_o = 0.026$ N	NE	E	SE	S	SW	W	NW	HOR
1	25.4	25.4	25.4	25.4	25.4	25.4	25.4	25.4	25.4	21.5
2	24.9	24.9	24.9	24.9	24.9	24.9	24.9	24.9	24.9	21.0
3	24.4	24.4	24.4	24.4	24.4	24.4	24.4	24.4	24.4	20.5
4	24.1	24.1	24.1	24.1	24.1	24.1	24.1	24.1	24.1	20.2
5	24.0	24.1	24.2	24.2	24.1	24.0	24.0	24.0	24.0	20.1
6	24.2	27.2	34.5	35.5	29.8	25.1	25.1	25.1	25.1	22.9
7	24.8	27.3	38.1	41.5	35.2	26.5	26.4	26.4	26.4	28.1
8	25.8	28.1	38.0	43.5	38.9	28.2	28.0	28.0	28.0	33.8
9	27.2	29.9	35.9	43.1	41.2	31.5	29.8	29.8	29.8	39.2
10	28.8	31.7	33.4	40.8	41.8	35.4	31.8	31.7	31.7	43.9
11	30.7	33.7	34.0	37.4	41.1	39.0	34.2	33.7	33.7	47.7
12	32.5	35.6	35.6	35.9	39.1	41.4	39.1	35.9	35.6	50.1
13	33.8	36.8	36.8	36.8	37.3	42.1	44.2	40.5	37.1	50.8
14	34.7	37.6	37.6	37.6	37.7	41.3	47.7	46.7	39.3	49.8
15	35.0	37.7	37.6	37.6	37.6	39.3	49.0	50.9	43.7	47.0
16	34.7	37.0	36.9	36.9	36.9	37.1	47.8	52.4	46.9	42.7
17	33.9	36.4	35.5	35.5	35.5	35.6	44.3	50.6	47.2	37.2
18	32.7	35.7	33.6	33.6	33.6	33.6	38.3	44.0	43.0	31.4
19	31.3	31.4	31.3	31.3	31.3	31.3	31.4	31.5	31.5	27.4
20	29.8	29.8	29.8	29.8	29.8	29.8	29.8	29.8	29.8	25.9
21	28.6	28.6	28.6	28.6	28.6	28.6	28.6	28.6	28.6	24.7
22	27.5	27.5	27.5	27.5	27.5	27.5	27.5	27.5	27.5	23.6
23	26.6	26.6	26.6	26.6	26.6	26.6	26.6	26.6	26.6	22.7
24	26.0	26.0	26.0	26.0	26.0	26.0	26.0	26.0	26.0	22.1
Avg.	**29.0**	**30.0**	**32.0**	**33.0**	**32.0**	**31.0**	**32.0**	**33.0**	**32.0**	**32.0**

Time	Air Temp. t_o, °C	Dark Colored Surface, $\alpha/h_o = 0.052$ N	NE	E	SE	S	SW	W	NW	HOR
1	25.4	25.4	25.4	25.4	25.4	25.4	25.4	25.4	25.4	21.5
2	24.9	24.9	24.9	24.9	24.9	24.9	24.9	24.9	24.9	21.0
3	24.4	24.4	24.4	24.4	24.4	24.4	24.4	24.4	24.4	20.5
4	24.1	24.1	24.1	24.1	24.1	24.1	24.1	24.1	24.1	20.2
5	24.0	24.2	24.4	24.3	24.1	24.0	24.0	24.0	24.0	20.2
6	24.2	30.2	44.7	46.7	35.4	26.0	26.0	26.0	26.0	25.5
7	24.8	29.7	51.5	58.2	45.6	28.2	28.0	28.0	28.0	35.4
8	25.8	30.5	50.1	61.2	52.1	30.7	30.1	30.1	30.1	45.8
9	27.2	32.5	44.5	58.9	55.1	35.8	32.3	32.3	32.3	55.1
10	28.8	34.5	38.0	52.8	54.9	42.0	34.7	34.5	34.5	62.8
11	30.7	36.8	37.2	44.0	51.5	47.4	37.7	36.8	36.8	68.5
12	32.5	38.7	38.7	39.3	45.7	50.4	45.7	39.3	38.7	71.6
13	33.8	39.9	39.9	39.9	40.8	50.5	54.6	47.1	40.3	71.6
14	34.7	40.4	40.4	40.4	40.6	47.9	60.8	58.7	43.9	68.7
15	35.0	40.3	40.1	40.1	40.1	43.6	62.9	66.7	52.3	62.9
16	34.7	39.4	39.0	39.0	39.0	39.6	61.0	70.1	59.0	54.7
17	33.9	38.8	37.1	37.1	37.1	37.3	54.7	67.3	60.6	44.5
18	32.7	38.7	34.5	34.5	34.5	34.5	43.9	55.2	53.2	34.0
19	31.3	31.5	31.3	31.3	31.3	31.3	31.4	31.6	31.7	27.5
20	29.8	29.8	29.8	29.8	29.8	29.8	29.8	29.8	29.8	25.9
21	28.6	28.6	28.6	28.6	28.6	28.6	28.6	28.6	28.6	24.7
22	27.5	27.5	27.5	27.5	27.5	27.5	27.5	27.5	27.5	23.6
23	26.6	26.6	26.6	26.6	26.6	26.6	26.6	26.6	26.6	22.7
24	26.0	26.0	26.0	26.0	26.0	26.0	26.0	26.0	26.0	22.1
Avg.	**29.0**	**32.0**	**35.0**	**37.0**	**37.0**	**34.0**	**37.0**	**37.0**	**35.0**	**40.0**

Note: Sol-air temperatures are calculated based on $\varepsilon\Delta R/h_o = -3.9$°C for horizontal surfaces and 0°C for vertical surfaces.

Table 7-3 SI Solar Intensity and Solar Heat Gain Factors for 40°N Latitude

Date	Solar Time	Direct Normal W/m²	Solar Heat Gain Factors, W/m² N	NNE	NE	ENE	E	ESE	SE	SSE	S	SSW	SW	WSW	W	WNW	NW	NNW	Hor.	Solar Time
Jan	8	446	17	17	55	223	350	417	420	358	236	68	17	17	17	17	17	17	44	4
	9	753	37	37	41	233	485	648	706	658	504	260	42	37	37	37	37	37	172	3
	10	865	51	51	51	97	390	627	761	776	671	460	161	53	51	51	51	51	303	2
	11	912	59	59	59	62	193	493	699	796	769	623	372	89	59	59	59	59	390	1
	12	926	62	62	62	62	66	283	563	739	802	739	563	283	66	62	62	62	419	12
HALF DAY TOTALS			194	194	231	627	1425	2315	2851	2941	2565	1770	860	318	196	194	194	194	1117	
Feb	7	175	6	10	71	127	160	167	150	107	43	6	6	6	6	6	6	6	11	5
	8	691	33	35	158	407	576	651	628	504	296	56	33	33	33	33	33	33	136	4
	9	856	52	52	70	337	587	738	773	688	496	209	55	52	52	52	52	52	52	3
	10	926	65	65	67	155	449	666	777	768	640	408	120	66	65	65	65	65	450	2
	11	957	73	73	73	77	224	503	690	768	729	579	325	86	73	73	73	73	538	1
	12	967	76	76	76	76	80	271	536	702	759	702	536	271	80	76	76	76	567	12
HALF DAY TOTALS			266	271	478	1139	2042	2887	3307	3201	2590	1601	789	360	269	276	266	266	1729	
Mar	7	540	27	92	295	440	514	509	425	271	69	26	26	26	26	26	26	26	83	5
	8	789	50	57	288	533	686	731	664	494	232	54	50	50	50	50	50	50	267	4
	9	888	67	70	147	428	639	749	743	624	404	127	69	67	67	67	67	67	450	3
	10	937	80	80	85	225	482	653	722	682	538	299	91	80	80	80	80	80	587	2
	11	960	88	88	88	94	247	475	623	672	622	473	244	94	88	88	88	88	672	1
	12	967	91	91	91	91	97	238	457	601	650	601	457	238	97	91	91	91	702	12
HALF DAY TOTALS			358	439	953	1775	2624	3261	3425	3052	2189	1269	693	416	359	357	357	357	2409	
Apr	6	282	36	144	228	275	279	241	164	56	16	15	15	15	15	15	15	15	34	6
	7	651	50	223	442	583	633	588	451	235	51	45	45	45	45	45	45	45	193	5
	8	794	69	140	402	600	705	703	593	391	130	69	67	67	67	67	67	67	389	4
	9	864	84	91	253	488	637	690	640	493	260	91	84	84	84	84	84	84	557	3
	10	901	96	99	117	291	480	589	608	538	380	177	101	96	96	96	96	96	684	2
	11	919	104	104	107	122	255	411	506	522	459	323	163	109	104	104	104	104	766	1
	12	925	106	106	106	109	114	196	341	448	486	448	341	196	114	109	106	106	793	12
HALF DAY TOTALS			486	835	1579	2389	3018	3312	3133	2464	1538	935	628	495	467	464	463	463	3018	
May	5	3	1	2	3	3	3	2	1	0	0	0	0	0	0	0	0	0	0	7
	6	452	113	284	403	458	445	363	223	56	33	33	33	33	33	33	33	35	96	6
	7	681	89	320	520	638	658	579	412	172	63	59	59	59	59	59	59	59	275	5
	8	787	86	230	470	629	693	654	518	294	92	80	80	80	80	80	80	80	460	4
	9	843	99	131	330	517	620	631	550	382	168	100	96	96	96	96	96	96	616	3
	10	874	107	114	171	332	467	529	512	418	262	127	111	107	107	107	107	107	736	2
	11	890	114	114	121	152	255	357	409	400	330	221	133	120	114	114	114	114	811	1
	12	895	117	117	117	121	126	171	257	329	355	329	257	171	126	121	117	117	835	12
HALF DAY TOTALS			679	1274	2100	2816	3228	3229	2775	1895	1128	779	629	568	553	550	549	552	3414	
Jun	5	68	32	54	68	70	63	46	20	5	4	4	4	4	4	4	4	7	8	7
	6	488	150	329	450	501	478	380	222	53	39	39	39	39	39	39	39	43	126	6
	7	681	118	355	543	647	654	562	385	145	68	65	65	65	65	65	65	67	306	5
	8	776	94	268	492	632	680	626	480	252	93	85	85	85	85	85	85	85	483	4
	9	829	105	160	358	524	606	601	507	332	142	104	100	100	100	100	100	100	633	3
	10	858	112	121	197	345	457	499	468	366	218	122	115	112	112	112	112	112	749	2
	11	874	119	123	128	166	254	332	367	347	279	188	130	124	119	119	119	119	821	1
	12	879	121	121	121	127	131	163	227	281	301	281	227	163	131	127	121	121	844	12
HALF DAY TOTALS			799	1482	2314	2967	3274	3150	2579	1649	995	743	642	602	592	588	587	594	3550	
Jul	5	7	3	5	7	7	6	5	2	0	0	0	0	0	0	0	0	1	1	7
	6	434	116	281	395	447	433	352	216	55	34	34	34	34	34	34	34	37	100	6
	7	656	95	321	513	625	643	564	400	166	66	62	62	62	62	62	62	62	278	5
	8	762	90	236	468	620	680	639	505	285	94	83	83	83	83	83	83	83	459	4
	9	818	102	138	333	513	610	618	537	371	165	104	99	99	99	99	99	99	611	3
	10	850	110	118	177	333	462	519	501	407	254	128	114	110	110	110	110	110	729	2
	11	866	117	120	125	157	256	352	400	389	321	217	135	123	117	117	117	117	802	1
	12	871	120	120	120	125	130	172	253	320	344	320	253	172	130	125	120	120	826	12
HALF DAY TOTALS			705	1296	2102	2791	3180	3164	2706	1842	1110	783	643	586	572	568	567	570	3395	
Aug	6	255	38	137	214	256	259	223	151	52	18	17	17	17	17	17	17	17	38	6
	7	603	55	223	426	557	602	557	426	222	55	49	49	49	49	49	49	49	196	5
	8	747	75	149	397	584	681	675	569	373	128	74	72	72	72	72	72	72	386	4
	9	819	89	97	259	481	621	669	618	475	251	97	89	89	89	89	89	89	549	3
	10	857	102	105	126	294	472	573	589	519	367	175	107	102	102	102	102	102	674	2
	11	876	109	109	113	130	257	403	492	505	443	313	165	116	109	109	109	109	753	1
	12	882	112	112	112	115	120	197	333	434	469	434	333	197	120	115	112	112	779	12
HALF DAY TOTALS			518	860	1571	2338	2928	2195	3014	2370	1495	932	647	523	496	492	492	492	2982	
Sep	7	471	28	87	265	395	460	456	381	244	66	27	27	27	27	27	27	27	80	5
	8	725	52	61	275	504	646	689	626	467	224	57	52	52	52	52	52	52	258	4
	9	830	71	73	148	413	613	717	712	599	390	129	73	71	71	71	71	71	434	3
	10	881	84	84	89	224	468	630	696	658	521	293	95	84	84	84	84	84	567	2
	11	906	92	92	92	99	245	463	604	652	603	461	242	99	92	92	92	92	650	1
	12	914	95	95	95	95	101	237	446	584	631	584	446	237	101	95	95	95	679	12
HALF DAY TOTALS			374	447	917	1683	2483	3091	3256	2917	2119	1250	699	432	376	373	373	373	2329	
Oct	7	152	6	10	64	113	142	148	132	94	38	7	6	6	6	6	6	6	12	5
	8	643	35	37	155	387	545	615	592	475	279	56	35	35	35	35	35	35	136	4
	9	811	54	54	73	329	567	710	742	661	476	202	57	54	54	54	54	54	305	3
	10	884	67	67	70	157	439	646	752	742	619	395	119	69	67	67	67	67	443	2
	11	917	76	76	76	80	223	491	670	745	707	562	317	89	76	76	76	76	529	1
	12	927	78	78	78	78	84	267	521	681	737	681	521	267	84	78	78	78	557	12
HALF DAY TOTALS			277	282	479	1105	1964	2770	3172	3073	2493	1555	780	369	279	277	277	277	1704	
Nov	8	429	17	17	55	217	339	404	406	346	228	66	18	17	17	17	17	17	44	4
	9	732	38	38	42	230	476	634	690	643	492	254	42	38	38	38	38	38	173	3
	10	846	52	52	52	99	385	616	748	762	658	451	159	54	52	52	52	52	303	2
	11	894	60	60	60	63	192	486	688	783	756	613	367	89	60	60	60	60	388	1
	12	907	63	63	63	63	67	280	555	728	789	728	555	280	67	63	63	63	417	12
HALF DAY TOTALS			197	197	235	623	1402	2271	2795	2882	2515	1737	849	319	199	97	197	197	1115	
Dec	8	279	9	9	25	129	212	259	264	230	157	52	10	9	9	9	9	9	20	4
	9	684	31	31	33	188	427	584	645	611	477	260	40	31	31	31	31	31	124	3
	10	824	45	45	45	78	357	594	732	755	661	462	173	47	45	45	45	45	243	2
	11	881	53	53	53	55	177	477	685	786	764	623	379	90	53	53	53	53	327	1
	12	897	56	56	56	56	60	281	560	736	798	736	560	281	60	56	56	56	356	12
HALF DAY TOTALS			165	165	178	461	1180	2045	2593	2735	2445	1757	869	298	167	165	165	165	891	
			N	NNW	NW	WNW	W	WSW	SW	SSW	S	SSE	SE	ESE	E	ENE	NE	NNE	Hor.	PM

Notes: 1. Clearness number = 1.00; Ground reflectance = 0.20. 2. Figures shown are for 21st day of each month.

Table 7-4 SI Shading Coefficients for Single and Insulating Glass

Glazing System		Center Glazing	Center Glazing	Glazing SHGC at Specified Incidence Angles						Total Window SHGC at Normal Incidence				Total Window VT at Normal Incidence	
				Normal					Hemis.	Aluminum		Other Frames		All Frames	
ID	Glass Thick, mm	VT	SC	0°	40°	50°	60°	70°	(Diffuse)	Operable	Fixed	Operable	Fixed	Operable	Fixed
Uncoated Single Glazing															
1a	3.2 Clear	0.90	1.00	0.86	0.85	0.83	0.78	0.67	0.78	0.75	0.78	0.63	0.75	0.65	0.78
1b	6.4 Clear	0.89	0.94	0.81	0.80	0.77	0.73	0.62	0.73	0.71	0.74	0.60	0.71	0.65	0.78
1c	3.2 Bronze	0.68	0.85	0.73	0.71	0.69	0.64	0.55	0.65	0.64	0.67	0.54	0.64	0.49	0.59
1d	6.4 Bronze	0.55	0.73	0.62	0.60	0.58	0.54	0.46	0.55	0.55	0.57	0.46	0.54	0.40	0.48
1e	3.2 Green	0.82	0.82	0.71	0.68	0.66	0.62	0.53	0.63	0.62	0.65	0.53	0.62	0.60	0.71
1f	6.4 Green	0.74	0.68	0.58	0.56	0.54	0.51	0.44	0.52	0.51	0.53	0.43	0.51	0.54	0.64
1g	3.2 Gray	0.62	0.82	0.70	0.68	0.66	0.61	0.53	0.63	0.61	0.64	0.52	0.61	0.45	0.54
1h	6.4 Gray	0.43	0.65	0.56	0.53	0.51	0.48	0.41	0.49	0.50	0.51	0.42	0.49	0.31	0.37
1i	6.4 Bluegreen	0.75	0.72	0.62	0.59	0.57	0.54	0.46	0.55	0.55	0.57	0.46	0.54	0.54	0.65
Reflective Single Glazing															
1j	6.4 SS on CLR 8%	0.08	0.22	0.19	0.19	0.18	0.17	0.15	0.17	0.18	0.18	0.15	0.17	0.06	0.07
1k	6.4 SS on CLR 14%	0.14	0.29	0.25	0.25	0.24	0.23	0.20	0.23	0.23	0.24	0.19	0.22	0.10	0.12
1l	6.4 SS on CLR 20%	0.20	0.36	0.31	0.30	0.30	0.28	0.24	0.28	0.28	0.29	0.24	0.27	0.15	0.17
1m	6.4 SS on GRN 14%	0.12	0.29	0.25	0.25	0.24	0.23	0.20	0.23	0.23	0.24	0.19	0.22	0.09	0.10
1n	6.4 TI on CLR 20%	0.20	0.34	0.29	0.29	0.28	0.26	0.23	0.27	0.27	0.27	0.22	0.26	0.15	0.17
1o	6.4 TI on CLR 30%	0.30	0.45	0.39	0.38	0.37	0.35	0.30	0.35	0.35	0.36	0.29	0.34	0.22	0.26
Uncoated Double Glazing															
5a	3.2 CLR CLR	0.81	0.87	0.75	0.73	0.70	0.63	0.49	0.65	0.66	0.68	0.55	0.66	0.59	0.71
5b	6.4 CLR CLR	0.78	0.81	0.70	0.68	0.65	0.58	0.45	0.60	0.61	0.64	0.52	0.61	0.57	0.68
5c	3.2 BRZ CLR	0.62	0.72	0.62	0.59	0.57	0.51	0.39	0.53	0.55	0.57	0.46	0.54	0.45	0.54
5d	6.4 BRZ CLR	0.48	0.59	0.50	0.47	0.45	0.40	0.31	0.42	0.45	0.46	0.37	0.44	0.35	0.42
5e	3.2 GRN CLR	0.74	0.70	0.60	0.57	0.55	0.49	0.38	0.51	0.53	0.55	0.45	0.53	0.54	0.64
5f	6.4 GRN CLR	0.66	0.54	0.47	0.44	0.42	0.38	0.30	0.40	0.42	0.43	0.35	0.41	0.48	0.57
5g	3.2 GRY CLR	0.56	0.69	0.59	0.57	0.54	0.48	0.37	0.50	0.52	0.54	0.44	0.52	0.41	0.49
5h	6.4 GRY CLR	0.40	0.51	0.44	0.42	0.40	0.35	0.28	0.38	0.39	0.41	0.33	0.39	0.29	0.35
5i	6.4 BLUGRN CLR	0.67	0.58	0.50	0.47	0.45	0.40	0.32	0.43	0.45	0.46	0.37	0.44	0.49	0.58
5j	6.4 HI-P GRN CLR	0.59	0.46	0.39	0.37	0.35	0.31	0.25	0.33	0.35	0.36	0.29	0.34	0.43	0.51
Reflective Double Glazing															
5k	6.4 SS on CLR 8%,CLR	0.07	0.15	0.13	0.13	0.12	0.12	0.10	0.12	0.13	0.13	0.10	0.12	0.05	0.06
5l	6.4 SS on CLR 14%, CLR	0.13	0.20	0.17	0.17	0.16	0.15	0.12	0.15	0.17	0.16	0.13	0.15	0.09	0.11
5m	6.4 SS on CLR 20%, CLR	0.18	0.26	0.22	0.21	0.21	0.19	0.16	0.19	0.21	0.21	0.17	0.20	0.13	0.16
5n	6.4 SS on GRN 14%, CLR	0.11	0.18	0.16	0.16	0.15	0.14	0.12	0.14	0.16	0.16	0.13	0.14	0.08	0.10
5o	6.4 TI on CLR 20%, CLR	0.18	0.24	0.21	0.20	0.20	0.18	0.15	0.19	0.20	0.20	0.16	0.19	0.13	0.16
5p	6.4 TI on CLR 30%, CLR	0.27	0.33	0.29	0.28	0.27	0.25	0.20	0.25	0.27	0.27	0.22	0.26	0.20	0.24
Low-e Double Glazing, e = 0.2 on Surface 2															
17a	3.2 LE CLR	0.76	0.76	0.65	0.63	0.61	0.55	0.43	0.57	0.57	0.59	0.48	0.57	0.55	0.66
17b	6.4 LE CLR	0.73	0.70	0.60	0.58	0.56	0.51	0.40	0.52	0.53	0.55	0.45	0.53	0.53	0.64
Low-e Double Glazing, e = 0.2 on Surface 3															
17c	3.2 CLR LE	0.76	0.81	0.70	0.68	0.65	0.59	0.46	0.61	0.61	0.64	0.52	0.61	0.55	0.66
17d	6.4 CLR LE	0.73	0.75	0.65	0.63	0.60	0.54	0.42	0.56	0.57	0.59	0.48	0.57	0.53	0.64
17e	3.2 BRZ LE	0.58	0.66	0.57	0.54	0.52	0.46	0.36	0.48	0.50	0.52	0.42	0.50	0.42	0.51
17f	6.4 BRZ LE	0.45	0.52	0.45	0.42	0.40	0.35	0.27	0.37	0.40	0.41	0.34	0.40	0.33	0.39
17g	3.2 GRN LE	0.70	0.63	0.55	0.52	0.50	0.44	0.34	0.46	0.49	0.50	0.41	0.48	0.51	0.61
17h	6.4 GRN LE	0.61	0.48	0.42	0.39	0.37	0.33	0.25	0.35	0.38	0.39	0.32	0.37	0.44	0.53
17i	3.2 GRY LE	0.53	0.63	0.54	0.51	0.49	0.43	0.33	0.46	0.48	0.50	0.40	0.47	0.38	0.46
17j	6.4 GRY LE	0.37	0.46	0.39	0.36	0.34	0.31	0.24	0.33	0.35	0.36	0.29	0.34	0.27	0.32
17k	6.4 BLUGRN LE	0.62	0.52	0.45	0.42	0.40	0.35	0.27	0.37	0.40	0.41	0.34	0.40	0.45	0.54
17l	6.4 HI-P GRN LE	0.55	0.40	0.34	0.31	0.29	0.26	0.20	0.28	0.31	0.32	0.26	0.30	0.40	0.48
Low-e Double Glazing, e = 0.1 on Surface 2															
21a	3.2 LE CLR	0.75	0.62	0.54	0.52	0.49	0.44	0.34	0.46	0.48	0.50	0.40	0.47	0.54	0.65
21b	6.4 LE CLR	0.72	0.59	0.51	0.49	0.47	0.42	0.32	0.44	0.45	0.47	0.38	0.45	0.52	0.63
21l	6.4 HI-P GRN W/LE CLR	0.57	0.36	0.31	0.30	0.29	0.26	0.21	0.27	0.28	0.29	0.24	0.27	0.41	0.50
Low-e Double Glazing, e = 0.1 on Surface 3															
21c	3.2 CLR LE	0.75	0.69	0.60	0.58	0.56	0.51	0.41	0.53	0.53	0.55	0.45	0.53	0.54	0.65
21d	6.4 CLR LE	0.72	0.66	0.56	0.54	0.52	0.47	0.38	0.49	0.50	0.51	0.42	0.49	0.52	0.63
21e	3.2 BRZ LE	0.57	0.56	0.48	0.46	0.43	0.39	0.31	0.41	0.43	0.44	0.36	0.42	0.41	0.50
21f	6.4 BRZ LE	0.45	0.45	0.39	0.37	0.34	0.31	0.24	0.33	0.35	0.36	0.29	0.34	0.33	0.39
21g	3.2 GRN LE	0.68	0.57	0.49	0.47	0.44	0.40	0.31	0.42	0.44	0.45	0.37	0.43	0.49	0.59
21h	6.4 GRN LE	0.61	0.45	0.39	0.36	0.34	0.30	0.24	0.33	0.35	0.36	0.29	0.34	0.44	0.53
21i	3.2 GRY LE	0.52	0.53	0.46	0.44	0.41	0.37	0.29	0.39	0.41	0.42	0.34	0.41	0.38	0.45
21j	6.4 GRY LE	0.37	0.40	0.35	0.33	0.31	0.28	0.22	0.29	0.32	0.33	0.26	0.31	0.27	0.32
21k	6.4 BLUGRN LE	0.62	0.48	0.42	0.39	0.37	0.33	0.26	0.35	0.38	0.39	0.32	0.37	0.45	0.54

Table 7-4 SI Shading Coefficients for Single and Insulating Glass (*Continued*)

Glazing System					Glazing SHGC at Specified Incidence Angles						Total Window SHGC at Normal Incidence				Total Window VT at Normal Incidence	
			Center Glazing	Center Glazing	Normal					Hemis.	Aluminum		Other Frames		All Frames	
ID	Glass Thick, mm		VT	SC	0°	40°	50°	60°	70°	(Diffuse)	Operable	Fixed	Operable	Fixed	Operable	Fixed
Low-e Double Glazing, e = 0.05 on Surface 2																
25a	3.2	LE CLR	0.72	0.48	0.41	0.38	0.34	0.26	0.14	0.35	0.37	0.38	0.31	0.36	0.52	0.63
25b	6.4	LE CLR	0.70	0.43	0.37	0.34	0.31	0.24	0.13	0.32	0.33	0.34	0.28	0.33	0.51	0.61
25c	6.4	BRZ W/LE CLR	0.42	0.30	0.26	0.24	0.22	0.18	0.10	0.23	0.24	0.24	0.20	0.23	0.31	0.37
25d	6.4	GRN W/LE CLR	0.60	0.35	0.30	0.28	0.25	0.20	0.11	0.26	0.28	0.28	0.23	0.27	0.44	0.52
25e	6.4	GRY W/LE CLR	0.35	0.27	0.24	0.22	0.20	0.16	0.10	0.20	0.22	0.23	0.18	0.21	0.25	0.30
25f	6.4	BLUE W/LE CLR	0.45	0.32	0.27	0.25	0.23	0.18	0.10	0.23	0.25	0.25	0.21	0.24	0.33	0.39
25g	6.4	HI-P GRN W/LE CLR	0.53	0.31	0.27	0.26	0.25	0.23	0.18	0.24	0.00	0.00	0.22	0.25	0.38	0.46
Triple Glazing																
29a	3.2	CLR CLR CLR	0.74	0.78	0.67	0.65	0.61	0.53	0.39	0.57	0.59	0.61	0.50	0.59	0.54	0.64
29b	6.4	CLR CLR CLR	0.70	0.71	0.61	0.58	0.55	0.48	0.35	0.51	0.54	0.56	0.45	0.54	0.51	0.61
29c	6.4	HI-P GRN CLR CLR	0.53	0.39	0.34	0.31	0.29	0.25	0.19	0.27	0.31	0.32	0.26	0.30	0.38	0.46
Triple Glazing, e = 0.2 on Surface 2																
32a	3.2	LE CLR CLR	0.68	0.69	0.60	0.58	0.55	0.48	0.35	0.51	0.53	0.55	0.45	0.53	0.49	0.59
32b	6.4	LE CLR CLR	0.64	0.62	0.53	0.50	0.47	0.41	0.30	0.44	0.47	0.49	0.39	0.47	0.46	0.56
Triple Glazing, e = 0.2 on Surface 5														0.00	0.00	
32c	3.2	CLR CLR LE	0.68	0.72	0.62	0.60	0.56	0.49	0.36	0.52	0.55	0.57	0.46	0.54	0.49	0.59
32d	6.4	CLR CLR LE	0.64	0.65	0.56	0.53	0.50	0.44	0.32	0.47	0.50	0.51	0.42	0.49	0.46	0.56
Triple Glazing, e = 0.1 on Surface 2 and 5																
40a	3.2	LE CLR LE	0.62	0.52	0.45	0.43	0.40	0.36	0.26	0.38	0.40	0.41	0.34	0.40	0.45	0.54
40b	6.4	LE CLR LE	0.59	0.47	0.41	0.39	0.37	0.32	0.24	0.34	0.37	0.38	0.31	0.36	0.43	0.51
Triple Glazing, e = 0.05 on Surface 2 and 4								0.00	0.00							
40c	3.2	LE LE CLR	0.58	0.37	0.32	0.30	0.29	0.26	0.19	0.27	0.29	0.30	0.24	0.28	0.42	0.51
40d	6.4	LE LE CLR	0.55	0.36	0.31	0.29	0.28	0.25	0.19	0.26	0.28	0.29	0.24	0.27	0.40	0.48

KEY:

CLR = clear, GRN = green, GRY = gray, SS = stainless steel reflective coating, TI = titanium reflective coating

Reflective coating decsriptors include percent visible transmittance as x%.

Hi-P GRN = high performance green tinted glass, LE = glass with a low-emissivity coating with an emittance of *e* = 0.xx

Low-e coating with an emittance of 0.2 is a pyrolytic coating. Other low-e coatings are sputtered coatings.

VT is Visible Transmittance, SC is Shading Coefficient, SHGC, is Solar Heat Gain Coefficient, and HEMIS is the hemispherical SHGC

ID numberss refer to U-factors in Table 5

SHGC at 90° is 0.

Table 7-5 SI Shading Coefficients for Single Glass with Indoor Shading

Type of Glass	Nominal Thickness,[a] mm	Solar Transmittance[b]	Type of Shading: Venetian Blinds — Medium	Venetian Blinds — Light	Roller Shade: Opaque — Dark	Opaque — White	Translucent — Light
Clear	2.4[c]	0.87 to 0.80	0.74[d] (0.63)[e]	0.67[d] (0.58)[e]	0.81	0.39	0.44
Clear	6 to 13	0.80 to 0.71					
Clear pattern	3 to 13	0.87 to 0.79					
Heat-absorbing pattern	3	—					
Tinted	5, 5.5	0.74, 0.71					
Heat-absorbing[f]	5, 6	0.46					
Heat-absorbing pattern	5, 6	—	0.57	0.53	0.45	0.30	0.36
Tinted	3, 5.5	0.59, 0.45					
Heat-absorbing or pattern	—	0.44 to 0.30	0.54	0.52	0.40	0.28	0.32
Heat-absorbing[f]	10	0.34					
Heat-absorbing or pattern		0.29 to 0.15					
	—	0.24	0.42	0.40	0.36	0.28	0.31
Reflective coated glass	S.C. = 0.30[g]		0.25	0.23			
	= 0.40		0.33	0.29			
	= 0.50		0.42	0.38			
	= 0.60		0.50	0.44			

[a]Refer to manufacturers' literature for values.
[b]For vertical blinds with opaque white and beige louvers in the tightly closed position, SC is 0.25 and 0.29 when used with glass of 0.71 to 0.80 transmittance.
[c]Typical residential glass thickness.
[d]From Van Dyck and Konen (1982), for 45° open venetian blinds, 35° solar incidence, and 35° profile angle.
[e]Values for closed venetian blinds. Use these values only when operation is automated for solar gain reduction (as opposed to daylight use).
[f]Refers to gray, bronze, and green tinted heat-absorbing glass.
[g]SC for glass with no shading device.

Table 7-6 SI Shading Coefficients for Double Glass[a] with Indoor Shading

Type of Glass	Nominal Thickness, Each Light	Solar Transmittance[a] — Outer Pane	Solar Transmittance[a] — Inner Pane	Type of Shading: Venetian Blinds[b] — Medium	Venetian Blinds[b] — Light	Roller Shade: Opaque — Dark	Opaque — White	Translucent — Light
Clear out	2.4, 3 mm	0.87	0.87	0.62[c]	0.58[c]	0.71	0.35	0.40
Clear in				(0.63)[d]	(0.58)[d]			
Clear in	6 mm	0.80	0.80					
Heat-absorbing[e] out	6 mm	0.46	0.80	0.39	0.36	0.40	0.22	0.30
Clear in								
Reflective coated glass	SC = 0.20[f]			0.19	0.18			
	= 0.30			0.27	0.26			
	= 0.40			0.34	0.33			

Table refers to factory-fabricated units with 5, 6, or 13 mm air space, or to prime windows plus storm windows.

[a]Refer to manufacturers' literature for exact values.
[b]For vertical blinds with opaque white or beige louvers, tightly closed, SC is approximately the same as for opaque white roller shades.
[c]From Van Dyck and Konen (1982), for 45° open venetian blinds, 35° solar incidence, and 35° profile angle.
[d]Values for closed venetian blinds. Use these values only when operation is automated for solar gain reduction (as opposed to daylight use).
[e]Refers to bronze, or green tinted, heat-absorbing glass.
[f]SC for glass with no shading device.

Table 7-14 SI Rates of Heat Gain from Occupants[a,b,c]

Degree of Activity		Total Heat, W Adult Male	Total Heat, W Adjusted, M/F[a]	Sensible Heat, W	Latent Heat, W	% Sensible Heat that is Radiant[b] Low V	% Sensible Heat that is Radiant[b] High V
Seated at theater	Theater, matinee	115	95	65	30		
Seated at theater, night	Theater, night	115	105	70	35	60	27
Seated, very light work	Offices, hotels, apartments	130	115	70	45		
Moderately active office work	Offices, hotels, apartments	140	130	75	55		
Standing, light work; walking	Department store; retail store	160	130	75	55	58	38
Walking, standing	Drug store, bank	160	145	75	70		
Sedentary work	Restaurant[c]	145	160	80	80		
Light bench work	Factory	235	220	80	140		
Moderate dancing	Dance hall	265	250	90	160	49	35
Walking 4.8 km/h; light machine work	Factory	295	295	110	185		
Bowling[d]	Bowling alley	440	425	170	255		
Heavy work	Factory	440	425	170	255	54	19
Heavy machine work; lifting	Factory	470	470	185	285		
Athletics	Gymnasium	585	525	210	315		

Notes:
1. Tabulated values are based on 24°C room dry-bulb temperature. For 27°C room dry bulb, the total heat remains the same, but the sensible heat values should be decreased by approximately 20%, and the latent heat values increased accordingly.
2. Also refer to Table 4, Chapter 8, for additional rates of metabolic heat generation.
3. All values are rounded to nearest 5 W.

[a]Adjusted heat gain is based on normal percentage of men, women, and children for the application listed, with the postulate that the gain from an adult female is 85% of that for an adult male, and that the gain from a child is 75% of that for an adult male.

[b]Values approximated from data in Table 6, Chapter 8, where is air velocity with limits shown in that table.

[c]Adjusted heat gain includes 18 W for food per individual (9 W sensible and 9 W latent).

[d]Figure one person per alley actually bowling, and all others as sitting (117 W) or standing or walking slowly (231 W).

Table 7-15 SI Heat Gain from Typical Electric Motors

Motor Nameplate or Rated Horsepower	(kW)	Motor Type	Nominal rpm	Full Load Motor Efficiency, %	A: Motor in, Driven Equipment in, Watt	B: Motor out, Driven Equipment in, Watt	C: Motor in, Driven Equipment out, Watt
0.05	(0.04)	Shaded pole	1500	35	105	35	70
0.08	(0.06)	Shaded pole	1500	35	170	59	110
0.125	(0.09)	Shaded pole	1500	35	264	94	173
0.16	(0.12)	Shaded pole	1500	35	340	117	223
0.25	(0.19)	Split phase	1750	54	346	188	158
0.33	(0.25)	Split phase	1750	56	439	246	194
0.50	(0.37)	Split phase	1750	60	621	372	249
0.75	(0.56)	3-Phase	1750	72	776	557	217
1	(0.75)	3-Phase	1750	75	993	747	249
1.5	(1.1)	3-Phase	1750	77	1453	1119	334
2	(1.5)	3-Phase	1750	79	1887	1491	396
3	(2.2)	3-Phase	1750	81	2763	2238	525
5	(3.7)	3-Phase	1750	82	4541	3721	817
7.5	(5.6)	3-Phase	1750	84	6651	5596	1066
10	(7.5)	3-Phase	1750	85	8760	7178	1315
15	(11.2)	3-Phase	1750	86	13 009	11 192	1820
20	(14.9)	3-Phase	1750	87	17 140	14 913	2230
25	(18.6)	3-Phase	1750	88	21 184	18 635	2545
30	(22.4)	3-Phase	1750	89	25 110	22 370	2765
40	(30)	3-Phase	1750	89	33 401	29 885	3690
50	(37)	3-Phase	1750	89	41 900	37 210	4600
60	(45)	3-Phase	1750	89	50 395	44 829	5538
75	(56)	3-Phase	1750	90	62 115	55 962	6210
100	(75)	3-Phase	1750	90	82 918	74 719	8290
125	(93)	3-Phase	1750	90	103 430	93 172	10 342
150	(110)	3-Phase	1750	91	123 060	111 925	11 075
200	(150)	3-Phase	1750	91	163 785	149 135	14 738
250	(190)	3-Phase	1750	91	204 805	186 346	18 430

Location of Motor and Driven Equipment with Respect to Conditioned Space or Airstream: A, B, C as above.

Table 7-17 SI Heat Gain from Selected Restaurant Equipment[a]

		Energy Rate, W		Recommended Rate of Heat Gain,[a] W			
				Without Hood			With Hood
Appliance	**Size**	**Rated**	**Standby**	**Sensible**	**Latent**	**Total**	**Sensible**
Electric, No Hood Required							
Barbeque (pit), per kilogram of food capacity	36 to 136 kg	88	—	57	31	88	27
Barbeque (pressurized) per kilogram of food capacity	20 kg	210	—	71	35	106	33
Blender, per litre of capacity	1.0 to 3.8 L	480	—	310	160	470	150
Braising pan, per litre of capacity	102 to 133 L	110	—	55	29	84	40
Cabinet (large hot holding)	0.46 to 0.49 m^3	2080	—	180	100	280	85
Cabinet (large hot serving)	1.06 to 1.15 m^3	2000	—	180	90	270	82
Cabinet (large proofing)	0.45 to 0.48 m^3	2030	—	180	90	270	82
Cabinet (small hot holding)	0.09 to 0.18 m^3	900	—	80	40	120	37
Cabinet (very hot holding)	0.49 m^3	6150	—	550	280	830	250
Can opener		170	—	170	—	170	0
Coffee brewer	12 cup/2 brnrs	1660	—	1100	560	1660	530
Coffee heater, per boiling burner	1 to 2 brnrs	670	—	440	230	670	210
Coffee heater, per warming burner	1 to 2 brnrs	100	—	66	34	100	32
Coffee/hot water boiling urn, per litre of capacity	11 L	120	—	79	41	120	38
Coffee brewing urn (large), per litre of capacity	22 to 38 L	660	—	440	220	660	210
Coffee brewing urn (small), per litre of capacity	10 L	420	—	280	140	420	130
Cutter (large)	460 mm bowl	750	—	750	—	750	0
Cutter (small)	360 mm bowl	370	—	370	—	370	0
Cutter and mixer (large)	28 to 45 L	3730	—	3730	—	3730	0
Dishwasher (hood type, chemical sanitizing), per 100 dishes/h	950 to 2000 dishes/h	380	—	50	110	160	50
Dishwasher (hood type, water sanitizing), per 100 dishes/h	950 to 2000 dishes/h	380	—	56	123	179	56
Dishwasher (conveyor type, chemical sanitizing), per 100 dishes/h	5000 to 9000 dishes/h	340	—	41	97	138	44
Dishwasher (conveyor type, water sanitizing), per 100 dishes/h	5000 to 9000 dishes/h	340	—	44	108	152	50
Display case (refrigerated), per cubic metre of interior	0.17 to 1.9 m^3	1590	—	640	0	640	0
Dough roller (large)	2 rollers	1610	—	1610	—	1610	0
Dough roller (small)	1 roller	460	—	460	—	460	0
Egg cooker	12 eggs	1800	—	850	570	1420	460
Food processor	2.3 L	520	—	520	—	520	0
Food warmer (infrared bulb), per lamp	1 to 6 bulbs	250	—	250	—	250	250
Food warmer (shelf type), per square metre of surface	0.28 to 0.84 m^3	2930	—	2330	600	2930	820
Food warmer (infrared tube), per metre of length	1.0 to 2.1 m	950	—	950	—	950	950
Food warmer (well type), per cubic metre of well	20 to 70 L	37400	—	12400	6360	18760	6000
Freezer (large)	2.07 m^3	1340	—	540	—	540	0
Freezer (small)	0.51 m^3	810	—	320	—	320	0
Griddle/grill (large), per square metre of cooking surface	0.43 to 1.1 m^2	29000	—	1940	1080	3020	1080
Griddle/grill (small), per square metre of cooking surface	0.20 to 0.42 m^2	26200	—	1720	970	2690	940
Hot dog broiler	48 to 56 hot dogs	1160	—	100	50	150	48
Hot plate (double burner, high speed)		4900	—	2290	1590	3880	1830
Hot plate (double burner stockpot)		4000	—	1870	1300	3170	1490
Hot plate (single burner, high speed)		2800	—	1310	910	2220	1040
Hot water urn (large), per litre of capacity	53 L	130	—	50	16	66	21
Hot water urn (small), per litre of capacity	7.6 L	230	—	87	30	117	37
Ice maker (large)	100 kg/day	1090	—	2730	—	2730	0
Ice maker (small)	50 kg/day	750	—	1880	—	1880	0
Microwave oven (heavy duty, commercial)	20 L	2630	—	2630	—	2630	0
Microwave oven (residential type)	30 L	600 to 1400	—	600 to 1400	—	600 to 1400	0
Mixer (large), per litre of capacity	77 L	29	—	29	—	29	0
Mixer (small), per litre of capacity	11 to 72 L	15	—	15	—	15	0
Press cooker (hamburger)	300 patties/h	2200	—	1450	750	2200	700
Refrigerator (large), per cubic metre of interior space	0.71 to 2.1 m^3	780	—	310	—	310	0
Refrigerator (small) per cubic metre of interior space	0.17 to 0.71 m^3	1730	—	690	—	690	0
Rotisserie	300 hamburgers/h	3200	—	2110	1090	3200	1020
Serving cart (hot), per cubic metre of well	50 to 90 L	21200	—	7060	3530	10590	3390
Serving drawer (large)	252 to 336 dinner rolls	1100	—	140	10	150	45
Serving drawer (small)	84 to 168 dinner rolls	800	—	100	10	110	33
Skillet (tilting), per litre of capacity	45 to 125 L	180	—	90	50	140	66
Slicer, per square metre of slicing carriage	0.06 to 0.09 m^2	2150	—	2150	—	2150	680
Soup cooker, per litre of well	7 to 11 L	130	—	45	24	69	21
Steam cooker, per cubic metre of compartment	30 to 60 L	214000	—	17000	10900	27900	8120
Steam kettle (large), per litre of capacity	76 to 300 L	95	—	7	5	12	4
Steam kettle (small), per litre of capacity	23 to 45 L	260	—	21	14	35	10
Syrup warmer, per litre of capacity	11 L	87	—	29	16	45	14

Table 7-17 SI Heat Gain from Selected Restaurant Equipment[a] (*Continued*)

		Energy Rate, W		Recommended Rate of Heat Gain,[a] W			
				Without Hood			With Hood
Appliance	Size	Rated	Standby	Sensible	Latent	Total	Sensible
Toaster (bun toasts on one side only)	1400 buns/h	1500	—	800	710	1510	480
Toaster (large conveyor)	720 slices/h	3200	—	850	750	1600	510
Toaster (small conveyor)	360 slices/h	2100	—	560	490	1050	340
Toaster (large pop-up)	10 slice	5300	—	2810	2490	5300	1700
Toaster (small pop-up)	4 slice	2470	—	1310	1160	2470	790
Waffle iron	0.05 m^2	1640	—	700	940	1640	520
Electric, Exhaust Hood Required							
Broiler (conveyor infrared), per square metre of cooking area/minute	0.19 to 9.5 m^2	60800	—	—	—	—	12100
Broiler (single deck infrared), per square metre of broiling area	0.24 to 0.91 m^2	34200	—	—	—	—	6780
Charbroiler, per linear metre of cooking surface	0.6 to 2.4 m	10600	8900	—	—	—	2700
Fryer (deep fat)	15 to 23 kg oil	14000	850	—	—	—	350
Fryer (pressurized), per kilogram of fat capacity	6 to 15 kg	1010	—	—	—	—	38
Griddle, per linear metre of cooking surface	0.6 to 2.4 m	18800	3000	—	—	—	1350
Oven (full-szie convection)		12000	5000	—	—	—	850
Oven (large deck baking with 15.2 m^3 decks), per cubic metre of oven spacer	0.43 to 1.3 m^3	17300	—	—	—	—	710
Oven (roasting), per cubic metre of oven space	0.22 to 0.66 m^3	28300	—	—	—	—	1170
Oven (small convection), per cubic metre of oven space	0.04 to 0.15 m^3	107000	—	—	—	—	1520
Oven (small deck baking with 7.7 m^3 decks), per cubic metre of oven space	0.22 to 0.66 m^3	28700	—	—	—	—	1170
Open range (top), per 2 element section	2 to 10 elements	4100	1350	—	—	—	620
Range (hot top/fry top), per square metre of cooking surface	0.36 to 0.74 m^2	22900	—	—	—	—	8500
Range (oven section), per cubic metre of oven space	0.12 to 0.32 m^3	40600	—	—	—	—	1660
Gas, No Hood Required							
Broiler, per square metre of broiling area	0.25	46600	190[b]	16800	9030	25830	3840
Cheese melter, per square metre of cooking surface	0.23 to 0.47	32500	190[b]	11600	3400	15000	2680
Dishwasher (hood type, chemical sanitizing), per 100 dishes/h	950 to 2000 dishes/h	510	190[b]	150	59	209	67
Dishwasher (hood type, water sanitizing), per 100 dishes/h	950 to 2000 dishes/h	510	190[b]	170	64	234	73
Dishwasher (conveyor type, chemical sanitizing), per 100 dishes/h	5000 to 9000 dishes/h	400	190[b]	97	21	118	38
Dishwasher (conveyor type, water sanitizing), per 100 dishes/h	5000 to 9000 dishes/h	400	190[b]	110	23	133	41
Griddle/grill (large), per square metre of cooking surface	0.43 to 1.1 m^2	53600	1040	3600	1930	5530	1450
Griddle/grill (small), per square metre of cooking surface	0.23 to 0.42 m^2	45400	1040	3050	1610	4660	1260
Hot plate	2 burners	5630	390[b]	3430	1020	4450	1000
Oven (pizza), per square metre of hearth	0.59 to 1.2 m^2	14900	190[b]	1970	690	2660	270
Gas, Exhaust Hood Required							
Braising pan, per litre of capacity	102 to 133 L	3050	190[b]	—	—	—	750
Broiler, per square metre of broiling area	0.34 to 0.36 m^3	68900	1660	—	—	—	5690
Broiler (large conveyor, infrared), per square metre of cooking area/minute	0.19 to 9.5 m^2	162000	6270	—	—	—	16900
Broiler (standard infrared), per square metre of broiling area	0.22 to 0.87 m^2	61300	1660	—	—	—	5040
Charbroiler (large), per linear metre of cooking area	0.6 to 2.4 m	34600	21000	—	—	—	3650
Fryer (deep fat)	15 to 23 kg	23500	1640	—	—	—	560
Oven (bake deck), per cubic metre of oven space	0.15 to 0.46 m^3	79400	190[b]	—	—	—	1450
Griddle, per linear metre of cooling surface	0.6 to 2.4 m	24000	6060	—	—	—	1540
Oven (full-size convection)		20500	8600	—	—	—	1670
Oven (pizza), per square metre of oven hearth	0.86 to 2.4 m^2	22800	190[b]	—	—	—	410
Oven (roasting), per cubic metre of oven space	0.26 to 0.79 m^3	44500	190[b]	—	—	—	800
Oven (twin bake deck), per cubic metre of oven space	0.31 to 0.61 m^3	45400	190[b]	—	—	—	810
Range (burners), per 2 burner section	2 to 10 burners	9840	390	—	—	—	1930
Range (hot top or fry top), per square metre of cooking surface	0.26 to 0.74 m^3	37200	1040	—	—	—	10700
Range (large stock pot)	3 burners	29300	580	—	—	—	5740
Range (small stock pot)	2 burners	11700	390	—	—	—	2290
Range top, open burner (per 2 element section)	2 to 6 elements	11700	4000	—	—	—	640
Steam							
Compartment steamer, per kilogram of food capacity/h	21 to 204 kg	180	—	14	9	23	7
Dishwasher (hood type, chemical sanitizing), per 100 dishes/h	950 to 2000 dishes/h	920	—	260	110	370	120
Dishwasher (hood type, water sanitizing), per 100 dishes/h	950 to 2000 dishes/h	920	—	290	120	410	130
Dishwasher (conveyor, chemical sanitizing), per 100 dishes/h	5000 to 9000 dishes/h	350	—	41	97	138	44
Dishwasher (conveyor, water sanitizing), per 100 dishes/h	5000 to 9000 dishes/h	350	—	44	108	152	50
Steam kettle, per litre of capacity	12 to 30 L	160	—	12	8	20	6

[a]In some cases, heat gain data are given per unit of capacity. In those cases, the heat gain is calculated by: q = (recommended heat gain per unit of capacity) * (capacity)

[b]Standby input rating is given for entire appliance regardless of size.

Table 7-18 SI Heat Gain from Selected Office and Hospital Equipment

Appliance	Size	Maximum Input Rating, W	Standby Input Rating, W	Recommended Rate of Heat Gain, W
Check processing workstation	12 pockets	4800	2460	2460
Computer devices				
Card puncher	—	800 to 1800	640 to 1410	640 to 1410
Card reader	—	2200	1520	1520
Communication/transmission	—	1800 to 4600	1640 to 2810	1640 to 2810
Disk drives/mass storage	—	1000 to 10000	1000 to 6570	1000 to 6570
Magnetic ink reader	—	960 to 4700	760 to 4220	760 to 4220
Microcomputer	16 to 640 Kbyte[a]	100 to 600	90 to 530	90 to 530
Minicomputer	—	2200 to 6600	2200 to 6600	2200 to 6600
Optical reader	—	3000 to 6000	2350 to 4980	2350 to 4980
Plotters	—	75	37	63
Printers				
Letter quality	30 to 45 char/min	350	175	292
Line, high speed	5000 or more lines/min	1000 to 5300	500 to 2550	730 to 3810
Line, low speed	300 to 600 lines/min	450	225	376
Tape drives	—	1200 to 6500	1000 to 4700	1000 to 4700
Terminal	—	90 to 200	80 to 180	80 to 180
Copiers/Duplicators				
Blue print	—	1150 to 12500	500 to 5000	1150 to 12500
Copiers (large)	30 to 67[a] copies/min	1700 to 6600	900	1700 to 6600
Copiers (small)	6 to 30[a] copies/min	460 to 1700	300 to 900	460 to 1700
Feeder	—	30	—	30
Microfilm printer	—	450	—	450
Sorter/collator	—	60 to 600	—	60 to 600
Electronic equipment				
Cassette recorders/players	—	60	—	60
Receiver/tuner	—	100	—	100
Signal analyzer	—	60 to 650	—	60 to 650
Mailprocessing				
Folding machine	—	125	—	80
Inserting machine	3600 to 6800 pieces/h	600 to 3300	—	390 to 2150
Labeling machine	1500 to 30000 pieces/h	600 to 6600	—	390 to 4300
Postage meter	—	230	—	150
Wordprocessors/Typewriters				
Letter quality printer	30 to 45 char/min	350	175	292
Phototypesetter	—	1725	—	1520
Typewriter	—	80	—	67
Wordprocessor	—	100 to 600	—	88 to 530
Vending machines				
Cigarette	—	72	15 to 25	72
Cold food/beverage	—	1150 to 1920	—	575 to 960
Hot beverage	—	1725	—	862
Snack	—	240 to 275	—	240 to 275
Miscellaneous				
Barcode printer	—	440	—	370
Cash registers	—	60	—	48
Coffee maker	10 cups	1500	—	1050 sens., 450 latent
Microfiche reader	—	85	—	85
Microfilm reader	—	520	—	520
Microfilm reader/printer	—	1150	—	1150
Microwave oven	28 L	600	—	400
Paper shredder	—	250 to 3000	—	200 to 2420
Water cooler	30 L/h	700	—	1750

[a]Input is not proportional to capacity.

Table 7-18 SI Heat Gain from Selected Office and Hospital Equipment (*Concluded*)

Appliance Type	Size	Maximum Input Rating, Watts	Recommended Rate of Heat Gain, Watts[a]
Autoclave (bench)	0.02 m^3	1250	140
Bath, hot or cold circulating, small	3.7 to 36.7 litres, −30 to 100°C	750 to 1800	130 to 310 (sensible) 250 to 590 (latent)
Blood analyzer	120 samples/h	735	735
Blood analyzer with CRT screen	115 samples/h	1500	1500
Centrifuge (large)	8 to 24 places	1100	1050
Centrifuge (small)	4 to 12 places	150	140
Chromatograph	—	2000	2000
Cytometer (cell sorter/analyzer)	1000 cells/s	21 460	21 460
Electrophoresis power supply	—	400	250
Freezer, blood plasma, medium	0.37 m^3, down to −40°C	3530[b]	1410[b]
Hot plate, concentric ring	4 holes, 100°C	1100	870
Incubator, CO_2	0.14 to 0.28 m^3, up to 55°C	2830	1410
Incubator, forced draft	0.28 m^3, 27 to 60°C	720	360
Incubator, general application	0.04 to 0.31 m^3, up to 70°C	1660 to 2260[b]	850 to 1130[b]
Magnetic stirrer	—	600	600
Microcomputer	16 to 256 kbytes[c]	100 to 600	88 to 528
Minicomputer	—	2200 to 6000	2200 to 6600
Oven, general purpose, small	0.04 to 0.08 m^3, 240°C	21 900[b]	2970[b]
Refrigerator, laboratory	0.63 to 3.0 m^3, 4°C	880[d]	350[d]
Refrigerator, blood, small	0.20 to 0.56 m^3, 4°C	2680[b]	1060[b]
Spectrophotometer	—	500	500
Sterilizer, freestanding	0.11 m^3, 100 to 132°C	20 900	2370
Ultrasonic cleaner, small	0.04 m^3	120	120
Washer, glassware	0.22 m^3 load area	4460	2930
Water still	19 to 57 litres	1120[e]	25[e]

Source: Alereza and Breen (1984).
[a]For hospital equipment installed under a hood, the heat gain is assumed to be zero.
[b]Heat gain per cubic metre of interior space.
[c]Input is not proportional to memory size.
[d]Heat gain per 10 m^3 of interior space.
[e]Heat gain per litre of capacity.

Table 7-20 SI July Cooling Load Temperature Differences for Calculating Cooling Load from Flat Roofs at 40° North Latitude

Roof No.	Hour 1	2	3	4	5	6	7	8	9	10	11	12	13	14	15	16	17	18	19	20	21	22	23	24
1	0	−1	−2	−3	−3	−3	0	7	16	25	33	41	46	49	49	46	41	33	24	14	8	5	3	1
2	1	0	−1	−2	−3	−3	−2	2	9	18	27	34	41	46	48	47	44	39	31	22	14	8	5	3
3	7	4	3	1	0	−1	0	3	7	13	19	26	32	37	40	41	41	37	33	27	21	17	13	9
4	9	6	4	2	1	−1	−2	−2	0	4	9	16	23	30	36	41	43	43	41	37	31	25	19	13
5	12	9	7	4	3	2	1	1	3	7	12	17	23	28	33	37	38	38	36	33	28	23	19	15
8	16	13	12	9	8	7	6	6	7	9	12	16	19	23	27	29	31	32	31	29	27	24	21	18
9	18	14	12	9	7	5	3	2	2	4	7	11	15	20	25	29	33	35	36	35	32	29	25	21
10	21	18	15	13	11	8	7	6	5	6	7	9	13	17	21	24	28	31	32	32	31	29	26	23
13	19	17	16	14	12	11	10	9	9	9	11	13	16	18	21	23	26	27	27	27	26	24	22	21
14	19	18	17	15	14	13	12	11	11	11	12	13	16	18	20	22	23	24	25	25	24	23	22	21

Note: 1. Direct application of data
- Dark surface
- Indoor temperature of 25.5°C
- Outdoor maximum temperature of 35°C with mean temperature of 29.5°C and daily range of 11.6°C
- Solar radiation typical of clear day on 21st day of month
- Outside surface film resistance of 0.059 $m^2 \cdot K/W$
- With or without suspended ceiling but no ceiling plenum air return systems
- Inside surface resistance of 0.121 $m^2 \cdot K/W$

Note: 2. Adjustments to table data
- Design temperatures : Corr. CLTD = CLTD + $(25.5 - t_r) + (t_m - 29.4)$

where

t_r = inside temperature and t_m = mean outdoor temperature

t_m = maximum outdoor temperature − (daily range)/2

- No adjustment recommended for color
- No adjustment recommended for ventilation of air space above a ceiling

Table 7-21 SI Roof Numbers Used In Table 7-20 SI

Mass Location**	Suspended Ceiling	R-Value, $m^2 \cdot K/W$	B7, Wood 25 mm	C12, HW Concrete 50 mm	A3, Steel Deck	Attic-Ceiling Combination
Mass inside the insulation	Without	0 to 0.9	*	2	*	*
		0.9 to 1.8	*	2	*	*
		1.8 to 2.6	*	4	*	*
		2.6 to 3.5	*	4	*	*
		3.5 to 4.4	*	5	*	*
		4.4 to 5.3	*	*	*	*
	With	0 to 0.9	*	5	*	*
		0.9 to 1.8	*	8	*	*
		1.8 to 2.6	*	13	*	*
		2.6 to 3.5	*	13	*	*
		3.5 to 4.4	*	14	*	*
		4.4 to 5.3	*	*	*	*
Mass evenly placed	Without	0 to 0.9	1	2	1	1
		0.9 to 1.8	2	*	1	2
		1.8 to 2.6	2	*	1	2
		2.6 to 3.5	4	*	2	2
		3.5 to 4.4	4	*	2	4
		4.4 to 5.3	*	*	*	*
	With	0 to 0.9	*	3	1	*
		0.9 to 1.8	4	*	1	*
		1.8 to 2.6	5	*	2	*
		2.6 to 3.5	9	*	2	*
		3.5 to 4.4	10	*	4	*
		4.4 to 5.3	10	*	*	*
Mass outside the insulation	Without	0 to 0.9	*	2	*	*
		0.9 to 1.8	*	3	*	*
		1.8 to 2.6	*	4	*	*
		2.6 to 3.5	*	5	*	*
		3.5 to 4.4	*	5	*	*
		4.4 to 5.3	*	*	*	*
	With	0 to 0.9	*	3	*	*
		0.9 to 1.8	*	3	*	*
		1.8 to 2.6	*	4	*	*
		2.6 to 3.5	*	5	*	*
		3.5 to 4.4	*	*	*	*
		4.4 to 5.3	*	*	*	*

*Denotes a roof that is not possible with the chosen parameters.

**The 50-mm concrete is considered massive and the others nonmassive.

Table 7-22 SI July Cooling Load Temperature Differences for Calculating Cooling Load from Sunlit Walls 40° North Latitude

Wall Number 1

Wall Face	Hour 1	2	3	4	5	6	7	8	9	10	11	12	13	14	15	16	17	18	19	20	21	22	23	24
N	1	0	–1	–1	–2	–1	4	6	6	7	9	12	14	15	16	16	16	16	15	9	6	4	3	2
NE	1	0	–1	–1	–2	1	13	23	26	24	19	16	15	16	16	16	15	13	11	8	6	4	3	2
E	1	0	–1	–1	–1	1	16	28	34	36	33	27	20	17	17	17	16	14	11	8	6	4	3	2
SE	1	0	–1	–1	–2	0	8	18	26	31	32	31	27	22	18	17	16	14	11	8	6	4	3	2
S	1	0	–1	–1	–2	–1	0	2	6	12	18	24	28	29	28	24	19	15	11	8	6	4	3	2
SW	1	0	–1	–1	–1	–1	0	2	4	7	9	14	22	29	36	39	38	34	25	13	7	4	3	2
W	1	1	–1	–1	–1	–1	1	2	4	7	9	12	15	23	33	41	44	44	34	18	9	5	3	2
NW	1	0	–1	–1	–1	–1	0	2	4	7	9	12	14	16	21	28	34	36	31	16	8	5	3	2

Wall Number 2

Wall Face	Hour 1	2	3	4	5	6	7	8	9	10	11	12	13	14	15	16	17	18	19	20	21	22	23	24
N	3	2	1	0	–1	–1	–1	2	4	5	6	8	10	12	13	14	15	16	16	15	12	9	7	4
NE	3	2	1	0	–1	–1	1	7	14	20	22	21	18	17	16	16	16	16	14	13	10	8	6	4
E	3	2	1	0	–1	–1	1	8	18	26	31	32	29	24	21	19	18	17	15	13	11	8	6	4
SE	3	2	1	0	–1	–1	0	4	11	18	24	28	29	28	25	22	19	17	16	13	11	8	6	4
S	3	2	1	0	–1	–1	–1	–1	1	4	8	13	18	23	26	27	26	22	18	15	12	8	6	4
SW	4	2	1	1	0	–1	–1	0	1	3	5	7	11	17	23	29	34	36	34	29	22	15	9	6
W	4	3	2	1	0	–1	–1	0	1	3	5	7	9	13	18	26	33	38	41	37	28	19	12	8
NW	4	2	1	1	–1	–1	–1	–1	1	3	5	7	9	12	14	18	23	28	32	30	23	16	11	7

Wall Number 3

Wall Face	Hour 1	2	3	4	5	6	7	8	9	10	11	12	13	14	15	16	17	18	19	20	21	22	23	24
N	4	3	2	1	1	0	1	3	4	4	6	8	9	11	13	13	14	14	15	13	11	9	7	6
NE	4	3	2	1	0	0	4	9	14	17	18	17	17	16	16	16	16	16	14	12	10	8	7	5
E	4	3	2	1	1	1	4	12	18	23	26	26	24	22	21	19	18	17	16	13	11	9	7	6
SE	4	3	2	1	1	0	2	7	12	18	22	24	26	24	23	21	19	18	16	13	11	9	7	6
S	4	3	2	1	1	0	0	1	2	5	9	13	17	21	23	23	22	20	17	14	12	9	8	6
SW	7	5	3	2	1	1	1	1	2	3	5	8	12	17	22	27	31	32	30	25	20	16	12	9
W	8	6	4	3	2	1	1	1	2	3	5	7	9	13	19	25	31	35	35	30	24	18	14	11
NW	7	4	3	2	1	1	0	1	2	3	5	7	9	11	14	18	22	27	28	24	19	15	12	9

Wall Number 4

Wall Face	Hour 1	2	3	4	5	6	7	8	9	10	11	12	13	14	15	16	17	18	19	20	21	22	23	24
N	6	4	3	2	1	0	0	1	2	3	4	6	7	9	11	12	13	14	15	15	14	12	11	8
NE	6	4	3	2	1	0	0	2	7	12	16	18	18	18	17	17	17	16	16	14	13	11	9	7
E	6	4	3	2	1	1	1	3	8	15	21	25	27	26	24	22	21	19	18	16	14	12	9	8
SE	6	4	3	2	1	1	0	1	4	9	15	20	24	26	26	24	23	21	19	17	14	12	10	8
S	6	4	3	2	1	1	0	1	0	1	3	7	11	16	19	23	24	23	22	19	17	13	11	8
SW	10	7	5	3	2	1	0	0	0	1	3	4	7	10	15	20	26	29	32	32	28	23	18	14
W	12	8	6	4	2	1	1	0	1	1	3	4	6	8	12	17	22	28	33	36	33	28	22	17
NW	10	7	5	3	2	1	0	0	0	1	2	4	6	8	11	13	17	21	25	27	27	23	18	14

Wall Number 5

Wall Face	Hour 1	2	3	4	5	6	7	8	9	10	11	12	13	14	15	16	17	18	19	20	21	22	23	24
N	7	6	4	3	3	2	1	2	3	3	4	5	7	8	9	11	12	13	13	13	13	12	10	8
NE	7	6	4	3	3	2	2	4	8	11	14	15	16	16	16	16	16	16	15	14	13	12	10	8
E	8	6	5	4	3	2	2	4	9	14	18	22	22	22	21	21	19	19	18	16	14	13	11	9
SE	8	7	5	4	3	2	2	3	6	10	14	18	21	22	22	21	21	19	18	17	15	13	11	9
S	8	7	5	4	3	2	2	1	2	2	4	7	11	14	17	19	20	20	19	18	16	13	12	10
SW	12	10	8	6	4	3	3	2	2	3	3	5	7	9	14	18	22	26	27	27	24	21	18	14
W	14	11	9	7	6	4	3	2	2	3	4	5	6	8	11	16	21	25	29	30	28	24	21	17
NW	12	9	7	6	4	3	2	2	2	2	3	4	6	8	9	12	15	19	22	23	22	19	17	14

Wall Number 6

Wall Face	Hour 1	2	3	4	5	6	7	8	9	10	11	12	13	14	15	16	17	18	19	20	21	22	23	24
N	7	6	5	4	3	3	2	3	3	4	4	6	7	8	9	10	11	12	12	13	12	11	9	8
NE	8	7	6	4	3	3	3	6	8	11	13	14	14	14	14	15	15	15	14	14	13	12	10	9
E	9	7	6	5	4	3	4	6	10	14	17	19	20	20	19	19	19	18	17	16	14	13	12	10
SE	9	8	6	5	4	3	3	4	7	10	13	16	18	19	20	19	19	18	18	16	15	13	12	10
S	9	7	6	5	4	3	3	2	2	3	5	7	10	13	16	17	18	18	17	16	15	13	12	10
SW	13	11	9	8	6	5	4	3	3	4	4	6	7	10	13	17	21	23	24	24	22	19	17	15
W	14	12	10	8	7	6	4	4	4	4	4	6	7	8	11	15	19	23	26	27	25	22	19	17
NW	12	10	8	7	6	4	4	3	3	3	4	5	6	8	9	12	14	18	20	21	20	18	16	14

Table 7-22 SI July Cooling Load Temperature Differences for Calculating Cooling Load from Sunlit Walls 40° North Latitude (*Continued*)

Wall Number 7

Wall Face	Hour 1	2	3	4	5	6	7	8	9	10	11	12	13	14	15	16	17	18	19	20	21	22	23	24
N	7	7	6	5	4	3	3	4	4	4	5	6	7	8	9	9	10	11	11	11	11	10	9	8
NE	8	7	6	6	5	4	5	7	9	11	12	13	13	13	13	14	14	14	13	13	12	11	10	9
E	9	8	7	7	6	5	6	9	12	14	17	18	18	18	18	18	17	17	16	15	14	13	12	11
SE	9	8	7	7	6	5	5	7	9	12	14	16	17	18	18	18	17	17	16	15	14	13	12	11
S	9	8	7	6	6	4	4	4	4	5	7	8	11	13	14	16	16	16	16	14	13	12	11	10
SW	13	11	10	9	7	7	6	6	6	6	6	7	8	11	14	17	19	21	22	21	19	17	16	14
W	14	12	11	9	8	7	7	6	6	6	7	7	8	9	12	16	19	22	23	23	21	19	17	16
NW	11	10	9	8	7	6	5	5	5	5	6	6	7	8	9	12	14	17	18	18	17	16	14	13

Wall Number 9

Wall Face	Hour 1	2	3	4	5	6	7	8	9	10	11	12	13	14	15	16	17	18	19	20	21	22	23	24
N	9	8	7	6	5	4	3	2	2	2	3	4	4	6	7	8	9	11	12	12	13	13	12	11
NE	10	8	7	6	5	4	3	3	3	6	9	11	13	14	14	15	15	16	16	15	14	14	13	11
E	11	9	8	7	6	4	3	3	4	7	11	14	18	20	21	21	21	20	19	18	17	16	14	13
SE	11	9	8	7	6	4	3	3	3	5	7	11	14	17	19	20	21	20	19	19	18	16	14	13
S	12	10	8	7	6	4	3	3	2	2	2	3	6	8	11	14	16	18	19	19	18	17	15	13
SW	17	14	12	10	8	7	5	4	3	3	3	3	4	6	8	11	14	18	22	24	25	24	22	20
W	19	17	14	12	9	8	6	4	4	3	3	4	4	6	7	9	12	17	21	24	27	27	25	23
NW	16	14	12	9	8	6	5	4	3	3	3	3	4	5	6	8	10	12	16	19	21	21	20	18

Wall Number 10

Wall Face	Hour 1	2	3	4	5	6	7	8	9	10	11	12	13	14	15	16	17	18	19	20	21	22	23	24
N	9	8	7	6	5	4	3	3	3	3	3	4	4	6	7	8	9	10	11	12	12	12	12	11
NE	10	9	7	6	5	4	3	3	4	7	9	11	12	13	14	14	15	15	15	15	14	13	12	11
E	11	9	8	7	6	4	4	4	6	8	11	14	17	19	19	20	20	19	19	18	17	16	14	13
SE	12	10	8	7	6	4	4	3	4	6	8	11	14	17	18	19	19	19	19	18	17	16	14	13
S	12	10	8	7	6	5	4	3	2	2	3	4	6	8	11	13	16	17	18	18	17	16	14	13
SW	17	15	13	11	9	7	6	4	4	3	3	4	4	6	8	11	14	18	21	23	23	23	21	19
W	19	17	14	12	10	8	7	5	4	4	4	4	4	6	7	9	13	17	21	23	25	25	23	22
NW	16	13	12	10	8	7	6	4	3	3	3	3	4	6	7	8	10	13	16	18	19	20	19	17

Wall Number 11

Wall Face	Hour 1	2	3	4	5	6	7	8	9	10	11	12	13	14	15	16	17	18	19	20	21	22	23	24
N	9	8	7	7	6	5	4	4	4	4	4	5	6	6	7	8	8	9	10	11	11	11	10	9
NE	10	9	8	7	7	6	5	5	6	8	9	11	12	12	13	13	13	13	14	14	13	13	12	11
E	12	11	9	9	8	7	6	6	7	9	12	14	16	17	17	17	17	17	17	17	16	15	14	13
SE	12	11	9	9	8	7	6	6	6	8	9	12	13	15	16	17	17	17	17	17	16	15	14	13
S	11	10	9	8	7	6	6	5	4	4	4	6	7	9	11	13	14	15	16	16	15	14	13	12
SW	16	14	13	11	10	9	8	7	6	6	6	6	7	8	9	12	14	17	18	20	20	19	18	17
W	17	16	14	12	11	10	9	8	7	7	6	7	7	7	8	11	13	16	18	21	22	21	20	18
NW	14	13	11	10	9	8	7	6	6	5	5	6	6	7	7	8	10	12	14	16	17	17	16	15

Wall Number 12

Wall Face	Hour 1	2	3	4	5	6	7	8	9	10	11	12	13	14	15	16	17	18	19	20	21	22	23	24
N	9	8	7	7	6	6	4	4	4	4	4	5	6	6	7	8	8	9	9	10	11	11	10	9
NE	10	9	8	8	7	6	6	6	7	8	9	11	12	12	12	13	13	13	13	13	13	12	12	11
E	12	11	10	9	8	7	7	7	8	9	12	14	16	16	17	17	17	17	17	16	16	15	14	13
SE	12	11	10	9	8	7	7	6	7	8	9	12	13	14	16	16	17	17	17	16	16	15	14	13
S	11	11	9	8	8	7	6	6	5	5	5	6	7	9	11	12	13	14	14	14	14	14	13	12
SW	15	14	13	12	11	9	8	8	7	7	7	7	7	8	9	11	13	16	18	19	19	19	18	17
W	17	16	14	13	12	11	9	8	8	7	7	7	7	8	9	11	13	15	18	19	21	20	19	18
NW	13	12	11	11	9	8	7	7	6	6	6	6	6	7	7	8	10	12	14	16	16	16	16	14

Table 7-22 SI July Cooling Load Temperature Differences for Calculating Cooling Load from Sunlit Walls 40° North Latitude (*Concluded*)

Wall Number 13

Wall Face	Hour 1	2	3	4	5	6	7	8	9	10	11	12	13	14	15	16	17	18	19	20	21	22	23	24
N	9	8	7	7	6	6	4	4	4	4	4	5	6	6	7	8	8	9	9	10	11	11	10	9
NE	10	9	8	8	7	6	6	6	7	8	9	11	12	12	12	13	13	13	13	13	13	12	12	11
E	12	11	10	9	8	7	7	7	8	9	12	14	16	16	17	17	17	17	17	16	16	15	14	13
SE	12	11	10	9	8	7	7	6	7	8	9	12	13	14	16	16	17	17	17	16	16	15	14	13
S	11	11	9	8	8	7	6	6	5	5	5	6	7	9	11	12	13	14	14	14	14	14	13	12
SW	15	14	13	12	11	9	8	8	7	7	7	7	7	8	9	11	13	16	18	19	19	19	18	17
W	17	16	14	13	12	11	9	8	8	7	7	7	7	8	9	11	13	15	18	19	21	20	19	18
NW	13	12	11	11	9	8	7	7	6	6	6	6	6	7	7	8	10	12	14	16	16	16	16	14

Wall Number 14

Wall Face	Hour 1	2	3	4	5	6	7	8	9	10	11	12	13	14	15	16	17	18	19	20	21	22	23	24
N	8	8	8	7	7	6	6	6	6	6	6	6	6	6	7	7	8	8	8	9	9	9	9	9
NE	11	10	9	9	8	8	7	7	8	8	9	10	11	11	11	12	12	12	12	12	12	12	12	11
E	13	12	12	11	10	9	9	8	9	10	12	13	14	14	15	15	16	16	16	16	15	14	14	13
SE	13	12	11	11	10	9	8	8	8	9	10	11	12	13	14	14	15	15	15	15	14	14	14	13
S	11	11	10	9	9	8	8	7	7	7	7	7	8	8	9	11	12	12	13	13	13	13	12	12
SW	14	14	13	12	12	11	10	9	9	8	8	8	8	9	9	11	12	14	15	16	17	17	16	16
W	16	15	14	13	13	12	11	10	9	9	9	9	9	9	9	11	12	13	15	17	18	18	17	17
NW	13	12	12	11	10	9	9	8	8	7	7	7	7	8	8	8	9	11	12	13	14	14	14	13

Wall Number 15

Wall Face	Hour 1	2	3	4	5	6	7	8	9	10	11	12	13	14	15	16	17	18	19	20	21	22	23	24
N	11	10	9	8	7	6	5	4	3	3	3	3	4	4	5	6	7	8	9	11	11	12	12	11
NE	12	11	9	8	7	6	5	4	4	5	6	8	10	11	12	13	14	14	14	14	14	14	14	13
E	14	12	11	9	8	7	6	5	5	6	8	10	13	15	17	18	19	19	19	18	18	17	16	15
SE	14	12	11	9	8	7	6	5	4	4	6	8	10	12	14	17	18	18	19	18	18	17	17	15
S	14	12	11	9	8	7	6	5	4	3	3	3	4	6	7	9	12	14	16	17	17	17	16	15
SW	19	18	16	14	12	10	9	7	6	5	4	4	4	5	6	8	10	13	16	18	21	22	22	21
W	22	19	18	16	13	12	10	8	7	6	5	4	4	5	6	7	9	12	14	18	21	23	23	23
NW	17	16	14	13	11	9	8	7	6	4	4	4	4	4	5	6	7	9	11	14	16	18	18	18

Wall Number 16

Wall Face	Hour 1	2	3	4	5	6	7	8	9	10	11	12	13	14	15	16	17	18	19	20	21	22	23	24
N	10	9	9	8	7	6	6	5	4	4	4	4	4	5	6	6	7	8	9	9	10	11	11	11
NE	12	11	10	9	8	7	6	6	6	6	7	8	9	11	12	12	13	13	13	14	14	13	13	13
E	14	13	12	11	9	8	7	6	6	7	8	11	12	14	16	17	17	17	18	18	17	17	16	15
SE	14	13	12	11	9	8	7	6	6	6	7	8	10	12	14	15	16	17	17	17	17	17	16	15
S	13	12	11	10	9	8	7	6	5	4	4	4	5	6	8	9	11	13	14	15	15	15	15	14
SW	18	17	16	14	13	11	10	8	7	7	6	6	6	6	7	8	10	12	15	17	18	19	19	19
W	20	18	17	16	14	12	11	9	8	7	7	6	6	6	7	8	9	11	14	17	19	21	21	21
NW	16	15	14	13	11	10	9	8	7	6	6	5	5	6	6	7	8	9	11	13	15	16	17	17

Note 1. Direct application of data

- Dark surface
- Indoor temperature of 25.5°C
- Outdoor maximum temperature of 35°C with mean temperature of 29.5°C and daily range of 11.6°C
- Solar radiation typical of clear day on 21st day of month
- Outside surface film resistance of 0.059 $m^2 \cdot K/W$
- Inside surface resistance of 0.121 $m^2 \cdot K/W$

Note 2. Adjustments to table data

- Design temperatures

$$\text{Corr. CLTD} = \text{CLTD} + (25.5 - t_r) + (t_m - 29.4)$$

where

t_r = inside temperature and

t_m = maximum outdoor temperature − (daily range)/2

- No adjustment recommended for color

Table 7-23 SI Thermal Properties and Code Numbers of Layers Used in Wall and Roof Descriptions, for Use with Table 7-22 SI

Code Number	Description	Thickness and Thermal Properties					
		L	k	ρ	c_p	R	Mass
A0	Outside surface resistance	0	0.000	0	0.00	0.059	0.00
A1	25 mm Stucco	25	0.692	1858	0.84	0.037	47.34
A2	100 mm Face brick	100	1.333	2002	0.92	0.076	203.50
A3	Steel siding	2	44.998	7689	0.42	0.000	11.71
A4	12 mm Slag	13	0.190	1121	1.67	0.067	10.74
A5	Outside surface resistance	0	0.000	0	0.00	0.059	0.00
A6	Finish	13	0.415	1249	1.09	0.031	16.10
A7	100 mm Face brick	100	1.333	2002	0.92	0.076	203.50
B1	Air space resistance	0	0.000	0	0.00	0.160	0.00
B2	25 mm Insulation	25	0.043	32	0.84	0.587	0.98
B3	50 mm Insulation	51	0.043	32	0.84	1.173	1.46
B4	75 mm Insulation	76	0.043	32	0.84	0.207	2.44
B5	25 mm Insulation	25	0.043	91	0.84	0.587	2.44
B6	50 mm Insulation	51	0.043	91	0.84	1.173	4.88
B7	25 mm Wood	25	0.121	593	2.51	1.760	15.13
B8	65 mm Wood	63	0.121	593	2.51	0.524	37.58
B9	100 mm Wood	100	0.121	593	2.51	0.837	60.02
B10	50 mm Wood	51	0.121	593	2.51	0.420	30.26
B11	75 mm Wood	76	0.121	593	2.51	0.628	45.38
B12	75 mm Insulation	76	0.043	91	0.84	1.760	6.83
B13	100 mm Insulation	100	0.043	91	0.84	2.347	9.27
B14	125 mm Insulation	125	0.043	91	0.84	2.933	11.71
B15	150 mm Insulation	150	0.043	91	0.84	3.520	14.15
B16	4 mm Insulation	4	0.043	91	0.84	0.088	0.49
B17	8 mm Insulation	8	0.043	91	0.84	0.176	0.49
B18	12 mm Insulation	12	0.043	91	0.84	0.264	0.98
B19	15 mm Insulation	15	0.043	91	0.84	0.352	1.46
B20	20 mm Insulation	20	0.043	91	0.84	0.440	1.95
B21	35 mm Insulation	35	0.043	91	0.84	0.792	2.93
B22	42 mm Insulation	42	0.043	91	0.84	0.968	3.90
B23	60 mm Insulation	62	0.043	91	0.84	1.408	5.86
B24	70 mm Insulation	70	0.043	91	0.84	1.584	6.34
B25	85 mm Insulation	85	0.043	91	0.84	1.936	7.81
B26	92 mm Insulation	92	0.043	91	0.84	2.112	8.30
B27	115 mm Insulation	115	0.043	91	0.84	2.640	10.74
C1	100 mm Clay tile	100	0.571	1121	0.84	0.178	113.70
C2	100 mm low density concrete block	100	0.381	609	0.84	0.266	61.98
C3	100 mm high density concrete block	100	0.813	977	0.84	0.125	99.06
C4	100 mm Common brick	100	0.727	1922	0.84	0.140	195.20
C5	100 mm high density concrete	100	1.731	2243	0.84	0.059	227.90
C6	200 mm Clay tile	200	0.571	1121	0.84	0.352	227.90
C7	200 mm low density concrete block	200	0.571	609	0.84	0.352	123.46
C8	200 mm high density concrete block	200	1.038	977	0.84	0.196	198.62
C9	200 mm Common brick	200	0.727	1922	0.84	0.279	390.40
C10	200 mm high density concrete	200	1.731	2243	0.84	0.117	455.79
C11	300 mm high density concrete	300	1.731	2243	0.84	0.176	683.20
C12	50 mm high density concrete	50	1.731	2243	0.84	0.029	113.70
C13	150 mm high density concrete	150	1.731	2243	0.84	0.088	341.60
C14	100 mm low density concrete	100	0.173	641	0.84	0.587	64.90
C15	150 mm low density concrete	150	0.173	641	0.84	0.880	97.60
C16	200 mm low density concrete	200	0.173	641	0.84	1.173	130.30
C17	200 mm low density concrete block (filled)	200	0.138	288	0.84	1.467	58.56
C18	200 mm high density concrete block (filled)	200	0.588	849	0.84	0.345	172.75
C19	300 mm low density concrete block (filled)	300	0.138	304	0.84	2.200	92.72
C20	300 mm high density concrete block (filled)	300	0.675	897	0.84	0.451	273.28
E0	Inside surface resistance	0	0.000	0	0.00	0.121	0.00
E1	20 mm Plaster or gypsum	20	0.727	1602	0.84	0.026	30.74
E2	12 mm Slag or stone	12	1.436	881	1.67	0.009	11.22
E3	10 mm Felt and membrane	10	0.190	1121	1.67	0.050	10.74
E4	Ceiling air space	0	0.000	0	0.00	0.176	0.00
E5	Acoustic tile	19	0.061	481	0.84	0.314	9.27

L = thickness, mm
k = thermal conductivity, W/(m·K)
ρ = density, kg/m^3
c_p = specific heat, kJ/(kg·K)
R = thermal resistance, (m^2·K)/W
Mass = mass per unit area, kg/m^2

Table 7-24A SI Wall Types, Mass Located Inside Insulation, for Use with Table 7-22 SI

Secondary Material	R-Value $m^2 \cdot K/W$	Principal Wall Material**														
		A1	A2	B7	B10	B9	C1	C2	C3	C4	C5	C6	C7	C8	C17	C18
Stucco and/or plaster	0 to 0.35	*	*	*	*	*	*	*	*	*	*	*	*	*	*	*
	0.35 to 0.44	*	5	*	*	*	*	*	*	*	5	*	*	*	*	*
	0.44 to 0.53	*	5	*	*	*	3	*	2	5	6	*	*	5	*	*
	0.53 to 0.62	*	5	*	*	*	4	2	2	5	6	*	*	6	*	*
	0.62 to 0.70	*	5	*	*	*	4	2	3	6	6	10	4	6	*	5
	0.70 to 0.84	*	6	*	*	*	5	2	4	6	6	11	5	10	*	10
	0.84 to 0.97	*	6	*	*	*	5	2	4	6	6	11	5	10	*	10
	0.97 to 1.14	*	6	*	*	*	5	2	5	10	7	12	5	11	*	10
	1.14 to 1.36	*	6	*	*	*	5	4	5	11	7	16	10	11	*	11
	1.36 to 1.59	*	6	*	*	*	5	4	5	11	7	*	10	11	*	11
	1.59 to 1.89	*	6	*	*	*	5	4	5	11	7	*	10	11	4	11
	1.89 to 2.24	*	6	*	*	*	5	4	5	11	11	*	10	11	4	11
	2.24 to 2.64	*	10	*	*	*	10	4	5	11	11	*	10	11	9	12
	2.64 to 3.08	*	10	*	*	*	10	5	5	11	11	*	11	12	10	16
	3.08 to 3.52	*	11	*	*	*	10	5	9	11	11	*	15	16	10	16
	3.52 to 4.05	*	11	*	*	*	10	9	9	16	11	*	15	16	10	16
	4.05 to 4.76	*	*	*	*	*	*	*	*	*	*	*	16	*	15	*
Steel or other light-weight siding	0 to 0.35	*	*	*	*	*	*	*	*	*	*	*	*	*	*	*
	0.35 to 0.44	*	3	*	*	*	*	*	2	3	5	*	*	*	*	*
	0.44 to 0.53	*	5	*	*	*	2	*	2	5	3	*	*	5	*	*
	0.53 to 0.62	*	5	*	*	*	3	1	2	5	5	*	*	5	*	*
	0.62 to 0.70	*	5	*	*	*	3	2	2	5	5	6	3	5	*	5
	0.70 to 0.84	*	6	*	*	*	4	2	2	5	5	10	4	6	*	5
	0.84 to 0.97	*	6	*	*	*	5	2	2	6	6	11	5	6	*	6
	0.97 to 1.14	*	6	*	*	*	5	2	3	6	6	11	5	6	*	6
	1.14 to 1.36	*	6	*	*	*	5	2	3	6	6	11	5	6	*	10
	1.36 to 1.59	*	6	*	*	*	5	2	3	6	6	12	5	6	*	11
	1.59 to 1.89	*	6	*	*	*	5	2	3	6	6	12	5	6	4	11
	1.89 to 2.24	*	6	*	*	*	5	2	3	6	7	12	6	11	4	11
	2.24 to 2.64	*	6	*	*	*	5	2	4	6	7	12	10	11	5	11
	2.64 to 3.08	*	10	*	*	*	6	4	4	10	7	*	10	11	9	11
	3.08 to 3.52	*	10	*	*	*	10	4	4	10	11	*	10	11	10	11
	3.52 to 4.05	*	11	*	*	*	10	4	5	11	11	*	10	11	10	16
	4.05 to 4.76	*	*	*	*	*	*	*	*	*	*	*	10	*	11	16
Face brick	0 to 0.35	*	*	*	*	*	*	*	*	*	*	*	*	*	*	*
	0.35 to 0.44	3	*	*	*	*	*	*	*	*	11	*	*	*	*	*
	0.44 to 0.53	5	11	*	*	*	*	*	6	11	12	*	*	*	*	*
	0.53 to 0.62	5	12	5	*	*	11	*	11	12	12	*	*	12	*	*
	0.62 to 0.70	5	12	6	*	*	12	6	12	12	13	*	*	12	*	*
	0.70 to 0.84	6	13	6	10	*	13	10	12	12	13	*	11	*	*	16
	0.84 to 0.97	6	13	6	11	*	*	11	12	13	13	*	16	*	*	*
	0.97 to 1.14	6	13	6	11	*	*	11	12	13	13	*	*	*	*	*
	1.14 to 1.36	6	13	6	11	*	*	11	13	*	13	*	*	*	*	*
	1.36 to 1.59	6	13	10	16	*	*	11	13	*	13	*	*	*	*	*
	1.59 to 1.89	6	14	10	16	*	*	11	13	*	14	*	*	*	16	*
	1.89 to 2.24	6	14	10	16	*	*	11	13	*	14	*	*	*	16	*
	2.24 to 2.64	6	*	11	16	*	*	12	13	*	*	*	*	*	*	*
	2.64 to 3.08	10	*	11	*	*	*	12	13	*	*	*	*	*	*	*
	3.08 to 3.52	10	*	11	*	*	*	16	*	*	*	*	*	*	*	*
	3.52 to 4.05	11	*	15	*	*	*	16	*	*	*	*	*	*	*	*
	4.05 to 4.76	*	*	*	*	*	*	16	*	*	*	*	*	*	*	*

*Denotes a wall that is not possible with the chosen set of parameters.
**See Table 11 for definition of Code letters

Table 7-24B SI Wall Types, Mass Evenly Distributed, for Use with Table 7-22 S

Secondary Material	R-Value $m^2 \cdot K/W$	Principal Wall Material** A1	A2	B7	B10	B9	C1	C2	C3	C4	C5	C6	C7	C8	C17	C18
Stucco and/or plaster	0 to 0.35	1	3	*	*	*	*	*	1	3	3	*	*	*	*	*
	0.35 to 0.44	1	3	1	*	*	2	*	2	4	4	*	*	5	*	*
	0.44 to 0.53	1	4	1	*	*	2	2	2	4	4	*	*	5	*	*
	0.53 to 0.62	1	*	1	*	*	2	2	*	*	*	10	4	5	*	4
	0.62 to 0.70	1	*	1	2	*	*	4	*	*	*	10	4	*	*	4
	0.70 to 0.84	1	*	1	2	*	*	*	*	*	*	10	4	*	*	4
	0.84 to 0.97	1	*	1	2	*	*	*	*	*	*	*	*	*	*	*
	0.97 to 1.14	1	*	2	4	10	*	*	*	*	*	*	*	*	*	*
	1.14 to 1.36	1	*	2	4	11	*	*	*	*	*	*	*	*	*	*
	1.36 to 1.59	1	*	2	4	16	*	*	*	*	*	*	*	*	*	*
	1.59 to 1.89	1	*	2	4	16	*	*	*	*	*	*	*	*	4	*
	1.89 to 2.24	1	*	2	5	*	*	*	*	*	*	*	*	*	4	*
	2.24 to 2.64	2	*	2	5	*	*	*	*	*	*	*	*	*	*	*
	2.64 to 3.08	2	*	2	5	*	*	*	*	*	*	*	*	*	*	*
	3.08 to 3.52	2	*	2	9	*	*	*	*	*	*	*	*	*	*	*
	3.52 to 4.05	2	*	4	9	*	*	*	*	*	*	*	*	*	*	*
	4.05 to 4.76	*	*	*	9	*	*	*	*	*	*	*	*	*	*	*
Steel or other light-weight siding	0 to 0.35	1	3	*	*	*	*	*	1	3	2	*	*	*	*	*
	0.35 to 0.44	1	3	1	*	*	2	*	1	3	2	*	*	3	*	*
	0.44 to 0.53	1	4	1	*	*	2	1	2	4	4	*	*	3	*	*
	0.53 to 0.62	1	*	1	*	*	4	1	*	*	*	5	2	4	*	4
	0.62 to 0.70	1	*	1	2	*	*	2	*	*	*	5	2	*	*	4
	0.70 to 0.84	1	*	1	2	*	*	*	*	*	*	10	4	*	*	4
	0.84 to 0.97	1	*	1	2	*	*	*	*	*	*	*	*	*	*	*
	0.97 to 1.14	1	*	1	2	10	*	*	*	*	*	*	*	*	*	*
	1.14 to 1.36	1	*	1	4	11	*	*	*	*	*	*	*	*	*	*
	1.36 to 1.59	1	*	2	4	16	*	*	*	*	*	*	*	*	*	*
	1.59 to 1.89	1	*	2	4	16	*	*	*	*	*	*	*	*	2	*
	1.89 to 2.24	1	*	2	4	*	*	*	*	*	*	*	*	*	4	*
	2.24 to 2.64	1	*	2	5	*	*	*	*	*	*	*	*	*	*	*
	2.64 to 3.08	1	*	2	5	*	*	*	*	*	*	*	*	*	*	*
	3.08 to 3.52	1	*	2	5	*	*	*	*	*	*	*	*	*	*	*
	3.52 to 4.05	2	*	4	9	*	*	*	*	*	*	*	*	*	*	*
	4.05 to 4.76	*	*	*	9	*	*	*	*	*	*	*	*	*	*	*
Face brick	0 to 0.35	3	6	*	*	*	*	*	*	*	6	*	*	*	*	*
	0.35 to 0.44	3	10	*	*	*	*	*	5	10	10	*	*	*	*	*
	0.44 to 0.53	4	10	5	*	*	5	*	5	10	11	*	*	10	*	*
	0.53 to 0.62	*	11	5	*	*	10	5	5	11	11	15	10	10	*	10
	0.62 to 0.70	*	11	5	10	*	10	5	5	11	11	16	10	16	*	10
	0.70 to 0.84	*	11	*	11	*	10	5	5	16	11	*	10	16	*	16
	0.84 to 0.97	*	11	*	11	*	10	5	10	16	16	*	10	16	*	16
	0.97 to 1.14	*	16	*	*	*	10	9	10	16	11	*	11	16	*	16
	1.14 to 1.36	*	16	*	*	*	11	9	10	16	16	*	16	16	*	*
	1.36 to 1.59	*	16	*	*	*	15	9	10	16	*	*	15	16	*	*
	1.59 to 1.89	*	16	*	*	*	15	10	10	*	16	*	16	*	10	*
	1.89 to 2.24	*	16	*	*	*	16	10	10	*	*	*	16	*	15	*
	2.24 to 2.64	*	16	*	*	*	16	10	10	*	16	*	*	*	15	*
	2.64 to 3.08	*	*	*	*	*	16	10	15	*	*	*	*	*	16	*
	3.08 to 3.52	*	*	*	*	*	16	15	15	*	*	*	*	*	16	*
	3.52 to 4.05	*	*	*	*	*	*	15	16	*	*	*	*	*	*	*
	4.05 to 4.76	*	*	*	*	*	*	15	*	*	*	*	*	*	*	*

*Denotes a wall that is not possible with the chosen set of parameters.
**See Table 11 for definition of Code letters

Table 7-24C SI Wall Types, Mass Located Outside Insulation, for Use with Table 7-22 SI

Secondary Material	R-Value, m²·K/W	Principal Wall Material**														
		A1	A2	B7	B10	B9	C1	C2	C3	C4	C5	C6	C7	C8	C17	C18
Stucco and/or plaster	0 to 0.35	*	*	*	*	*	*	*	*	*	*	*	*	*	*	*
	0.35 to 0.44	*	3	*	*	*	*	*	2	3	5	*	*	*	*	*
	0.44 to 0.53	*	3	*	*	*	2	*	2	4	5	*	*	5	*	*
	0.53 to 0.62	*	3	*	*	*	2	2	2	5	5	*	*	5	*	*
	0.62 to 0.70	*	3	*	*	*	2	2	2	5	5	10	4	6	*	5
	0.70 to 0.84	*	4	*	*	*	4	2	2	5	5	10	4	6	*	9
	0.84 to 0.97	*	4	*	*	*	4	2	2	5	6	11	5	10	*	10
	0.97 to 1.14	*	5	*	*	*	4	2	2	5	6	11	5	10	*	10
	1.14 to 1.36	*	5	*	*	*	4	2	2	5	6	11	5	10	*	10
	1.36 to 1.59	*	5	*	*	*	5	2	4	5	6	16	10	10	*	10
	1.59 to 1.89	*	5	*	*	*	5	4	4	5	6	16	10	10	4	11
	1.89 to 2.24	*	5	*	*	*	5	4	4	10	6	16	10	10	9	11
	2.24 to 2.64	*	5	*	*	*	5	4	4	10	10	*	10	11	9	11
	2.64 to 3.08	*	5	*	*	*	5	4	4	10	10	*	10	11	10	16
	3.08 to 3.52	*	5	*	*	*	9	4	4	10	10	*	10	15	10	16
	3.52 to 4.05	*	9	*	*	*	9	9	9	15	10	*	10	15	15	16
	4.05 to 4.76	*	*	*	*	*	*	*	*	*	*	*	15	*	15	16
Steel or other light-weight siding	0 to 0.35	*	*	*	*	*	*	*	*	*	*	*	*	*	*	*
	0.35 to 0.44	*	3	*	*	*	*	*	2	3	2	*	*	*	*	*
	0.44 to 0.53	*	3	*	*	*	2	*	2	3	2	*	*	*	*	*
	0.53 to 0.62	*	3	*	*	*	2	1	2	4	3	*	*	4	*	*
	0.62 to 0.70	*	3	*	*	*	2	2	2	4	3	5	2	5	*	4
	0.70 to 0.84	*	3	*	*	*	2	2	2	4	3	10	3	5	*	5
	0.84 to 0.97	*	3	*	*	*	2	2	2	5	3	10	4	5	*	5
	0.97 to 1.14	*	4	*	*	*	2	2	2	5	3	10	4	5	*	5
	1.14 to 1.36	*	4	*	*	*	2	2	2	5	4	11	5	5	*	6
	1.36 to 1.59	*	5	*	*	*	2	2	2	5	4	11	5	5	*	6
	1.59 to 1.89	*	5	*	*	*	2	2	2	5	4	11	5	5	4	10
	1.89 to 2.24	*	5	*	*	*	4	2	2	5	5	11	5	5	4	10
	2.24 to 2.64	*	5	*	*	*	4	2	2	5	5	11	5	10	5	10
	2.64 to 3.08	*	5	*	*	*	4	2	4	5	5	16	9	10	9	10
	3.08 to 3.52	*	5	*	*	*	4	4	4	9	5	16	9	10	10	10
	3.52 to 4.05	*	9	*	*	*	4	4	4	9	9	16	10	10	10	11
	4.05 to 4.76	*	*	*	*	*	*	*	*	*	*	16	10	*	10	15
Face brick	0 to 0.35	*	*	*	*	*	*	*	*	*	*	*	*	*	*	*
	0.35 to 0.44	3	*	*	*	*	*	*	*	*	11	*	*	*	*	*
	0.44 to 0.53	3	10	*	*	*	*	*	5	10	11	*	*	*	*	*
	0.53 to 0.62	3	11	5	*	*	10	*	5	11	11	*	*	11	*	*
	0.62 to 0.70	3	11	5	*	*	10	5	6	11	11	*	*	11	*	*
	0.70 to 0.84	3	11	5	10	*	10	5	10	11	11	*	10	11	*	16
	0.84 to 0.97	3	12	5	10	*	10	9	10	11	12	*	11	16	*	16
	0.97 to 1.14	4	12	5	10	*	10	10	10	12	12	*	15	16	*	16
	1.14 to 1.36	4	12	5	10	*	11	10	10	12	12	*	16	*	*	16
	1.36 to 1.59	5	12	5	15	*	11	10	10	16	12	*	16	*	*	*
	1.59 to 1.89	5	12	9	15	*	11	10	10	16	12	*	16	*	15	*
	1.89 to 2.24	5	12	10	15	*	11	10	10	*	12	*	16	*	15	*
	2.24 to 2.64	5	*	10	16	*	11	10	11	*	*	*	16	*	15	*
	2.64 to 3.08	5	*	10	16	*	15	10	11	*	*	*	16	*	*	*
	3.08 to 3.52	5	*	10	16	*	16	15	15	*	*	*	*	*	*	*
	3.52 to 4.05	9	*	15	16	*	16	15	15	*	*	*	*	*	*	*
	4.05 to 4.76	*	*	*	*	*	*	15	*	*	*	*	*	*	*	*

*Denotes a wall that is not possible with the chosen set of parameters.
**See Table 11 for definition of Code letters

Table 7-25 SI Cooling Load Temperature Differences (CLTD) for Conduction Through Glass

Solar Time, h	CLTD, °C	Solar Time, h	CLTD, °C
0100	1	1300	7
0200	0	1400	7
0300	−1	1500	8
0400	−1	1600	8
0500	−1	1700	7
0600	−1	1800	7
0700	−1	1900	6
0800	0	2000	4
0900	1	2100	3
1000	2	2200	2
1100	4	2300	2
1200	5	2400	1

Corrections: The values in the table were calculated for an inside temperature of 25.5°C and an outdoor maximum temperature of 35°C with an outdoor daily range of 11.6°C. The table remains approximately correct for other outdoor maximums 33 to 39°C and other outdoor daily ranges 9 to 19°C, provided the outdoor daily average temperature remains approximately 29.5°C. If the room air temperature is different from 25.5°C and/or the outdoor daily average temperature is different from 29.5°C see note 2, Table 32.

Table 7-26 SI Zone Types for Use With CLF Tables, Interior Rooms

Zone Parameters[a]				Zone Type	
Room Location	Middle Floor	Ceiling Type	Floor Covering	People and Equipment	Lights
Single story	N/A	N/A	Carpet	C	B
	N/A	N/A	Vinyl	D	C
Top floor	65 mm Concrete	With	Carpet	D	C
	65 mm Concrete	With	Vinyl	D	D
	65 mm Concrete	Without	b	D	B
	25 mm Wood	b	b	D	B
Bottom floor	65 mm Concrete	With	Carpet	D	C
	65 mm Concrete	b	Vinyl	D	D
	65 mm Concrete	Without	Carpet	D	D
	25 mm Wood	b	Carpet	D	C
	25 mm Wood	b	Vinyl	D	D
Mid-floor	65 mm Concrete	N/A	Carpet	D	C
	65 mm Concrete	N/A	Vinyl	D	D
	25 mm Wood	N/A	b	C	B

[a]A total of 14 zone parameters is fully defined in Table 20. Those not shown in this table were selected to achieve an error band of approximately 10%.

[b]The effect of this parameter is negligible in this case.

Table 7-27 SI July Solar Cooling Load For Sunlit Glass 40° North Latitude

Zone Type A

Glass Face	Hour 1	2	3	4	5	6	7	8	9	10	11	12	13	14	15	16	17	18	19	20	21	22	23	24
												Solar Time												
N	0	0	0	0	3	79	85	88	101	110	120	126	126	123	113	98	98	113	38	19	9	3	3	0
NE	0	0	0	0	6	268	406	422	353	236	173	151	139	126	117	101	82	57	22	9	6	3	0	0
E	0	0	0	0	6	293	495	583	576	485	334	211	167	142	123	104	82	57	22	9	6	3	0	0
SE	0	0	0	0	3	148	299	413	473	473	413	306	198	154	129	107	85	57	22	9	6	3	0	0
S	0	0	0	0	0	28	54	79	129	202	268	306	302	265	198	132	98	63	25	13	6	3	0	0
SW	0	0	0	0	0	28	54	76	95	110	123	202	318	419	476	479	419	293	110	54	25	13	6	3
W	3	0	0	0	0	28	54	76	95	110	120	126	205	359	498	589	605	491	180	85	41	19	9	6
NW	3	0	0	0	0	28	54	76	95	110	120	126	126	158	265	381	450	410	145	69	35	16	9	3
Hor	0	0	0	0	0	76	217	378	532	665	759	810	816	772	684	554	394	221	91	44	22	9	6	3

Zone Type B

Glass Face	Hour 1	2	3	4	5	6	7	8	9	10	11	12	13	14	15	16	17	18	19	20	21	22	23	24
												Solar Time												
N	6	6	3	3	3	69	72	76	88	101	110	117	120	117	110	101	98	110	50	32	22	16	13	9
NE	6	3	3	3	6	230	343	365	318	230	183	164	151	142	129	113	95	72	41	28	19	16	9	9
E	6	6	3	3	6	252	419	501	510	450	331	233	198	173	151	129	107	79	47	32	22	16	13	9
SE	6	6	3	3	3	126	255	353	413	422	384	302	217	183	154	132	110	82	47	32	25	19	13	9
S	6	6	3	3	3	25	47	66	113	176	233	271	274	249	198	145	117	85	50	35	25	19	13	9
SW	19	16	13	9	6	28	50	69	85	98	113	183	280	369	425	435	397	296	145	98	66	47	35	25
W	25	19	16	13	9	28	50	69	85	98	110	117	186	318	438	523	545	463	208	135	95	66	47	35
NW	19	16	13	9	6	28	50	69	85	98	107	117	117	145	239	340	403	375	161	104	69	50	35	25
Hor	25	19	16	13	9	69	189	328	463	583	674	734	753	731	668	567	432	284	167	117	85	60	44	35

Zone Type C

Glass Face	Hour 1	2	3	4	5	6	7	8	9	10	11	12	13	14	15	16	17	18	19	20	21	22	23	24
												Solar Time												
N	16	16	13	13	13	76	72	76	85	95	104	107	110	107	101	91	91	107	44	32	25	22	19	19
NE	22	19	19	16	19	236	334	337	277	192	154	148	142	135	126	113	98	79	50	41	35	32	28	25
E	28	25	25	22	25	261	410	466	457	391	280	195	176	164	148	135	117	95	63	54	47	41	38	35
SE	28	25	22	19	19	142	258	337	381	381	337	258	186	161	148	132	113	91	60	50	44	41	35	32
S	22	22	19	16	16	38	57	72	113	170	221	249	249	221	170	126	104	82	50	41	38	32	28	25
SW	44	38	35	32	28	47	66	82	91	104	113	180	271	347	391	394	350	252	117	88	72	63	54	47
W	54	47	41	38	35	54	69	85	98	107	113	117	186	309	416	482	491	403	158	110	88	76	66	60
NW	38	35	32	28	25	44	63	79	91	101	107	113	113	139	230	321	372	337	123	82	66	54	47	41
Hor	76	66	60	54	50	107	214	337	454	551	627	668	677	652	595	504	387	261	167	139	120	107	95	85

Zone Type D

Glass Face	Hour 1	2	3	4	5	6	7	8	9	10	11	12	13	14	15	16	17	18	19	20	21	22	23	24
												Solar Time												
N	25	22	19	19	19	66	66	66	76	85	91	98	101	98	95	88	91	101	54	44	38	35	32	28
NE	35	32	28	25	28	198	274	284	243	183	154	151	145	139	132	123	110	91	69	60	54	47	44	38
E	47	41	38	35	35	221	337	387	391	347	268	205	189	180	167	151	135	117	91	79	69	63	57	50
SE	44	41	35	32	32	123	214	284	321	328	299	246	189	173	161	148	132	110	85	76	66	60	54	50
S	35	32	28	25	22	38	54	66	101	145	186	211	217	198	164	129	113	95	69	60	54	47	44	38
SW	66	60	54	47	44	57	69	79	88	98	107	161	233	296	334	343	315	246	142	117	104	91	82	72
W	79	72	63	57	54	66	76	88	95	104	107	110	167	265	353	410	425	365	180	145	123	110	98	88
NW	57	50	47	41	38	54	66	76	85	95	101	104	107	129	202	274	318	296	132	104	91	79	69	63
Hor	117	104	95	85	76	120	202	299	391	473	539	583	602	592	554	491	403	302	227	198	176	158	142	129

Notes:

1. Values are in W/m^2.
2. Apply data directly to standard double strength glass with no inside shade.
3. Data applies to 21st day of July.
4. For other types of glass and internal shade, use shading coefficients as multiplier. See text. For externally shaded glass, use north orientation. See text.

Table 7-32 SI CLTD Values for Single Family Residence[a]

Daily Temperature Range[b]	Design Temperature, °C											
	29		32			35			38		41	43
	L	M	L	M	H	L	M	H	M	H	M	H
All walls and doors												
North	4	2	7	4	2	10	7	4	10	7	10	13
NE and NW	8	5	11	8	5	13	11	8	13	11	13	16
East and West	10	7	13	10	7	16	13	10	16	13	16	18
SE and SW	9	6	12	9	6	14	12	9	14	12	14	17
South	6	3	9	6	3	12	9	6	12	9	12	14
Roofs and ceilings												
Attic or flat built-up	23	21	26	23	21	28	26	23	28	26	28	31
Floors and ceilings												
Under conditioned space, over unconditioned room, over crawl space	5	2	7	5	2	8	7	5	8	7	8	11
Partitions												
Inside or shaded	5	2	7	5	2	8	7	5	8	7	8	11

[a]Cooling load temperature differences (CLTDs) for single-family detached houses, duplexes, or multifamily, with both east and west exposed walls or only north and south exposed walls, K.

[b]L denotes low daily range, less than 9 K; M denotes medium daily range, 9 to 14 K; and H denotes high daily range, greater than 14 K.

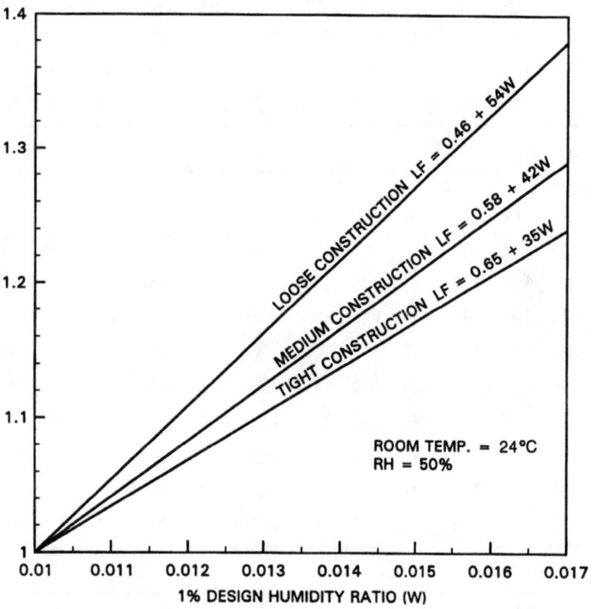

Fig. 7-6 SI Effect of Infltration on Latent Load Factor

Table 7-33 SI CLTD Values for Multifamily Residences[a]

Daily Temperature Range[b]		Design Temperature, °C											
		29		32			35			38		41	43
		L	M	L	M	H	L	M	H	M	H	M	H
Walls and doors[c]													
N	Low	8	6	11	9	7	13	12	9	14	12	15	18
	Medium	7	6	10	8	6	13	11	9	14	12	14	17
	High	5	3	8	6	4	11	9	7	12	9	12	15
NE	Low	13	9	16	12	9	18	15	12	18	14	17	20
	Medium	11	8	14	11	9	17	14	12	16	14	16	19
	High	9	7	12	9	7	14	12	10	14	12	14	17
E	Low	18	15	21	18	15	24	21	18	23	21	23	26
	Medium	17	13	19	16	13	22	19	16	22	18	22	24
	High	13	10	16	13	10	19	16	13	18	16	18	21
SE	Low	17	15	19	17	14	23	21	17	23	21	23	26
	Medium	16	12	18	15	12	21	18	15	21	18	21	24
	High	12	9	14	12	9	18	15	12	17	15	18	21
S	Low	14	12	16	14	12	19	17	14	20	18	21	24
	Medium	12	10	14	12	10	17	14	12	17	15	18	21
	High	9	6	11	9	7	14	12	9	14	12	15	18
SW	Low	22	20	24	22	19	28	26	22	28	26	29	32
	Medium	18	16	21	19	16	24	22	19	25	22	26	29
	High	13	10	16	13	11	20	17	14	19	17	20	23
W	Low	24	23	27	25	22	30	28	26	31	29	32	35
	Medium	21	18	23	21	18	26	23	21	27	24	27	31
	High	14	12	17	15	13	21	18	15	21	18	21	24
NW	Low	18	17	21	19	17	24	22	19	24	22	25	28
	Medium	16	14	18	16	13	21	18	16	22	19	22	25
	High	11	9	14	11	9	17	14	12	17	14	18	21
Roof and ceiling													
Attic or flat built-up	Light	32	29	36	33	31	39	36	33	39	36	40	43
Flat built-up	Medium or heavy	12	10	13	12	10	14	13	12	14	13	14	16
Floors and ceiling													
Under or over unconditioned space, crawl space		5	2	7	5	2	8	7	5	8	7	8	11
Partitions													
Inside or shaded		5	2	7	5	2	8	7	5	8	7	8	11

[a]Cooling load temperature differences (CLTDs) for multifamily low-rise or single-family detached if zoned with separate temperature control for each zone, K.

[b]L denotes low daily range, less than 9 K; M denotes medium daily range, 9 to 14 K; and H denotes high daily range, greater than 14 K.

[c]Low denotes low-density; medium denotes medium-density; and high denotes high-density construction.

Table 7-34 SI Window Glass Load Factors (GLFs) for Single-Family Residences[a]

Design Temperature, °C	Regular Single Glass						Regular Double Glass						Heat-Absorbing Double Glass						Clear Triple Glass		
	29	32	35	38	41	43	29	32	35	38	41	43	29	32	35	38	41	43	29	32	35
No inside shading																					
North	107	114	129	148	151	158	95	95	107	117	120	129	63	63	73	79	82	88	85	85	95
NE and NW	199	205	221	237	243	262	173	177	186	196	199	208	114	117	123	132	139	139	158	158	167
East and West	278	284	300	315	322	337	243	246	255	265	268	278	161	161	170	177	186	186	221	221	230
SE and SW[b]	249	255	271	287	290	309	218	221	230	240	243	252	142	145	155	161	170	170	196	199	205
South[b]	167	173	189	205	211	227	145	148	158	167	170	180	98	98	107	114	123	123	132	132	142
Horizontal skylight	492	492	508	524	527	539	432	435	442	451	454	464	284	287	293	300	303	309	391	394	401
Draperies, venetian blinds, translucent roller shades, fully drawn																					
North	57	60	73	85	91	104	50	50	60	69	73	82	41	44	50	57	60	66	47	50	57
NE and NW	101	104	120	132	136	148	91	95	101	110	114	123	76	76	85	91	91	101	88	88	95
East and West	142	145	158	170	173	186	126	129	139	145	148	158	104	104	114	120	120	129	123	123	129
SE and SW[b]	126	129	145	155	161	173	114	117	123	132	136	145	91	95	101	107	110	117	110	114	120
South[b]	85	88	104	117	120	132	76	79	88	98	98	107	63	66	73	79	82	88	73	76	82
Horizontal skylight	246	249	262	271	274	284	224	224	233	240	243	249	183	186	192	199	199	205	218	218	224
Opaque roller shades, fully drawn																					
North	44	47	63	73	79	91	41	44	54	60	63	73	38	38	47	54	54	63	41	41	47
NE and NW	79	82	98	107	114	126	73	76	85	95	95	104	66	69	76	82	85	91	73	73	82
East and West	107	114	126	139	142	155	101	104	114	120	123	132	91	95	101	107	110	117	101	101	110
SE and SW[b]	98	101	114	126	132	145	91	95	104	110	114	123	82	85	91	98	101	107	91	91	98
South[b]	66	69	85	95	101	114	63	63	73	82	85	95	57	60	66	73	76	82	60	63	69
Horizontal skylight	189	192	202	214	218	227	180	180	189	196	199	205	164	164	173	180	180	186	177	180	186

[a]Glass load factors (GLFs) for single-family detached houses, duplexes, or multifamily residences, with both east and west exposed walls or only north and south exposed walls, W/m^2.

[b]Correct by +30% for latitude of 48° and by −30% for latitude of 32°. Use linear interpolation for latitude from 40 to 48 and from 40 to 32°.

To obtain GLF for other combinations of glass and/or inside shading: $GLF_a = (SC_a/SC_t)(GLF_t - U_tD_t) + U_aD_t$, where the subscripts a and t refer to the alternate and table values, respectively. SC_t and U_t are given in Table 5. $D_t = (t_a - 24)$, where $t_a = t_o - (DR/2)$; t_o is the outdoor design temperature and DR is the daily range.

Table 7-35 SI Window Glass Load Factors (GLFs) for Multifamily Residences[a]

Design Temperature, °C	Regular Single Glass						Regular Double Glass						Heat-Absorbing Double Glass						Clear Triple Glass		
	29	32	35	38	41	43	29	32	35	38	41	43	29	32	35	38	41	43	29	32	35
No inside shading																					
North	126	139	155	170	183	202	107	114	123	132	139	148	73	76	82	91	95	104	95	101	107
NE	278	281	287	300	306	315	246	249	252	262	265	268	164	164	167	173	173	180	224	224	230
East	429	432	438	448	454	464	378	382	385	394	397	401	249	249	255	262	262	265	344	344	350
SE	407	410	423	438	445	454	344	356	366	375	378	385	227	237	243	249	249	255	312	325	331
South[b]	278	287	303	319	331	347	240	246	255	265	271	281	158	164	170	177	183	189	214	221	227
SW	486	501	517	533	549	565	423	432	442	451	457	467	281	287	293	300	306	312	382	388	394
West	549	561	577	593	606	621	476	486	495	505	511	520	315	322	328	334	341	347	432	438	445
NW	388	401	416	432	445	464	337	344	353	363	369	382	224	227	237	243	249	255	303	309	315
Horizontal	785	795	807	823	833	845	688	694	703	713	719	725	454	460	467	473	479	486	624	631	637
Draperies, venetian blinds, translucent roller shades, fully drawn																					
North	66	79	91	104	114	126	57	66	73	82	88	98	47	54	60	66	73	79	54	60	66
NE	136	139	145	158	161	164	123	126	129	139	142	145	104	104	107	114	114	117	123	123	126
East	211	214	221	233	237	240	192	196	199	205	208	211	158	158	161	170	170	173	189	189	192
SE	202	205	218	230	233	243	183	186	192	199	202	208	151	151	158	164	164	170	180	180	186
South[b]	142	151	164	177	186	199	126	132	139	148	155	164	104	107	114	123	126	132	120	126	132
SW	249	262	274	287	296	309	221	227	237	246	252	262	180	186	196	202	208	214	214	218	224
West	281	290	303	315	325	337	249	255	265	271	278	287	205	208	218	224	227	237	240	246	252
NW	199	208	221	233	243	255	177	183	192	199	208	214	145	151	158	164	170	177	170	173	180
Horizontal	397	404	416	426	432	445	356	363	369	378	382	391	293	296	303	309	315	322	347	350	356
Opaque roller shades, fully drawn																					
North	54	66	79	91	101	114	47	54	63	73	79	88	44	47	57	63	69	76	47	50	57
NE	104	107	110	123	126	132	98	101	104	114	110	117	91	88	95	101	101	107	101	98	104
East	161	164	167	180	192	205	151	155	158	167	164	173	142	142	145	151	151	155	155	155	158
SE	155	158	167	180	183	192	145	148	155	164	164	173	132	136	142	148	148	155	145	145	151
South[b]	110	120	132	145	155	167	101	107	117	126	132	132	91	98	104	110	117	123	101	104	110
SW	192	205	218	230	243	255	180	186	196	205	211	221	164	170	177	183	189	196	177	183	189
West	214	224	237	252	262	274	202	208	214	224	230	240	183	189	196	202	208	214	199	202	208
NW	155	164	177	189	199	211	142	148	158	167	173	183	129	136	142	148	155	161	142	145	151
Horizontal	306	312	322	334	341	350	287	293	300	306	312	322	262	268	274	281	284	290	284	290	293

[a]Glass load factors (GLFs) for multifamily low-rise or single-family detached residences if zoned with separate temperature control for each zone, W/m^2.

[b]Correct by +30% for latitude of 48° and by −30% for latitude of 32°. Use linear interpolation for latitude from 40 to 48 and from 40 to 32°.

To obtain GLF for other combinations of glass and/or inside shading: $GLF_a = (SC_a/SC_t)(GLF_t - U_tD_t) + U_aD_t$, where the subscripts a and t refer to the alternate and table values, respectively. SC_t and U_t are given in Table 5. $D_t = (t_a - 24)$, where $t_a = t_o - (DR/2)$; t_o is the outdoor design temperature and DR is the daily range.

Table 7-36 SI Shading Coefficients and U-Factors for Residential Windows

	Inside Shade					
	None		Drapery, Venetian Blind, or Translucent Roller Shade		Opaque Roller Shade	
Glass Type	SC	*U*	SC	*U*	SC	*U*
Single	1.00	5.91	0.50	4.60	0.38	4.60
Double	0.88	3.46	0.45	3.12	0.36	3.12
Heat-absorbing	0.58	2.56	0.37	2.50	0.33	2.50
Triple	0.80	2.50	0.44	2.27	0.36	2.27

Note: *U* is in W/(m^2·K).

Table 7-37 SI Shade Line Factors (SLFs)

Direction Window Faces	Latitude, Degrees N						
	24	32	36	40	44	48	52
East	0.8	0.8	0.8	0.8	0.8	0.8	0.8
SE	1.8	1.6	1.4	1.3	1.1	1.0	0.9
South	9.2	5.0	3.4	2.6	2.1	1.8	1.5
SW	1.8	1.6	1.4	1.3	1.1	1.0	0.9
West	0.8	0.8	0.8	0.8	0.8	0.8	0.8

Note: Shadow length below the overhang equals the shade line factor times the overhang width. Values are averages for the 5 h of greatest solar intensity on August 1.

Table 7-38 SI Summer Exchange Rates (ACH) as Function of Airtightness

Class	Outdoor Design Temperature, °C					
	29	32	35	38	41	43
Tight	0.33	0.34	0.35	0.36	0.37	0.38
Medium	0.46	0.48	0.50	0.52	0.54	0.56
Loose	0.68	0.70	0.72	0.74	0.76	0.78

Note: Values are for 3.4 m/s (12 km/h) wind and indoor temperature of 24 °C.

Table 7-39 SI Summary of Procedures for Residential Cooling Load Calculations

Load Source	Equation	Tables and Notes
Glass and window areas	$q = (\text{GLF})A$	Glass load factors may be found in Tables 3 and 4 according to window orientation, type of glass, type of interior shading, and outdoor design temperature. The GLF includes effects of both transmission and solar radiation. Glass shaded by overhangs is treated as north glass. Table 6 gives shade line factors.
Doors	$q = U_d A(\text{CLTD})$	Door CLTD values are in Tables 1 and 2 according to orientation, outdoor design temperature, and design daily temperature range.
Above-grade exterior walls	$q = U_w A(\text{CLTD})$	Wall CLTD values are in Tables 1 and 2 based on the outdoor design temperature, daily range, and orientation.
Partitions to unconditioned space	$q = U_p A \Delta t$	Where Δt is the temperature difference across the partition.
Ceilings and roofs	$q = U_r A(\text{CLTD})$	Tables 1 and 2 for CLTD, based on outdoor design temperature and daily range.
Exposed floors	$q = U_f A(\text{CLTD})$	Tables 1 and 2 for CLTD, based on outdoor design temperature and daily range.
Infiltration	$q = 1.2Q\Delta t$ $Q = \text{ACH} \times (\text{room volume}) \times 1000/3600$	Air exchange rates are given in Tables 7 and 8.
Internal loads— People, appliances, lights	Plan 67 W per person.	Divide occupants evenly among rooms not used as bedrooms. If number of occupants is not known, assume two people for first bedroom and one person for each additional bedroom. The appliance and light load of 470 W is divided between the kitchen and adjoining room and the laundry and adjoining room. Use 350 W for multifamily units.
Total loads	Total cooling load = LF × (Sum of individual sensible cooling load components)	Load factors are from Figure 1 according to outdoor design humidity ratio and airtightness classification.

q = sensible cooling load, W
Δt = design temperature difference between outside and inside air, K
A = area of applicable surface, m^2
U = U-factors for appropriate construction, W/(m^2·K)
Q = volumetric airflow rate, L/s
ACH = air changes per hour, 1/h
GLF = glass load factor, W/m^2
CLTD = cooling load temperature difference, K
LF = latent load multiplier

Chapter 8

ENERGY ESTIMATING METHODS

This chapter discusses general techniques, as well as several simplified methods, for estimating the energy consumption of heating and cooling systems, including the variable-base degree-day and the bin concepts. Details of the more complete and sophisticated procedures may be found in Chapter 30, Energy Estimating and Modeling Methods, of the 1997 *ASHRAE Handbook—Fundamentals*.

8.1 General Considerations

The energy requirements and fuel consumption of building HVAC systems have a direct impact on the cost of operating a building and an indirect impact on the environment. This chapter takes an introductory look at methods for estimating energy use as a guide in design, for standards/code compliance, and for economic optimization. These energy estimating methods can provide quantitative energy and cost comparisons among design alternatives. A primary objective of building energy analysis is economic—to determine which of the available options has the lowest total (life cycle) cost. Several building energy codes and standards allow the use of an energy analysis to demonstrate compliance with the energy performance goals in the code. In fact, this use of energy analysis programs may be more prevalent than actual comparative energy studies. The large number of uncontrolled and/or unknown factors related to actual building use and HVAC system control generally preclude the use of such methods for determining absolute energy consumption and should not be used to predict future energy bills.

Often, the energy requirements and fuel consumption of environmental control systems must be estimated for either short- or long-term operation. The most direct and reliable energy estimating procedure requires hourly integration of various loads as a function of weather, use schedules, and control systems.

Although the procedures used for estimating energy requirements vary widely in their degree of complexity, they share three elements. These elements are the calculation of: (1) space load; (2) secondary equipment load; and (3) primary equipment energy requirements. *Secondary* refers to equipment that distributes the heating, cooling, or ventilating medium to the conditioned spaces; *primary* refers to the central plant equipment that converts fuel or electric energy for heating or cooling.

The **first step** in calculating energy requirements is to determine the **space load**, which is the amount of energy that must be added to or extracted from a space to maintain thermal comfort. The simplest procedures assume that the energy required to maintain comfort is a function of a single parameter—the outdoor dry-bulb temperature. More accurate methods consider solar effects, internal gains, heat storage in the walls and interiors, and the effects of wind on both the building envelope heat transfer and infiltration. The most sophisticated procedures are based on hourly profiles for climatic conditions and operational characteristics for a number of typical days of the year or a full 8760 hours of operation.

The **second step** translates the space load into a load on the **secondary system** equipment. This step must include calculation of all forms of energy required by the secondary system, which may include electrical energy to operate fans and/or pumps, as well as energy in the form of heated or chilled water.

The **third step** calculates the fuel and energy required by the **primary equipment** to meet these loads. It considers efficiencies and part-load characteristics of the equipment. Often, the different forms of energy, such as electricity, natural gas, or oil, must be tracked. In some cases where calculations are done to assure compliance with codes or standards, these energies must be converted to the energy source or resource consumed, as opposed to that delivered to the building boundary.

Energy calculations often lead to an economic analysis that aims to establish the cost effectiveness of conservation measures. Thus, a thorough energy analysis provides intermediate data, such as time of energy usage and maximum demand, so that utility charges can be accurately estimated. Although not part of the energy calculations, estimated capital equipment costs should be included in the complete analysis.

The sophistication of the calculation procedure used can often be inferred from the number of separate ambient conditions and/or time increments used in the calculations. A simple procedure may use only one measure, such as annual degree-days, and is appropriate only for simple systems and applications. Such methods are called *single-method measures*. Improved accuracy may be obtained by using more information, such as the number of hours anticipated under particular conditions of operation. These methods, of which the *bin method* is the most well known, are called *simplified multiple-measure methods*. The most elaborate methods perform energy balance calculations at each hour over some period of analysis, typically one year. These *detailed simulation methods* require hourly weather data, as well as hourly estimates of internal loads such as lighting and occupants.

Because systems that consume energy in buildings are nonlinear, dynamic, and very complex, few methods other than **computer modeling** are available for accurately calculating energy consumption. The most accurate methods for calculating building energy consumption are the most costly because of their intense computational requirements and high degree of user expertise. However, the cost of the computer facilities and the software itself are typically a small fraction of the total cost of running a building energy analysis. The major costs are for learning to use the program and for the time involved in using it.

8.2 Component Modeling and Loads

8.2.1 Loads

After peak loads have been evaluated, equipment with capacity sufficient to offset these loads must be selected. Air supplied to the space must be at the proper conditions to satisfy both the sensible and latent loads. However, peak load occurs but a few times each year, whereas partial load operation exists most of the time. With operation predominately at part load, partial load analysis for energy use and fuel cost is often as important as the sizing procedure.

Calculating instantaneous space load is a key step in any building energy simulation. The **heat balance method** and the **weighing factor method** are two methods used for these calculations. The weighing factor method and the heat balance method use conduction transfer functions (or their equivalents) to calculate transmission heat gain or loss. The principal difference is in the methods used to calculate the subsequent internal heat transfers to the room. Experience with both methods has indicated largely the same results, provided the weighing factors are determined for the specific building under analysis.

8.2.2 Secondary System Components

Secondary HVAC systems generally include all elements of the overall building energy system between a central heating and cooling plant and the building zones. The precise definition depends heavily on the building design. A secondary system typically includes air handling equipment, air distribution systems with the associated ductwork, dampers, fans, and heating, cooling, and humidity conditioning equipment. Secondary systems also include the liquid distribution systems between the central plant and the zone and air handling equipment, including piping, valves, and pumps.

To the extent that the secondary system consumes energy and transfers energy between the building and central plant, and energy analysis can be performed by characterizing the energy consumption of the individual components and the energy transferred among system components. In fact, few of the secondary components consume energy directly, except fans, pumps, furnaces, direct-expansion air-conditioning package units with gas fired heaters, and inline heaters. Secondary components are divided into two categories: distribution components and heat and mass transfer components.

The distribution system of an HVAC system affects energy consumption in two ways. First fans and pumps consume electrical energy directly, based on the flow and pressures under which the device operates. Ducts and dampers, or pipes and valves, and the system control strategies affect the flow and pressures at the fan. Second, thermal energy is often transferred to (or from) the fluid due to heat transfer through pipes and ducts and due to the electrical input to fans and pumps. The analysis of system components should, therefore, account for both direct electrical energy consumption and thermal energy transfer.

Strictly speaking, performance calculations of the fan and air distribution systems in a building require a detailed pressure balance on the entire network.

While a detailed analysis of a distribution system requires flow and pressure balancing among the components, nearly all commercially-available energy analysis methods approximate the effect of the interactions with part-load performance curves. This procedure eliminates the need to calculate pressure drop through the distribution system at off-design conditions. The exact shape of the part-load curve depends on the effect of flow control on the pressure and fan efficiency, and may be calculated using a detailed analysis.

8.2.3 Primary System Components

Primary HVAC systems consume energy and deliver heating and cooling to a building, usually through secondary systems. Primary equipment generally includes chillers, boilers, cooling towers, cogeneration equipment, and plant-level thermal storage equipment. In particular, primary equipment generally represents the major energy-consuming equipment of a building, so accurate characterization of building energy use relies on accurate modeling of primary equipment energy consumption.

The energy consumption characteristics of primary equipment generally depend on equipment design, load conditions, environmental conditions, and equipment control strategies. For example, chiller performance depends on the basic equipment design features (e.g., heat exchange surfaces, compressor design), the temperatures and flow through the condenser and evaporator, and the methods for controlling the chiller at different loads and operating conditions (e.g., inlet guide vane control on centrifugal chillers to maintain leaving chilled water temperature setpoint). In general, these variables that dictate energy consumption vary constantly and require calculations on an hourly basis.

While many secondary components are readily described by fundamental engineering principles (e.g., heat exchangers, valves), the complex nature of most primary equipment has discouraged the use of first-principle models for energy calculations. Instead, the energy consumption characteristics of primary equipment have traditionally been modeled using simple equations developed by running regression and analyses on manufacturers' published design data. Because published data are generally only available for full-load design conditions, additional correction functions are used to correct the full-load data to part-load conditions. The functional form of the regression equations and correction functions take many forms, including exponentials, Fourier series, and, most of the time, second or third-order polynomials. The selection of an appropriate functional form depends on the behavior of the equipment. In some cases, energy consumption is calculated using direct interpolation from tables of data. However, this method often requires excessive data input and computer memory.

8.3 Overall Modeling Strategies

In developing a simulation model for building energy prediction, two basic issues must be considered—modeling of components or subsystems, and the overall modeling strategy. Modeling of components, results in sets of equations describing the individual components. Overall modeling strategy refers to the *sequence* and *procedures* used to solve these equations. The accuracy of results and the computer resources required to achieve these results depend on the modeling strategy.

In most building energy programs, the load models are executed for every space for every hour of the simulation period. (Practically all models use one hour as the time-step, which excludes any information on phenomena occurring in a shorter time span.) The load model is followed by running models for every secondary system, one at a time, for every hour of the simulation. Finally, the plant simulation model is executed again for the entire period. Each sequential execution processes the *fixed* output of the preceding step.

This procedure is illustrated in Fig. 8-1. The solid lines represent data passed from one model to the next. The dashed lines represent information, usually provided by the user, about one model to the preceding model.

Because of this loads-systems-plants sequence, certain phenomena cannot be modeled precisely. For example, if the heat balance method for computing loads is used and some component in the system simulation model cannot meet the load, the program can only report the current load. In actuality, the space temperature should readjust until the load matches the equipment capacity, but this cannot be modeled because the loads have been precalculated and fixed. If the weighting factor method is used for loads, this problem is partially overcome, because loads are continually readjusted during the system simulation. However, the weighting factor

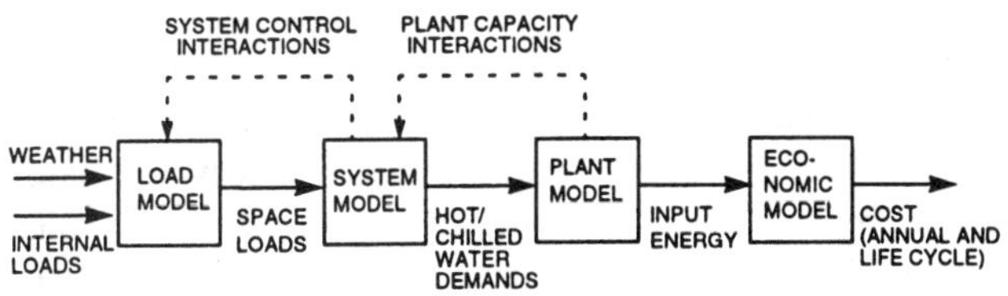

Fig. 8-1 Overall Modeling Strategy

technique is based on linear mathematics, and wide departures of room temperatures from those used during execution of the load program can introduce errors.

A similar problem arises in plant simulation. For example, in an actual building, as the load on the central plant varies the supply, chilled water temperature also varies. This variation in turn affects the capacity of the secondary system equipment. In an actual building, when the central plant becomes overloaded, space temperatures should rise to reduce the load. However, in most energy estimating programs, this condition cannot occur; thus, only the overload condition can be reported. These are some of the penalties associated with decoupling of the load, system, and plant models.

An alternative strategy, in which all calculations are performed at each time step, is conceivable. Here the load, system, and plant equations are solved simultaneously at each time interval. With this strategy, unmet loads and imbalances cannot occur; conditions at the plant are immediately reflected to the secondary system and then to the load model, forcing them to readjust to the instantaneous conditions throughout the building. The results of this modeling strategy are superior to those currently available, although the magnitude and importance of the improvement are uncertain.

The principal disadvantage of the alternative approach, and the reason that it has not been widely used, is that it demands more computing resources.

An economic model, as included in Fig. 8-1, calculates energy costs (and sometimes capital costs) based on the estimated required input energy. Thus, the simulation model calculates energy usage and cost for any given input weather and internal loads. By applying this model (i.e., determining output for given inputs) at each hour (or other suitable interval), the hour-by-hour energy consumption and cost can be determined. Maintaining running sums of these quantities yields monthly or annual energy usage and costs.

These models only compare design alternatives; a large number of uncontrolled and unknown factors usually rules out such models for accurate prediction of utility bills.

Traditionally, most energy analysis programs include a set of preprogrammed models that represent various systems, such as variable air volume, terminal reheat, multizone, etc. In this scheme, the equations for each system are arranged so they can be solved sequentially. If this is not possible, then the smallest number of equations that must be solved simultaneously is solved using an appropriate technique. Furthermore, individual equations may vary from hour to hour in the simulation, depending on controls and operating conditions. For example, a dry coil uses different equations than a wet coil.

The primary disadvantage of this scheme is that it is relatively inflexible—in order to modify a system, the program source code may have to be modified and recompiled. Alternative strategies have viewed the system as a series of components (e.g. fan, coil, pump, duct, pipe, damper, thermostat)

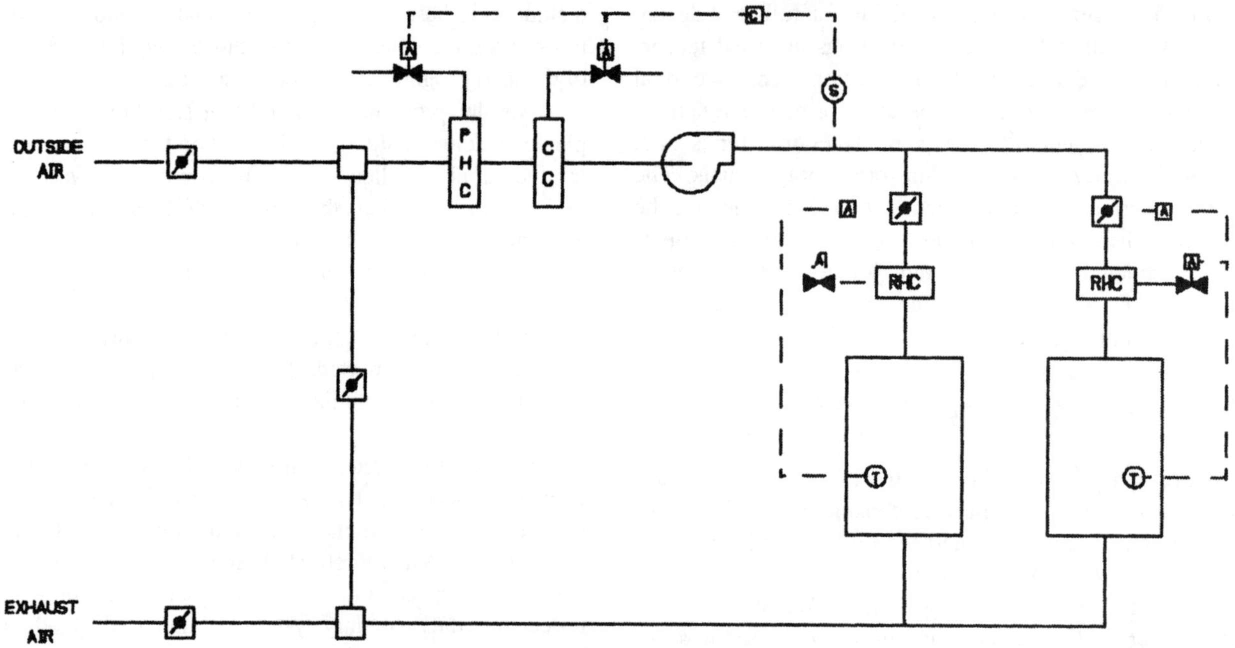

Fig. 8-2 Schematic of Variable Air Volume System with Reheat

that may be organized in a component library. Users of the program specify the connections between the components. The program then resolves the specification of components and connections into a set of simultaneous equations.

8.4 Integration of System Models

Energy calculations for secondary systems involve construction of the complete system from the set of HVAC components. For example, a VAV system is a single path system that controls zone temperature by modulating the airflow while maintaining a constant supply air temperature. VAV terminal units, located at each zone, adjust the quantity of air reaching each zone depending on its load requirements. Reheat coils may be included to provide required heating for perimeter zones.

This VAV system simulation consists of a central air handling unit and a VAV terminal unit with reheat coil located at each zone, as shown in Fig. 8-2. The central air handling unit includes a tan cooling coil, preheat coil, and an outside air economizer. The supply air leaving the air handling unit is controlled to a fixed setpoint. The VAV terminal unit at each zone varies the airflow to meet the cooling load. As the zone cooling load decreases, the VAV terminal unit decreases the zone airflow until the unit reaches its minimum position. If the cooling load continues to decrease the reheat coil will be activated to meet the zone load. As the supply air volume leaving the unit decreases the fan power consumption will also be reduced. A variable speed drive is used to control the supply fan.

The simulation is based on system characteristics and zone design requirements. For each zone, the inputs include the sensible and latent loads, the zone set point temperature, and the minimum zone supply air mass flow. System characteristics include the supply air temperature setpoint, the entering water temperature of the reheat, preheat and cooling coils, the minimum mass flow of outside air, and the economizer temperature/enthalpy set point for minimum airflow.

The algorithm for performing the calculations for this VAV system is shown in Fig. 8-3. The algorithm directs sequential calculations of system performance. Calculations proceed from the zones forward along the return air path to the cooling coil inlet and back through the supply air path to the cooling oil discharge.

This basic algorithm for simulation of a VAV system might be used in conjunction with a heat-balance type of load calculation. For a weighting factor approach, it would have to be modified to allow zone temperatures to vary and a consequent readjustment of zone loads. It should also be enhanced to allow for possible limits on reheat temperature and/or cooling coil limits, zone humidity limits, outside air control (economizers), and/or heat-recovery devices, zone exhaust, return air fan, heat gain in the return air path because of lights, the presence of baseboard-type heaters, and more realistic control profiles. Most current building energy programs incorporate these and other features as user options, as well as algorithms for other types of systems.

The method chosen to analyze a building's energy use is determined by the purpose for the investigation.

Forward modeling begins with a description of the building system or component of interest and defines the building being modeled according to its physical description. For example, the building geometry, geographical location, type of HVAC system, wall insulation, etc. may be defined. The primary benefits of this method are that it based on sound engineering principles and it has widespread accep-

```
BEGIN LOOP Calculate zone related design requirements
    •  Calculate required supply airflow to meet zone load
    •  Sum actual zone mass air flow rate
    •  Sum zone latent loads
  IF zone equals last zone THEN Exit Loop
END LOOP
•  Calculate system return air temperature from zone temps
•  Assume an initial cooling coil leaving air humidity ratio

BEGIN LOOPIterate on cooling coil leaving air humidity ratio
    •  Calculate return air humidity ratio from latent loads
    •  Calculate supply fan power consumption and
       entering fan air temperature
    •  Calculate mixed air temperature and humidity
       ratio using an economizer cycle
  IF mixed air temperature is less than design
       supply air temperature THEN
       •  Calculate preheat coil load
  ELSE
       •  Calculate cooling coil load and leaving air
          humidity ratio
  ENDIF
  IF cooling coil leaving air humidity ratio converged
  THEN Exit Loop
END LOOP

BEGIN LOOP Calculate the zone reheat coil loads
  IF zone supply air temperature is greater than system
  design supply air temperature THEN
       •  Calculate reheat coil load
          (Subroutine: COILINV/HCDET)
  ENDIF
    •  Sum reheat coil loads for all zones
  IF zone equals last zone THEN Exit Loop
END LOOP
```

Fig. 8-3 Algorithm for Calculating Performance of VAV with Reheat System

tance and use in major public domain simulation codes (e.g., BLAST and DOE-2). Figure 8-4 is a flow chart that illustrates the ordering of the analysis that is typically performed by a building energy simulation program.

Inverse modeling is based on the empirical behavior of the building as it relates to one or more driving forces. This approach is referred to as a system identification, parameter identification, or inverse modeling. In this modeling approach a structure or physical configuration of the building or system is assumed first and then important parameters are identified by a statistical analysis.

8.5 Degree-day Methods

Degree-day methods are the simplest methods for energy analysis and are appropriate if the building use and the efficiency of the HVAC equipment are constant. Where efficiency or conditions of use vary with outdoor temperature, the consumption can be calculated for different values of outdoor temperature and multiplied by the corresponding number of hours; this approach is used in various bin methods. When the indoor temperature is allowed to fluctuate or

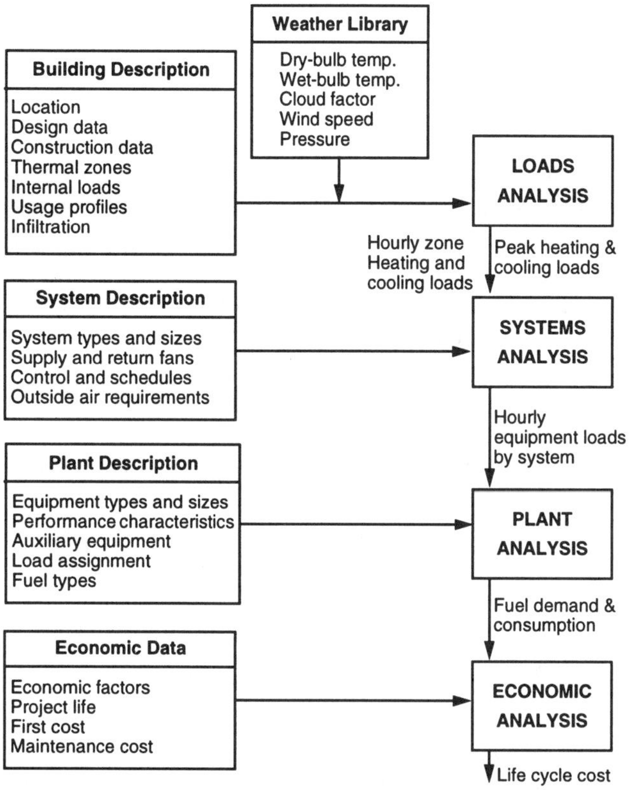

Fig. 8-4 Flow Chart for Building Energy Simulation Program
(Ayres and Stamper 1995)

when interior gains vary, models other than simple steady-state models must be used.

Single-measure methods for estimating cooling energy are less established than those for heating, primarily because the indoor-outdoor temperature difference during cooling is typically much smaller than under heating conditions. As a result, cooling loads depend more on such factors as solar gain and internal loads (besides temperature) than do heating loads. Since these loads largely depend on specific building features, attempts to correlate cooling energy requirements against a single climate parameter have not been very successful. Nonetheless, a companion to the heating degree-day procedure has emerged, the *cooling degree-day method*, and is widely used.

Even in an age when computers can easily calculate the energy consumption of a building, the concepts of degree-days and balance point temperature remain valuable tools. The severity of a climate can be characterized concisely in terms of degree-days. Also, the degree-day method and its generalizations can provide a simple estimate of annual loads, which can be accurate if the indoor temperature and internal gains are relatively constant and if the heating or cooling systems are to operate for a complete season. Thus, basic steady-state methods continue to be important.

Virtually all the energy-consumption estimating techniques used prior to the last few years are based on an assumed or measured set of average conditions taken from a relatively small sampling of buildings. These techniques use steady-state models based on monthly average weather and operating conditions and, for the degree-day method in particular, assume that energy use depends only on the difference between indoor and outdoor dry-bulb temperature. Thus, the degree-day method is restricted to small structures in which the heating and cooling loads are envelope-dominated. Other methods should be used for larger commercial or industrial buildings, where internal, cooling only zones are prevalent or where cooling loads are not linearly dependent on the outdoor-to-indoor temperature difference.

Any estimating method produces a more reliable result over a long period of operation than over a short period. Nearly all of the methods in use give reasonable results over a full annual heating season, but estimates for shorter periods, such as a month, may produce inaccurate results. As the period of the estimate shortens, there is more chance that some factor not directly taken into account in the estimating method will deviate from its long-term average value, and thus lead to an error in the predicted energy requirement.

8.5.1 Balance Point Temperature and Degree-Days

The *balance-point temperature* is the average outdoor temperature at which the building requires neither heating nor cooling from the HVAC system. The degree-day procedure recognizes that the heating equipment needs to meet only the heating not covered by internal sources such as lights, equipment, occupants, and solar gain. In other words, these sources provide heat down to the balance-point temperature, and below that, energy requirements of the space are proportional to the difference between the balance-point and the outside temperature.

The balance point temperature for heating t_{bal} of a building is defined as that value of the outdoor temperature t_o at which, for the specified value of the interior temperature t_i, the total heat gain q_{gain} is equal to all space heat gains from sun, occupants, lights, and so forth.

The steady-state heating requirements of a building q_h can be expressed as:

$$q_h = K(t_i - t_o) - q_{gain} \tag{8-1}$$

where

- K = building loss coefficient (design heat loss divided by the design temperature difference)
- t_i = indoor temperature
- t_o = outdoor temperature
- q_{gain} = all space heat gains not attributed to the space-conditioning system

The balance temperature is determined by setting $q_H = 0$ and solving for $t_o = t_{bal}$, so

$$t_{bal} = t_i - q_{gain}/K \tag{8-2}$$

Heating is needed only when to drops below t_{bal}.

With $t_{o,av}$ being the daily average value of the outdoor temperature for a particular day, the heating degree-days $DD_h(t_{bal})$ for that day are obtained as $(t_{bal} - t_{o,av})$ and for any particular period as

$$DD_h(t_{bal}) = (1\text{ day})\Sigma(t_{bal} - t_{o,av}) \tag{8-3}$$

where the summation may extend over a month, the heating season, or the entire year. In connection with degree-days, the balance temperature is also known as the base of the degree-days.

Cooling degree-days can be calculated using an expression analogous to heating degree-days:

$$DD_c(t_{bal}) = (1\text{ day})\Sigma(t_o - t_{bal}) \tag{8-4}$$

While the definition of the balance point temperature is the same as that for heating, in a given building its numerical value for cooling is generally different from that for heating because q_{gain}, K, and/or t_i can be different.

8.5.2 Seasonal Efficiency

The seasonal efficiency of heating equipment η depends on such factors as steady-state efficiency, sizing, cycling effects, and energy conservation devices installed. Sometimes it is much lower than and other times it is comparable to steady-state efficiency. Expressions have been developed from information supplied by the National Institute of Standards and Technology which estimate the seasonal efficiency for a variety of furnaces if information on rated input and output is available. For the case where heat loss from the ducting is neglected, the series of equations is

$$\eta = \eta_{ss} CF_{pl} \tag{8-5}$$

where η_{ss} is the steady-state efficiency (rated output/input).

The term CF_{pl} is a trait of the part-load efficiency of the heating equipment, which may be calculated as follows:

Gas-forced air furnaces

With pilot:

$$CF_{pl} = 0.6328 + 0.5738RLC - 0.3323(RLC)^2$$

With intermittent ignition:

$$CF_{pl} = 0.7791 + 0.1983RLC - 0.0711(RLC)^2$$

Oil furnaces without stack damper

$$CF_{pl} = 0.7092 + 0.6515RLC - 0.4711(RLC)^2$$

Resistance electric furnaces

$$CF_{pl} = 1.0$$

RLC is defined as follows:

$$RLC = \frac{K(t_{bal} - t_{od})}{CHT}$$

where

K = building loss coefficient
t_{od} = outside design temperature
CHT = rated output of equipment

8.5.3 Heating Degree-Day Method

The degree-day procedure for estimating heating energy requirements is based on the assumption that, on a long-term average, solar and internal gains offset heat loss when the mean daily outdoor temperature is equal to the balance point temperature, and that fuel consumption is proportional to the difference between the mean daily temperature and the balance point temperature. In other words, if the balance point temperature is 60°F, then on a day when the mean temperature is 50°F (10°F below 60°F), 10 times as much fuel is consumed as on days when the mean temperature is 59°F (1°F below 60°F). This basic concept can be represented in an equation stating that energy consumption is directly proportional to the number of degree-days in the estimation period with the heat loss per degree difference being constant.

Estimating the theoretical seasonal energy requirement of a conventional heating system (gas furnace, oil furnace, electrical furnace, and so forth) using the degree-day method is simple because the efficiency of the system is assumed to be constant regardless of outdoor temperature. The theoretical heating requirement is calculated as

$$\frac{\text{Design heat loss (Btu/h)} \times 24 \times \text{degree-days}}{\text{Design temperature difference}}$$

The general form of the degree-day equation is

$$E = \frac{q_L(\text{DD})24}{\eta(\text{HV})\Delta t} C_D \tag{8-6}$$

where

E = fuel or energy consumption for the estimate period, units of fuel
q_L = design heat loss, including infiltration and ventilation, Btu/h
DD = number of degree-days for the estimate period
Δt = design temperature difference, °F
η = efficiency of heating system [Eq. (8-5)], also designated on an annual basis as the annual fuel utilization efficiency (AFUE)
HV = heating value of fuel, Btu/unit of fuel
C_D = 1 if DD are based on t_{bal}
= 0.77 if 65°F is arbitrarily assumed as the balance temperature

Typical heating values HV are given in Table 8-1; additional values for η are provided in Chapter 19.

Heating degree-days or degree-hours for a balance point temperature of 65°F have been widely tabulated based on the observation that this has represented average conditions in typical buildings in the **past**. Today, use of the 65°F base will considerably overestimate the energy consumption due to improved building construction as well as increased internal loads in recent years. The errors inherent in the established base of 65°F (18.3°C) may be adjusted by using an empirical correction factor C_D. The best single value for C_D is taken from the DOE HSPF methodology, which uses the correction factor 0.77 as the multiplier for the design heat loss per degree to provide a more appropriate building loss coefficient K to account for internal heat gains in energy estimation. However, the best approach is to avoid the arbitrary 65°F base, using the variable base degree-day approach instead.

Table 8-1 Heating Values

Fuel	Heating Value of Fuel
Natural gas	1050 Btu/ft^3 (39 MJ/m^3)
Propane	90,000 Btu/gal (25 GJ/m^3)
No. 2 fuel oil	140,000 Btu/gal (39 GJ/m^3)

Example 8-1 A residence located in St. Joseph, Missouri, has a design heating load of 84,000 Btu/h. Determine

(a) Gallons of No. 2 fuel oil used for heating season with warm air system
(b) Electrical energy used for heating if electric baseboard units are used

Solution:

From Equation (8-6) [with η = 1 and HV = 1],

$$E = \frac{84{,}000 \times 5435 \times 24}{[72-(-1)]} 0.77$$
$$= 115{,}600{,}000 \text{ Btu/h}$$

$$\text{(a) No. 2 fuel oil} = \frac{115.6 \times 10^6}{140{,}000 \times 0.75} = 1100 \text{ gallons}$$

$$\text{(b) Heating electrical energy} = \frac{115.6 \times 10^6}{3413} = 34{,}200 \text{ kWh}$$

8.5.4 Variable Base Heating Degree-Day

The variable base degree-day method (VBDD) is a generalization of the degree-day method. It retains the original degree-day concept, but counts degree-days based on the actual balance-point temperature rather than the now outdated 65°F.

The degree-day method, like any steady-state method, is unreliable for estimating the consumption during mild weather. Despite such problems, the degree-day method (using an appropriate base temperature) can give remarkably accurate results for the annual heating energy of single-zone buildings dominated by gains through the walls and roof and/or ventilation.

Table 8-2 provides the degree-days in °F to several bases for various locations in the United States. Annual degree-day tabulations for seven base temperatures in °C at 1195 stations in Canada are in Canadian Climate Normals (Atmospheric Environment Service 1981).

Table 8-2 Degree-Days to Several Bases (in °F) for Various U.S. Locations

STATE	HEATING					COOLING				
	BASE					BASE				
	65	60	55	50	45	65	60	55	50	45
ALABAMA										
Birmingham	2844	1995	1333	838	488	1928	2916	4073	5403	6877
Huntsville	3302	2414	1670	1103	686	1808	2747	3828	5090	6492
Mobile	1684	1062	619	330	148	2577	3780	5162	6698	8342
Montgomery	2269	1508	945	547	232	2238	3302	4568	5991	7551
ALASKA										
Anchorage AP	10911	9122	7492	6081	4896	0	36	224	647	1279
Annette AP	7053	5315	3773	2513	1543	14	98	386	940	1803
Barrow AP	20265	18440	16615	14803	13009	0	0	0	13	44
Barter Island AP	19994	18169	16344	14528	12733	0	0	0	9	44
Bethel AP	13203	11404	9695	8140	6835	0	26	142	411	938
Bettles AP	15925	14180	12548	11060	9718	17	97	289	626	1110
Big Delta AP	13698	11985	10410	8977	7735	34	145	395	787	1370
Cold Bay AP	9865	8040	6230	4532	3095	0	0	16	138	533
Fairbanks AP	14345	12661	11115	9714	8451	52	196	467	898	1468
Gulkana	13938	12162	10507	8985	7648	9	63	228	537	1027
Homer	10364	8539	6745	5133	3840	0	0	24	240	777
Juneau AP	9007	7222	5557	4107	2925	0	39	197	573	1219
King Salmon AP	11582	9773	8047	6563	5304	0	12	112	456	1023
Kodiak	8860	7049	5327	3819	2593	0	7	117	436	1032
Kotzebue AP	16039	14237	12491	10852	9337	0	23	102	258	598
McGrath AP	14487	12736	11107	9634	8348	14	88	284	642	1184
Nome AP	14325	12503	10721	9047	7528	0	0	46	197	503
St. Paul Island AP	11119	9294	7469	5667	4021	0	0	0	24	199
Shemya AP	9735	7910	6085	4298	2693	0	0	0	30	254
Summit FAA AP	14368	12556	10790	9146	7640	0	10	71	253	578
Talkeetna	11708	9934	8306	6848	5609	6	57	254	620	1207
Unalakleet	14027	12238	10515	8943	7565	0	31	138	391	842
Yakutat AP	9533	7711	5942	4420	3181	0	0	56	362	947
ARIZONA										
Flagstaff	7322	5776	4421	3267	2299	140	416	894	1562	2418
Phoenix	1552	899	431	165	45	3508	4680	6039	7596	9297
Prescott FAA AP	4456	3303	2321	1507	883	882	1560	2400	3414	4612
Tucson	1752	1050	541	229	65	2314	3937	5253	6765	8431
Winslow	4733	3623	2683	1882	1249	1203	1921	2802	3828	5018
Yuma	1005	507	211	59	8	4195	5518	7045	8719	10498
ARKANSAS										
Fort Smith	3336	2442	1687	1075	613	2022	2949	4015	5239	6595
Little Rock	3354	2442	1687	1075	624	1925	2843	3908	5128	6496
CALIFORNIA										
Bakersfield	2185	1367	760	371	147	2179	3185	4400	5835	7437
Bishop	4313	3179	2230	1437	848	1037	1728	2603	3641	4875
Blue Canyon	5704	4271	3037	2015	1206	302	698	1283	2079	3106
Daggett FAA AP	2203	1420	824	410	166	2729	3765	5004	6415	7996
Eureka	4679	2925	1494	607	194	0	55	460	1414	2816
Fresno	2650	1724	995	493	205	1671	2563	3667	4986	6525
Long Beach	1606	772	292	70	8	985	1982	3325	4928	6696
Los Angeles INTL	1819	833	295	66	7	615	1464	2755	4348	6115
Los Angeles Civic Ctr	1245	522	158	26	0	1185	2289	3747	5442	7244
Mount Shasta	5890	4458	3215	2177	1338	286	680	1263	2045	3035
Oakland	2909	1570	714	263	61	128	622	1598	2963	4587
Red Bluff	2688	1762	1018	505	208	1904	2803	3895	5196	6727
Sacramento	2843	1837	1043	493	186	1159	1971	3011	4286	5812
Sacramento City	2587	1627	893	406	148	1291	2158	3249	4584	6151
Sandberg	4427	3177	2107	1250	622	800	1374	2123	3100	4293
San Diego	1507	648	213	42	9	722	1694	3084	4746	6532
San Francisco	3042	1668	769	289	67	108	550	1496	2832	4438
San Francisco Fed Bldg	3080	1576	608	169	25	39	368	1230	2619	4298
Santa Maria	3053	1624	690	229	42	84	484	1377	2738	4380
Stockton	2806	1835	1072	537	219	1259	2100	3167	4455	5968
COLORADO										
Alamosa	8609	7029	5654	4473	3457	88	329	780	1428	2227
Colorado Springs	6473	5131	3954	2949	2089	461	945	1592	2417	3383
Denver - Stapleton	6016	4723	3601	2653	1852	625	1159	1857	2739	3759
Denver - City	5505	4246	3175	2271	1533	742	1312	2071	2993	4074
Eagle AP	8426	6864	5505	4319	3317	117	385	845	1487	2313
Grand Junction	5605	4441	3425	2551	1814	1140	1810	2619	3565	4653
Pueblo	5394	4221	3220	2351	1628	981	1632	2456	3412	4514
CONNECTICUT										
Bridgeport	5461	4264	3216	2321	1583	735	1362	2140	3064	4152
Hartford	6350	5085	3971	3005	2173	584	1143	1855	2715	3706

Table 8-2 Degree-Days to Several Bases (in °F) for Various U.S. Locations (*Continued*)

STATE	HEATING BASE 65	60	55	50	45	COOLING BASE 65	60	55	50	45
DC										
Wash DC-Dulles Apt	5005	3881	2898	2054	1380	940	1636	2474	3458	4616
Wash DC-Natl Apt	4211	3182	2293	1563	984	1415	2210	3152	4237	5489
DELAWARE										
Wilmington Ncastle	4940	3824	2839	2003	1330	992	1697	2537	3525	4675
FLORIDA										
Apalachicola	1361	792	426	189	67	2663	3930	5377	6967	8669
Daytona Beach	897	480	215	71	25	2919	4321	5881	7563	9341
Fort Myers	457	189	56	9	0	3711	5265	6958	8741	10553
Jacksonville	1327	788	429	194	70	2596	3890	5349	6938	8641
Key West	59	7	0	0	0	4888	6660	8474	10299	12124
Lakeland	678	330	128	40	7	3298	4774	6398	8135	9927
Miami	206	54	8	0	0	4038	5715	7494	9306	11131
Orlando	733	370	151	48	9	3226	4686	6291	8016	9806
Pensacola	1578	991	575	302	135	2695	3932	5341	6893	8551
Tallahassee	1563	996	550	279	116	2563	3792	5200	6755	8415
Tampa	718	364	151	50	14	3366	4836	6447	8172	9963
West Palm Beach	299	88	27	0	0	3786	5408	7159	8960	10785
GEORGIA										
Athens	2975	2084	1370	830	462	1722	2661	3767	5052	6508
Atlanta	3095	2189	1461	911	524	1589	2511	3604	4880	6316
Augusta	2547	1729	1106	652	348	1995	2999	4204	5573	7094
Columbus	2378	1600	1010	593	313	2143	3188	4429	5831	7375
Macon	2240	1492	934	536	271	2294	3373	4643	6068	7626
Rome	3342	2422	1653	1068	637	1615	2514	3576	4816	6210
Savannah	1952	1258	751	413	185	2317	3444	4766	6248	7851
HAWAII										
Hilo	0	0	0	0	0	3066	4887	6712	8537	10362
Honolulu	0	0	0	0	0	4221	6046	7871	9696	11521
Kahului	0	0	0	0	0	3732	5555	7380	9205	11030
Lihue AP	0	0	0	0	0	3719	5535	7360	9185	11010
IDAHO										
Boise	5833	4533	3399	2434	1626	714	1233	1929	2793	3811
Idaho Falls	8619	7129	5800	4609	3590	237	573	1064	1703	2511
Lewiston	5464	4168	3050	2112	1366	657	1186	1886	2780	3856
Pocatello	7063	5687	4454	3401	2504	437	883	1477	2252	3177
ILLINOIS										
Cairo	3833	2895	2090	1447	925	1806	2687	3710	4893	6197
Chicago Midway AP	6127	4952	3912	2998	2219	925	1575	2361	3272	4317
Chicago O'Hare AP	6497	5245	4163	3220	2404	664	1243	1986	2863	3872
Decatur	5344	4247	3293	2461	1778	1197	1925	2797	3791	4932
Moline	6395	5202	4170	3263	2462	893	1530	2324	3236	4262
Peoria	6098	4930	3910	3013	2239	968	1631	2431	3360	4412
Rockford	6845	5600	4507	3555	2713	714	1298	2032	2899	3883
Springfield	5558	4437	3468	2615	1913	1116	1821	2670	3654	4772
INDIANA										
Evansville	4624	3578	2685	1929	1327	1364	2139	3064	4140	5367
Fort Wayne	6209	4992	3930	2996	2193	748	1358	2117	3008	4030
Indianapolis	5577	4430	3431	2568	1856	974	1653	2478	3441	4554
South Bend	6462	5213	4118	3156	2333	695	1271	2002	2865	3867
IOWA										
Burlington Radio KBUR	6149	4988	3970	3077	2308	994	1657	2466	3396	4447
Des Moines	6710	5521	4470	3546	2728	928	1561	2335	3235	4243
Dubuque	7277	5992	4871	3893	3028	606	1146	1850	2697	3657
Mason City AP	7901	6586	5430	4425	3529	580	1088	1763	2581	3508
Sioux City	6953	5745	4674	3738	2898	932	1545	2298	3182	4177
Spencer	7770	6474	5329	4334	3448	641	1171	1857	2685	3620
Waterloo	7415	6153	5040	4070	3199	675	1236	1950	2806	3760
KANSAS										
Concordia	5623	4498	3509	2646	1912	1302	1998	2832	3795	4886
Dodge City	5046	3963	3011	2184	1512	1411	2153	3022	4025	5176
Goodland	6119	4891	3804	2857	2041	925	1515	2253	3131	4139
Russell FAA AP	5312	4220	3259	2423	1735	1485	2219	3081	4076	5210
Topeka	5243	4152	3203	2378	1700	1361	2093	2974	3974	5112
Wichita	4687	3654	2750	1977	1346	1673	2464	3386	4438	5638
KENTUCKY										
Covington	5070	3965	3001	2189	1527	1080	1798	2654	3672	4834
Lexington	4729	3652	2743	1963	1350	1197	1941	2858	3904	5120
Louisville	4640	3584	2676	1906	1303	1268	2032	2942	4005	5227

Table 8-2 Degree-Days to Several Bases (in °F) for Various U.S. Locations (*Continued*)

STATE	HEATING BASE 65	60	55	50	45	COOLING BASE 65	60	55	50	45
LOUISIANA										
Alexandria	2200	1443	880	490	234	2193	3260	4525	5958	7531
Baton Rouge	1670	1036	582	295	120	2585	3775	5150	6685	8340
Lake Charles	1498	908	500	240	91	2739	3978	5391	6956	8638
New Orleans, Aud. Park	1343	805	439	202	82	2876	4165	5622	7215	8916
New Orleans, N O	1465	893	492	239	96	2706	3960	5383	6956	8638
Shreveport	2167	1438	883	490	233	2538	3634	4906	6335	7903
MAINE										
Bangor	7950	6496	5222	4103	3122	268	640	1194	1896	2740
Caribou	9632	8044	6634	5409	4319	128	365	784	1379	2116
Old Town FAA AP	8648	7133	5800	4628	3589	209	519	1016	1660	2454
Portland	7498	6035	4764	3658	2705	252	616	1169	1890	2758
MARYLAND										
Baltimore	4729	3631	2682	1873	1236	1108	1840	2708	3728	4918
MASSACHUSETTS										
Blue Hill	6335	5020	3885	2895	2071	457	968	1659	2493	3498
Boston	5621	4383	3313	2405	1659	661	1250	2000	2920	4000
Nantucket AP	5929	4520	3323	2311	1513	284	708	1332	2143	3170
Worcester	6848	5498	4326	3296	2421	387	863	1514	2303	3259
MICHIGAN										
Alpena	8518	6982	5635	4473	3464	208	497	981	1642	2459
Detroit	6419	5167	4072	3113	2280	654	1227	1961	2823	3815
Flint	7041	5705	4540	3529	2640	438	923	1586	2399	3335
Grand Rapids	6801	5514	4383	3396	2524	575	1108	1807	2646	3598
Houghton Lake	8347	6861	5579	4455	3486	250	590	1132	1832	2689
Lansing	6904	5608	4464	3470	2595	535	1059	1747	2578	3528
Marquette	8351	6835	5517	4379	3378	216	531	1031	1725	2549
Muskegon	6890	5550	4390	3373	2482	469	953	1620	2428	3360
Sault Ste Marie	9193	7614	6215	5017	3971	139	386	816	1443	2217
Traverse City AP	7698	6272	5035	3953	3013	376	773	1362	2101	2989
MINNESOTA										
Duluth	9756	8185	6793	5581	4540	176	425	864	1482	2259
Intnl Falls	10547	8995	7623	6413	5348	176	454	908	1523	2283
Minn. - St. Paul	8159	6842	5677	4668	3765	585	1097	1758	2575	3491
Rochester	8227	6868	5682	4643	3733	474	943	1579	2370	3280
St. Cloud	8868	7481	6255	5187	4241	426	862	1468	2220	3098
MISSISSIPPI										
Jackson	2300	1548	988	590	319	2316	3394	4664	6086	7639
Meridian	2388	1621	1042	623	339	2231	3289	4538	5940	7483
MISSOURI										
Columbia Region	5078	3997	3064	2259	1605	1269	2009	2901	3919	5089
Kansas City	5161	4089	3157	2351	1694	1421	2169	3061	4085	5249
St Louis	4750	3701	2798	2031	1419	1475	2252	3174	4232	5445
St Joseph	5435	4341	3378	2544	1847	1334	2064	2925	3911	5046
Springfield	4570	3517	2611	1844	1235	1382	2149	3068	4126	5342
MONTANA										
Billings	7265	5898	4697	3641	2766	498	951	1581	2354	3298
Butte	9719	8059	6557	5225	4078	58	222	545	1038	1718
Cut Bank AP	9033	7474	6096	4907	3886	140	406	856	1489	2299
Dillon AP	8354	6821	5457	4255	3237	199	492	953	1570	2382
Glasgow	8969	7572	6329	5238	4302	438	867	1449	2185	3074
Great Falls	7652	6248	5022	3965	3074	339	760	1365	2132	3066
Havre	8687	7282	6073	5005	4104	395	818	1432	2191	3113
Helena	8190	6710	5389	4247	3258	256	606	1105	1786	2629
Kalispell	8554	6959	5542	4304	3233	117	348	755	1342	2096
Lewistown FAA AP	8586	7038	5676	4487	3467	192	468	933	1567	2379
Miles City AP	7889	6562	5392	4369	3479	752	1252	1905	2706	3641
Missoula	7931	6410	5066	3884	2876	188	497	970	1616	2428
NEBRASKA										
Grand Island	6420	5224	4166	3239	2434	1036	1662	2428	3326	4345
Lincoln AP	6218	5062	4040	3139	2362	1148	1809	2611	3536	4585
Lincoln	6012	4875	3870	2993	2234	1187	1865	2685	3634	4701
Norfolk	6981	5745	4663	3710	2863	925	1520	2263	3131	4118
North Platte	6743	5470	4345	3354	2509	802	1359	2060	2898	3874
Omaha - Eppley	6049	4907	3911	3037	2290	1173	1862	2691	3637	4715
Omaha - North	6601	5400	4349	3427	2624	949	1573	2346	3249	4270
Scottsbluff	6774	5473	4304	3289	2415	666	1188	1845	2653	3605
Valentine	7300	6006	4859	3847	2956	736	1267	1945	2758	3692
NEVADA										
Elko	7483	6027	4714	3586	2625	342	706	1228	1910	2785
Ely	7814	6327	5004	3826	2829	207	550	1052	1694	2526

Table 8-2 Degree-Days to Several Bases (in °F) for Various U.S. Locations (*Continued*)

STATE	HEATING BASE 65	60	55	50	45	COOLING BASE 65	60	55	50	45
Las Vegas	2601	1770	1120	625	306	2946	3938	5114	6443	7950
Lovelock FAA	5990	4695	3550	2579	1747	684	1217	1894	2743	3740
Reno	6022	4612	3387	2360	1534	329	739	1344	2150	3140
Tonopah	5900	4610	3492	2532	1723	631	1167	1869	2739	3753
Winnemucca	6629	5241	3994	2931	2015	407	845	1423	2185	3096
NEW HAMPSHIRE										
Concord	7360	5967	4757	3682	2762	349	781	1394	2150	3051
Mount Washington	13878	12053	10253	8534	6960	0	0	25	132	379
NEW JERSEY										
Atlantic City	4946	3783	2784	1941	1267	864	1533	2349	3339	4485
Atlantic City Marina	4693	3534	2530	1713	1076	835	1503	2317	3333	4517
Newark	5034	3911	2920	2074	1391	1024	1721	2543	3533	4677
Trenton	4947	3818	2832	1996	1323	968	1661	2493	3482	4634
NEW MEXICO										
Albuquerque	4292	3234	2330	1557	963	1316	2080	2996	4053	5288
Clayton	5207	3999	2966	2089	1374	767	1380	2176	3120	4231
Roswell	3697	2729	1898	1226	706	1560	2417	3412	4566	5872
Truth or Consequences	3392	2447	1636	1007	542	1558	2429	3447	4647	6008
Tucumcari FAA	4047	3015	2135	1415	858	1357	2148	3096	4200	5467
Zuni FAA	5815	4507	3381	2437	1648	473	983	1685	2567	3605
NEW YORK										
Albany	6888	5596	4451	3457	2595	574	1111	1787	2619	3583
Binghamton	7285	5908	4714	3677	2767	369	820	1452	2231	3151
Buffalo	6927	5591	4429	3403	2508	437	928	1590	2388	3319
Massena FAA	8237	6827	5596	4510	3552	343	759	1352	2088	2958
New York Cntrl Park	4848	3739	2771	1958	1299	1068	1784	2636	3653	4814
New York JFK INTL AP	5184	4023	2994	2130	1422	861	1520	2321	3278	4395
New York LaGuardia	4909	3787	2806	1980	1311	1048	1752	2587	3589	4740
Oswego East	6792	5444	4274	3243	2376	435	915	1570	2360	3319
Rochester	6719	5417	4285	3291	2434	531	1062	1750	2580	3549
Syracuse	6678	5379	4250	3267	2429	551	1081	1778	2621	3607
NORTH CAROLINA										
Asheville	4237	3129	2224	1488	937	872	1587	2508	3595	4868
Cape Hatteras	2731	1846	1166	702	380	1550	2485	3635	4991	6500
Charlotte	3218	2300	1552	984	585	1596	2503	3579	4842	6263
Greensboro	3825	2811	1984	1324	825	1341	2158	3149	4318	5640
Raleigh-Durham	3514	2542	1744	1123	670	1394	2242	3273	4482	5850
Wilmington	2433	1632	1028	610	321	1964	2995	4225	5622	7162
NORTH DAKOTA										
Bismarck	9044	7656	6425	5326	4374	487	928	1518	2248	3116
Fargo	9271	7891	6663	5573	4615	473	919	1515	2251	3122
Minot FAA	9407	7964	6685	5564	4573	370	758	1299	2002	2837
Williston	9161	7753	6504	5387	4450	422	841	1415	2128	3011
OHIO										
Akron-Canton	6224	4971	3883	2936	2129	634	1205	1943	2820	3839
Cincinnati Abbe Obs	4844	3763	2830	2040	1412	1188	1931	2819	3864	5060
Cincinnati AP	5070	3965	3001	2189	1527	1080	1798	2654	3672	4834
Cleveland	6154	4901	3819	2876	2079	613	1183	1926	2807	3836
Columbus	5702	4513	3480	2597	1846	809	1449	2244	3183	4257
Dayton	5641	4483	3468	2600	1866	936	1603	2414	3370	4460
Mansfield	5818	4618	3573	2679	1917	818	1445	2225	3152	4219
Toledo Express	6381	5136	4049	3091	2274	685	1268	2001	2870	3877
Youngstown	6426	5145	4032	3054	2232	518	1065	1774	2621	3623
OKLAHOMA										
Oklahoma City	3695	2760	1962	1326	809	1876	2768	3788	4980	6289
Tulsa	3680	2750	1950	1306	778	1949	2850	3865	5052	6347
OREGON										
Astoria	5295	3620	2233	1215	570	13	159	596	1415	2598
Burns	7212	5740	4436	3299	2343	289	649	1168	1851	2724
Eugene	4739	3313	2141	1226	607	239	638	1286	2201	3417
Meacham	7863	6249	4817	3556	2495	103	317	712	1275	2034
Medford	4930	3614	2496	1577	882	562	1077	1779	2685	3813
North Bend AP	4688	2985	1642	756	292	0	131	597	1553	2913
Pendleton	5240	3968	2868	1970	1264	656	1211	1935	2858	3982
Portland	4792	3385	2234	1333	708	300	711	1378	2309	3520
Redmond AP	6643	5106	3767	2621	1680	170	459	943	1620	2512
Salem	4852	3424	2246	1317	667	232	620	1272	2169	3355
Sexton Summit	6430	4859	3477	2311	1374	137	381	837	1499	2386

Table 8-2 Degree-Days to Several Bases (in °F) for Various U.S. Locations (*Continued*)

STATE	HEATING BASE 65	60	55	50	45	COOLING BASE 65	60	55	50	45
PACIFIC										
Guam	0	0	0	0	0	5011	6836	8661	10486	12311
Johnston AP	0	0	0	0	0	5086	6911	8736	10561	12386
Koror	0	0	0	0	0	6008	7833	9658	11483	13308
Kwajalein AP	0	0	0	0	0	6164	7989	9814	11639	13464
Majuro AP	0	0	0	0	0	5904	7729	9554	11379	13204
Pago Pago AP	0	0	0	0	0	5325	7150	8975	10800	12625
Ponape	0	0	0	0	0	5652	7477	9302	11127	12952
Truk, Moen I, AP	0	0	0	0	0	5888	7713	9538	11363	13188
Wake	0	0	0	0	0	5455	7280	9105	10930	12755
Yap AP	0	0	0	0	0	5916	7741	9566	11391	13216
PENNSYLVANIA										
Allentown	5827	4618	3550	2633	1843	772	1392	2150	3053	4088
Bradford AP	7804	6294	5006	3894	2931	170	482	1022	1735	2596
Erie	6851	5485	4304	3283	2411	373	832	1482	2282	3235
Harrisburg	5224	4087	3097	2238	1541	1025	1711	2545	3511	4644
Philadelphia	4865	3753	2788	1965	1312	1104	1817	2671	3679	4849
Pittsburgh City	5278	4135	3138	2294	1603	948	1630	2456	3440	4573
Pittsburgh AP	5930	4694	3637	2720	1938	647	1240	2004	2914	3961
W-Barre-Scranton	6277	5018	3928	2972	2149	608	1181	1909	2778	3783
Williamsport	5981	4757	3695	2764	1971	698	1299	2059	2952	3986
RHODE ISLAND										
Block Island	5771	4432	3289	2306	1517	359	844	1523	2368	3409
Providence	5972	4682	3565	2599	1803	532	1067	1774	2625	3662
SOUTH CAROLINA										
Charleston AP	2146	1406	864	496	240	2078	3163	4454	5903	7478
Charleston City	1904	1230	741	412	188	2354	3502	4839	6334	7937
Columbia	2598	1783	1154	686	374	2087	3094	4292	5647	7159
Florence	2566	1748	1127	676	374	1952	2960	4171	5538	7060
Grnvle-Spartenburg	3163	2246	1493	921	519	1573	2477	3552	4809	6229
SOUTH DAKOTA										
Aberdeen	8617	7267	6078	5014	4087	566	1046	1678	2440	3337
Huron	8055	6751	5600	4582	3678	711	1239	1912	2714	3641
Pierre AP	7677	6401	5271	4273	3409	858	1406	2102	2928	3889
Rapid City	7324	5982	4799	3762	2868	661	1148	1786	2575	3511
Sioux Falls	7838	6543	5401	4394	3498	719	1253	1933	2746	3681
TENNESSEE										
Bristol	4306	3255	2373	1646	1093	1107	1880	2823	3922	5197
Chattanooga	3505	2574	1785	1180	737	1636	2526	3566	4791	6169
Knoxville	3478	2557	1775	1187	744	1569	2475	3518	4753	6135
Memphis	3227	2352	1624	1058	640	2029	2984	4077	5339	6744
Nashville	3696	2758	1964	1338	852	1694	2576	3613	4812	6151
Oak Ridge	3944	2955	2119	1445	933	1367	2202	3187	4338	5656
TEXAS										
Abilene	2610	1801	1162	664	342	2466	3481	4670	5995	7498
Amarillo	4183	3156	2278	1548	976	1433	2230	3177	4274	5527
Austin	1737	1097	620	316	127	2903	4095	5443	6962	8600
Brownsville	650	336	146	54	19	3874	5385	7020	3753	10543
Corpus Christi	930	514	243	98	28	3474	4880	6438	8111	9872
Dallas	2290	1544	949	526	250	2755	3835	5073	6467	8016
Del Rio	1523	923	494	230	80	3363	4596	5986	7548	9222
El Paso	2678	1833	1149	653	326	2098	3077	4229	5548	7048
Fort Worth	2382	1616	1007	562	274	2587	3642	4862	6239	7775
Galveston	1224	704	369	157	54	3004	4312	5800	7413	9139
Houston	1434	864	471	215	81	2889	4147	5576	7150	8835
Laredo No. 2	876	481	230	87	32	4137	5568	7143	8824	10593
Lubbock	3545	2603	1807	1163	666	1647	2535	3559	4745	6068
Lufkin AP	1940	1253	731	385	163	2592	3730	5033	6512	8114
Midland	2621	1808	1159	656	333	2245	3258	4434	5757	7258
Port Arthur	1518	924	504	238	86	2798	4028	5431	6990	8669
San Angelo	2240	1498	918	493	227	2702	3789	5031	6432	7993
San Antonio	1570	956	518	242	92	2994	4206	5594	7146	8818
Victoria	1227	702	364	150	51	3140	4440	5925	7537	9262
Waco	2058	1357	807	437	195	2863	3988	5271	6717	8303
Wichita Falls	2904	2061	1384	832	451	2611	3594	4741	6015	7458
UTAH										
Blanding	6163	4869	3732	2757	1912	600	1129	1827	2670	3646
Bryce Canyon AP	9133	7459	5949	4616	3480	41	193	505	1005	1686
Cedar City AP	6137	4833	3690	2717	1897	615	1130	1813	2671	3678
Milford	6412	5109	3957	2969	2121	688	1212	1885	2721	3704
Salt Lake City	5983	4733	3633	2676	1864	927	1502	2221	3094	4108

Table 8-2 Degree-Days to Several Bases (in °F) for Various U.S. Locations (*Continued*)

STATE	HEATING BASE 65	60	55	50	45	COOLING BASE 65	60	55	50	45
Wendover, Utah	5760	4558	3511	2621	1870	1137	1760	2538	3475	4547
VERMONT										
Burlington	7876	6488	5270	4190	3246	396	833	1440	2180	3066
VIRGINIA										
Lynchburg	4233	3172	2269	1536	966	1100	1861	2783	3873	5128
Norfolk	3488	2516	1710	1100	663	1441	2284	3315	4530	5918
Richmond	3939	2916	2061	1388	866	1353	2157	3127	4276	5580
Roanoke	4307	3234	2326	1580	1011	1030	1778	2690	3771	5029
Wallops Island	4240	3170	2268	1531	978	1107	1865	2788	3881	5149
WASHINGTON										
Olympia	5530	3970	2653	1617	854	101	365	880	1657	2731
Omak	6858	5476	4253	3230	2355	522	965	1573	2367	3324
Quillayute	5951	4232	2750	1603	813	8	116	458	1137	2172
Seattle-Tacoma	5185	3657	2386	1416	731	129	423	984	1832	2981
Seattle (Urban)	4727	3269	2091	1194	602	183	549	1197	2127	3358
Spokane	6835	5420	4173	3088	2188	388	797	1377	2120	3040
Stampede Pass	9400	7643	6006	4532	3256	16	83	274	623	1176
Walla Walla	4835	3616	2600	1760	1126	862	1471	2279	3260	4457
Yakima	6009	4655	3483	2502	1688	479	945	1604	2452	3455
PUERTO RICO										
San Juan	0	0	0	0	0	4982	6807	8632	10457	12282
WEST INDIES										
Swan Island	0	0	0	0	0	5809	7634	9459	11284	13109
WEST VIRGINIA										
Beckley	5615	4356	3279	2390	1652	490	1061	1809	2745	3833
Charleston	4590	3500	2590	1809	1216	1055	1790	2699	3750	4981
Elkins	5975	4659	3533	2616	1834	389	905	1601	2508	3555
Huntington	4624	3533	2624	1843	1249	1098	1829	2746	3790	5020
Parkersburg	4817	3720	2786	1987	1363	1045	1770	2657	3686	4888
WISCONSIN										
Eau Claire AP	8388	7033	5832	4786	3860	459	928	1554	2331	3231
Green Bay	8098	6689	5473	4405	3478	386	805	1411	2168	3066
La Crosse AP	7417	6158	5050	4088	3219	695	1264	1978	2841	3798
Madison	7730	6373	5188	4156	3250	460	923	1572	2361	3279
Milwaukee	7444	6080	4898	3860	2946	450	911	1554	2342	3252
WYOMING										
Casper	7555	6167	4914	3813	2857	458	895	1468	2193	3061
Cheyenne	7255	5825	4562	3452	2512	327	734	1288	2003	2886
Lander	7869	6471	5207	4080	3140	383	814	1376	2078	2965
Rock Springs AP	8410	6922	5592	4412	3393	227	563	1059	1703	2515
Sheridan	7708	6298	5024	3935	3000	446	860	1411	2147	3037

8.5.5 Cooling Degree-Day Method

Cooling degree-days are also available to several base temperatures as provided in Table 8-2.

Cooling energy is predicted in a similar fashion as described for heating earlier:

$$E_C = \frac{q_g(\text{CDD})24}{1000(\text{SEER})\Delta t_d} \tag{0-1}$$

where

E_C = energy consumed for cooling, kWh
q_g = design cooling load, Btu/h (kW)
CDD = cooling degree-days
Δt_d = design temperature difference, °F (°C)
SEER = seasonal energy efficiency ratio, (Btu/h)/W (W/W)

The variable base cooling degree-day procedure for estimating cooling energy requirements is similar to the procedure for heating. If no cooling is done by ventilation, the balance temperature t_{bal} is calculated in the same way as the balance temperature for heating, except that summer values for cooling set temperature t_i, total heat gains q_g, and loss coefficient K must be used. The only significant difference from heating in the calculation procedure is that q_g customarily includes a latent term q_l for cooling.

The degree-day method assumes that t_{bal} is constant, which is not well satisfied in practice. Solar gains are zero at night, and internal gains tend to be highest during the evening. Also, during the intermediate season, heat gains can be eliminated, and the onset of mechanical cooling can be postponed by opening windows or increasing the ventilation. Therefore, cooling degree-hours can be used to better represent the period when equipment is operating than cooling degree-days, because degree-days assume uninterrupted equipment operation as long as there is a cooling load.

Example 8-2 For a residence located in El Paso, Texas, the design cooling load is 10.7 kW (36,500 Btu/h). Determine

(a) Annual energy requirements for cooling
(b) Cost of this energy if a unit having an SEER of 11.5 is selected and the electric rate is 6.9¢/kWh

Solution:

Table 8-2: Cooling degree-days = 2678
Summer design = 98°F

(a) Using cooling degree method,

$$\text{Cooling} = [36{,}500/(98-78)] \times 2678 \times 24$$
$$= 117{,}300{,}000 \text{ Btu}$$

$$E_C = 117{,}300{,}000/(1000 \times 11.5) = 10{,}200 \text{ kWh}$$

(b) Cost = 10,200 kWh × \$0.069/kWh = \$704

Example 8-3 A small dental office, 30 ft by 100 ft, located in downtown Chicago, Illinois, has design heating and cooling loads of 240,000 Btu/h and 85,000 Btu/h, respectively. Design conditions of 72°F inside and −3°F outside were used for winter while 78°F inside and 91°F outside were used for summer. The average interior heat gain during the winter has been estimated at 8 kW. Estimate the annual heating and cooling energy requirements and the corresponding energy costs using the national average rates given in the table below, if

(a) Electric baseboard heating units and a "high-efficiency" air conditioner (SEER = 14) are used.
(b) A condensing gas furnace and the same air conditioner are used.

Unit Fuel Prices

Natural gas	\$0.62/therm
No. 2 fuel oil	\$1.06/gallon
Electricity	\$0.072/kWh

Solution:

The heat loss per °F, K = 240,000/[72 − (−3)] = 3200

The balance temperature with an internal gain of 8 kW is determined from Eq. 8-2 as

$$t_{bal} = 72 - (8 \times 3413)/3200$$
$$= 72 - 8.5 = 63.5\text{°F}$$

From Table 8-2, the degree-days to this base can be obtained by interpolation to be 5775. For summer, the CDD to base 65 are found from Table 8-2 to be 713.

(a) From Eq. 8-6, the heating energy requirements are

$$E_H = \frac{240{,}000 \times 5775 \times 24}{0.95 \times 3413 \times 75} = 129{,}900 \text{ kWh}$$

(assuming 5% loss from baseboard units through wall)

Heating cost = 129,900 × \$0.072 = \$9350

From Eq. 8-7, the cooling energy is determined:

$$E_C = \frac{85{,}000 \times 713 \times 24}{1000 \times 14 \times (91-78)} = 7990 \text{ kWh}$$

Cooling cost = 7990 × \$0.072 = \$575

(b) From Eq. 8-6, the heating energy requirements are

$$E_H = \frac{240{,}000 \times 5775 \times 24}{0.93 \times 100{,}000 \times 75} = 4770 \text{ therm}$$

(with 1 therm = 100,000 Btu and assuming 93% AFUE from Chapter 19)

Heating cost = 4770 × \$0.062 = \$2960

8.6 Bin Method (Heating and Cooling)

For many applications, the degree-day method should not be used, even with the variable base method, because the heat loss coefficient K the efficiency η of the HVAC system, or the balance point temperature may not be sufficiently constant. The efficiency of a heat pump, for example, varies strongly with outdoor temperature; or the efficiency of the HVAC equipment may be affected indirectly by t_o when the efficiency varies with the load, which is a common situation for boilers and chillers. Furthermore, in most commercial buildings, the occupancy has a pronounced pattern, which affects heat gain, indoor temperature, and ventilation rate.

Table 8-3 Hourly Weather Occurrences

LOCATION	Outdoor Temperature, °F 72	67	62	57	52	47	42	37	32	27	22	17	12	7	2	−3	−8	−13	−18
Albany, NY	588	733	740	708	652	625	647	769	793	574	404	278	184	110	63	32	10	5	4
Albuquerque, NM	767	831	719	651	687	734	741	689	552	346	154	66	21	4	1	1			
Atlanta, GA	1185	926	823	784	735	676	598	468	271	112	44	19	8	2					
Bakersfield, CA	831	898	966	977	908	746	541	247	77	7									
Birmingham, AL	1138	908	805	742	668	614	528	433	292	143	69	17	6	3					
Bismark, ND	454	566	614	606	563	520	518	604	653	550	474	371	338	292	278	208	131	77	80
Boise, ID	492	575	643	702	786	798	878	829	522	307	148	53	26	14	6	2			
Boston, MA	676	819	804	781	766	757	828	848	674	429	256	151	74	35	4	9	1		
Buffalo, NY	646	772	760	700	666	624	647	756	849	602	426	267	170	81	5	24	2		
Burlington, VT	573	670	703	694	655	603	637	716	752	561	491	336	272	216	135	81	39	17	8
Casper, WY	423	532	592	642	606	670	782	831	806	683	495	325	200	116	73	45	30	15	5
Charleston, SC	1267	1090	889	787	651	576	434	321	192	79	27	5							
Charleston, WV	912	949	767	689	661	667	607	633	630	356	252	135	73	22	7	1			
Charlotte, NC	1115	908	839	752	730	684	634	515	360	166	64	23	5	2					
Chattanooga, TN	1021	895	775	722	713	679	642	553	414	228	113	45	4	4	2				
Chicago, IL	762	769	653	592	569	543	591	800	822	551	335	196	117	85	59	25	12	3	
Cincinnati, OH	879	843	726	639	611	599	627	698	711	460	249	131	68	44	18	8	2		
Cleveland, OH	763	831	723	641	638	607	620	754	806	578	355	201	111	47	22	11	2		
Columbus, OH	774	820	720	648	622	603	658	772	730	502	280	169	94	40	20	10	4	1	
Corpus Christi, TX	1175	1041	748	551	444	302	180	83	27	9	3								
Dallas, TX	831	795	693	656	629	576	504	371	231	91	34	17	4	1					
Denver, CO	549	684	783	731	678	704	692	717	721	553	359	216	119	78	36	22	6	1	1
Des Moines, IA	707	751	681	600	585	512	510	627	747	557	405	281	211	152	104	59	23	8	1
Detroit, MI	721	783	695	633	592	566	595	808	884	618	377	248	131	61	17	4	1		
El Paso, TX	933	839	749	760	687	611	494	369	233	34	104	10	2						
Ft. Wayne, IN	728	777	699	608	569	552	601	725	905	596	381	205	124	69	40	19	6	1	
Fresno, CA	709	803	921	1006	1036	952	673	426	168	34									
Grand Rapids, MI	634	739	712	647	571	565	554	742	938	690	469	293	172	78	31	10	1	1	
Great Falls, MT	407	520	636	754	822	830	832	813	698	533	355	218	167	136	118	101	68	51	62
Harrisburg, PA	807	824	737	692	635	659	722	888	749	427	222	125	52	18	4	1			
Hartford, CT	617	755	751	752	649	575	683	807	825	552	370	233	153	77	33	11	3	2	
Houston, TX	1172	980	772	681	570	452	291	141	64	18	4	2							
Indianapolis, IN	821	815	722	585	586	579	605	712	791	551	293	152	97	60	35	13	3	2	
Jackson, MS	1168	922	790	677	618	605	484	367	224	103	41	6	2	2	1				
Jacksonville, FL	1334	975	879	692	530	355	288	154	83	24	2								
Kansas City, MO	761	723	601	572	553	562	628	591	625	407	265	175	99	51	21	4			
Knoxville, TN	1056	889	746	675	672	689	648	590	456	217	101	41	21	7	2				
Las Vegas, NV	651	644	699	786	769	716	591	396	194	44	7	1							
Little Rock, AR	940	803	725	672	638	669	605	509	363	172	50	25	5	1					
Los Angeles, CA	881	1654	2193	1904	1054	428	107	10											
Louisville, KY	869	758	693	654	619	634	649	703	631	332	169	97	45	25	8	3	1		
Lubbock, TX	833	829	688	700	642	618	620	546	490	346	180	86	33	7	5	1			
Memphis, TN	977	798	715	690	618	633	614	532	374	196	74	25	10	4					
Miami, FL	1705	810	452	277	147	71	26	4											
Milwaukee, WI	597	753	749	634	585	591	611	774	913	659	421	285	176	116	83	47	18	4	3
Minneapolis, MN	621	690	695	602	588	482	500	560	632	609	514	383	311	246	186	119	62	31	16
Mobile, AL	1411	1038	882	698	609	506	377	214	109	49	7	3							
Nashville, TN	933	838	738	697	637	619	627	565	463	263	132	67	28	9	3	1	1		
New Orleans, LA	1189	987	850	692	621	449	282	128	47	9	2								
New York, NY	926	877	754	745	722	796	838	858	603	330	188	82	26	10	1				
Oklahoma City, OK	881	769	717	173	643	645	611	641	570	468	287	77	36	12	3	1			
Omaha, NB	726	721	606	558	539	543	543	655	663	511	390	287	189	135	93	40	15	1	
Philadelphia, PA	863	809	735	710	663	701	758	818	654	335	189	100	32	9					
Phoenix, AZ	762	776	767	769	659	540	391	182	57	8									
Pittsburgh, PA	722	910	799	678	637	587	631	688	569	774	360	233	159	60	30	7	1		
Portland, ME	407	627	780	808	760	748	722	839	820	599	408	293	190	109	60	29	15	5	1
Portland, OR	373	581	1001	1316	1274	1271	1238	772	343	123	40	10	4	1					
Raleigh, NC	1087	937	848	762	707	672	638	527	410	236	103	38	11	1					
Reno, NV	418	477	572	690	845	909	890	829	733	530	387	277	101	37	15	4	1		
Richmond, VA	953	850	784	745	690	673	699	632	478	285	138	67	19	2	1				
Sacramento, CA	630	773	1071	1329	1298	1049	701	355	93	8									
Salt Lake City, UT	569	615	614	635	682	685	755	831	798	564	328	158	80	41	16	2			
San Antonio, TX	1086	943	789	669	569	445	387	190	94	31	11	4	1	1					
San Francisco, CA	285	665	1264	2341	2341	1153	449	99	10										
Seattle, WA	258	448	750	1272	1462	1445	1408	914	427	104	39	20	3						
Shreveport, LA	1063	886	772	679	619	609	516	361	200	72	23	6	2						
Sioux Falls, SD	566	684	669	605	522	498	501	625	712	585	520	448	293	208	152	102	59	43	18
St. Louis, MO	823	728	646	575	585	578	620	671	650	411	219	134	77	40	15	7	1		
Syracuse, NY	627	735	723	717	656	641	651	729	830	547	392	282	190	102	55	23	5	2	2
Tampa, FL	1387	1187	877	570	345	216	137	48	10	1									
Waco, TX	909	830	701	622	651	558	501	354	216	84	24	3	1						
Washington, DC	960	766	740	673	690	684	790	744	542	254	138	54	17	2					
Wichita, KS	758	709	641	603	589	592	611	584	607	426	273	161	85	45	14	3	1		

In such cases, a steady-state calculation can yield good results for the annual energy consumption if different temperature intervals and time periods are evaluated separately. This approach is known as the *bin method*, because the energy consumption E_{bin} is calculated for several values of the outdoor temperature t_o and multiplied by the number of hours N_{bin} in the temperature interval (bin) centered around that temperature:

$$E_{bin} = N_{bin}K_{tot}(t_{bal} - t_o)/\eta \quad (0\text{-}2)$$

This equation is evaluated for each bin, and the total energy consumption is the sum of E_{bin} over all bins:

$$E = \Sigma E_{bin}$$

In the United States, the necessary data are widely available. The bins are usually in 5°F increments and are often collected in three daily 8-h shifts. Mean coincident wet-bulb temperature data (for each dry-bulb bin) are used to calculate latent cooling loads from infiltration and ventilation. The bin method considers both occupied and unoccupied building conditions and gives credit for internal loads by adjusting the balance point. For many applications, the number of calculations can be minimized. A residential heat pump (heating mode) could be evaluated using only the bins below the balance point without the three-shift breakdown.

The data included in Table 8-3 are annual totals for various cities in the United States. ASHRAE (1984) and USAF (1978) include monthly data and data further separated into time intervals throughout the day.

Modified Bin Method. Various refinements, such as the seasonal variation of solar gains, can be included in a bin calculation. If a separate calculation is done for each month, the heat gain could be based on the average solar heat gain of the month. The diurnal variation of solar gains can be accounted for by calculating the average solar gain for each of the hourly time periods of the bin method. If such a detailed calculation of solar gains is not necessary, a linear correlation of monthly average solar heat gains with monthly average outdoor temperature could be assumed. Using bin data for the corresponding periods, the calculation can also account for the operating schedules of commercial buildings.

The modified bin method has the advantage of allowing the use of diversified (part-load) rather than peak load values to establish the load as a function of outdoor dry-bulb temperature. This method also allows both secondary and primary (plant) HVAC equipment effects to be included in the energy calculation. The modified bin method permits the user to predict more accurately effects such as reheat and heat recovery that can only be guessed at with the degree-day or conventional bin methods.

In the modified bin method, average solar gain profiles, average equipment and lighting use profiles, and cooling load temperature difference (CLTD) values are used to characterize time-dependent diversified loads. The CLTDs approximate the transient effects of building mass. Time dependencies resulting from scheduling are averaged over a selected period, or multiple calculation periods are established. The duration of a calculation period determines the number of bin hours included. Normally, two calculation periods, representing occupied and unoccupied hours, are sufficient. The method can be further refined by making calculations on a monthly, not annual, basis.

Degree-Day Data from Bin Data. To calculate degree-days from hourly bin data, the base or balance temperature must first be determined. When t_{bal} is known, the following summation can be used for any time scale, either monthly or annually, or for several periods of a day on either a monthly or annual basis.

$$DD_h(t_{bal}) = [\Sigma(t_{bal} - t_{bin})N_{bin}]/24$$

where

t_{bin} = temperature at center of bin
N_{bin} = number of hours in bin at t_{bin}

Cooling degree-days are calculated analogously from

$$DD_c(t_{bal}) = [\Sigma(t_{bin} - t_{bal})N_{bin}]/24$$

This method generally produces degree-day values slightly higher than published values from NOAA or the National Climatic Data Center. This small but systematic deviation can be suppressed by ignoring degree-days during the swing seasons when totals are less than a minimum, e.g., 50 to 100 Fahrenheit degree-days per month.

Weather data for use with the bin method are available from ASHRAE and in *Engineering Weather Data* (U.S. Air Force Manual 88-29 1978). Copies may be obtained from the Superintendent of Documents, Government Printing Office, Washington, D.C. 26402. When time-of-occurrence bin data are not required, the hourly weather occurrence information in Table 8-3 may be used.

The basic data form for making a bin analysis is provided in Table 8-4.

Example 8-4 Estimate the energy requirements for a residence in Nashville, TN, with a design heat loss of 11,700 W at 30°C design temperature difference. Inside design temperature is 21°C. It is estimated that internal heat gains average 1250 W. Weather data in terms of hours for each bin is included as Table 8-5. Assume the selection of a 10.5 kW heat pump having the characteristics given in Columns E and H of Table 8-6 and Figure 8-5. Figure 8-5 shows the relationship between the heat loss and the integrated heat pump capacity. At temperatures below the balance point, supplemental heat is required, and at higher temperatures, the heat pump cycles on and off.

Solution:

The design heat loss is based on no internal generation. To compute the heat pump system energy input, compute the net heat requirements of the space, i.e., envelope loss minus internal heat generation. The net heat loss per degree and the heating/cooling balance temperature may be computed:

Table 8-4 Bin Data Form

Climate			House	Heat Pump							Supplemental		
A Temp. Bin, °F	B Temp. Diff. $t_{bal} - t_{bin}$	C Weather Data Bin, hours	D Heat Loss Rate, 1000 Btu/h	E Heat Pump Integrated Heating Capacity, 1000 Btu/h	F Cycling Capacity Adjustment Factor[a]	G Adjusted Heat Pump Capacity, 1000 Btu/h[b]	H Rated Electric Input, kW	I Operating Time Fraction[c]	J Heat Pump Supplied Heating, 10^6 Btu[d]	K Seasonal Heat Pump Elec. Consumption, kWh[e]	L Space Load, 10^6 Btu[f]	M Supplemental Heating Required, kWh[g]	N Total Electric Energy Consumption
62													
57													
52													
47													
42													
37													
32													
27													
22													
17													
12													
7													
2													
−3													
									TOTALS:				

a Cycling Capacity Adjustment Factor = 1 − $Cd(1 - x)$, where Cd = degradation coefficient (default = 0.25 unless part load factor is known) and x = building heat loss per unit capacity at temperature bin. Cycling capacity = 1 at the balance point and below.

b Col G = Col E × Col F

c Operating Time Factor equals smaller of 1 or Col D/Col G

d Col J = (Col I × Col G × Col C)/1000

e Col K = Col I × Col H × Col C

f Col L = Col C × Col D/1000

g Col M = (Col L − Col J) × 10^6/3413

h Col N = Col K + Col M

$$HL/\Delta t = 11{,}700/30 = 390 \text{ W/K}$$

$$t_{bal} = 21 - (1250/390) = 17.8°C$$

Table 8-6 is then computed resulting in an estimate of total electrical energy consumption for heat pump and supplemental heating of 7618 kWh.

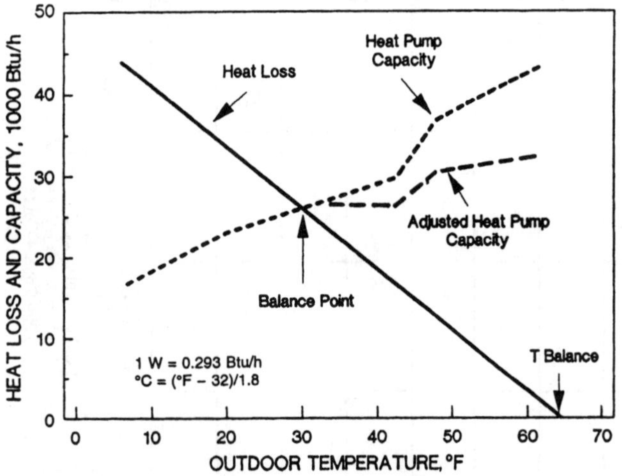

Fig. 8-5 Heat Pump Capacity and Building Load

8.7 Problems

8.1 The total design heating load on a residence in New York City is 32.8 kW (112,000 Btu/h) for an indoor temperature of 72°F. The furnace is *off* from June through September. Estimate

(a) The annual energy requirement for heating

(b) The annual heating cost if electric heat is used with the single rate of 16¢/kWh, \$/yr

(c) The maximum savings effected if the thermostat is set back to 65°F between 10 P.M. and 6 A.M., \$/yr

8.2 Determine the cost per 1000 Btu of supplying heat in your territory for (a) oil, (b) gas, (c) direct electric heating, and (d) an air-source heat pump. In calculating gas and oil costs, assume heating plant efficiencies of 80% and 75%, respectively. In calculating heat pump costs, assume a condensing refrigerant temperature of 110°F, an evaporating refrigerant temperature 10°F below the local average winter outdoor air temperature, and an actual COP 70% of that for the reversed Carnot cycle. Assume a compressor mechanical efficiency of 80%, with the compressor located in the airstream being heated.

Table 8-5 Hourly Weather Occurrences for Example 8-4

City	Bin																				
	39/ 41	36/ 38	33/ 35	30/ 32	27/ 29	24/ 26	21/ 23	18/ 20	15/ 17	12/ 14	9/ 11	6/ 8	3/ 5	0/ 2	−3/ −1	−6/ −4	−9/ −7	−12/ −10	−15/ −13	−18/ −16	−21/ −19
Chicago			74	176	431	512	960	660	591	780	510	770	686	1671	380	304	125	66	49	11	4
Dallas/Ft Worth	4	170	322	511	922	1100	1077	750	803	870	581	728	418	464	37	3					
Denver			81	217	406	390	570	726	712	902	809	783	750	1467	446	216	106	85	52	44	8
Los Angeles	4	10	9	16	56	194	1016	1874	2280	2208	843	227	23								
Miami			14	648	2147	2581	1852	734	390	202	100	76	14	2							
Nashville		4	82	366	717	756	1291	831	693	801	670	858	6 39	793	141	89	29				
Seattle				10	88	139	330	497	898	1653	1392	1844	1127	715	40	26	1				

Table 8-6 Sample Bin Data for Example 8-4

Climate			House	Heat Pump							Supplemental		
A	B	C	D	E	F	G	H	I	J	K	L	M	N
Temp. Bin, °C	Temp. Diff., $t_{bal}-t_{bin}$	Weather Data Bin, h	Heat Loss Rate, kW	Heat Pump Integrated Heating Capacity, kW	Cycling Capacity Adjustment Factor[a]	Adjusted Heat Pump Capacity, kW[b]	Rated Electric Input, kW	Operating Time Fraction[c]	Heat Pump Supplied Heating, kWh[d]	Seasonal Heat Pump Electric Consumption, kWh[e]	Space Load, kWh[f]	Supplemental Heating Required, kWh[g]	Total Electric Energy Consumption, kWh[h]
16	1.8	693	0.70	12.80	0.764	9.78	3.74	0.072	488	187	485	—	187
13	4.8	801	1.87	12.01	0.789	9.48	3.63	0.197	1496	573	1497	—	573
10	7.8	670	3.04	11.22	0.818	9.18	3.52	0.331	2036	781	2037	—	781
7	10.8	858	4.21	9.80	0.857	8.40	3.40	0.501	3611	1462	3612	—	1462
4	13.8	639	5.38	8.49	0.908	7.71	3.18	0.698	3439	1418	3438	—	1418
1	16.8	793	6.55	7.98	0.955	7.62	3.10	0.860	5196	2114	5195	—	2114
−2	19.8	141	7.72	7.47	1.000	7.47	3.02	1.000	1053	426	1089	36	462
−5	22.8	89	8.89	6.95	1.000	6.95	2.93	1.000	618	261	791	173	434
−8	25.8	29	10.06	6.48	1.000	6.48	2.85	1.000	188	83	292	104	187
−11	28.8	0	11.23	5.69	1.000	—	—	—	—	—	—	—	—
								TOTALS:	18125	7305	18436	313	7618

8.3 A home is located in Cleveland, Ohio, and has a design heat loss of 112,000 Btu/h at an inside design temperature of 72°F and an outside design temperature of 0°F. The home has an oil-fired furnace. Find the savings in gallons of fuel oil if the owner lowers the temperature in the home to 68°F between 10 P.M. and 6 A.M. every day during January.

[Ans: 13.2 gal (50 L)]

8.4 The total design heating load on a residence in Kansas City, Missouri, is 32.8 kW (112,000 Btu/h). The furnace is *off* during June through September. Estimate

(a) Annual energy requirement for heating
(b) Annual heating cost if No. 2 fuel oil is used in a furnace with an efficiency of 80% (assume fuel oil costs 47¢/L)
(c) Maximum savings effected if the thermostat is set back from 22.2 to 18.3°C (72 to 65°F) between 10 P.M. and 6 A.M. in $/yr

8.5 A residence located in Tulsa, Oklahoma has a design heating load of 20 kW and a design cooling load of 9.4 kW. Determine the following:

(a) Heating energy requirements, kWh
(b) Litres of No. 2 fuel oil per season if used as heating fuel
(c) Litres of natural gas per season if used as heating fuel
(d) kWh of electric energy if used as heating fuel with baseboard units
(e) kWh of electric energy if used for air-conditioning system having $COP_{seasonal} = 3.4$
(f) Total airflow rate in L/s if a warm air system is used
(g) Total steam flow in kg/s if a steam system is used

8.6 As a move to conserve energy, underground houses have been designed. One such house has walls, floor, and roof/ceiling which are all 10-in. thick concrete. The roof is covered with 6 in. of soil having a thermal conductivity of 9.0 Btu·in/h·ft²·°F. Outdoor air design temperature is 0°F. The house is overall 70 ft by 28 ft by 8 ft, interior dimensions. Two air changes per hour are provided. Determine the furnace size required and the energy requirements for a 5900 degree-days heating season. The groundwater is 50°F.

[Ans: 122,000 Btu/h, 2.3×10^8 Btu/yr]

8.7 Repeat Problem 8.6 with R-30 insulation added to the ceiling.

8.8 A general office building located in Rolla, Missouri, has a winter sensible space heating load of 1,150,000 Btu/h for design conditions of 75°F and −5°F. The heating system operates with 25% outside air mixed with return air.

(a) Draw schematically the flow diagram and label including temperatures and flow rates at each location.
(b) Specify the necessary furnace size.
(c) Determine:
  (1) Annual energy requirements for heating, Btu
  (2) Annual fuel cost using No. 2 fuel oil with heating value of 140,000 Btu/gal at 99.9¢/gal
  (3) Percentage savings in fuel if a 60°F set-back is used between 6 P.M. and 6 A.M., Monday through Thursday, and over the weekend

8.9 Estimate the annual energy costs for heating and cooling a residence located in Cleveland, Ohio, having design loads of 65,000 Btu/h (heating) and 30,000 Btu/h (cooling) based on a 75°F indoor temperature. In winter the thermostat is set back to 60°F for 10 h each night. The furnace is on from October 1 through May 31. Electric baseboard heat is used. The air conditioner has an SEER of 7.3 (Btu/h)/W. Electricity costs 0.0725 $/kWh year round.

[Ans: $2414]

8.10 A residence in St. Joseph, Missouri, has a design heating load of 68,000 Btu/h when design indoor and outdoor temperatures are 75°F and 3°F, respectively. The furnace is *off* from June through September. Determine the fuel and energy requirements for heating in

(a) Btu
(b) Gallons of No. 2 fuel oil/yr
(c) Cubic feet of natural gas/yr
(d) kWh
(e) Total airflow rate in cfm if a warm air system is used
(f) Total steam flow in lb/h if a steam system is used
(g) Total water flow rate in gpm if a hydronic system is used
(h) Total electric power in kW if electric heating is used

8.11 For a residence located in New Orleans, Louisiana, the design cooling load is 12 kW (41,000 Btu/h). Determine

(a) Annual energy requirements for cooling, kWh
(b) Cost of this energy if the electric rate is 6.5¢/kWh

8.12 An office building located in Springfield, Missouri, has a heat loss of 2,160,000 Btu/h for design condition of 75°F inside and 10°F outside. The heating system is operational between October 1 and April 30. Determine

(a) Annual energy usage for heating
(b) Estimated fuel cost if No. 2 fuel oil is used having a heating value of 140,000 Btu/gal and costing 98.9¢/gal

[Ans: 3.0 × 109 Btu; $30,400]

8.13 A small football promotion office is being designed for Jacksonville, Florida. The design heating and cooling loads are 61,200 and 55,400 Btu/h, respectively, based on 97-1/2% and 2-1/2% outdoor design dry bulb temperatures. Balance point has been estimated as 65°F.

(a) Select an appropriate heat pump from the XYZ Corporation models listed on the next page and estimate the energy costs for summer and winter if electricity is 8¢/kWh.
(b) Compare the heating energy cost for the heat pump to that for a condensing gas furnace with natural gas costing $0.49 per therm.

8.14 A 1980 ft² residence located in Cincinnati, Ohio, has design heating and cooling loads of 74,000 Btu/h and 35,000 Btu/h, respectively. Determine

HEAT PUMP MODELS—XYZ CORPORATION for *Problem* 8.13—
Performance Data at ARI Standard Conditions

Model Numbers	COOLING CAPACITY — Design Conditions: ARI Rating Temperatures 80°F.D.B., 67°F.W.B. Indoor, Return Air; 95°F.D.B. Outdoor.							HEATING CAPACITY (70°F Indoor Air) — Outside Air 47°F.D.B./43°F.W.B. DOE High Temperature			HEATING CAPACITY (70°F Indoor Air) — Outside Air 17°F.D.B./15°F.W.B. DOE Low Temperature			DOE Region IV
	ARI Std. Cap. BTU/Hr.	Net Sens. Cooling Cap.	Net. Lat. BTU/Hr.	Single Phase SEER	Single Phase Total Watts	ARI Noise Rating	Approx. CFM	BTU/Hr.	Power Input Watts	COP	BTU/Hr.	Power Input Watts	COP	HSPF BTU/Watt-Hr.
A018	18.200	13.700	4.500	11.20	1820	7.0	650	18.400	1671	3.25	9.700	1255	2.25	8.15
A024	24.200	18.000	6.200	10.80	2513	7.0	850	24.800	2162	3.35	14.400	1718	2.45	8.85
A030	30.000	22.000	8.000	10.60	3151	7.2	1050	31.800	2885	3.25	18.600	2263	2.40	8.65
A036	36.800	25.500	10.300	10.50	3837	7.4	1250	39.000	3590	3.15	22.000	2763	2.35	8.25
A042	42.500	31.900	10.600	11.20	4250	7.6	1450	43.500	3803	3.35	24.600	2929	2.45	8.85
A048	49.500	36.800	12.700	10.50	5269	7.6	1650	51.000	4596	3.25	30.000	3578	2.45	8.80
A060	60.000	43.700	16.300	10.50	6250	7.8	2050	66.000	6050	3.20	37.000	4612	2.35	8.50

A-030 HEATING
INDOOR AIR CONDITIONS 70°F D.B.

OUTDOOR TEMPERATURE	BTUH	WATT	COP	EER
−18	8900	1800	1.45	4.94
−13	9700	1830	1.55	5.30
−8	10600	1880	1.65	5.64
−3	11800	1940	1.78	6.08
2	13200	2010	1.92	6.57
7	14800	2090	2.07	7.08
12	16600	2170	2.24	7.65
17	18600	2260	2.41	8.23
22	20500	2360	2.55	8.69
27	22700	2470	2.69	9.19
32	24900	2570	2.84	9.69
37	27300	2690	2.97	10.15
42	29600	2800	3.10	10.57
47	31800	2890	3.22	11.00
52	34500	3020	3.35	11.42
57	37000	3140	3.45	11.78
62	39400	3250	3.55	12.12
67	41800	3350	3.66	12.48
72	44100	3450	3.75	12.78
77	46400	3550	3.83	13.07
82	48600	3640	3.91	13.35

A-036 HEATING
INDOOR AIR CONDITIONS 70°F D.B.

OUTDOOR TEMPERATURE	BTUH	WATT	COP	EER
−18	9300	2150	1.27	4.33
−13	10300	2210	1.37	4.66
−8	11700	2270	1.51	5.15
−3	13300	2350	1.66	5.66
2	15100	2440	1.81	6.19
7	17200	2550	1.98	6.75
12	19500	2650	2.15	7.33
17	22000	2760	2.34	7.97
22	24500	2910	2.47	8.42
27	27300	3050	2.62	8.95
32	30100	3190	2.76	9.44
37	33100	3330	2.91	9.94
42	36100	3480	3.04	10.37
47	39000	3610	3.17	10.80
52	42200	3770	3.28	11.19
57	45200	3910	3.39	11.56
62	48300	4050	3.49	11.93
67	51200	4190	3.58	12.22
72	54100	4310	3.68	12.55
77	56900	4440	3.75	12.82
82	59600	4550	3.84	13.10

A-048 HEATING
INDOOR AIR CONDITIONS 70°F D.B.

OUTDOOR TEMPERATURE	BTUH	WATT	COP	EER
−18	10900	2780	1.15	3.92
−13	13200	2860	1.35	4.62
−8	15700	2950	1.56	5.32
−3	18400	3060	1.76	6.01
2	21200	3180	1.95	6.67
7	24200	3310	2.14	7.31
12	27300	3450	2.32	7.91
17	30000	3580	2.46	8.38
22	33000	3760	2.63	8.99
27	37300	3930	2.78	9.49
32	40800	4100	2.92	9.95
37	44400	4280	3.04	10.37
42	48000	4460	3.15	10.76
47	51000	4600	3.25	11.09
52	55400	4810	3.37	11.52
57	59200	4990	3.48	11.86
62	63000	5160	3.58	12.21
67	66700	5330	3.67	12.51
72	70500	5490	3.76	12.84
77	74200	5640	3.85	13.16
82	78000	5790	3.95	13.47

A-060 HEATING
INDOOR AIR CONDITIONS 70°F D.B.

OUTDOOR TEMPERATURE	BTUH	WATT	COP	EER
−18	16800	3360	1.46	5.00
−13	18300	3470	1.55	5.27
−8	20400	3600	1.66	5.67
−3	23000	3760	1.79	6.12
2	26000	3940	1.93	6.60
7	29400	4130	2.09	7.12
12	33200	4350	2.24	7.63
17	37000	4610	2.35	8.03
22	41700	4810	2.54	8.67
27	46300	5050	2.69	9.17
32	51000	5300	2.82	9.62
37	56000	5560	2.95	10.07
42	61000	5810	3.08	10.50
47	66000	6050	3.20	10.91
52	71200	6320	3.30	11.27
57	76300	6560	3.41	11.63
62	81300	6790	3.51	11.97
67	85200	7020	3.60	12.28
72	91000	7230	3.69	12.59
77	95600	7420	3.78	12.88
82	99900	7600	3.85	13.14

(a) Heating energy requirements, Btu
(b) Gallons of No. 2 fuel oil if 75% efficient oil-fired warm air system is used
(c) Therms of natural gas if 88% efficient gas-fired warm air system is used
(d) kWh of electricity if 98% efficient baseboard units are used
(e) Required airflow, cfm, for warm air systems
(f) kWh of electricity if heat pump system (WA-36 specifications follow) including supplementary electric resistance heat is used
(g) kWh of electricity for cooling for air conditioner with SEER of 8.5 using degree-day estimation
(h) Required airflow, cfm, for air conditioning

Performance Data for Model WA-36 Heat Pump

Air Temperature, °F	Heat Pump Output, 1000 Btu	Heat Pump Input, kW
62	44	4.5
57	43	4.4
52	41	4.3
47	39	4.1
42	36	4.0
37	33	3.9
32	30	3.7
27	27	3.6
22	24	3.5
17	22	3.3
12	19	3.2
7	17	3.1
2	15	2.9
−3	13	2.8

8.15 A small commercial building located in Oklahoma City, Oklahoma, has design loads of 245,000 Btu/h, *heating*, and 162,000 Btu/h, *cooling*. Balance point for the building has been estimated at 65°F. Determine:

(a) Annual energy requirements for heating, Btu
(b) Fuel cost using LPG at 83¢/gallon, $
(c) Fuel cost using electric baseboard units with electricity at 6.7¢/kWh, $
(d) Savings if setback to 55°F is effected between 10 P.M. and 6 A.M., Monday through Saturday, and all day Sunday, %
(e) Cooling season energy cost using cooling degree-days if conditioner has SEER of 11.5 and electricity is 7¢/kWh

8.16 A small commercial building in Indianapolis, Indiana, has design heating and cooling loads of 98,000 Btu/h and 48,000 Btu/h, respectively. Internal heat gains throughout the winter are relatively steady at 4.5 kW. Electricity costs 7.1¢/kWh. Estimate

(a) Annual heating cost if baseboard electric resistance units are used.
(b) Annual cooling cost with a conventional vapor compression air-cooled unit, using your choice of method.

Select a heat pump system for the building from the XYZ Corporation models. Determine the

(a) Annual heating cost and
(b) Annual cooling cost.

8.17 A small (2200 ft^2) food mart store located in Charlotte, NC, has design heating and cooling loads of 94,500 Btu/h and 57,400 Btu/h, respectively, based on inside design temperatures of 72°F (winter) and 78°F (summer). The store is open 24 h a day and has a relatively constant internal load due to lights, food cases, people, etc., of 3.3 W/ft^2. Select a suitable heat pump for the XYZ Corporation and estimate its operating energy costs for both summer and winter if the price of electricity is 7.4 ¢/kWh.

8.8 Bibliography

ASHRAE. 1995. *Bin and degree hour weather data for simplified energy calculations*, ASHRAE, Atlanta, GA.

USAF. 1978. Engineering weather data. U.S. Air Force *Manual* 88-29. Superintendent of Documents, Government Printing Office, Washington, D.C. 26402

Chapter 9

DUCT AND PIPE SIZING

This chapter discusses the design of systems for conveying air and water. Chapter 32 of the 1997 *ASHRAE Handbook—Fundamentals* has further details on the design of duct systems. Chapter 31 from the same source gives details on space air diffusion. Chapter 33 of the 1997 *ASHRAE Handbook—Fundamentals* has additional details on pipe sizing while Chapters 18, 38, and 40 in the 1996 *ASHRAE Handbook—Systems and Equipment* has further information on fans, pumps, pipes, tubes, and fittings.

9.1 Duct Systems

An air-conditioning system must not only condition air, it must also distribute conditioned air throughout the space. Usually the conditioning fluid is distributed from a central equipment location to the individual spaces requiring environment control. For example, a fan and duct system distributes air, and a pump and piping system distributes water. Conditioned air is distributed into the room by air diffusers or grilles.

An objective of duct system design is to provide a system that, within prescribed limits of velocities, noise intensity, and space available for ducts, efficiently transmits the required flow rate of air to each space, while maintaining a proper balance between investment and operating cost. When the heating, cooling, or ventilation load is established, the total flow rate of air required can be determined by methods shown in Chapters 27 and 28 of the 1997 *ASHRAE Handbook—Fundamentals*. The size of the duct system governs frictional losses and thereby the size of fan and power required to operate the duct system.

9.1.1 Pressure Changes

Resistance to airflow imposed by the supply duct system must be overcome by mechanical energy, which is ordinarily supplied by a fan. Resistance also is imposed by the return-air system which must also be overcome by the fan. In air-conditioning and ventilating work, the pressure differences are ordinarily so small that the equations for incompressible flow can be applied. Additional simplification is obtained by considering the air to be at the standard density of 0.075 lb/ft^3 (1.2 kg/m^3).

At any cross-section in a duct, the total pressure p_t is the sum of the static pressure ps and the velocity pressure p_v.

$$p_t = p_s + p_v \tag{9-1}$$

Pressures are normally expressed in inches of water (Pa). The velocity pressure is then given by:

$$p_v = \left(\frac{V}{cf_1}\right)^2 \tag{9-2}$$

where V is defined by the equation:

$$V = cf_2(Q/A) \tag{9-3}$$

where

p_v = velocity pressure, in. of water (Pa)
= mean velocity of fluid, ft/min (m/s)
Q = airflow rate, ft/min (L/s)
A = cross-sectional area of duct, in^2 (mm^2)
cf_1 = conversion factor, 4005 (1.29)
cf_2 = conversion factor, 144 (1000)

The following table relates the air velocity to the velocity pressure for a range of velocities which might be encountered in HVAC duct systems. These values were calculated from Equation (9-2) assuming a standard density of air as 0.075 lb$_m$/ft^3.

V fpm	**P$_v$** in. water	**V** fpm	**P$_v$** in. water	**V** fpm	**P$_v$** in. water
500	0.016	1800	0.202	4400	1.21
600	0.022	2000	0.249	4600	1.32
700	0.031	2200	0.302	4800	1.44
800	0.040	2400	0.359	5000	1.56
900	0.050	2600	0.421	5200	1.69
1000	0.062	2800	0.489	5400	1.82
1100	0.075	3000	0.561	5600	1.96
1200	0.090	3200	0.638	5800	2.10
1300	0.105	3400	0.721	6000	2.24
1400	0.122	3600	0.808	6200	2.40
1500	0.140	3800	0.900	6400	2.55
1600	0.160	4000	0.998	6600	2.72
1700	0.180	4200	1.10	6800	2.88

If the air is not at this standard density, Equation (9-4) may be used in place of Equation (9-2):

$$p_v = \rho\left(\frac{V}{cf_3}\right)^2 \tag{9-4}$$

where

ρ = air density, lb/ft^3 (kg/m^3)
V = fluid mean velocity, ft/min (m/s)
p_v = velocity pressure, in. of water (Pa)
cf_3 = conversion factor, 1097 (1.414)

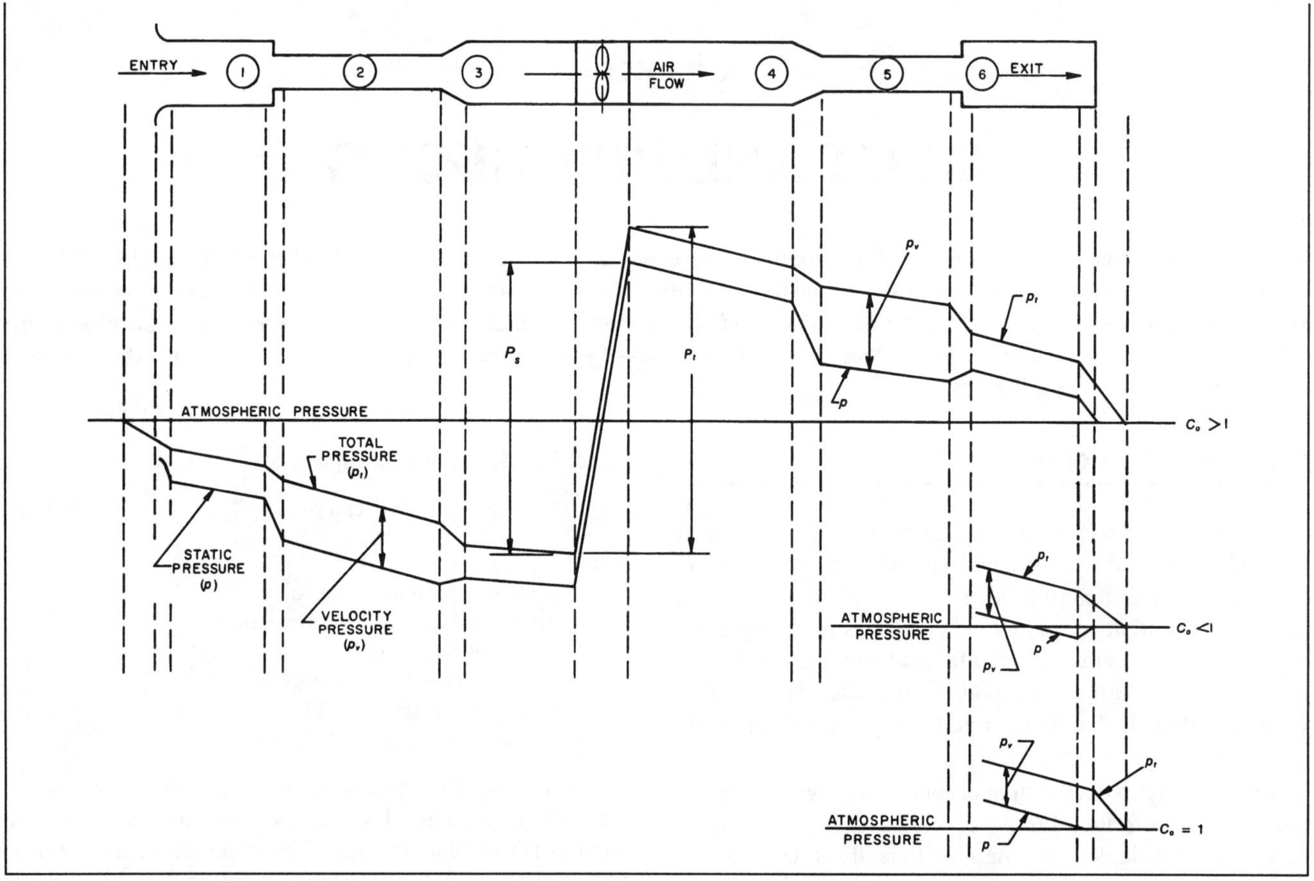

Fig. 9-1 Pressure Changes During Flow in Ducts

The total pressure p_t is a measure of the total available energy at a cross section. In any duct system, the total pressure always decreases in the direction of the airflow. Static and velocity pressure are mutually convertible and either increase or decrease in the flow direction.

Total and static pressure changes in a simplified fan/duct system are shown in Figure 9-1. This illustrative system consists of a fan with both supply and return air duct work. Also shown are the total and static pressure gradients referenced to atmospheric pressure.

For all constant-area sections, such as ducts and elbows, the total and static pressure losses are equal. In the case of ducts, the losses are entirely frictional, while the losses in constant-area fitting are frictional and dynamic.

At diverging sections 3 and 6, the velocity pressure decreases, the absolute value of the total pressure decreases, and the absolute value of the static pressure may increase. The increase in static pressure as shown at these sections is known as **static regain**.

At converging sections 1 and 4, the velocity pressure increases in the direction of airflow, and the absolute value of both the total and static pressure decreases. The static or total pressure loss from upstream to downstream is the difference in total/static pressure between the two sections.

At the exit, total pressure loss depends on the shape of the fitting and the flow characteristics. Exit loss coefficients can be greater than, less than, or equal to, one. For this variation of coefficients, the total and static pressure grade lines are shown in Figure 9-1. Note that when the loss coefficient is less than one, the static pressure upstream of the exit is less than atmospheric pressure (negative). The static pressure upstream of the discharge fitting can be calculated by subtracting the upstream velocity pressure from the upstream total pressure.

The entry loss also depends on the shape of the fitting. The total pressure immediately downstream of the entrance equals the difference between the upstream pressure, which is zero (atmospheric pressure), and the loss through the fitting. The static pressure at the entrance is zero, and immediately downstream, the difference between static pressure is negative, algebraically equal to the total pressure (negative) and the velocity pressure (always positive), or $p_s = p_t - p_v$.

The total system resistance to airflow is noted by p_t in Figure 9-1. The fan inlet and outlet system effect factors due to the interaction of the fan and system are not shown; only system resistances are shown. To obtain the fan static pressure p_s requirement for selecting a fan, knowing the systems' total pressure, use:

$$p_s = p_t - p_{v,o} \tag{9-5}$$

where the subscript *o* refers to the discharge area of the fan.

Static pressure is used as the basis for system design; total pressure determines the actual mechanical energy that must be supplied to the system. Total pressure always decreases in the direction of flow. Note, however, in Figure 9-1, the static pressure decreases and then increases in the direction of flow. Moreover, it can even become negative (below atmospheric). Therefore, in dealing with static pressure, distinction must always be made between static pressure **loss** and static pressure **change** as a result of conversion of velocity pressure.

9.1.2 Circular Equivalents of Rectangular Ducts

An air-handling system is usually sized first for round ducts. Then, if rectangular ducts are desired, duct sizes are selected to provide flow rates equivalent to those of the round ducts originally selected.

Rectangular ducts of aspect ratios not exceeding 8:1 usually have the same friction pressure loss for equal lengths and mean velocities of flow as do circular ducts of the same hydraulic diameter. When duct sizes are expressed in terms of hydraulic diameter (4 times area divided by perimeter), and when equations for friction loss in round and rectangular ducts are equated for equal flow rate and equal length, Equation (9-6), giving the circular equivalent of a rectangular duct, is obtained.

$$d_c = \frac{1.30ab^{0.625}}{(a+b)^{0.250}} \qquad (9\text{-}6)$$

where

a = length of one side of rectangular duct, in. (mm)

b = length of adjacent side of rectangular duct, in. (mm)

d_c = circular equivalent of a rectangular duct for equal friction and capacity, in. (mm)

The circular equivalents of rectangular ducts for equal friction and flow rate for aspect ratios not greater than 8:1, based on Equation (9-6), are given in Table 9-1. Note that the mean velocity in a rectangular duct is less than its circular equivalent.

Multiplying or dividing the length of each side of a duct by a constant is the same as multiplying or dividing the equivalent round size by the same constant. Thus, if the circular equivalent of an 80 in. by 24 in. duct is required, it is twice that of a 40 in. by 12 in. duct, or 2 × 23.0 = 46.0 in.

9.1.3 Friction Losses

Pressure drop in a straight duct is caused by surface friction. This friction loss can be calculated by using the Air Friction Charts (Figure 9-2). The charts were built from the basic flow equation for pressure loss in circular ducts:

$$\Delta p_{fr} = f_D\,(cf_4\,L/D)\,p_v \qquad (9\text{-}7)$$

where

Δp_{fr} = friction loss in terms of total pressure, in. of water (Pa)

f_D = dimensionless friction factor, which for air-conditioning work depends on Reynolds number and relative roughness of the conduit. Approximate values of f were taken from Moody (1944) where e = 0.0003 ft (0.09 mm). It numerically equals the reciprocal of the number of duct diameters required to cause a pressure loss equal to one velocity pressure.

L = length of duct, ft (m)

D = inside diameter of duct, in. (mm)

p_v = velocity pressure of mean velocity, in. of water (Pa)

cf_4 = conversion factor, 12 (1).

The air friction chart is based on air with a density of 0.075 lb/ft^3 (1.2 kg/m^3), flowing through average, clean, round, galvanized metal ducts with beaded slip couplings on 48-in. (1220 mm) centers.

Variations in air temperature of the order of ±20°F from 70°F (±11°C from 20°C) have little effect on duct friction. Therefore, Figure 9-2 may be used for all air systems with temperatures from 50 to 90°F (10 to 32°C). However, the values found in the charts must be corrected for systems carrying air at much higher temperatures. To determine the friction loss in such systems, the actual flow rate or velocity existing at the nonstandard conditions must be used. For duct materials other than those indicated, and for significant variations in temperature and barometric pressure/elevation, correction factors should be applied to the Air Friction Chart values. Details concerning these correction factors can be found in Chapter 32 of the 1997 *ASHRAE Handbook—Fundamentals*.

9.1.4 Dynamic Losses

Wherever eddying flow is present, a greater loss in total pressure takes place than would occur in steady flow through a similar length of straight duct having a uniform cross section. The amount of this loss in excess of straight duct friction is termed **dynamic loss**.

Dynamic losses result from flow disturbances caused by fittings that change the airflow path's direction and/or area. These fittings include entries, exits, transitions, and junctions. Idelchik (1986) discusses parameters affecting fluid resistance of fittings and presents loss coefficients in three forms: tables, curves, and equations.

The following dimensionless coefficient is used for fluid resistance, since this coefficient has the same value in dynamically similar streams, i.e., streams with geometrically similar stretches, equal values of Reynolds number, and equal values of other criteria necessary for dynamic similarity. The fluid resistance coefficient represents the ratio of total pressure loss to velocity pressure at the referenced cross section.

$$C = \frac{\Delta p_j}{\rho(V/1097)^2} = \frac{\Delta p_j}{p_v} \qquad (9\text{-}8\ \text{I-P})$$

Table 9-1 Equivalent Rectangular Duct Dimension
(Table 2, Chapter 32 of the 1997 *ASHRAE Handbook—Fundamentals*)

Duct Diameter, in.		Aspect Ratio 1.00	1.25	1.50	1.75	2.00	2.25	2.50	2.75	3.00	3.50	4.00	5.00	6.00	7.00	8.00
		Rectangular Size, in.														
6	Width	—	6													
	Height	—	5													
7	Width	6	8													
	Height	6	6													
8	Width	7	9	9	11											
	Height	7	7	6	6											
9	Width	8	9	11	11	12	14									
	Height	8	7	7	6	6	6									
10	Width	9	10	12	12	14	14	15	17							
	Height	9	8	8	7	7	6	6	6							
11	Width	10	11	12	14	14	16	18	17	18	21					
	Height	10	9	8	8	7	7	7	6	6	6					
12	Width	11	13	14	14	16	16	18	19	21	21	24				
	Height	11	10	9	8	8	7	7	7	7	6	6				
13	Width	12	14	15	16	18	18	20	19	21	25	24	30			
	Height	12	11	10	9	9	8	8	7	7	7	6	6			
14	Width	13	14	17	18	18	20	20	22	24	25	28	30	36		
	Height	13	11	11	10	9	9	8	8	8	7	7	6	6		
15	Width	14	15	17	18	20	20	23	25	24	28	28	35	36	42	
	Height	14	12	11	10	10	9	9	9	8	8	7	7	6	6	
16	Width	15	16	18	19	20	23	23	25	27	28	32	35	42	42	48
	Height	15	13	12	11	10	10	9	9	9	8	8	7	7	6	6
17	Width	16	18	20	21	22	25	25	28	27	32	32	35	42	49	48
	Height	16	14	13	12	11	11	10	10	9	9	8	7	7	7	6
18	Width	16	19	21	23	24	25	28	28	30	32	36	40	42	49	56
	Height	16	15	14	13	12	11	11	10	10	9	9	8	7	7	7
19	Width	17	20	21	23	24	27	28	30	30	35	36	40	48	49	56
	Height	17	16	14	13	12	12	11	11	10	10	9	8	8	7	7
20	Width	18	20	23	25	26	27	30	30	33	35	40	45	48	56	56
	Height	18	16	15	14	13	12	12	11	11	10	10	9	8	8	7
21	Width	19	21	24	26	28	29	30	33	33	39	40	45	54	56	64
	Height	19	17	16	15	14	13	12	12	11	11	10	9	9	8	8
22	Width	20	23	26	26	28	32	33	36	36	39	44	50	54	56	64
	Height	20	18	17	15	14	14	13	13	12	11	11	10	9	8	8
23	Width	21	24	26	28	30	32	35	36	39	42	44	50	54	63	64
	Height	21	19	17	16	15	14	14	13	13	12	11	10	9	9	8
24	Width	22	25	27	30	32	34	35	39	39	42	48	55	60	63	72
	Height	22	20	18	17	16	15	14	14	13	12	12	11	10	9	9
25	Width	23	25	29	30	32	36	38	39	42	46	48	55	60	70	72
	Height	23	20	19	17	16	16	15	14	14	13	12	11	10	10	9
26	Width	24	26	30	32	34	36	38	41	42	46	52	55	66	70	72
	Height	24	21	20	18	17	16	15	15	14	13	13	11	11	10	9
27	Width	25	28	30	33	36	38	40	41	45	49	52	60	66	70	80
	Height	25	22	20	19	18	17	16	15	15	14	13	12	11	10	10
28	Width	26	29	32	35	36	38	43	44	45	49	56	60	66	77	80
	Height	26	23	21	20	18	17	17	16	15	14	14	12	11	11	10
29	Width	27	30	33	35	38	41	43	44	48	53	56	65	72	77	88
	Height	27	24	22	20	19	18	17	16	16	15	14	13	12	11	11
30	Width	27	31	35	37	40	43	45	47	48	53	60	65	72	77	88
	Height	27	25	23	21	20	19	18	17	16	15	15	13	12	11	11
31	Width	28	31	35	39	40	43	45	50	51	56	60	70	78	84	88
	Height	28	25	23	22	20	19	18	18	17	16	15	14	13	12	11
32	Width	29	33	36	39	42	45	48	50	54	56	60	70	78	84	96
	Height	29	26	24	22	21	20	19	18	18	16	15	14	13	12	12
33	Width	30	34	38	40	44	47	50	52	54	60	64	75	78	91	96
	Height	30	27	25	23	22	21	20	19	18	17	16	15	13	13	12
34	Width	31	35	39	42	44	47	50	52	57	60	64	75	84	91	96
	Height	31	28	26	24	22	21	20	19	19	17	16	15	14	13	12
35	Width	32	36	39	42	46	50	53	55	57	63	68	75	84	91	104
	Height	32	29	26	24	23	22	21	20	19	18	17	15	14	13	13
36	Width	33	36	41	44	48	50	53	55	60	63	68	80	90	98	104
	Height	33	29	27	25	24	22	21	20	20	18	17	16	15	14	13
38	Width	35	39	44	47	50	54	58	61	63	67	72	85	96	105	112
	Height	35	31	29	27	25	24	23	22	21	19	18	17	16	15	14

*Shaded area not recommended.

Table 9-1 Equivalent Rectangular Duct Dimension (*Concluded*)

(Table 2, Chapter 32 of the 1997 *ASHRAE Handbook—Fundamentals*)

Duct Diameter, in.		Aspect Ratio 1.00	1.25	1.50	1.75	2.00	2.25	2.50	2.75	3.00	3.50	4.00	5.00	6.00	7.00	8.00
		Rectangular Size, in.														
40	Width	37	41	45	49	52	56	60	63	66	70	76	90	96	105	120
	Height	37	33	30	28	26	25	24	23	22	20	19	18	16	15	15
42	Width	38	43	48	51	56	59	63	66	69	74	80	90	102	112	120
	Height	38	34	32	29	28	26	25	24	23	21	20	18	17	16	15
44	Width	40	45	50	54	58	61	65	69	72	81	84	95	108	119	128
	Height	40	36	33	31	29	27	26	25	24	23	21	19	18	17	16
46	Width	42	48	53	56	60	65	68	72	75	84	88	100	114	126	136
	Height	42	38	35	32	30	29	27	26	25	24	22	20	19	18	17
48	Width	44	49	54	60	62	68	70	74	78	88	92	105	120	126	136
	Height	44	39	36	34	31	30	28	27	26	25	23	21	20	18	17
50	Width	46	51	57	61	66	70	75	77	81	91	96	110	120	133	144
	Height	46	41	38	35	33	31	30	28	27	26	24	22	20	19	18
52	Width	48	54	59	63	68	72	78	83	84	95	100	115	126	140	152
	Height	48	43	39	36	34	32	31	30	28	27	25	23	21	20	19
54	Width	49	55	62	67	70	77	80	85	90	98	104	120	132	147	160
	Height	49	44	41	38	35	34	32	31	30	28	26	24	22	21	20
56	Width	51	58	63	68	74	79	83	88	93	102	108	125	138	147	160
	Height	51	46	42	39	37	35	33	32	31	29	27	25	23	21	20
58	Width	53	60	66	70	76	81	85	91	96	105	112	130	144	154	168
	Height	53	48	44	40	38	36	34	33	32	30	28	26	24	22	21
60	Width	55	61	68	74	78	83	90	94	99	109	116	130	144	161	
	Height	55	49	45	42	39	37	36	34	33	31	29	26	24	23	
62	Width	57	64	71	75	82	88	93	96	102	112	120	135	150	168	
	Height	57	51	47	43	41	39	37	35	34	32	30	27	25	24	
64	Width	59	65	72	79	84	90	95	99	105	116	124	140	156		
	Height	59	52	48	45	42	40	38	36	35	33	31	28	26		
66	Width	60	68	75	81	86	92	98	105	108	119	128	145	162		
	Height	60	54	50	46	43	41	39	38	36	34	32	29	27		
68	Width	62	70	77	82	90	95	100	107	111	123	132	150	168		
	Height	62	56	51	47	45	42	40	39	37	35	33	30	28		
70	Width	64	71	80	86	92	99	105	110	114	126	136	155			
	Height	64	57	53	49	46	44	42	40	38	36	34	31			
72	Width	66	74	81	88	94	101	108	113	117	130	140	160			
	Height	66	59	54	50	47	45	43	41	39	37	35	32			
74	Width	68	76	84	91	98	104	110	116	123	133	144	165			
	Height	68	61	56	52	49	46	44	42	41	38	36	33			
76	Width	70	78	86	93	100	106	113	118	126	137	148	165			
	Height	70	62	57	53	50	47	45	43	42	39	37	33			
78	Width	71	80	89	95	102	110	115	121	129	140	152				
	Height	71	64	59	54	51	49	46	44	43	40	38				
80	Width	73	83	90	98	104	113	118	124	132	144	156				
	Height	73	66	60	56	52	50	47	45	44	41	39				
82	Width	75	84	93	100	108	115	123	129	135	147	160				
	Height	75	67	62	57	54	51	49	47	45	42	40				
84	Width	77	86	95	103	110	117	125	132	138	151	164				
	Height	77	69	63	59	55	52	50	48	46	43	41				
86	Width	79	88	98	105	112	119	128	135	141	154	168				
	Height	79	70	65	60	56	53	51	49	47	44	42				
88	Width	80	90	99	107	116	124	130	138	144	158					
	Height	80	72	66	61	58	55	52	50	48	45					
90	Width	82	93	102	110	118	126	133	140	147	161					
	Height	82	74	68	63	59	56	53	51	49	46					
92	Width	84	94	104	112	120	128	138	143	150	165					
	Height	84	75	69	64	60	57	55	52	50	47					
94	Width	86	96	107	116	124	131	140	146	153	168					
	Height	86	77	71	66	62	58	56	53	51	48					
96	Width	88	99	108	117	126	135	143	151	159						
	Height	88	79	72	67	63	60	57	55	53						
98	Width	90	100	111	119	128	137	145	154	162						
	Height	90	80	74	68	64	61	58	56	54						
100	Width	91	103	113	123	132	140	148	157	165						
	Height	91	82	75	70	66	62	59	57	55						
102	Width	93	105	116	124	134	142	153	160	168						
	Height	93	84	77	71	67	63	61	58	56						

*Shaded area not recommended.

$$C = \frac{\Delta p_j}{\rho(V^2/2)} = \frac{\Delta p_j}{p_v} \quad \text{(9-8 SI)}$$

where

C = local loss coefficient, dimensionless

Δp_j = fitting total pressure loss, in. of water (Pa)

ρ = density, lb_m/ft^3 (kg/m^3)

V = velocity, fpm (m/s)

p_v = velocity pressure, in. of water (Pa)

Dynamic losses occur along a duct length and cannot be separated from frictional losses. For ease of calculation, dynamic losses are assumed to be concentrated at a section (local) and to exclude friction. Frictional losses must be considered only for relatively long fittings. Generally, fitting friction losses are accounted for by measuring duct lengths from the centerline of one fitting to that of the next fitting. For fittings closely coupled (less than six hydraulic diameters apart), the flow pattern entering subsequent fittings differs from the flow pattern used to determine loss coefficients. Adequate data for these situations are unavailable.

For all fittings, except junctions, calculate the total pressure loss Δp_j at a section by:

$$\Delta p_j = C_o p_{v,o} \quad \text{(9-9)}$$

where the subscript *o* is the cross section at which the velocity pressure is referenced. The dynamic loss is based on the actual velocity in the duct, not the velocity in an equivalent noncircular duct. Where necessary (unequal area fittings), convert a loss coefficient from section *o* to section *i* by Equation (9-10), where *V* is the velocity at the respective sections.

$$C_i = \frac{C_o}{(V_i/V_o)^2} \quad \text{(9-10)}$$

For converging and diverging flow junctions, total pressure losses through the straight (main) section are calculated as:

$$\Delta p_j = C_{c,s} p_{v,c} \quad \text{(9-10a)}$$

For total pressure losses through the branch section:

$$\Delta p_j = C_{c,b} p_{v,c} \quad \text{(9-10b)}$$

where $P_{v,c}$ is the velocity pressure at the common section *c*, and $C_{c,s}$ and $C_{c,b}$ are losses for the straight (main) and branch flow paths, respectively, each referenced to the velocity pressure at section *c*. To convert junction local loss coefficients referenced to straight and branch velocity pressures, use Equation (9-10c).

$$C_i = \frac{C_{c,i}}{(V_i/V_c)^2} \quad \text{(9-10c)}$$

where

C_i = local loss coefficient referenced to section being calculated (see subscripts), dimensionless

$C_{c,i}$ = straight ($C_{c,s}$) or branch ($C_{c,b}$) local loss coefficient referenced to dynamic pressure at the common section, dimensionless

V_i = velocity at section to which C_i is being referenced

V_c = velocity at common section

Subscripts:

b = branch

s = straight (main) section

c = common section

The junction of two parallel streams moving at different velocities is characterized by turbulent mixing of the streams, accompanied by pressure losses. In the course of this mixing, an exchange of momentum takes place between the particles moving at different velocities, finally resulting in the equalization of the velocity distributions in the common stream. The jet with higher velocity loses a part of its kinetic energy by transmitting it to the slower moving jet. The loss in total pressure before and after mixing is always large and positive for the higher velocity jet and increases with an increase in the amount of energy transmitted to the lower velocity jet. Consequently, the local loss coefficient, defined by Equation (9-8), will always be positive. The energy stored in the lower velocity jet increases as a result of mixing. The loss in total pressure and the local loss coefficient can, therefore, also have negative values for the lower velocity jet (Idelchik 1986).

9.1.5 Ductwork Sectional Losses

Total pressure loss in a duct section is calculated by combining Equations (9-7) and (9-8) in terms of Δp, where ΣC is the sum of local loss coefficients within the duct section. Each fitting loss coefficient must be referenced to that section's velocity pressure.

$$\Delta p = \left(\frac{12fL}{D} + \Sigma C\right)\rho(V/1097)^2 \quad \text{(9-11 I-P)}$$

$$\Delta p = \left(\frac{1000fL}{D} + \Sigma C\right)\rho(V^2/2) \quad \text{(9-11 SI)}$$

9.1.6 System Analysis

Since $p_t = p_s + p_v$:

$$\Delta p_t = p_{t,1} - p_{t,2} \quad \text{(9-12)}$$

where Δp_t is the change in total pressure in the direction of airflow between stations 1 and 2. For all main and branch ducts in a system, including both supply and return air ductwork, Equation (9-12) may be used for any fitting/duct or section of ductwork. The path with the greatest resistance to flow, usually the longest and most complicated, is known as the critical path. The minimum total pressure to be developed by the fan is the summation of duct/fitting losses

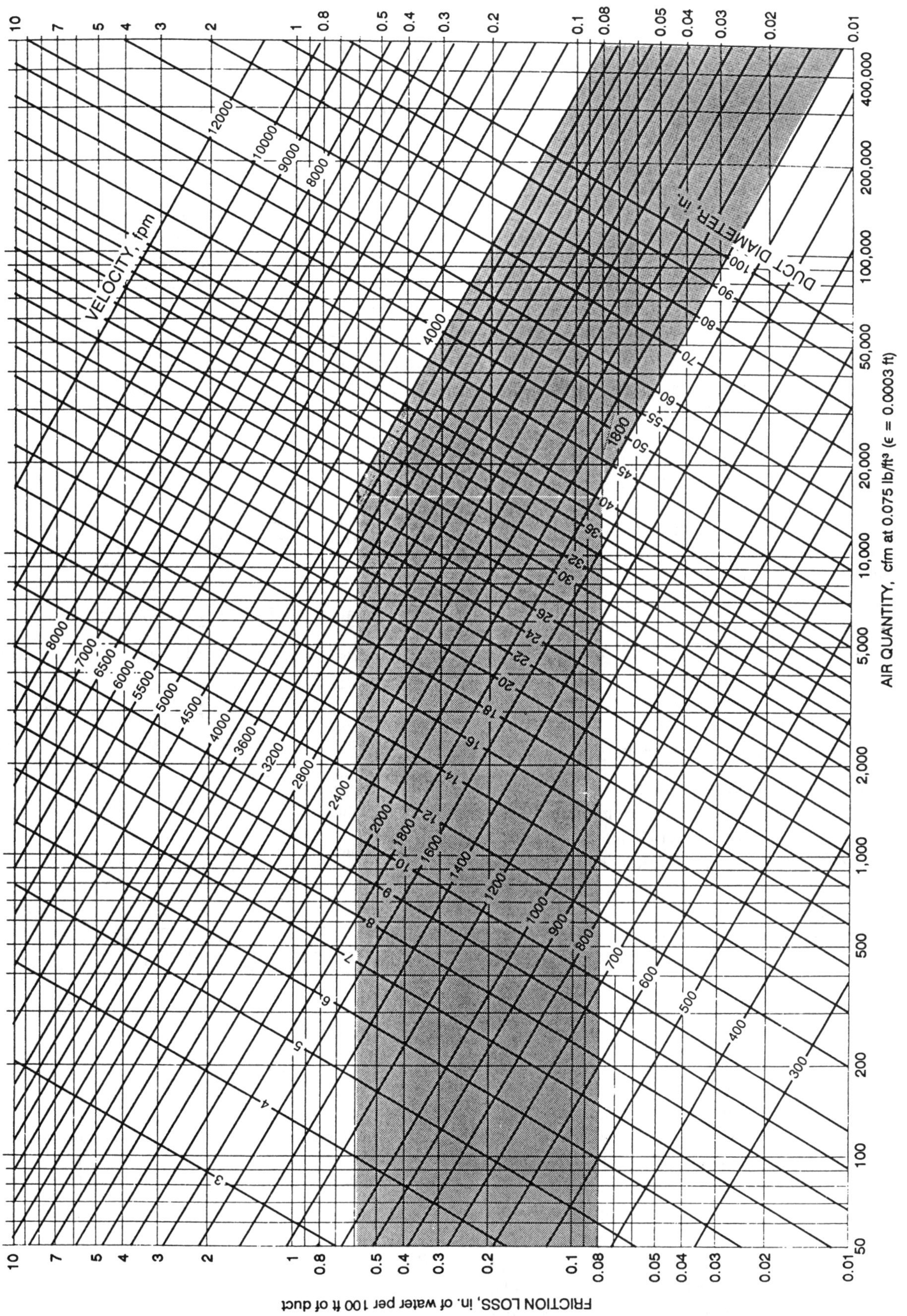

Fig. 9-2 Friction Chart for Round Duct ($\rho = 0.075\ lb_m/ft^3$ *and* $e = 0.0003\ ft$)

throughout the **critical path** of the system, plus the fan system effect factors.

Thus:

$$\Delta p_t = \sum_{i=1}^{n} \Delta p_i + SEF_s + SEF_d \qquad (9\text{-}13)$$

where

Δp_t = fan's total pressure, in. of water (Pa)
Δp_i = component total pressure loss, in. of water (Pa)
n = number of ducts/fittings in critical path of system
SEF_s = system effect factor due to fan inlet conditions, in. of water (Pa)
SEF_d = system effect due to fan outlet conditions, in. of water (Pa)

For some simple systems, SEF_s and SEF_d can be negligible. However, for typical systems, these quantities must be estimated. Also, duct heat transfer must be considered in duct system design. Information concerning these items is given in Chapter 32 of the 1997 *ASHRAE Handbook—Fundamentals.*

9.1.7 Duct Design

This discussion refers to central station ducts for commercial and industrial heating, ventilating, and air-conditioning systems. The equal friction and static regain methods given yield the static pressure required to overcome the resistance of the ductwork, including the supply outlets and return intakes. The fan selected for the duct system must produce not only this pressure but also the additional pressure required by the central equipment such as washers or spray chambers, heating or cooling coils, and filters. Pressure losses of these components should be obtained from the manufacturers' catalogs.

Rules that should be followed in the design of ducts are:

1. Convey air as directly as possible at the permissible velocities to obtain the desired results with minimum noise and greatest economy of power, material, and space.
2. Avoid sudden changes in air direction or velocity. When sudden changes are necessary at bends, use turning vanes to minimize the pressure loss.
3. Where the greatest air-carrying capacity per unit area of sheet metal is desired, make rectangular ducts as nearly square as possible. Avoid aspect ratios (ratio of width to depth) greater than 8 to 1. Where possible, maintain a ratio of 4 to 1 or less.
4. Ducts should be constructed of smooth material, such as steel or aluminum sheet metal. For ducts made from other materials, allow for the change in roughness.
5. A reasonable estimate of the flow resistances offered by the system can be obtained through the following design procedures. However, in actual installations, resistances may vary considerably from the calculated values because of variation in the smoothness of materials, types of joints used, and the ability to fabricate the system in accordance with the design. Select fans and motors to provide at least a slight factor of safety, and install dampers in each branch outlet for balancing the system.
6. Avoid obstructing ducts with piping, conduits, or structural members. Unavoidable duct obstructions must be streamlined with an easement or a tear-drop, the length of which should be at least three times the thickness of the tear-drop.

9.1.8 Design Velocities

It is impossible to give specific rules for selecting duct velocities and duct shapes (rectangular, round, or oval) without considering cost and system constraints. An ideal design has minimum owning and operating costs when all constraints on the design are considered. The velocity and friction loss rate ranges indicated in Figure 9-2 are offered as preliminary design values. In the constant velocity design method, ignore the limits on friction loss rate. Do not use Figure 9-2 indiscriminately, as noise generation throughout a system increases as the velocity increases.

A summary of recommended velocities for HVAC components encountered in built-up systems is presented in Table 9-2. In most cases, the values are abstracted from the 1996 *ASHRAE Handbook—Systems and Equipment*, and

Table 9-2 Recommended Duct Velocities and Typical Velocities and Pressure Losses of Various HVAC Components

	Recommended Velocities, fpm		
Designation	**Residences**	**Schools, Theaters, Public Buildings**	**Industrial Buildings**
Main ducts	700-900	1000-1300	1200-1800
Branch ducts	600	600-900	800-1000
Branch risers	500	600-700	800
	Maximum Velocities, fpm		
Main ducts	800-1200	1100-1600	1300-2200
Branch ducts	700-1000	800-1300	1000-1800
Branch risers	650-800	800-1200	1000-1600
Components			
Outdoor air intakes	500	500	500
Filters	250	300	350
Heating coils	450	500	600
Cooling coils	450	500	600
Air washers	500	500	500
Fan outlets	1000-1600	1300-2000	1600-2400

High Velocity Systems

Airflow Carried by Duct, cfm	Maximum Velocity, fpm
60,000 to 40,000	6000
40,000 to 25,000	5000
25,000 to 15,000	4500
15,000 to 10,000	4000
10,000 to 6,000	3500
6,000 to 3,000	3000
3,000 to 1,000	2500

Component	Static pressure loss, in. w.g.
Static regain supply duct	0.30
Supply plenum	0.50
HEPA	0.70
Supply grille	0.05
Raised floor perforations	0.05
Return plenum	0.05
Ducted return	0.40
30/30 prefilters	0.30
Bag filters	0.80
Cooling coil	0.35

final component selection should be based on data in these chapters or from manufacturers.

9.1.9 Design Methods

The transmission of air at high velocities has gained wide acceptance in comfort air-conditioning and ventilation systems. This acceptance is due partly to improved fans and special sound attenuation and control equipment, and partly to improved design and installation methods based on a better understanding of the design and installation of high velocity air-conditioning systems.

The design of high velocity duct systems involves a compromise between reduction of duct size and the consequent need for higher fan power. While the duct size and air velocities are governed in large part by the space available, the maximum velocities (given later in this section) should not be exceeded without carefully examining all factors.

The following principles and laws apply to all duct systems regardless of the design method used or the numerical values obtained.

1. The measure of the amount of energy required to move air from one location to another is the change (decrease) in the total pressure within the system.
2. The total pressure pt at any location within a system is a measure of the total mechanical energy at that location. It is the sum of the static pressure and the velocity pressure.
3. In any duct system, the total pressure always decreases in the direction of airflow.
4. In any system having two or more branches, the losses in total pressure between the fan and the end of each branch are the same.
5. Static pressure and velocity pressure are mutually convertible and can either increase or decrease in the direction of flow. For example, in a straight run of duct, the static pressure decreases, the velocity pressure remains constant, and the total pressure (their sum) decreases. In a gradually diverging section (area increase), the velocity pressure decreases, the static pressure increases, and the total pressure remains the same (neglecting the small friction loss).

The most common methods of air duct design are (1) equal friction; (2) velocity reduction; and (3) static regain and variations such as total pressure. No single duct design method automatically produces the most economical duct system for all conditions; the system design with the minimum owning and operating cost depends on both the application and ingenuity of the designer.

Equal Friction Method. The principle of this method is to size a system's ductwork for a constant pressure loss per unit length of duct. At higher airflow rates, it may be necessary to limit the velocity so as not to generate objectionable noises. For an initial design, the friction loss per unit length of duct for the corresponding recommended velocities is given in Figure 9-2.

Once the system is sized, the total pressure losses for the main and branch sections from junction-to-junction/fan/terminal may be calculated and the total pressure grade line plotted. To optimize a system, additional designs are necessary to establish the annual system and power cost curves, and to find the minimum point on the total owning and operating cost curve. For system costs, only the incremental differences due to the redesign need to be considered.

After the system has been designed and the total pressure grade line plotted, sections of ductwork may be redesigned to achieve an approximate balance at the junctions without relying entirely on balancing dampers.

Velocity Reduction Method. This method consists of selecting the velocity at the fan discharge, and designing for progressively lower velocities in the main duct at each junction or branch duct. For the selected velocities and known airflow rates, the various duct diameters may be read directly from Figure 9-2 and the equivalent rectangular sizes obtained from Equation (9-6). The return air ductwork is sized similarly, starting with the highest velocity at the fan suction and decreasing progressively in the direction of the return intakes. With the ducts sized and the fittings known, the total pressure losses can be calculated, the pressure gradients plotted, and the maximum pressure loss or critical path of the system established.

A refinement of this method involves sizing the branch ducts to dissipate the pressure available at the entrance to each. The pressure loss of the ductwork between the fan and first branch take-off is subtracted from the total fan pressure to obtain the available pressure at the first junction. Through trial, a branch velocity is found that results in the branch pressure loss being equal to or less than the pressure available. The procedure is repeated for each branch.

If the fan is specified so that the total pressure available for the system is known, the method consists of finding, through trial, the velocities in the main and branch ducts that will result in a pressure loss equal to or less than the pressure available. The branch ducts are sized as discussed previously.

Static Regain Method. In the static regain method, the ducts are sized so that the increase in static pressure (static regain) at each take-off offsets the pressure loss of the succeeding section of ductwork. This method is especially suited for high velocity installations having long runs with many take-offs or terminal units. Approximately the same static pressure exists at the entrance to each branch, which simplifies outlet or terminal unit selection and system balancing. With the ductwork sized by this method, the system's total pressure losses can be calculated. A disadvantage of this method is that excessively large ducts (low velocities) result at the ends of long duct runs.

The total pressure design method is an adaptation of the static regain method. This method is advantageous since the intermediate system pressures and control of duct sizes and velocities are known.

9.1.10 Duct Design Procedures

The general procedure for duct design is as follows:

1. Study the plans of the building and arrange the supply return outlets to provide proper distribution of air within each space. Adjust calculated actual air quantities for duct heat gains or losses and duct leakage. Adjust the suply, return, and/or exhaust air quantities to meet space pressurization requirements.
2. Select outlet sizes from manufacturers' data. (Refer to Chapter 31, Space Air Diffusion, of the 1997 *ASHRAE Handbook—Fundamentals*.)
3. Sketch the duct system, connect the supply outlets and return intakes with the central station apparatus, and avoid all structural obstructions and equipment. Be aware of system space allocations. Use round duct whenever feasible.
4. Divide the system into sections and number each section. A duct system should be divided at all points where flow, size, or shape changes. Assign fittings to the section toward the supply and return (or exhaust) terminals.
5. Size ducts by the selected design method. Calculate system total pressure loss; then select the fan (refer to Chapter 18 in the 1996 *ASHRAE Handbook—Systems and Equipment*).
6. Lay out the system in detail. If duct routing and fittings vary significantly from the original design, recalculate the pressure losses. Reselect the fan if necessary.
7. Resize duct sections to approximately balance pressures at each junction.
8. Analyze the design for objectionable noise levels and specify sound attenuators as necessary.

9.1.11 Fitting Loss Coefficients

A duct fitting database (ASHRAE 1994), which includes 225 round and rectangular fittings with the provision to include flat oval fittings, is available from ASHRAE in electronic form with the capability to be linked to duct design programs. The fittings are numbered (coded) as shown in Table 9-3.

For convenience, a selection of dynamic loss coefficients for common duct fittings are given in Table 9-4. These coefficients are taken from Chapter 32 of the 1997 *ASHRAE Handbook—Fundamentals*.

Table 9-3 Duct Fitting Codes

Fitting Function	Geometry	Category	Sequence Number
S: Supply	D: round (Diameter)	1. Entries 2. Exits	1,2,3,...*n*
E: Exhaust/ Return	R: Rectangular	3. Elbows 4. Transitions	
	O: flat Oval	5. Junctions	
C: Common (supply and return)		6. Obstructions 7. Fan and system interactions 8. Duct-mounted equipment 9. Dampers 10. Hoods 11. Straight duct	

9.1.12 Automated Duct Design

Duct design calculations have been automated by computers. Automated duct design offers features such as: (1) standardization of duct design; (2) stored loss coefficients for fittings; (3) stored duct construction and thermal insulation standards; (4) balancing analysis; (5) noise analysis; (6) duct heat gain or loss analysis; (7) material takeoffs; and (8) documentation. For available duct design programs and hardware requirements, refer to Chapter 32 of the 1997 *ASHRAE Handbook—Fundamentals* and the annual classified section in the *ASHRAE Journal*.

Table 9-4 Fitting Loss Coefficients

ENTRIES

1-1 Duct Mounted in Wall (Hood, Nonenclosing, Flanged, and Unflanged) (Idelchik 1986, Diagram 3-1)

General. If entry has a screen, use Fitting 6-7 to calculate screen resistance.

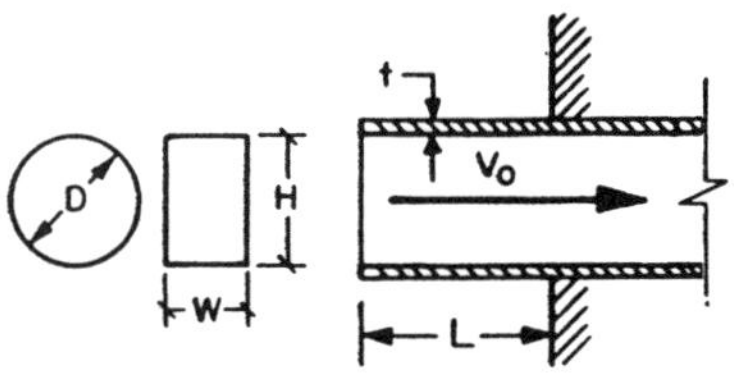

Rectangular: $D = 2HW/(H + W)$

	C_o						
	L/D						
t/D	0	0.002	0.01	0.05	0.2	0.5	≥1.0
≈0	0.50	0.57	0.68	0.80	0.92	1.0	1.0
0.02	0.50	0.51	0.52	0.55	0.66	0.72	0.72
≥0.05	0.50	0.50	0.50	0.50	0.50	0.50	0.50

1-2 Smooth Converging Bellmouth without End Wall (Idelchik 1986, Diagram 3-4)

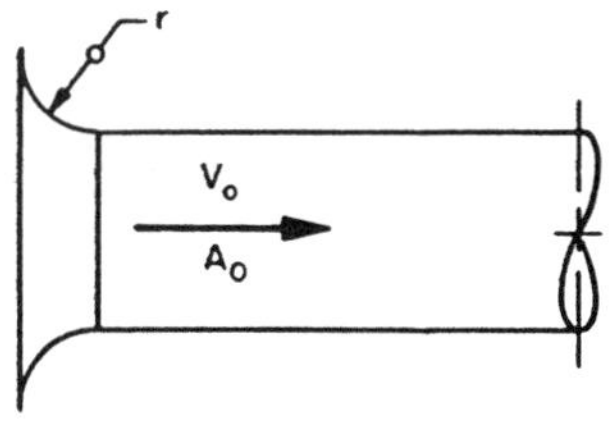

r/D	0	0.01	0.02	0.03	0.04	0.05
C_o	1.0	0.87	0.74	0.61	0.51	0.40
r/D	0.06	0.08	0.10	0.12	0.16	≥ 0.20
C_o	0.32	0.20	0.15	0.10	0.06	0.03

1-3 Smooth Converging Bellmouth with End Wall (Idelchik 1986, Diagram 3-4)

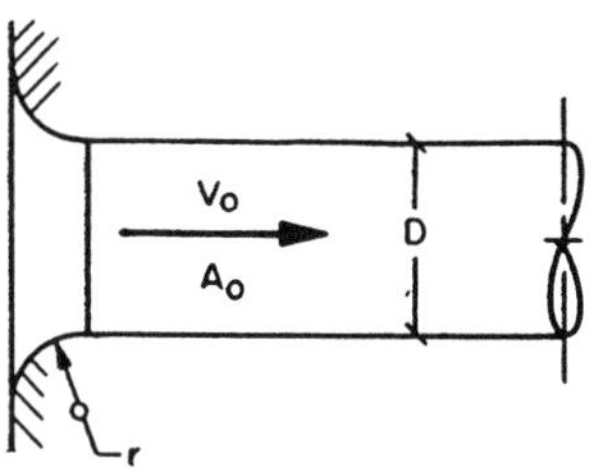

r/D	0	0.01	0.02	0.03	0.04	0.05
C_o	0.50	0.44	0.37	0.31	0.26	0.22
r/D	0.06	0.08	0.10	0.12	0.16	≥ 0.20
C_o	0.20	0.15	0.12	0.09	0.06	0.03

1-4 Conical Converging Bellmouth without End Wall, Round and Rectangular

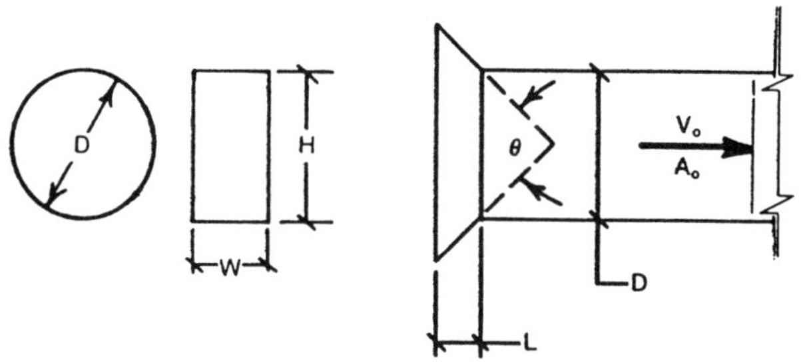

Rectangular: $D = 2HW/(H + W)$

	C_o									
	θ, degrees									
L/D	0	10	20	30	45	60	90	120	150	180
0.025	1.0	0.96	0.93	0.90	0.85	0.80	0.72	0.64	0.57	0.50
0.05	1.0	0.93	0.86	0.80	0.73	0.67	0.60	0.56	0.52	0.50
0.10	1.0	0.80	0.67	0.55	0.46	0.41	0.41	0.43	0.46	0.50
0.25	1.0	0.68	0.45	0.30	0.21	0.17	0.21	0.28	0.38	0.50
0.60	1.0	0.46	0.27	0.18	0.14	0.13	0.19	0.27	0.37	0.50
1.0	1.0	0.32	0.20	0.14	0.11	0.10	0.16	0.24	0.35	0.50

1-5 Conical Converging Bellmouth with End Wall, Round and Rectangular (Idelchik 1986, Diagram 3-7)

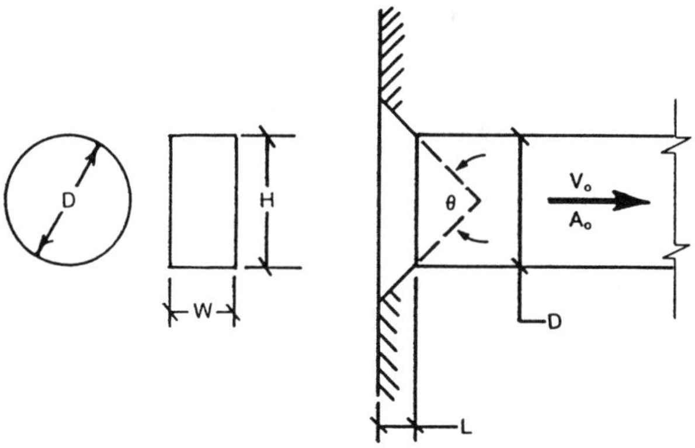

Rectangular: $D = 2HW/(H + W)$

	C_o									
	θ, degrees									
L/D	0	10	20	30	45	60	90	120	150	180
0.025	0.50	0.47	0.45	0.43	0.41	0.40	0.42	0.44	0.46	0.50
0.05	0.50	0.45	0.41	0.36	0.32	0.30	0.34	0.39	0.44	0.50
0.075	0.50	0.42	0.35	0.30	0.25	0.23	0.28	0.35	0.43	0.50
0.10	0.50	0.39	0.32	0.25	0.21	0.18	0.25	0.33	0.41	0.50
0.15	0.50	0.37	0.27	0.20	0.16	0.15	0.23	0.31	0.40	0.50
0.60	0.50	0.27	0.18	0.13	0.11	0.12	0.20	0.30	0.40	0.50

1-6 Intake Hood (Idelchik 1986, Diagram 3-18)

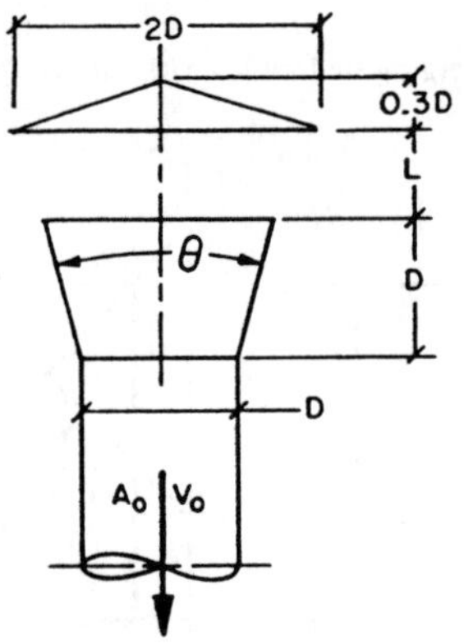

	C_o								
	L/D								
θ, deg	**0.1**	**0.2**	**0.3**	**0.4**	**0.5**	**0.6**	**0.8**	**1.0**	**4.0**
0	2.63	1.83	1.53	1.39	1.31	1.19	1.08	1.06	1.0
15	1.32	0.77	0.60	0.48	0.41	0.30	0.28	0.25	0.25

1-7 Hood, Tapered, Flanged or Unflanged (Brandt 1946)

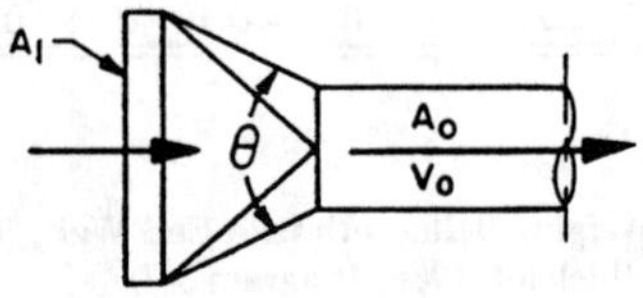

$A_1 \geq 2A_o$

θ is major angle for rectangular hoods

	Hood Shape: Round									
θ, deg.	0	20	40	60	80	100	120	140	160	180
C_o	1.0	0.11	0.06	0.09	0.14	0.18	0.27	0.32	0.43	0.50
	Hood Shape: Square or Rectangular									
θ, deg.	0	20	40	60	80	100	120	140	160	180
C_o	1.0	0.19	0.13	0.16	0.21	0.27	0.33	0.43	0.53	0.62

1-8 Orifice, Sharp-Edged, Inlet Duct (Idelchik 1986; Diagrams 3-12, 3-14, and 4-19)

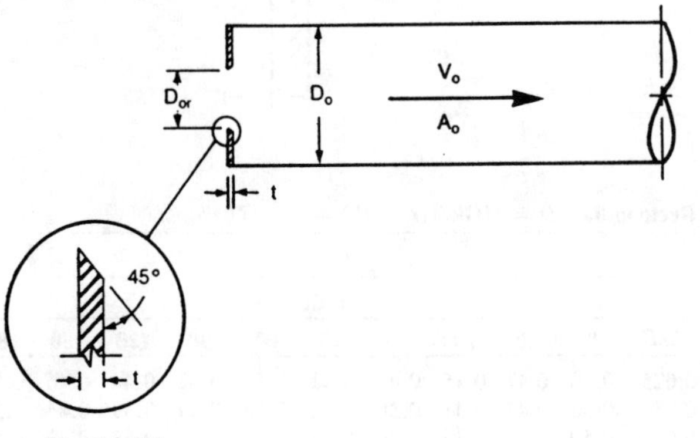

$t/D_{or} \leqslant 0.015$

$\text{Re} = D_o V_o / \nu$

A_{or}: orifice area

	C_o							
	A_{or}/A_o							
Re × 10⁻³	**0.2**	**0.3**	**0.4**	**0.5**	**0.6**	**0.7**	**0.8**	**0.9**
4	45	18	7.9	3.9	2.3	1.3	0.83	0.51
10	49	20	9.2	4.4	2.7	1.5	0.96	0.59
20	50	21	9.3	4.9	2.9	1.6	1.1	0.65
100	55	23	11.0	5.6	3.3	1.9	1.2	0.75

EXITS

General. If exit has a screen, use Fitting 6-7 to calculate screen resistance.

2-1 Exit, Abrupt, Round and Rectangular (Idelchik 1986, Diagram 11-1)

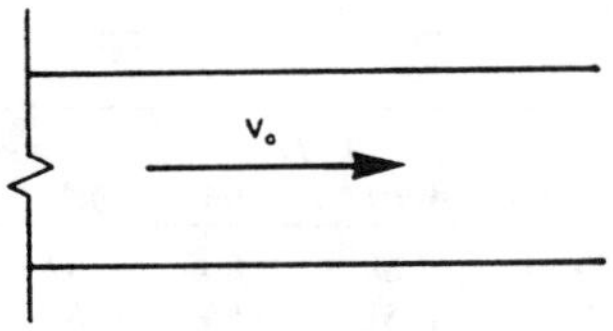

Uniform Velocity Distribution

$C_o = 1.0$

Exponential, Sinusoidal, Asymmetrical, and Parabolic Velocity Distribution

C_o varies from 1.0 to 3.67. For details, consult Idelchik (1986), Diagram 11-1.

2-2 Exit, Abrupt, Round and Rectangular, with End Idelchik 1986, Diagrams 5-2 and 5-4)

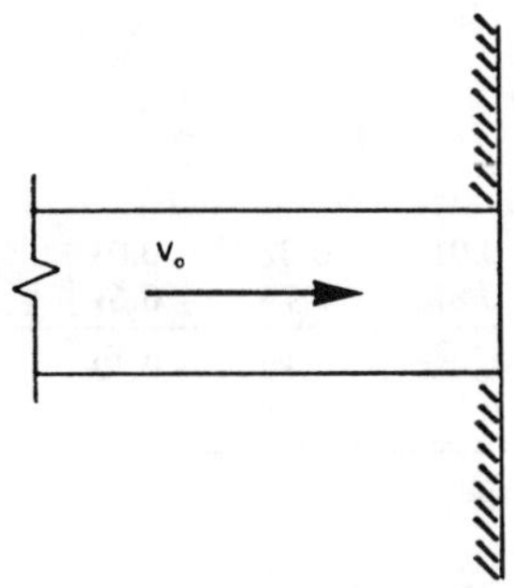

$C_o = 0.88$

2-3 Exit, Duct Flush with Wall, Flow along Wall (Idelchik 1986, Diagram 11-2)

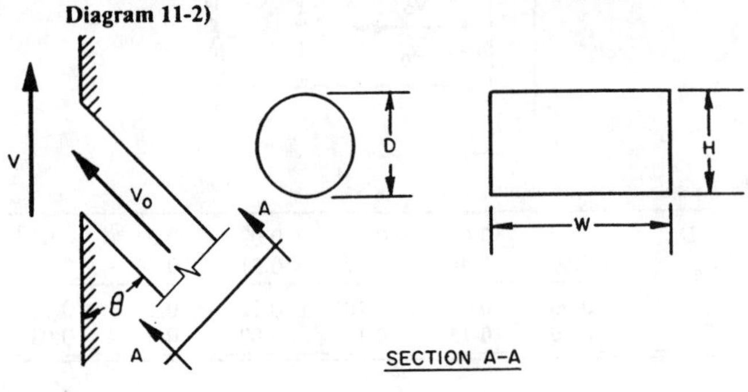

Round

	C_o				
	V/V_o				
θ, deg	0	0.5	1.0	1.5	2.0
⩽ 45	1.0	1.0	1.1	1.3	1.6
60	1.0	0.90	1.1	1.4	1.6
90	1.0	0.80	0.95	1.4	1.7
120	1.0	0.80	0.95	1.3	1.7
150	1.0	0.82	0.83	1.0	1.3

Rectangular

		C_o				
Aspect Ratio		V/V_o				
(H/W	θ, deg	0	0.5	1.0	1.5	2.0
⩽ 0.2	⩽ 90	1.0	0.95	1.2	1.5	1.8
	120	1.0	0.92	1.1	1.4	1.9
	150	1.0	0.75	0.95	1.4	1.8
0.5-2.0	⩽ 45	1.0	1.0	1.1	1.3	1.6
	60	1.0	0.90	1.1	1.4	1.6
	90	1.0	0.80	0.95	1.4	1.7
	120	1.0	0.80	0.95	1.3	1.7
	150	1.0	0.82	0.83	1.0	1.3
⩾ 5	45	1.0	0.92	0.93	1.1	1.3
	60	1.0	0.87	0.87	1.0	1.3
	90	1.0	0.82	0.80	0.97	1.2
	120	1.0	0.80	0.76	0.90	0.98

2-4 Exit, Round, Diverging (Idelchik 1986, Diagram 11-3)

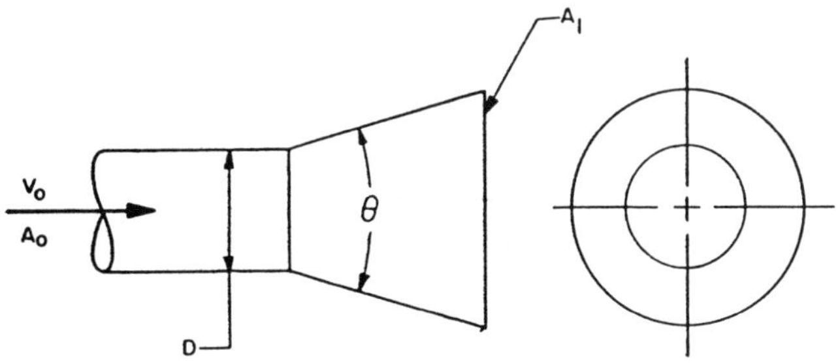

	C_o						
	θ, degrees						
A_1/A_o	8	10	14	20	30	45	⩾ 60
2	0.36	0.33	0.37	0.51	0.90	1.0	1.0
4	0.24	0.21	0.28	0.40	0.70	0.99	1.0
6	0.20	0.19	0.26	0.37	0.67	0.99	1.0
10	0.18	0.16	0.24	0.36	0.68	0.99	1.0
16	0.16	0.16	0.20	0.36	0.66	0.99	1.0

2-5 Exit, Round, with End Wall Transition (Idelchik 1986, Diagram 5-8)

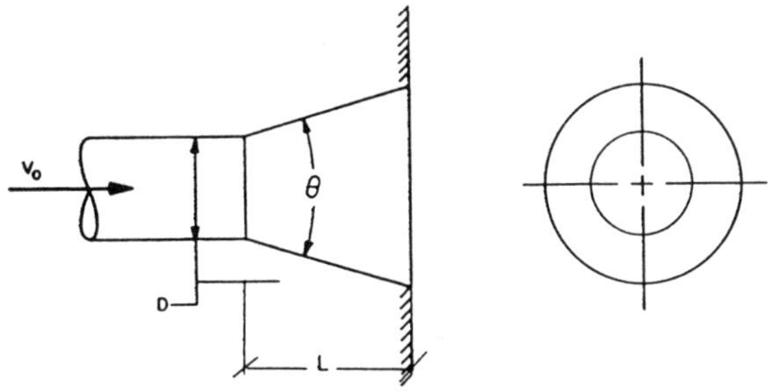

θ = optimum angle

L/D	0.5	1.0	2.0	3.0	4.0	5.0	6.0	8.0	10	12	14
θ	34	24	16	13	11	10	9	8	7	6	6
C_o	0.41	0.32	0.24	0.20	0.17	0.15	0.14	0.12	0.11	0.11	0.10

2-6 Exit, Rectangular, Two Sides Parallel, Diverging, Symmetrical (Idelchik 1986, Diagram 11-6)

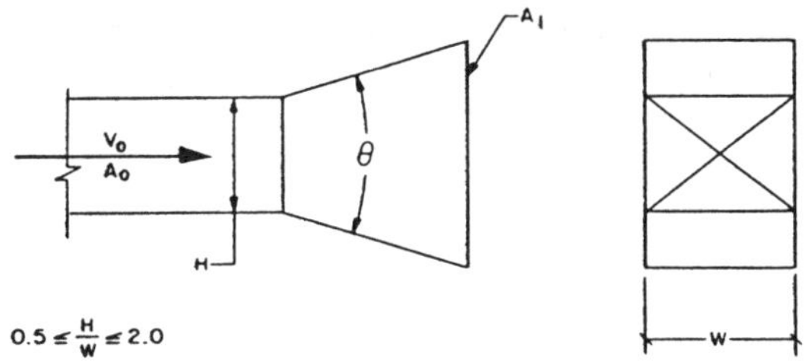

$0.5 \leqslant H/W \leqslant 2$

	C_o						
	θ, degrees						
A_1/A_o	8	10	14	20	30	45	⩾ 60
2	0.50	0.51	0.56	0.63	0.80	0.96	1.0
4	0.34	0.38	0.48	0.63	0.76	0.91	1.0
6	0.32	0.34	0.41	0.56	0.70	0.84	0.96

2-7 Exit, Rectangular, with Wall, Two Sides Parallel, Symmetrical, Diverging (Idelchik 1986, Diagram 5-10)

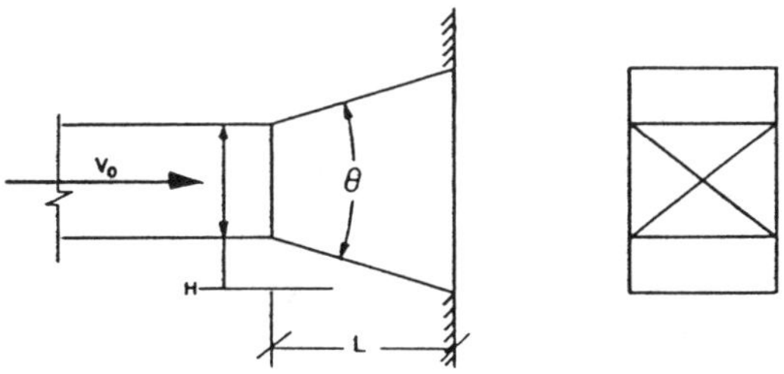

θ = optimum angle

L/H	0.5	1.0	2.0	3.0	4.0	5.0	6.0	8.0	10	12	14
θ	50	35	25	21	18	16	15	13	12	11	10
C_o	0.53	0.44	0.35	0.31	0.28	0.25	0.24	0.22	0.20	0.19	0.19

2-8 Exit, Rectangular, Pyramidal, Diverging (Idelchik 1986, Diagram 11-5)

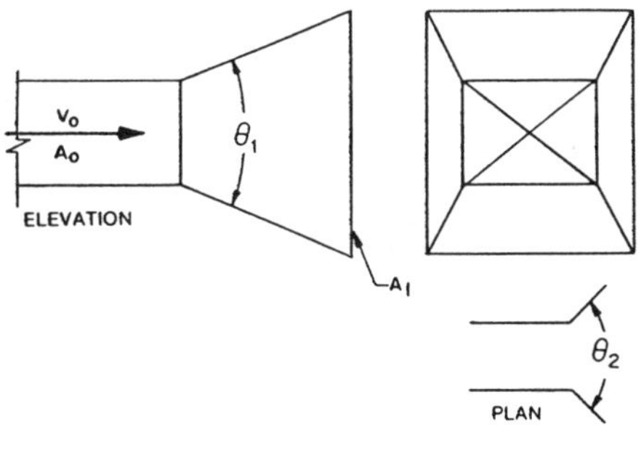

θ is larger of θ_1 and θ_2

	C_o						
	θ, degrees						
A_1/A_o	8	10	14	20	30	45	≥60
2	0.65	0.68	0.74	0.82	0.92	1.1	1.1
4	0.53	0.60	0.69	0.78	0.90	1.0	1.1
6	0.50	0.57	0.66	0.77	0.91	1.0	1.1
10	0.45	0.53	0.64	0.74	0.85	0.97	1.1

2-9 Exit, Rectangular, with Wall, Pyramidal, Diverging (Idelchik 1986, Diagram 5-9)

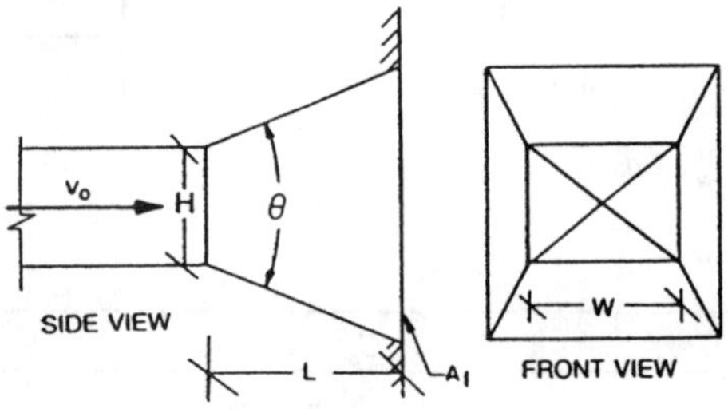

$D = 2HW/(H + W)$
θ = optimum angle

L/D	0.5	1.0	2.0	3.0	4.0	5.0	6.0	8.0	10	12	14
θ	26	19	13	11	9	8	7	6	6	5	5
C_o	0.49	0.40	0.30	0.26	0.23	0.21	0.19	0.17	0.16	0.15	0.14

2-10 Exit, Discharge to Atmosphere from a 90° Elbow, Rectangular and Round (Note: Elbow Loss Included) (Idelchik 1986, Diagram 11-14)

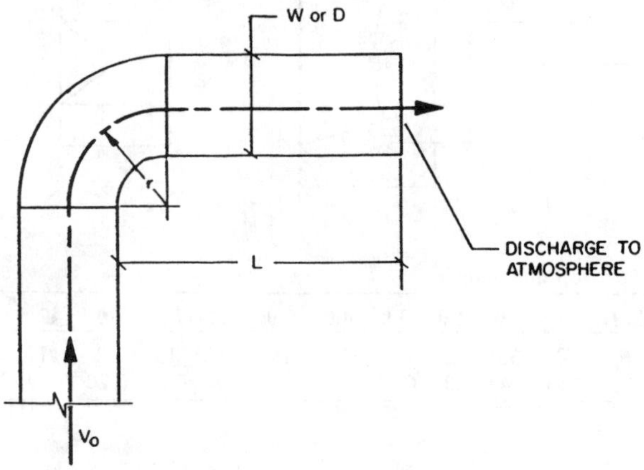

Rectangular

	C_o									
	L/W									
$\frac{r}{W}$	0	0.5	1.0	1.5	2.0	3.0	4.0	6.0	8.0	12.0
0	3.0	3.1	3.2	3.0	2.7	2.4	2.2	2.1	2.1	2.0
0.75	2.2	2.2	2.1	1.8	1.7	1.6	1.6	1.5	1.5	1.5
1.0	1.8	1.5	1.4	1.4	1.3	1.3	1.2	1.2	1.2	1.2
1.5	1.5	1.2	1.1	1.1	1.1	1.1	1.1	1.1	1.1	1.1
2.5	1.2	1.1	1.1	1.0	1.0	1.0	1.0	1.0	1.0	1.0

Round (r/D = 1.0)

L/D	0.9	1.3
C_o	1.5	1.4

2-11 Exhaust Hood (Idelchik 1986, Diagram 11-16)

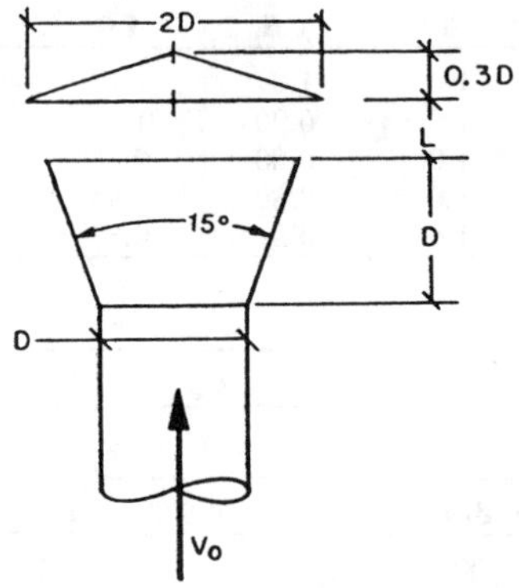

Poor design—should not be used (see Chapter 14, Figure 13)

L/D	0.1	0.2	0.25	0.3	0.35	0.4	0.5	0.6	0.8	1.0
C_o	2.6	1.2	1.0	0.80	0.70	0.65	0.60	0.60	0.60	0.60

2-12 Stackhead (Idelchik 1986, Diagram 11-23)

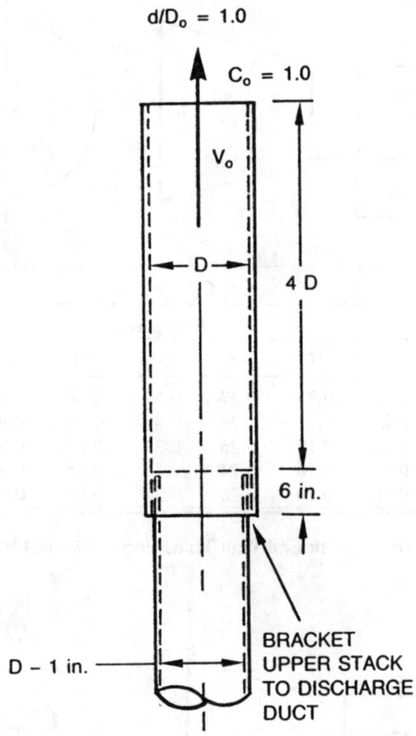

d/D	0.3	0.4	0.5	0.6	0.7	0.8	0.9	1.0
C_o	130	41	17	8.1	4.4	2.6	1.6	1.0

ELBOWS

3-1 Elbow, Smooth Radius (Die Stamped), Round (Locklin 1950, Eq. A-10)

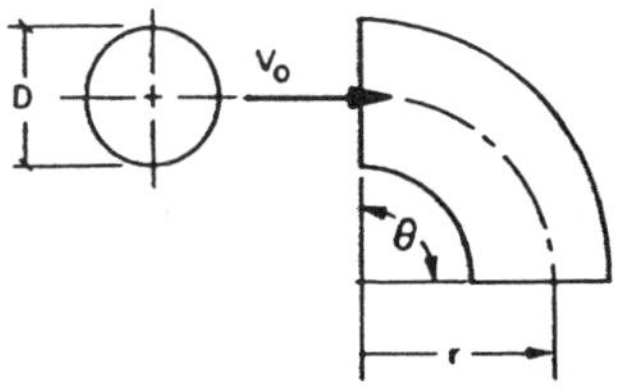

$C_o = K_\theta C_o'$

Coefficients for 90° Elbows

r/D	0.5	0.75	1.0	1.5	2.0	2.5
C_o'	0.71	0.33	0.22	0.15	0.13	0.12

Angle Correction Factors K_θ (Idelchik 1986, Diagram 6-1):

θ	0	20	30	45	60	75	90	110	130	150	180
K_θ	0	0.31	0.45	0.60	0.78	0.90	1.00	1.13	1.20	1.28	1.40

3-2 Elbows; 3, 4, and 5-Pieces, Round (Locklin 1950, Fig. 10)

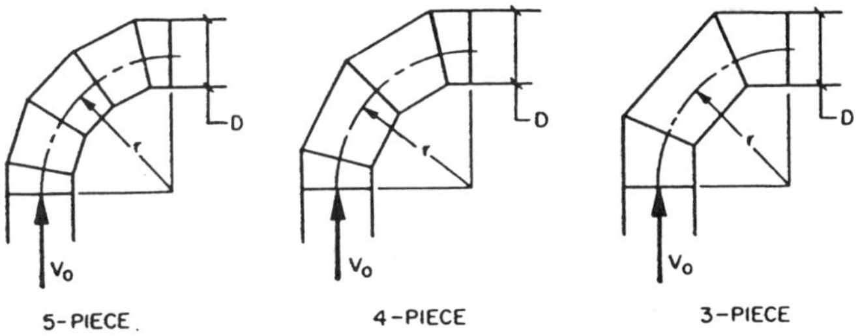

$C_o = K_\theta C_o'$

Coefficients for 90° Elbows (C_o')

No. of Pieces	r/D 0.75	1.0	1.5	2.0
5	0.46	0.33	0.24	0.19
4	0.50	0.37	0.27	0.24
3	0.54	0.42	0.34	0.33

Angle Correction Factors K_θ (Idelchik 1986, Diagram 6-1)

θ	0	20	30	45	60	75	90	110	130	150	180
K_θ	0	0.31	0.45	0.60	0.78	0.90	1.00	1.13	1.20	1.28	1.40

3-3 Elbow, Mitered, Round (Idelchik 1986, Diagram 6-5)

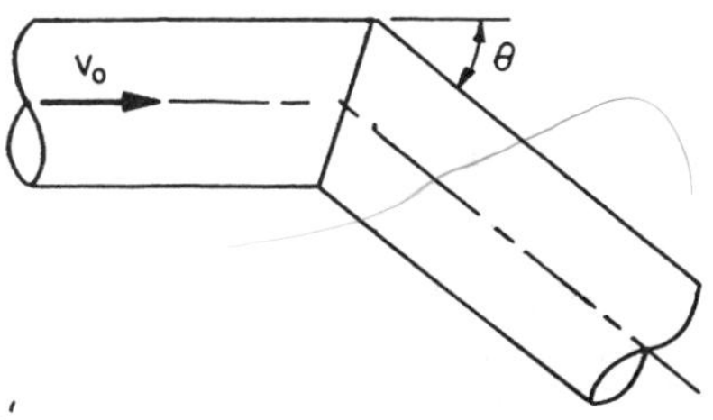

$C_o = K_{Re} C_o'$

θ, deg	20	30	45	60	75	90
C_o'	0.08	0.16	0.34	0.55	0.81	1.2

Reynolds Number Correction factors: M/hc

$Re \times 10^{-4}$	1	2	3	4	6	8	10	≥ 14
K_{Re}	1.40	1.26	1.19	1.14	1.09	1.06	1.04	1.0

3-4 Elbows, 30° Z-Shaped, Round

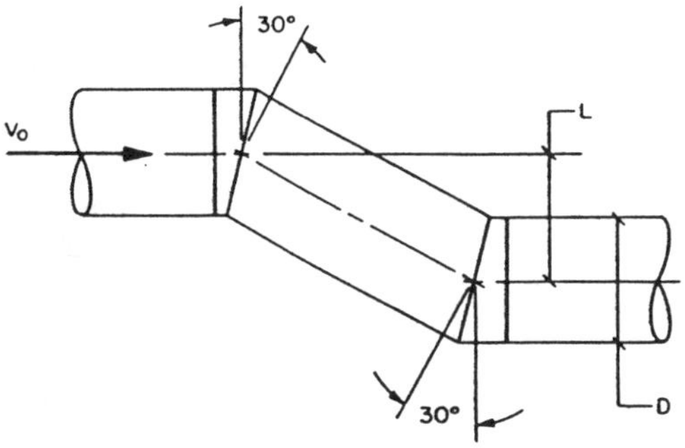

$C_o = K_{Re} C_o'$

L/D	0	0.5	1.0	1.5	2.0	2.5	3.0
C_o'	0	0.15	0.15	0.16	0.16	0.16	0.16

Reynolds Number Correction Factors

$Re \times 10^{-4}$	1	2	3	4	6	8	10	≥
K_{Re}	1.40	1.26	1.19	1.14	1.09	1.06	1.04	1.0

3-5 Elbow, without Vanes, Rectangular (Idelchik 1986, Diagram 6-1)

Smooth Radius

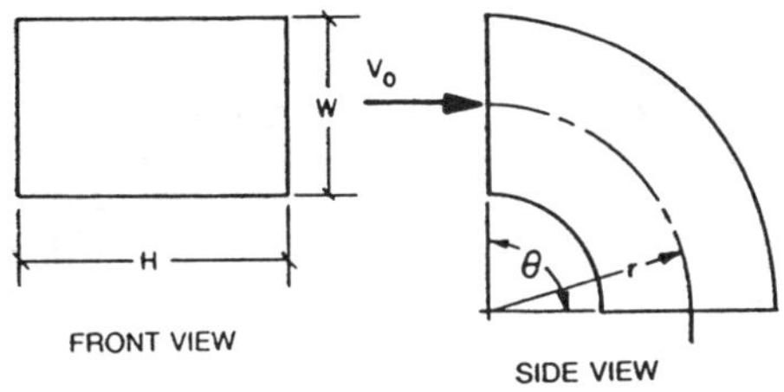

$C_o = K_\theta K_{Re} C_o'$

90°, Sharp Throat Radius Heel (r/W = 0.5)

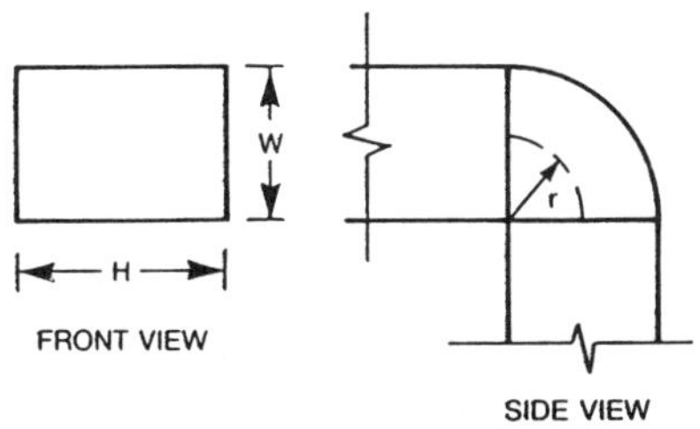

$C_o = K_{Re} C_o'$

Coefficients for 90° Elbows (C_o')

	H/W										
r/W	0.25	0.5	0.75	1.0	1.5	2.0	3.0	4.0	5.0	6.0	8.0
0.5	1.3	1.3	1.2	1.2	1.1	1.0	1.0	1.1	1.1	1.2	1.2
0.75	0.57	0.52	0.48	0.44	0.40	0.39	0.39	0.40	0.42	0.43	0.44
1.0	0.27	0.25	0.23	0.21	0.19	0.18	0.18	0.19	0.20	0.21	0.21
1.5	0.22	0.20	0.19	0.17	0.15	0.14	0.14	0.15	0.16	0.17	0.17
2.0	0.20	0.18	0.16	0.15	0.14	0.13	0.13	0.14	0.14	0.15	0.15

Angle Correction Factor

θ	0	20	30	45	60	75	90	110	130	150	180
K_θ	0	0.31	0.45	0.60	0.78	0.90	1.00	1.13	1.20	1.28	1.40

Reynolds Number Correction Factor (K_{Re})

	Re × 10^{-4}							
r/W	1	2	3	4	6	8	10	14	≥ 20
0.5	1.40	1.26	1.19	1.14	1.09	1.06	1.04	1.0	1.0
≥0.75	2.0	1.77	1.64	1.56	1.46	1.38	1.30	1.15	1.0

3-6 Elbow, Mitered, Rectangular (Idelchik 1986, Diagram 6-5)

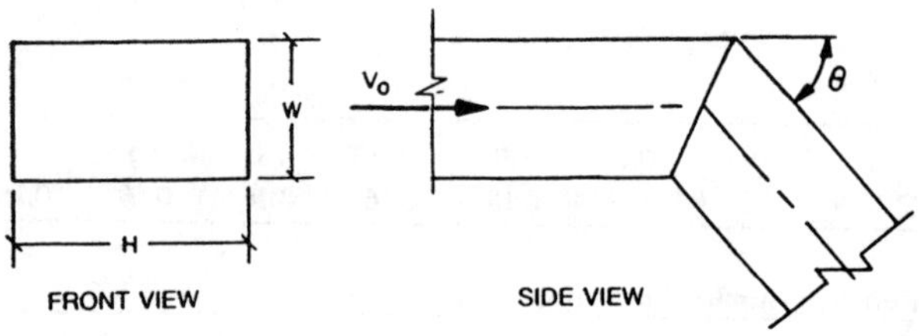

$$C_o = K_{Re} C_o'$$

	C_o'										
	H/W										
θ, deg	0.25	0.5	0.75	1.0	1.5	2.0	3.0	4.0	5.0	6.0	8.0
20	0.08	0.08	0.08	0.07	0.07	0.07	0.06	0.06	0.05	0.05	0.05
30	0.18	0.17	0.17	0.16	0.15	0.15	0.13	0.13	0.12	0.12	0.11
45	0.38	0.37	0.36	0.34	0.33	0.31	0.28	0.27	0.26	0.25	0.24
60	0.60	0.59	0.57	0.55	0.52	0.49	0.46	0.43	0.41	0.39	0.38
75	0.89	0.87	0.84	0.81	0.77	0.73	0.67	0.63	0.61	0.58	0.57
90	1.3	1.3	1.2	1.2	1.1	1.1	0.98	0.92	0.89	0.85	0.83

Reynolds number corrections factors

Re × 10^{-4}	1	2	3	4	6	8	10	≥ 14
K_{Re}	1.40	1.26	1.19	1.14	1.09	1.06	1.04	1.0

3-7 Elbow, Smooth Radius with Splitter Vanes, Rectangular (Locklin 1950, Eq. 10; Madison and Parker 1936)

One Splitter Vane

$$C_o = K_\theta C_o'$$
$$R_1 = R/CR$$

where

R = throat radius
R_1 = splitter vane radius
CR = 'CURVE RATIO' (values from Table below)
K_θ = angle factor (see Fitting 3-1 for values)

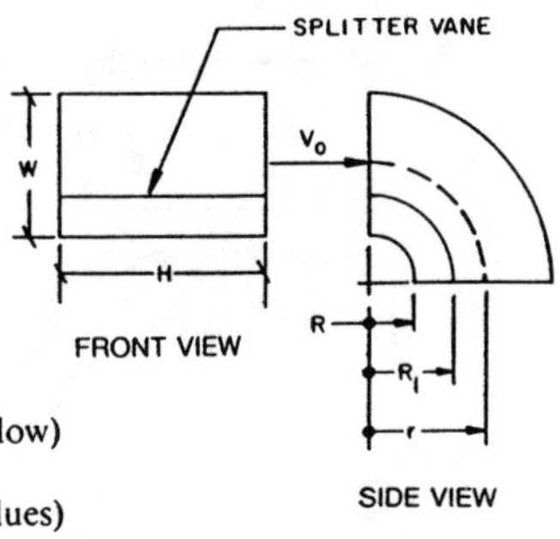

Table 3-7.a Coefficients for elbows with 1 splitter vane:

			C_o'										
			H/W										
R/W	r/W	CR	0.25	0.5	1.0	1.5	2.0	3.0	4.0	5.0	6.0	7.0	8.0
0.05	0.55	0.218	0.52	0.43	0.43	0.45	0.55	0.66	0.75	0.84	0.93	1.0	1.1
0.10	0.60	0.302	0.36	0.27	0.25	0.28	0.30	0.35	0.39	0.42	0.46	0.49	0.52
0.15	0.65	0.361	0.28	0.21	0.18	0.19	0.20	0.22	0.25	0.26	0.28	0.30	0.32
0.20	0.70	0.408	0.22	0.16	0.14	0.14	0.15	0.16	0.17	0.18	0.19	0.20	0.21
0.25	0.75	0.447	0.18	0.13	0.11	0.11	0.11	0.12	0.13	0.14	0.14	0.15	0.15
0.30	0.80	0.480	0.15	0.11	0.09	0.09	0.09	0.09	0.10	0.10	0.11	0.11	0.12
0.35	0.85	0.509	0.13	0.09	0.08	0.07	0.07	0.08	0.08	0.08	0.08	0.09	0.09
0.40	0.90	0.535	0.11	0.08	0.07	0.06	0.06	0.06	0.06	0.07	0.07	0.07	0.07
0.45	0.95	0.557	0.10	0.07	0.06	0.05	0.05	0.05	0.05	0.05	0.06	0.06	0.06
0.50	1.00	0.577	0.09	0.06	0.05	0.05	0.04	0.04	0.04	0.05	0.05	0.05	0.05

b. 2 Splitter Vanes

$$C_o = K_\theta C_o'$$
$$R_1 = R/CR$$
$$R_2 = R_1/CR = R/CR^2$$

where

R = throat radius
R_1 = splitter vane #1 radius
R_2 = splitter vane #2 radius
CR = 'CURVE RATIO' (values from Table 3.7.b)
K_θ = angle factor (see Note 3 for values)

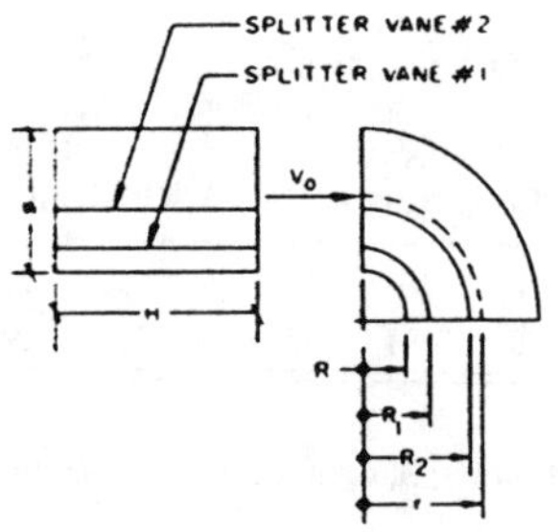

Table 3-7.b Coefficients for elbows with 2 splitter vanes:

			C_o'										
			H/W										
R/W	r/W	CR	0.25	0.5	1.0	1.5	2.0	3.0	4.0	5.0	6.0	7.0	8.0
0.05	0.55	0.362	0.26	0.20	0.22	0.25	0.28	0.33	0.37	0.41	0.45	0.48	0.51
0.10	0.60	0.450	0.17	0.13	0.11	0.12	0.13	0.15	0.16	0.17	0.19	0.20	0.21
0.15	0.65	0.507	0.12	0.09	0.08	0.08	0.08	0.09	0.10	0.10	0.11	0.11	0.11
0.20	0.70	0.550	0.09	0.07	0.06	0.05	0.06	0.06	0.06	0.06	0.07	0.07	0.07
0.25	0.75	0.585	0.08	0.05	0.04	0.04	0.04	0.04	0.05	0.05	0.05	0.05	0.05
0.30	0.80	0.613	0.06	0.04	0.03	0.03	0.03	0.03	0.03	0.03	0.04	0.04	0.04

c. 3 Splitter Vanes

$$C_o = K_\theta C_o'$$
$$R_1 = R/CR$$
$$R_2 = R_1/CR = R/CR^2$$
$$R_3 = R_2/CR = R/CR^3$$

where

R = throat radius
R_1 = splitter vane #1 radius
R_2 = splitter vane #2 radius
R_3 = splitter vane #3 radius
CR = 'CURVE RATIO' (values from Table 3.7.c)
K_θ = angle factor (see Note 3 for values)

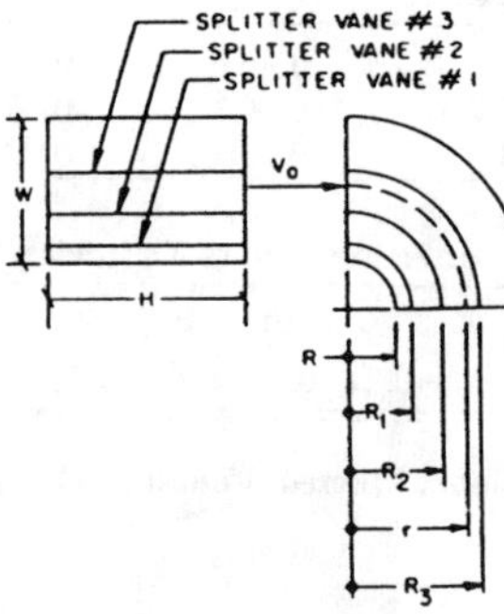

Coefficients for elbow with 3 splitter vanes (C_o')

			H/W										
R/W	r/W	CR	0.25	0.5	1.0	1.5	2.0	3.0	4.0	5.0	6.0	7.0	8.0
0.05	0.55	0.467	0.11	0.10	0.12	0.13	0.14	0.16	0.18	0.19	0.21	0.22	0.23
0.10	0.60	0.549	0.07	0.05	0.06	0.06	0.06	0.07	0.07	0.08	0.08	0.08	0.09

3-8 Elbow, Mitered, with Single-Thickness Vanes, Rectangular (Rozell 1974)

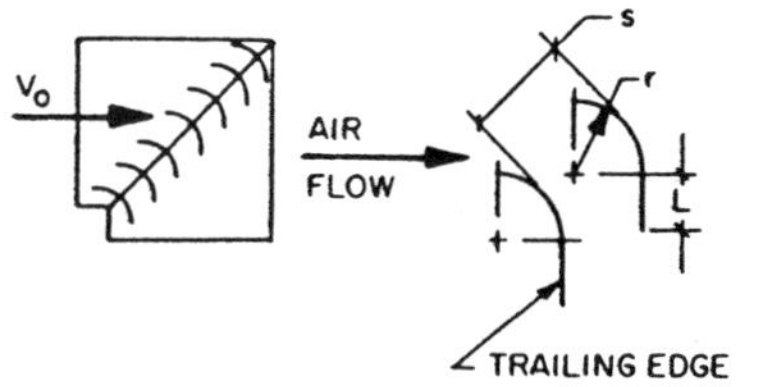

Design No.	Dimensions, in. r	s	L	C_o
1[a]	2.0	1.5	0.75	0.12
2	4.5	2.25	0	0.15
3	4.5	3.25	1.60	0.18

[a]When extension of trailing edge is not provided for this vane, losses are approximately unchanged for single elbows, but increase considerably for elbows in series.

3-9 Elbow, Mitered, with Double-Thickness Vanes, Rectangular (Rozell 1974)

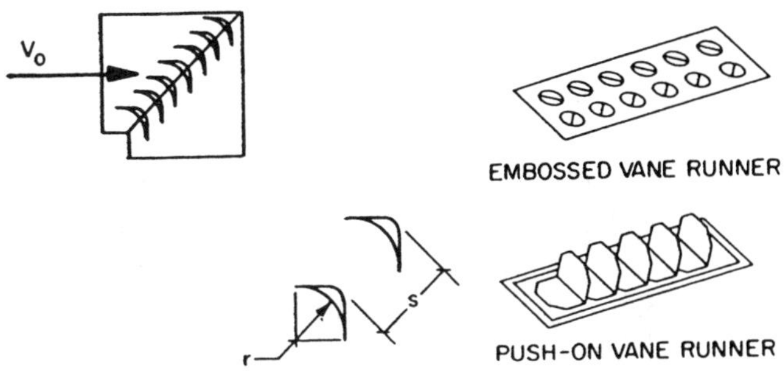

Design No.	Dimensions, in. r	s	C_o Velocity V_o, fpm 1000	2000	3000	4000	Remarks
1	2.0	1.5	0.27	0.22	0.19	0.17	Embossed Vane Runner
2	2.0	1.5	0.33	0.29	0.26	0.23	Push-On Vane Runner
3	2.0	2.13	0.38	0.31	0.27	0.24	Embossed Vane Runner
4	4.5	3.25	0.26	0.21	0.18	0.16	Embossed Vane Runner

3-10 Elbow, Variable Inlet/Outlet Areas, Rectangular (Idelchik 1986, Diagram 6-4)

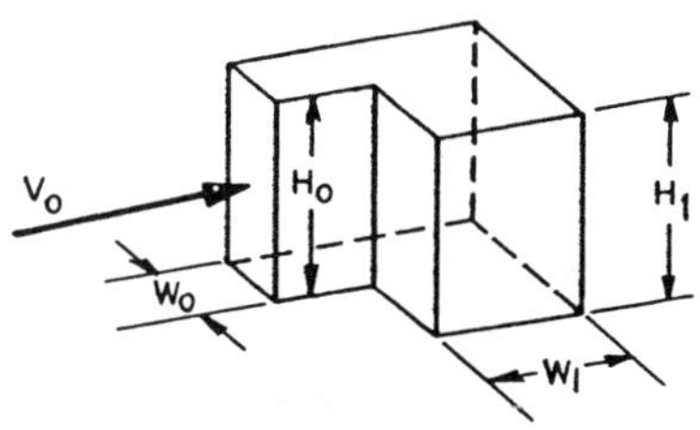

$C_o = K_{Re} C_o'$

H_o/W_o	C_o' W_1/W_o 0.6	0.8	1.2	1.4	1.6	2.0
0.25	1.8	1.4	1.1	1.1	1.1	1.1
1.0	1.7	1.4	1.0	0.95	0.90	0.84
4.0	1.5	1.1	0.81	0.76	0.72	0.66
∞	1.5	1.0	0.69	0.63	0.60	0.55

Reynolds number correction factor

Re × 10^{-4}	1	2	3	4	6	8	10	≥ 14
K_{Re}	1.40	1.26	1.19	1.14	1.09	1.06	1.04	1.0

3-11 Elbows, 90°, Z-Shaped, Rectangular (Idelchik 1986, Diagram 6-11)

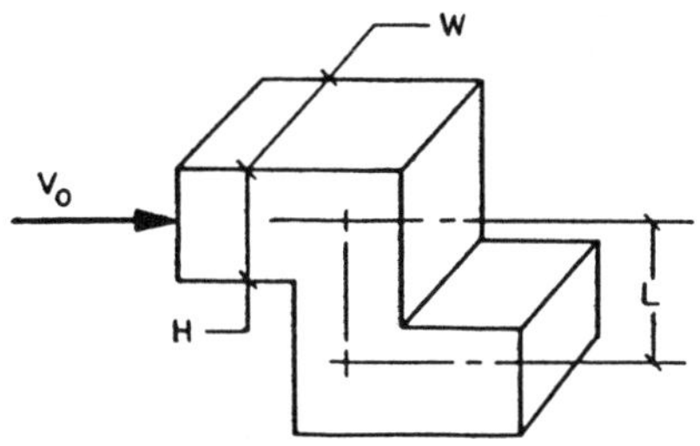

$C = K K_{Re} C_o'$

Coefficients for $W/H = 1.0$

L/H	0	0.4	0.6	0.8	1.0	1.2	1.4	1.6	1.8	2.0
C_o'	0	0.62	0.90	1.6	2.6	3.6	4.0	4.2	4.2	4.2
L/H	2.4	2.8	3.2	4.0	5.0	6.0	7.0	9.0	10.0	∞
C_o'	3.7	3.3	3.2	3.1	2.9	2.9	2.8	2.7	2.5	2.3

For W/H values other than 1.0, apply the following factor

W/H	0.25	0.50	0.75	1.0	1.5	2.0	3.0	4.0	6.0	8.0
K	1.10	1.07	1.04	1.0	0.95	0.,90	9.83	0.78	0.72	0.70

Reynolds Number Correction Factor

Re × 10^{-4}	1	2	3	4	6	8	10	≥14
K_{Re}	1.40	1.26	1.19	1.14	1.09	1.06	1.04	1.0

3-12 Combined 90° Elbows Lying in Different Planes, Rectangular (Idelchik 1986, Diagram 6-11)

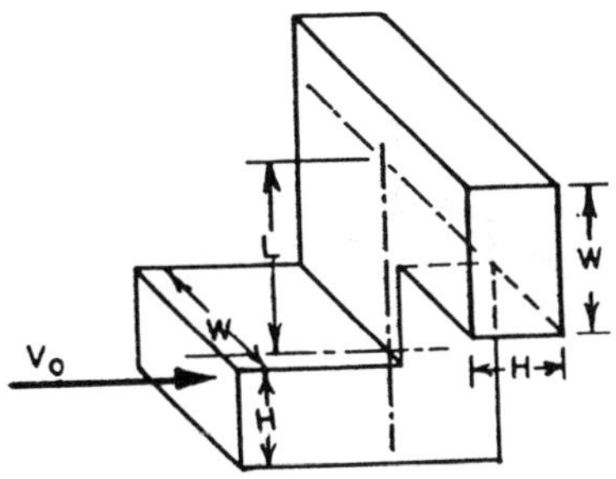

$C_o = K K_{Re} C_o'$

Coefficients for Square Ducts

L/W	0	0.4	0.6	0.8	1.0	1.2	1.4	1.6	1.8	2.0
C_o'	1.2	2.4	2.9	3.3	3.4	3.4	3.4	3.3	3.2	3.1
L/W	2.4	2.8	3.2	4.0	5.0	6.0	7.0	9.0	10.0	∞
C_o'	3.2	3.2	3.2	3.0	2.9	2.8	2.7	2.5	2.4	2.3

Apply the following factor for other than $H/W = 1.0$

H/W	0.25	0.50	0.75	1.0	1.5	2.0	3.0	4.0	6.0	8.0
K	1.10	1.07	1.04	1.0	0.95	0.90	0.83	0.78	0.72	0.70

Reynolds Number Correction Factor

$Re \times 10^{-4}$	1	2	3	4	6	8	10	≥14
K_{Re}	1.40	1.26	1.19	1.14	1.09	1.06	1.04	1.0

3-13 Offset, S-Shaped (Gooseneck), Rectangular and Round (Idelchik 1986, Diagram 6-16)

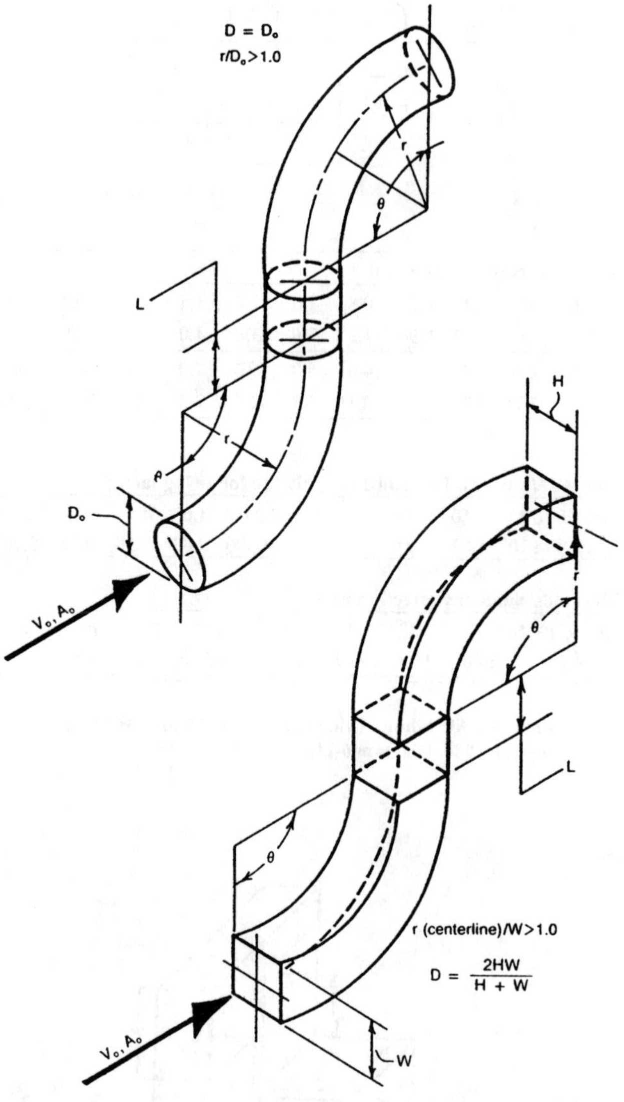

$$C_o = K\,C_o'$$

where

C_o = offset loss coefficient
C_o' = single elbow loss coefficient (see Fittings 3-1, 3-2, and 3-5)

θ, deg	K, L/D = 0	1	2	3	4	6	8	10
15	0.20	0.42	0.60	0.78	0.94	1.16	1.20	1.15
30	0.40	0.65	0.88	1.16	1.20	1.18	1.12	1.06
45	0.60	1.06	1.20	1.23	1.20	1.08	1.03	1.08
60	1.05	1.38	1.37	1.28	1.15	1.06	1.16	1.30
75	1.50	1.58	1.46	1.30	1.27	1.30	1.37	1.47
90	1.70	1.67	1.40	1.37	1.38	1.47	1.55	1.63

θ, deg	K, L/D = 12	14	16	18	20	25	≥40
15	1.08	1.05	1.02	1.00	1.10	1.25	2.0
30	1.06	1.15	1,28	1.40	1.50	1.70	2.0
45	1.17	1.30	1.42	1.55	1.65	1.80	2.0
60	1.42	1.54	1.66	1.76	1.85	1.95	2.0
75	1.57	1.68	1.75	1.80	1.88	1.97	2.0
90	1.70	1.76	1.82	1.88	1.92	1.98	2.0

3-14 Offset, S-Shaped in Two Planes 90° Apart, Rectangular and Round (Idelchik 1986, Diagram 6-16)

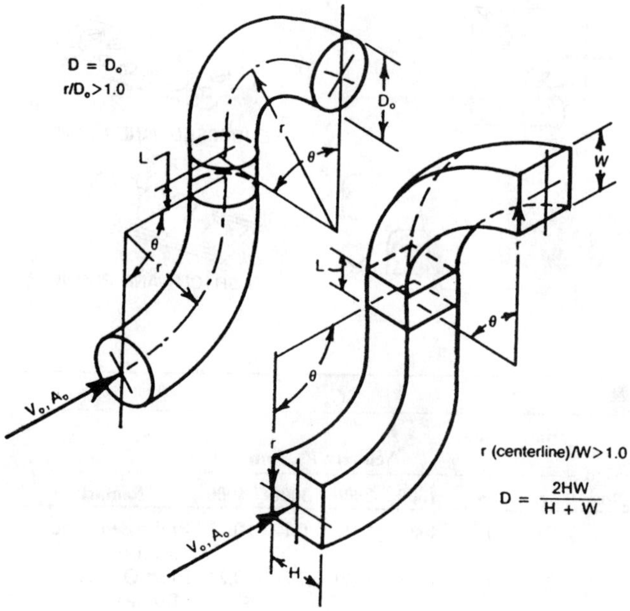

$$C_o = K\,C_o'$$

where

C_o = offset loss coefficient
C_o' = single elbow loss coefficient (see Fittings 3-1, 3-2, and 3-5)

θ, deg	K, L/D = 0	1	2	3	4	6	8
60	2.0	1.90	1.50	1.35	1.30	1.20	1.25
90	2.0	1.80	1.60	1.55	1.55	1.65	1.80

θ, deg	K, L/D = 10	12	14	20	25	40
60	1.50	1.63	1.73	1.85	1.95	2.0
90	1.90	1.93	1.98	2.0	2.0	2.0

3-15 Elbows (4), 45°, Smooth Radius, Rectangular, Arranged to Go Around an Obstruction (SMACNA 1981, Table 6-14K)

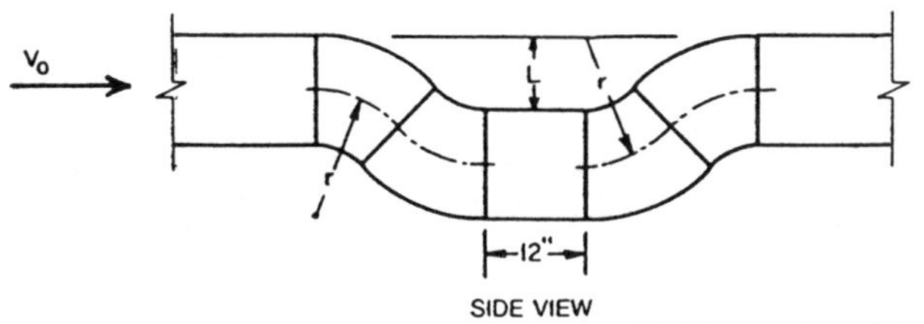

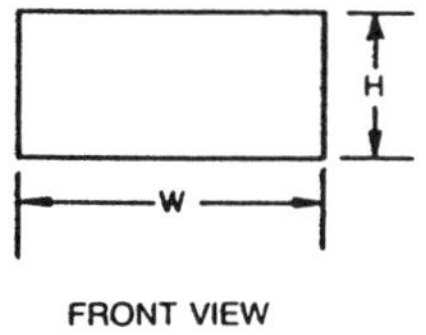

$W/H = 4$, $r/H = 1.5$, $L = 1.5H$

V_o, fpm	800	1200	1600	2000	2400
C_o	0.18	0.22	0.24	0.25	0.26

TRANSITIONS

4-1 Transition, Round (Idelchik 1986, Diagrams 5-2 and 5-22)

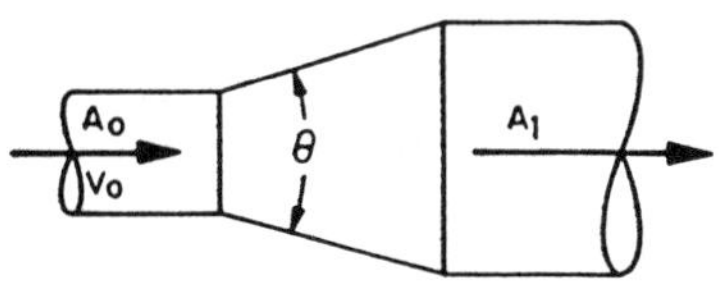

$A_o/A_1 < 1$

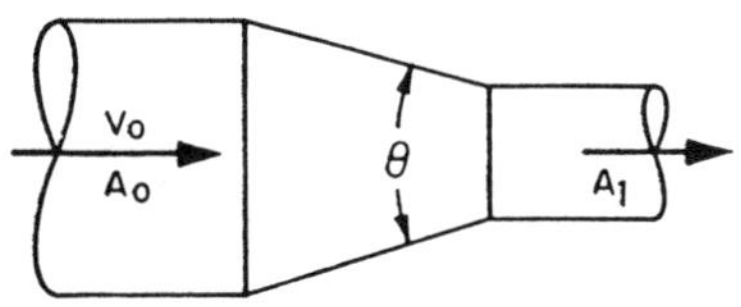

$A_o/A_1 > 1$

	C_o									
	θ, degrees									
A_o/A_1	10	15	20	30	45	60	90	120	150	180
0.06	0.21	0.29	0.38	0.60	0.84	0.88	0.88	0.88	0.88	0.88
0.1	0.21	0.28	0.38	0.59	0.76	0.80	0.83	0.84	0.83	0.83
0.25	0.16	0.22	0.30	0.46	0.61	0.68	0.64	0.63	0.62	0.62
0.5	0.11	0.13	0.19	0.32	0.33	0.33	0.32	0.31	0.30	0.30
1	0	0	0	0	0	0	0	0	0	0
2	0.20	0.20	0.20	0.20	0.22	0.24	0.48	0.72	0.96	1.0
4	0.80	0.64	0.64	0.64	0.88	1.1	2.7	4.3	5.6	6.6
6	1.8	1.4	1.4	1.4	2.0	2.5	6.5	10	13	15
10	5.0	5.0	5.0	5.0	6.5	8.0	19	29	37	43

4-2 Transition, Rectangular, Two Sides Parallel, Symmetrical (Idelchik 1986, Diagram 5-5)[a]

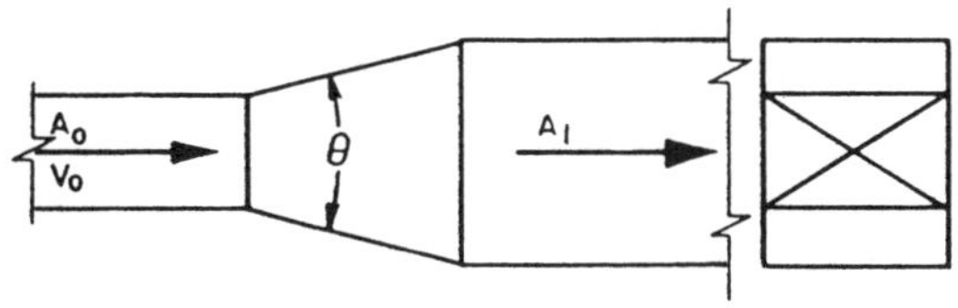

	C_o									
	θ, degrees									
A_o/A_1	10	15	20	30	45	60	90	120	150	180
0.06	0.26	0.27	0.40	0.56	0.71	0.86	1.00	0.99	0.98	0.98
0.1	0.24	0.26	0.36	0.53	0.69	0.82	0.93	0.93	0.92	0.91
0.25	0.17	0.19	0.22	0.42	0.60	0.68	0.70	0.69	0.67	0.66
0.5	0.14	0.13	0.15	0.24	0.35	0.37	0.38	0.37	0.36	0.35
1	0	0	0	0	0	0	0	0	0	0
2	0.23	0.20	0.20	0.20	0.24	0.28	0.54	0.78	1.0	1.1
4	0.81	0.64	0.64	0.64	0.88	1.1	2.8	4.4	5.7	6.6
6	1.8	1.4	1.4	1.4	2.0	2.5	6.6	10	13	15
10	5.0	5.0	5.0	5.0	6.5	8.0	19	29	37	43

[a] $A_o/A_1 > 1$ is tentative (adapted from Fitting 4-1 data).

4-3 Transition, Rectangular, Three Sides Straight[a]

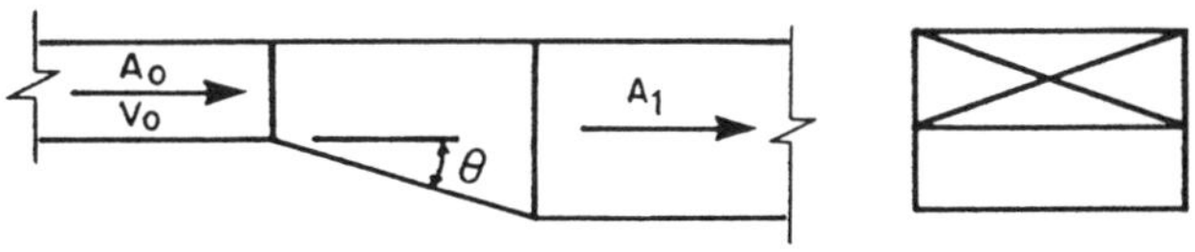

	C_o						
	θ, degrees						
A_o/A_1	10	15	20	30	45	60	90
0.06	0.26	0.27	0.40	0.56	0.71	0.86	1.00
0.1	0.24	0.26	0.36	0.53	0.69	0.82	0.93
0.25	0.17	0.19	0.22	0.42	0.60	0.68	0.70
0.5	0.14	0.13	0.15	0.24	0.35	0.37	0.38
1	0	0	0	0	0	0	0
2	0.23	0.20	0.20	0.20	0.24	0.28	0.54
4	0.81	0.64	0.64	0.64	0.88	1.1	2.8
6	1.8	1.4	1.4	1.4	2.0	2.5	6.6
10	5.0	5.0	5.0	5.0	6.5	8.0	19

[a] Tentative (assumed same as Fitting 4-2 data).

4-4 Transition, Rectangular, Pyramidal (Idelchik 1986, Diagram 5-4)[a]

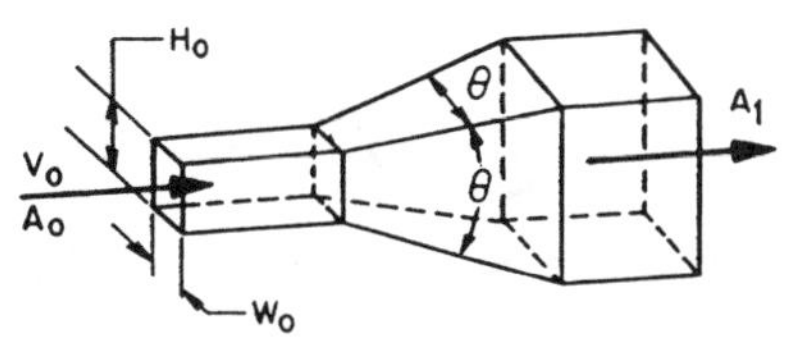

	C_o									
	θ, degrees									
A_o/A_1	10	15	20	30	45	60	90	120	150	180
0.06	0.26	0.30	0.44	0.54	0.53	0.65	0.77	0.88	0.95	0.98
0.1	0.24	0.30	0.43	0.50	0.53	0.64	0.75	0.84	0.89	0.91
0.25	0.20	0.25	0.34	0.36	0.45	0.52	0.58	0.62	0.64	0.64
0.5	0.14	0.15	0.20	0.21	0.25	0.30	0.33	0.33	0.33	0.32
1	0	0	0	0	0	0	0	0	0	0
2	0.23	0.22	0.21	0.20	0.22	0.2	0.49	0.74	0.99	1.1
4	0.84	0.68	0.68	0.64	0.88	1.1	2.7	4.3	5.6	6.6
6	1.8	1.5	1.5	1.4	2.0	2.5	6.5	10	13	15
10	5.0	5.0	5.1	5.0	6.5	8.0	19	29	37	43

[a] $A_o/A_1 > 1$ is tentative (adapted from Fitting 4-1 data).

4-5 Transition, Round/Rectangular (Idelchik 1986, Diagram 5-27)

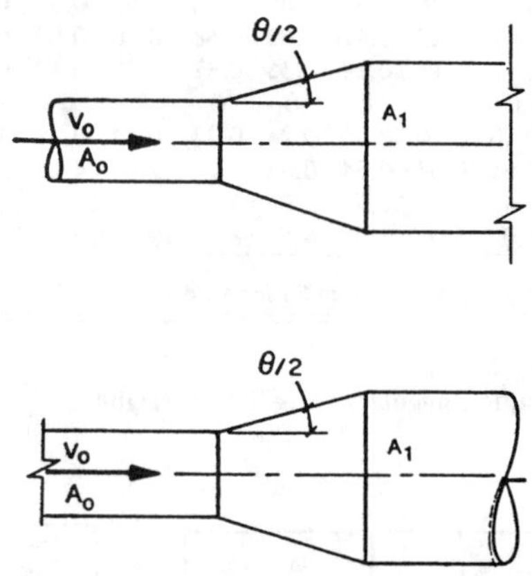

	C_o								
	θ, degrees								
A_1/A_o	8	10	14	20	30	45	60	90	180
2	0.14	0.15	0.20	0.25	0.30	0.33	0.33	0.33	0.30
4	0.20	0.25	0.34	0.45	0.52	0.58	0.62	0.64	0.64
6	0.21	0.30	0.42	0.53	0.63	0.72	0.78	0.79	0.79
≥ 10	0.24	0.30	0.43	0.53	0.64	0.75	0.84	0.89	0.88

4-6 Transition, Rectangular to Round (Idelchik 1986, Diagram 5-26)

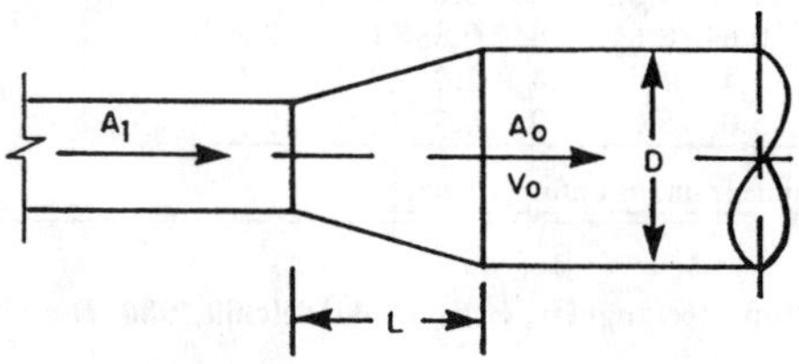

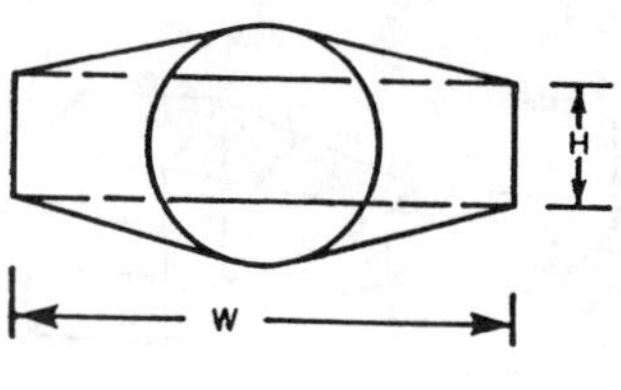

$$Re = DV_o/\nu$$

$$B = \frac{W}{H}\left(\frac{A_o}{A_1}\right)^2$$

C_o for $A_o > A_1$ and $H < D$

		B							
Re × 10^{-4}	L/D	0.1	0.5	1	2	5	10	20	50
1	1	0.46	0.48	0.50	0.55	0.70	0.94	1.4	2.9
	1.5	0.46	0.47	0.49	0.53	0.64	0.82	1.2	2.3
	2	0.46	0.47	0.48	0.50	0.58	0.71	0.98	1.8
	3	0.45	0.46	0.46	0.48	0.51	0.57	0.69	1.0
	4	0.45	0.46	0.46	0.46	0.48	0.51	0.56	0.73
	5	0.45	0.46	0.46	0.47	0.49	0.53	0.61	0.84
2	1	0.41	0.43	0.46	0.51	0.66	0.90	1.4	2.9
	1.5	0.41	0.43	0.45	0.48	0.59	0.78	1.1	2.2
	2	0.41	0.42	0.44	0.46	0.54	0.67	0.93	1.7
	3	0.41	0.42	0.42	0.43	0.47	0.53	0.64	0.99
	4	0.41	0.41	0.41	0.42	0.44	0.46	0.52	0.69
	5	0.41	0.41	0.42	0.43	0.45	0.49	0.57	0.80
5	1	0.31	0.33	0.35	0.40	0.55	0.79	1.3	2.8
	1.5	0.31	0.32	0.34	0.38	0.49	0.67	1.0	2.1
	2	0.31	0.32	0.33	0.36	0.43	0.57	0.83	1.6
	3	0.30	0.31	0.31	0.33	0.36	0.42	0.54	0.88
	4	0.30	0.31	0.31	0.31	0.33	0.36	0.41	0.58
	5	0.30	0.31	0.31	0.32	0.34	0.38	0.46	0.70
10	1	0.19	0.21	0.23	0.28	0.43	0.68	1.2	2.6
	1.5	0.19	0.20	0.22	0.26	0.37	0.55	0.92	2.0
	2	0.19	0.20	0.21	0.24	0.31	0.45	0.71	1.5
	3	0.19	0.19	0.20	0.21	0.24	0.30	0.42	0.77
	4	0.18	0.19	0.19	0.19	0.21	0.24	0.29	0.46
	5	0.18	0.19	0.19	0.20	0.22	0.26	0.34	0.58
20	1	0.07	0.09	0.12	0.17	0.31	0.56	1.1	2.5
	1.5	0.07	0.09	0.10	0.14	0.25	0.43	0.80	1.9
	2	0.07	0.08	0.09	0.12	0.20	0.33	0.59	1.4
	3	0.07	0.07	0.08	0.09	0.13	0.18	0.30	0.65
	4	0.07	0.07	0.07	0.08	0.10	0.12	0.18	0.34
	5	0.07	0.07	0.08	0.08	0.11	0.15	0.22	0.46
50	1	0.01	0.03	0.05	0.10	0.25	0.30	0.99	2.5
	1.5	0.01	0.02	0.04	0.08	0.19	0.37	0.74	1.8
	2	0.01	0.02	0.03	0.06	0.13	0.27	0.53	1.3
	3	0	0.01	0.02	0.03	0.06	0.12	0.24	0.58
	4	0	0.01	0.01	0.01	0.03	0.06	0.11	0.28
	5	0	0.01	0.01	0.02	0.04	0.08	0.16	0.40

C_o for $A_o < A_1$ and $H < D$

		B					
Re × 10^{-4}	L/D	0.1	1	5	10	20	50
1	1	0.27	0.27	0.28	0.29	0.31	0.37
	3	0.27	0.27	0.28	0.29	0.30	0.33
	4	0.27	0.27	0.28	0.28	0.29	0.32
	5	0.27	0.27	0.27	0.27	0.27	0.27
2	1	0.25	0.25	0.26	0.27	0.29	0.35
	3	0.25	0.25	0.25	0.26	0.28	0.33
	4	0.25	0.25	0.25	0.26	0.27	0.30
	5	0.25	0.25	0.25	0.25	0.25	0.25
5	1	0.18	0.18	0.19	0.20	0.22	0.28
	3	0.18	0.18	0.19	0.20	0.22	0.27
	4	0.18	0.18	0.19	0.19	0.20	0.23
	5	0.18	0.18	0.18	0.18	0.18	0.18
10	1	0.11	0.11	0.12	0.13	0.15	0.21
	3	0.11	0.11	0.12	0.13	0.14	0.19
	4	0.11	0.11	0.12	0.12	0.13	0.16
	5	0.11	0.11	0.11	0.11	0.11	0.11
20	1	0.04	0.04	0.05	0.06	0.08	0.14
	3	0.04	0.04	0.05	0.06	0.07	0.12
	4	0.04	0.04	0.05	0.05	0.06	0.09
	5	0.04	0.04	0.04	0.04	0.04	0.04
50	1	0	0	0.01	0.02	0.04	0.10
	3	0	0	0.01	0.02	0.04	0.09
	4	0	0	0.01	0.01	0.02	0.05
	5	0	0	0	0	0	0

4-7 Transition, Rectangular to Round, Stepped, Conical (Idelchik 1986, Diagram 4-9)

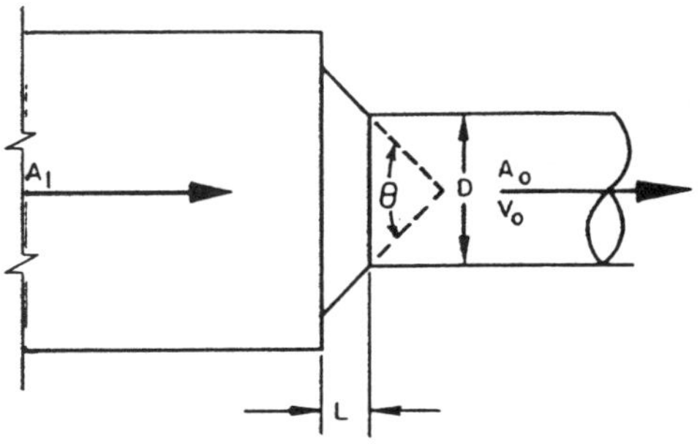

A_o/A_1	L/D	C_o θ, degrees 0	10	20	30	45	60	90	120	150	180
0.1	0.025	0.46	0.43	0.42	0.40	0.38	0.37	0.38	0.40	0.43	0.46
	0.05	0.46	0.42	0.38	0.33	0.30	0.28	0.31	0.36	0.41	0.46
	0.075	0.46	0.39	0.32	0.28	0.23	0.21	0.26	0.32	0.39	0.46
	0.1	0.46	0.36	0.30	0.23	0.19	0.17	0.23	0.30	0.38	0.46
	0.15	0.46	0.34	0.25	0.18	0.15	0.14	0.21	0.29	0.37	0.46
	0.3	0.46	0.31	0.22	0.16	0.13	0.13	0.20	0.28	0.37	0.46
	0.6	0.46	0.25	0.17	0.12	0.10	0.11	0.19	0.27	0.36	0.46
0.25	0.025	0.40	0.38	0.36	0.35	0.33	0.32	0.33	0.35	0.37	0.40
	0.05	0.40	0.36	0.33	0.29	0.26	0.24	0.27	0.31	0.35	0.40
	0.075	0.40	0.34	0.28	0.24	0.20	0.19	0.23	0.28	0.34	0.40
	0.1	0.40	0.31	0.26	0.20	0.17	0.14	0.20	0.26	0.33	0.40
	0.15	0.40	0.30	0.22	0.16	0.13	0.12	0.18	0.25	0.32	0.40
	0.3	0.40	0.27	0.19	0.14	0.11	0.11	0.18	0.25	0.32	0.40
	0.6	0.40	0.22	0.14	0.10	0.09	0.10	0.16	0.24	0.32	0.40
0.5	0.025	0.30	0.28	0.27	0.25	0.24	0.24	0.25	0.26	0.27	0.30
	0.05	0.30	0.27	0.24	0.21	0.19	0.18	0.20	0.23	0.26	0.30
	0.075	0.30	0.25	0.21	0.18	0.15	0.14	0.17	0.21	0.25	0.30
	0.1	0.30	0.23	0.19	0.15	0.12	0.11	0.15	0.19	0.24	0.30
	0.15	0.30	0.22	0.16	0.12	0.09	0.09	0.13	0.18	0.24	0.30
	0.3	0.30	0.20	0.14	0.10	0.08	0.08	0.13	0.18	0.24	0.30
	0.6	0.30	0.16	0.11	0.08	0.07	0.07	0.12	0.17	0.23	0.30
0.8	0.025	0.15	0.14	0.13	0.13	0.12	0.12	0.12	0.13	0.14	0.15
	0.05	0.15	0.13	0.12	0.11	0.10	0.09	0.10	0.12	0.13	0.15
	0.075	0.15	0.13	0.10	0.09	0.08	0.07	0.08	0.10	0.13	0.15
	0.1	0.15	0.12	0.10	0.07	0.06	0.05	0.07	0.10	0.12	0.15
	0.15	0.15	0.11	0.08	0.06	0.05	0.04	0.07	0.09	0.12	0.15
	0.3	0.15	0.10	0.07	0.05	0.04	0.04	0.07	0.09	0.12	0.15
	0.6	0.15	0.08	0.05	0.04	0.03	0.04	0.06	0.09	0.12	0.15

JUNCTIONS (Tees, Wyes, Crosses)

5-1 Wye, 30°, Converging (Idelchik 1986, Diagram 7-1)

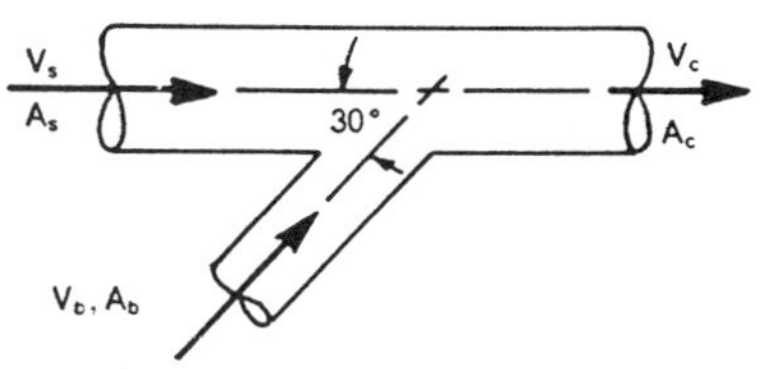

$A_S = A_C$

Branch, $C_{c,b}$

Q_b/Q_c	A_b/A_c 0.1	0.2	0.3	0.4	0.6	0.8	1.0
0	−1.0	−1.0	−1.0	−0.9	−0.9	−0.9	−0.9
0.1	0.21	−0.46	−0.57	−0.51	−0.53	−0.54	−0.54
0.2	3.1	0.37	−0.06	−0.16	−0.23	−0.24	−0.28
0.3	7.6	1.5	0.50	0.15	−0.04	−0.06	−0.08
0.4	14	3.0	1.2	0.42	0.19	0.13	0.12
0.5	21	4.6	1.8	0.53	0.24	0.19	0.15
0.6	30	6.4	2.6	0.77	0.35	0.25	0.17
0.7	41	8.5	3.4	0.99	0.42	0.28	0.22
0.8	54	12	4.2	1.2	0.47	0.29	0.25
0.9	58	14	5.3	1.4	0.49	0.29	0.22
1.0	84	17	6.3	1.6	0.49	0.21	0.15

Main, $C_{c,s}$

Q_b/Q_c	A_b/A_c 0.1	0.2	0.3	0.4	0.6	0.8	1.0
0	0	0	0	0	0	0	0
0.1	0.02	0.11	0.13	0.15	0.16	0.17	0.17
0.2	− 0.33	0.01	0.13	0.19	0.24	0.27	0.29
0.3	− 1.1	−0.25	−0.01	0.10	0.22	0.30	0.35
0.4	− 2.2	−0.75	−0.30	−0.05	0.17	0.26	0.36
0.5	− 3.6	−1.4	−0.70	−0.35	0	0.21	0.32
0.6	− 5.4	−2.4	−1.3	−0.70	−0.20	0.06	0.25
0.7	− 7.6	−3.4	−2.0	−1.2	−0.50	−0.15	0.10
0.8	−10	−4.6	−2.7	−1.8	−0.90	−0.43	−0.15
0.9	−13	−6.2	−3.7	−2.6	−1.4	−0.80	−0.45
1.0	−16	−7.7	−4.8	−3.4	−1.9	−1.2	−0.75

5-2 Wye, 45°, Converging, Round (Idelchik 1986, Diagram 7-2)

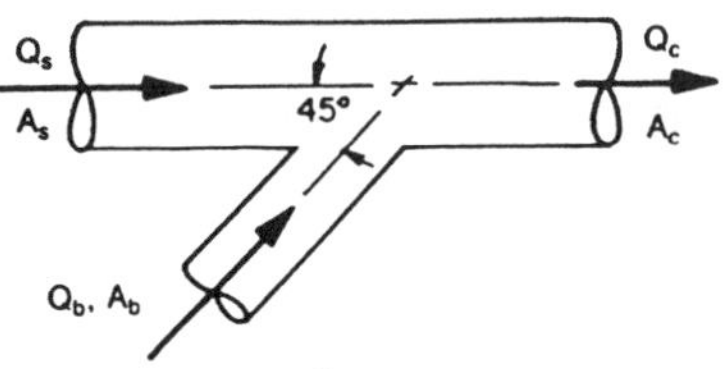

$A_S = A_C$

$C_{c,b}$

Q_b/Q_c	A_b/A_c 0.1	0.2	0.3	0.4	0.6	0.8	1.0
0	− 1.0	− 1.0	−1.0	−0.90	−0.90	−0.90	−0.90
0.1	0.24	− 0.45	−0.56	−0.50	−0.52	−0.53	−0.53
0.2	3.2	0.54	−0.02	−0.14	−0.21	−0.23	−0.23
0.3	8.0	1.6	0.60	0.23	0.06	0	−0.02
0.4	14	3.2	1.3	0.52	0.25	0.18	0.15
0.5	22	5.0	2.1	0.65	0.33	0.25	0.22
0.6	32	7.0	3.0	0.91	0.81	0.61	0.51
0.7	43	9.2	3.9	1.2	0.56	0.39	0.33
0.8	56	12	4.9	1.5	0.66	0.39	0.36
0.9	71	15	6.2	1.8	0.72	0.44	0.35
1.0	87	19	7.4	2.0	0.78	0.44	0.32

$C_{c,s}$

Q_b/Q_c	A_b/A_c 0.1	0.2	0.3	0.4	0.6	0.8	1.0
0	0	0	0	0	0	0	0
0.1	0.05	0.12	0.14	0.16	0.17	0.17	0.17
0.2	− 0.20	0.17	0.22	0.27	0.27	0.29	0.31
0.3	− 0.76	−0.13	0.08	0.20	0.28	0.32	0.40
0.4	− 1.7	−0.50	−0.12	0.08	0.26	0.36	0.41
0.5	− 2.8	−1.0	−0.49	−0.13	0.16	0.30	0.40
0.6	− 4.3	−1.7	−0.87	−0.45	−0.04	0.20	0.33
0.7	− 6.1	−2.6	−1.4	−0.85	−0.25	0.08	0.25
0.8	− 8.1	−3.6	−2.1	−1.3	−0.55	−0.17	0.06
0.9	−10	−4.8	−2.8	−1.9	−0.88	−0.40	−0.18
1.0	−13	−6.1	−3.7	−2.6	−1.4	−0.77	−0.42

5-3 Tee, Converging, Round (Idelchik 1986, Diagram 7-4)

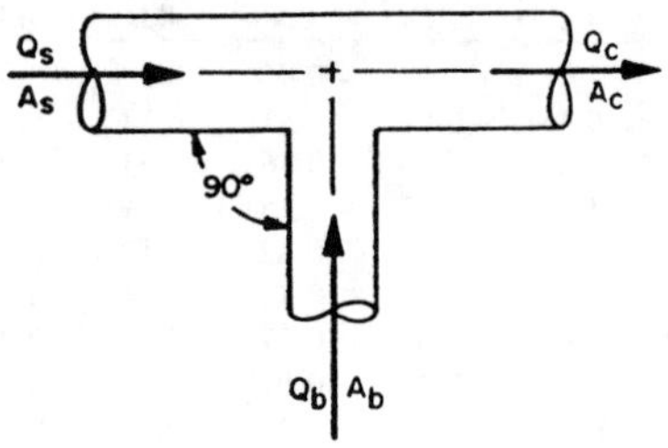

$A_s = A_c$

Branch, $C_{c,b}$

Q_b/Q_c	A_b/A_c 0.1	0.2	0.3	0.4	0.6	0.8	1.0
0	– 1.0	– 1.0	– 1.0	−0.90	−0.90	−0.90	−0.90
0.1	0.40	– 0.37	– 0.51	−0.46	−0.50	−0.51	−0.52
0.2	3.8	0.72	0.17	−0.02	−0.14	−0.18	−0.24
0.3	9.2	2.3	1.0	0.44	0.21	0.11	−0.08
0.4	16	4.3	2.1	0.94	0.54	0.40	0.32
0.5	26	6.8	3.2	1.1	0.66	0.49	0.42
0.6	37	9.7	4.7	1.6	0.92	0.69	0.57
0.7	43	13	6.3	2.1	1.2	0.88	0.72
0.8	65	17	7.9	2.7	1.5	1.1	0.86
0.9	82	21	9.7	3.4	1.8	1.2	0.99
1.0	101	26	12	4.0	2.1	1.4	1.1

Main

Q_b/Q_c	0	0.1	0.2	0.3	0.4	0.5	0.6	0.7	0.8	0.9	1.0
$C_{c,s}$	0	0.16	0.27	0.38	0.46	0.53	0.57	0.59	0.60	0.59	0.55

5-4 Wye, 30°, Converging, Round, Conical Main (Sepsy 1973)

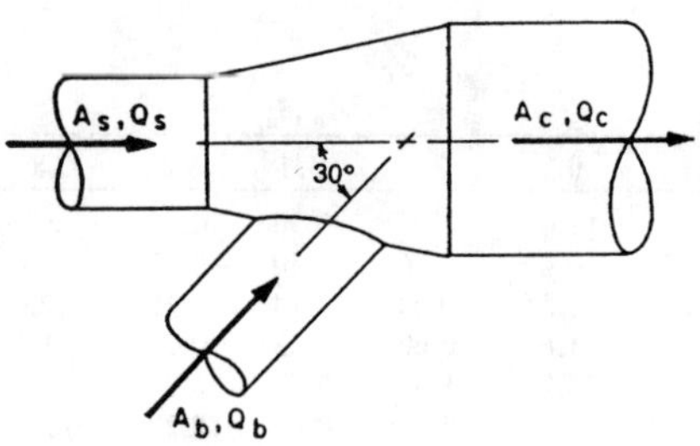

Branch, $C_{c,b}$

A_s/A_c	A_b/A_c	Q_b/Q_s 0.2	0.4	0.6	0.8	1.0	1.2	1.4	1.6	1.8	2.0
0.3	0.2	−2.4	−.11	1.8	3.4	4.8	6.0	7.1	8.0	8.9	9.7
	0.3	−2.8	−1.3	0.14	0.72	1.4	2.0	2.4	2.8	3.2	3.5
0.4	0.2	−1.4	0.61	2.3	3.8	5.2	6.3	7.3	8.3	9.1	9.8
	0.3	−1.8	−.54	0.42	1.2	1.8	2.3	2.7	3.1	3.4	3.7
	0.4	−1.9	−.89	−.17	0.36	0.76	1.1	1.3	1.5	1.7	1.9
0.5	0.2	−.82	0.97	2.6	4.0	5.3	6.4	7.4	8.3	9.1	9.9
	0.3	−1.2	−.15	0.71	1.4	2.0	2.5	2.9	3.3	3.6	3.9
	0.4	−1.4	−.54	0.06	0.50	0.85	1.1	1.3	1.5	1.7	1.8
	0.5	−1.4	−.66	−.15	0.21	0.48	0.68	0.84	0.97	1.1	1.2
0.6	0.2	−.52	1.2	2.7	4.1	5.3	6.4	7.4	8.3	9.1	9.9
	0.3	−.93	0.06	0.85	1.5	2.1	2.6	3.0	3.4	3.7	4.0
	0.4	−1.1	−.37	0.16	0.55	0.86	1.1	1.3	1.4	1.6	1.8
	0.5	−1.1	−.49	−.06	0.25	0.48	0.66	0.79	0.90	1.0	1.1
	0.6	−1.2	−.55	−.15	0.12	0.31	0.45	0.56	0.65	0.71	0.77
0.8	0.2	−.27	1.3	2.7	4.0	5.2	6.3	7.3	8.2	9.0	9.7
	0.3	−.67	0.18	0.90	1.5	2.0	2.5	2.9	3.3	3.6	4.0
	0.4	−.85	−.27	0.16	0.49	0.75	0.97	1.2	1.3	1.4	1.6
	0.5	−.90	−.40	−.07	0.18	0.36	0,50	0.61	0.70	0.78	0.84
	0.6	−.92	−.46	−.16	0.04	0.18	0.29	0.37	0.44	0.49	0.53
	0.7	−.93	−.49	−.21	−.03	0.10	0.19	0.25	0.30	0.34	0.37
	0.8	−.93	−.50	−.24	−.07	0.05	0.13	0.19	0.23	0.27	0.29
1.0	0.2	−.26	1.2	2.6	3.9	5.1	6.1	7.1	8.0	8.8	9.5
	0.3	−.65	0.12	0.79	1.4	1.9	2.4	2.8	3.1	3.5	3.8
	0.4	−.83	−.34	0.04	0.33	0.58	0.78	0.95	1.1	1.2	1.3
	0.5	−.89	−.48	−.20	0	0.15	0.27	0.37	0.45	0.51	0.57
	0.6	−.91	−.54	−.31	−.14	−.03	0.06	0.12	0.18	0.22	0.25
	0.8	−.93	−.59	−.38	−.25	−.16	−.10	−.06	−.03	−.01	0.01
	1.0	−.93	−.60	−40	−.28	−.20	−.14	−.11	−.08	−.07	−.06

Main, $C_{c,s}$

A_s/A_c	A_b/A_c	Q_b/Q_s 0.2	0.4	0.6	0.8	1.0	1.2	1.4	1.6	0.8	2.0
0.3	0.2	4.5	2.8	1.5	0.56	−.17	−.74	−1.2	−1.6	−1.9	−2.1
	0.3	4.6	3.1	2.0	1.2	0.57	0.08	−.30	−.62	−.89	−1.1
0.4	0.2	1.6	0.85	0.16	−.43	−.92	−1.3	−1.7	−1.9	−2.2	−2.4
	0.3	1.7	1.1	0.58	0.13	−.24	−.56	−.82	−1.1	−1.3	−1.4
	0.4	1.8	1.3	0.80	0.42	0.11	−.15	−.37	−.55	−.72	−.86
0.5	0.2	0.67	0.18	−.33	−.79	−1.2	−1.5	−1.8	−2.1	−2.3	−2.5
	0.3	0.75	0.42	0.07	−.25	−.54	−.80	−1.0	−1.2	−1.4	−1.5
	0.4	0.80	0.55	0.28	0.03	−.20	−.40	−.57	−.73	−.86	−.98
	0.5	0.82	0.62	0.41	0.20	0.02	−.15	−.29	−.42	−.53	−.63
0.6	0.2	0.26	−.11	−.54	−.95	−1.3	−1.6	−1.9	−2.1	−2.4	−2.5
	0.3	0.34	0.13	−.14	−42	−.67	−.90	−1.1	−1.3	−1.4	−1.6
	0.4	0.39	0.25	0.06	−.14	−.33	−.51	−.66	−.80	−.93	−1.0
	0.5	0.41	0.32	0.18	0.03	−1.2	−.26	−.38	−.50	−.60	−.69
	0.6	0.43	0.37	0.26	0.14	0.02	−.09	−.19	−.29	−.37	−.45
0.8	0.2	−.01	−.30	−.67	−1.1	−1.4	−1.7	−2.0	−2.2	−2.4	−2.6
	0.3	0.07	−.07	−.29	−.58	−.76	−.97	−1.2	−1.3	−1.5	−1.6
	0.4	0.11	0.05	−.09	−.26	−.42	−.58	−.72	−.85	−.97	−1.1
	0.5	0.14	0.12	0.03	−.09	−.21	−.34	−.45	−.55	−.64	−.73
	0.6	0.15	0.17	0.11	0.02	−.07	−.17	−.26	−.34	−.42	−.49
	0.7	0.17	0.21	0.17	0.11	0.03	−.05	−.12	−.19	−.26	−.32
	0.8	0.17	0.23	0.22	0.17	0.11	0.05	−.02	−.07	−.13	−.18
1.0	0.2	−.05	−.33	−.70	−1.1	−1.4	−1.7	−2.0	−2.2	−2.4	−2.6
	0.3	0.03	−.10	−.31	−.55	−.78	−.98	−1.2	−1.3	−1.5	−1.6
	0.4	0.07	0.02	−.12	−.28	−.44	−.59	−.73	−.86	−.98	−1.1
	0.5	0.09	0.09	0.01	−.11	−.23	−.35	−.46	−.56	−.65	−.74
	0.6	0.11	0.14	0.09	0	−.09	−.18	−.27	−.35	−.43	−.50
	0.8	0.13	0.20	0.19	0.15	0.09	0.03	−.03	−.08	−.14	−.19
	1.0	0.14	0.24	0.25	0.24	0.20	0.16	0.12	0.08	0.04	0

5-5 Wye, 45°, Converging, Round, Conical Main (Sepsy 1973)

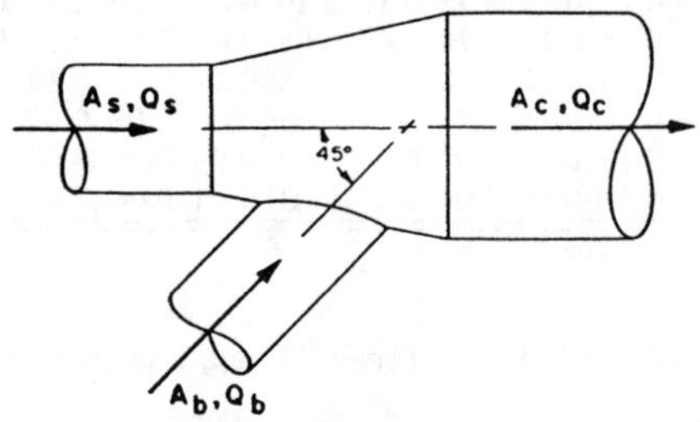

Branch, $C_{c,b}$

A_s/A_c	A_b/A_c	Q_b/Q_s 0.2	0.4	0.6	0.8	1.0	1.2	1.4	1.6	1.8	2.0
0.3	0.2	−2.4	−.01	2.0	3.8	5.3	6.6	7.8	8.9	9.8	11
	0.3	−2.8	−1.2	0.12	1.1	1.9	2.6	3.2	3.7	4.2	4.6
0.4	0.2	−1.2	0.93	2.8	4.5	5.9	7.2	8.4	9.5	10	11
	0.3	−1.6	−.27	0.81	1.7	2.4	3.0	3.6	4.1	4.5	4.9
	0.4	−1.8	−.72	0.07	0.66	1.1	1.5	1.8	2.1	2.3	2.5
0.5	0.2	−.46	1.5	3.3	4.9	6.4	7.7	8.8	9.9	11	12
	0.3	−.94	0.25	1.2	2.0	2.7	3.3	3.8	4.2	4.7	5.0
	0.4	−1.1	−.24	0.42	0.92	1.3	1.6	1.9	2.1	2.3	2.5
	0.5	−1.2	−.38	0.18	0.58	0.88	1.1	1.3	1.5	1.6	1.7

Branch, $C_{c,b}$

A_s/A_c	A_b/A_c	Q_b/Q_s 0.2	0.4	0.6	0.8	1.0	1.2	1.4	1.6	1.8	2.0
0.6	0.2	–.55	1.3	3.1	4.7	6.1	7.4	8.6	9.6	11	12
	0.3	–1.1	0	0.88	1.6	2.3	2.8	3.3	3.7	4.1	4.5
	0.4	–1.2	–.48	0.10	0.54	0.89	1.2	1.4	1.6	1.8	2.0
	0.5	–1.3	–.62	–.14	0.21	0.47	0.68	0.85	0.99	1.1	1.2
	0.6	–1.3	–.69	–.26	0.04	0.26	0.42	0.57	0.66	0.75	0.82
0.8	0.2	0.06	1.8	3.5	5.1	6.5	7.8	8.9	10	11	12
	0.3	–.52	0.35	1.1	1.7	2.3	2.8	3.2	3.6	3.9	4.2
	0.4	–.67	–.05	0.43	0.80	1.1	1.4	1.6	1.8	1.9	2.1
	0.6	–.75	–.27	0.05	0.28	0.45	0.58	0.68	0.76	0.83	0.88
	0.7	–.77	–.31	–.02	0.18	0.32	0.43	0.50	0.56	0.61	0.65
	0.8	–.78	–.34	–.07	0.12	0.24	0.33	0.39	0.44	0.47	0.50
1.0	0.2	0.40	2.1	3.7	5.2	6.6	7.8	9.0	11	11	12
	0.3	–.21	0.54	1.2	1.8	2.3	2.7	3.1	3.7	3.7	4.0
	0.4	–.33	0.21	0.62	0.96	1.2	1.5	1.7	2.0	2.0	2.1
	0.5	–.38	0.05	0.37	0.60	0.79	0.93	1.1	1.2	1.2	1.3
	0.6	–.41	–.02	0.23	0.42	0.55	0.66	0.73	0.80	0.85	0.89
	0.8	–.44	–.10	0.11	0.24	0.33	0.39	0.43	0.46	0.47	0.48
	1.0	–.46	–.14	0.05	0.16	0.23	0.27	0.29	0.30	0.30	0.29

Main, $C_{c,s}$

A_s/A_c	A_b/A_c	Q_b/Q_s 0.2	0.4	0.6	0.8	1.0	1.2	1.4	1.6	1.8	2.0
0.3	0.2	5.3	–.01	2.0	1.1	0.34	–.20	–.61	–.93	–1.2	–1.4
	0.3	5.4	3.7	2.5	1.6	1.0	0.53	0.16	–.14	–.38	–.58
0.4	0.2	1.9	1.1	0.46	–.07	–.49	–.83	–1.1	–1.3	–1.5	–1.7
	0.3	2.0	1.4	0.81	0.42	0.08	–.20	–.43	–.62	–.78	–.92
	0.4	2.0	1.5	1.0	0.68	0.39	0.16	–.04	–.21	–.35	–.47
0.5	0.2	0.77	0.34	–.09	–.48	–.81	–1.1	–1.3	–1.5	–1.7	–1.8
	0.3	0.85	0.56	0.25	–.03	–.27	–.48	–.67	–.82	–.96	–1.1
	0.4	0.88	0.66	0.43	0.21	0.02	–.15	–.30	–.42	–.54	–.64
	0.5	0.91	0.73	0.54	0.36	0.21	0.06	–.06	–.17	–.26	–.35
0.6	0.2	0.30	0	–.34	–.67	–.96	–1.2	–1.4	–1.6	–1.8	–1.9
	0.3	0.37	0.21	–.02	–.24	–.44	–.63	–.79	–.93	–1.1	–1.2
	0.4	0.40	0.31	0.16	–0.1	–.16	–.30	–.43	–.54	–.64	–.73
	0.5	0.43	0.37	0.26	0.14	0.02	–.09	–.20	–.29	–.37	–.45
	0.6	0.44	0.41	0.33	0.24	0.14	0.05	–.03	–.11	–.18	–.25
0.8	0.2	–.06	–.27	–.57	–.86	–1.1	–1.4	–1.6	–1.7	–1.9	–2.0
	0.3	0	–.08	–.25	–.43	–.62	–.78	–.93	–1.1	–1.2	–1.3
	0.4	0.04	0.02	–.08	–.21	–.34	–.46	–.57	–.67	–.77	–.85
	0.5	0.06	0.08	0.02	–.06	–.16	–.25	–.34	–.42	–.50	–.57
	0.6	0.07	0.12	0.09	0.03	–.04	–.11	–.18	–.25	–.31	–.37
	0.7	0.08	0.15	0.14	0.10	0.05	–.01	–.07	–.12	–.17	–.22
	0.8	0.09	0.17	0.18	0.16	0.11	0.07	0.02	–.02	–.07	–.11
1.0	0.2	–.19	–.39	–.67	–.96	–1.2	–1.5	–1.6	–1.8	–2.0	–2.1
	0.3	–.12	–.19	–.35	–.54	–.71	–.87	–1.0	–1.2	–1.3	–1.4
	0.4	–.09	–.10	–.19	–.31	–.43	–.55	–.66	–.77	–.86	–.94
	0.5	–.07	–.04	–.09	–.17	–.26	–.35	–.44	–.52	–.59	–.66
	0.6	–.06	0	–.02	–.07	–.14	–.21	–.28	–.34	–.40	–.46
	0.8	–.04	0.06	0.07	0.05	0.02	–.03	–.07	–.12	–.16	–.20
	1.0	–0.3	0.09	0.13	0.13	0.11	0.08	0.06	0.03	–.01	–.03

5-6 Tee, Converging, Rectangular (Idelchik 1986, Diagram 7-11)

$r/w_b = 1$

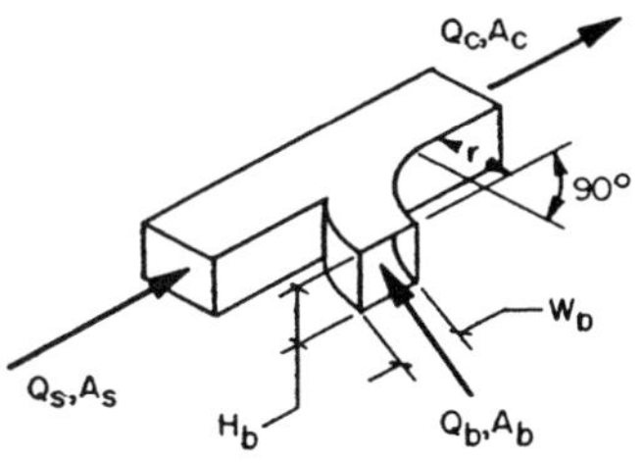

Branch, $C_{c,b}$

A_b/A_s	A_b/A_c	Q_b/Q_c 0.1	0.2	0.3	0.4	0.5	0.6	0.7	0.8	0.9
0.33	0.25	–1.2	–.40	0.40	1.6	3.0	4.8	6.8	8.9	11
0.5	0.5	–.50	–.20	0	0.25	0.45	0.70	1.0	1.5	2.0
0.67	0.5	–1.0	–.60	–.20	0.10	0.30	0.60	1.0	1.5	2.0
1.0	0.5	–2.2	–1.5	–.95	–.50	0	0.40	0.80	1.3	1.9
1.0	1.0	–.60	–.30	–.10	–.04	0.13	0.21	0.29	0.36	0.42
1.33	1.0	–1.2	–.80	–.40	–.20	0	0.16	0.24	0.32	0.38
2.0	1.0	–2.1	–1.4	–.90	–.50	–.20	0	0.20	0.25	0.30

Main, $C_{c,s}$

A_b/A_s	A_b/A_c	Q_b/Q_c 0.1	0.2	0.3	0.4	0.5	0.6	0.7	0.8	0.9
0.33	0.25	0.30	0.30	0.20	–.10	–.45	–.92	–1.5	–2.0	–2.6
0.5	0.5	0.17	0.16	0.10	0	–0.08	–.18	–.27	–.37	–.46
0.67	0.5	0.27	0.35	0.32	0.25	0.12	–.03	–.23	–.42	–.58
1.0	0.5	1.2	1.1	0.90	0.65	0.35	0	–.40	–.80	–1.3
1.0	1.0	0.18	0.24	0.27	0.26	0.23	0.18	0.10	0	–.12
1.33	1.0	0.75	0.36	0.38	0.35	0.27	0.18	0.05	–.08	–.22
2.0	1.0	0.80	0.87	0.80	0.68	0.55	0.40	0.25	0.08	–.10

5-7 Tee, Converging, Round Tap to Rectangular Main (SMACNA 1981, Table 6-9C)

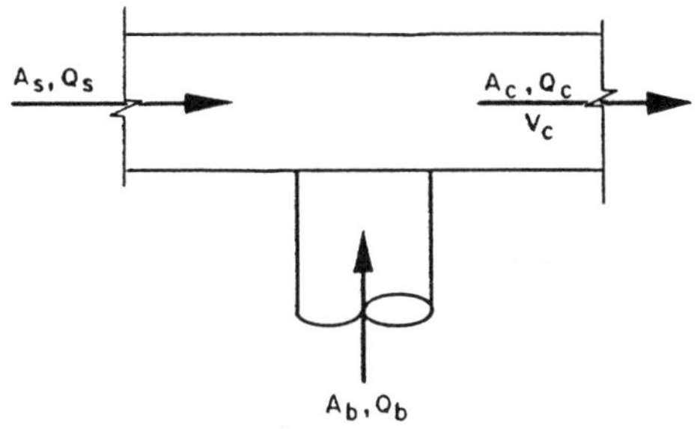

A_b/A_s	A_s/A_c	A_b/A_c
0.5	1.0	0.5

Branch, $C_{c,b}$

V_c (fpm)	Q_b/Q_c 0.1	0.2	0.3	0.4	0.5	0.6	0.7	0.8	0.9	1.0
<1200	–.63	–.55	0.13	0.23	0.78	1.30	1.93	3.10	4.88	5.60
>1200	–.49	–.21	0.23	0.60	1.27	2.06	2.75	3.70	4.93	5.95

For main coefficient ($C_{c,s}$), see Fitting 5-3.

5-8 Tee, Converging, Rectangular Main and Tap (SMACNA 1981, Table 6-9D)

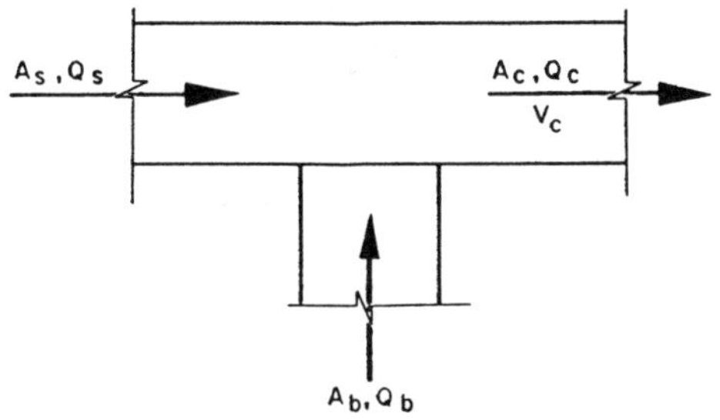

A_b/A_s	A_s/A_c	A_b/A_c
0.5	1.0	0.5

Branch, $C_{c,b}$

V_c (fpm)	Q_b/Q_c 0.1	0.2	0.3	0.4	0.5	0.6	0.7	0.8	0.9	1.0
<1200	–.75	–.53	–.03	0.33	1.03	1.10	2.15	2.93	4.18	4.78
>1200	–.69	–.21	0.23	0.67	1.17	1.66	2.67	3.36	3.93	5.13

For main coefficient ($C_{c,s}$), see Fitting 5-3.

5-9 Converging, Rectangular Main and Tap (45° Entry) (SMACNA 1981, Table 6-9F)

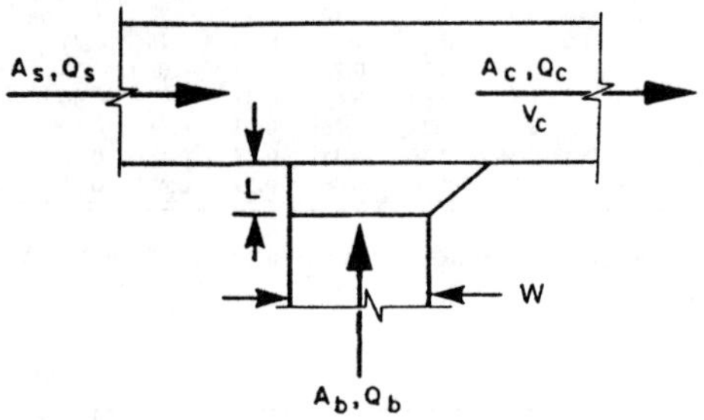

$L = 0.25\ W$, 3 in. min.

A_b/A_s	A_s/A_c	A_b/A_c
0.5	1.0	0.5

V_c	Branch, $C_{c,b}$									
	Q_b/Q_c									
(fpm)	0.1	0.2	0.3	0.4	0.5	0.6	0.7	0.8	0.9	1.0
<1200	−.83	−.68	−.30	0.28	0.55	1.03	1.50	1.93	2.50	3.03
>1200	−.72	−.52	−.23	0.34	0.76	1.14	1.83	2.01	2.90	3.63

For main coefficient ($C_{c,s}$), see Fitting 5-3.

5-10 Tee, Diverging, Round, Conical Branch (Jones 1969, Fig. 12)

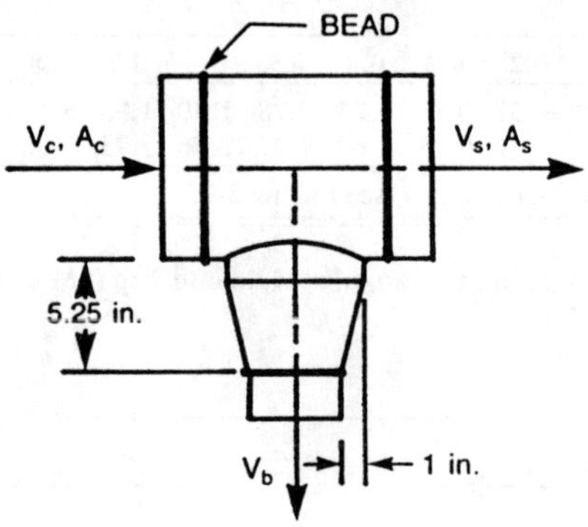

$A_c = A_s$

Branch											
V_b/V_c	0	0.2	0.4	0.6	0.8	1.0	1.2	1.4	1.6	1.8	2.0
$C_{c,b}$	1.0	0.85	0.74	0.62	0.52	0.42	0.36	0.32	0.32	0.37	0.52

For main loss coefficient ($C_{c,s}$), see Fitting 5-23.

5-11 Wye, 45°, Diverging, Round, Conical Branch (Jones 1969, Fig. 14)

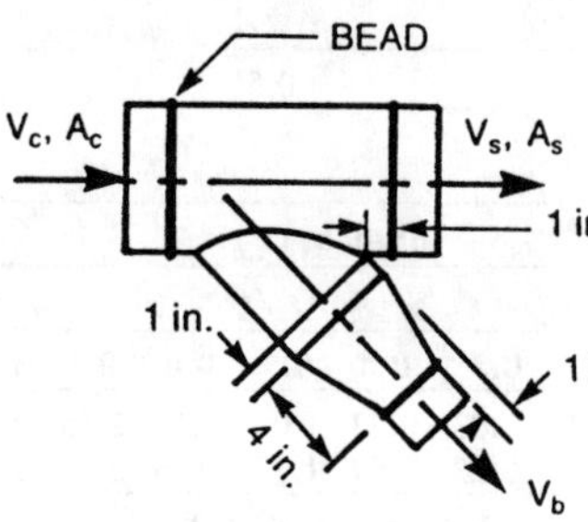

$A_c = A_s$

Branch											
V_b/V_c	0	0.2	0.4	0.6	0.8	1.0	1.2	1.4	1.6	1.8	2.0
$C_{c,b}$	1.0	0.84	0.61	0.41	0.27	0.17	0.12	0.12	0.14	0.18	0.27

For main loss coefficient ($C_{c,s}$), see Fitting 5-23.

5-12 Tee, Diverging, Round, with 90° Elbow, Branch 90° to Main (Jones 1969, Fig. 17)

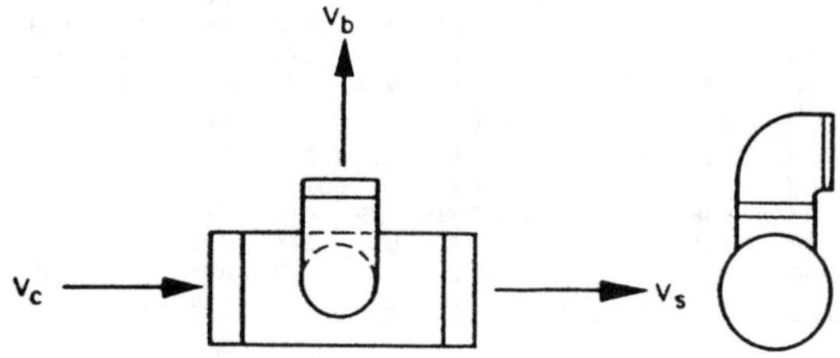

$A_c = A_s$

Branch											
V_b/V_c	0	0.2	0.4	0.6	0.8	1.0	1.2	1.4	1.6	1.8	2.0
$C_{c,b}$	1.0	1.03	1.08	1.18	1.33	1.56	1.86	2.2	2.6	3.0	3.4

For main loss coefficient ($C_{c,s}$), see Fitting 5-23.

5-13 Tee, Diverging, Round, with 45° Elbow, Branch 90° to Main (Jones 1969, Fig. 18)

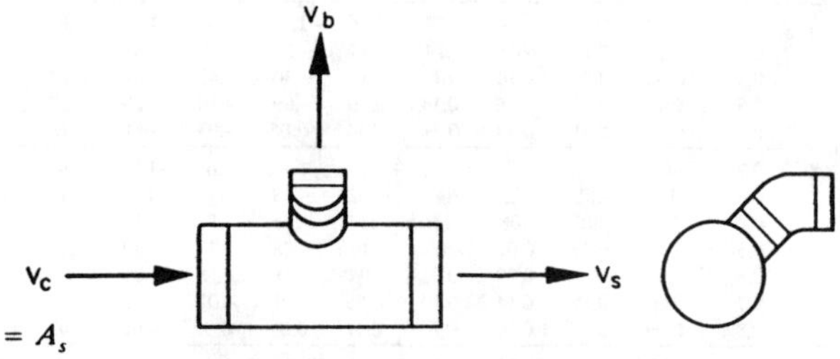

$A_c = A_s$

Branch											
V_b/V_c	0	0.2	0.4	0.6	0.8	1.0	1.2	1.4	1.6	1.8	2.0
$C_{c,b}$	1.0	1.32	1.51	1.60	1.65	1.74	1.87	2.0	2.2	2.5	2.7

For main loss coefficient ($C_{c,s}$), see Fitting 5-23.

5-14 Tee, Diverging, Round (Conical Branch), with 45° Elbow, Branch 90° to Main (Jones 1969, Fig. 19)

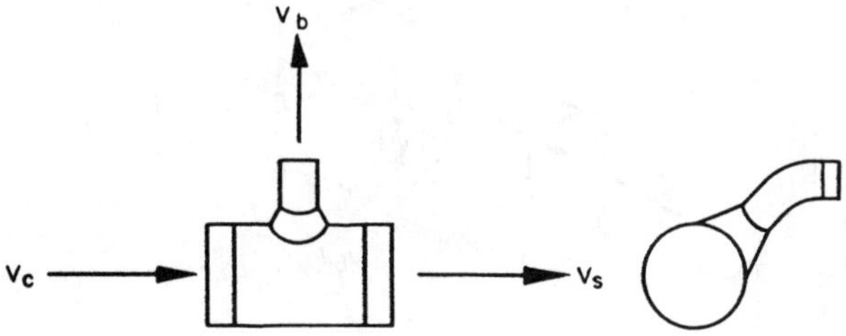

For tee geometry, see Fitting 5-10.

$A_c = A_s$

Branch											
V_b/V_c	0	0.2	0.4	0.6	0.8	1.0	1.2	1.4	1.6	1.8	2.0
$C_{c,b}$	1.0	0.94	0.88	0.84	0.80	0.82	0.84	0.87	0.90	0.95	1.02

For main loss coefficient ($C_{c,s}$), see Fitting 5-23.

5-15 Wye, 45°, Round, with 60° Elbow, Branch 90° to Main (Jones 1969, Fig. 3)

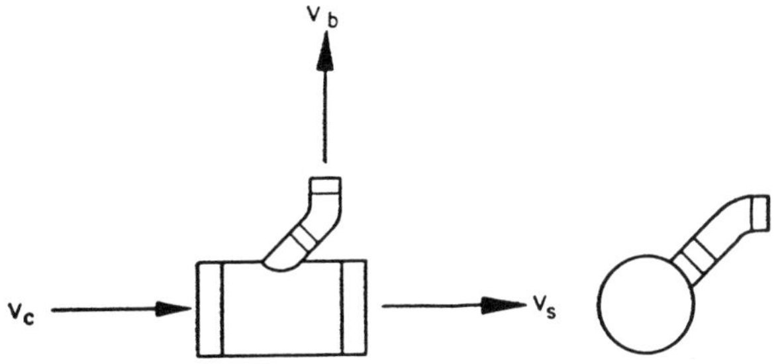

$A_c = A_s$

Branch											
V_b/V_c	0	0.2	0.4	0.6	0.8	1.0	1.2	1.4	1.6	1.8	2.0
$C_{c,b}$	1.0	0.88	0.77	0.68	0.65	0.69	0.73	0.88	1.14	1.54	2.2

For main loss coefficient ($C_{c,s}$), see Fitting 5-23.

5-16 Wye, 45°, Diverging, Round (Conical Branch), with 60° Elbow, Branch 90° to Main (Jones 1969, Fig. 20)

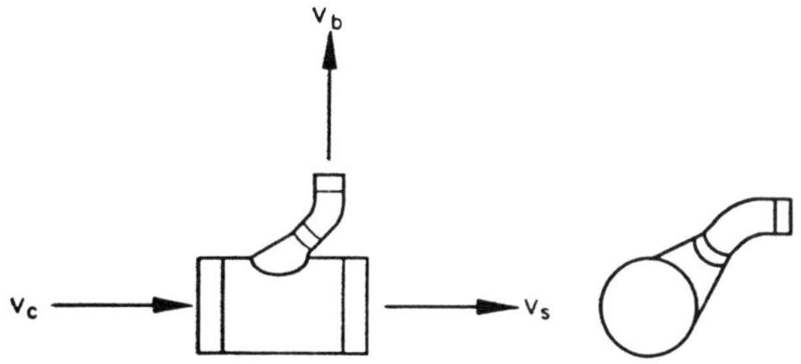

For wye geometry, see Fitting 5-11.

$A_c = A_s$

Branch											
V_b/V_c	0	0.2	0.4	0.6	0.8	1.0	1.2	1.4	1.6	1.8	2.0
$C_{c,b}$	1.0	0.82	0.63	0.52	0.45	0.42	0.41	0.40	0.41	0.45	0.56

For main loss coefficient ($C_{c,s}$), see Fitting 5-23.

5-17 Wye, 48°, Diverging, Conical Main and Branch, with 45° Elbow, Branch 90° to Main (Idelchik 1986, Diagram 7-19)

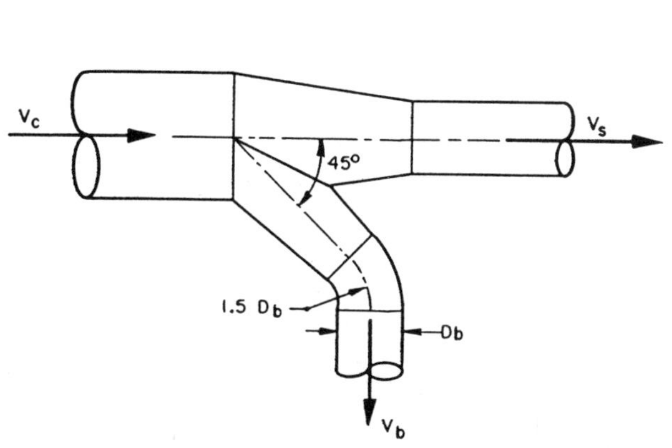

Branch									
V_b/V_c	0.2	0.4	0.6	0.7	0.8	0.9	1.0	1.1	1.2
$C_{c,b}$	0.76	0.60	0.52	0.50	0.51	0.52	0.56	0.61	0.68
V_b/V_c	1.4	1.6	1.8	2.0	2.2	2.4	2.6	2.8	3.0
$C_{c,b}$	0.86	1.1	1.4	1.8	2.2	2.6	3.1	3.7	4.2

Main										
V_s/V_c	0.2	0.4	0.6	0.8	1.0	1.2	1.4	1.6	1.8	2.0
$C_{c,s}$	0.14	0.06	0.05	0.09	0.18	0.30	0.46	0.64	0.84	1.0

5-18 Tee, Diverging, Round, with 60° Elbow, Branch 45° to Main (Jones 1969, Fig. 22)

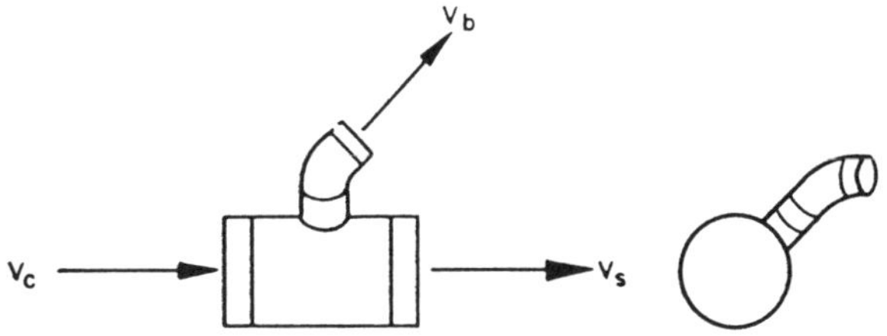

$A_c = A_s$

Branch											
V_b/V_c	0	0.2	0.4	0.6	0.8	1.0	1.2	1.4	1.6	1.8	2.0
$C_{c,b}$	1.0	1.06	1.15	1.29	1.45	1.65	1.89	2.2	2.5	2.9	3.3

For main loss coefficient ($C_{c,s}$), see Fitting 5-23.

5-19 Tee, Diverging, Round (Conical Branch), with 60° Elbow, Branch 45° to Main (Jones 1969, Fig. 23)

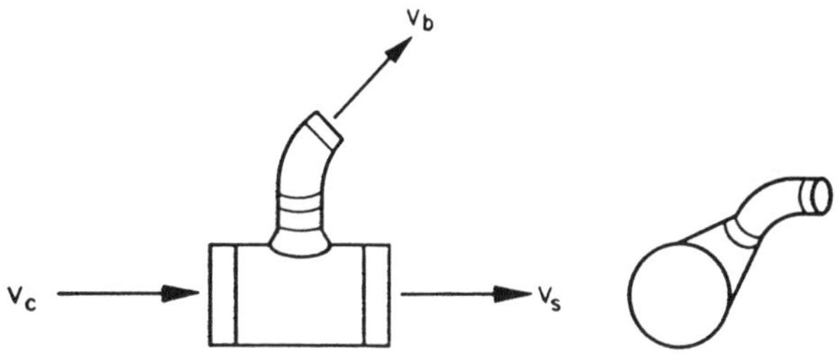

For tee geometry, see Fitting 5-10.

$A_c = A_s$

Branch											
V_b/V_c	0	0.2	0.4	0.6	0.8	1.0	1.2	1.4	1.6	1.8	2.0
$C_{c,b}$	1.0	0.95	0.90	0.86	0.81	0.79	0.79	0.81	0.86	0.96	1.10

For main loss coefficient ($C_{c,s}$), see Fitting 5-23.

5-20 Wye, 45°, Diverging, Round, with 30° Elbow, Branch 45° to Main (Jones 1969, Fig. 2)

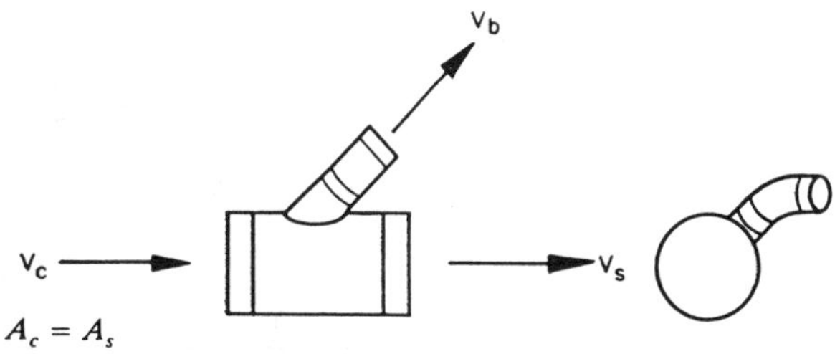

$A_c = A_s$

Branch											
V_b/V_c	0	0.2	0.4	0.6	0.8	1.0	1.2	1.4	1.6	1.8	2.0
$C_{c,b}$	1.0	0.84	0.72	0.62	0.54	0.50	0.56	0.71	0.92	1.22	1.66

For main loss coefficient ($C_{c,s}$), see Fitting 5-23.

5-21 Wye, 45°, Diverging, Round (Conical Branch), with 30° Elbow, Branch 45° to Main (Jones 1969, Fig. 24)

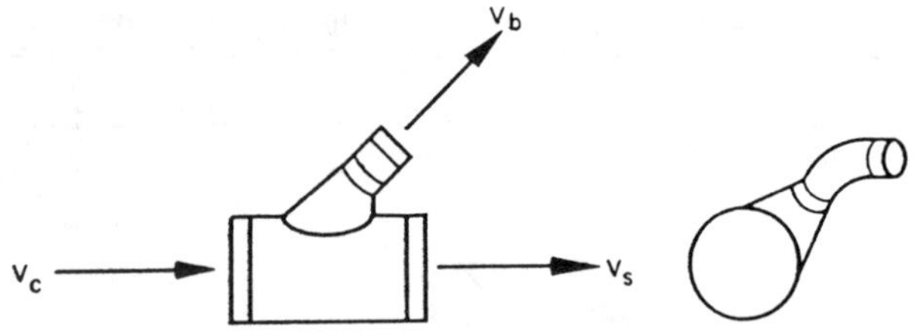

For wye geometry, see Fitting 5-11.

$A_c = A_s$

Branch											
V_b/V_c	0	0.2	0.4	0.6	0.8	1.0	1.2	1.4	1.6	1.8	2.0
$C_{c,b}$	1.0	0.93	0.71	0.55	0.44	0.42	0.42	0.44	0.47	0.54	0.62

For main loss coefficient ($C_{c,s}$), see Fitting 5-23.

5-22 Tee, Diverging, Rectangular (Idelchik 1986, Diagram 7-21)

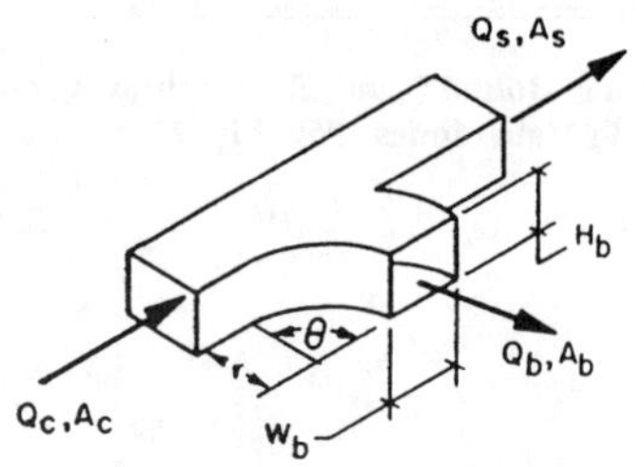

$\theta = 90°$

$r/W_b = 1.0$

Branch $C_{c,b}$

A_b/A_s	A_b/A_c	Q_b/Q_c 0.1	0.2	0.3	0.4	0.5	0.6	0.7	0.8	0.9
0.25	0.25	0.55	0.50	0.60	0.85	1.2	1.8	3.1	4.4	6.0
0.33	0.25	0.35	0.35	0.50	0.80	1.3	2.0	2.8	3.8	5.0
0.5	0.5	0.62	0.48	0.40	0.40	0.48	0.60	0.78	1.1	1.5
0.67	0.5	0.52	0.40	0.32	0.30	0.34	0.44	0.62	0.92	1.4
1.0	0.5	0.44	0.38	0.38	0.41	0.52	0.68	0.92	1.2	1.6
1.0	1.0	0.67	0.55	0.46	0.37	0.32	0.29	0.29	0.30	0.37
1.33	1.0	0.70	0.60	0.51	0.42	0.34	0.28	0.26	0.26	0.29
2.0	1.0	0.60	0.52	0.43	0.33	0.24	0.17	0.15	0.17	0.21

Main, $C_{c,s}$

A_b/A_s	A_b/A_c	Q_b/Q_c 0.1	0.2	0.3	0.4	0.5	0.6	0.7	0.8	0.9
0.25	0.25	−.01	−.03	−.01	0.05	0.13	0.21	0.29	0.38	0.46
0.33	0.25	0.08	0	−.02	−.01	0.02	0.08	0.16	0.24	0.34
0.5	0.5	−.03	−.06	−.05	0	0.06	0.12	0.19	0.27	0.35
0.67	0.5	0.04	−.02	−.04	−.03	−.01	0.04	0.12	0.23	0.37
1.0	0.5	0.72	0.48	0.28	0.13	0.05	0.04	0.09	0.18	0.30
1.0	1.0	−.02	−.04	−.04	−.01	0.06	0.13	0.22	0.30	0.38
1.33	1.0	0.10	0	0.01	−.03	−.01	0.03	0.10	0.20	0.30
2.0	1.0	0.62	0.38	0.23	0.23	0.08	0.05	0.06	0.10	0.20

5-23 Wye, Diverging, Rectangular and Round (Idelchik 1986, Diagrams 7-15 and 7-17)

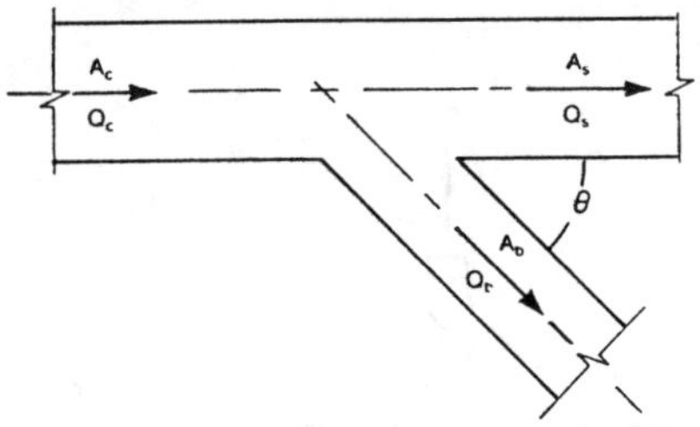

$A_c = A_s$; $H_b = H_c$, where H is height of rectangular duct

$\theta = 30°$

Branch, $C_{c,b}$

A_b/A_c	Q_b/Q_c 0.1	0.2	0.3	0.4	0.5	0.6	0.7	0.8	0.9
0.8	0.75	0.55	0.40	0.28	0.21	0.16	0.15	0.16	0.19
0.7	0.72	0.51	0.36	0.25	0.18	0.15	0.16	0.20	0.26
0.6	0.69	0.46	0.31	0.21	0.17	0.16	0.20	0.28	0.39
0.5	0.65	0.41	0.26	0.19	0.18	0.22	0.32	0.47	0.67
0.4	0.59	0.33	0.21	0.20	0.27	0.40	0.62	0.92	1.3
0.3	0.55	0.28	0.24	0.38	0.76	1.3	2.0	3.0	4.1
0.2	0.40	0.26	0.58	1.3	2.5	4.1	6.1	8.6	11.0
0.1	0.28	1.5	4.3	8.3	15.0	—	—	—	—

$\theta = 45°$

Branch, $C_{c,b}$

A_b/A_c	Q_b/Q_c 0.1	0.2	0.3	0.4	0.5	0.6	0.7	0.8	0.9
0.8	0.78	0.62	0.49	0.40	0.34	0.31	0.32	0.35	0.40
0.7	0.77	0.59	0.47	0.38	0.34	0.32	0.35	0.41	0.50
0.6	0.74	0.56	0.44	0.37	0.35	0.36	0.43	0.54	0.68
0.5	0.71	0.52	0.41	0.38	0.40	0.45	0.59	0.78	1.0
0.4	0.66	0.47	0.40	0.43	0.54	0.69	0.95	1.3	1.7
0.3	0.66	0.48	0.52	0.73	1.2	1.8	2.7	3.7	4.9
0.2	0.56	0.56	1.0	1.8	3.2	4.9	7.1	9.6	13.0
0.1	0.60	2.1	5.1	9.3	16.0	—	—	—	—

$\theta = 60°$

Branch, $C_{c,b}$

A_b/A_c	Q_b/Q_c 0.1	0.2	0.3	0.4	0.5	0.6	0.7	0.8	0.9
0.8	0.83	0.71	0.62	0.56	0.52	0.50	0.53	0.60	0.68
0.7	0.82	0.69	0.61	0.56	0.54	0.54	0.60	0.70	0.82
0.6	0.81	0.68	0.60	0.58	0.58	0.61	0.72	0.87	1.1
0.5	0.79	0.66	0.61	0.62	0.68	0.76	0.94	1.2	1.5
0.4	0.76	0.65	0.65	0.74	0.89	1.1	1.4	1.8	2.3
0.3	0.80	0.75	0.89	1.2	1.8	2.6	3.5	4.6	6.0
0.2	0.77	0.96	1.6	2.5	4.0	6.0	8.3	11.0	—
0.1	1.0	2.9	6.2	10.0	—	—	—	—	—

$\theta = 90°$

Branch, $C_{c,b}$

A_b/A_c	Q_b/Q_c 0.1	0.2	0.3	0.4	0.5	0.6	0.7	0.8	0.9
0.8	0.95	0.92	0.92	0.93	0.94	0.95	1.1	1.2	1.4
0.7	0.95	0.94	0.95	0.98	1.0	1.1	1.2	1.4	1.6
0.6	0.96	0.97	1.0	1.1	1.1	1.2	1.4	1.7	2.0
0.5	0.97	1.0	1.1	1.2	1.4	1.5	1.8	2.1	2.5
0.4	0.99	1.1	1.3	1.5	1.7	2.0	2.4	3.0	3.6
0.3	1.1	1.4	1.8	2.3	3.2	4.3	5.5	6.9	8.5
0.2	1.3	1.9	2.9	4.1	6.2	8.5	11.0	—	—
0.1	2.1	4.8	8.9	14.0	—	—	—	—	—

Main									
V_s/V_c	0	0.1	0.2	0.3	0.4	0.5	0.6	0.8	1.0
$C_{c,s}$	0.40	0.32	0.26	0.20	0.14	0.10	0.06	0.02	0

5-24 Diverging Wye, Rectangular (Idelchik 1986, Diagrams 7-16 and 7-17)

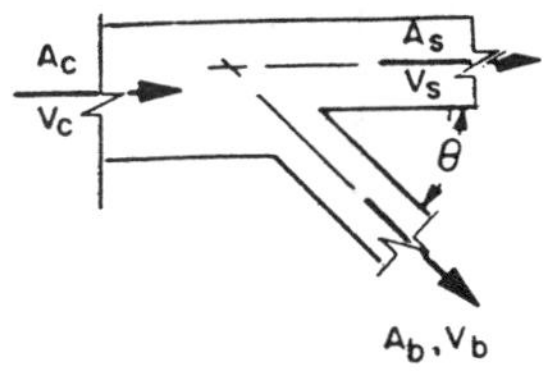

$\theta = 15°$ to $90°$ and $A_c = A_s + A_b$

Branch, $C_{c,b}$													
θ,	V_b/V_c												
deg	**0.1**	**0.2**	**0.3**	**0.4**	**0.5**	**0.6**	**0.8**	**1.0**	**1.2**	**1.4**	**1.6**	**1.8**	**2.0**
15	0.81	0.65	0.51	0.38	0.28	0.20	0.11	0.06	0.14	0.30	0.51	0.76	1.0
30	0.84	0.69	0.56	0.44	0.34	0.26	0.19	0.15	0.15	0.30	0.51	0.76	1.0
45	0.87	0.74	0.63	0.54	0.45	0.38	0.29	0.24	0.23	0.30	0.51	0.76	1.0
60	0.90	0.82	0.79	0.66	0.59	0.53	0.43	0.36	0.33	0.39	0.51	0.76	1.0
90	1.0	1.0	1.0	1.0	1.0	1.0	1.0	1.0	1.0	1.0	1.0	1.0	1.0

Main, $C_{c,s}$						
θ, deg	**15–60**	**90**				
$\frac{V_s}{V_c}$		A_s/A_c				
	0–1.0	**0–0.4**	**0.5**	**0.6**	**0.7**	**≥0.8**
0	1.0	1.0	1.0	1.0	1.0	1.0
0.1	0.81	0.81	0.81	0.81	0.81	0.81
0.2	0.64	0.64	0.64	0.64	0.64	0.64
0.3	0.50	0.50	0.52	0.52	0.50	0.50
0.4	0.36	0.36	0.40	0.38	0.37	0.36
0.5	0.25	0.25	0.30	0.28	0.27	0.25
0.6	0.16	0.16	0.23	0.20	0.18	0.16
0.8	0.04	0.04	0.17	0.10	0.07	0.04
1.0	0	0	0.20	0.10	0.05	0
1.2	0.07	0.07	0.36	0.21	0.14	0.07
1.4	0.39	0.39	0.79	0.59	0.39	—
1.6	0.90	0.90	1.4	1.2	—	—
1.8	1.8	1.8	2.4	—	—	—
2.0	3.2	3.2	4.0	—	—	—

5-25 Tee, Diverging, Rectangular Main to Round Tap (SMACNA 1981, Table 6-10T)

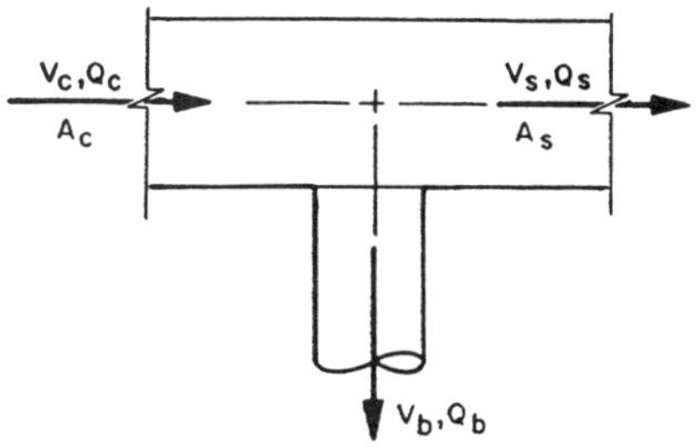

$A_c = A_s$

Branch, $C_{c,b}$									
	Q_b/Q_c								
V_b/V_c	**0.1**	**0.2**	**0.3**	**0.4**	**0.5**	**0.6**	**0.7**	**0.8**	**0.9**
0.2	1.00								
0.4	1.01	1.07							
0.6	1.14	1.10	1.08						
0.8	1.18	1.31	1.12	1.13					
1.0	1.30	1.38	1.20	1.23	1.26				
1.2	1.46	1.58	1.45	1.31	1.39	1.48			
1.4	1.70	1.82	1.65	1.51	1.56	1.64	1.71		
1.6	1.93	2.06	2.00	1.85	1.70	1.76	1.80	1.88	
1.8	2.06	2.17	2.10	2.13	2.06	1.98	1.99	2.00	2.07

For main coefficient ($C_{c,s}$), see Fitting 5-23.

5-26 Tee, Diverging, Rectangular Main to Round Tap (Conical) (Inoue 1980, Korst 1950)

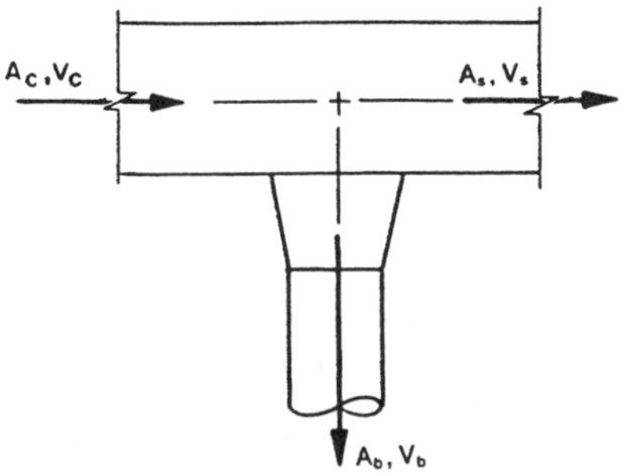

$A_c = A_s$

Branch						
V_b/V_c	0.40	0.50	0.75	1.0	1.3	1.5
$C_{c,b}$	0.80	0.83	0.90	1.0	1.1	1.4

For main coefficient ($C_{c,s}$), see Fitting 5-23.

5-27 Tee, Diverging, Rectangular Main, and Tap (45° Entry) (SMACNA 1981, Table 6-10N)

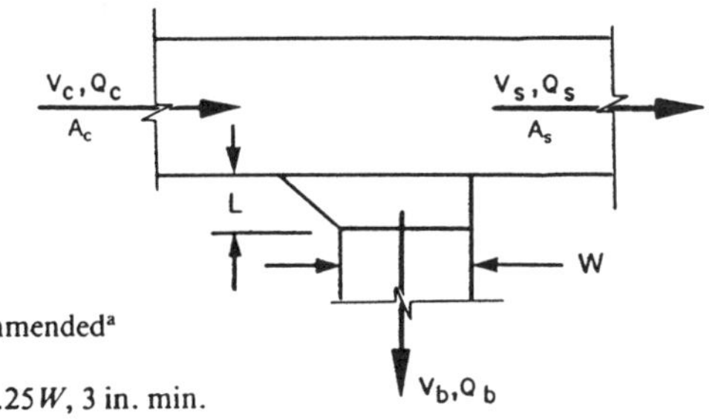

Recommended[a]

$L = 0.25W$, 3 in. min.

$A_c = A_s$

Branch, $C_{c,b}$									
	Q_b/Q_c								
V_b/V_c	**0.1**	**0.2**	**0.3**	**0.4**	**0.5**	**0.6**	**0.7**	**0.8**	**0.9**
0.2	0.91								
0.4	0.81	0.79							
0.6	0.77	0.72	0.70						
0.8	0.78	0.73	0.69	0.66					
1.0	0.78	0.98	0.85	0.79	0.74				
1.2	0.90	1.11	1.16	1.23	1.03	0.86			
1.4	1.19	1.22	1.26	1.29	1.54	0.25	0.92		
1.6	1.35	1.42	1.55	1.59	1.63	1.50	1.31	1.09	
1.8	1.44	1.50	1.75	1.74	1.72	2.24	1.63	1.40	1.17

For main coefficient ($C_{c,s}$), see Fitting 5-23.

[a] For performance study, see SMACNA (1987).

5-28 Tee, Diverging, Rectangular Main, and Tap[a] (SMACNA 1981, Table 10Q)

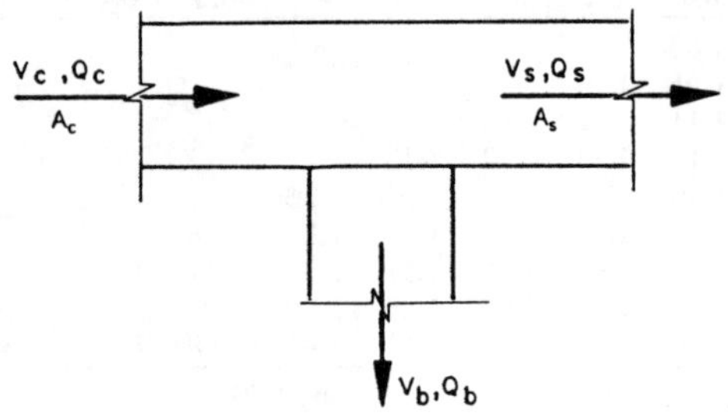

$A_c = A_s$

	Branch, $C_{c,b}$								
	Q_b/Q_c								
V_b/V_c	0.1	0.2	0.3	0.4	0.5	0.6	0.7	0.8	0.9
0.2	1.03								
0.4	1.04	1.01							
0.6	1.11	1.03	1.05						
0.8	1.16	1.21	1.17	1.12					
1.0	1.38	1.40	1.30	1.36	1.27				
1.2	1.52	1.61	1.68	1.91	1.47	1.66			
1.4	1.79	2.01	1.90	2.31	2.28	2.20	1.95		
1.6	2.07	2.28	2.13	2.71	2.99	2.81	2.09	2.20	
1.8	2.32	2.54	2.64	3.09	3.72	2.48	2.21	2.29	2.57

For main coefficient ($C_{c,s}$), see Fitting 5-23.

[a] For performance study, see SMACNA (1987).

5-29 Tee, Diverging, Rectangular Main and Tap (45° Entry), with Damper (SMACNA 1981, Table 6-10P)

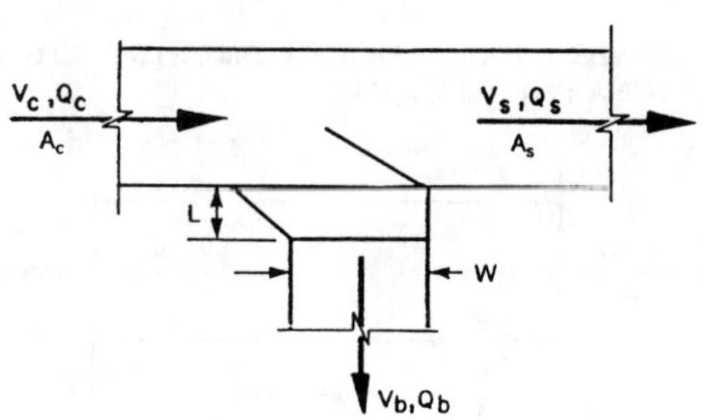

Poor; should not be used.[a]

$L = 0.25W$, 3 in. min.

$A_c = A_s$

	Branch, $C_{c,b}$								
	Q_b/Q_c								
V_b/V_c	0.1	0.2	0.3	0.4	0.5	0.6	0.7	0.8	0.9
0.2	0.61								
0.4	0.46	0.61							
0.6	0.43	0.50	0.54						
0.8	0.39	0.43	0.62	0.53					
1.0	0.34	0.57	0.77	0.73	0.68				
1.2	0.37	0.64	0.85	0.98	1.07	0.83			
1.4	0.57	0.71	1.04	1.16	1.54	1.36	1.18		
1.6	0.89	1.08	1.28	1.30	1.69	2.09	1.81	1.47	
1.8	1.33	1.34	2.04	1.78	1.90	2.40	2.77	2.23	1.92

For main coefficient ($C_{c,s}$), see Fitting 5-31.

[a] For performance study, see SMACNA (1987).

5-30 Tee, Diverging, Rectangular Main and Tap, with Damper (SMACNA 1981, Table 6-10R)

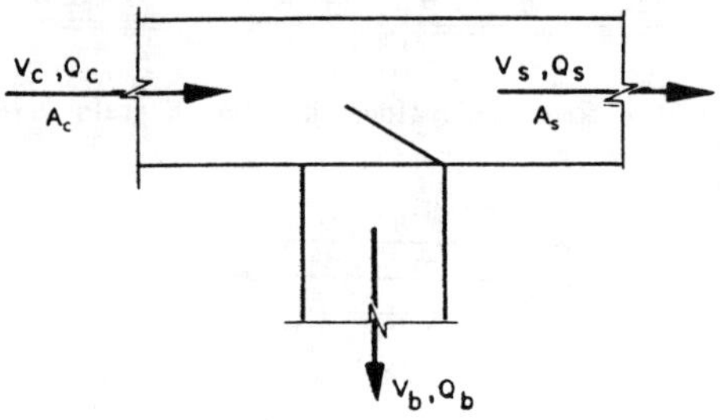

Poor; should not be used.[a]

$A_c = A_s$

	Branch, $C_{c,b}$								
	Q_b/Q_c								
V_b/V_c	0.1	0.2	0.3	0.4	0.5	0.6	0.7	0.8	0.9
0.2	0.58								
0.4	0.67	0.64							
0.6	0.78	0.76	0.75						
0.8	0.88	0.98	0.81	1.01					
1.0	1.12	1.05	1.08	1.18	1.29				
1.2	1.49	1.48	1.40	1.51	1.70	1.91			
1.4	2.10	2.21	2.25	2.29	2.32	2.48	2.53		
1.6	2.72	3.30	2.84	3.09	3.30	3.19	3.29	3.16	
1.8	3.42	4.58	3.65	3.92	4.20	4.15	4.14	4.10	4.05

For main coefficient ($C_{c,s}$), see Fitting 5-31.

[a] For performance study, see SMACNA (1987).

5-31 Tee, Diverging, Rectangular, with Extractor (SMACNA 1981, Table 6-10S)

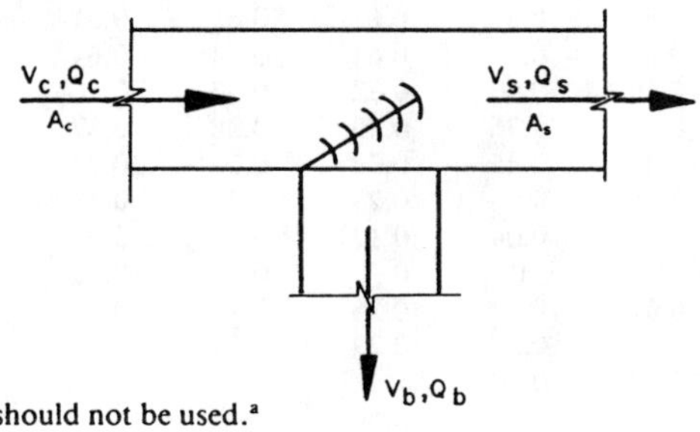

Poor; should not be used.[a]

$A_c = A_s$

	Branch, $C_{c,b}$								
	Q_b/Q_c								
V_b/V_c	0.1	0.2	0.3	0.4	0.5	0.6	0.7	0.8	0.9
0.2	0.60								
0.4	0.62	0.69							
0.6	0.74	0.80	0.82						
0.8	0.99	1.10	0.95	0.90					
1.0	1.48	1.12	1.41	1.24	1.21				
1.2	1.91	1.33	1.43	1.52	1.55	1.64			
1.4	2.47	1.67	1.70	2.04	1.86	1.98	2.47		
1.6	3.17	2.40	2.33	2.53	2.31	2.51	3.13	3.25	
1.8	3.85	3.37	2.89	3.23	3.09	3.03	3.30	3.74	4.11

Main									
V_b/V_c	0.2	0.4	0.6	0.8	1.0	1.2	1.4	1.6	1.8
$C_{c,s}$	0.03	0.04	0.07	0.12	0.13	0.14	0.27	0.30	0.25

[a] For performance study, see SMACNA (1987).

5-32 Symmetrical Wye, Dovetail, Rectangular (Idelchik 1986, Diagram 7-24)

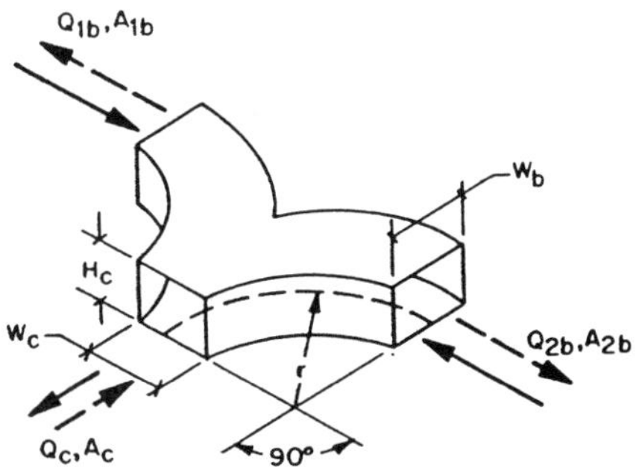

$r/W_c = 1.5$

$Q_{1b}/Q_c = Q_{2b}/Q_c = 0.5$

Converging

A_{1b}/A_c or A_{2b}/A_c	0.50	1.0
$C_{c,1b}$ or $C_{c,2b}$	0.23	0.07

Diverging

A_{1b}/A_c or A_{2b}/A_c	0.50	1.0
$C_{c,1b}$ or $C_{c,2b}$	0.30	0.25

5-33 Wye, Rectangular and Round (Idelchik 1986, Diagram 7-30)

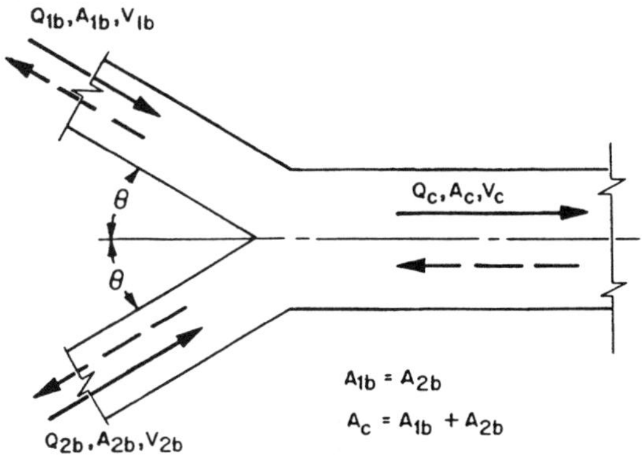

Converging — $C_{c,1b}$ or $C_{c,2b}$

θ, deg	Q_{1b}/Q_c or Q_{2b}/Q_c: 0	0.1	0.2	0.3	0.4	0.5	0.6	0.7	0.8	0.9	1.0
15	−2.6	−1.9	−1.3	−.77	−.30	0.10	0.41	0.67	0.85	0.97	1.0
30	−2.1	−1.5	−1.0	−.53	−.10	0.28	0.69	0.91	1.1	1.4	1.6
45	−1.3	−.93	−.55	−.16	0.20	0.56	0.92	1.3	1.6	2.0	2.3

Diverging — $C_{c,1b}$ or $C_{c,2b}$

θ, deg	V_{1b}/V_c or V_{2b}/V_c: 0.1	0.2	0.3	0.4	0.5	0.6	0.8	1.0	1.2	1.4	1.6	1.8	2.0
15	0.81	0.65	0.51	0.38	0.28	0.20	0.11	0.06	0.14	0.30	0.51	0.76	1.0
30	0.84	0.69	0.56	0.44	0.34	0.26	0.19	0.15	0.15	0.30	0.51	0.76	1.0
45	0.87	0.74	0.63	0.54	0.45	0.38	0.29	0.24	0.23	0.30	0.51	0.76	1.0
60	0.90	0.82	0.79	0.66	0.59	0.53	0.43	0.36	0.33	0.39	0.51	0.76	1.0
90	1.0	1.0	1.0	1.0	1.0	1.0	1.0	1.0	1.0	1.0	1.0	1.0	1.0

5-34 Wye (Double), 45°, Rectangular and Round (Idelchik 1986, Diagram 7-27)

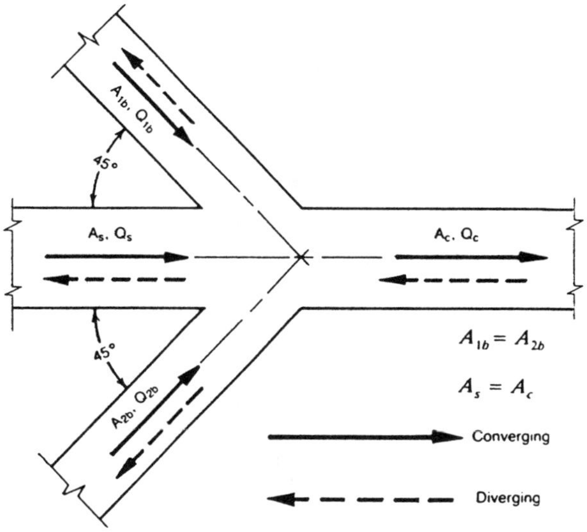

Converging Flow

Branch, $C_{c,b}$

Q_{2b}/Q_{1b}	Q_{1b}/Q_c: 0	0.1	0.2	0.3	0.4	0.5	0.6
			$A_{1b}/A_c = 0.2$				
0.5	−1.0	−.36	0.59	1.8	3.2	4.9	6.8
1.0	−1.0	−.24	0.63	1.7	2.6	3.7	—
2.0	−1.0	−.19	0.21	0.04	—	—	—
			$A_{1b}/A_c = 0.4$				
0.5	−1.0	−.48	−.02	0.58	0.92	1.3	16
1.0	−1.0	−.36	0.17	0.55	0.72	0.78	—
2.0	−1.0	−.18	0.16	−.06	—	—	—
			$A_{1b}/A_c = 0.6$				
0.5	−1.0	−.50	−.07	0.31	0.60	0.82	0.92
1.0	−1.0	−.37	0.12	0.55	0.60	0.52	—
2.0	−1.0	−.18	0.26	0.16	—	—	—
			$A_{1b}/A_c = 1.0$				
0.5	−1.0	−.51	−.09	0.25	0.50	0.65	0.64
1.0	−1.0	−.37	0.13	0.46	0.61	0.54	—
2.0	−1.0	−.15	0.38	0.42	—	—	—

Main, $C_{c,s}$

Q_{2b}/Q_{1b}	Q_s/Q_c: 0	0.1	0.2	0.3	0.4	0.5	0.6	0.7	0.8	0.9	1.0
					$A_{1b}/A_c = 0.2$						
0.5 & 2.0	−2.9	−1.9	−1.3	−.80	−.56	−.23	−.01	0.16	0.22	0.15	0
1.0	−2.5	−1.9	−1.3	−.80	−.42	−.12	0.08	0.20	0.22	0.15	0
					$A_{1b}/A_c = 0.4$						
0.5 & 2.0	−.98	−.61	−.30	−.05	0.14	0.26	0.33	0.34	0.28	0.17	0
1.0	−.77	−.44	−.16	0.05	0.21	0.31	0.36	0.35	0.29	0.17	0
					$A_{1b}/A_c = 0.6$						
0.5 & 2.0	−.32	0.08	0.11	0.27	0.37	0.43	0.44	0.40	0.31	0.18	0
1.0	−.18	−.04	0.21	0.34	0.42	0.46	0.46	0.41	0.31	0.18	0
					$A_{1b}/A_c = 1.0$						
0.5 & 2.0	0.11	0.36	0.46	0.53	0.57	0.56	0.52	0.44	0.33	0.18	0
1.0	0.29	0.42	0.51	0.57	0.58	0.58	0.54	0.45	0.33	0.18	0

Diverging Flow: Use Fitting 5-23.

5-35 Cross, 90°, Rectangular and Round (Idelchik 1986, Diagram 7-29)

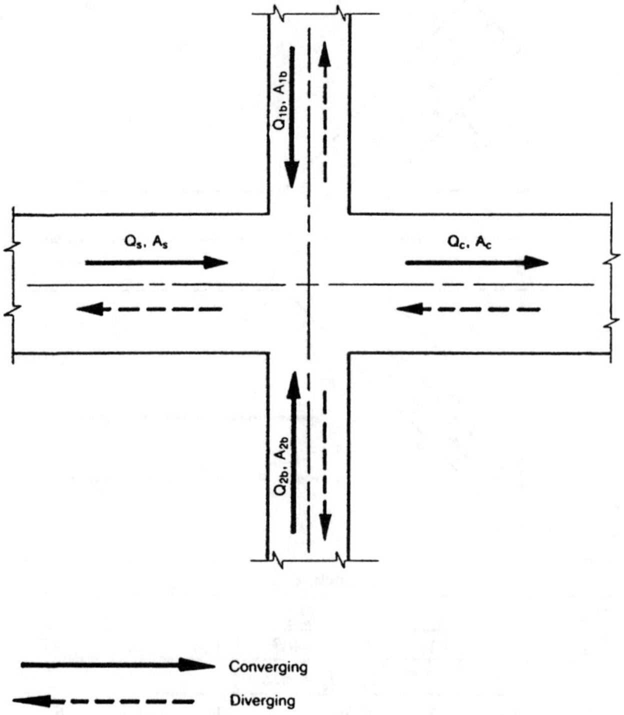

$A_{1b} = A_{2b}$

$A_s = A_c$

Converging Flow

Q_{2b}/Q_{1b}	Branch, $C_{c,b}$: Q_{1b}/Q_c or Q_{2b}/Q_c = 0	0.1	0.2	0.3	0.4	0.5	0.6
	$A_{1b}/A_c = 0.2$						
0.5	−.85	−.10	1.1	2.7	4.8	7.3	10
1.0	−.85	−.05	1.4	3.1	5.1	7.4	—
2.0	−.85	−.31	1.8	3.4	—	—	—
	$A_{1b}/A_c = 0.4$						
0.5	−.85	−.29	0.34	1.0	1.8	2.6	3.4
1.0	−.85	−.14	0.60	1.3	2.1	2.7	—
2.0	−.85	0.12	1.0	1.7	—	—	—
	$A_{1b}/A_c = 0.6$						
0.5	−.85	−.32	0.20	0.72	1.2	1.7	2.1
1.0	−.85	−.18	0.46	1.0	1.5	1.9	—
2.0	−.85	0.09	0.88	1.4	—	—	—
	$A_{1b}/A_c = 0.8$						
0.5	−.85	−.33	0.13	0.61	1.0	1.4	1.7
1.0	−.85	−.18	0.41	0.91	1.3	1.5	—
2.0	−.85	0.08	0.83	1.3	—	—	—
	$A_{1b}/A_c = 1.0$						
0.5	−.85	−.34	0.13	0.56	0.93	1.3	1.5
1.0	−.85	−.19	0.39	0.86	1.2	1.4	—
2.0	−.85	0.07	0.81	1.2	—	—	—

Main

Q_s/Q_c	0	0.1	0.2	0.3	0.4	0.5
$C_{c,s}$	1.2	1.2	1.2	1.1	1.1	0.96
Q_s/Q_c	0.6	0.7	0.8	0.9	1.0	
$C_{c,s}$	0.85	0.72	0.56	0.39	0.20	

Diverging Flow: Use Fitting 5-23.

OBSTRUCTIONS

6-1 Damper, Butterfly, Round (Idelchik 1986, Diagram 9-16; Zolotov 1967)

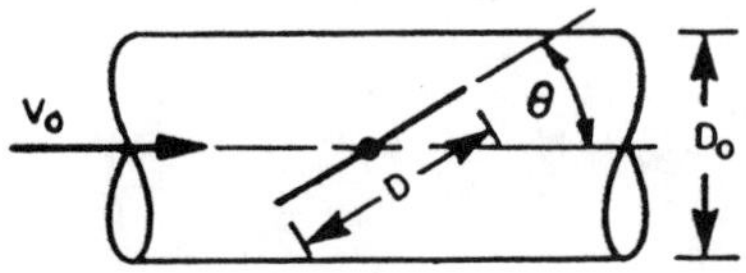

D/D_o	C_o, θ, degrees: 0	10	20	30	40	50	60	70	75	80	85
0.5	0.19	0.27	0.37	0.49	0.61	0.74	0.86	0.96	0.99	1.0	1.0
0.6	0.19	0.32	0.48	0.69	0.94	1.2	1.5	1.7	1.8	1.9	1.9
0.7	0.19	0.37	0.64	1.0	1.5	2.1	2.8	3.5	3.7	3.9	4.1
0.8	0.19	0.45	0.87	1.6	2.6	4.1	6.1	8.4	9.4	10	10
0.9	0.19	0.54	1.2	2.5	5.0	9.6	17	30	38	45	50
1.0	0.19	0.67	1.8	4.4	11	32	113	—	—	—	—

6-2 Damper, Butterfly, Rectangular (Idelchik 1986, Diagram 9-17; Zolotov 1967)

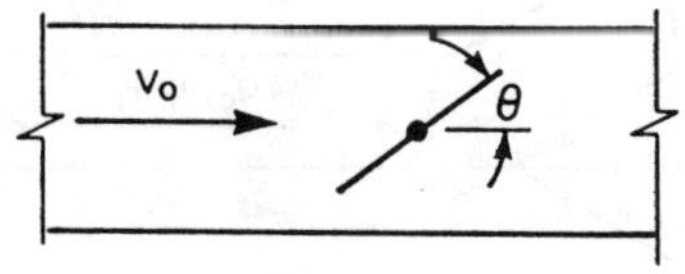

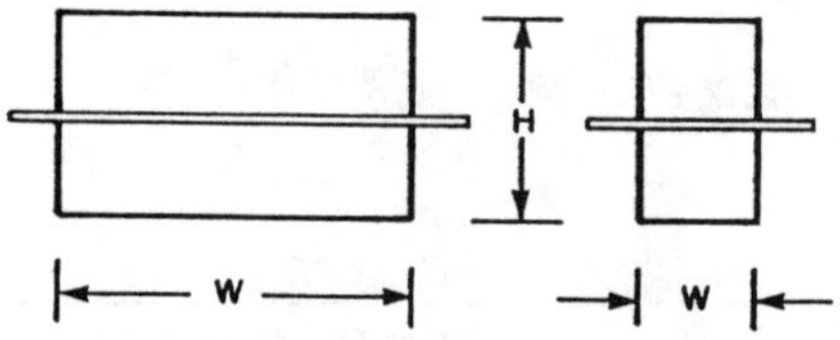

TYPE 1 (Axis parallel to long side) **TYPE 2** (Axis parallel to short side)

Type	H/W	C_o, θ, degrees: 0	10	20	30	40	50	60	65	70
1	<0.25	0.04	0.30	1.1	3.0	8.0	23	60	100	190
1	0.25–1.0	0.08	0.33	1.2	3.3	9.0	26	70	128	210
2	>1.0	0.13	0.35	1.3	3.6	10	29	80	155	230

6-3 Damper, Gate, Round (Idelchik 1986, Diagram 9-5)

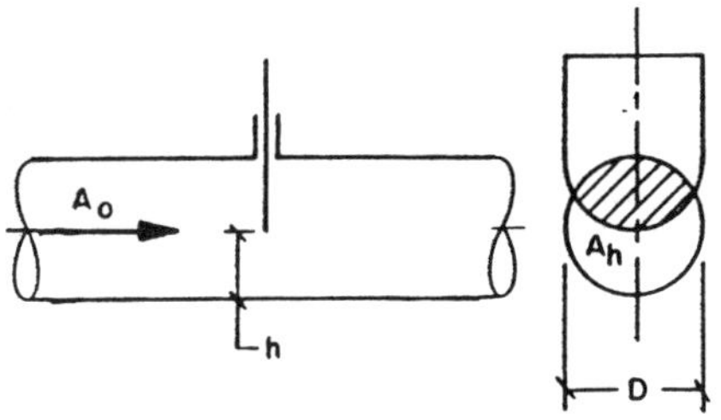

h/D	0.2	0.3	0.4	0.5	0.6	0.7	0.8	0.9
A_h/A_o	0.25	0.38	0.50	0.61	0.71	0.81	0.90	0.96
C_o	35	10	4.6	2.1	0.98	0.44	0.17	0.06

6-4 Damper, Gate, Rectangular (Idelchik 1986, Diagram 9-5)

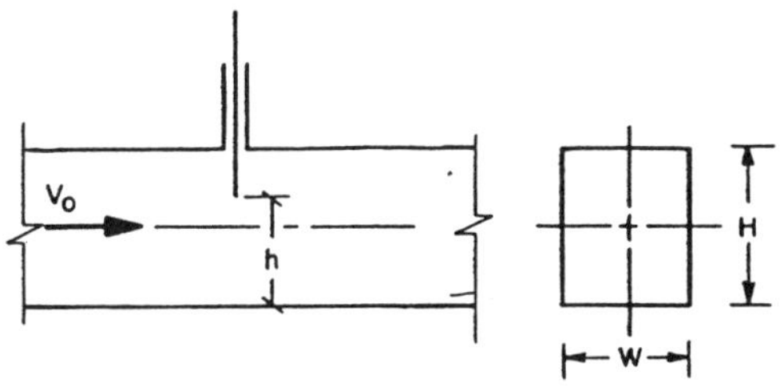

	h/H						
H/W	0.3	0.4	0.5	0.6	0.7	0.8	0.9
0.5	14	6.9	3.3	1.7	0.83	0.32	0.09
1.0	19	8.8	4.5	2.4	1.2	0.55	0.17
1.5	20	9.1	4.7	2.7	1.2	0.47	0.11
2.0	18	8.8	4.5	2.3	1.1	0.51	0.13

6-5 Damper, Rectangular, Parallel Blades (Brown 1957)

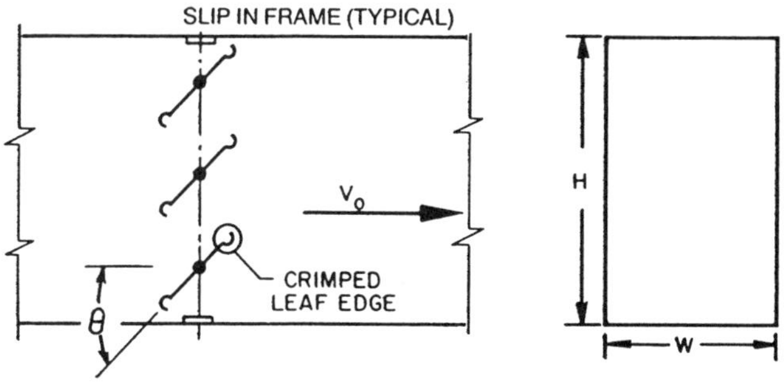

$$L/R = \frac{NW}{2(H + W)}$$

where

N = number of damper blades
W = duct dimension parallel to blade axis, in.
H = duct height, in.
L = sum of damper blade lengths, in.
R = perimeter of duct, in.

	C_o							
$\frac{L}{R}$	θ, degrees							
	0	10	20	30	40	50	60	70
0.3	0.52	0.79	1.4	2.3	5.0	9	14	32
0.4	0.52	0.85	1.5	2.4	5.0	9	16	38
0.5	0.52	0.92	1.5	2.4	5.0	9	18	45
0.6	0.52	0.92	1.5	2.4	5.4	9	21	45
0.8	0.52	0.92	1.5	2.5	5.4	9	22	55
1.0	0.52	1.0	1.6	2.6	5.4	10	24	65
1.5	0.52	1.0	1.6	2.7	5.4	10	28	102

6-6 Damper, Rectangular, Opposed Blades (Brown 1957)

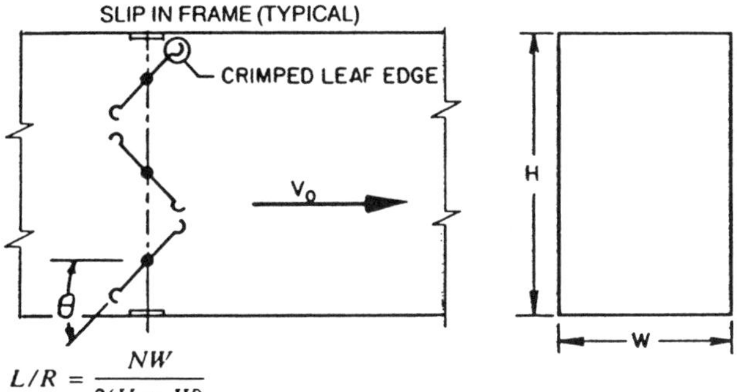

$$L/R = \frac{NW}{2(H + W)}$$

See Fitting 6-5 for definition of terms.

	C_o							
$\frac{L}{R}$	θ, degrees							
	0	10	20	30	40	50	60	70
0.3	0.52	0.85	2.1	4.1	9	21	73	284
0.4	0.52	0.92	2.2	5.0	11	28	100	332
0.5	0.52	1.0	2.3	5.4	13	33	122	377
0.6	0.52	1.0	2.3	6.0	14	38	148	411
0.8	0.52	1.1	2.4	6.6	18	54	188	495
1.0	0.52	1.2	2.7	7.3	21	65	245	547
1.5	0.52	1.4	3.2	9.0	28	107	361	677

6-7 Obstruction, Screen, Round and Rectangular (Idelchik 1986, Diagram 8-6)

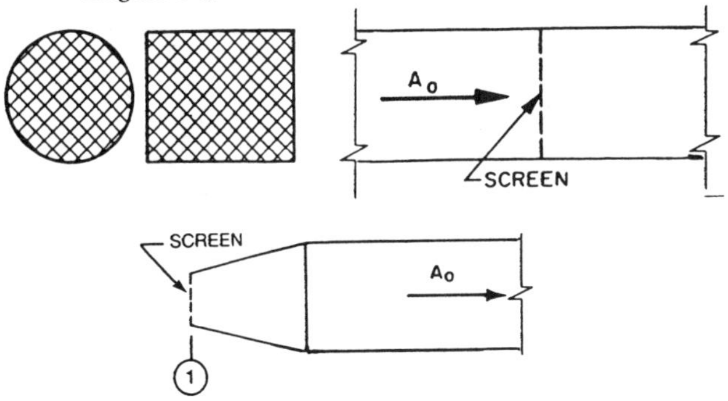

n = free area ratio of screen
A_o = area of duct
A_1 = cross-sectional area of duct or fitting where screen is located

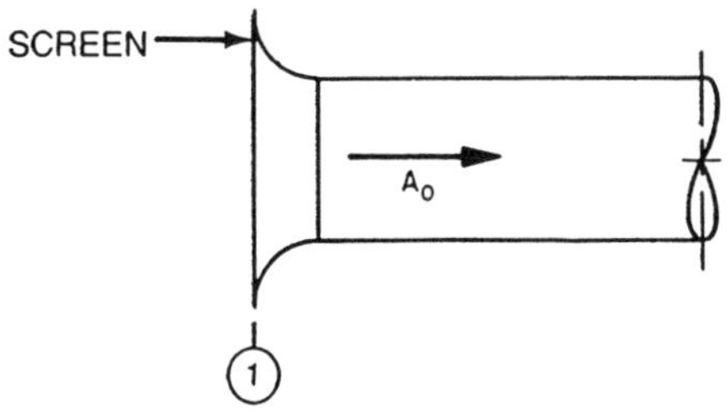

	C_o							
A_1/A_o	n							
	0.3	0.4	0.5	0.6	0.7	0.8	0.9	1.0
0.2	155	75	42	24	15	8.0	3.5	0
0.3	69	33	19	11	6.4	3.6	1.6	0
0.4	39	19	10	6.1	3.6	2.0	0.88	0
0.6	17	8.3	4.7	2.7	1.6	0.89	0.39	0
0.8	9.7	4.7	2.7	1.5	0.91	0.50	0.22	0
1.0	6.2	3.0	1.7	0.97	0.58	0.32	0.14	0
1.2	4.3	2.1	1.2	0.67	0.40	0.22	0.10	0
1.4	3.2	1.5	0.87	0.49	0.30	0.16	0.07	0
1.6	2.4	1.2	0.66	0.38	0.23	0.12	0.05	0
2.0	1.6	0.75	0.43	0.24	0.15	0.08	0.04	0
2.5	0.99	0.48	0.27	0.16	0.09	0.05	0.02	0
3.0	0.69	0.33	0.19	0.11	0.06	0.04	0.02	0
4.0	0.39	0.19	0.11	0.06	0.04	0.02	0.01	0
6.0	0.17	0.08	0.05	0.03	0.02	0.01	0	0

6-8 Obstruction, Perforated Plate, Thick, Round and Rectangular (Idelchik 1986, Diagram 8-6)

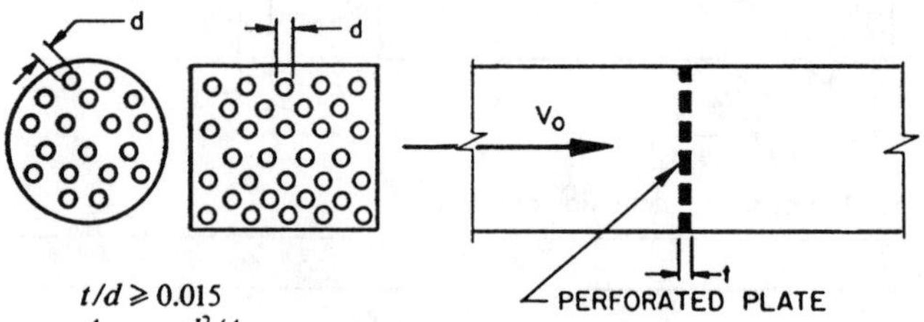

$t/d \geqslant 0.015$
$A_{or} = \pi d^2/4$
$n = \Sigma A_{or}/A_o$

where

A_o = area of duct
A_{or} = orifice area
d = diameter of perforated hole
n = free area ratio of plate, dimensionless
t = plate thickness

	C_o								
	n								
t/d	0.20	0.25	0.30	0.40	0.50	0.60	0.70	0.80	0.90
0.015	52	30	18	8.3	4.0	2.0	0.97	0.42	0.13
0.2	48	28	17	7.7	3.8	1.9	0.91	0.40	0.13
0.4	46	27	17	7.4	3.6	1.8	0.88	0.39	0.13
0.6	42	24	15	6.6	3.2	1.6	0.80	0.36	0.13

6-9 Obstruction, Smooth Cylinder in Round and Rectangular Ducts (Idelchik 1986, Diagram 10-1)

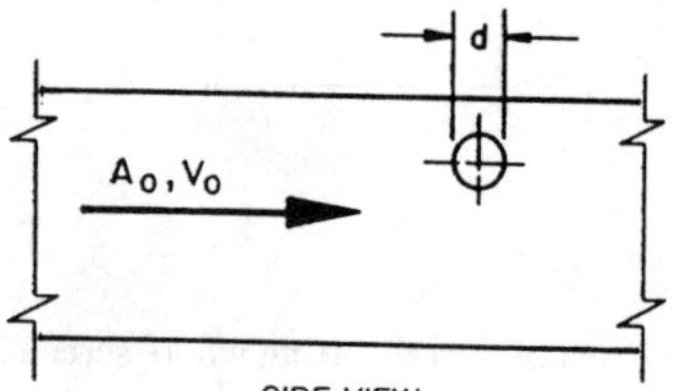

SIDE VIEW

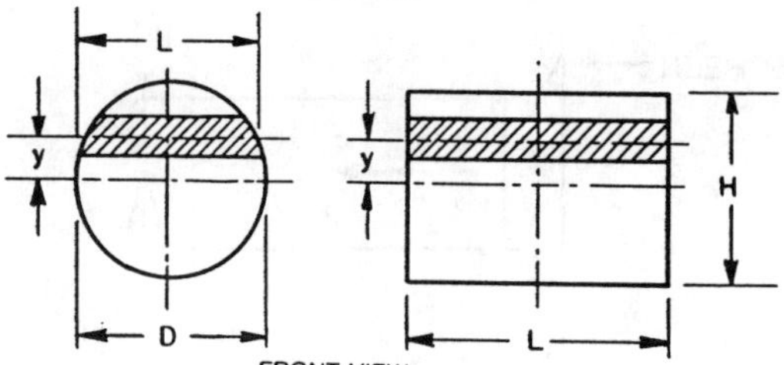

FRONT VIEW

$S_m/A_o < 0.3$
$S_m = dL$
$Re' = dV_0/\nu$ [To calculate Re′, see Equation (27).]
$C_o = KC_o'$

	C_o'			
	S_m/A_o			
Re	0.05	0.10	0.15	0.20
0.1	3.9	8.4	14	19
0.5	1.5	3.2	5.2	7.1
1	0.66	1.4	2.3	3.2
5	0.30	0.64	1.1	1.4
10	0.17	0.38	0.62	0.84
50	0.11	0.24	0.38	0.52
100	0.10	0.21	0.35	0.47
500 to 200 000	0.07	0.15	0.24	0.33
3×10^5	0.07	0.16	0.26	0.35
4×10^5	0.05	0.11	0.19	0.25
5×10^5	0.04	0.09	0.14	0.19
6×10^5 to 10^6	0.02	0.05	0.07	0.10

For obstruction offset from the centerline, use the following factors:

y/D or y/H	0	0.05	0.10	0.15	0.20	0.25	0.30	0.35	0.40
K	1.0	0.97	0.93	0.89	0.84	0.79	0.74	0.67	0.58

6-10 Round Duct, Depressed to Avoid an Obstruction (SMACNA 1981, Table 6-14I)

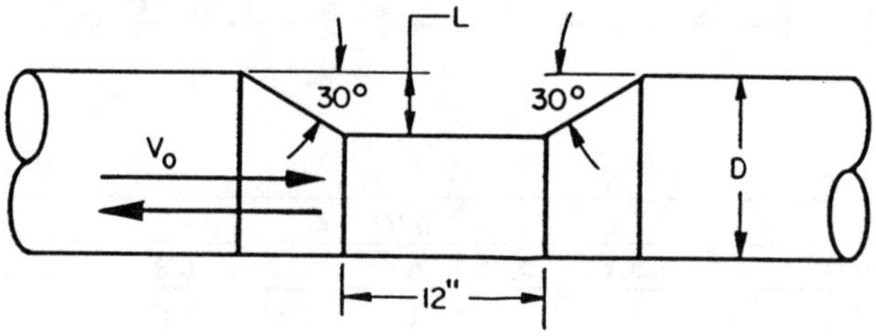

$L/D = 0.33$
$C_o = 0.24$

6-11 Rectangular Duct, Depressed to Avoid an Obstruction (SMACNA 1981, Table 6-14J)

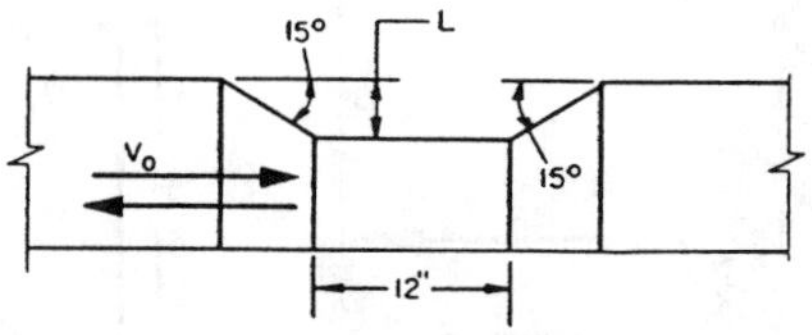

SIDE VIEW

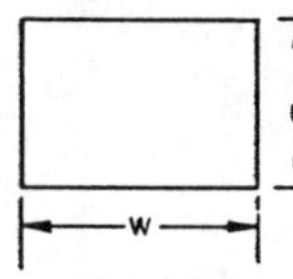

FRONT VIEW

	C_o			
	L/H			
W/H	0.125	0.15	0.25	0.30
1.0	0.26	0.30	0.33	0.35
4.0	0.10	0.14	0.22	0.30

FAN-SYSTEM CONNECTIONS

7-1 Fans Discharging into a Plenum (ACMA 1973, Fig. 19)

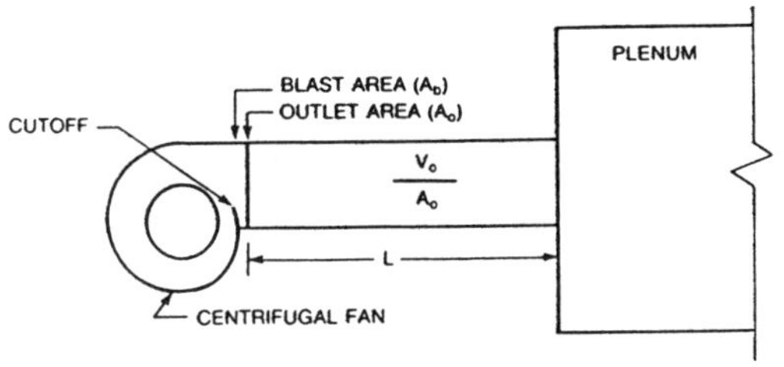

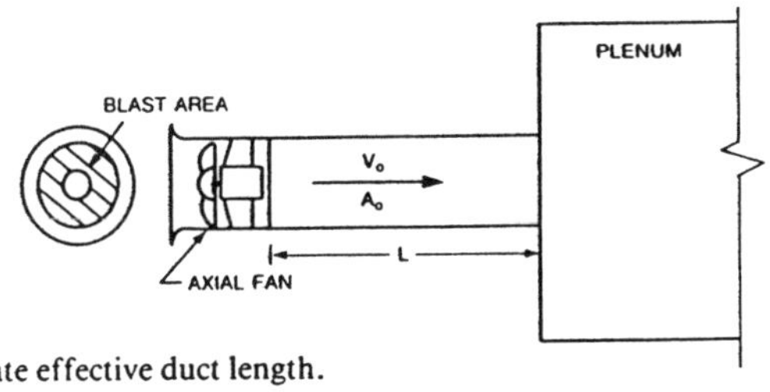

Calculate effective duct length.

$V_o > 2500$ fpm: $L_e = V\sqrt{A_o}/10{,}600$

$V_o \leqslant 2500$ fpm: $L_e = \sqrt{A_o}/4.3$

where

V_o = duct velocity, fpm
L_e = effective duct length, ft
A_o = duct area, in^2

	C_o				
	L/L_e				
A_b/A_o	0	0.12	0.25	0.5	⩾ 1.0
0.4	2.0	1.0	0.40	0.18	0
0.5	2.0	1.0	0.40	0.18	0
0.6	1.0	0.66	0.33	0.14	0
0.7	0.8	0.40	0.14	0	0
0.8	0.47	0.22	0.10	0	0
0.9	0.22	0.14	0	0	0
1.0	0	0	0	0	0

7-2 Single Width Single Inlet (SWSI) Fan with an Outlet Duct Elbow (AMCA 1973, Fig. 22)

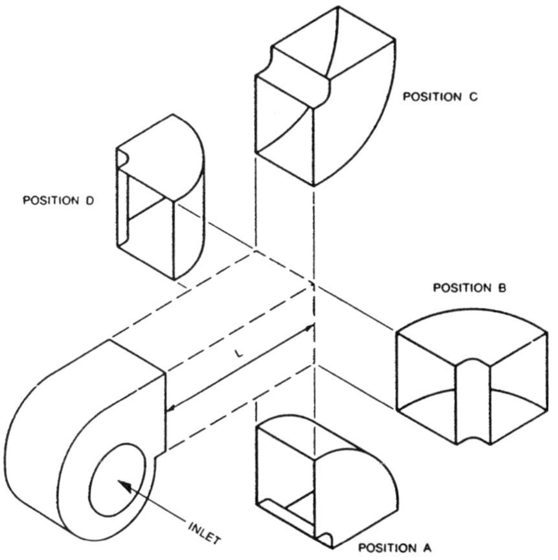

SWSI CENTRIFUGAL FAN

A_b = centrifugal fan blast area (see Fitting 7-1)
A_o = duct/outlet area (see Fitting 7-1)

To calculate effective duct length L_e, see Fitting 7-1.

		C_o				
	Outlet Elbow	L/L_e				
A_b/A_o	Position	0	0.12	0.25	0.5	⩾ 1.0
0.4	A	3.2	2.7	1.8	0.84	0
	B	4.0	3.3	2.2	1.0	0
	C	5.8	4.8	3.2	1.5	0
	D	5.8	4.8	3.2	1.5	0
0.5	A	2.3	1.9	1.3	0.60	0
	B	2.8	2.4	1.6	0.72	0
	C	4.0	3.3	2.2	1.0	0
	D	4.0	3,3	2.2	1.0	0
0.6	A	1.6	1.3	0.88	0.40	0
	B	2.0	1.7	1.1	0.52	0
	C	2.9	2.4	1.6	0.76	0
	D	2.9	2.4	1.6	0.76	0
0.7	A	1.1	0.88	0.60	0.28	0
	B	1.3	1.1	0.72	0.36	0
	C	2.0	1.6	1.1	0.52	0
	D	2.0	1.6	1.1	0.52	0
0.8	A	0.76	0.64	0.44	0.20	0
	B	0.96	0.80	0.52	0.24	0
	C	1.4	1.2	0.76	0.36	0
	D	1.4	1.2	0.76	0.36	0
0.9	A	0.60	0.48	0.32	0.16	0
	B	0.76	0.64	0.44	0.20	0
	C	1.1	0.92	0.64	0.28	0
	D	1.1	0.92	0.64	0.28	0
1.0	A	0.56	0.48	0.32	0.16	0
	B	0.68	0.56	0.36	0.16	0
	C	1.0	0.84	0.56	0.26	0
	D	1.0	0.84	0.56	0.28	0

7-3 Double Width Double Inlet (DWDI) Fan with an Outlet Duct Elbow (ACMA 1973, Fig. 22)

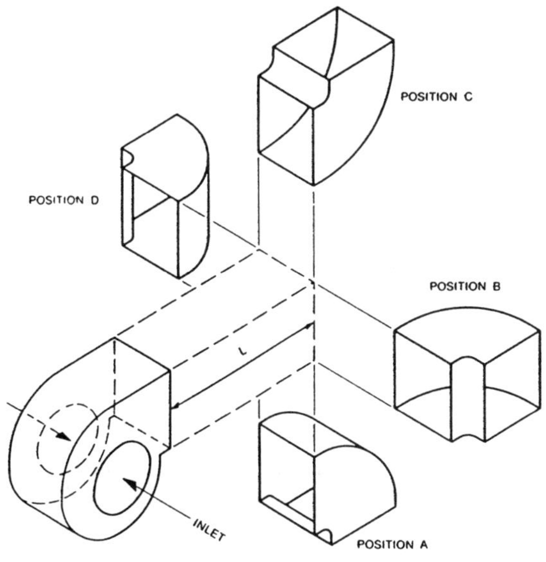

DWDI CENTRIFUGAL FAN

A_b = centrifugal fan blast area (see Fitting 7-1)
A_o = duct/outlet area (see Fitting 7-1)

To calculate *effective* duct length L_e, see Fittings 7-1.

A_b/A_o	Outlet Elbow Position	C_o				
		L/L_e				
		0	0.12	0.25	0.5	≥ 1.0
0.4	A	3.2	2.7	1.8	0.84	0
	B	5.0	4.2	2.8	1.3	0
	C	5.8	4.8	3.2	1.5	0
	D	4.9	4.1	2.7	1.3	0
0.5	A	2.3	1.9	1.3	0.60	0
	B	3.6	3.0	2.0	0.90	0
	C	4.0	3.3	2.2	1.0	0
	D	3.4	2.8	1.9	0.88	0
0.6	A	1.6	1.3	0.88	0.40	0
	B	2.5	2.1	1.4	0.65	0
	C	2.9	2.4	1.6	0.76	0
	D	2.5	2.1	1.4	0.65	0
0.7	A	1.1	0.88	0.60	0.28	0
	B	1.7	1.4	0.90	0.45	0
	C	2.0	1.6	1.1	0.52	0
	D	1.7	1.4	0.92	0.44	0
0.8	A	0.76	0.64	0.44	0.20	0
	B	1.2	1.0	0.65	0.30	0
	C	1.4	1.2	0.76	0.36	0
	D	1.2	0.99	0.65	0.31	0
0.9	A	0.60	0.48	0.32	0.16	0
	B	0.95	0.80	0.55	0.25	0
	C	1.1	0.92	0.64	0.28	0
	D	0.95	0.78	0.54	0.24	0
1.0	A	0.56	0.48	0.32	0.16	0
	B	0.85	0.70	0.45	0.20	0
	C	1.0	0.84	0.56	0.28	0
	D	0.85	0.71	0.48	0.24	0

7-4 Nonuniform Elbow into a Fan Inlet Induced by a 90° Round Smooth Radius Elbow without Vanes (ACMA 1973, Fig. 27)

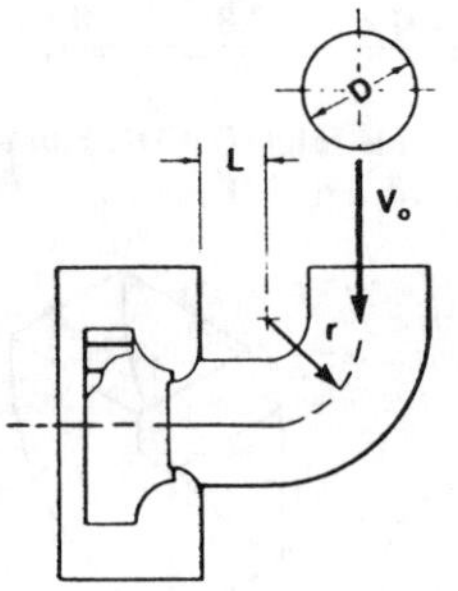

$\frac{r}{D}$	C_o		
	L/D		
	0	2.0	≥ 5.0
0.75	1.4	0.80	0.40
1.0	1.2	0.66	0.33
1.5	1.1	0.60	0.33
2.0	1.0	0.53	0.33
3.0	0.66	0.40	0.22

7-5 Nonuniform Elbow into a Fan Inlet Induced by 90° Mitered and Multipiece Elbows without Vanes (ACMA 1973, Fig. 29)

Mitered

L/D	0	2.0	≥ 5.0
C_o	3.2	2.0	1.0

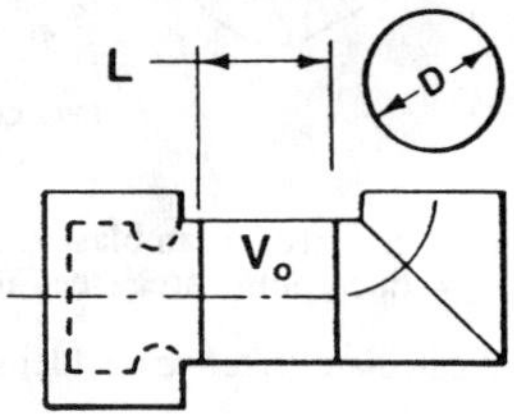

3-Piece

r/D	C_o		
	L/D		
	0	2.0	≥ 5.0
0.50	2.5	1.6	0.80
0.75	1.6	1.0	0.47
1.0	1.2	0.66	0.33
1.5	1.1	0.60	0.33
2.0	1.0	0.53	0.33
3.0	0.80	0.47	0.26

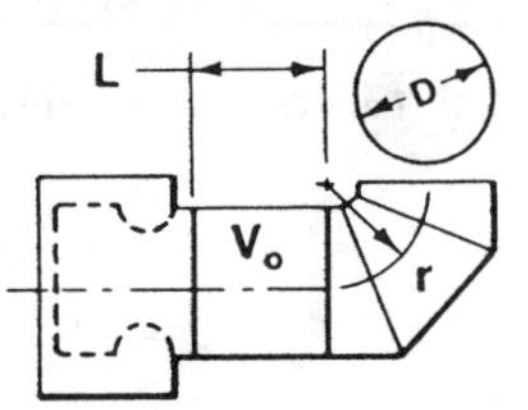

4-Piece or more

r/D	C_o		
	L/D		
	0	2.0	≥ 5.0
0.50	1.8	1.0	0.53
0.75	1.4	0.80	0.40
1.0	1.2	0.66	0.33
1.5	1.1	0.60	0.33
2.0	1.0	0.53	0.33
3.0	0.66	0.40	0.22

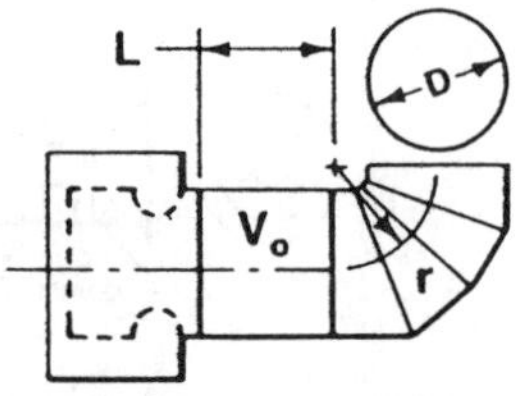

7-6 Nonuniform Elbow into a Fan Inlet Induced by a 90° Square Smooth Radius Elbow (ACMA 1973, Fig. 35A)

Square Elbow with an Inlet Transition,[a] No Vanes

r/D	C_o		
	L/H		
	0	2.5	≥ 6.0
0.50	2.5	1.6	0.80
0.75	2.0	1.2	0.66
1.0	1.2	0.66	0.33
1.5	1.0	0.57	0.30
2.0	0.8	0.47	0.26

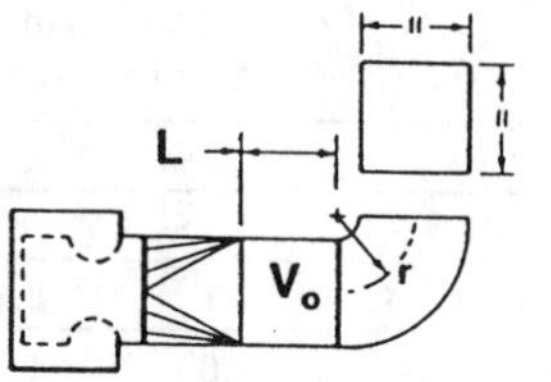

Square Elbow with an Inlet Transition,[a] Full Radius Vanes Equally Spaced

r/D	C_o		
	L/H		
	0	2.5	≥ 6.0
0.50	0.80	0.47	0.26
1.0	0.53	0.33	0.18
1.5	0.40	0.28	0.16
2.0	1.26	0.22	0.14

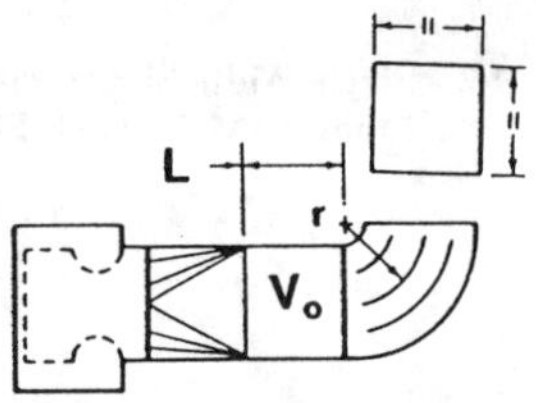

Square Elbow with an Inlet Transition,[a] Short Vanes per Fitting 3-8

r/D	C_o		
	L/H		
	0	2.5	≥ 6.0
0.50	0.80	0.47	0.26
1.0	0.53	0.33	0.18
1.5	0.40	0.28	0.16
2.0	0.26	0.22	0.14

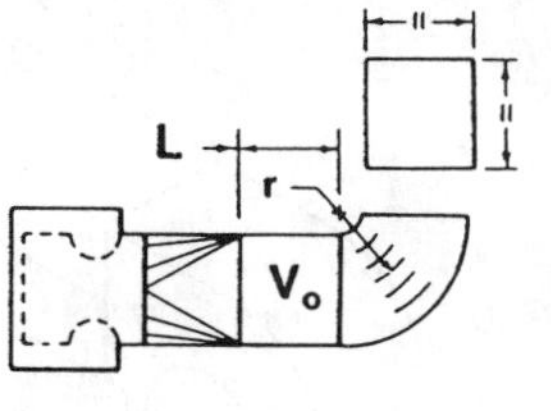

[a] The inside area of the square duct ($H \times H$) is equal to the inside area circumscribed by the fan inlet collar. The maximum angle of any converging element of the transition is 15° and for a diverging element, 7.5°.

7-7 Fans Located in Plenums and Cabinet Enclosures (AMCA 1973, Fig. 35A)

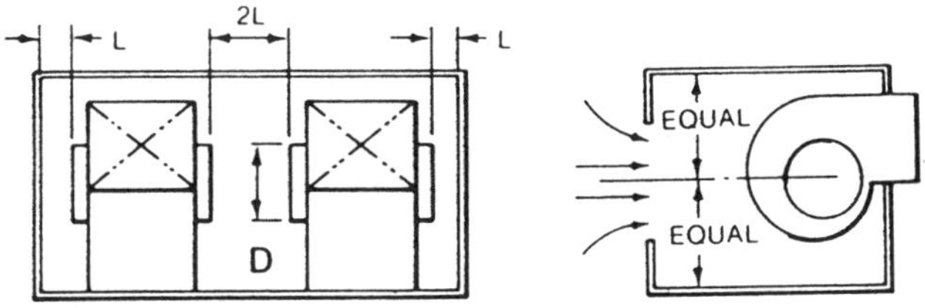

L	C_o
0.75 D	0.22
0.5 D	0.40
0.4 D	0.53
0.3 D	0.80
0.2 D	1.2

7-8 Fan Without an Outlet Diffuser (AMCA 1973, Fig. 19)

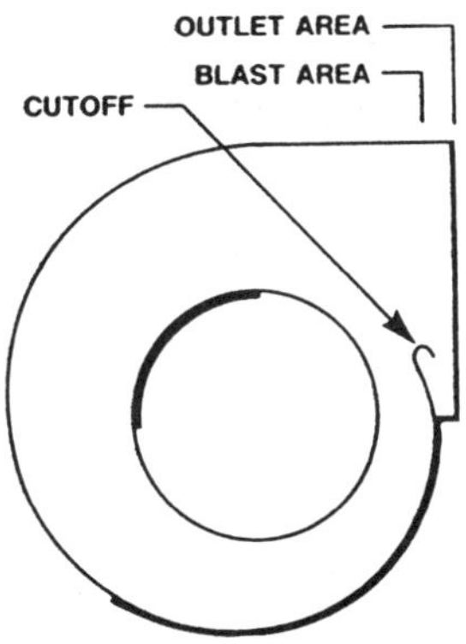

Poor; should not be used.

A_b/A_o	0.4	0.5	0.6	0.7	0.8	0.9	1.0
C_o	2.0	2.0	1.0	0.80	0.47	0.22	0

7-9 Plane Asymmetric Diffuser at Fan Outlet Without Ductwork (Idelchik 1986, Diagram 11-11)

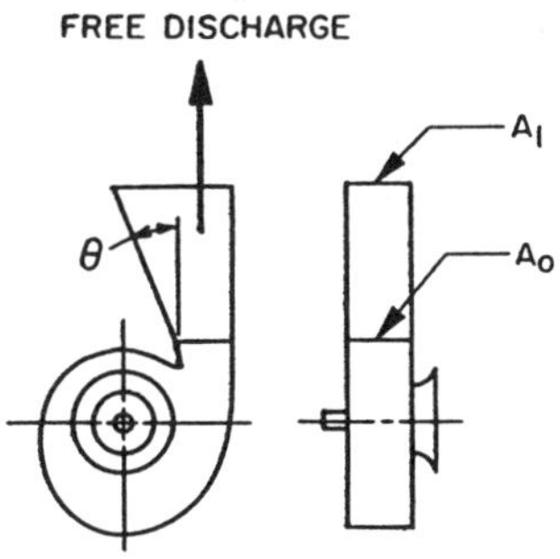

	C_o					
θ,	A_1/A_o					
deg	1.5	2.0	2.5	3.0	3.5	4.0
10	0.51	0.34	0.25	0.21	0.18	0.17
15	0.54	0.36	0.27	0.24	0.22	0.20
20	0.55	0.38	0.31	0.27	0.25	0.24
25	0.59	0.43	0.37	0.35	0.33	0.33
30	0.63	0.50	0.46	0.44	0.43	0.42
35	0.65	0.56	0.53	0.52	0.51	0.50

If diffuser has a screen, use Fitting 6-7 to calculate screen resistance.

7-10 Pyramidal Diffuser at Fan Outlet Without Ductwork (Idelchik 1986, Diagram 11-11)

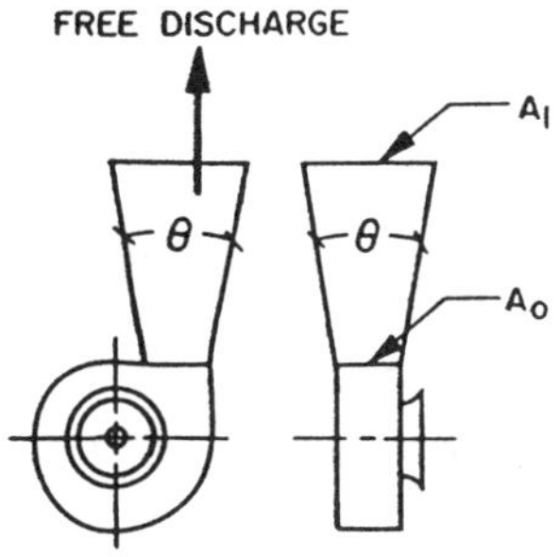

	C_o					
θ,	A_1/A_o					
deg	1.5	2.0	2.5	3.0	3.5	4.0
10	0.54	0.42	0.37	0.34	0.32	0.31
15	0.67	0.58	0.53	0.51	0.50	0.51
20	0.75	0.67	0.65	0.64	0.64	0.65
25	0.80	0.74	0.72	0.70	0.70	0.72
30	0.85	0.78	0.76	0.75	0.75	0.76

If diffuser has a screen, use Fitting 6-7 to calculate screen resistance.

7-11 Plane Symmetric Diffuser at Fan Outlet with Ductwork (Idelchik 1986, Diagram 5-12)

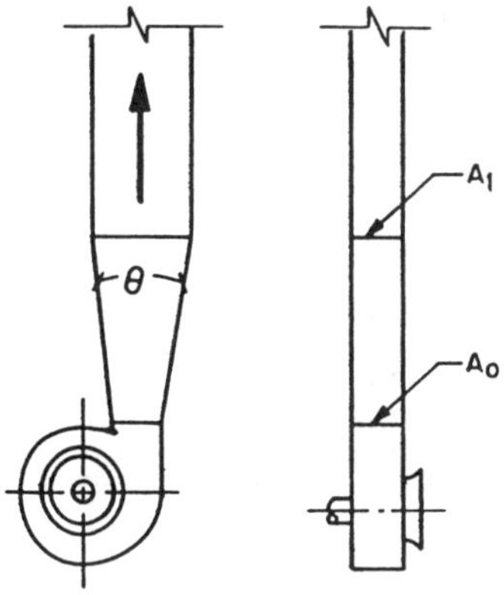

	C_o					
θ,	A_1/A_o					
deg	1.5	2.0	2.5	3.0	3.5	4.0
10	0.05	0.07	0.09	0.10	0.11	0.11
15	0.06	0.09	0.11	0.13	0.13	0.14
20	0.07	0.10	0.13	0.15	0.16	0.16
25	0.08	0.13	0.16	0.19	0.21	0.23
30	0.16	0.29	0.39	0.32	0.34	0.35
35	0.24	0.34	0.39	0.44	0.48	0.50

7-12 Plane Asymmetric Diffuser at Fan Outlet with Ductwork (Idelchik 1986, Diagram 5-13)

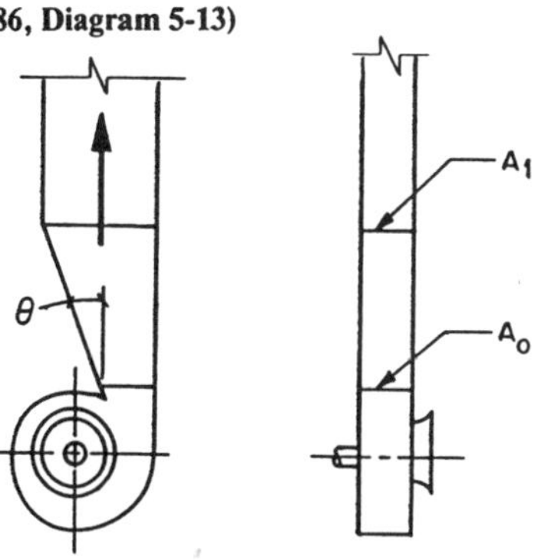

θ, deg	C_o					
	A_1/A_o					
	1.5	2.0	2.5	3.0	3.5	4.0
10	0.08	0.09	0.10	0.10	0.11	0.11
15	0.10	0.11	0.12	0.13	0.14	0.15
20	0.12	0.14	0.15	0.16	0.17	0.18
25	0.15	0.18	0.21	0.23	0.25	0.26
30	0.18	0.25	0.30	0.33	0.35	0.35
35	0.21	0.31	0.38	0.41	0.43	0.44

7-13 Plane Asymmetric Diffuser at Fan Outlet with Ductwork (Idelchik 1986, Diagram 5-14)

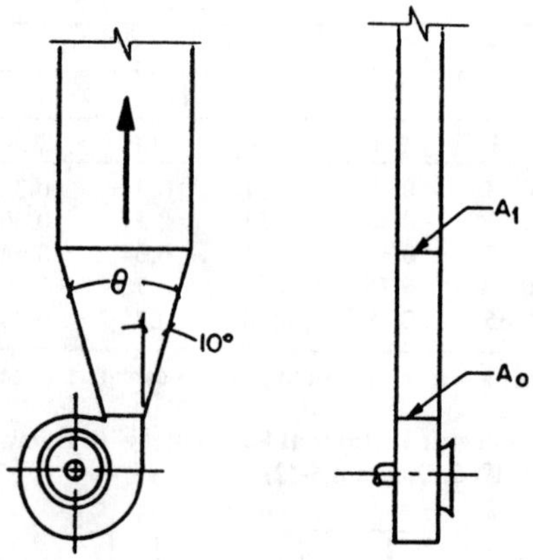

θ, deg	C_o					
	A_1/A_o					
	1.5	2.0	2.5	3.0	3.5	4.0
10	0.05	0.08	0.11	0.13	0.13	0.14
15	0.06	0.10	0.12	0.14	0.15	0.15
20	0.07	0.11	0.14	0.15	0.16	0.16
25	0.09	0.14	0.18	0.20	0.21	0.22
30	0.13	0.18	0.23	0.26	0.28	0.29
35	0.15	0.23	0.28	0.33	0.35	0.36

7-14 Plane Asymmetric Diffuser at Fan Outlet with Ductwork (Idelchik 1986, Diagram 5-15)

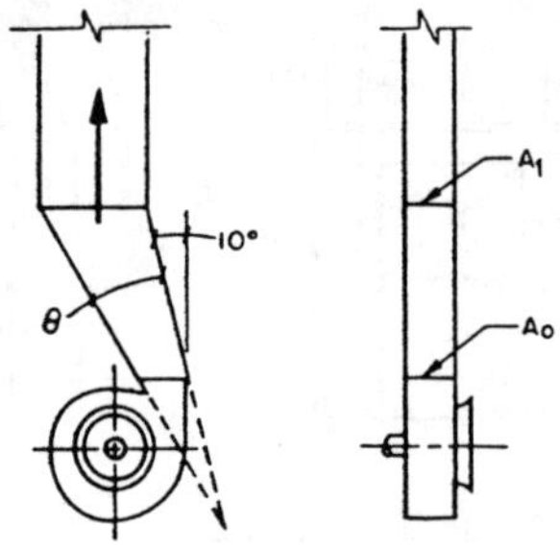

θ, deg	C_o					
	A_1/A_o					
	1.5	2.0	2.5	3.0	3.5	4.0
10	0.11	0.13	0.14	0.14	0.14	0.14
15	0.13	0.15	0.16	0.17	0.18	0.18
20	0.19	0.22	0.24	0.26	0.28	0.30
25	0.29	0.32	0.35	0.37	0.39	0.40
30	0.36	0.42	0.46	0.49	0.51	0.51
35	0.44	0.54	0.61	0.64	0.66	0.66

7-15 Pyramidal Diffuser at Fan Outlet with Ductwork (Idelchik 1986, Diagram 5-16)

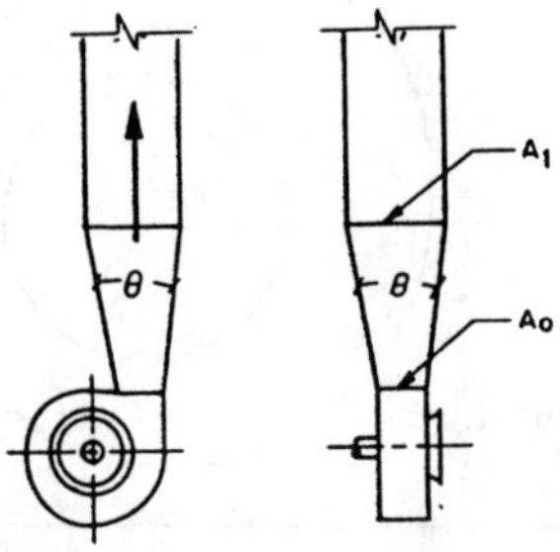

θ, deg	C_o					
	A_1/A_o					
	1.5	2.0	2.5	3.0	3.5	4.0
10	0.10	0.18	0.21	0.23	0.24	0.25
15	0.23	0.33	0.38	0.40	0.42	0.44
20	0.31	0.43	0.48	0.53	0.56	0.58
25	0.36	0.49	0.55	0.58	0.62	0.64
30	0.42	0.53	0.59	0.64	0.67	0.69

Example 9.1. The supply duct system for the 100% outside makeup air system of a clean room as shown in the following sketch is to use rectangular, galvanized ducting throughout. An air velocity of 500 fpm is to be used. The following data are known about the components: (a) elbows are mitered, design 2 type (3-8), (b) the flow split is accomplished with a symmetrical wye (5-32), (c) the loss coefficient for the combination of transition section and outlet diffuser C_c is 1.86, (d) the HEPA filter is to be 99.9% efficient, and (e) the coil is a 4-row Series 56 with 12 fins per inch. Data for the filter and coil can be obtained from the given data.

Size each duct and determine the total pressure drop for the supply duct.

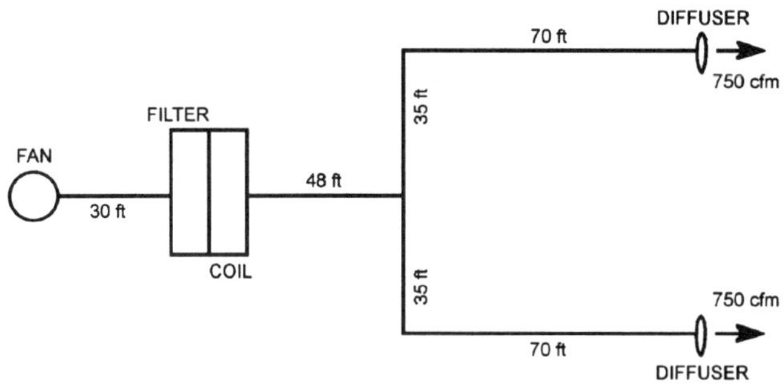

Pressure Losses, Inches of Water

Filter Pressure Losses	Velocity, fpm 250 (Clean / Dirty)*	500 (Clean / Dirty)*
Panel 2 in. pleated 30% efficiency	0.08 / 0.90	0.28 / 0.90
Panel 4 in. pleated 30% efficiency	0.07 / 0.90	0.27 / 0.90
Bag 22 in. deep 60-65% efficiency	0.12 / 1.00	0.30 / 1.00
Bag 22 in. deep 80-85% efficiency	0.28 / 1.00	.045 / 1.00
Bag 22 in. deep 90-95% efficiency	0.50 / 1.50	0.70 / 1.50
Cartridge 12 in. deep 60-65% efficiency	0.15 / 1.50	0.29 / 1.50
Cartridge 12 in. deep 80-85% efficiency	0.27 / 1.50	0.50 / 1.50
Cartridge 12 in. deep 90-95% efficiency	0.34 / 1.50	0.68 / 1.50
HEPA 12 in. deep, 99.97% DOP**	0.60 / 2.00	1.20 / 2.00

* Unit air flow performance should be selected halfway between initial (clean) and final (firty) filter pressure loss, or as specified.
** HEPA's shown are high flow capacity; rated for 500 fpm face velocity.

Fin Type	Fins per inch	Face Velocity, fpm 200	300	400	500	600	700
Series 56 (5/8 in. tubes)	8	0.050	0.092	0.140	0.196	0.257	0.324
	10	0.063	0.112	0.170	0.234	0.304	0.379
	12	0.075	0.133	0.199	0.271	0.360	0.435

Solution:

$$P_v = \left(\frac{500}{4005}\right)^2 = 0.156 \text{ in. wg.}$$

Main Duct: 78 ft long, 1500 cfm, 500 fpm

$$A = \frac{1500}{500} = 3 \text{ ft}^2 = \frac{\pi D_e^{\,2}}{4}$$

D_e = 1.95 ft = 23.5 in.

equivalent rectangular = 32 × 16 to 48 × 12

Select 32 × 16 (lower aspect ratio and easier to match with coil face)

From Fig. 9.2 Δp/100 ft = 0.013 in. w.g.

$$\Delta p_M = 0.013 \times \frac{78}{100} = 0.010 \text{ in. w.g.}$$

Branches: 105 feet, 750 cfm, 500 fpm

$$750/500 = 1.5 \text{ ft}^2$$

D_e = 1.38 ft = 16.6 in.
equivalent rectangular = 16 × 16 to 32 × 8
From Fig. 9.2 Δp/100 ft = 0.022

$$\Delta p_B = 0.022 \times \frac{105}{100} = 0.023 \text{ in. wg.}$$

Elbows: (type 3-8-2) $C_o = 0.15$ $\Delta p_e = C_o\, p_v$

$$\Delta p_e = 0.15\ (0.0156 \text{ in. w.g.}) = 0.0023 \text{ in. w.g.}$$

Wye: (type 5-32) $C_o = 0.30$

$$\Delta p_Y = 0.30\ (0.0156) = 0.0047 \text{ in. w.g.}$$

Diffusers: $C_o = 1.86$

$$\Delta p_D = 1.86\ (0.0156) = 0.029 \text{ in. w.g.}$$

$$\begin{aligned}\Delta p_{TOTAL} &= \Delta p_M + \Delta p_F + \Delta p_C + \Delta p_Y \\ &\quad + \Delta p + \Delta p + \Delta p_D \\ &= 0.010 + 1.60(\text{avg}) + (4 \times 0.271) + 0.0047 \\ &\quad + 0.023 + 0.0023 + 0.029 \\ &= 2.75 \text{ in. w.g.}\end{aligned}$$

Example 9.2. Find the total pressure loss in the straight-through section of a 90° cylindrical tee. The velocity in the main upstream section is 2000 fpm and in the main downstream is 1500 fpm. The velocity in the tee branch is 1060 fpm. Also, calculate the total pressure loss between the straight through section and the branch. The value of A_b/A_c is 0.6.

Solution:

(a) For the straight-through section:

$$V_c = 2000 \text{ fpm } V_s = 1500 \text{ fpm } V_b = 1060 \text{ fpm}$$

From Equation (9-2),

$$p_{vc} = (2000/4005)^2 = 0.25 \text{ in. of water}$$

For Fitting 5-23, Table 9-4, with θ = 90°, and $V_s/V_c = 0.75$:

$$c_{c,s} = 0.03$$

By Equation (9-10a),

$$\Delta p_t = C_{c,s}$$

$$\Delta p_t = 0.03\ (0.25) = 0.0075 \text{ in. of water (negligible)}$$

(b) For the branch section for θ = 90° and $V_b/V_c = 0.53$ and $A_b/A_c = 0.06$, for Fitting 5-23, Table 9-4:

$$c_{c,b} = 1.01$$

By Equation (9-10b),

$$\Delta p_1 = C_{c,b}$$

$$\Delta p_t = 1.01\ (0.25) = 0.25 \text{ in. w.g.}$$

9.2 Fans

A fan is an air pump, a machine that creates a pressure difference and causes airflow. The impeller imparts to the air static and kinetic energy, which varies in proportion, depending on the type of fan.

Fans are classified as centrifugal fans or axial flow fans, according to the direction of airflow through the impeller. The general configuration of a centrifugal fan is shown in Figure 9-3. A similar description of an axial flow fan is shown in Figure 9-4. In addition to these two types, there are several subdivisions of each of the general types. A comparison of typical characteristics of some fan types is shown in Table 9-5.

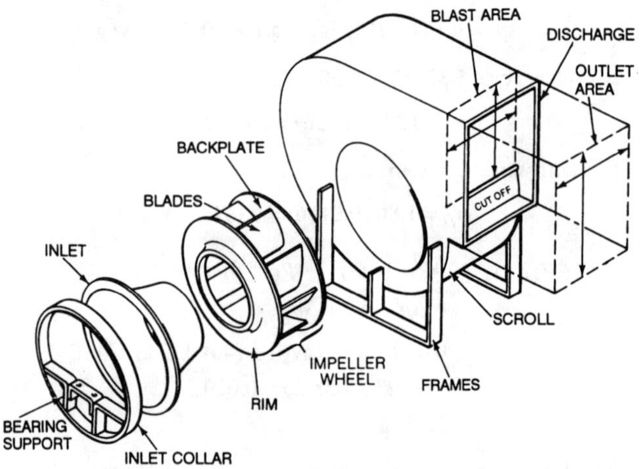

Fig. 9-3 Centrifugal Fan Components

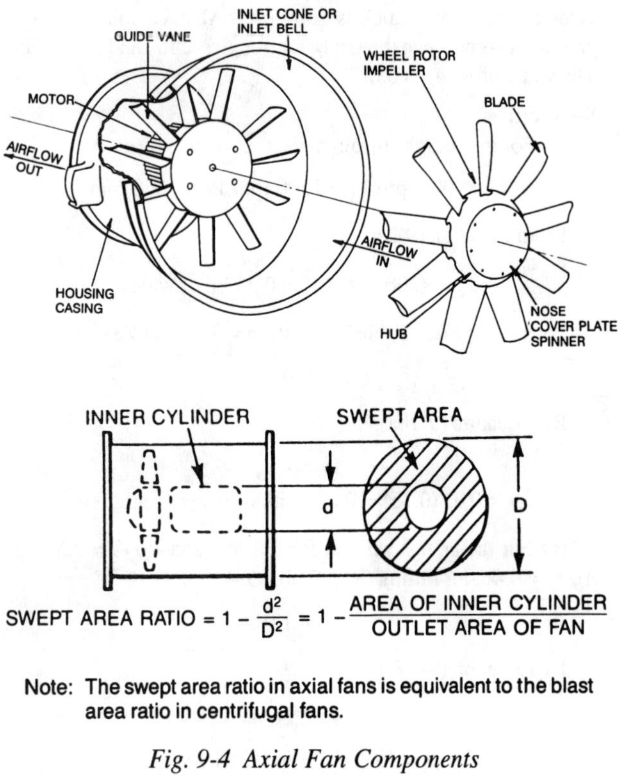

$$\text{SWEPT AREA RATIO} = 1 - \frac{d^2}{D^2} = 1 - \frac{\text{AREA OF INNER CYLINDER}}{\text{OUTLET AREA OF FAN}}$$

Note: The swept area ratio in axial fans is equivalent to the blast area ratio in centrifugal fans.

Fig. 9-4 Axial Fan Components

9.2.1 Principles of Operation

Centrifugal fan impellers produce pressure from two related sources: (1) the centrifugal force created by rotating the air column enclosed between the blades; and (2) the kinetic energy imparted to the air by its velocity leaving the impeller. This velocity is a combination of rotative velocity of the impeller and air speed relative to the impeller. When the blades are inclined forward, these two velocities are cumulative, when backward, oppositional. The forward-curved fans depend less on centrifugal force for pressure and more on velocity pressure conversion in the scroll. Conversely, fans with backward-curved blades build up more pressure by centrifugal force and less by velocity conversion in the scroll. However, since the buildup of pressure by centrifugal force is a more efficient form of energy transfer than the conversion of velocity, backward-curved blade fans generally are more efficient than forward-curved blade fans.

Axial flow fans produce all of their static pressure from the change in velocity of the air passing through the impeller. These fans are divided into three subtypes. Propeller fans, customarily used at free delivery, are of relatively simple construction. The impellers usually have a small hub-to-tip ratio and are mounted in an orifice plate or inlet ring. Tubeaxial fans are mounted in a cylindrical tube. They have reduced running clearance and operate at higher tip speeds, which give the tubeaxial fan a higher static pressure capability than the propeller fan. Vaneaxial fans are essentially tubeaxial fans with guide vanes which give improved pressure characteristics and efficiency.

9.2.2 Definitions

Volume flow rate handled by the fan is the number of cubic feet of air per minute expressed at fan inlet conditions.

Fan total pressure rise is the fan total pressure at outlet minus the fan total pressure at inlet, in. of water.

Fan velocity pressure is the pressure corresponding to the average velocity determined from the volume flow rate and fan outlet area, in. of water.

Fan static pressure rise is the fan total pressure rise dimin ished by the fan velocity pressure. The fan inlet velocity head is assumed equal to zero for fan rating purposes, in. of water.

Power output of a fan is expressed as horsepower and is based on the fan volume flow rate and the fan total pressure.

Power input of a fan is expressed as horsepower and is measured as power delivered to the fan shaft.

Mechanical efficiency (or fan total efficiency) of a fan is the ratio of power output to power input.

Static efficiency of a fan is the mechanical efficiency multiplied by the ratio of fan static pressure to fan total pressure.

Point of rating may be any point on the fan performance. curve. For each case, the particular point on the curve must be specifically defined.

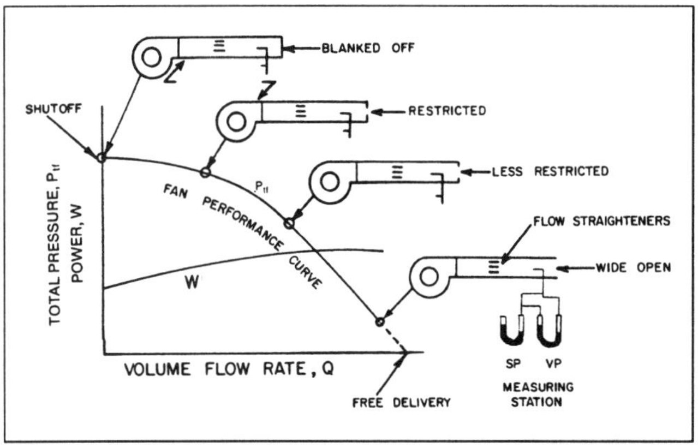

Fig. 9-6 Method of Obtaining Fan Performance Curve

9.2.3 Fan Testing

The pilot tube duct traverse can be used to explain the procedure by which a constant speed fan performance curve can be obtained (Figure 9-5). Fans are tested in accordance with *ASHRAE Standard* 51 and *AMCA Standard* 210.

The fan is tested from **shutoff** conditions to nearly **free delivery** conditions. At shutoff, the duct is completely blanked off; at free delivery, the outlet resistance is reduced to zero. Between these two conditions, various flow restrictions are placed on the end of the duct to simulate various conditions on the fan. Sufficient points are obtained to define the curve between the shutoff point and free delivery conditions.

Fans designed for duct systems are tested with a length of duct between the fan and the measuring station. This length of duct smoothes the flow of the fan and provides stable, uniform flow conditions at the plane of measurement. The measured pressures are corrected back to fan outlet conditions. Fans designed for use without ducts are tested without ductwork.

Not all sizes are tested for rating. Test information may be used to calculate the performance of larger fans which are geometrically similar, but it should not be extrapolated to smaller fans. For the performance of one fan to be determined from the known performance of another, the two fans must be dynamically similar. Strict dynamic similarity requires that the important nondimensional parameters vary in only insignificant ways. These nondimensional parameters include those which affect the aerodynamic characteristics, such as Mach number, Reynolds number, surface roughness, and gap size. (For more specific information, the manufacturer's application manual or engineering data should be consulted.)

9.2.4 Fan Laws

Fan laws relate the performance variables for any geometrically similar series of fans (Table 9-6). The variables involved are fan size D, rotational speed N, gas density ρ, volume flow rate Q, pressure p_t or p_s, power H (either air or shaft), and mechanical efficiency η_1.

Fan laws mathematically express the fact that when two fans are both members of a geometrically similar series, their performance curves are homologous. At the same point of rating, i.e., at the same relative point on the fan performance curve, efficiencies are equal. Point of rating is sometimes expressed as a stated percent of free delivery airflow. Another method of describing point of rating is the static pressure-velocity pressure ratio p_s/p_v.

Table 9-5 Fan Laws

(Table 2, Chapter 18, 1996 *ASHRAE Handbook—Systems and Equipment*)

Law No.	Dependent Variables				Independent Variables
1a	Q_1	=	Q_2	×	$(D_1/D_2)^3\,(N_1/N_2)$
1b	p_1	=	p_2	×	$(D_1/D_2)^2\,(N_1/N_2)^2\,\rho_1/\rho_2$
1c	W_1	=	W_2	×	$(D_1/D_2)^5\,(N_1/N_2)^3\,\rho_1/\rho_2$
2a	Q_1	=	Q_2	×	$(D_1/D_2)^2\,(p_1/p_2)^{1/2}\,(\rho_2/\rho_1)^{1/2}$
2b	N_1	=	N_2	×	$(D_2/D_1)\,(p_1/p_2)^{1/2}\,(\rho_2/\rho_1)^{1/2}$
2c	W_1	=	W_2	×	$(D_1/D_2)^2\,(p_1/p_2)^{3/2}\,(\rho_2/\rho_1)^{1/2}$
3a	N_1	=	N_2	×	$(D_2/D_1)^3\,(Q_1/Q_2)$
3b	p_1	=	p_2	×	$(D_2/D_1)^4\,(Q_1/Q_2)^2\,\rho_1/\rho_2$
3c	W_1	=	W_2	×	$(D_2/D_1)^4\,(Q_1/Q_2)^3\,\rho_1/\rho_2$

Notes:
1. Subscript 1 denotes the variable for the fan under consideration. Subscript 2 denotes the variable for the tested fan.
2. For all fans laws $(\eta_t)_1 = (\eta_t)_2$ and (Point of rating)$_1$ = (Point of rating)$_2$.
3. p equals either p_{tf} or p_{sf}.

Unless otherwise identified, fan performance data are based on a standard air density of 0.075 lb/ft^3 (1.2 kg/m^3). With constant size and speed, the power and pressure varies directly as the ratio of gas density to standard air density.

The application of the fan laws for a change in fan speed N to a specific size fan is illustrated in Figure 9-6. The computed P curve is derived from the base curve. For example, point E (N_1 = 650) is computed from point D (N_2 = 600) as follows:

At D, Q_2 = 6000 and p_{tf2} = 1.13

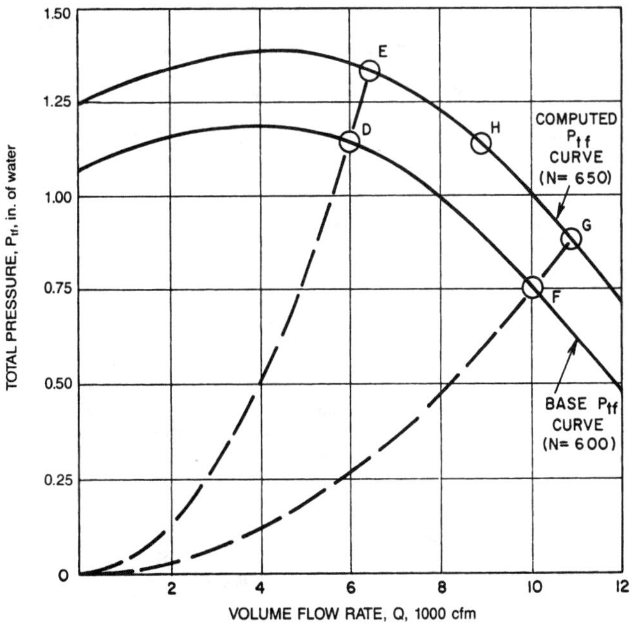

Fig. 9-7 Example Application of Fan Laws

Table 9-5 Types of Fans

	TYPE	IMPELLER DESIGN	HOUSING DESIGN
CENTRIFUGAL FANS	AIRFOIL	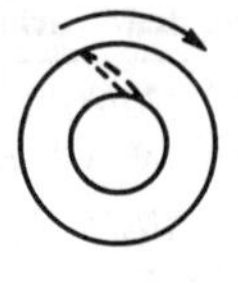 • Highest efficiency of all centrifugal fan designs. • Ten to 16 blades of airfoil contour curved away from direction of rotation. Deep blades allow for efficient expansion within blade passages. • Air leaves impeller at velocity less than tip speed. • For given duty, has highest speed of centrifugal fan designs.	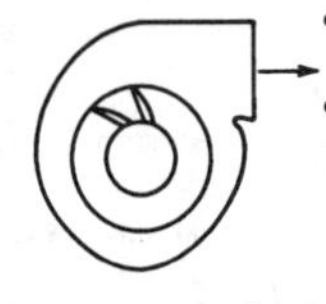 • Scroll-type design for efficient conversion of velocity pressure to static pressure. • Maximum efficiency requires close clearance and alignment between wheel and inlet.
CENTRIFUGAL FANS	BACKWARD-INCLINED BACKWARD-CURVED	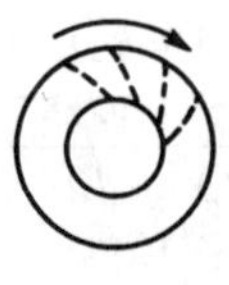 • Efficiency only slightly less than airfoil fan. • Ten to 16 single-thickness blades curved or inclined away from direction of rotation. • Efficient for same reasons as airfoil fan.	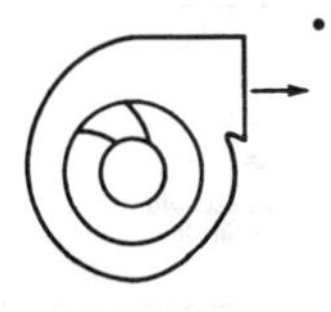 • Uses same housing configuration as airfoil design.
CENTRIFUGAL FANS	RADIAL	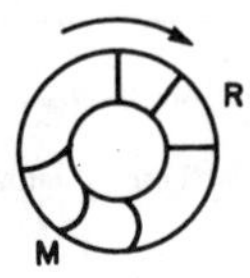 • Higher pressure characteristics than airfoil, backward-curved, and backward-inclined fans. • Curve may have a break to left of peak pressure and fan should not be operated in this area. • Power rises continually to free delivery.	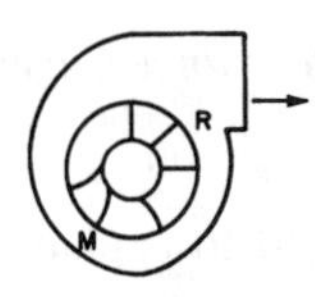 • Scroll. Usually narrowest of all centrifugal designs. • Because wheel design is less efficient, housing dimensions are not as critical as for airfoil and backward-inclined fans.
CENTRIFUGAL FANS	FORWARD-CURVED	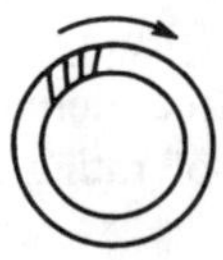 • Flatter pressure curve and lower efficiency than the airfoil, backward-curved, and backward-inclined. • Do not rate fan in the pressure curve dip to the left of peak pressure. • Power rises continually toward free delivery. Motor selection must take this into account.	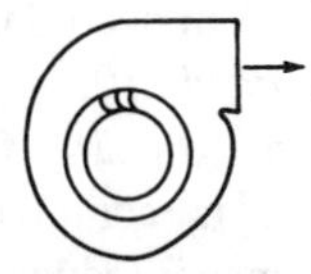 • Scroll similar to and often identical to other centrifugal fan designs. • Fit between wheel and inlet not as critical as for airfoil and backward-inclined fans.
AXIAL FANS	PROPELLER	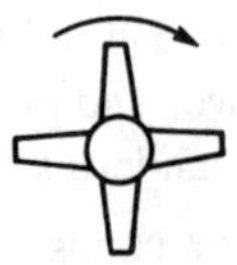 • Low efficiency. • Limited to low-pressure applications. • Usually low cost impellers have two or more blades of single thickness attached to relatively small hub. • Primary energy transfer by velocity pressure.	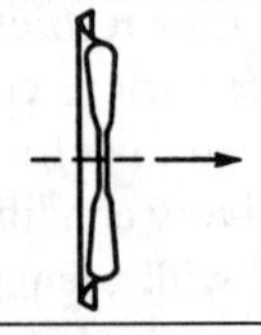 • Simple circular ring, orifice plate, or venturi. • Optimum design is close to blade tips and forms smooth airfoil into wheel.
AXIAL FANS	TUBEAXIAL	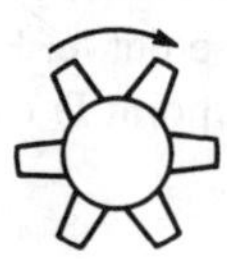 • Somewhat more efficient and capable of developing more useful static pressure than propeller fan. • Usually has 4 to 8 blades with airfoil or single-thickness cross section. • Hub usually less than transfer by velocity pressure.	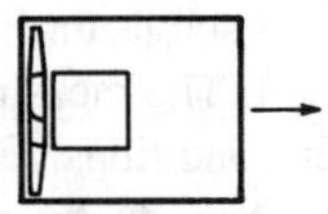 • Cylindrical tube with close clearance to blade tips.
AXIAL FANS	VANEAXIAL	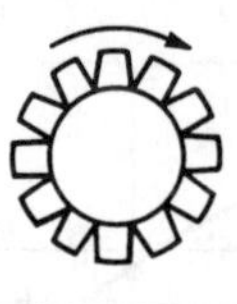 • Good blade design gives medium- to high-pressure capability at good efficiency. • Most efficient of these fans have airfoil blades. • Blades may have fixed, adjustable, or controllable pitch. • Hub is usually greater than half fan tip diameter.	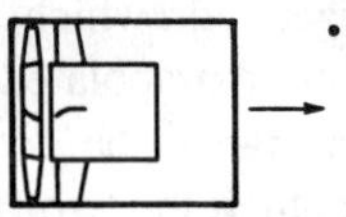 • Cylindrical tube with close clearance to blade tips. • Guide vanes upstream or downstream from impeller increase pressure capability and efficiency.
SPECIAL DESIGNS	TUBULAR CENTRIFUGAL	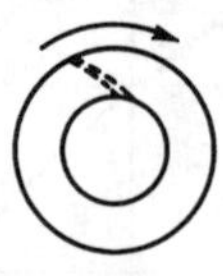 • Performance similar to backward-curved fan except capacity and pressure are lower. • Lower efficiency than backward-curved fan. • Performance curve may have a dip to the left of peak pressure.	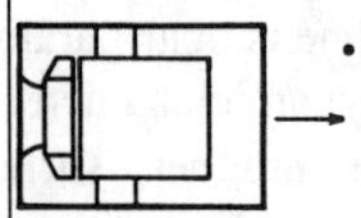 • Cylindrical tube similar to vaneaxial fan, except clearance to wheel is not as close. • Air discharges radially from wheel and turns 90° to flow through guide vanes.
SPECIAL DESIGNS	POWER ROOF VENTILATORS — CENTRIFUGAL	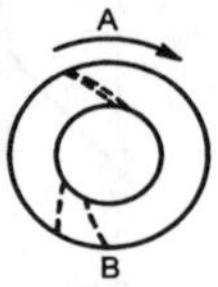 • Low-pressure exhaust systems such as general factory, kitchen, warehouse, and some commercial installations. • Provides positive exhaust ventilation, which is an advantage over gravity-type exhaust units. • Centrifugal units are slightly quieter than axial units.	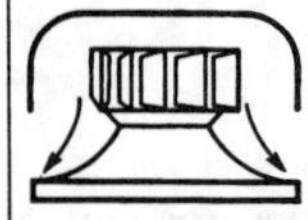 • Normal housing not used, since air discharges from impeller in full circle. • Usually does not include configuration to recover velocity pressure component.
SPECIAL DESIGNS	POWER ROOF VENTILATORS — AXIAL	 • Low-pressure exhaust systems such as general factory, kitchen, warehouse, and some commercial installations. • Provides positive exhaust ventilation, which is an advantage over gravity-type exhaust units.	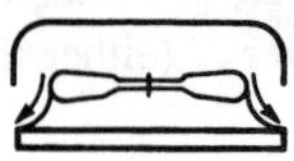 • Essentially a propeller fan mounted in a supporting structure. • Hood protects fan from weather and acts as safety guard. • Air discharges from annular space at bottom of weather hood.

Table 9-5 Types of Fans (*Concluded*)

PERFORMANCE CURVES[a]	PERFORMANCE CHARACTERISTICS	APPLICATIONS
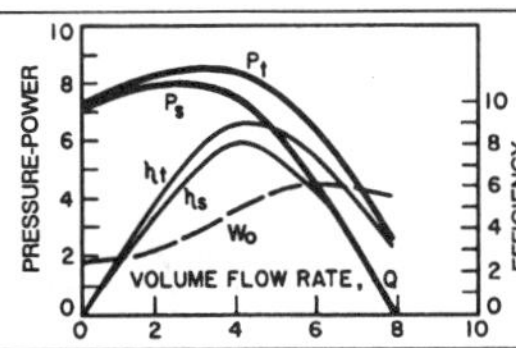	• Highest efficiencies occur at 50 to 60% of wide open volume. This volume also has good pressure characteristics. • Power reaches maximum near peak efficiency and becomes lower, or self-limiting, toward free delivery.	• General heating, ventilating, and air-conditioning applications. • Usually only applied to large systems, which may be low-, medium-, or high-pressure applications. • Applied to large, clean-air industrial operations for significant energy savings.
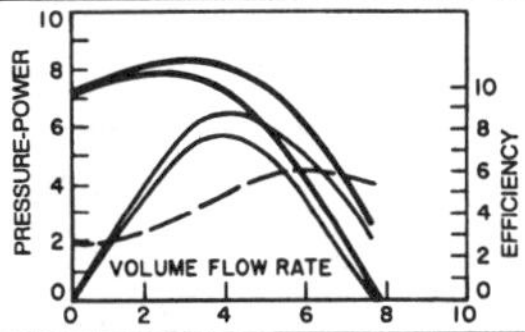	• Similar to airfoil fan, except peak efficiency slightly lower.	• Same heating, ventilating, and air-conditioning applications as airfoil fan. • Used in some industrial applications where airfoil blade may corrode or erode due to environment.
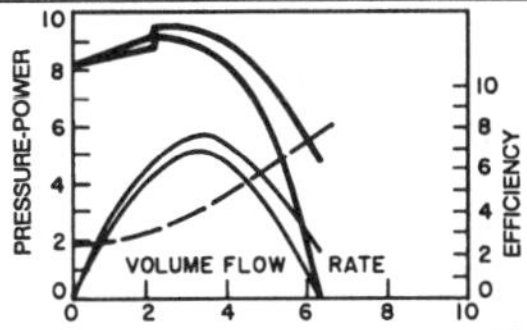	• Higher pressure characteristics than airfoil and backward-curved fans. • Pressure may drop suddenly at left of peak pressure, but this usually causes no problems. • Power rises continually to free delivery.	• Primarily for materials handling in industrial plants. Also for some high-pressure industrial requirements. • Rugged wheel is simple to repair in the field. Wheel sometimes coated with special material. • Not common for HVAC applications.
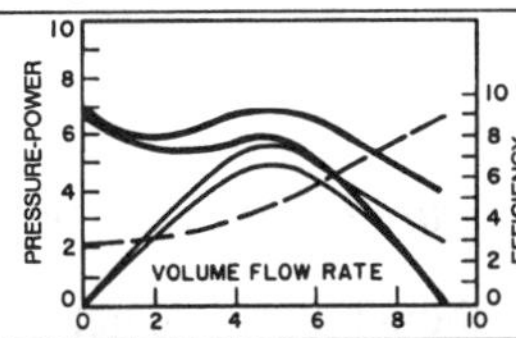	• Pressure curve less steep than that of backward-curved fans. Curve dips to left of peak pressure. • Highest efficiency to right of peak pressure at 40 to 50% of wide open volume. • Rate fan to right of peak pressure. • Account for power curve, which rises continually toward free delivery, when selecting motor.	• Primarily for low-pressure HVAC applications, such as residential furnaces, central station units, and packaged air conditioners.
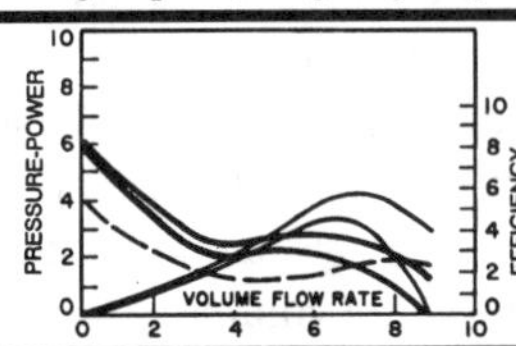	• High flow rate, but very low-pressure capabilities. • Maximum efficiency reached near free delivery. • Discharge pattern circular and airstream swirls.	• For low-pressure, high-volume air moving applications, such as air circulation in a space or ventilation through a wall without ductwork. • Used for makeup air applications.
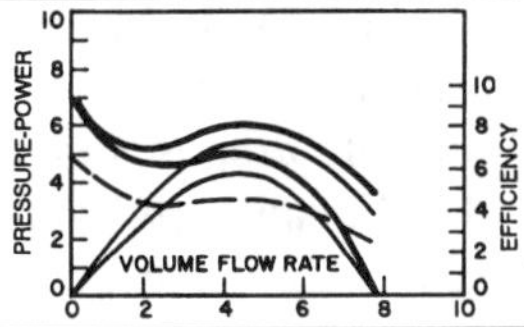	• High flow rate, medium-pressure capabilities. • Performance curve dips to left of peak pressure. Avoid operating fan in this region. • Discharge pattern circular and airstream rotates or swirls.	• Low- and medium-pressure ducted HVAC applications where air distribution downstream is not critical. • Used in some industrial applications, such as drying ovens, paint spray booths, and fume exhausts.
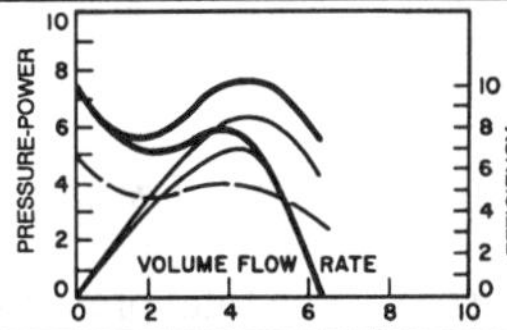	• High-pressure characteristics with medium-volume flow capabilities. • Performance curve dips to left of peak pressure due to aerodynamic stall. Avoid operating fan in this region. • Guide vanes correct circular motion imparted by wheel and improve pressure characteristics and efficiency of fan.	• General HVAC systems in low-, medium-, and high-pressure applications where straight-through flow and compact installation are required. • Has good downstream air distribution. • Used in industrial applications in place of tubeaxial fans. • More compact than centrifugal fans for same duty.
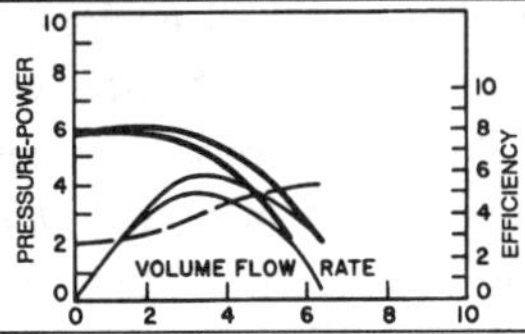	• Performance similar to backward-curved fan, except capacity and pressure is lower. • Lower efficiency than backward-curved fan because air turns 90°. • Performance curve of some designs is similar to axial flow fan and dips to left of peak pressure.	• Primarily for low-pressure, return air systems in HVAC applications. • Has straight-through flow.
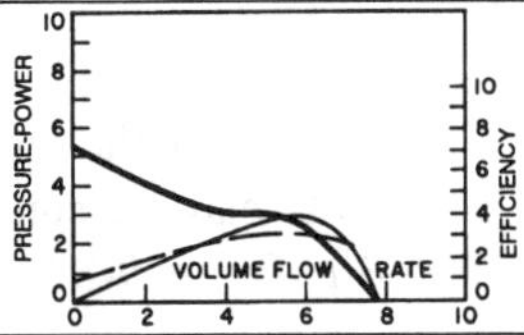	• Usually operated without ductwork; therefore, operates at very low pressure and high volume. • Only static pressure and static efficiency are shown for this fan.	• Low-pressure exhaust systems, such as general factory, kitchen, warehouse, and some commercial installations. • Low first cost and low operating cost give an advantage over gravity flow exhaust systems. • Centrifugal units are somewhat quieter than axial flow units.
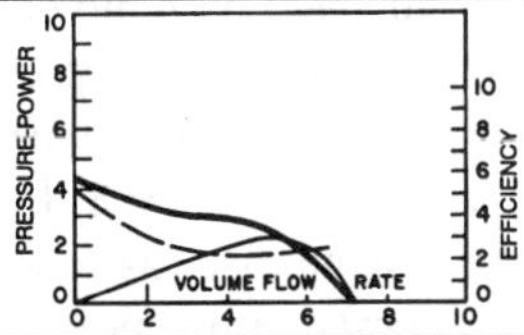	• Usually operated without ductwork; therefore, operates at very low pressure and high volume. • Only static pressure and static efficiency are shown for this fan.	• Low-pressure exhaust systems, such as general factory, kitchen, warehouse, and some commercial installations. • Low first cost and low operating cost give an advantage over gravity flow exhaust systems.

[a] These performance curves reflect general characteristics of various fans as commonly applied. They are not intended to provide complete selection criteria, since other parameters, such as diameter and speed, are not defined.

Using Fan Law 1a at Point E:

$$Q_1 = 6000\ (650/600) = 6500$$

Using Fan Law 1b:

$$p_{t1} = 1.13\ (650/600)^2 = 1.33$$

Therefore, the completed P_{tf1}, $N = 650$ curve may be generated by computing additional points from data on the base curve, such as point G from point F. If equivalent points of rating are joined, as illustrated by the dotted lines in Figure 9-6, they will lie on parabolas.

Each point on the base P_{tf} curve determines only one point on the computed curve. For example, there is no way to calculate point H from either point D or point F. It is totally unrelated to either one of these points. Point H is, however, related to some point between these two points on the base P_{tf} curve, and only that point can be used to locate point H. Furthermore, there is no way that point D can be used to calculate the position of point F on the base P_{tf} curve. The entire base curve must be defined by test.

9.2.5 Duct System Characteristics

A simplified duct system with three 90° elbows is shown in Figure 9-7. These elbows represent the resistance offered by the ductwork, heat exchangers, cabinets, dampers, grilles, and other system components. A given rate of airflow through a given system requires a definite total pressure in the system. The resulting total pressure varies as the volume flow rate squared.

The following Equation (9-14) is true for turbulent airflow systems. Heating, ventilating, and air-conditioning systems generally follow this law closely, and no serious error is introduced by its use.

$$\frac{\Delta p_2}{\Delta p_1} = \left(\frac{Q_1}{Q_2}\right)^2 \qquad (9\text{-}14)$$

The discussion in this chapter is limited to turbulent flow, which is the flow regime in which most fans operate. In some systems, particularly constant or variable volume air conditioning, the air handling devices and associated controls may produce system resistance curves that deviate

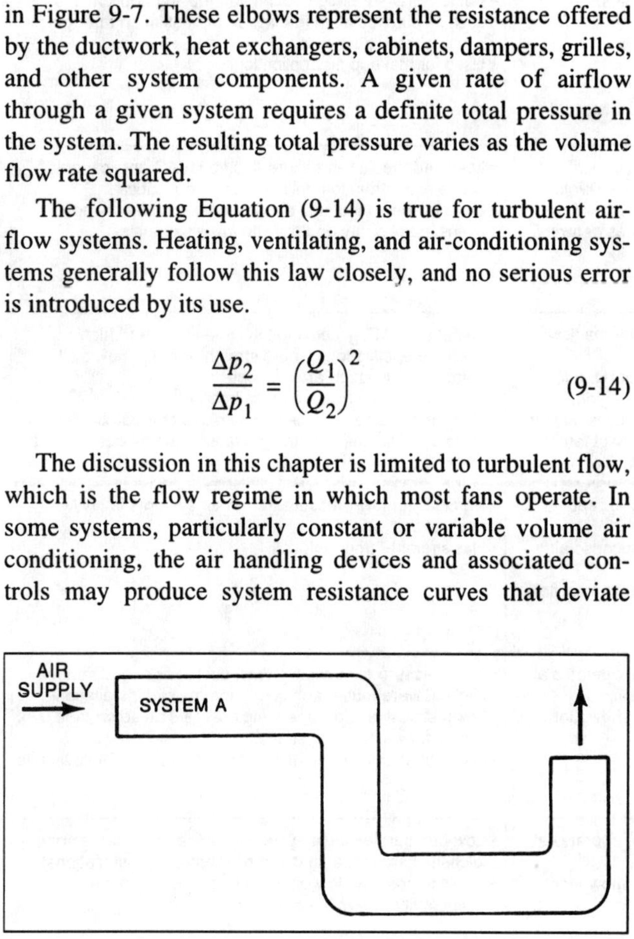

Fig. 9-7 Simplified Duct System with Resistance to Flow Represented by Three 90° Elbows

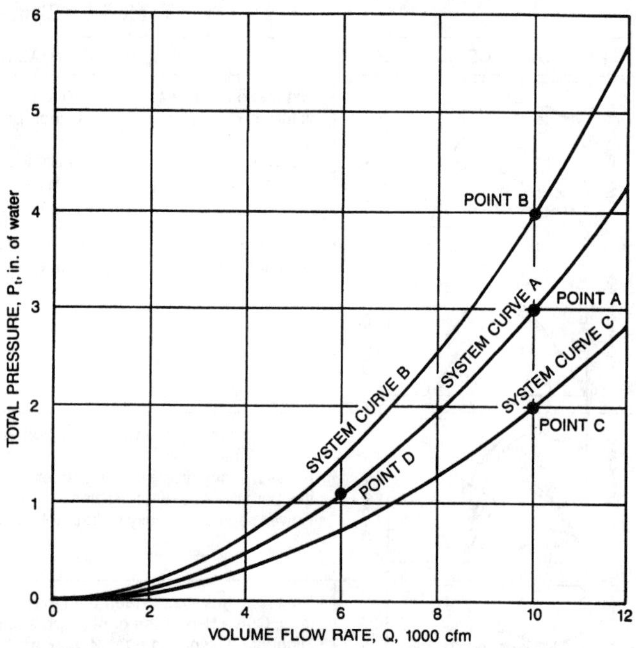

Fig. 9-8 Example System Total Pressure Loss (Δp) Curves

widely from Equation (9-14), even though each element of the system may be described by this equation.

Note that Equation (9-14) permits plotting a turbulent flow system's pressure loss (Δp) curve from one known operating condition (see Figure 9-5). The fixed system must operate at some point on this system curve as the volume flow rate changes. As an example, at point A, curve A, Figure 9-8, when the flow rate through a duct system such as shown in Figure 9-7 is 10,000 cfm, the total pressure drop is 3 in. of water. If these values are substituted in Equation (9-14) for Δp_1 and Q_1, other points of the system's Δp curve can be determined.

For 6000 cfm:

$$\Delta p_2 = 3 \text{ in. of water } (6000/10{,}000)^2 = 1.08 \text{ in. of water}$$

If a change is made in the system so that the total pressure at design flow rate is increased, the system will no longer operate on the previous Δp curve; a new curve will be defined.

For example, in Figure 9-9, an additional elbow has been added to the schematic duct system shown in Figure 9-7, which increases the total pressure of the system. If the total pressure at 10,000 cfm is increased by 1.0 in. of water, the system total pressure drop at this point will now be 3.0 in. of water, as shown by point B in Figure 9-8. Following the procedure outlined above, a series of Δp points may be computed and a new curve plotted (Δp curve B in Figure 9-8).

If the system in Figure 9-7 is now changed by removing one of the schematic elbows, the resulting system total pressure drops below the total pressure resistance (Figure 9-10). The new Δp curve is shown in Curve C of Figure 9-8. For curve C, a total pressure reduction of 1.0 in. has been assumed when 10,000 cfm flows through the system; thus, the point of operation is at 2.0 in. of water as shown by point C. These

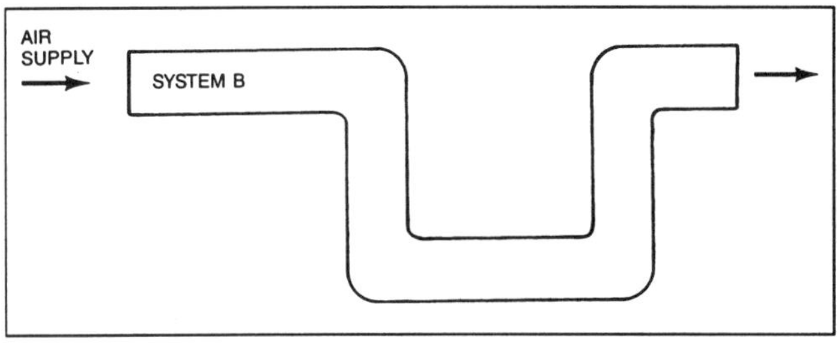

Fig. 9-9 Resistance Added to System of Figure 9-7

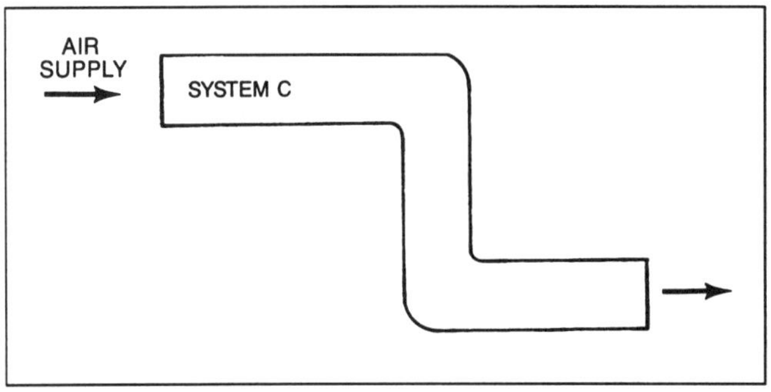

Fig. 9-10 Resistance Removed from that of Figure 9-7

three AP curves all follow the relationship expressed in Equation (9-14). Note also that these curves result from changes within the system itself and do not change the fan performance. During the design phase, such system total pressure changes may be due to studies of alternate duct routing, studies of differences in duct sizes, allowance for future duct extensions, or the effect of the design safety factor being applied to the system.

In an actual operating system, these three Δp curves could represent three system characteristic lines that result from three different positions of a throttling control damper. Curve C is the most open position, and curve B is the most closed position of the three positions illustrated. A control damper actually forms a continuous series of these Δp curves as it moves from a wide open position to a completely closed position and covers a much wider range of operation than illustrated here. Such curves could also represent the clogging of turbulent flow filters in a system.

9.2.6 Fan Selection

After the system pressure loss curve of the air distribution system has been defined, a fan can be selected to meet the system's requirements. Fan manufacturers present performance data in either the tabular (multirating table) or the graphic (curve) as in Figure 9-11a, which shows the performance of a fan of a fixed size running at fixed speed. Figure 9-11b is an example of a manufacturers fan table.

Multirating tables usually provide only performance data within the recommended (safe) operating range. The optimum selection area or peak efficiency point is identified in various ways by the different manufacturers. Performance data in the usual fan tables are based on arbitrary increments of flow rate and pressure. In these tables, adjacent data,

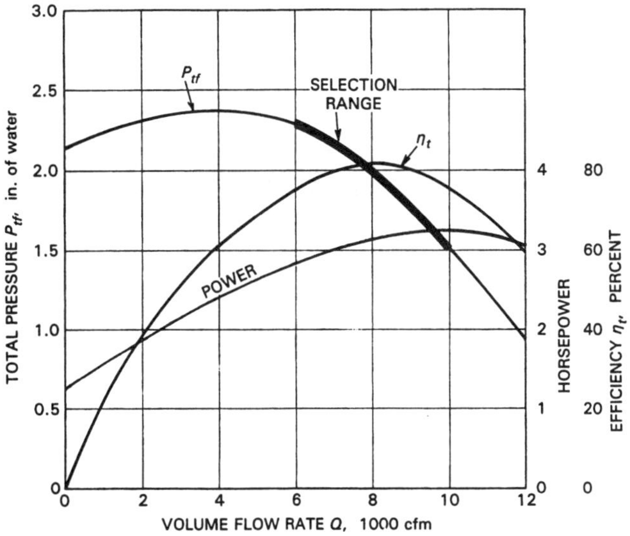

Fig. 9-11a Typical Manufacturer's Fan Performance Curve

either horizontally or vertically, represent different points of operation (i.e., different points of rating) on the fan performance curve. These points of rating depend solely on the fan's characteristics; they cannot be obtained one from the other by use of the Fan Laws. However, these points are usually close together, so intermediate points may be interpolated arithmetically with accuracy adequate for fan selection.

The selection of a fan for a particular air distribution system requires the fan pressure characteristics to fit the system pressure characteristics. Thus, the total system must be evaluated and the flow requirements and resistances existing at the fan inlet and outlet must be known. The direct effect that certain types of installations have on fan performance must also be considered. Performance pressure changes, known as system effect factors, are a direct effect that must be added to the system resistance before fan selection.

Fan speed and power requirements are then calculated using one of the methods available from fan manufacturers. These may consist of the multirating tables as mentioned or of single- or multispeed performance curves or graphs.

The point of operation selected must be at a desirable point on the fan curve, so that maximum efficiency and resistance to stall and pulsation can be attained (Figure 9-12). On systems where more than one point of operation is encountered during operation, the range of performance must be evaluated to determine how the selected fan will react within this complete range. This is particularly true in variable volume systems, where the fan not only experiences a change in performance, but the entire system does not follow the relationship defined in Equation (9-14). In these cases, actual losses in the system at performance extremes must be evaluated.

9.3 Air-Diffusing Equipment

Supply air outlets and diffusing equipment introduce air into a conditioned space to obtain a desired indoor atmo-

SIZE 273

Wheel diameter: 27"

Fan outlet area: 4.19 sq. ft.

$$\text{Maximum BHP} = 2.87 \left(\frac{\text{RPM}}{1000}\right)^3$$

CFM	OV	½" SP		1" SP		1½" SP		2" SP		2½" SP		3" SP		4" SP		5" SP		6" SP		7" SP		8" SP	
		RPM	BHP	RPM	BHP	RPM	BHP	RPM	BHP	RPM	BHP	RPM	BHP	RPM	BHP	RPM	BHP	RPM	BHP	RPM	BHP	RPM	BHP
3351	800	487	0.33	643	0.68	783	1.11	904	1.57	1010	2.07	1108	2.61	1280	3.74	1430	4.96	1568	6.29	1692	7.68	1809	9.15
3770	900	511	0.38	652	0.75	784	1.19	904	1.68	1010	2.21	1107	2.76	1279	3.95	1432	5.25	1566	6.61	1694	8.07	1808	9.56
4189	1000	539	0.44	665	0.82	788	1.27	904	1.78	1011	2.34	1106	2.92	1279	4.17	1429	5.51	1567	6.93	1691	8.41	1809	10.0
4608	1100	569	0.51	683	0.91	797	1.37	908	1.91	1011	2.47	1107	3.08	1278	4.38	1430	5.77	1568	7.27	1691	8.79	1808	10.4
5027	1200	601	0.58	705	1.01	810	1.48	915	2.02	1015	2.62	1108	3.24	1278	4.61	1429	6.04	1567	7.58	1691	9.17	1810	10.8
5446	1300	634	0.67	730	1.11	828	1.61	925	2.16	1020	2.77	1110	3.41	1279	4.82	1429	6.31	1566	7.91	1691	9.56	1808	11.2
5865	1400	668	0.77	758	1.23	847	1.74	939	2.31	1027	2.92	1115	3.59	1279	5.02	1429	6.58	1566	8.22	1692	9.94	1809	11.7
6284	1500	704	0.88	787	1.36	871	1.88	955	2.46	1040	3.11	1122	3.77	1282	5.26	1431	6.86	1565	8.53	1692	10.3	1809	12.1
6703	1600	739	1.01	818	1.51	896	2.05	975	2.64	1054	3.28	1133	3.98	1288	5.51	1431	7.13	1566	8.87	1691	10.7	1808	12.5
7541	1800	813	1.28	884	1.84	953	2.42	1022	3.05	1092	3.72	1163	4.44	1303	6.01	1440	7.71	1568	9.51	1692	11.4	1806	13.4
8379	2000	887	1.62	952	2.22	1015	2.86	1077	3.52	1140	4.23	1203	4.97	1329	6.58	1455	8.34	1578	10.2	1696	12.2	1809	14.3
9217	2200	962	2.01	1024	2.69	1081	3.36	1138	4.07	1194	4.81	1252	5.61	1367	7.27	1482	9.08	1595	11.0	1708	13.0	1816	15.2
10055	2400	1039	2.49	1096	3.21	1149	3.94	1202	4.71	1253	5.47	1306	6.31	1411	8.05	1515	9.88	1622	11.8	1726	13.9	1829	16.2
10893	2600	1115	3.01	1170	3.81	1220	4.59	1268	5.41	1317	6.23	1364	7.08	1460	8.87	1558	10.8	1654	12.8	1753	15.0	1850	17.3
11731	2800	1192	3.62	1244	4.49	1293	5.35	1337	6.18	1382	7.07	1427	7.96	1517	9.87	1606	11.8	1696	13.9	1787	16.1	1878	18.4
12569	3000	1270	4.32	1319	5.25	1364	6.14	1408	7.07	1451	8.01	1492	8.95	1576	10.9	1658	12.9	1741	15.0	1826	17.3	1912	19.8
13407	3200	1349	5.13	1395	6.11	1438	7.06	1480	8.05	1520	9.03	1559	10.0	1637	12.0	1714	14.1	1793	16.4	1870	18.7	1952	21.2
14245	3400	1427	6.02	1472	7.07	1513	8.09	1553	9.12	1591	10.1	1628	11.2	1703	13.3	1774	15.5	1850	17.9	1923	20.3	1997	22.7

SIZE 303

Wheel diameter: 30"

Fan outlet area: 5.17 sq. ft.

$$\text{Maximum BHP} = 4.83 \left(\frac{\text{RPM}}{1000}\right)^3$$

CFM	OV	½" SP		1" SP		1½" SP		2" SP		2½" SP		3" SP		4" SP		5" SP		6" SP		7" SP		8" SP	
		RPM	BHP	RPM	BHP	RPM	BHP	RPM	BHP	RPM	BHP	RPM	BHP	RPM	BHP	RPM	BHP	RPM	BHP	RPM	BHP	RPM	BHP
4135	800	438	0.41	579	0.84	704	1.36	813	1.94	910	2.56	997	3.21	1151	4.61	1286	6.12	1410	7.76	1523	9.47	1628	11.2
4652	900	460	0.47	586	0.92	705	1.46	813	2.07	910	2.72	996	3.41	1150	4.87	1288	6.47	1409	8.14	1524	9.96	1629	11.8
5169	1000	484	0.54	598	1.01	710	1.58	814	2.21	909	2.88	996	3.61	1150	5.14	1288	6.81	1410	8.55	1524	10.4	1628	12.3
5686	1100	512	0.62	614	1.11	717	1.69	817	2.34	910	3.05	996	3.81	1150	5.41	1286	7.12	1411	8.96	1524	10.8	1630	12.9
6203	1200	541	0.72	634	1.23	730	1.83	823	2.51	913	3.23	996	4.01	1150	5.67	1286	7.45	1409	9.35	1524	11.3	1628	13.4
6720	1300	571	0.83	657	1.37	744	1.98	832	2.66	917	3.41	998	4.21	1151	5.94	1286	7.79	1409	9.74	1522	11.7	[illegible]	13.9
7237	1400	601	0.95	682	1.51	762	2.14	844	2.85	926	3.62	1003	4.43	1152	6.22	1286	8.12	1409	10.1	1522	12.2	1628	14.4
7754	1500	633	1.08	709	1.68	783	2.32	860	3.05	935	3.83	1011	4.67	1154	6.48	1287	8.46	1409	10.5	1522	12.7	1628	15.0
8271	1600	665	1.23	736	1.85	806	2.53	877	3.26	949	4.06	1020	4.92	1158	6.78	1288	8.79	1409	10.9	1522	13.1	1626	15.5
9305	1800	731	1.58	795	2.27	857	2.98	920	3.77	983	4.59	1046	5.48	1172	7.41	1295	9.51	1413	11.7	1522	14.1	1628	16.6
10339	2000	798	1.99	857	2.74	913	3.53	970	4.37	1025	5.22	1083	6.15	1197	8.14	1311	10.3	1420	12.6	1528	15.1	1628	17.6
11373	2200	866	2.48	922	3.32	972	4.14	1023	5.02	1074	5.93	1126	6.91	1230	8.96	1333	11.2	1437	13.6	1537	16.1	1636	18.8
12407	2400	935	3.07	986	3.96	1034	4.86	1081	5.79	1129	6.79	1175	7.78	1270	9.92	1364	12.2	1459	14.6	1553	17.2	1646	20.1
13441	2600	1003	3.72	1053	4.71	1097	5.67	1141	6.65	1184	7.68	1227	8.72	1313	10.9	1402	13.3	1488	15.8	1577	18.5	1665	21.3
14475	2800	1072	4.46	1119	5.53	1163	6.59	1204	7.66	1244	8.71	1283	9.82	1365	12.1	1445	14.6	1526	17.1	1608	19.9	1689	22.8
15509	3000	1142	5.33	1187	6.47	1227	7.57	1267	8.72	1305	9.88	1343	11.0	1417	13.4	1491	15.9	1568	18.7	1642	21.4	1720	24.4
16543	3200	1213	6.32	1255	7.53	1294	8.71	1331	9.92	1368	11.1	1402	12.3	1473	14.8	1544	17.5	1613	20.2	1685	23.2	1756	26.1
17577	3400	1284	7.42	1324	8.72	1361	9.98	1397	11.2	1431	12.5	1465	13.8	1532	16.4	1598	19.2	1664	22.0	1730	25.0	1797	28.1

SIZE 363

Wheel diameter: 36½"

Fan outlet area: 7.66 sq. ft.

$$\text{Maximum BHP} = 12.8 \left(\frac{\text{RPM}}{1000}\right)^3$$

CFM	OV	½" SP		1" SP		1½" SP		2" SP		2½" SP		3" SP		4" SP		5" SP		6" SP		7" SP		8" SP	
		RPM	BHP	RPM	BHP	RPM	BHP	RPM	BHP	RPM	BHP	RPM	BHP	RPM	BHP	RPM	BHP	RPM	BHP	RPM	BHP	RPM	BHP
6127	800	360	0.58	475	1.21	578	1.97	669	2.81	750	3.69	823	4.64	953	6.68	1065	8.84	1166	11.1	1260	13.6	1348	16.1
6893	900	377	0.67	481	1.33	580	2.11	668	2.99	748	3.93	821	4.93	952	7.08	1063	9.33	1166	11.7	1261	14.3	1348	17.0
7659	1000	397	0.78	491	1.46	582	2.26	669	3.18	747	4.16	820	5.21	950	7.46	1064	9.86	1166	12.3	1260	15.0	1347	17.8
8425	1100	419	0.91	504	1.61	589	2.44	670	3.37	748	4.41	819	5.49	948	7.82	1061	10.3	1165	12.9	1260	15.7	1347	18.6
9191	1200	442	1.03	520	1.77	598	2.63	675	3.59	749	4.64	819	5.77	946	8.21	1060	10.7	1164	13.5	1258	16.4	1346	19.4
9957	1300	466	1.19	539	1.97	611	2.85	682	3.82	752	4.89	820	6.06	945	8.55	1058	11.2	1162	14.1	1257	17.1	1345	20.2
10723	1400	491	1.36	559	2.18	626	3.09	693	4.09	758	5.18	823	6.36	946	8.96	1058	11.7	1160	14.6	1255	17.7	1344	20.9
11489	1500	517	1.55	580	2.41	643	3.35	705	4.37	767	5.49	829	6.69	947	9.34	1057	12.1	1158	15.2	1253	18.4	1340	21.6
12255	1600	543	1.76	603	2.67	662	3.64	719	4.69	778	5.82	836	7.05	950	9.73	1058	12.6	1157	15.7	1252	19.0	1339	22.4
13787	1800	596	2.23	651	3.26	703	4.31	754	5.41	806	6.61	859	7.88	962	10.6	1062	13.6	1158	16.9	1251	20.3	1336	23.9
15319	2000	650	2.81	701	3.93	748	5.08	795	6.27	842	7.52	888	8.84	981	11.6	1075	14.8	1166	18.1	1253	21.7	1338	25.4
16851	2200	704	3.47	752	4.71	796	5.96	838	7.21	881	8.55	923	9.92	1009	12.8	1094	16.0	1178	19.4	1261	23.1	1342	27.0
18383	2400	759	4.24	804	5.61	845	6.93	885	8.31	924	9.71	963	11.1	1041	14.2	1119	17.5	1197	21.0	1274	24.7	1351	28.7
19915	2600	815	5.13	857	6.61	869	8.08	934	9.54	971	11.0	1007	12.6	1078	15.7	1150	19.1	1221	22.7	1294	26.6	1364	30.5
21447	2800	871	6.15	911	7.75	948	9.33	984	10.9	1017	12.4	1051	14.1	1119	17.4	1184	20.9	1252	24.7	1319	28.6	1386	32.7
22979	3000	926	7.27	966	9.05	1000	10.7	1035	12.4	1066	14.0	1098	15.7	1162	19.3	1223	22.9	1286	26.8	1348	30.8	1410	35.0
24511	3200	984	8.61	1020	10.4	1053	12.2	1086	14.0	1117	15.8	1147	17.6	1206	21.3	1266	25.2	1324	29.2	1381	33.2	1440	37.5
26043	3400	1040	10.0	1075	12.0	1108	14.0	1138	15.8	1168	17.7	1197	19.7	1253	23.6	1309	27.6	1363	31.6	1418	35.9		

BHP shown does not include belt drive losses.
Performance shown is for General Purpose Fans with outlet ducts and with or without inlet ducts.
Selection within tinted area renders most efficient. quietest operation.

Fig. 9-11b Manufacturer's Fan Performance Table

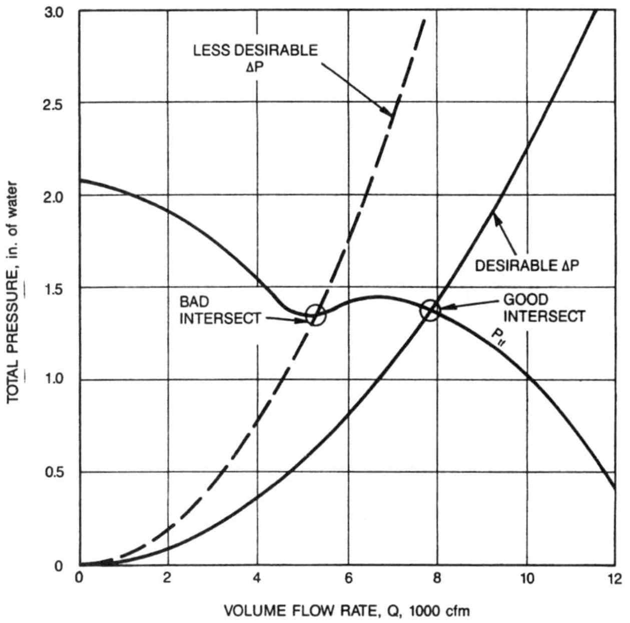

Fig. 9-12 Desirable Combination of p_{tf} and Δp Curves

spheric environment. Return and exhaust air are removed from the space through return and exhaust inlets. Various types of diffusing equipment are available as standard manufactured products. Refer to Chapter 31 of the 1997 *ASHRAE Handbook—Fundamentals* and Chapter 17 of the 1996 *ASHRAE Handbook—Systems and Equipment* for additional details concerning space air distribution.

Air diffusion in warm air heating, ventilating, and air-conditioning systems should create the proper combination of temperature, humidity, and air motion in the occupied zone of the conditioned room [floor to 6 ft (1.8 m) above floor level]. Standard limits have been established as **acceptable, effective draft temperature**. This term comprises air temperature, air motion, relative humidity, and their physiological effect on the human body. Any variation from accepted standards of one of these elements results in discomfort to the occupants. Such discomfort may arise due to excessive room air temperature variations (horizontally, vertically, or both), excessive air motion (draft), failure to deliver or distribute the air according to the load requirements at the different locations, or overly rapid fluctuation of room temperature.

To define the difference θ in effective draft temperature between any point in the occupied zone and the control condition, investigators have used the following equation:

$$\theta = (t_x - t_c) - a(V_x - b) \tag{9-15}$$

where

t_x = local airstream dry-bulb temperature, °F.
V_x = local airstream velocity, ft/min
t_c = average room dry-bulb temperature, °F
b = 30
a = 0.07

Equation (9-15) accounts for the feeling of coolness produced by air motion. It also shows that a 1.8°F temperature change is equal to a 25 fpm velocity change. In summer, the local airstream temperature t_x is below the control temperature. Hence, both temperature and velocity terms are negative when the velocity V_x is greater than 30 fpm, and both of them add to the feeling of coolness. If, in winter, t_x is above the control temperature, any air velocity above 30 fpm subtracts from the feeling of warmth produced by t_x. Therefore, it is usually possible to have zero difference in effective temperature between location "x" and the control point in winter, but not in summer.

Conditioned air is normally supplied to air outlets at velocities much higher than would be acceptable in the occupied zone. The conditioned air temperature may be above, below, or equal to the temperature of the air in the occupied zone. Proper air distribution, therefore, calls for: (1) entrainment of room air by the primary airstream outside the zone of occupancy so that air motion and temperature differences are reduced to acceptable limits before the air enters the occupied zone; and (2) counteraction of the natural convection and radiation effects within the room.

9.3.1 Supply Air Outlets

The correct types of outlets, properly sized and properly located, control the air pattern within the space to obtain proper air motion and temperature equalization in the occupied zone. Four types of supply outlets are commonly available: (1) grille outlets, (2) slot diffuser outlets, (3) ceiling diffuser outlets, and (4) perforated ceiling panels. These outlets have different construction features and physical configurations and differ in their performance characteristics (air pattern).

9.3.2 Outlet Selection and Location Procedure

The following procedure is generally used in selecting outlet locations and types of outlets:

1. Determine the amount of air to be supplied to each room. Refer to Chapter 3 to determine air quantities for heating and cooling. Determine the amount of outdoor air to be introduced according to ventilation requirements of appropriate codes.
2. Select the type and quantity of outlets for each room, considering such factors as air quantity required, distance available for throw or radius of diffusion, structural characteristics, and architectural concepts. Table 9-7 is based on experience and typical ratings of various types of outlets. It may be used as a guide to the types of outlets applicable to various room air loadings. Special conditions such as ceiling heights greater than 8 to 12 ft (2.4 to 3.6 m), exposed duct mounting, and so forth, as well as product modifications and unusual conditions of room occupancy can all modify the information in this table. Manufacturers' rating data should be consulted to determine the suitability of the specific outlets.
3. Locate outlets to distribute the air as uniformly as possible throughout the room. Outlets may be sized and located to distribute air in various portions of the room in proportion to the heat gain or loss in those areas.

Table 9-7 Guide to Use of Various Outlets

Type of Outlet	Air Loading of Floor Space, cfm/ft² [L/(s·m²)]	Approximate Maximum Air Changes per hour for 10 ft (3 m) Ceiling
Grille	0.6 to 1.2 (3 to 6)	7
Slot	0.8 to 2.0 (4 to 10)	12
Perforated panel	0.9 to 3.0 (5 to 15)	18
Ceiling diffuser	0.9 to 5.0 (5 to 25)	30
Perforated ceiling	1.0 to 10 (5 to 50)	60

4. Select proper outlet size from manufacturers' ratings according to the air quantities, discharge velocities, distribution patterns, and sound levels. Note manufacturers' recommendations with regard to use, method of installation, minimum velocities, maximum temperature differentials, and any air distribution characteristics that may limit the performance of the outlet. Give special attention to obstructions to the normal air-distribution pattern.

9.3.3 Noise Control

Sound at an outlet is composed of the sound generation of the outlet (a function of the discharge velocity) and the transmission of systemic noise (a function of the size of the outlet). Higher-frequency sounds are caused by excessive outlet velocity, but they may also be the result of sounds generated in the duct by the moving air stream. Lower-pitched sounds are generally caused by mechanical equipment noise transmitted through the duct system and outlet. The cause of high-frequency sounds can be pinpointed as outlet or system sounds by removing the outlet during operation. A reduction in sound level indicates that the outlet is causing noise. If the sound level remains essentially unchanged, then the system is at fault.

Example 9.3. Calculate the maximum throw for an outlet grille with a core area 12 in. by 18.75 in., $R_{fa} = 0.90$, $C_d = 0.80$, $K' = 5.0$ (see Table 3, Chapter 31 of the 1997 *ASHRAE Handbook—Fundamentals*) and the discharge flow rate is 600 cfm. If this outlet is circular, what is the total volume flow rate at the maximum throw?

Solution:

(a) Use Equation (10), Chapter 31 of the 1997 *ASHRAE Handbook—Fundamentals*, to calculate the maximum throw for an outlet.

$$L = \frac{K'Q}{50Z\sqrt{A_c}}$$

$$A_c = 12 \times 18.75/144 = 1.56 \text{ ft}^2$$

$$Z = \sqrt{C_d R_{fa}} = \sqrt{0.8 \times 0.9} = 0.848$$

$$L = \frac{5(600)}{50(0.848)\sqrt{1.56}} = 56.7 \text{ ft}$$

(b) Use Equation (13), Chapter 31 of the 1997 *ASHRAE Handbook—Fundamentals*, to estimate the entrainment ratio:

$$Q_x/Q_o = 2V_o/V_x \text{ or,}$$

$$V_o = (V_c/C_d)R_{fa}$$

$$V_c = Q/A_c = 600/1.56 = 384.6 \text{ fpm}$$

$$V_o = 384.6/(0.8 \times 0.9) = 534 \text{ fpm}$$

Therefore:

$$Q_x/Q_o = 2(534/50) = 21.36$$

$$Q_x = 21.36(600) = 12{,}800 \text{ cfm}$$

Example 9.4. At point A (1.5 m above the floor) in a room, the temperature is 26°C and the velocity is 0.15 m/s. At point B (150 mm above the floor) in the same room, the temperature is 21.5°C and the velocity is 0.40 m/s. The control temperature for the room is 24°C. Determine if either of these locations are considered to be drafty.

Solution:

Use Equation (1), Chapter 31 of the 1997 *ASHRAE Handbook—Fundamentals*, to calculate the difference in effective temperature Δt. At point A:

$$\Delta t = (t_x - 24) - 8(V_x - 0.15)$$

$$\Delta t = (26 - 24) - 8(0.150 - 0.15) = 2°\text{C}$$

From Figure 9, Chapter 31 of the 1997 *ASHRAE Handbook—Fundamentals*, for the neck region, most people would feel a sense of warmth. It would probably not feel drafty.

At point B:

$$\Delta t = (t_x - 24) - 8(V_x - 0.15)$$

$$\Delta t = (21.5 - 24) - 8(0.40 - 0.15) = -2.5 - 1.2 = -3.7°\text{C}$$

Figure 9 indicates that for the ankle region, more than half of the occupants would feel a draft at this point. If point A is above point B, the air distribution system is probably ineffective since a person would feel warm at the head and cool at the feet.

9.4 Pipe, Tube, and Fittings

9.4.1 Selection and Application

Listed in Tables 9-8 and 9-9 are the common sizes and dimensions for pipes and tubing used in the HVAC&R industry. Regulatory codes and voluntary standards of such organizations as the American Society of Mechanical Engineers (ASME) and American Society for Testing and Materials (ASTM) should be considered when selecting and applying these components.

9.4.2 Materials

Table 9-10 is a guide to materials used in heating and air conditioning. While steel, iron, and copper materials are most commonly used, iron and steel alloys, copper alloys, nickel and nickel alloys, and non-metallic pipe are finding increasing applications.

Codes, dimensional standards, and material specifications cover service requirements, which consider such effects as corrosion, scale, thermal or mechanical fatigue, and metallurgical instability at high temperatures. Copper and red

Table 9-8 Steel Pipe Data

(Table 2, Chapter 40, 1996 *ASHRAE Handbook—Systems and Equipment*)

Nominal Size, in.	Pipe OD, in.	Schedule Number or Weight[a]	Wall Thickness *t*, in.	Inside Diameter *d*, in.	Surface Area: Outside, ft²/ft	Surface Area: Inside, ft²/ft	Cross Section: Metal Area, in²	Cross Section: Flow Area, in²	Weight: Pipe, lb/ft	Weight: Water, lb/ft	Working Pressure[c] ASTM A53 B to 400°F: Mfr. Process	Joint Type[b]	psig
1/4	0.540	40 ST	0.088	0.364	0.141	0.095	0.125	0.104	0.424	0.045	CW	T	188
		80 XS	0.119	0.302	0.141	0.079	0.157	0.072	0.535	0.031	CW	T	871
3/8	0.675	40 ST	0.091	0.493	0.177	0.129	0.167	0.191	0.567	0.083	CW	T	203
		80 XS	0.126	0.423	0.177	0.111	0.217	0.141	0.738	0.061	CW	T	820
1/2	0.840	40 ST	0.109	0.622	0.220	0.163	0.250	0.304	0.850	0.131	CW	T	214
		80 XS	0.147	0.546	0.220	0.143	0.320	0.234	1.087	0.101	CW	T	753
3/4	1.050	40 ST	0.113	0.824	0.275	0.216	0.333	0.533	1.13	0.231	CW	T	217
		80 XS	0.154	0.742	0.275	0.194	0.433	0.432	1.47	0.187	CW	T	681
1	1.315	40 ST	0.133	1.049	0.344	0.275	0.494	0.864	1.68	0.374	CW	T	226
		80 XS	0.179	0.957	0.344	0.251	0.639	0.719	2.17	0.311	CW	T	642
1-1/4	1.660	40 ST	0.140	1.380	0.435	0.361	0.669	1.50	2.27	0.647	CW	T	229
		80 XS	0.191	1.278	0.435	0.335	0.881	1.28	2.99	0.555	CW	T	594
1-1/2	1.900	40 ST	0.145	1.610	0.497	0.421	0.799	2.04	2.72	0.881	CW	T	231
		80 XS	0.200	1.500	0.497	0.393	1.068	1.77	3.63	0.765	CW	T	576
2	2.375	40 ST	0.154	2.067	0.622	0.541	1.07	3.36	3.65	1.45	CW	T	230
		80 XS	0.218	1.939	0.622	0.508	1.48	2.95	5.02	1.28	CW	T	551
2-1/2	2.875	40 ST	0.203	2.469	0.753	0.646	1.70	4.79	5.79	2.07	CW	W	533
		80 XS	0.276	2.323	0.753	0.608	2.25	4.24	7.66	1.83	CW	W	835
3	3.500	40 ST	0.216	3.068	0.916	0.803	2.23	7.39	7.57	3.20	CW	W	482
		80 XS	0.300	2.900	0.916	0.759	3.02	6.60	10.25	2.86	CW	W	767
4	4.500	40 ST	0.237	4.026	1.178	1.054	3.17	12.73	10.78	5.51	CW	W	430
		80 XS	0.337	3.826	1.178	1.002	4.41	11.50	14.97	4.98	CW	W	695
6	6.625	40 ST	0.280	6.065	1.734	1.588	5.58	28.89	18.96	12.50	ERW	W	696
		80 XS	0.432	5.761	1.734	1.508	8.40	26.07	28.55	11.28	ERW	W	1209
8	8.625	30	0.277	8.071	2.258	2.113	7.26	51.16	24.68	22.14	ERW	W	526
		40 ST	0.322	7.981	2.258	2.089	8.40	50.03	28.53	21.65	ERW	W	643
		80 XS	0.500	7.625	2.258	1.996	12.76	45.66	43.35	19.76	ERW	W	1106
10	10.75	30	0.307	10.136	2.814	2.654	10.07	80.69	34.21	34.92	ERW	W	485
		40 ST	0.365	10.020	2.814	2.623	11.91	78.85	40.45	34.12	ERW	W	606
		XS	0.500	9.750	2.814	2.552	16.10	74.66	54.69	32.31	ERW	W	887
		80	0.593	9.564	2.814	2.504	18.92	71.84	64.28	31.09	ERW	W	1081
12	12.75	30	0.330	12.090	3.338	3.165	12.88	114.8	43.74	49.68	ERW	W	449
		ST	0.375	12.000	3.338	3.141	14.58	113.1	49.52	48.94	ERW	W	528
		40	0.406	11.938	3.338	3.125	15.74	111.9	53.48	48.44	ERW	W	583
		XS	0.500	11.750	3.338	3.076	19.24	108.4	65.37	46.92	ERW	W	748
		80	0.687	11.376	3.338	2.978	26.03	101.6	88.44	43.98	ERW	W	1076
14	14.00	30 ST	0.375	13.250	3.665	3.469	16.05	137.9	54.53	59.67	ERW	W	481
		40	0.437	13.126	3.665	3.436	18.62	135.3	63.25	58.56	ERW	W	580
		XS	0.500	13.000	3.665	3.403	21.21	132.7	72.04	57.44	ERW	W	681
		80	0.750	12.500	3.665	3.272	31.22	122.7	106.05	53.11	ERW	W	1081
16	16.00	30 ST	0.375	15.250	4.189	3.992	18.41	182.6	62.53	79.04	ERW	W	421
		40 XS	0.500	15.000	4.189	3.927	24.35	176.7	82.71	76.47	ERW	W	596
18	18.00	ST	0.375	17.250	4.712	4.516	20.76	233.7	70.54	101.13	ERW	W	374
		30	0.437	17.126	4.712	4.483	24.11	230.3	81.91	99.68	ERW	W	451
		XS	0.500	17.000	4.712	4.450	27.49	227.0	93.38	98.22	ERW	W	530
		40	0.562	16.876	4.712	4.418	30.79	223.7	104.59	96.80	ERW	W	607
20	20.00	20 ST	0.375	19.250	5.236	5.039	23.12	291.0	78.54	125.94	ERW	W	337
		30 XS	0.500	19.000	5.236	4.974	30.63	283.5	104.05	122.69	ERW	W	477
		40	0.593	18.814	5.236	4.925	36.15	278.0	122.82	120.30	ERW	W	581

[a] Numbers are schedule numbers per ASME *Standard* B36.10M; ST = Standard Weight; XS = Extra Strong.

[b] T = Thread; W = Weld

[c] Working pressures were calculated per ASME B31.9 using furnace butt-weld (continuous weld, CW) pipe through 4 in. and electric resistance weld (ERW) thereafter. The allowance A has been taken as

(1) 12.5% of *t* for mill tolerance on pipe wall thickness, *plus*

(2) An arbitrary corrosion allowance of 0.025 in. for pipe sizes through NPS 2 and 0.065 in. from NPS 2½ through 20, *plus*

(3) A thread cutting allowance for sizes through NPS 2.

Because the pipe wall thickness of threaded standard pipe is so small after deducting the allowance A, the mechanical strength of the pipe is impaired. It is good practice to limit standard weight threaded pipe pressure to 90 psig for steam and 125 psig for water.

Table 9-9 Copper Tube Data

(Table 3, Chapter 40, 1996 *ASHRAE Handbook—Systems and Equipment*)

Nominal Diameter, in.	Type	Wall Thickness t, in.	Diameter: Outside D, in.	Diameter: Inside d, in.	Surface Area: Outside, ft^2/ft	Surface Area: Inside, ft^2/ft	Cross Section: Metal Area, in^2	Cross Section: Flow Area, in^2	Weight: Tube, lb/ft	Weight: Water, lb/ft	Working Pressure[a,b,c] ASTM B88 to 250°F: Annealed, psig	Working Pressure[a,b,c] ASTM B88 to 250°F: Drawn, psig
1/4	K	0.035	0.375	0.305	0.098	0.080	0.037	0.073	0.145	0.032	851	1596
	L	0.030	0.375	0.315	0.098	0.082	0.033	0.078	0.126	0.034	730	1368
3/8	K	0.049	0.500	0.402	0.131	0.105	0.069	0.127	0.269	0.055	894	1676
	L	0.035	0.500	0.430	0.131	0.113	0.051	0.145	0.198	0.063	638	1197
	M	0.025	0.500	0.450	0.131	0.118	0.037	0.159	0.145	0.069	456	855
1/2	K	0.049	0.625	0.527	0.164	0.138	0.089	0.218	0.344	0.094	715	1341
	L	0.040	0.625	0.545	0.164	0.143	0.074	0.233	0.285	0.101	584	1094
	M	0.028	0.625	0.569	0.164	0.149	0.053	0.254	0.203	0.110	409	766
5/8	K	0.049	0.750	0.652	0.196	0.171	0.108	0.334	0.418	0.144	596	1117
	L	0.042	0.750	0.666	0.196	0.174	0.093	0.348	0.362	0.151	511	958
3/4	K	0.065	0.875	0.745	0.229	0.195	0.165	0.436	0.641	0.189	677	1270
	L	0.045	0.875	0.785	0.229	0.206	0.117	0.484	0.455	0.209	469	879
	M	0.032	0.875	0.811	0.229	0.212	0.085	0.517	0.328	0.224	334	625
1	K	0.065	1.125	0.995	0.295	0.260	0.216	0.778	0.839	0.336	527	988
	L	0.050	1.125	1.025	0.295	0.268	0.169	0.825	0.654	0.357	405	760
	M	0.035	1.125	1.055	0.295	0.276	0.120	0.874	0.464	0.378	284	532
1-1/4	K	0.065	1.375	1.245	0.360	0.326	0.268	1.217	1.037	0.527	431	808
	L	0.055	1.375	1.265	0.360	0.331	0.228	1.257	0.884	0.544	365	684
	M	0.042	1.375	1.291	0.360	0.338	0.176	1.309	0.682	0.566	279	522
	DWV	0.040	1.375	1.295	0.360	0.339	0.168	1.317	0.650	0.570	265	497
1-1/2	K	0.072	1.625	1.481	0.425	0.388	0.351	1.723	1.361	0.745	404	758
	L	0.060	1.625	1.505	0.425	0.394	0.295	1.779	1.143	0.770	337	631
	M	0.049	1.625	1.527	0.425	0.400	0.243	1.831	0.940	0.792	275	516
	DWV	0.042	1.625	1.541	0.425	0.403	0.209	1.865	0.809	0.807	236	442
2	K	0.083	2.125	1.959	0.556	0.513	0.532	3.014	2.063	1.304	356	668
	L	0.070	2.125	1.985	0.556	0.520	0.452	3.095	1.751	1.339	300	573
	M	0.058	2.125	2.009	0.556	0.526	0.377	3.170	1.459	1.372	249	467
	DWV	0.042	2.125	2.041	0.556	0.534	0.275	3.272	1.065	1.416	180	338
2-1/2	K	0.095	2.625	2.435	0.687	0.637	0.755	4.657	2.926	2.015	330	619
	L	0.080	2.625	2.465	0.687	0.645	0.640	4.772	2.479	2.065	278	521
	M	0.065	2.625	2.495	0.687	0.653	0.523	4.889	2.026	2.116	226	423
3	K	0.109	3.125	2.907	0.818	0.761	1.033	6.637	4.002	2.872	318	596
	L	0.090	3.125	2.945	0.818	0.771	0.858	6.812	3.325	2.947	263	492
	M	0.072	3.125	2.981	0.818	0.780	0.691	6.979	2.676	3.020	210	394
	DWV	0.045	3.125	3.035	0.818	0.795	0.435	7.234	1.687	3.130	131	246
3-1/2	K	0.120	3.625	3.385	0.949	0.886	1.321	8.999	5.120	3.894	302	566
	L	0.100	3.625	3.425	0.949	0.897	1.107	9.213	4.291	3.987	252	472
	M	0.083	3.625	3.459	0.949	0.906	0.924	9.397	3.579	4.066	209	392
4	K	0.134	4.125	3.857	1.080	1.010	1.680	11.684	6.510	5.056	296	555
	L	0.110	4.125	3.905	1.080	1.022	1.387	11.977	5.377	5.182	243	456
	M	0.095	4.125	3.935	1.080	1.030	1.203	12.161	4.661	5.262	210	394
	DWV	0.058	4.125	4.009	1.080	1.050	0.741	12.623	2.872	5.462	128	240
5	K	0.160	5.125	4.805	1.342	1.258	2.496	18.133	9.671	7.846	285	534
	L	0.125	5.125	4.875	1.342	1.276	1.963	18.665	7.609	8.077	222	417
	M	0.109	5.125	4.907	1.342	1.285	1.718	18.911	6.656	8.183	194	364
	DWV	0.072	5.125	4.981	1.342	1.304	1.143	19.486	4.429	8.432	128	240
6	K	0.192	6.125	5.741	1.603	1.503	3.579	25.886	13.867	11.201	286	536
	L	0.140	6.125	5.845	1.603	1.530	2.632	26.832	10.200	11.610	208	391
	M	0.122	6.125	5.881	1.603	1.540	2.301	27.164	8.916	11.754	182	341
	DWV	0.083	6.125	5.959	1.603	1.560	1.575	27.889	6.105	12.068	124	232
8	K	0.271	8.125	7.583	2.127	1.985	6.687	45.162	25.911	19.542	304	570
	L	0.200	8.125	7.725	2.127	2.022	4.979	46.869	19.295	20.280	224	421
	M	0.170	8.125	7.785	2.127	2.038	4.249	47.600	16.463	20.597	191	358
	DWV	0.109	8.125	7.907	2.127	2.070	2.745	49.104	10.637	21.247	122	229
10	K	0.338	10.125	9.449	2.651	2.474	10.392	70.123	40.271	30.342	304	571
	L	0.250	10.125	9.625	2.651	2.520	7.756	72.760	30.054	31.483	225	422
	M	0.212	10.125	9.701	2.651	2.540	6.602	73.913	25.584	31.982	191	358
12	K	0.405	12.125	11.315	3.174	2.962	14.912	100.554	57.784	43.510	305	571
	L	0.280	12.125	11.565	3.174	3.028	10.419	105.046	40.375	45.454	211	395
	M	0.254	12.125	11.617	3.174	3.041	9.473	105.993	36.706	45.863	191	358

[a] When using soldered or brazed fittings, the joint determines the limiting pressure.

[b] Working pressures were calculated using ASME *Standard* B31.9 allowable stresses. A 5% mill tolerance has been used on the wall thickness. Higher tube ratings can be calculated using the allowable stress for lower temperatures.

[c] If soldered or brazed fittings are used on hard drawn tubing, use the annealed ratings. Full-tube allowable pressures can be used with suitably rated flare or compression-type fittings.

Table 9-10 Application of Pipe, Fitting and Valves for Heating and Air-Conditioning
(Table 5, Chapter 40, 1996 *ASHRAE Handbook—Systems and Equipment*)

Application	Pipe Material	Weight	Joint Type	Fitting Class	Fitting Material	System Temperature, °F	System Maximum Pressure at Temperature[a], psig
Recirculating Water 2 in. and smaller	Steel (CW)	Standard	Thread	125	Cast iron	250	125
	Copper, hard	Type L	Braze or silver solder[b]		Wrought copper	250	150
	PVC	Sch 80	Solvent	Sch 80	PVC	75	
	CPVC	Sch 80	Solvent	Sch 80	CPVC	150	
	PB	SDR-11	Heat fusion		PB	160	
			Insert crimp		Metal	160	
2.5 to 12 in.	A53 B ERW Steel	Standard	Weld	Standard	Wrought steel	250	400
			Flange	150	Wrought steel	250	250
			Flange	125	Cast iron	250	175
			Flange	250	Cast iron	250	400
			Groove		MI or ductile iron	230	300
	PB	SDR-11	Heat fusion		PB	160	
Steam and Condensate 2 in. and smaller	Steel (CW)	Standard[c]	Thread	125	Cast iron		90
			Thread	150	Malleable iron		90
	A53 B ERW Steel	Standard[c]	Thread	125	Cast iron		100
			Thread	150	Malleable iron		125
	A53 B ERW Steel	XS	Thread	250	Cast iron		200
			Thread	300	Malleable iron		250
2.5 to 12 in.	Steel	Standard	Weld	Standard	Wrought steel		250
			Flange	150	Wrought steel		200
			Flange	125	Cast iron		100
	A53 B ERW Steel	XS	Weld	XS	Wrought steel		700
			Flange	300	Wrought steel		500
			Flange	250	Cast iron		200
Refrigerant	Copper, hard	Type L or K	Braze		Wrought copper		
	A53 B SML Steel	Standard	Weld		Wrought steel		
Underground Water							
Through 12 in.	Copper, hard	Type K	Braze or silver solder[b]		Wrought copper	75	350
Through 6 in.	Ductile iron	Class 50	MJ	MJ	Cast iron	75	250
	PB	SDR 9, 11	Heat fusion		PB	75	
		SDR 7, 11.5	Insert crimp		Metal	75	
Potable Water, Inside Building	Copper, hard	Type L	Braze or silver solder[b]		Wrought copper	75	350
	Steel, galvanized	Standard	Thread	125	Galv. cast iron	75	125
				150	Galv. mall. iron	75	125
	PB	SDR-11	Heat fusion		PB	75	
			Insert crimp		Metal	75	

[a] Maximum allowable working pressures have been derated in this table. Higher system pressures can be used for lower temperatures and smaller pipe sizes. Pipe, fittings, joints, and valves must all be considered.

[b] Lead- and antimony-based solders should not be used for potable water systems. Brazing and silver solders should be employed.

[c] Extra strong pipe is recommended for all threaded condensate piping to allow for corrosion.

brass pipe have always been used in heating, ventilating, refrigeration, and water supply installations because of their corrosion resistance. However, copper and brass are not compatible with ammonia and should not be used in ammonia refrigeration systems.

Plastic pipe has become popular in heating and air-conditioning installations because its flexibility in handling, lower labor costs, and resistance to corrosive fluids. Pressure and temperature are the basic limitations to be considered. Basically, two kinds of plastics are used:

1. **Thermoplastic**, which melts under heat, hardens when cooled, and can be melted and reworked again and again.
2. **Thermoset**, which hardens and fuses under heat and pressure into a permanent shape and cannot be remelted.

Some thermoplastics remain flexible and have moderate strength for water service where temperature and pressures are moderate. Thermoplastics may be joined by solvent welding and hot-gas welding. Both pipe and fittings are available in IPS sizes.

Epoxy or polyester resins, usually reinforced with glass fibers, are the major ingredient of thermosetting piping. They are available in commercial pipe sizes, joined by either standard screwed or socket-type fittings. Commercial polyester pipe is suitable for temperatures up to 250°F (120°C).

9.4.3 Pipe Fittings

Metal pipe is joined by welding one length to another, or by using fittings. Pipe fittings are made in such forms as elbows, tees, couplings, reducers, and unions; they may be screwed, flanged, or welded. The type of fitting used is determined by the pressure of the fluid being carried, or by the intended use of the pipeline. The materials generally used are steel, cast iron, malleable iron (heat treated cast iron), copper, brass, stainless steel, alloy steel, or bronze. The material used also depends upon the pressure and fluid characteristics.

Fittings are designated and sized in accordance with ANSI specifications and are identified by their nominal pipe sizes. In the case of reducing tees, crosses, and Y-branches (laterals), the size of the largest run opening is given first, followed by the size of the opening at the opposite end of the run. Where the fitting is a tee or Y-branch (lateral), the size of the outlet is given last. Where the fitting is a cross, the largest side outlet opening is the third dimension given followed by the opening opposite. Where an external thread is wanted, the word male follows the size of that opening; female indicates an internal thread.

9.4.4 Pipe Sizing

Specific procedures for sizing various fluid flow systems using piping or tubing are given in Chapter 33 of the 1997 *ASHRAE Handbook—Fundamentals*.

Example 9.5. Select the design pipe sizes for the two-pipe, forced circulation hot water system shown in the figure below. A 20°F drop in the water temperature has been selected and the water leaves the boiler at 190°F. The numbers in parentheses are the measured linear runs of pipe. The dashed line is the return line pipe. The piping in the system is to be Type L copper tube.

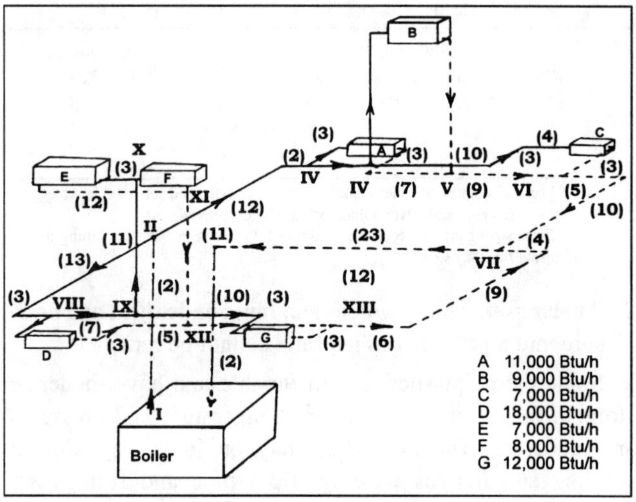

The pressure loss through each convector is given as:

A 1600 millinches	E 1425 millinches
B 1500 millinches	F 1450 millinches
C 1450 millinches	G 1550 millinches
D 1600 millinches	

Solution:

First, calculate the gallons per minute circulated through each circuit of the system. For the ABC circuit, the total heat delivered is:

$$11{,}000 + 9000 + 7000 = 27{,}000 \text{ Btu/h}$$

The relation between heat flow and flow rate is:

$$q = 60\ Wc_p(t_{in} - t_{out}), \text{ or}$$

$$q = 490\ Q(t_{in} - t_{out})$$

where

q = output of the convectors, Btu/h
Q = flow rate, gpm
$(t_{in} - t_{out})$ = temperature drop of the water across convector

For this circuit:

$$Q = 27{,}000/(490 \times 20) = 2.76 \text{ gpm}$$

For circuit DEFG:

$$q = 45{,}000 \text{ Btu/h}$$

and:

$$Q = 45{,}000/(490 \times 20) = 4.59 \text{ gpm}$$

Next, select a design friction loss for the system. Assume a design value of 2.5 ft/100 ft (0.3 in/ft). Now the pipe can be sized for each branch in the system, using Figure 2, Chapter 33 of the 1997 *ASHRAE Handbook—Fundamentals*, on the supply side:

for I-II	at 7.34 gpm (72,000 Btu/h), use 1-1/4 in.
II-III	at 2.75 gpm (27,000 Btu/h), use 3/4 in.
III-IV	at 1.63 gpm (16,000 Btu/h), use 5/8 in.
Convector A	at 1.12 gpm (11,000 Btu/h), use 5/8 in.
Convector B	at 0.92 gpm (0,000 Btu/h), use 1/2 in.
Convector C	at 0.71 gpm (7,000 Btu/h), use 1/2 in.
II-VIII	at 4.59 gpm (45,000 Btu/h), use 1 in.
VIII-IX	at 2.75 gpm (27,000 Btu/h), use 3/4 in.
IX-X	at 1.53 gpm (15,000 Btu/h), use 5/8 in.
Convector D	at 1.84 gpm (18,000 Btu/h), use 3/4 in.
Convector E	at 0.71 gpm (7,000 Btu/h), use 1/2 in.
Convector F	at 0.82 gpm (8,000 Btu/h), use 1/2 in.
Convector G	at 1.22 gpm (12,000 Btu/h), use 5/8 in.

and on the return side:

for V-VI	at 2.04 gpm (20,000 Btu/h), use 3/4 in.
VI-VII	at 2.75 gpm (27,000 Btu/h), use 3/4 in.
XI-XII	at 1.53 gpm (15,000 Btu/h), use 5/8 in.
XII-XIII	at 3.34 gpm (33,000 Btu/h), use 1 in.
XIII-VII	at 4.59 gpm (45,000 Btu/h), use 1 in.
VII-I	at 7.34 gpm (72,000 Btu/h), use 1-1/4 in.

Next, find the longest run in the system. Apparently, this is the circuit from I-II-IX-X-Convector E-XI-XII-I. The other possible longest run could be one that includes convector F or one that includes convector B. Both should be checked. Assume here that the convector E run is the longest. The pressure or head loss is found from Figure 2, Chapter 33 of the 1997 *ASHRAE Handbook—Fundamentals*. For example, for 7.34 gpm in a 1-1/4 in. pipe, the friction loss is 1.46 ft/100 ft.

For *section I-II* the loss is 2 × 1.46 = 2.92 ft/100 ft. The friction losses in the other straight sections are found in a similar manner:

I-II	2.92 ft/100 ft
II-VIII	24.66 ft/100 ft
VII-IX	17.50 ft/100 ft
IX-X	22.92 ft/100 ft
X-Convector	4.37 ft/100 ft
Convector-XI	17.50 ft/100 ft
XI-XII	23.83 ft/100 ft
XII-XIII	12.0 ft/100 ft
XIII-VII	15.0 ft/100 ft
VII-I	33.5 ft/100 ft
Total =	174.2 ft/100 ft

The friction losses for the fittings are as follows:

Elbow (Using Figure 2 and Table 4, Chapter 33 of the 1997 *ASHRAE Handbook—Fundamentals*)

2.5 × 1.66	= 4.17 ft/100 ft
2 × 1.2 × 1.46	= 3.50 ft/100 ft
2 × 2.5 × 1.66	= 8.3 ft/100 ft
1.0 × 3.3 × 1.46	= 4.83 ft/100 ft
Total	= 20.8 ft/100 ft

Tees (Using Figure 2, Figure 4, and Table 4, Chapter 33 of the 1997 *ASHRAE Handbook—Fundamentals*) at

II	8.3 ft/100 ft
IX	8.17 ft/100 ft
X	3.50 ft/100 ft
XI	8.83 ft/100 ft
XII	4.83 ft/100 ft
XIII	8.0 ft/100 ft
VII	10.4 ft/100 ft
Total	= 57.5 ft/100 ft

Convector loss = 1425 millinch (1.425 in. of water per foot of pipe or 11.87 ft/100 ft)

Total fitting losses

$$= 20.8 + 57.5 + 11.87 = 90.2 \text{ ft/100 ft}$$

The total friction loss for the longest run is then:

$$174.2 + 90.2 = 264.4 \text{ ft/100 ft}$$

Select a boiler and pump combination that will supply 72,000 Btu/h and circulate 7.62 gpm with a developed head of 264.4 ft/100 ft (friction loss).

***Notes*:**

(a) Some friction loss will occur through the boiler, which must be added to the total friction loss of the system.

(b Balancing cocks will need to be placed in the various circuits to balance the flow to each convector. Include the friction loss for these balancing cocks (valves) in the calculation.

(c) Air vent valves, as well as drain valves, should also be put into the system. Also include the friction loss due to these fittings.

9.5 Pumps

Pumps can be classified into three broad categories: (1) reciprocating, (2) rotary, and (3) centrifugal. Both reciprocating and rotary pumps are **positive displacement** pumps. They discharge a fixed amount of liquid for a given speed. The primary moving element of a reciprocating pump is a piston or plunger, while for a rotary pump, it is a rotor. Rotary pumps include gear pumps, vane pumps, lobe pumps, screw pumps, and cam action pumps.

Centrifugal pumps can be classified by the style of impeller: single or double suction, closed or open, radial, Francis, axial; as well as the casing: volute, diffuser, and concentric.

In pumps with radial or Francis impellers, centrifugal force develops the pressure energy and is a function of the impeller peripheral velocity. The liquid enters at the eye of the impeller and energy is added to the liquid by the impeller. The casing collects the liquid as it leaves the impeller and guides it out the discharge of the pump.

In the heating, ventilating, and air-conditioning industry, the most frequently used pump has a radial or Francis enclosed impeller, a volute casing, and is single stage.

9.5.1 Pump Laws

Approximate centrifugal pump performance comparisons of flow, head, and power, depending on impeller diameter, speed, and liquid density are given in Table 9-11.

Table 9-11 Affinity Laws for Pumps

Impeller Diameter	Speed	Density	To Correct For	Multiply By
			Flow	$\left(\frac{\text{New Speed}}{\text{Old Speed}}\right)$
Constant	Variable	Constant	Head	$\left(\frac{\text{New Speed}}{\text{Old Speed}}\right)^2$
			Power	$\left(\frac{\text{New Speed}}{\text{Old Speed}}\right)^3$
			Flow	$\left(\frac{\text{New Speed}}{\text{Old Speed}}\right)$
Variable	Constant	Constant	Head	$\left(\frac{\text{New Speed}}{\text{Old Speed}}\right)^2$
			Power	$\left(\frac{\text{New Speed}}{\text{Old Speed}}\right)^3$
Constant	Constant	Variable	Power	$\left(\frac{\text{New Density}}{\text{Old Density}}\right)$

9.5.2 Pump Performance Curves

Performance of a pump is commonly shown graphically, as in Figure 9-13, which relates the flow (gpm and L/s), the pressure produced (ft and Pa), the power required (bhp and kW), the hydraulic efficiency in percent, the shaft speed (rpm and r/s), and the net positive suction head (ft and Pa, absolute) required for normal operation of the pump with various impeller diameters. Pump curves present the average results obtained from testing several pumps of the same design under standardized test conditions. Manufacturers should be consulted for pump applications that differ considerably from ordinary practice.

The maximum efficiency of a pump is not always the most important feature in making a selection. If the pump is to operate at its peak efficiency, system resistance must also

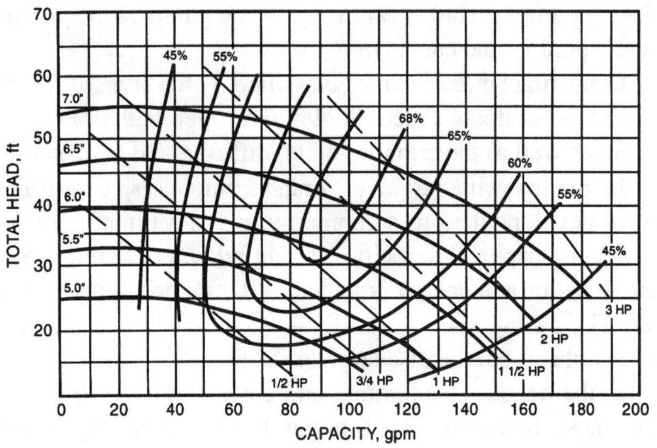

Fig. 9-13 Typical Pump Performance Curves

be considered. Systems with no corrosion and systems protected against corrosion should not be designed from pipe friction loss tables containing high corrosion allowances. Such tables show excessive pressure losses, which require selecting a larger pump than necessary. Pumps for systems using liquids for heating and cooling should be hydraulically and mechanically designed for quiet operation, durability, simple service, minimum maintenance, and minimum suction requirements rather than for minimum cost or size.

9.5.3 Hydronic System Characteristics

Hydronic systems in HVAC are all of the loop type (open or closed); the water is circulated through the system and returned to the pumps. No appreciable amount of water is lost from the system, except in the cooling tower, where evaporative cooling occurs.

Hydronic systems are either full flow or throttling flow. Full flow systems are usually found on residential or small commercial systems where pump motors are small and the energy waste caused by constant flow is not appreciable. Larger systems use flow control valves. These valves control flow in the system in accordance with the heating or cooling load imposed on the system. Hydronic systems can also operate continuously or intermittently. Most hot water or chilled water systems are in continuous operation as long as a heating or cooling load exists on the system. Condensate and boiler feed pumps are often of the intermittent type, starting and stopping as the water level changes in condensate tanks or boilers.

Pumps move water through hydronic systems, overcoming the friction caused by liquid flow through equipment, piping, fittings, and valves. The system head curve graphically describes the flow-head relationship for a hydronic system from minimum to maximum flow (Figure 9-14). The total head consists of the independent head and the system friction head. The independent head is unaffected by the total flow in the system. Typical **independent heads** are: (1) static rise to the top of a cooling tower in condenser water systems; (2) boiler pressure in condensate and boiler feed systems; and (3) control valve and heating or cooling coil friction in hot and chilled water systems.

The head loss of a control valve and its coil is independent of total flow in a system because these head losses can occur at any time, regardless of the total flow on the system; i.e., a particular coil may require its maximum flow and, therefore, maximum head loss for the coil and its valve, even though the total flow in the entire system is at a minimum with minimum system friction head.

The other component, **system friction head**, depends on total system flow, increasing or decreasing with total system flow.

Plotting the system head against the system flow produces a curve as shown in Figure 9-14. If no independent head exists in a hydronic system, the system friction curve becomes the system curve as shown in Figure 9-15. Domestic and small commercial heating and cooling systems without control valves are typical systems without independent head. In actual operation, since flow is not throttled, flow occurs at only one point in the system-at the intersection of the pump head-capacity curve and the system curve (Figure 9-15).

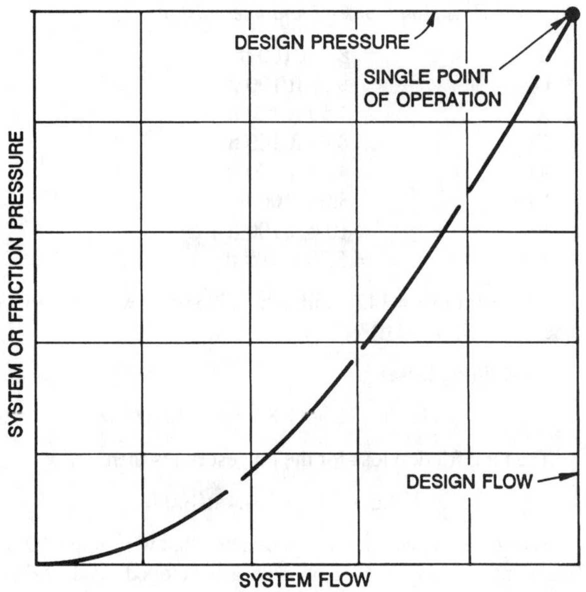

Fig. 9-14 Typical System Curve

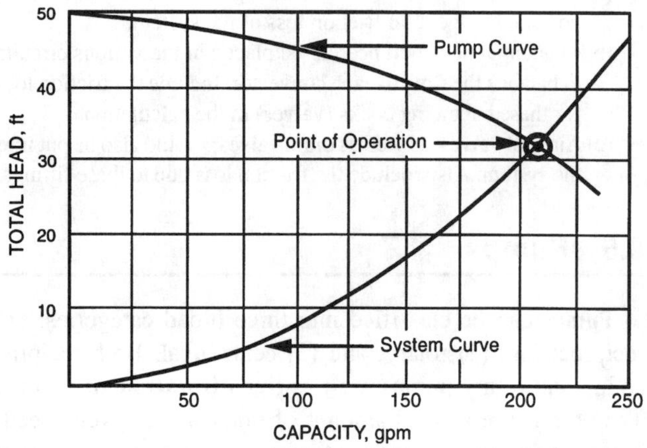

Fig. 9-15 System and Pump Curves

Additional data concerning pump design, selection, and operation can be found in Chapter 38 of the 1996 *ASHRAE Handbook—Systems and Equipment.*

9.6 Problems

9.1 The air velocity in a human occupied zone should not exceed (a) 10 to 25 ft/min, (b) 25 to 40 ft/min, (c) 40 to 64 ft/min, (d) None of the above.

9.2 You are to select the type of outlets for a home to be constructed in Houston, Texas. Discuss your selection of outlets and locations for each of the following combinations: (a) Group A or Group C, (b) Group B or Group E.

9.3 What velocity of air is necessary at a location in a room such that most people will feel neither cool nor warm? Assume that the local temperature is equal to the control temperature of 24.4°C. [Ans: 0.152 m/s]

9.4 The choice of air distribution for a new home is left to your judgment as the customer finalizes the design with the architect. The house is a rambling, one-story ranch with full basement, unfinished attic, 4 bedrooms, 3 1/2 baths, and 3-car garage on a 6-acre wooded plot five miles from Alfred, New York. The customer indicates no intention of installing air-conditioning equipment, but wants the air distribution sized for and suitable for air conditioning to be added. (a) What type of air-distribution system would you recommend? (b) Identify it by group. (c) Why did you choose this type?

9.5 Air leaves a two-dimensional plane opening at a velocity of 105 fpm. The jet is a long slot, 1 in. wide and 8 ft long. Find the maximum throw and spread (angle of divergence = 22° of the jet and label these on a sketch.

9.6 An outlet has dimensions of 14 in. by 19 in. with R_{fa} = 0.87 and C_d = 0.72. For this grille, the K' value is 4.1. Calculate the discharge velocity for a V_x of 75 fpm with a throw of 42 ft. [Ans: 447 fpm]

9.7 A 10 ft by 12 ft bedroom with 8-ft ceiling has a heat loss of 6400 Btu/h. The total heat loss of the house is 47,000 Btu/h and the fan discharges 1140 cfm. Determine the size and location of the supply grilles for this room.

9.8 For the air jet in *Problem 9.5*, calculate the total volume flow rate at the maximum throw.

9.9 Air leaves a circular grille at 250 fpm. The grille has a 12 in. diameter and a K' value of 5.1. Plot the velocity profile at a distance of 10 ft from the grille, for a circular jet, $x = r_{0.5}/0.0847$.

9.10 In *Problem 9.9*, what is the entrainment volume at the specified location? At what radius will the velocity be less than 70 fpm? [Ans: 869 fpm]

9.11 Air leaves a two-dimensional plane opening at a velocity of 0.5 m/s. The jet is a long slot 30 mm wide and 2.5 m long. Find the maximum throw and spread (angle of divergence = 22°) of the jet and label these on a sketch. [Ans: 1.68 m, 0.69 m]

9.12 Solve the following problems.

(a) Find the airflow through a 12 in. by 24 in. (305 mm by 610 mm) duct if the static pressure is measured at 0.5 in. of water (125 Pa) and total pressure is measured at 0.54 in. of water (135 Pa)

(b) The pressure difference available to a 60 ft (18.3 m) length of circular duct is 0.2 in. of water (50 Pa). The duct has an ID of 12 in. (305 mm). What rate of airflow is expected?

9.13 For a residential air-conditioning system, one branch duct must supply 207 cfm to one of the rooms. The branch duct has a run of 16 ft. (a) Determine the branch duct size and the pressure drop from the main duct to the room, and (b) specify the supply and return grille sizes for the room.

9.14 How large of a duct is required to carry 20,000 cfm (9400 L/s) of air if the velocity is not to exceed 1600 fpm (8.1 m/s)? [Ans: 48 in. (1220 mm)]

9.15 Given the duct system shown below, plot p_v, Δp_s, and Δp_t for the flow through the system.

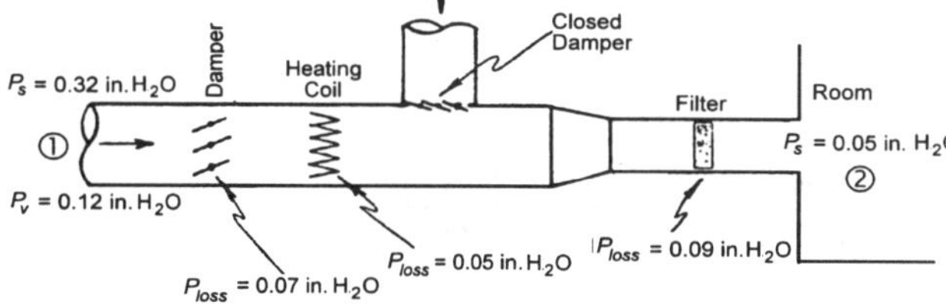

9.16 Solve the following.

(a) For *Problem 9.15*, find the frictional pressure loss between points (1) and (2).

(b) How can the static pressure be increased in a duct system as the air moves away from the fan?

9.17 Determine the dynamic loss of total pressure that occurs in an abrupt expansion from a 1-ft^2 (0.093-m^2) duct to a 2-ft^2 (0.186 m^2) duct carrying 1000 cfm (470 L/s) of air. [Ans: 0.02 in. of water (5 Pa)]

9.18 Determine the friction loss when circulating 20,000 cfm (9430 L/s) of air at 75°F (23.9°C) through 150 ft (45.7 m) of 36 in. (0.914 m) diameter galvanized steel duct.

9.19 If in *Problem 9.18*, the duct is very rough, find the total friction loss in pressure. If the duct is made of aluminum instead of galvanized steel, what is the total friction pressure loss?

9.20 Determine the friction pressure loss for the duct of *Problem 9.18*; however, it is carrying air at 40°F (4.4°C). [Ans: 0.37 in. of water (92 Pa)]

9.21 Find the equivalent rectangular duct for equal friction and capacity for the duct in:

(a) *Problem 9.14*, one side is 26 in.

(b) *Problem 9.20*, one side is 20 in.

9.22 Find the pressure loss between points A and D for the 12 in. by 12 in. duct shown below. Air at standard conditions is being supplied at the rate of 2000 cfm in galvanized duct of average construction. Elbows No. 1 and No. 2 have center line radii of 13 in. and 24 in., respectively.

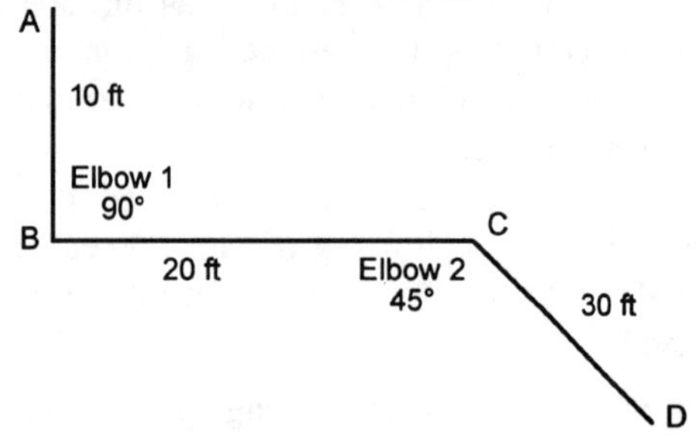

9.23 High velocities in duct systems allow use of smaller ducts, but the pressure friction loss is increased. Describe the relationship between velocity change and change in pressure friction loss. [Ans: $\Delta p \propto V^2$]

9.24 Analyze the air-handling system shown in the following diagram. Determine if a damper is needed in either section (d) or (b), and if so, in what section. There is a damper located in section (u) so that the proper static pressure can be maintained in section (u). If a damper is needed, what is the pressure loss across the damper?

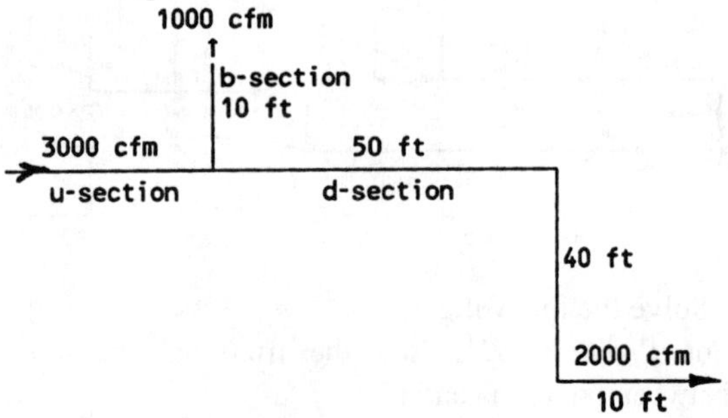

$\rho = 0.075$ lb/ft^3 $\quad f = 0.02$

$D = 12$ in. $\quad (R/D)_{elbows} = 1$

9.25 A 1-ft high by 3-ft wide main duct carries 2000 cfm of air to a branch where 1500 cfm continues in the 1 ft by 2 ft straight through section and 500 cfm goes into the branch. Find the actual static pressure regain and the total pressure loss in the straight through section if the static regain coefficient is 0.80. If the branch take off is a 45° cylindrical Y, find the static pressure loss in this section.

9.26 Determine the entering air temperature and heat loss for a duct 12 in. (305 mm) in diameter and 50 ft (15.2 m) long. The duct is insulated with 1 in. (25.4 mm) of insulation having a conductivity of 0.31 Btu/h·ft^2·°F/in. (0.0447 W/m·K). The duct carries air moving at 1500 fpm (7.6 m/s) at a temperature of 130°F (54.4°C). The air surrounding the insulated duct is at 30°F (−1.1°C). [Ans: 134°F (56.7°C), 4368 Btu/h (1.28 kW)]

9.27 What can be said about the relationship between the total pressure drop in branch BC and branch BD in the schematic of an air distribution system shown below?

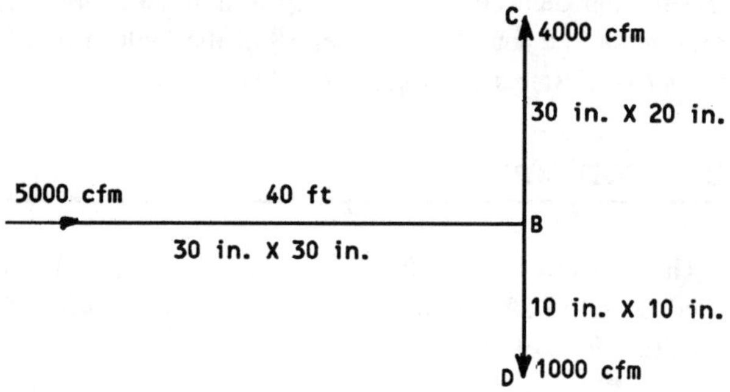

9.28 The supply ductwork for an office space is shown in the following diagram. Size the ductwork by the equal-friction method and calculate the pressure drop. Assume a maximum duct depth of 12 in. and that all duct take-offs are straight rectangular take-offs.

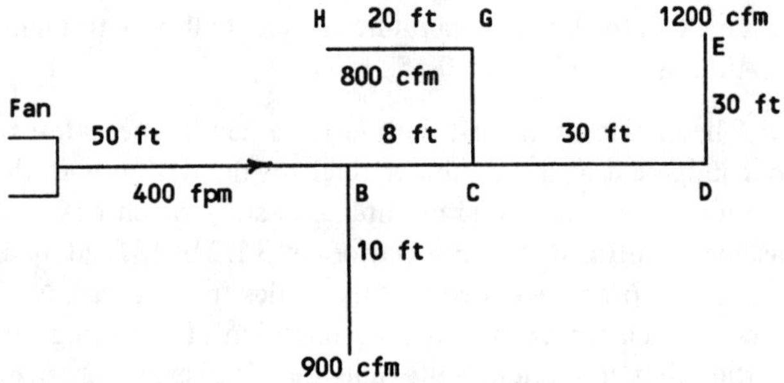

9.29 The following duct system contains circular, galvanized duct. The velocity in the ducts is to be 2000 fpm, and each outlet is to handle 2000 cfm. Each outlet grille has a pressure loss of 0.12 in. of water. Estimate the required pressure increase of the fan. [Ans: 0.97 in. of water]

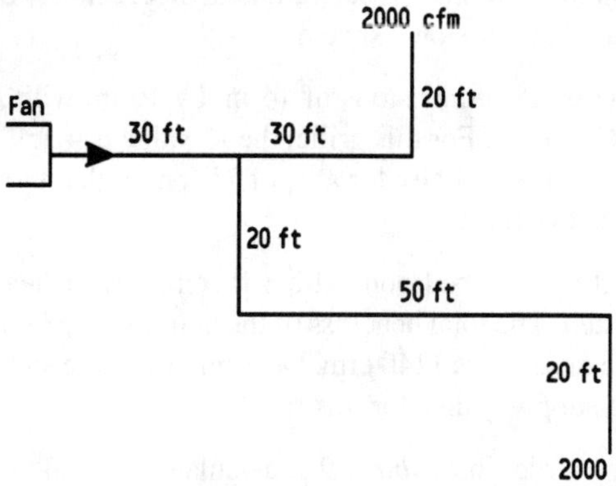

9.30 Select a fan for the following system. The radius ratio of the elbows is 1.0 and the elbows are 3 piece. The pipe is circular. Calculate the frictional pressure loss for the system and the total capacity required by the fan.

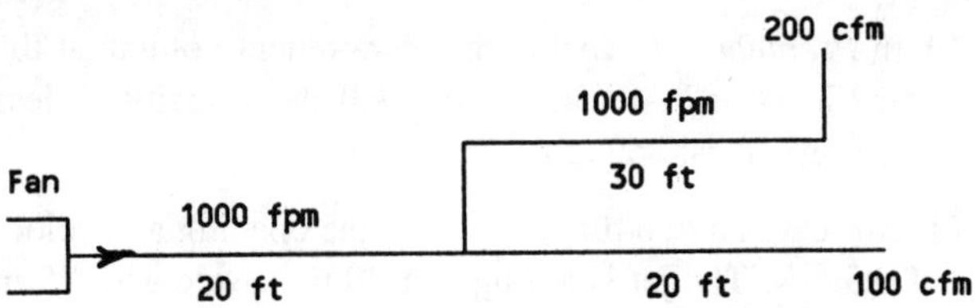

9.31 (a) Estimate the total pressure loss between points (1) and (2) and between (1) and (3) in the following take-off.

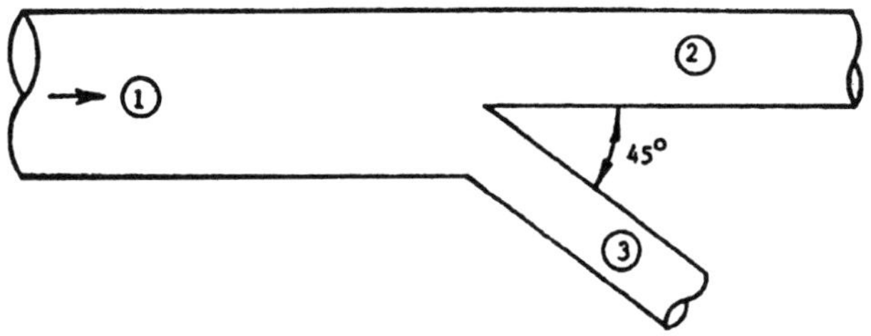

when:

$V_1 = 8.12$ m/s $Q_1 = 1510$ L/s
$V_2 = 6.1$ m/s $Q_2 = 1227$ L/s
$V_3 = 3.05$ m/s $Q_3 = 283$ L/s

The duct is rectangular, of commercial fabrication, and has mastic tape joints.

(b) Estimate the static pressure at (3) if the static pressure at (1) is 1.0 in. of water.

9.32 For the duct configuration shown below, size the ducts between A and B, and B and C for equal static pressure in each branch of 1 in. of water. Assume spiral pipe will be used and start at A with a static pressure of 1 in. of water. Also, start with a 50-in. round duct with the velocity at 4000 fpm. [Ans: 45 in., 40 in.]

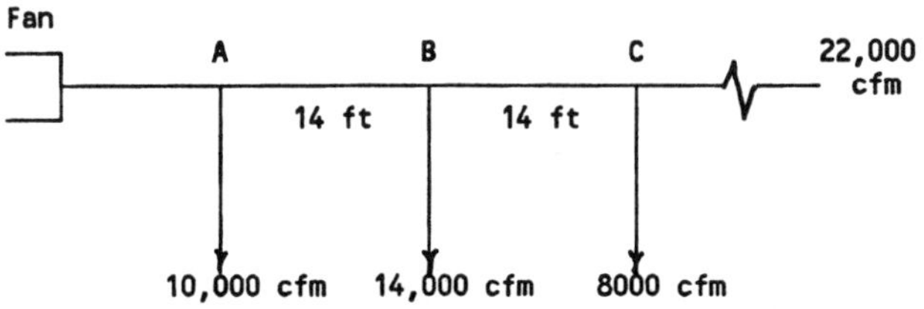

9.33 Design the following duct system to be perfectly balanced without the aid of dampers:

Room A (conference room) requires 3000 cfm.
Room B (lunchroom) requires 5000 cfm.
Both rooms are at atmospheric pressure.

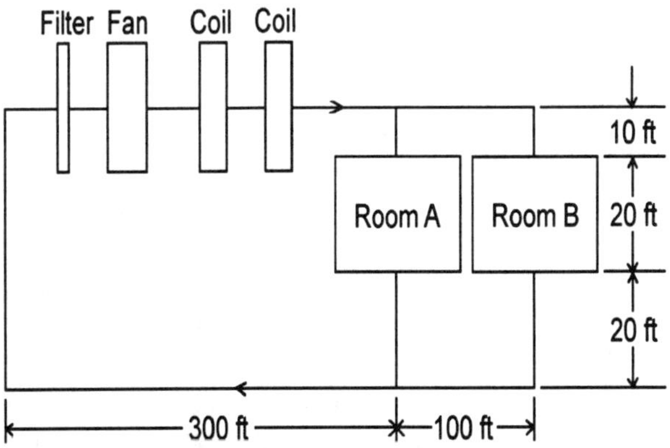

The design should include:

(a) duct sizes (assume round) and duct velocities
(b) capacity and static pressure required of the fan
(c) Does balancing, here, without a damper create a possible noise problem?
(d) If the noise problem were to be eliminated by reducing velocities, what A_{pf} of the damper would be required, and where should it be located?

9.34 Solve the following problems:

(a) What is the expected approximate frictional pressure from (1) to (2) in the following length of duct. Assume round ducts, clean sheet metal, and air at standard temperature and pressure.

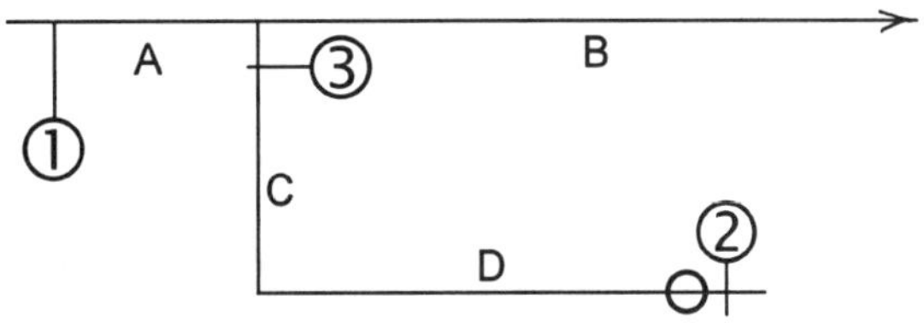

Elbow Radius = 36 in.
Grille loss = 0.1 in w.g. at 600 fpm

Duct	cfm	Vel., fpm	length
A	2000	1000	40 ft
B	1000	600	–
C	1000	600	30 ft
D	1000	600	30 ft

(b) If the static pressure at (3) is 0.350 in. of water, what friction drop will be required of a damper at 68°F?
(c) What size duct would be required (for ducts C and D) if the damper is eliminated? What is the velocity in the line? Assume a temperature of 68°F. Assume that the static pressure at (3) is still 0.35 in. of water and that the *R*/*D* of the elbow is 2. Also assume that the grille loss is linear with velocity.

9.35 Determine the following duct size by the static regain method:

$V_1 = 1600$ fpm $Q_1 = 2000$ cfm
$V_3 = 500$ fpm $Q_3 = 500$ cfm
$V_2 = ?$ fpm $Q_2 = 1500$ cfm
$V_4 = 500$ fpm $Q_4 = 500$ cfm

Find D_1, D_2, D_3, and D_4.
[Ans: 15.2 in., 13 in., 13.6 in., 13.6 in.]

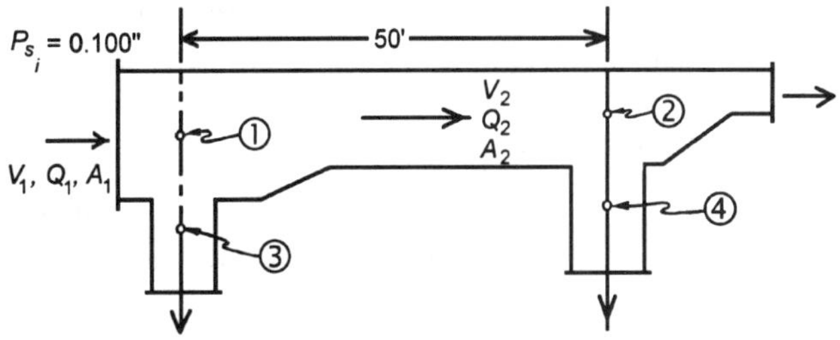

9.36 The pressure (energy) loss between A-B, A-C, A-D, and A-E must be equal if a proper air balance is to be achieved. The static pressure required in the duct at points B, C, D, and E to produce the proper flow from the air diffusing terminal units (ceiling diffusers) is assumed to be uniform and to be

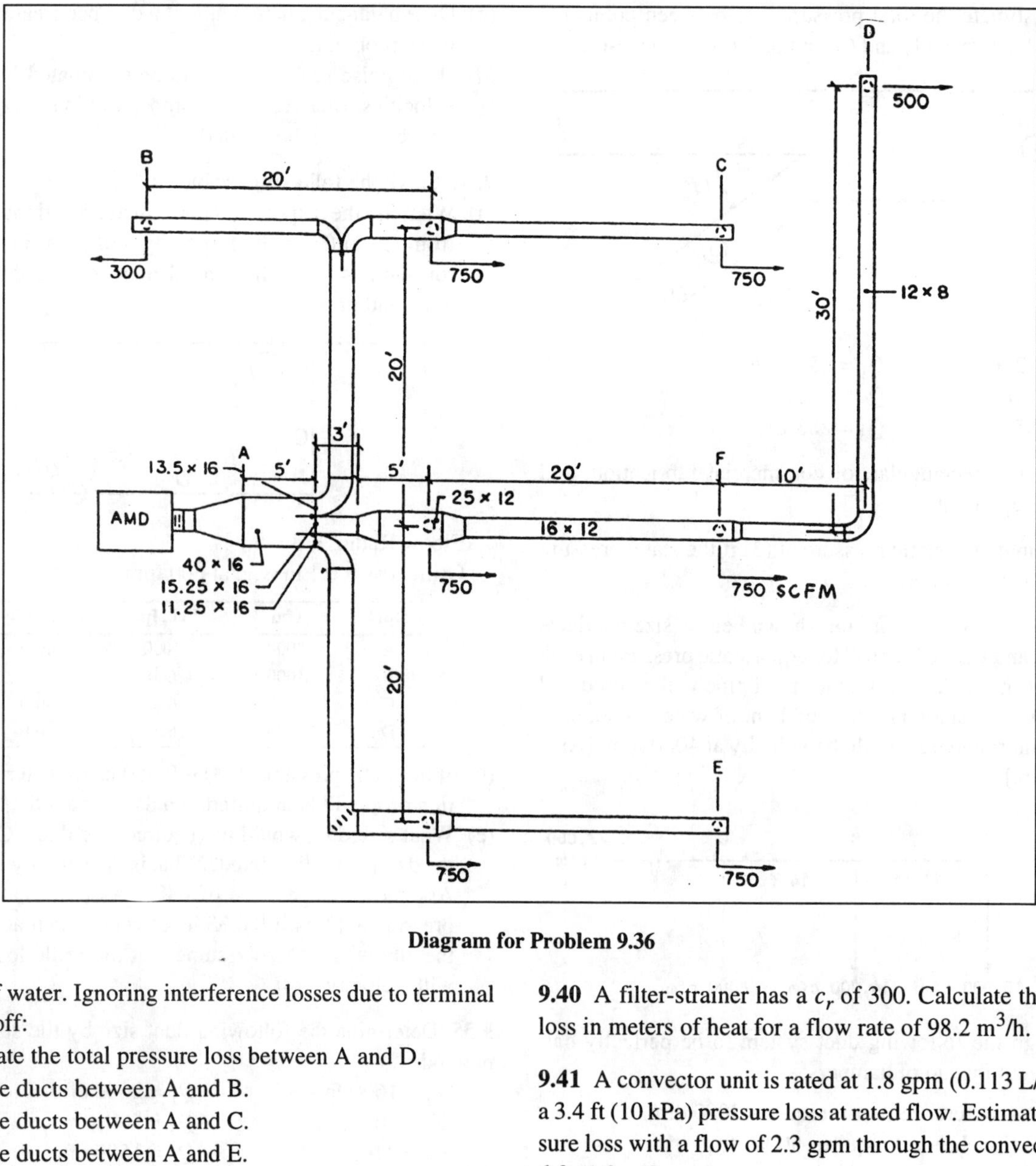

Diagram for Problem 9.36

0.10 in. of water. Ignoring interference losses due to terminal unit take off:

1. Calculate the total pressure loss between A and D.
2. Size the ducts between A and B.
3. Size the ducts between A and C.
4. Size the ducts between A and E.
5. What would the static pressure be at F?

Note: In practical application, minor static pressure imbalances up to 0.05 in. of water can be absorbed by adjustment of dampers installed in air-diffusing terminal units and further minor adjustments of diverting dampers, in branch fittings. For greater imbalances, duct sizing must be modified and/or butterfly dampers installed in the branch ducts.

9.37 Determine the equivalent feet of pipe for a 2-in. (50 mm) open gate valve and a 2-in. (50 mm) open globe valve at a flow velocity of 5 fps (1.5 m/s).

9.38 Determine the through-the-main equivalent pipe length and the side branch equivalent length for a 2-in. (50 mm) tee with 30% of the flow being diverted.

9.39 A filter-strainer has a C_v of 300. Calculate the pressure loss in feet of head for a flow rate of 432 gpm (27.3 L/s).

9.40 A filter-strainer has a c_r of 300. Calculate the pressure loss in meters of heat for a flow rate of 98.2 m^3/h.

9.41 A convector unit is rated at 1.8 gpm (0.113 L/s) and has a 3.4 ft (10 kPa) pressure loss at rated flow. Estimate the pressure loss with a flow of 2.3 gpm through the convector. [Ans: 6 ft (1.8 m)]

9.42 Size the system shown in *Example 9.5* for a 10°F temperature drop.

9.43 Size the system shown in *Example 9.5* for 30°F temperature drop.

9.44 Size the system shown for iron pipe. The water leaves the boiler at 200°F and has a 20°F temperature drop. The convectors have a loss given by the equation: Loss (millinches) = 0.3 ((Btu/h output). Note: 1 millinch = 0.001 in. of water.

Assume a 3-ft rise is needed to get to the convectors and then a 3-ft drop to return to the boiler. What head must be developed by the pump and what flow rate (gpm) is required?

9.45 Rework *Problem 9.44* using Type L copper tubing.

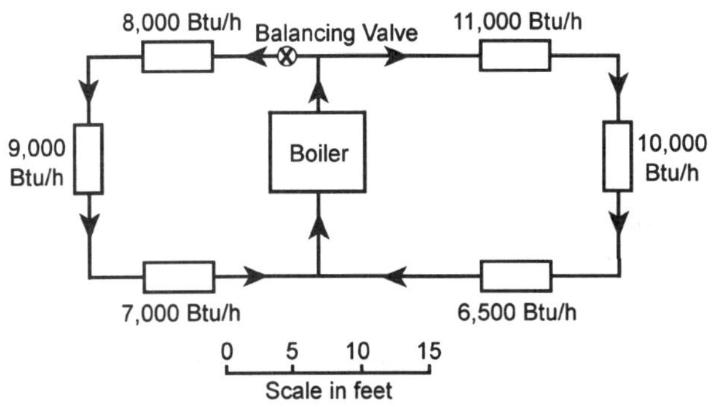

9.46 Calculate the friction pressure loss in the following hot-water circuit. Assume that the water leaves the boiler at 200°F and that the total temperature drop is 30°F. Assume that all of the piping is 5/8-in. copper tube. [Ans: 4.14 ft]

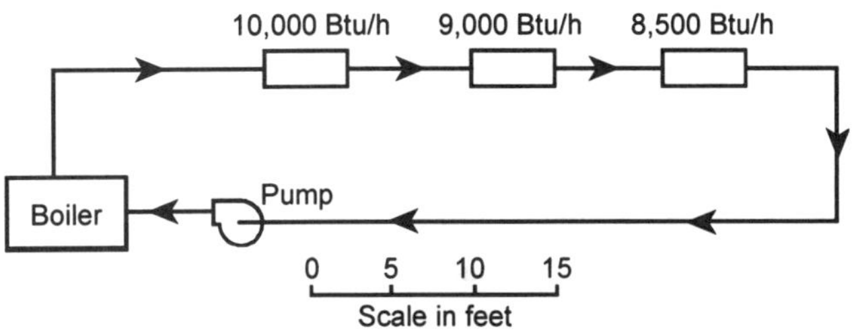

9.47 What pressure drop should be used for the steam piping of a system if the measured length of the longest run is 400 ft (121.0 m) and the initial pressure is not to be over 5 psig (35 kPa)? [Ans: 1.5 psig (10 kPa)]

9.48 A steam system requires 15,000 lb/h of steam at an initial pressure of 120 psig. The design pressure drop is to be 6 psi per 100 ft. Determine the size of schedule 40 pipe required and the velocity in the steam pipe.

9.49 Solve the following problems:

(a) The water quantity required to circulate in a hot water heating system with a heating load of 70,000 Btu/h and water leaving the boiler at 180°F and entering the boiler at 160°F is ____________?

(b) If the greatest pressure drop in a system was a series loop in (a), which includes 100 ft total actual length and 150 ft total equivalent length of 3/4-in. copper pipe (including 40,000 Btu/h capacity of 3/4-in. pipe size baseboard convectors), how would the required capability of the pump required be stated?

(c) How can the user affect the heat supplied (reduce the heat output) of a particular room heater of such a system if only one thermostat is used for all four rooms of that zone?

9.50 Hot water heating systems should be designed for velocities between 24 in/s and 48 in/s for pipe sizes 2 in. or under (but 36 to 48 ips for downfeed pipes), and about 500 mill-inches per ft (0.5 in. of water/ft) for piping over 2-in. nominal pipe size. Indicate for each situation described below, the pipe size necessary for that situation and why or from where?

(a) 6 gpm in iron pipe

(b) 6 gpm in copper pipe

(c) 40,000 Btu/h in iron pipe (20°F Δt)

(d) 40,000 Btu/h in copper pipe (20°F Δt)

(e) 70 gpm in copper tube

(f) 3 million Btu/h conveyed at 20°F Δt in iron pipe
[Ans: 1 in., 1 in., 3/4 in., 1 in., 3 in., 6 in.]

9.51 Assume a minimum street main pressure of 76 psig (517 kPa) for water to a building. The height of the topmost fixture (a flush valve urinal) is 60 ft (18.3 m) above the street main. The developed pipe length from the water main to the highest fixture is 120 ft (36.6 m). The total load on the system is 65 fixtures which are flush valve operated. Estimate the required size of the supply main.

9.52 Estimate the water consumption for your family for a typical week during the winter and for a typical week during the summer.

9.53 A garden hose is connected to a sill cock and is passing 5 gpm (0.31 L/s). The pressure at the entrance to the hose is found to be 18 psig (124 kPa). If this is 1/2-in. ID (13 mm) hose, estimate the length of the hose. [Ans: 45 ft (13.7 m)]

9.54 Determine the pipe sizes for the refrigeration systems shown in the following figure.

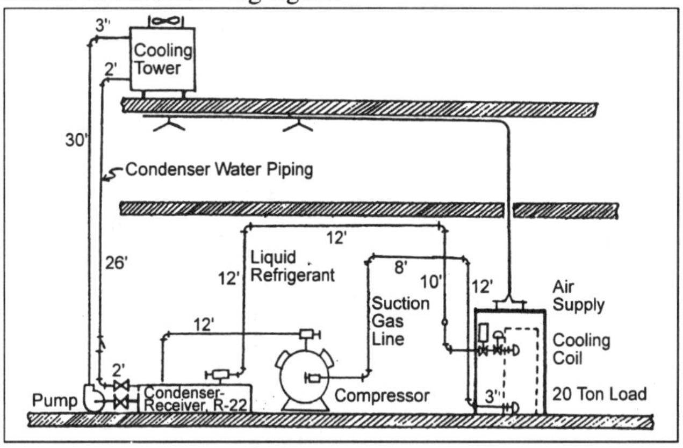

Diagram for Problem 9.54

(a) Refrigerant lines using R-22

(b) Condenser water lines

9.55 A gas appliance has an input rating of 80,000 Btu/h and is operated with natural gas (specific gravity = 0.60) having a heating value of 1050 Btu/ft^3. What size of supply pipe is necessary when the equivalent length is 70 ft and a pressure loss of 0.3 in. of water is allowable?

9.56 Find the pressure loss in an oil fuel line which is 3/8-in. OD (10 mm) tubing carrying 80 gal/h (84 mL/s) of No. 4 fuel oil at 40°F (4.4°C).

9.57 In a reduced size branch tee (50 to 25 mm), calculate the side branch equivalent length for 9.1 m^3/h and 22.75 m^3/h entering the tee.

9.58 A fan operating at 1200 rpm has been delivering 6500 cfm against a static head of 3.25 in. of water and a total head of 5.25 in. of water. The air temperature is 130°F, gage temperature, 90°F, and the input power is 6.1 kW. During a time of power difficulty, the operator notices that the static head is now 2.36 in. of water. There has been no change in the system. Find:

(a) New capacity in cfm
(b) New power input in kW
(c) Original efficiency of the fan (%)
[Ans: 5570 cfm, 3.82 kw, 65.5%]

9.59 A certain damper design introduces a head loss of 0.5 velocity heads when wide open. A damper of this design is to be installed in a 12 in. by 30 in. duct that handles 3000 cfm. The pressure drop in the undampered system is 1.5 in. of water. If the pressure drop through the damper when wide open is to be 5% of the total system resistance, how much cross-sectional area in the duct should the damper occupy?

9.60 What effect on the following parameters does a variation in air density have for a fan operating in a system:
(a) flow rate
(b) developed head
(c) horsepower

9.61 Should fans be placed before or after air heaters? Why?

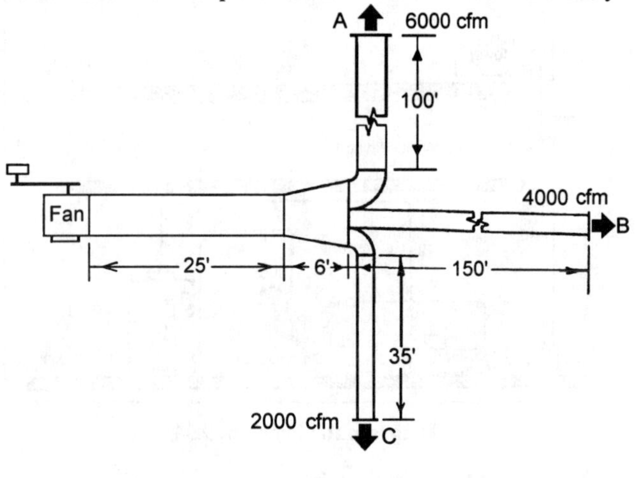

9.62 A fan delivers 1500 cfm (708 L/s) of dry air at 65°F (18.3°C) against a static pressure of 0.20 in. of water (50 Pa) and requires 0.10 bhp. Find the volume circulated, the static pressure, and the bhp required to deliver the same weight of air when the air temperature is increased to 165°F (73.9°C). (Note: Atmospheric pressure is constant.)

9.63 A 40 in. by 24 in. rectangular duct conveying 12,000 cfm of standard air divides into 3 branches (see figure). Branch A carries 6000 cfm for 100 ft, B carries 4000 cfm for 150 ft, and C carries 2000 for 35 ft.

(a) Size each branch for equal total friction of 0.15 in. of water. Do not exceed upper velocity limit of 2000 fpm.

(b) What is the total friction loss if the same quantity of air, 12,000 cfm of air at 150°F and 14.0 psia, is passed through the same system as part (a)?

(c) Assuming a fan is selected for part (a), at what percentage of the speed in part (a) must the fan run to satisfy part (b)?

9.64 A fan operating at N_1 rpm on a system with CFM_1, density d_1, and static pressure p_1 is to operate at the same static pressure at a lower density d_2 on the same system. Determine the relationship between N_1 and N_2.

9.65 A centrifugal fan operating at 2400 rpm delivers 20,000 cfm of air through a 32-in. diameter duct against a static pressure of 4.8 in. of water. The air is 40°F. The barometer is 29.0 in. Hg. Determine the horsepower input if the efficiency is 70%. If the fan size, gas density, and duct system remain the same, calculate the horsepower required if operated at 3200 rpm. [Ans: 60 hp]

9.66 Compute the efficiency of Fan 303 (Fig. 9-11b) when delivering 15,500 cfm at 4″ static pressure (SP).

9.67 Develop and explain the following relations for fan performance:
(a) $HP = CFM \times \Delta P/6350\eta_f$
(b) $kWH = HP\ (0.746)\ Hours/\eta_m$
(c) $\Delta t_f = \Delta P(0.371)/\eta_f$
(d) $HP \sim CFM^3$

9.68 A water pump develops a total head of 200 ft. The pump efficiency is 80% and the motor efficiency is 87.5%. If the power rate is 1.5 cents per kilowatt-hour, what is the power cost for pumping 1000 gallons? [Ans: 1.35 cents in 1 hr]

9.69 For a certain system it is required to select a pump that will deliver 2400 gpm (150 L/s) at a total head of 360 ft (110 m), and a pump shaft speed of 2400 rpm. What type of pump would you suggest? [Ans: centrifugal]

9.70 A pump delivers 1400 gpm of water. The inlet pipe is 4 in. nominal and the outlet pipe is 2 in. nominal standard pipe. The water temperature is 40°F. The surface of the inlet supply is 40 ft higher than the pump centerline. The discharge gage, which is 22 ft above the pump centerline, reads 180 psi. If the pump and motor combined efficiency is 60%, calculate the necessary input to the motor in kilowatts. [Ans: 290 kW]

9.71 A pump is required to force 9250 lb/h (4200 kg/h) of water at 165°F (74°C) through a heating system against a total resistance of 82,300 millinches of water (20.5 kPa). If the mechanical efficiency of the pump is 65%, find the required horsepower input.

9.72 How many horsepower are required to pump 66 gpm (4.16 L/s) against 60 ft (18.3 m) of head assuming 75% efficiency?

9.73 Solve the following problems:
(a) A certain system is found to have losses due to frictional effects according to the equation $H = 0.001\ (gpm)^2$ where H is in ft of water. The system is handling water at 160°F. For a design capacity of 300 gpm, what is the head devel-

oped by the pump and the bhp if the pump efficiency is 80%?

(b) What would be the theoretical maximum length of suction in order to prevent cavitation if the level of the supply tank is below the centerline of the pump? Assume atmospheric pressure to be 14.7 psi.

(c) If a capacity of 400 gpm is desired, what would be the speed ratio n_2/n_1 for the same pump, density of fluid, and system?

(d) Should a backward- or forward-curved blade pump be chosen? Would you make arrangements for a priming system for the pump? [Ans: 90 ft, 8.4 hp, 23.6 ft, 1.33]

9.7 References

ASHRAE. 1996 *ASHRAE Handbook—HVAC Systems and Equipment.*

ASHRAE. 1997 *ASHRAE Handbook—Fundamentals.*

ASHRAE. 1994. Duct fitting database.

Idelchik, I.E., G.R. Malyavskaya, O.G. Martynenko, and E. Fried. 1986. Handbook of Hydraulic Resistance, 2nd ed. Hemisphere Publishing Corp., New York.

Moody, L.F. 1944. Friction factors for pipe flow. *ASME Transactions* 66:671.

SI Figures and Tables

Table 9-1 SI Equivalent Rectangular Duct Dimension[a]

(Table 2, Chapter 32, 1997 *ASHRAE Handbook—Fundamentals*, SI version)

Length of One Side of Rectangular Duct (a), mm — Circular Duct Diameter, mm

Lgth Adj.[b]	100	125	150	175	200	225	250	275	300	350	400	450	500	550	600	650	700	750	800	900
100	109																			
125	122	137																		
150	133	150	164																	
175	143	161	177	191																
200	152	172	189	204	219															
225	161	181	200	216	232	246														
250	169	190	210	228	244	259	273													
275	176	199	220	238	256	272	287	301												
300	183	207	229	248	266	283	299	314	328											
350	195	222	245	267	286	305	322	339	354	383										
400	207	235	260	283	305	325	343	361	378	409	437									
450	217	247	274	299	321	343	363	382	400	433	464	492								
500	227	258	287	313	337	360	381	401	420	455	488	518	547							
550	236	269	299	326	352	375	398	419	439	477	511	543	573	601						
600	245	279	310	339	365	390	414	436	457	496	533	567	598	628	656					
650	253	289	321	351	378	404	429	452	474	515	553	589	622	653	683	711				
700	261	298	331	362	391	418	443	467	490	533	573	610	644	677	708	737	765			
750	268	306	341	373	402	430	457	482	506	550	592	630	666	700	732	763	792	820		
800	275	314	350	383	414	442	470	496	520	567	609	649	687	722	755	787	818	847	875	
900	289	330	367	402	435	465	494	522	548	597	643	686	726	763	799	833	866	897	927	984
1000	301	344	384	420	454	486	517	546	574	626	674	719	762	802	840	876	911	944	976	1037
1100	313	358	399	437	473	506	538	569	598	652	703	751	795	838	878	916	953	988	1022	1086
1200	324	370	413	453	490	525	558	590	620	677	731	780	827	872	914	954	993	1030	1066	1133
1300	334	382	426	468	506	543	577	610	642	701	757	808	857	904	948	990	1031	1069	1107	1177
1400	344	394	439	482	522	559	595	629	662	724	781	835	886	934	980	1024	1066	1107	1146	1220
1500	353	404	452	495	536	575	612	648	681	745	805	860	913	963	1011	1057	1100	1143	1183	1260
1600	362	415	463	508	551	591	629	665	700	766	827	885	939	991	1041	1088	1133	1177	1219	1298
1700	371	425	475	521	564	605	644	682	718	785	849	908	964	1018	1069	1118	1164	1209	1253	1335
1800	379	434	485	533	577	619	660	698	735	804	869	930	988	1043	1096	1146	1195	1241	1286	1371
1900	387	444	496	544	590	663	674	713	751	823	889	952	1012	1068	1122	1174	1224	1271	1318	1405
2000	395	453	506	555	602	646	688	728	767	840	908	973	1034	1092	1147	1200	1252	1301	1348	1438
2100	402	461	516	566	614	659	702	743	782	857	927	993	1055	1115	1172	1226	1279	1329	1378	1470
2200	410	470	525	577	625	671	715	757	797	874	945	1013	1076	1137	1195	1251	1305	1356	1406	1501
2300	417	478	534	587	636	683	728	771	812	890	963	1031	1097	1159	1218	1275	1330	1383	1434	1532
2400	424	486	543	597	647	695	740	784	826	905	980	1050	1116	1180	1241	1299	1355	1409	1461	1561
2500	430	494	552	606	658	706	753	797	840	920	996	1068	1136	1200	1262	1322	1379	1434	1488	1589
2600	437	501	560	616	668	717	764	810	853	935	1012	1085	1154	1220	1283	1344	1402	1459	1513	1617
2700	443	509	569	625	678	728	776	822	866	950	1028	1102	1173	1240	1304	1366	1425	1483	1538	1644
2800	450	516	577	634	688	738	787	834	879	964	1043	1119	1190	1259	1324	1387	1447	1506	1562	1670
2900	456	523	585	643	697	749	798	845	891	977	1058	1135	1208	1277	1344	1408	1469	1529	1586	1696

Length of One Side of Rectangular Duct (a), mm — Circular Duct Diameter, mm

Lgth Adj.[b]	1000	1100	1200	1300	1400	1500	1600	1700	1800	1900	2000	2100	2200	2300	2400	2500	2600	2700	2800	2900
1000	1093																			
1100	1146	1202																		
1200	1196	1256	1312																	
1300	1244	1306	1365	1421																
1400	1289	1354	1416	1475	1530															
1500	1332	1400	1464	1526	1584	1640														
1600	1373	1444	1511	1574	1635	1693	1749													
1700	1413	1486	1555	1621	1684	1745	1803	1858												
1800	1451	1527	1598	1667	1732	1794	1854	1912	1968											
1900	1488	1566	1640	1710	1778	1842	1904	1964	2021	2077										
2000	1523	1604	1680	1753	1822	1889	1952	2014	2073	2131	2186									
2100	1558	1640	1719	1793	1865	1933	1999	2063	2124	2183	2240	2296								
2200	1591	1676	1756	1833	1906	1977	2044	2110	2173	2233	2292	2350	2405							
2300	1623	1710	1793	1871	1947	2019	2088	2155	2220	2283	2343	2402	2459	2514						
2400	1655	1744	1828	1909	1986	2060	2131	2200	2266	2330	2393	2453	2511	2568	2624					
2500	1685	1776	1862	1945	2024	2100	2173	2243	2311	2377	2441	2502	2562	2621	2678	2733				
2600	1715	1808	1896	1980	2061	2139	2213	2285	2355	2422	2487	2551	2612	2672	2730	2787	2842			
2700	1744	1839	1929	2015	2097	2177	2253	2327	2398	2466	2533	2598	2661	2722	2782	2840	2896	2952		
2800	1772	1869	1961	2048	2133	2214	2292	2367	2439	2510	2578	2644	2708	2771	2832	2891	2949	3006	3061	
2900	1800	1898	1992	2081	2167	2250	2329	2406	2480	2552	2621	2689	2755	2819	2881	2941	3001	3058	3115	3170

[a]Table based on $D_e = 1.30(ab)^{0.625}/(a+b)^{0.25}$.

[b]Length of adjacent side of rectangular duct (b), mm.

Table 9-8 SI Steel Pipe Data

(Table 2, Chapter 40, 1996 *ASHRAE Handbook—Systems and Equipment*, SI version)

U.S. Nominal Size, in.	Nominal Size, mm	Schedule[a]	Wall Thickness t, mm	Inside Diameter d, mm	Surface Area: Outside, m²/m	Surface Area: Inside, m²/m	Cross Section: Metal Area, mm²	Cross Section: Flow Area, mm²	Mass: Pipe, kg/m	Mass: Water, kg/m	Working Pressure[c] ASTM A53 B to 200°C: Mfr. Process	Joint Type[b]	kPa (gage)
1/4	8	40 ST	2.24	9.25	0.043	0.029	80.6	67.1	0.631	0.067	CW	T	1296
		80 XS	3.02	7.67	0.043	0.024	101.5	46.2	0.796	0.046	CW	T	6006
3/8	10	40 ST	2.31	12.52	0.054	0.039	107.7	123.2	0.844	0.123	CW	T	1400
		80 XS	3.20	10.74	0.054	0.034	140.2	90.7	1.098	0.091	CW	T	5654
1/2	15	40 ST	2.77	15.80	0.067	0.050	161.5	196.0	1.265	0.196	CW	T	1476
		80 XS	3.73	13.87	0.067	0.044	206.5	151.1	1.618	0.151	CW	T	5192
3/4	20	40 ST	2.87	20.93	0.084	0.066	214.6	344.0	1.68	0.344	CW	T	1496
		80 XS	3.91	18.85	0.084	0.059	279.7	279.0	2.19	0.279	CW	T	4695
1	25	40 ST	3.38	26.64	0.105	0.084	318.6	557.6	2.50	0.558	CW	T	1558
		80 XS	4.55	24.31	0.105	0.076	412.1	464.1	3.23	0.464	CW	T	4427
1-1/4	32	40 ST	3.56	35.05	0.132	0.110	431.3	965.0	3.38	0.965	CW	T	1579
		80 XS	4.85	32.46	0.132	0.102	568.7	827.6	4.45	0.828	CW	T	4096
1-1/2	40	40 ST	3.68	40.89	0.152	0.128	515.5	1 313	4.05	1.313	CW	T	1593
		80 XS	5.08	38.10	0.152	0.120	689.0	1 140	5.40	1.140	CW	T	3972
2	50	40 ST	3.91	52.50	0.190	0.165	690.3	2 165	5.43	2.165	CW	T	1586
		80 XS	5.54	49.25	0.190	0.155	953	1 905	7.47	1.905	CW	T	3799
2 -1/2	65	40 ST	5.16	62.71	0.229	0.197	1 099	3 089	8.62	3.089	CW	W	3675
		80 XS	7.01	59.00	0.229	0.185	1 454	2 734	11.40	2.734	CW	W	5757
3	80	40 ST	5.49	77.93	0.279	0.245	1 438	4 769	11.27	4.769	CW	W	3323
		80 XS	7.62	73.66	0.279	0.231	1 946	4 261	15.25	4.261	CW	W	5288
4	100	40 ST	6.02	102.26	0.359	0.321	2 048	8 213	16.04	8.213	CW	W	2965
		80 XS	8.56	97.18	0.359	0.305	2 844	7 417	22.28	7.417	CW	W	4792
6	150	40 ST	7.11	154.05	0.529	0.484	3 601	18 639	28.22	18.64	ERW	W	4799
		80 XS	10.97	146.33	0.529	0.460	5 423	16 817	42.49	16.82	ERW	W	8336
8	200	30	7.04	205.0	0.688	0.644	4 687	33 000	36.73	33.01	ERW	W	3627
		40 ST	8.18	202.7	0.688	0.637	5 419	32 280	42.46	32.28	ERW	W	4433
		80 XS	12.70	193.7	0.688	0.608	8 234	29 460	64.51	29.46	ERW	W	7626
10	250	30	7.80	257.5	0.858	0.809	6 498	52 060	50.91	52.06	ERW	W	3344
		40 ST	9.27	254.5	0.858	0.800	7 683	50 870	60.20	50.87	ERW	W	4178
		XS	12.70	247.7	0.858	0.778	10 388	48 170	81.39	48.17	ERW	W	6116
		80	15.06	242.9	0.858	0.763	12 208	46 350	95.66	46.35	ERW	W	7453
12	300	30	8.38	307.1	1.017	0.965	8 307	74 060	65.09	74.06	ERW	W	3096
		ST	9.53	304.8	1.017	0.958	9 406	72 970	73.70	72.97	ERW	W	3641
		40	10.31	303.2	1.017	0.953	10 158	72 190	79.59	72.21	ERW	W	4020
		XS	12.70	298.5	1.017	0.938	12 414	69 940	97.28	69.96	ERW	W	5157
		80	17.45	289.0	1.017	0.908	16 797	65 550	131.62	65.57	ERW	W	7419
14	350	30 ST	9.53	336.6	1.117	1.057	10 356	88 970	81.15	88.96	ERW	W	3316
		40	11.10	333.4	1.117	1.047	12 013	87 290	94.13	87.30	ERW	W	3999
		XS	12.70	330.2	1.117	1.037	13 681	85 610	107.21	85.63	ERW	W	4695
		80	19.05	317.5	1.117	0.997	20 142	79 160	157.82	79.17	ERW	W	7453
16	400	30 ST	9.53	387.4	1.277	1.217	11 876	117 800	93.06	117.8	ERW	W	2903
		40 XS	12.70	381.0	1.277	1.197	15 708	114 000	123.09	114.0	ERW	W	4109
18	450	ST	9.53	438.2	1.436	1.376	13 396	150 800	104.98	150.8	ERW	W	2579
		30	11.10	435.0	1.436	1.367	15 556	148 600	121.90	148.6	ERW	W	3110
		XS	12.70	431.8	1.436	1.357	17 735	146 450	138.97	146.4	ERW	W	3654
		40	14.27	428.7	1.436	1.347	19 863	144 300	155.65	144.3	ERW	W	4185
20	500	20 ST	9.53	489.0	1.596	1.536	14 916	187 700	116.88	187.4	ERW	W	2324
		30 XS	12.70	482.6	1.596	1.516	19 762	182 900	154.85	182.9	ERW	W	3289
		40	15.06	477.9	1.596	1.501	23 325	179 400	182.78	179.4	ERW	W	4006

[a] Numbers are schedule numbers per ASME *Standard* B36.10M; ST = Standard; XS = Extra Strong.

[b] T = Thread; W = Weld

[c] Working pressures were calculated per ASME B31.9 using furnace butt-weld (continuous weld, CW) pipe through 100 mm and electric resistance weld (ERW) thereafter. The allowance A has been taken as

(1) 12.5% of t for mill tolerance on pipe wall thickness, *plus*

(2) An arbitrary corrosion allowance of 0.64 mm for pipe sizes through NPS 2 and 1.65 mm from NPS 2½ through 20, *plus*

(3) A thread cutting allowance for sizes through NPS 2.

Because the pipe wall thickness of threaded standard pipe is so small after deducting the allowance A, the mechanical strength of the pipe is impaired. It is good practice to limit standard threaded pipe pressure to 620 kPa (gage) for steam and 860 kPa (gage) for water.

Table 9-9 SI Copper Tube Data

(Table 3, Chapter 40, 1996 *ASHRAE Handbook—Systems and Equipment*, SI version)

U.S. Nominal Size, in.	Type	Wall Thick-ness *t*, mm	Diameter		Surface Area		Cross Section		Mass		Working Pressure[a,b,c] ASTM B88 to 120°C MPa (gage)	
			Outside *D*, mm	Inside *d*, mm	Outside, m^2/m	Inside, m^2/m	Metal Area, mm^2	Flow Area, mm^2	Tube, kg/m	Water, kg/m	Annealed	Drawn
1/4	K	0.89	9.53	7.75	0.030	0.0244	24	47	0.216	0.047	5.868	11.004
	L	0.76	9.53	8.00	0.030	0.0250	21	50	0.188	0.050	5.033	9.432
3/8	K	1.24	12.70	10.21	0.040	0.0320	45	82	0.400	0.082	6.164	11.556
	L	0.89	12.70	10.92	0.040	0.0344	33	94	0.295	0.094	4.399	8.253
	M	0.64	12.70	11.43	0.040	0.0360	24	103	0.216	0.103	3.144	5.895
1/2	K	1.24	15.88	13.39	0.050	0.0421	57	141	0.512	0.141	4.930	9.246
	L	1.02	15.88	13.84	0.050	0.0436	48	151	0.424	0.151	4.027	7.543
	M	0.71	15.88	14.45	0.050	0.0454	34	164	0.302	0.164	2.820	5.282
5/8	K	1.24	19.05	16.56	0.060	0.0521	70	215	0.622	0.215	4.109	7.702
	L	1.07	19.05	16.92	0.060	0.0530	60	225	0.539	0.225	3.523	6.605
3/4	K	1.65	22.23	18.92	0.070	0.0594	106	281	0.954	0.281	4.668	8.757
	L	1.14	22.23	19.94	0.070	0.0628	75	312	0.677	0.312	3.234	6.061
	M	0.81	22.23	20.60	0.070	0.0646	55	333	0.488	0.333	2.303	4.309
1	K	1.65	28.58	25.27	0.090	0.0792	139	502	1.249	0.502	3.634	6.812
	L	1.27	28.58	26.04	0.090	0.0817	109	532	0.973	0.532	2.792	5.240
	M	0.89	28.58	26.80	0.090	0.0841	77	564	0.691	0.564	1.958	3.668
1-1/4	K	1.65	34.93	31.62	0.110	0.0994	173	785	1.543	0.785	2.972	5.571
	L	1.40	34.93	32.13	0.110	0.1009	147	811	1.316	0.811	2.517	4.716
	M	1.07	34.93	32.79	0.110	0.1030	114	845	1.015	0.845	1.924	3.599
	DWV	1.02	34.93	32.89	0.110	0.1033	108	850	0.967	0.850	1.827	3.427
1-1/2	K	1.83	41.28	37.62	0.130	0.1183	226	1 111	2.025	1.111	2.786	5.226
	L	1.52	41.28	38.23	0.130	0.1201	190	1 148	1.701	1.148	2.324	4.351
	M	1.24	41.28	38.79	0.130	0.1219	157	1 181	1.399	1.182	1.896	3.558
	DWV	1.07	41.28	39.14	0.130	0.1228	135	1 203	1.204	1.203	1.627	3.048
2	K	2.11	53.98	49.76	0.170	0.1564	343	1 945	3.070	1.945	2.455	4.606
	L	1.78	53.98	50.42	0.170	0.1585	292	1 997	2.606	1.997	2.069	3.951
	M	1.47	53.98	51.03	0.170	0.1603	243	2 045	2.171	2.045	1.717	3.220
	DWV	1.07	53.98	51.84	0.170	0.1628	177	2 111	1.585	2.111	1.241	2.331
2-1/2	K	2.41	66.68	61.85	0.209	0.1942	487	3 004	4.35	3.004	2.275	4.268
	L	2.03	66.68	62.61	0.209	0.1966	413	3 079	3.69	3.079	1.917	3.592
	M	1.65	66.68	63.37	0.209	0.1990	337	3 154	3.02	3.154	1.558	2.917
3	K	2.77	79.38	73.84	0.249	0.2320	666	4 282	5.96	4.282	2.193	4.109
	L	2.29	79.38	74.80	0.249	0.2350	554	4 395	4.95	4.395	1.813	3.392
	M	1.83	79.38	75.72	0.249	0.2378	446	4 503	3.98	4.503	1.448	2.717
	DWV	1.14	79.38	77.09	0.249	0.2423	281	4 667	2.51	4.667	0.903	1.696
3-1/2	K	3.05	92.08	85.98	0.289	0.2701	852	5 806	7.62	5.806	2.082	3.903
	L	2.54	92.08	87.00	0.289	0.2733	714	5 944	6.39	5.944	1.738	3.254
	M	2.11	92.08	87.86	0.289	0.2761	596	6 063	5.33	6.063	1.441	2.703
4	K	3.40	104.78	97.97	0.329	0.3078	1084	7 538	9.69	7.538	2.041	3.827
	L	2.79	104.78	99.19	0.329	0.3115	895	7 727	8.00	7.727	1.675	3.144
	M	2.41	104.78	99.95	0.329	0.3139	776	7 846	6.94	7.846	1.448	2.717
	DWV	1.47	104.78	101.83	0.329	0.3200	478	8 144	4.27	8.144	0.883	1.655
5	K	4.06	130.18	122.05	0.409	0.3834	1610	11 699	14.39	11.70	1.965	3.682
	L	3.18	130.18	123.83	0.409	0.3889	1266	12 042	11.32	12.04	1.531	2.875
	M	2.77	130.18	124.64	0.409	0.3917	1108	12 201	9.91	12.20	1.338	2.510
	DWV	1.83	130.18	126.52	0.409	0.3975	737	12 572	6.59	12.57	0.883	1.655
6	K	4.88	155.58	145.82	0.489	0.4581	2309	16 701	20.64	16.70	1.972	3.696
	L	3.56	155.58	148.46	0.489	0.4663	1698	17 311	15.18	17.31	1.434	2.696
	M	3.10	155.58	149.38	0.489	0.4694	1484	17 525	13.27	17.53	1.255	2.351
	DWV	2.11	155.58	151.36	0.489	0.4755	1016	17 993	9.09	17.99	0.855	1.600
8	K	6.88	206.38	192.61	0.648	0.6050	4314	29 137	38.56	29.14	2.096	3.930
	L	5.08	206.38	196.22	0.648	0.6163	3212	30 238	28.71	30.24	1.544	2.903
	M	4.32	206.38	197.74	0.648	0.6212	2741	30 710	24.50	30.71	1.317	2.468
	DWV	2.77	206.38	200.84	0.648	0.6309	1771	31 680	15.83	31.62	0.841	1.579
10	K	8.59	257.18	240.00	0.808	0.7541	6705	45 241	59.93	45.15	2.096	3.937
	L	6.35	257.18	244.48	0.808	0.7681	5004	46 942	44.73	46.94	1.551	2.910
	M	5.38	257.18	246.41	0.808	0.7742	4259	47 686	38.07	47.69	1.317	2.468
12	K	10.29	307.98	287.40	0.968	0.9028	9621	64 873	85.99	64.87	2.103	3.937
	L	7.11	307.98	293.75	0.968	0.9229	6722	67 771	60.09	67.77	1.455	2.724
	M	6.45	307.98	295.07	0.968	0.9269	6112	68 382	54.63	68.38	1.317	2.468

[a] When using soldered or brazed fittings, the joint determines the limiting pressure.

[b] Working pressures were calculated using ASME *Standard* B31.9 allowable stresses. A 5% mill tolerance has been used on the wall thickness. Higher tube ratings can be calculated using the allowable stress for lower temperatures.

[c] If soldered or brazed fittings are used on hard drawn tubing, use the annealed ratings. Full-tube allowable pressures can be used with suitably rated flare or compression-type fittings.

Table 9-10 SI Application of Pipe, Fittings, and Valves for Heating and Air Conditioning
(Table 5, Chapter 40, 1996 *ASHRAE Handbook—Systems and Equipment*, SI version)

				Fitting		System	
Application	**Pipe Material**	**Type**	**Joint Type**	**Class**	**Material**	**Temperature, °C**	**Maximum Pressure at Temperature[a], kPa (gage)**
Recirculating Water 50 mm and smaller	Steel (CW)	Standard	Thread	125	Cast iron	120	860
	Copper, hard	Type L	Braze or silver solder[b]		Wrought copper	120	1030
	PVC	Sch 80	Solvent	Sch 80	PVC	24	
	CPVC	Sch 80	Solvent	Sch 80	CPVC	65	
	PB	SDR-11	Heat fusion		PB	70	
			Insert crimp		Metal	70	
65 to 300 mm	A53 B ERW Steel	Standard	Weld	Standard	Wrought steel	120	2760
			Flange	150	Wrought steel	120	1720
			Flange	125	Cast iron	120	1200
			Flange	250	Cast iron	120	2760
			Groove		MI or ductile iron	110	2070
	PB	SDR-11	Heat fusion		PB	70	
Steam and Condensate 50 mm and smaller	Steel (CW)	Standard[c]	Thread	125	Cast iron		620
			Thread	150	Malleable iron		620
	A53 B ERW Steel	Standard[c]	Thread	125	Cast iron		690
			Thread	150	Malleable iron		860
	A53 B ERW Steel	XS	Thread	250	Cast iron		1380
			Thread	300	Malleable iron		1720
65 to 300 mm	Steel	Standard	Weld	Standard	Wrought steel		1720
			Flange	150	Wrought steel		1380
			Flange	125	Cast iron		690
	A53 B ERW Steel	XS	Weld	XS	Wrought steel		4830
			Flange	300	Wrought steel		3450
			Flange	250	Cast iron		1380
Refrigerant	Copper, hard	Type L or K	Braze		Wrought copper		
	A53 B SML Steel	Standard	Weld		Wrought steel		
Underground Water							
Through 300 mm	Copper, hard	Type K	Braze or silver solder[b]		Wrought copper	24	2410
Through 150 mm	Ductile iron	Class 50	MJ	MJ	Cast iron	24	1720
	PB	SDR 9, 11	Heat fusion		PB	24	
		SDR 7, 11.5	Insert crimp		Metal	24	
Potable Water, Inside Building	Copper, hard	Type L	Braze or silver solder[b]		Wrought copper	24	2410
	Steel, galvanized	Standard	Thread	125	Galv. cast iron	24	860
				150	Galv. mall. iron	24	860
	PB	SDR-11	Heat fusion		PB	24	
			Insert crimp		Metal	24	

[a] Maximum allowable working pressures have been derated in this table. Higher system pressures can be used for lower temperatures and smaller pipe sizes. Pipe, fittings, joints, and valves must all be considered.

[b] Lead- and antimony-based solders should not be used for potable water systems. Brazing and silver solders should be employed.

[c] Extra strong pipe is recommended for all threaded condensate piping to allow for corrosion.

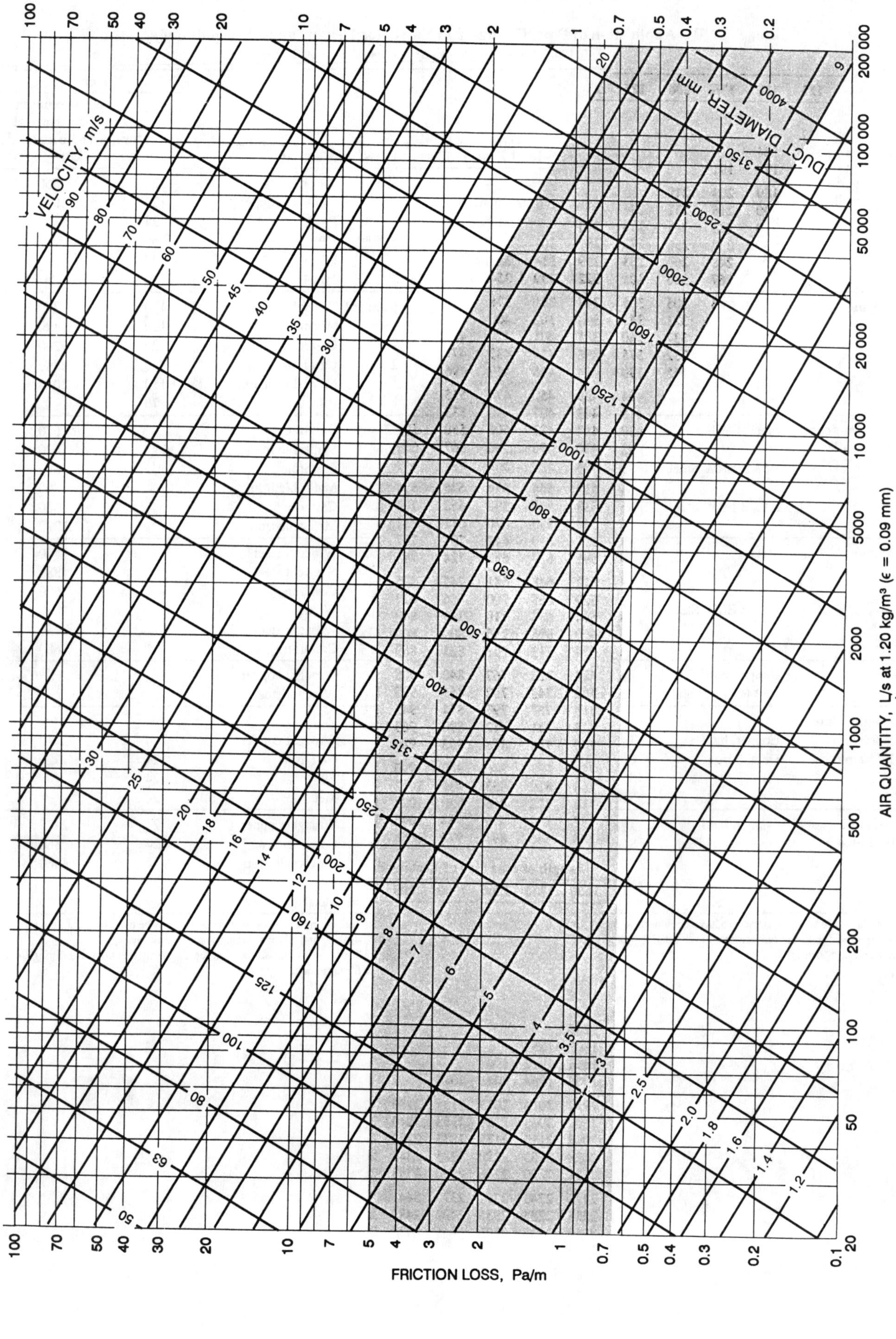

Fig. 9-2 SI Friction of Air in Straight Ducts

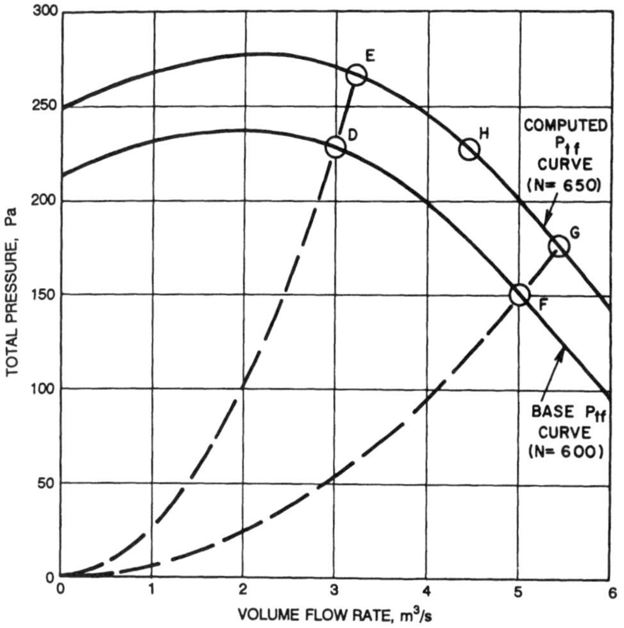

Fig. 9-6 SI Application of Fan Laws

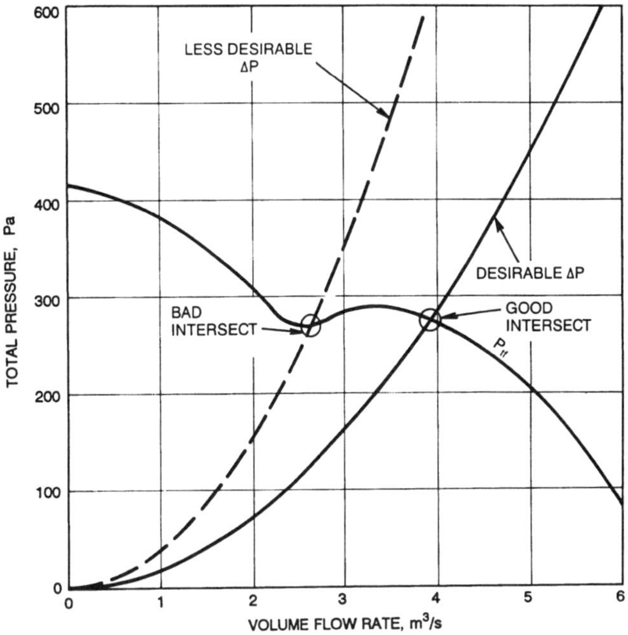

Fig. 9-12 SI Desirable Combination of p_{tf} and Δp Curves

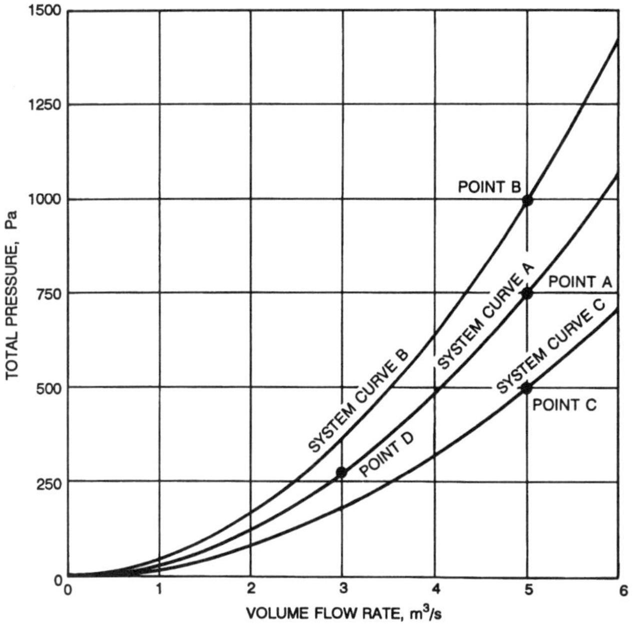

Fig. 9-8 SI System Total Pressure Loss (Δp) Curves

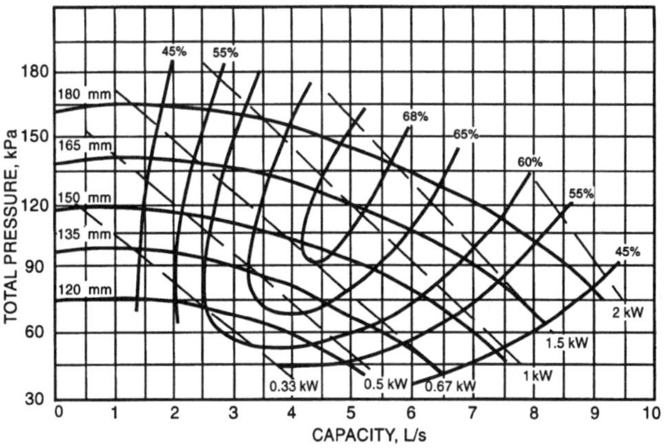

Fig. 9-13 SI Pump Performance Curves

Chapter 10

LIFE-CYCLE COSTS

This chapter presents the fundamentals for doing a simple engineering economic analysis for heating and air-conditioning systems and refrigeration installations. Additional information and more extensive analysis procedures are given in Chapter 33 of the 1995 *ASHRAE Handbook—HVAC Applications*.

10.1 General Concepts

A properly engineered HVAC system must also be economical. The selection of any system is often based on a compromise between its performance and economic merits. The system selected is usually determined by the user's needs, the designer's experience, local building codes, first costs, most efficient use of source energy, and the projected operating costs. Any one of the above factors may alter the choice of the system. However, when the choice is between alternatives that give equal results, the system with the lowest life-cycle costs should be chosen. This does not imply the lowest initial cost system; instead, it directs a decision toward a system with the lowest long-term costs. This overall cost may be divided into two main categories: owning costs and operating costs. These may be further subdivided as follows:

Owning Costs:
- Capital recovery and interes
- Taxes
- Insurance

Operating Costs:
- Energy and fuels
- Operating and maintenance services
- Materials and supplies

A representative form for assembling and tabulating these costs is shown in Table 10-1. Table 10-2 is an initial cost checklist to help identify the items that should be considered in the initial cost analysis. Additional information is given in Chapter 33 of the 1995 *ASHRAE Handbook—HVAC Applications.*

Life-cycle costs consider expenses that are experienced over an extended period. Many economic procedures can be used for life-cycle costing; they all project long-term costs so that comparisons can be made between systems having different initial and long-term operating costs. To be accurate, any procedure must include all cost factors relevant to the specific investment, such as initial costs, service life, interest, energy costs, taxes, operating expenses, and cost escalation.

Life-cycle cost techniques or procedures commonly used include (1) present worth, (2) uniform annual owning and operating costs, (3) rate of return, (4) rate of return of investment, (5) benefit cost analysis, (6) years to pay back, and (7) cash flow. Sophisticated systems, such as cash flow, are used by owners and investors to meet their particular objectives. Simpler techniques, such as benefit cost analysis and years to pay back, meet some needs, but can lead to improper decisions since important financial information is often neglected.

10.2 Owning Costs

Owning costs occur even if there is no activity in the facility. They can be expressed as annual costs that are distributed over an extended period, or as an equivalent total value, which is called **present worth**. Owning costs include initial costs, salvage value, property taxes, rents, and insurance.

10.2.1 Initial Costs

The first significant step in analyzing a system is to determine the first or initial costs. Initial costs include construction costs of the system and additional building costs attributed to the system. Costs to design, administer construction, and raise capital can also be included.

Interest. Money has a true value since it must be borrowed, obtained from equity or investors, or diverted from other uses. The cost of borrowed capital (interest) is a proper and important part of the life-cycle cost of an installation. Interest is also referred to as **cost of capital** or **discount rate**.

Time Period. The time period used by owners and engineers to analyze the system can be defined using several terms such as those following.

Depreciation period allocates the first cost of the asset over its estimated useful life. The period is the basis for a deduction against income in calculating income taxes. Various methods are allowed by the Internal Revenue Service, including straight line or the more accelerated procedures, such as declining balance or sum of the years.

Amortization period is the period n selected to perform economic comparisons. It is a time over which periodic payments of monies are made to discharge a debt. The amortization period used is often arbitrarily selected to meet the needs of the project.

Service life is a time value that reflects the expected life of a specific component. Service life should not be confused with **useful life** or **depreciation period**, as used for income tax purposes. It is the life expectancy of system components. Equipment life is highly variable due to diverse equipment applications, the preventive maintenance given, the environment, technical advancements of new equipment, and personal opinions. The values in Table 10-3 describe the replacement time of the components. Service life can be used to establish an amortization period; or, if an amortization period is given, service life can give insight into adjusting the maintenance costs of components.

Capital recovery factor (CRF) is calculated using interest i and amortization period n that determines the uniform annual cost needed to repay a debt or initial cost. The factor is determined by the following equation:

$$\text{CRF} = \frac{i(1+i)^n}{(1+i)^n - 1} \tag{10-1}$$

CRF values are listed in Table 10-4. As an example, if a $1000 expenditure is to be amortized over 20 years at 8%, the CRF factor is 0.10185. Multiplying the expenditure by the CRF factor gives $101.85. This is then the uniform annual owning cost necessary when 20 years is required to repay the debt.

Present Worth. The initial cash required (or present worth) is the current value of monies to be spent over the selected amortization period. In essence, it is the money necessary today for initial investment plus all the monies necessary for all future costs remaining.

Present worth factor, uniform annual series (PW_{uas}) is given in standard discount tables and is used to calculate the present worth when given a uniform annual cost. It is the reciprocal of CRF. The term does not consider escalation nor those costs which are not uniform or annual. PW is obtained by multiplying annual cost by PW_{uas} or by l/CRF.

Series compound amount factor, uniform annual series (SCAF) is used to determine a future sum of money when a uniform annual payment is made. The factor is determined by the following equation:

$$\text{SCAF} = \frac{(1+i)^n - 1}{i} \tag{10-2}$$

The actual sum is determined by multiplying the annual cost by SCAF. The reciprocal of SCAF is called the sinking fund factor (SFF) and is used to calculate a uniform annual cost from a given value at the end of an amortization period n.

Present worth factor, single payment (PWF_{sp}) is used to calculate the present worth of a future one-time cost. The PWF_{sp} is determined by the following equation:

$$PWF_{sp} = \frac{1}{(1+i)^n} \tag{10-3}$$

This factor, when multiplied by the actual costs, gives the present worth of a one-time cost, such as major overhaul or equipment replacement. The reciprocal is called the compound amount factor, single payment.

10.2.2 Property Tax

Property tax is included as an owning cost and is levied as a percentage of the market value of buildings. It varies with localities. The engineer must evaluate the effects of appreciation or depreciation of property values with time and the variation of the property tax rate. Tax incentives for energy conservation items may be an important consideration in determining justifiable long-term investment.

10.2.3 Insurance

Insurance is the means by which a property owner can be reimbursed for a financial loss from property damage that requires repair or replacement. Financial recovery may also include the recovery for loss of income, rents, or profits resulting from the property damage.

Each state regulates the activities of insurance companies doing business in the state and determines the premium rates that may be charged for the various forms of property insured. Some factors that influence the premium include building size, construction material, amount and size of mechanical equipment, the policy's liability limits, nature of the owner's business, and the amount of the deductibles. The selection of insurance is complex and is best determined by the owner and an insurance specialist.

10.2.4 Salvage Value

Terminal values of equipment occur at the end of life or amortization periods. These values are often assumed to be zero for many building components, as replacement takes place only when the equipment is practically worthless or costs as much to remove as its market value. Where such an assumption cannot be made, a salvage value should be included in the calculation.

10.3 Operating Costs

Annual expenses resulting from the actual use of the system are called operating costs. They include costs for energy, wages, supplies, water, material, maintenance, parts, and services.

10.3.1 Energy

Utility costs usually require a monthly calculation considering energy consumption and peak demands. Utilities then apply demand cost and step rate schedules to establish actual cost. Costs and service policies should be reviewed so that the most advantageous selection of energy type, systems, and system operation can be made. The most reliable energy cost-estimating procedure requires hourly integration of calculated energy use of each building component as a function of weather, internal loads, building heat gains and losses, and ventilation. The peak and total of these hourly consumption rates should reveal the comparative cost features of alternative control systems, distribution systems, energy sources, and other design options.

Table 10-1 Owning and Operating Cost Data Summary
(Table 1, Chapter 33, 1995 *ASHRAE Handbook—HVAC Applications*)

OWNING COSTS

I. Initial Cost of System

- A. Equipment (see Table 2 for items included) ______
- B. Control systems—Complete ______
- C. Wiring and piping costs attributable to system ______
- D. Any increase in building construction cost attributable to system ______
- E. Any decrease in building construction cost attributable to system ______
- F. Installation costs ______

TOTAL INITIAL COST ______

II. Annual Fixed Charges

- A. Equivalent uniform annual cost ______
- B. Income taxes ______
- C. Property taxes ______
- D. Insurance ______
- E. Rent ______

TOTAL ANNUAL FIXED CHARGES ______

OPERATING COSTS

III. Annual Maintenance Allowances

- A. Replacement or servicing of oil, air, or water filters ______
- B. Contracted maintenance service ______
- C. Lubricating oil and grease ______
- D. General housekeeping cost ______
- E. Replacement of worn parts (labor and material) ______
- F. Refrigerant ______

TOTAL ANNUAL MAINTENANCE ALLOWANCE ______

IV. Annual Energy, Fuel, and Water Costs

- A. Electric Energy Costs
  - 1. Chiller or compressor ______
  - 2. Pumps
    - a) Chilled water ______
    - b) Heating water ______
    - c) Condenser or tower water ______
    - d) Potable hot water recirculation ______
    - e) Well water ______
    - f) Boiler auxiliaries (including fuel oil heaters) ______
  - 3. Fans
    - a) Condenser or tower ______
    - b) Inside air handling ______
    - c) Exhaust ______
    - d) Makeup air ______
    - e) Boiler auxiliaries and equipment room ventilation ______

IV. Annual Energy, Fuel and Water Costs (*Continued*)

  - 4. Resistance heaters (primary or supplementary) ______
  - 5. Heat pump ______
  - 6. Domestic water heating ______
  - 7. Lighting ______
  - 8. Cooking and food service equipment ______
  - 9. Miscellaneous (e.g., elevators, escalators, and computers) ______
- B. Gas, Oil, Coal, or Purchased Steam Costs
  - 1. On-site generation of the electrical power requirements under A of this section ______
  - 2. Heating
    - a) Direct heating ______
    - b) Ventilation
      - (1) Preheaters ______
      - (2) Reheaters ______
    - c) Supplementary heating (i.e., oil preheating) ______
    - d) Other ______
  - 3. Domestic water heating ______
  - 4. Cooking and food service equipment ______
  - 5. Air conditioning
    - a) Absorption ______
    - b) Chiller or compressor
      - (1) Gas/Diesel engine driven ______
      - (2) Gas turbine driven ______
      - (3) Steam turbine driven ______
  - 6. Miscellaneous ______
- C. Water
  - 1. Condenser makeup water ______
  - 2. Sewer charges ______
  - 3. Chemicals ______
  - 4. Miscellaneous ______

TOTAL ANNUAL FUEL, ENERGY, AND WATER COSTS ______

V. **ANNUAL WAGES OF ENGINEERS AND OPERATORS** ______

SUMMARY

- II. Total Annual Fixed Charges ______
- III. Total Annual Maintenance Allowance ______
- IV. Total Annual Energy, Fuel, and Water Costs ______
- V. Annual Wages of Engineers and Operators ______

TOTAL ANNUAL OWNING AND OPERATING COSTS ______

Table 10-2 Initial Cost Checklist
(Table 2, Chapter 33, 1995 *ASHRAE Handbook—HVAC Applications*)

Energy and Fuel Service Costs
Fuel service, storage, handling, piping, and distribution costs
Electrical service entrance and distribution equipment costs
Total energy plant
Heat-Producing Equipment
Boilers and furnaces
Steam-water converters
Heat pumps or resistance heaters
Make-up air heaters
Heat-producing equipment auxiliaries
Refrigeration Equipment
Compressors, chillers, or absorption units
Cooling towers, condensers, well water supplies
Refrigeration equipment auxiliaries
Heat Distribution Equipment
Pumps, reducing valves, piping, piping insulation, etc.
Terminal units or devices
Cooling Distribution Equipment
Pumps, piping, piping insulation, condensate drains, etc.
Terminal units, mixing boxes, diffusers, grilles, etc.
Air Treatment and Distribution Equipment
Air heaters, humidifiers, dehumidifiers, filters, etc.
Fans, ducts, duct insulation, dampers, etc.
Exhaust and return systems
System and Controls Automation
Terminal or zone controls
System program control
Alarms and indicator system
Building Construction and Alteration
Mechanical and electric space
Chimneys and flues
Building insulation
Solar radiation controls
Acoustical and vibration treatment
Distribution shafts, machinery foundations, furring

Although cost escalation is difficult to establish, it can be applied to most annual costs. In the long run, investors expect to be compensated for purchasing power declines caused by inflation, plus a little extra. The difference between interest and inflation is called the **real return**. Historically, real returns are in the 1 to 5% range. Escalation values affect life-cycle costing and thereby influence the selection of equipment to be used, even when initial costs are greater.

The present worth of an annual cost over a selected time period n, using an interest of money i, and a cost escalation j, is the present worth escalation factor (PWEF). The following simplified, one-step calculation works when the interest and fuel cost rises are not equal:

$$\text{PWEF} = \frac{[(1+j)/(1+i)]^n - 1}{1-(1+i)/(1+j)} \qquad (10\text{-}4)$$

10.3.2 Maintenance

Expenses for labor and material necessary to make repairs, as well as for cleaning, painting, inspection, testing, and so forth, are important in determining total operating costs. Generally, an operating engineer or staff handles routine maintenance. If the responsibility extends to facilities beyond the equipment discussed here, only an equitable share of the group's time should be charged to maintenance on the system being evaluated. Extraordinary repairs are often handled by maintenance divisions and the expense is charged to the system's maintenance costs. In other cases, some or all maintenance is handled by outside service firms and it is considered as maintenance cost. These costs vary considerably with the type of system and the proficiency of the servicing organization. The annual maintenance allowance should be based on the entire amortization period under study. If annual costs are expected to rise or fall at a rate different from interest, present worth should be recalculated using escalation.

Dohrmann and Alereza (1986) developed a technique for estimating building HVAC maintenance costs for various equipment combinations. Using data from Table 10-5, the following method may be used; however, manufacturers and other industry sources should be consulted for current information on new types of equipment. Several important limitations of the data presented here should be noted:

- Only selected data from Dohrmann and Alereza (1986) are presented here.
- Data were collected for office buildings only.
- Data measure total HVAC building maintenance costs and do not measure the costs associated with maintaining particular items or individual pieces of equipment.
- The cost data are not intended for use in selecting new HVAC equipment or systems. This information is for equipment and systems already in place and may not be representative of the maintenance costs expected with newer equipment.

The premise of this method assumes that the base HVAC system in the building consists of fire-tube boilers for heating equipment, centrifugal chillers for cooling equipment, and variable-air-volume (VAV) distribution systems. The total building HVAC maintenance cost for this system is 33.38 ¢/ft². Adjustment factors from Table 10-5 are then applied to this base cost to account for building age and variations on type of HVAC equipment as follows:

C = Total building HVAC maintenance cost (¢/ft²)
= Base system maintenance costs
+ (Age adjustment factor) × (Age in years n)
+ Heating system adjustment factor h
+ Cooling system adjustment factor c
+ Distribution system adjustment factor d

or, in equation form,

$$C = 33.38 + 0.18n + h + c + d \qquad (10\text{-}5)$$

Example 10-1 Estimate the total building HVAC maintenance costs per square foot for a building that is 10 years old and has an electric boiler, a reciprocating chiller, and a constant volume distribution system.

Table 10-3 Estimates of Equipment Service Life[a]
(Table 3, Chapter 33, 1995 *ASHRAE Handbook—HVAC Applications*)

Equipment Item	Median Years	Equipment Item	Median Years	Equipment Item	Median Years
Air conditioners		Air terminals		Air-cooled condensers	20
Window unit	10	Diffusers, grilles, and registers	27	Evaporative condensers	20
Residential single or split package	15	Induction and fan-coil units	20	Insulation	
Commercial through-the-wall	15	VAV and double-duct boxes	20	Molded	20
Water-cooled package	15	Air washers	17	Blanket	24
Heat pumps		Ductwork	30	Pumps	
Residential air-to-air	15[b]	Dampers	20	Base-mounted	20
Commercial air-to-air	15	Fans		Pipe-mounted	10
Commercial water-to-air	19	Centrifugal	25	Sump and well	10
Roof-top air conditioners		Axial	20	Condensate	15
Single-zone	15	Propeller	15	Reciprocating engines	20
Multizone	15	Ventilating roof-mounted	20	Steam turbines	30
Boilers, hot water (steam)		Coils		Electric motors	18
Steel water-tube	24 (30)	DX, water, or steam	20	Motor starters	17
Steel fire-tube	25 (25)	Electric	15	Electric transformers	30
Cast iron	35 (30)	Heat Exchangers		Controls	
Electric	15	Shell-and-tube	24	Pneumatic	20
Burners	21	Reciprocating compressors	20	Electric	16
Furnaces		Package chillers		Electronic	15
Gas- or oil-fired	18	Reciprocating	20	Valve actuators	
Unit heaters		Centrifugal	23	Hydraulic	15
Gas or electric	13	Absorption	23	Pneumatic	20
Hot water or steam	20	Cooling towers		Self-contained	10
Radiant heaters		Galvanized metal	20		
Electric	10	Wood	20		
Hot water or steam	25	Ceramic	34		

Source: Data obtained from a survey of the United States by ASHRAE Technical Committee TC 1.8 (Akalin 1978).

[a]See Lovvorn and Hiller (1985) and Easton Consultants (1986) for further information.
[b]Data updated by TC 1.8 in 1986.

Table 10-4 Annual Capital Recovery Factors
(Table 5, Chapter 33, 1995 *ASHRAE Handbook—HVAC Applications*)

	Rate of Return or Interest Rate, % per Year								
Years	3.5	4.5	6	8	10	12	15	20	25
2	0.52640	0.53400	0.54544	0.56077	0.57619	0.59170	0.61512	0.65455	0.69444
4	0.27225	0.27874	0.28859	0.30192	0.31547	0.32923	0.35027	0.38629	0.42344
6	0.18767	0.19388	0.20336	0.21632	0.22961	0.24323	0.26424	0.30071	0.33882
8	0.14548	0.15161	0.16104	0.17401	0.18744	0.20130	0.22285	0.26061	0.30040
10	0.12024	0.12638	0.13587	0.14903	0.16275	0.17698	0.19925	0.23852	0.28007
12	0.10348	0.10967	0.11928	0.13270	0.14676	0.16144	0.18448	0.22526	0.26845
14	0.09157	0.09782	0.10758	0.12130	0.13575	0.15087	0.17469	0.21689	0.26150
16	0.08268	0.08902	0.09895	0.11298	0.12782	0.14339	0.16795	0.21144	0.25724
18	0.07582	0.08224	0.09236	0.10670	0.12193	0.13794	0.16319	0.20781	0.25459
20	0.07036	0.07688	0.08718	0.10185	0.11746	0.13388	0.15976	0.20536	0.25292
25	0.06067	0.06744	0.07823	0.09368	0.11017	0.12750	0.15470	0.20212	0.25095
30	0.05437	0.06139	0.07265	0.08883	0.10608	0.12414	0.15230	0.20085	0.25031
35	0.05000	0.05727	0.06897	0.08580	0.10369	0.12232	0.15113	0.20034	0.25010
40	0.04683	0.05434	0.06646	0.08386	0.10226	0.12130	0.15056	0.20014	0.25006

$$C = 33.38 + 0.18(10) - 2.67 - 4.0 + 8.81$$
$$= 37.32\ \text{¢/ft}^2 \text{ in 1983 dollars}$$

This estimate can be adjusted by multiplying the maintenance cost estimate by the current Consumer Price Index (CPI) divided by the CPI in July 1983, which was 100.1. Monthly CPI statistics are recorded in Survey of Current Business, a U.S. Department of Commerce publication. This estimating method is limited to one equipment variable per situation. That is, the method can estimate maintenance costs for a building having either a centrifugal chiller or a reciprocating chiller, but not both. Assessing the effects of combining two or more types of equipment in a single category requires a more complex statistical analysis.

Table 10-5 HVAC Maintenance Cost Adjustment Factors (In ¢/ft², 1983 U.S. Dollars)

(Table 4, Chapter 33, 1995 *ASHRAE Handbook—HVAC Applications*)

Age Adjustment	0.18 n
Heating Equipment h	
Water tube boiler	+0.77
Cast iron boiler	+0.94
Electric boiler	−2.67
Heat pump	−9.69
Electric resistance	−13.3
Cooling Equipment c	
Reciprocating chiller	−4.0
Absorption chiller (single stage)[a]	+19.25
Water-source heat pump	−4.72
Distribution System d	
Single zone	+8.29
Multizone	−4.66
Dual duct	−0.29
Constant volume	+8.81
Two-pipe fan coil	−2.77
Four-pipe fan coil	+5.80
Induction	+6.82

[a]These results pertain to buildings with older, single-stage absorption chillers. The data from the survey are not sufficient to draw inferences about the costs of HVAC maintenance in buildings equipped with new absorption chillers.

10.3.3 Labor for Operations

System operators are often necessary due to the scope of the facility or because of local ordinances. Building personnel may have functions unrelated to the system; thus, charges should be properly allocated.

10.3.4 Water Costs

Heat from a cooling system may be rejected either to purchased water or by means of cooling towers. Water conservation equipment must often be used regardless of economics because of local regulations intended to conserve the existing supply. Water treatment costs represent a significant operating expense. Lack of proper treatment can cause high energy consumption and operating problems.

10.3.5 Income Tax

Income taxes can be considered an operating cost in performing life-cycle cost analysis. The tax rate used in the calculation is the marginal rate, that is, the tax to be paid on the next dollar to be earned rather than the average tax rate. The allowances for depreciation and other deductions used in calculating income taxes strongly influence investments by reducing life-cycle costs. In the private sector this should not be ignored. Significant tax credits are often available for investments and should be included in life-cycle costs.

10.4 Life-Cycle Cost Techniques

10.4.1 Present Worth

The most commonly used life-cycle cost technique is present worth. This technique compares the equivalent cash needed on hand to own and operate a system over an entire selected time. It produces a single investment value in dollars.

Example 10-2 Calculate the future value of a system presently valued at \$10,000 in 10 years at 10% per year interest.

$$F = P(1+i)^n = \$10{,}000(1+0.1)^{10} = \$25{,}937.42$$

Example 10-3 Using the present worth factor for 10% per year interest and an analysis period of 10 years, calculate the present value of a future sum of money valued at \$10,000. (Another way of stating this problem is to determine what sum of money must be invested today at 10% per year interest to yield an amount of \$10,000 ten years from now.)

$$P = F \times \text{PWF}(i,n)_{sgl}$$

$$P = \frac{10{,}000 \times 1}{(1+0.1)^{10}} = \$3855.43$$

10.4.2 Uniform Annual Owning and Operating Costs

This technique compares the cost of both investment and annual costs on an annual base. Thus, the cost of owning the building or system is spread over the full amortization period.

In some cases, an economic analysis must be considered when a component has additional cost at some particular point in its life, as with replacements or major overhauls. This cost can be included in either owning or operating costs by multiplying the one-time expense by the single payment present worth factor determined by Equation (10-3).

In those economic cases where the components can be given different life expectancies, analysis is done by assigning the components different yearly maintenance costs or salvage values and keeping the same study or amortization period. Otherwise, separate amortization periods for each system that reflect the actual life expectancies of the equipment are used.

10.4.3 Rate of Return

The rate of return is the (average annual net benefits/original cost) × 100.

Example 10-4. An initial cost of \$800 in a unit will result in saving \$100/yr. The estimated life of the unit is 20 years. Determine the rate of return on the investment.

Solution:

$$\$100/\$800 = 0.125$$

The CRF is 0.125, and using the 20 year life and Table 10-4, the rate of return would be 10.92% by interpolation.

The **rate of return on investment** is the rate of return less the value of the money.

Example 10-5. For the case in Example 10-4, the interest rate is 8%. What is the rate of return on investment?

Solution:

$$\text{Rate of return on investment} = \text{Rate of return} - \text{Interest rate}$$

$$\text{Rate of return on investment} = 10.92 - 8 = 2.92\%$$

10.4.4 Benefit/Cost Analysis

This technique is a comparative procedure that provides the engineer and owner a ratio of cost versus saving. Both cost and saving must be converted to their present worth values or their uniform annual cost values.

Example 10-6. Using the same savings potential for a unit as given in Example 10-4 and an interest rate of 6%, determine the benefit/cost ratio excluding escalation.

Solution:

The present worth is calculated as

$$PW_{savings} = \text{Benefit} \times \frac{1}{CRF}$$

$$= \frac{100}{0.08718} = \$1147.05$$

The benefit/cost ratio is

$$B/C = PW_{benefit}/PW_{cost}$$

$$= PW_{savings}/\text{cost}$$

$$= \$1147.05/\$800 = 1.43$$

10.4.5 Years to Payback

Years to payback is similar to benefit cost analysis in that it does not look for system cost comparison at a specific life. As long as both engineer and owner agree that years to payback is reasonable and that life expectancy is not too different, it is a term that can be used in design concepts. Years to payback is determined by finding the years required for the present worth of the investment to equal the savings. A rigorous years to payback technique can be formulated by incorporating interest and cost escalation factors.

Example 10-7. Determine the simple payback period for a furnace air heater that costs \$10,000 to purchase and install and \$3,000 per year on the average to operate and maintain. By preheating the combustion air with this air heater it is expected to save an average of 10,000 therms of gas per year at \$0.64/therm.

Solution:

$$\text{Payback period} = \frac{\text{Present worth of investment}}{\text{Annual savings}}$$

$$= \frac{\$10{,}000}{[10,(000(\$0.64) - \$3000)]/\text{year}}$$

$$= 2.9 \text{ years}$$

Example 10-8 For the situation given in Example 10-4 (\$800 investment difference, first year savings of \$100, and interest rate of 6%) and assuming an escalation rate of 8%, determine the years to payback.

Solution:

The payback period PB occurs when the PW of the investment equals the PW of the savings. The PW of the savings can be adjusted for interest and escalation by use of Equation (10-4):

$$PW_{cost} = \text{Saving} \times \text{PWEF at year } n$$

$$\$800 = \$100 \times \frac{[(1+j)/(1+i)]^n - 1}{1-(1+i)/(1+j)}$$

$$\$800 = \$100 \times \frac{[(1.08)/(1.06)]^n - 1}{1-(1.06/1.08)} = 1.1480$$

$$1.1480 = 1.0189^n$$

Then

$$n = \ln 1.1480/\ln 1.0189$$

$$n = 7.37 \text{ years to payback}$$

10.4.6 Cash Flow

The **discounted cash flow approach** provides the owner with a technique to incorporate variable annual outlays and taxes, with the amount and year of the cash income. To evaluate the effect of interest and time, the net cash flow must be multiplied by the single payment present worth factor. The interest at which the summation of present worth of net cash flow is zero gives the rate of return. If this rate offers an acceptable rate of return to the investor, the proposal should be approved; otherwise, it should be rejected.

Another approach is to obtain an investment value at a given rate of return. This is accomplished by adding the present worth of the net cash flows, but not including the investment cost.

10.5 Problems

10.1 If \$1000 is invested at 8% interest, determine the value of this money in 10 years.

10.2 Find the present worth of money that will have a value of \$35,000 in 3 years with an interest rate of 9%.

10.3 \$1000 is invested at the end of each year for 10 years. Interest is 11%. Find the amount accumulated.

10.4 If \$100,000 is invested at 8% interest, find the yearly withdrawal that will use up the money in 20 years.

10.5 The cost of a new heat pump system is \$3000 with an expected lifetime of 20 years. Neglect energy and maintenance costs. Find the annual cost if the salvage value is \$0 and the interest rate is 8%.

10.6 A new heating system has a cost of \$15,000 and a salvage value of \$5000, independent of age. The new system saves \$1400 per year in fuel cost. Calculate the break-even point if $i = 9\%$. Neglect maintenance costs.

10.7 A new high-efficiency cooling system costs \$60,00 0 and saves \$7500 in energy costs each year. The system has a salvage value of \$10,000 in 20 years. Compute the rate of return. Neglect maintenance costs.

10.8 The costs of two small heat pump units A and B are \$1000 and \$1200 and the annual operating costs are \$110 and \$100, respectively. The interest rate is 8% and the amortization is selected as 20 years. Compare the systems on the basis of present worth.

10.9 Compare the units in *Problem* 10.8 on the basis of uniform annual costs.

10.6 References

ASHRAE. 1995 *Handbook—HVAC Applications.*

Dohrmann, D.R. and T. Alereza. 1986. Analysis of Survey Data on HVAC Maintenance Costs. *ASHRAE Transactions* 92(2A): 550-65.

Easton Consultants. 1986. Survey of Residential Heat Pump Service Life and Maintenance Issues. Catalog No. S-77126. American Gas Association, Arlington, VA.

Lovvorn, N.C. and C.C. Hiller. 1985. A Study of Heat Pump Service Life. *ASHRAE Transactions* 91(2B): 573-88.

Chapter 11

AIR-CONDITIONING SYSTEMS

An air-conditioning system maintains desired environmental conditions within a space. In almost every application there is a myriad of options available to the designer to satisfy the basic goal. It is in the selection and combination of these options that the engineer must consider all the parameters relating to the project.

Air-conditioning systems are categorized by how they control temperature in the conditioned area. They are also segregated to accomplish specific purposes by special equipment arrangement. This chapter considers elements that constitute the system. Chapter 12 describes those systems that are used to solve the psychrometric problem and control the environmental conditions of the occupied space, and Chapter 13 discusses the design of hot water and chilled water systems. Chapters 14 through 19 describe the various components of the air-conditioning system.

11.1 System Objectives and Categories

The two fundamental objectives of the air-conditioning system are to control the quality of the air in the conditioned space and the thermodynamic properties of the air. Additionally, in conjunction with other aspects of the space and system design, they become the major element in providing for the thermal comfort in the space.

11.1.1 Air Quality

Air quality is usually obtained through a process of ventilation combined with filtration. Ventilation consists of the removal of contaminants from the indoor air by replacing the contaminated air with non-contaminated air from the out of doors. This replacement is generally achieved through a process of dilution or, in rare cases—displacement. The amount of outdoor air required is determined by the rate and type of contaminant generation, generally as prescribed by ASHRAE *Standard* 62-1989 (or subsequent revisions thereof).

In many systems, the outdoor air is mixed with the return air from the space at the inlet to the air-conditioning system, and the mixture, then, conditioned to the thermodynamic state necessary to control the space temperature. However, this method need not be employed, and in many cases it is preferable to provide total thermodynamic conditioning of the outdoor ventilation air separate and apart from the space conditioning unit or directly to the space via a separate ventilating supply air system. The separate ventilating system, properly applied is preferable when using variable air volume systems because of the assurance of adequate ventilation at all conditions of load and improved humidity control in humid climates with most temperature control systems.

11.1.2 Thermodynamic Conditioning

The thermodynamic conditioning of the air is the process of simultaneously cooling and dehumidifying the air or heating (and sometimes humidifying) it to maintain comfort conditions within the space. In most systems designed for human comfort, the system control responds to dry bulb temperature, with the dehumidification being provided as a non-controlled by-product of the cooling process.

The fundamental equation describing a sensible cooling or heating process is:

$$q_s = 1.1Q\Delta t \tag{11-1}$$

where

q_s = heating or sensible cooling load, Btu/h
Q = flow quantity of supply air, ft³/min or cfm
1.1 = constant for standard air, Btu·min/h·°F·ft³
Δt = difference between room temp. and supply air temp.

For design conditions, i.e., for the airflow and temperature differential at the design system load (maximum system capacity), the sensible design load is calculated and Equation (11-1) is usually solved for Q, in which the designer selects a Δt. For cooling, the Δt is equal to $t_r - t_s$, where t_s is the supply air temperature, usually selected as the dewpoint temperature necessary to provide the latent cooling at design conditions.

Then, where the myriad of different types of air conditioning systems arise from is the different methods that are employed to change the capacity as the load reduces. Considering Equation (11-1), if the load q reduces (or changes) the only methods by which the equation can be kept in balance is by reducing either the Q or the Δt or some combination of the two. Thermodynamically four different methods are used to achieve these changes:

- Heat-Cool-Off
- Dual Stream
- Reheat
- Variable Air Volume

11.1.3 Heat-Cool-Off Systems

Heat-cool-off systems are any system which responds to the need for changes in capacity by varying the temperature of the air supplied by the unit, usually while maintaining a constant flow. There are many configurations of heat-cool-off systems, both two position and modulating, and although it is not common, they can be both variable flow rate Q or variable Δt, but are usually the latter. The essential feature that defines a heat-cool-off system is that it is limited to a *single* control zone.

11.1.4 Dual Stream Systems

Dual stream systems are applicable to cases in which multiple control zones are to be served from a single air conditioning unit. They are constant flow (Q), variable Δt systems. They achieve the variation in supply air temperature (from full cooling load to full heating load) by mixing a high temperature stream with a low temperature stream. The two most common dual stream systems are double duct and multi-zone systems. The induction system is another special configuration of a dual stream system.

11.1.5 Reheat Systems

Reheat systems also apply to cases in which multiple control zones are served from a single air-conditioning unit. However, single-zone units which function as heat-cool-off *can* be thermodynamically configured as reheat systems when applied to controlled dehumidifying requirements. This system is a constant flow, variable Δt system. In the multiple zoned reheat system (generally called **terminal reheat systems**) the central air handling system generally conditions the air to a fixed or controlled dewpoint temperature and the cool air is reheated to the temperature required to satisfy the space sensible load for each control zone.)

11.1.6 Variable Air Volume (VAV) Systems

These systems, like the dual stream and reheat systems apply to cases in which multiple control zones are served from a single air-conditioning unit. The main difference between variable-air-volume systems and other multiple zone systems, is that the VAV system varies the flow of the supply air rather than the temperature. Two characteristics of the VAV system become immediately evident.

- The VAV system can be either heat or cool at any given time, but it cannot do both at the same time. In order to both, it must be combined with one of the other systems (i.e., VAV-reheat, or VAV-dual stream).
- Conceptually, as the load reduces the air flow rate reduces and as the air flow rate reduces the fan power reduces, ideally as the cube of the flow.

Since, in most applications, the supply fan systems consume more energy annually than the refrigeration systems, the use of VAV systems offer significant potential benefits in energy conservation.

Most systems employ a combination of two or more of the above, such as dual stream/reheat, VAV/dual stream, VAV/reheat, heat-cool-off/reheat, etc. The following discussions will subdivide the system types into air systems and water systems consistent with the types discussed in the 1996 *ASHRAE Handbook—Systems and Equipment*. And, although the physical description and common name of the systems more closely describes their physical configuration, the designer is encouraged to always relate the system for purposes of modelling, diagnostics, or analyses to its generic thermodynamic type as described above.

11.2 System Selection and Design

An air-conditioning system maintains desired environmental conditions within a space. In almost every application, there are numerous options available to the designer to satisfy this basic goal. In the selection and combination of these options, the engineer must consider all the criteria defined by the functional requirements, or the design parameters.

In addition to the thermodynamic characteristics discussed above, air-conditioning systems are sometimes categorized by the method used to control cooling in the conditioned area. This chapter considers procedures for selecting the appropriate system for a given application. It also describes and defines the design concepts and characteristics of basic air-conditioning systems.

11.3 Design Parameters

The design engineer is responsible for considering various systems and selecting the one or more that will best satisfy all of the design parameters. It is imperative that the designer and the owner collaborate on identifying the goals of the design. Some of the parameters that should be considered are

- Load dynamics
- Performance requirements
- Availability of equipment
- Capacity
- Spatial requirements
- First cost
- Energy consumption
- Operating cost
- Simplicity
- Reliability
- Flexibility (short range and long range)
- Operations requirements
- Serviceability
- Maintainability
- Availability of service
- Availability of replacement components
- Environmental requirements of the space
- Environmental requirements of the community

The degree of success of the design of any system is directly related to the accuracy with which the designer (1) identifies the design parameters and (2) achieves them.

Because these factors are interrelated, the owner and system designer must consider how each factor affects the others. The relative impact of these parameters differs with different owners and often changes from one project to another for the same owner.

11.4 Performance Requirements

In addition to goals for providing the desired environment for human comfort, the designer must be aware of and account for other goals the owner may require. These goals may include

- Supporting a process, such as the operation of computer equipment
- Promoting an aseptic environment
- Increasing sales
- Increasing net rental income
- Increasing the salability of a property

Typical concerns of owners include first cost compared to operating cost, the extent and frequency of maintenance and whether that maintenance requires entering the occupied space, the expected frequency of failure of a system, the impact of a failure, and the time required to correct the failure. Each of these concerns has a different priority, depending on the owner's goals.

The owner can only make appropriate value judgments if the designer provides complete information on the advantages and disadvantages (i.e., the impact) of each option. Just as the owner does not usually know the relative advantages and disadvantages of different systems, the designer rarely knows all the owner's financial and functional goals. Hence, it is important to involve the owner in the selection of a system.

11.5 System Option Constraints

The first step in selecting a system is to determine and document constraints dictated by performance, capacity, available space, and any other parameters.

Few projects allow detailed quantitative evaluation of all alternatives. Common sense and subjective experience can be used to narrow choices to two or three potential systems.

11.5.1 Cooling Load

Establishing the cooling load often narrows the choice to systems that will satisfy all of the part load requirements, fit within the available space and are compatible with the building architecture. Chapter 7 covers determination of the magnitude and characteristics of the cooling load and its variation with time and operating conditions. By establishing the capacity requirement, the equipment size can be estimated. Then, the choice may be narrowed to those systems that work well on projects within a size range.

11.5.2 Zoning Requirements

Loads vary over time due to changes in the occupancy, weather, activities, and solar exposure. Each space with a different load dynamics requires a different control zone to maintain constant temperature. Some areas with special requirements in dry bulb or wet bulb control points may need individual control or individual systems, independent of the rest of the building. Variations in indoor conditions which are acceptable in one space, may be unacceptable in other areas of the same building. The extent of zoning, the degree of control required in each zone, and the space required for individual zones also narrow the system choices.

No matter how efficiently a particular system operates or how economical it may be to install, it cannot be considered if it (1) cannot maintain the desired interior environment within an acceptable tolerance under all conditions and occupant activities and (2) does not physically fit into the building without being objectionable and non-maintainable.

11.5.3 Heating and Ventilation

Cooling and humidity control are often the basis of sizing air-conditioning components and subsystems, but the system may also provide other functions, such as heating and ventilation. For example, if the system provides large quantities of outside air for ventilation or to replace air exhausted from the building, only systems that transport large air volumes need to be considered. In this situation, the ventilation system requires a large air-handling and duct distribution system, which may eliminate some systems.

Effective delivery of heat to an area may be an equally important factor in system selection. A distribution system that offers high efficiency and comfort for cooling may be a poor choice for heating. This performance compromise may be small for one application in one climate, but may be unacceptable in another that has more demanding heating requirements.

11.5.4 Architectural Constraints

Air-conditioning systems and the associated distribution systems often occupy a significant amount of space. Major components may also require special support from the structure. The size and appearance of terminal devices (whether they are diffusers, fan-coil units, or radiant panels) have an effect on the architectural design because they are visible from the occupied space.

Other factors that limit the selection of a system include (1) acceptable noise levels, (2) the space available to house equipment and its location relative to the occupied space, (3) the space available for distribution pipes and ducts, and (4) the acceptability of components obtruding into the occupied space, both physically and visually.

11.6 Narrowing the Choice

Chapter 12 covers the types of systems categorized by all-air systems, air-and-water systems, all-water systems, and unitary refrigerant-based systems. Each section includes an evaluation component, which briefly summarizes the positive and negative features of various systems. Comparing the features against the list of design parameters and their relative importance usually allows identification of two or three systems that best satisfy the project criteria. In making subjective choices, it is helpful to keep notes on all systems considered and the reasons for eliminating those that are unacceptable.

In most cases, two or three systems must be selected: a **secondary system** (or distribution system), which delivers heating or cooling to the occupied space, and a **primary system**, which converts energy from fuel or electricity and in some cases, an intermediate system which conveys energy between the primary system and the secondary system. Chapter 13 discusses the most common type of intermediate systems—water systems. The systems are, to a great extent, independent, so that several secondary systems may work with different primary and intermediate systems. In some cases, however, only one secondary system may be suitable for a particular primary system.

Once subjective analysis has identified two or three systems—and sometimes only one choice may remain—detailed quantitative evaluations of each system must be made. All systems considered should provide satisfactory performance to meet the design parameters goals. The owner then needs specific data on each system to make an informed choice. Chapter 8 outlines methods for estimating annual energy costs, and Chapter 10 describes life-cycle costing, which can be used to compare the overall economics of systems.

Example 11.1. A dual stream cooling system is a double-duct system with 55°F saturated air in the cold duct and 95°F db/60°F dewpoint air in the hot duct. The air in the cold duct is conditioned by cooling a mixed air stream (i.e., return air and outdoor air from 80°F db/66.8°F wb to 55°F saturated). The air in the hot duct is conditioned by heating the same mixed air stream to 95°F db with no addition or removal of water vapor. The room or space conditions are 75°F db/50% rh.

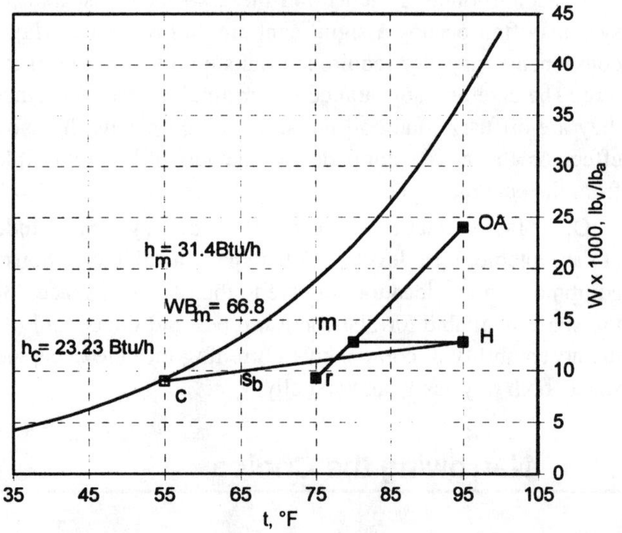

(a) A given zone has a sensible design cooling load of 12,960 Btu/h. What airflow (in cfm) must be supplied?

Solution: From Equation (11-1)

$$q_s = 1.1Q\Delta t$$

$$Q = \frac{q}{1.1(t_r - t_s)} = \frac{12960}{1.1(75-55)}$$

$$Q = 590 \text{ cfm}$$

(b) The load reduces, and when the space sensible load is 50% of design or 6480 Btu/h what is the condition of the supply air (dry bulb temperature and wet bulb temperature)?

Solution:

Dry-bulb temperature

From Equation (11-1)

$$t_{sdb} = t_r - \frac{q}{1.1Q} = 75 - \frac{6480}{1.1(590)}$$

$$t_s = 65\,°\text{F dry bulb}$$

Wet-bulb temperature

The wet-bulb temperature is determined where the mixing line between H (air at "m" heated to 95°F) and C on the psychrometric chart shown in the figure cross the 65°F db line. Thus

$$t_{swb} = 59.7°\text{F wet bulb}$$

(c) At the half load condition, approximately what airflow from the cold duct and the hot duct will be required?

Solution:

From the following equation for mixed air

$$t_m = t_c + \frac{m_H}{m_C + m_H}(t_H - t_C)$$

Solve for

$$\frac{Q_H}{Q_C} = \frac{m_H}{m_C + m_H} = \frac{t_m - t_C}{t_H - t_C} = \frac{65-55}{95-55} = 0.25$$

Then $Q_H = 0.25Q = 0.25(590) = 148$ cfm

$Q_C = 590 - 148 = 442$ cfm

(d) At thc half scnsiblc load condition, approximately what is the load on the cooling coil (in Btu/h) related to this zone?

Solution: From the following energy equation:

$$q_C = \dot{m}(h_m - h_C) = 60\rho_a Q(h_m - h_C)$$

$$q_C = 60(0.075)Q(31.4 - 23.23) = 4.5(442)(8.17)$$

$$= 16{,}250 \text{ Btu/h}$$

(e) At the half sensible load condition, approximately what is the load on the heating coil related to this zone?

Solution: From Equation (11-1):

$$q_H = 1.1(148)(95-65) = 4880 \text{ Btu/h}$$

(f) At full load condition, approximately what is the load on the cooling coil related to this zone? The heating coil?

Solution:

$$q_C = 4.5Q(h_m - h_C)$$

$$= 4.5(590)(31.4 - 23.23)$$

$$= 22690 \text{ Btu/h}$$

$$q_H = 0$$

11.7 Energy Considerations of Air Systems

Those systems which move energy from place to place within a building, such as the air distribution systems and liquid fluid circulation systems are called the energy transport systems. In first selecting, and then designing these systems, the power and energy required are seen to be two of the basic selection parameters.

The impact of the power is twofold. First, if the power is less, the first cost will be less because the machinery is smaller. And second, if the power is less the energy consumption will be less (other things being equal) because the energy consumed is simply the product of the power and the operating hours.

11.7.1 Air System Power and Energy

Equation (11-1), the heat capacity equation is the first consideration in the design of energy effective systems. It becomes evident that if the designer can do anything to reduce the load, which is a power term (Btu/h or tons of cooling) the system and machinery will be smaller, thus will cost less and use less energy when operated.

The fan power equation is:

$$P = \frac{Q\Delta p_t}{6350\eta_f} \qquad (11\text{-}2)$$

where

P = fan power, horsepower
Q = air circulation rate, ft³/min
Δp_t = fan total pressure rise, in. w.g.
η_f = fan efficiency, decimal

The equation shows that reducing the flow rate or the system pressure or increasing the fan efficiency will reduce the power. The flow rate can be reduced by, (1) reducing the load [Equation (11-1)], (2) by making a careful load analysis that does not include excessive or hidden uncertainty or "safety factors", or (3) by increasing the temperature difference between the supply and room air. [i.e., $(t_r - t_s)$].

The fan pressure equals the pressure loss requirement of the conditioner and the distribution system, a term which can be controlled by the system designer. Friction losses in the distribution system can be expressed by the Darcy-Weisbach equation which is:

$$\Delta h_f = f\frac{L}{D}\frac{V^2}{2g_c} \qquad (11\text{-}3)$$

where

Δh_f = friction loss, in. w.g.
f = friction factor, dimensionless
L = length of duct, ft
D = diameter of duct, ft
V = velocity of air in duct, ft/s
g_c = gravitational constant, $lb_f \cdot ft/s^2 \cdot lb_m$

The methods, then, to reduce the fan pressure requirement (fluid head loss) are:

- Limit the length of duct runs to the minimum possible
- Increase the diameter (or equivalent diameter)
- Reduce the velocity
- Reduce the roughness of interior surfaces which reduces the friction factor

Additionally, the duct fittings, in most systems, create a significant amount of the pressure losses. All fittings, in both the supply and return ductwork should be designed for minimum pressure losses, which are a function of the fitting construction and the velocity head $V^2/2g_c$. (See Chapter 32, 1997 *ASHRAE Handbook—Fundamentals*.) To assure continued operation with low pressure drops, any device such as a damper, coil, turning vanes, etc., which could result in a blockage to air flow should be provided with an inspection port.

An additional consideration regarding the pressure is the temperature rise across the fan. The temperature rise is expressed by the equation:

$$\Delta t_f = \frac{0.371\Delta p_t}{\eta_f} \qquad (11\text{-}4)$$

where

Δt_f = temperature rise across fan, °F
Δp_t = total pressure rise across fan, in. w.g.
η_f = fan efficiency, decimal

Equation (11-4) shows that if the fan efficiency is 74%, the temperature rise in °F would equal one half the pressure rise in in. w.g. For example, a 74% efficient fan producing 4 in. w.g. pressure would raise the air temperature 2°F. In most systems, this temperature rise becomes part of the cooling load, thus requiring the use of yet more energy.

Regarding fan efficiencies, fans should always be selected at the maximum efficiency point on their curves and it is highly recommended that a designer should always use a fan curve when selecting a fan so that the anticipated range of operation can be analyzed.

The fan energy equation is the power equation multiplied by the hours of operation and with the appropriate terms for motor efficiency and conversion of horsepower to kilowatts.

$$q_{fan} = \frac{Q\Delta p_t\theta}{8512\eta_f\eta_m} \qquad (11\text{-}5)$$

where

q_{fan} = fan energy, kWh
Q = air circulation rate, ft³/min
Δp_t = total fan pressure, in. w.g.
θ = time of operation, hours
η_f = fan efficiency
η_m = motor efficiency

The only variables that have been incorporated in this equation that were not included in the power Equation (11-2) are the hours of operation and the motor efficiency. In selecting and designing a system, accommodations should always be made to maintain an unoccupied building under controlled conditions while shutting down the major energy consuming devices, or operating them at a low energy consumption idle mode.

Regarding motor efficiencies, the use of high efficiency motors are always recommended for fan or pump drives.

Another form of the fan energy equation for *a fixed or given system* (i.e., the system curve is constant) is:

$$P_{fan} = \frac{Q^3}{6350\eta_f C_s^2} \quad (11\text{-}6)$$

$$q_{fan} = \frac{Q^3\theta}{8512\eta_f\eta_m C_s^2} \quad (11\text{-}7)$$

where C_s is the system constant in ft^3/[min (in w.g.)$^{0.5}$].

This equation shows that for a given system, if the air delivery rate can be reduced, the energy consumption is reduced as the cube of the flow rate (e.g. 20% flow reduction equates to 49% energy reduction, 50% flow reduction equates to 87.5% energy reduction, etc.). This characteristic explains one of the major benefits of using a variable flow system instead of a variable Δt system.

11.7.2 Water System Power and Energy

The relationships of power and energy consumption in water systems are similar to those in air systems, except for the change in the constants and dimensions. The fundamental power and energy equations for pumps in chilled and heating water systems are:

$$P_p = \frac{Q\Delta h}{3960\eta_p} \quad (11\text{-}8)$$

$$q_p = \frac{Q\Delta h\theta}{5308\eta_p\eta_m} \quad (11\text{-}9)$$

where

P_p = pump horsepower
q_p = pump energy, kWh
Q = water circulating rate, gallons/minute (gpm)
Δh = pump head, feet of water
θ = time of operation, hours
η_p = pump efficiency, decimal
η_m = motor efficiency, decimal

The principles of energy effective design discussed above for air systems apply equally to water systems.

Example 11.2. An air system is designed to handle 29,630 cfm at a total pressure of 6 in. w.g. If the ideal fan horsepower can be calculated by the use of Equation (11-2) with the fan efficiency term set at 100% efficiency,

(a) What is the ideal fan horsepower?

$$P = \frac{29630(6)}{6350} = 28.0 \text{ horsepower}$$

(b) If the fan were 70% efficient what would be the power requirement?

$$P = \frac{28.0}{0.70} = 40.0 \text{ hp}$$

(c) If the pressure required was reduced to 4 in. w.g. by modifying the distribution system, what power would be required?

$$P = \frac{29630(4)}{6350(0.70)} = 26.7 \text{ hp}$$

(d) If after installing the system, it was decided the load could be reduced 20% by reducing the fan speed, what would the power requirement be?

$$P = P_c\left(\frac{\text{New flow rate}}{\text{Original flow rate}}\right)^3$$

$$= 26.7(0.8)^3 = 13.7 \text{ hp}$$

11.8 Basic Central Air-Conditioning and Distribution System

The basic secondary system is an all-air, single-zone, air-conditioning system. It may be designed to supply a constant air volume or a variable air volume and for low-, medium-, or high-velocity air distribution. Normally, the equipment is located outside the conditioned area, in a basement, penthouse, or service area. It can, however, be installed within the area if conditions permit. The equipment can be adjacent to the primary heating and refrigeration equipment, or at considerable distance from it by circulating refrigerant, chilled water, hot water, or steam for energy transfer.

11.8.1 Applications

Some central system applications are (1) spaces with uniform loads, (2) small spaces requiring precision control, (3) multiple systems for large areas, (4) systems for complete environmental control, and (5) primary sources of conditioned air for other subsystems.

11.8.2 Spaces with Uniform Loads

Spaces with uniform loads are generally those with relatively large open areas and small external loads, such as theaters, auditoriums, department stores, and the public spaces of many buildings. Adjustment for minor variations in the air-conditioning load in parts of the space can be made by supplying more or less air in the original design and balance of the system.

In office buildings, the interior areas generally meet these criteria as long as local areas of relatively intense and variable heat sources, such as computer rooms and conference rooms, are treated separately. In these applications, dwarf partitions allow wider diffusion of the conditioned air and equalization of temperatures. These areas usually require year-round cooling, and any isolated spaces with limited occupancy may require special evaluation, as discussed in Chapter 3 of the 1995 *ASHRAE Handbook—Applications.*

In most single-room commercial applications, temperature variations up to 4°F at the outside walls are usually considered acceptable for tenancy requirements. However, these variations should be carefully determined and limited during design. If people sit or work near the outside walls, or if they are isolated by partitions, supplementary heating equipment may be required at the walls, depending on the outdoor design temperature in winter and the thermal characteristics of the wall. If the wall surface temperature is calculated to be more than 10°F below the room temperature, some special consideration must be given to the addition of heat at the perimeter.

11.8.3 Spaces Requiring Precise Control

These spaces are usually isolated rooms within a larger building (such as a computer room, auditorium, etc.) and have stringent requirements for such things as cleanliness, humidity, temperature control, and/or air distribution. Central system components can be selected and assembled to meet the exact requirements of the area.

11.8.4 Multiple Systems for Large Areas

In large buildings such as hangars, factories, large stores, office buildings, and hospitals, practical considerations sometimes require installation of multiple central single zone systems. The size of the individual system is usually determined by first cost, operating cost, and geometrical considerations.

11.8.5 Systems for Environmental Control

ASHRAE *Standard* 62 specifies ventilation rates for acceptable indoor air quality (IAQ). All-air systems often provide the necessary air supply to dilute the contaminants in the air in controlled spaces. These applications consist of combinations of supply systems and exhaust systems that circulate the diluting air through the space. The designer must consider the terminal systems used because establishing adequate dilution volumes is closely related to design criteria, occupancy type, air delivery, and scavenging methods. Indoor air quality is an essential consideration in the design of all systems.

Cleanliness of the air supply also relates directly to the level of environmental control desired. Suitable air filtration should be incorporated in the central system upstream from the air-moving and temperature control equipment. Some applications, such as hospitals, require downstream filtration as well.

Chapter 24 of the 1996 *ASHRAE Handbook—Systems and Equipment* has information on air cleaners.

11.8.6 Primary Sources for Other Systems

Systems for separate control of multiple zones are described in Chapter 12. These secondary systems may move a constant or variable supply of conditioned air for ventilation and temperature control and handle some or all of the air-conditioning load. Use of a secondary system may reduce the amount of conditioned air required to be delivered by the central system, thereby reducing the size of and the space required for ductwork. Ductwork size can be reduced further either by moving air at high velocities or by delivering air at reduced temperatures. However, high-velocity system design must consider the resultant high pressure, sound levels, and energy requirements. System design for low-temperature air delivery must consider the minimum required ventilation rates and insulation and condensation problems associated with lower temperatures as well as the additional refrigeration power.

11.8.7 Central System Performance

Figure 11.1 shows a typical draw-through central system that supplies conditioned air to a single zone or to multiple zones. A blow-through configuration may also be used if space or other conditions dictate. The quantity and quality of supplied air are fixed by space requirements and determined as indicated in Chapters 6 and 7. Air gains and loses heat by contacting heat transfer surfaces and by mixing with air of another condition. Some of this mixing is intentional, as at the outdoor air intake; for others, mixing is the result of the physical characteristics of a particular component as when untreated air passes without contacting the fins of a coil (bypass factor).

All treated and untreated air must be thoroughly mixed for maximum performance of heat transfer surfaces and for uniform temperatures in the airstream. Stratified, parallel paths of treated and untreated air must be avoided, particularly in the vertical plane of systems using double inlet or multiple-wheel fans. Because these fans do not completely mix the air, different temperatures can occur in branches coming from opposite sides of the supply duct.

11.9 Smoke Management

Air-conditioning systems are often used for smoke control during fires. Controlled air flow can provide smoke-free areas for occupant evacuation and fire fighter access. Space pressurization creates a low-pressure area at the smoke source, surrounding it with high-pressure spaces. For more information, see Chapter 48 of the 1995 *ASHRAE Handbook —Applications.* The publication, *Design of Smoke Management Systems* (ASHRAE 1992), has detailed information.

11.10 Components

11.10.1 Air-Conditioning Units

To determine a system's air-handling requirement, the designer must consider the function and physical characteristics of the space to be conditioned and the air volume and thermal exchange capacities required. Then, the various components may be selected and arranged by considering the fundamental requirements of the central system. Equip-

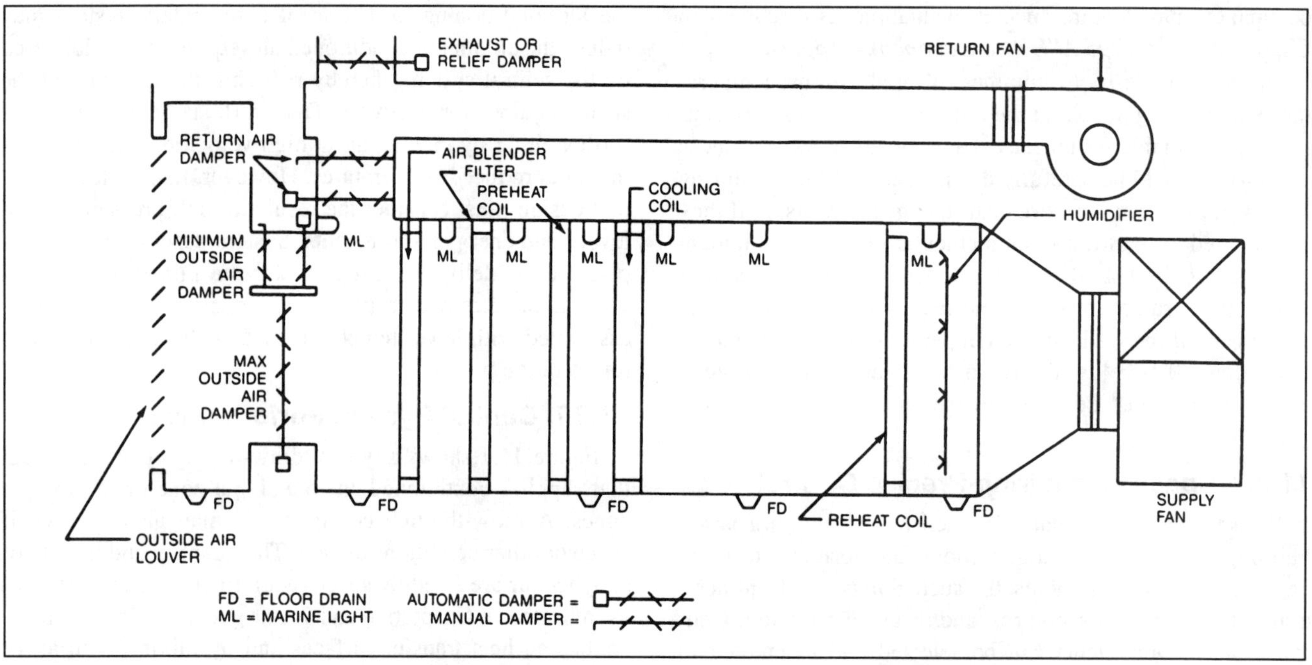

Fig. 11-1 Equipment Arrangement for Central System Draw-Through Unit

ment must be accessible for easy maintenance, and not too complex in arrangement and control to produce the required conditions.

Further, the designer should consider economics in component selection. Both initial cost and operating costs affect design decisions. The designer should not arbitrarily design for a 500 fpm face velocity, which has been common for selection of cooling coils and other components. Filter and coil selection at 300 to 400 fpm, with resultant lower pressure loss, could produce a substantial payback in constant volume systems.

Figure 11.1 shows a general arrangement of the components for a single-zone, all-air central system suitable for year-round air conditioning. With this arrangement, close control of temperature and humidity are possible. All these components are seldom used simultaneously in a comfort application. Although Figure 11.1 indicates a built-up system, most of the components are available from many manufacturers completely assembled or in subassembled sections that can be bolted together in the field. These units are called **air handling units**.

When selecting central system components, specific design parameters must be evaluated to balance cost, controllability, operating expense, maintenance, noise, and space. The sizing and selection of primary air-handling units substantially affect the results obtained in the conditioned space.

11.10.2 Return and Relief Air Fans

A return air fan is optional but is essential for the proper operation of a so-called air economizer or free cooling systems unless the excess intake air can be relieved directly from the space. It provides a positive return and exhaust from the conditioned area, preventing over pressurization of the space when mixing dampers provide cooling with outdoor air in intermediate seasons and winter.

The return air fan prevents excess ambient pressure in the conditioned space(s) when economizer cycles introduce more than the minimum quantity of outside air. It also reduces the static pressure the supply fan has to work against.

The supply fan(s) must be carefully matched with the return fans. The return air fan should handle a smaller amount of air to account for the building ventilation air requirements, and to ensure a slight positive pressure in the conditioned space.

In many situations, a relief (or exhaust) air fan may be used instead of a return fan. A relief air fan relieves ventilation air introduced during air economizer operation and operates only when this control cycle is in effect.

When a relief air fan is used, the supply fan must be designed for the total supply and return static pressure in the system and to operate without the relief air fan during the noneconomizer mode of operation. During the economizer mode of operation for a constant volume system, the relief fan must be controlled to exhaust at a rate that tracks the quantity of outside air introduced, to ensure a slight positive pressure in the conditioned space, as with the return air fan system cited previously.

When a mixing chamber and economizer system are utilized with a variable air volume system, special precautions must be taken in the control of the return air or relief air fans to assure that adequate ventilation air is provided at all times (see Chapter 12 for more discussion).

11.10.3 Automatic Dampers

Opposed blade dampers for the outdoor, return, and relief air-streams provides the highest degree of control. Section 11.10.7 on Mixing Plenums cover the conditions that dictate the use of parallel blade dampers.

Pressure relationships between various sections must be considered to ensure that automatic dampers are properly sized for wide open and modulating pressure drops.

11.10.4 Relief Openings

Relief openings in large buildings should be constructed similarly to outdoor air intakes, but they may require motorized or self-acting backdraft dampers to prevent high wind pressure or stack action from causing the airflow to reverse when the automatic dampers are open. The pressure loss through relief openings should be 0.10 in. w.g. or less. Low-leakage dampers, such as those for outdoor intakes, prevent rattling and minimize leakage.

Relief dampers sized for the same air velocity as the maximum outdoor air dampers facilitate control when an air economizer cycle is used. The relief air opening should be located so that the exhaust air does not short-circuit to the outdoor air intake.

11.10.5 Return Air Dampers

The negative pressure in the outdoor air intake plenum is a function of the resistance or static pressure loss through the outside air louvers, damper, and duct. The positive pressure in the relief air plenum is, likewise, a function of the static pressure loss through the exhaust or relief damper, the exhaust duct between the plenum and outside, and the relief louver. The pressure drop through the return air damper must accommodate the pressure difference between the positive-pressure relief air plenum and the negative-pressure outside air plenum. Proper sizing of this damper facilitates both air balancing and mixing. An additional manual damper may be required for proper air balancing.

11.10.6 Outdoor Air Intakes

Resistance through outdoor intakes varies widely, depending on construction. Frequently, architectural considerations dictate the type and style of louver. The designer should ensure that the louvers selected offer minimum pressure loss, preferable not more than 0.10 in. w.g. High-efficiency, low-pressure louvers that effectively limit carry over of rain are available. Flashing installed at the outside wall and weep holes or a floor drain will carry away rain and melted snow entering the intake. Cold regions may require a snow baffle to direct fine snow particles to a low-velocity area below the dampers. Outdoor dampers should be low-leakage types with special gasketed edges and special end treatment. **Separate damper sections with separate damper operators are strongly recommended for the minimum outdoor air needed for ventilation.** The maximum outdoor air needed for economizer cycles is then drawn through the entire outside air damper.

11.10.7 Mixing Plenum

To achieve effective mixing, many designers prefer to mix in the ductwork some distance upstream of the unit inlet. If a mixing plenum is employed careful consideration must be given to the objective of total mixing with no stratification under all conditions of operation.

If the equipment is alongside outdoor louvers in a wall, the minimum outdoor air damper should be located as close as possible to the return damper connection. An outside air damper sized for 1500 fpm usually provides acceptable control. The pressure difference between the relief plenum and outdoor intake plenum must be measured through the return damper section. A higher velocity through the return air damper—high enough to cause this loss at its full open position—enhances air balance and provides for better mixing. To create maximum turbulence and mixing, return air dampers should be set so that any deflection of air is toward the outside air. Parallel blade dampers may aid mixing.

When using a plenum or chamber, mixing dampers should be placed across the full width of the unit, even though the location of the return duct makes it more convenient to return air through the side. When return dampers are placed at one side, return air passes through one side of a double-inlet fan, and cold outdoor air passes through the other. If the air return must enter the side, some form of air blender or mixing device should be used.

Although opposed blade dampers offer better control, properly proportioned parallel blade dampers are more effective for mixing airstreams of different temperatures. If parallel blades are used, each damper should be mounted so that its partially opened blades direct the airstreams toward the other damper for maximum mixing.

Baffles that direct the two airstreams to impinge on each other at right angles and in multiple jets create the turbulence required to mix the air thoroughly. In some instances, unit heaters or propeller fans have been used for mixing, regardless of the final type and configuration of dampers. Otherwise, the preheat coil will waste heat, or the cooling coil may freeze. Low-leakage outdoor air dampers minimize leakage during shutdown.

Coil freezing can be a serious problem with chilled water coils. Full flow circulation of chilled water during freezing weather, or even reduced flow with a small recirculating pump, discourages coil freezing. Further, it can provide a source of off-season chilled water in air-and-water systems. Anti-freeze solutions or complete coil draining also prevent coil freezing. However, because it is difficult, if not impossible, to drain most cooling coils completely, caution should be exercised if this option is considered. (See Chapter 13.)

11.10.8 Filter Section

Control of air cleanliness depends heavily on the filter. Unless the filter is regularly maintained, system resistance is increased and airflow diminishes. Accessibility is a primary consideration in filter selection and location. In a built-up system, there should be minimum of 3 ft. between the upstream face of the filter bank and any obstruction. Other requirements for filters can be found in Chapters 24 and 25 of the 1996 *ASHRAE Handbook—Systems and Equipment*, and ASHRAE *Standard* 52.1-1992.

Good mixing of outdoor and return air is also necessary for good filter performance. A poorly placed outdoor air duct or a poor duct connection to the mixing plenum can cause uneven loading of the filter and poor distribution of air through the coil section.

11.10.9 Preheat Coil

The preheat coil should have relatively wide fin spacing, be accessible for easy cleaning, and be protected by filters. If the preheat coil is located in the minimum outdoor airstream rather than in the mixed airstream as shown in Figure 11-1, it should not heat the air to an exit temperature above 35 to 45°F; preferably, it should become inoperative at outdoor temperatures of 45°F. Inner distributing tube or integral face and bypass coils are preferable with steam. Hot water preheat coils should have a constant flow recirculating pump and should be piped for parallel heat flow so that the coldest air will contact the warmest coil surface first.

11.10.10 Cooling Coil

In this section, sensible and latent heat are removed from the air. In all finned coils, some air passes through without contacting (i.e., being thermally affected by) the fins or tubes. The amount of this bypass can vary from 30% for a four-row coil at 700 fpm to less than 2% for an eight-row coil at 300 fpm.

The dew point of the air mixture leaving a four-row coil might satisfy a comfort installation with 25% or less outdoor air, a small internal latent load, and sensible temperature control only. For close control of room conditions for precision work, a deeper coil is required.

A central station unit that is the primary source of conditioned air or ventilation air for other subsystems, such as in an air-and-water system, does not need to supply as much air to a space. In this case, the primary air furnishes outdoor air for ventilation and handles space dehumidification and some sensible cooling. This application normally requires deeper coils and can be provided with sprays.

11.10.11 Reheat Coil Section

Reheat is strongly discouraged, unless it is required to satisfy humidity control requirements. For energy conservation purposes, consideration may be given to using some form of recovered energy for a reheat source.

Heating coils located in the reheat position, as shown in Figure 11-1, in addition to being used for temperature control purposes, are frequently used for warm-up, although a coil in the preheat position is preferable for this purpose.

Hot water heating coils provide the highest degree of control. Oversized coils, particularly steam, can stratify the airflow; thus, where cost-effective, inner distributing coils are preferable for steam applications. Electric coils may also be used.

11.10.12 Humidifiers

For comfort installations not requiring close control, moisture can be added to the air by mechanical atomizers or point-of-use electric or ultrasonic humidifiers. Proper location of this equipment prevents stratification of moist air in the system.

Steam grid humidifiers with dew-point control usually are used for more accurate humidity control. In this application, the heat of evaporation should be replaced by heating the recirculated water, rather than by increasing the size of the preheat coil. It is not possible, of course, to add moisture to saturated air, even with a steam grid humidifier. Air in a laboratory or other application that requires close humidity control must be reheated after leaving a dehumidifier coil before moisture can be added. This requires reconsideration of air discharge temperatures and quantities.

The capacity of the humidifying equipment should not exceed the expected peak load by more than 10%. If the humidity is controlled from a sensor in the room or the return air, a limiting humidistat and fan interlock may be needed in the supply duct. This prevents condensation and mold or mildew growth within the ductwork when temperature controls call for cooler air. Many humidifiers add some sensible heat that should be accounted for in the psychrometric evaluation.

11.10.13 Supply Air Fan

Either axial flow, centrifugal, or plug fans may be chosen as supply air fans for straight-through flow applications. In factory-fabricated units, more than one centrifugal fan may be tied to the same shaft. If headroom permits, a single-inlet fan should be chosen when air enters at right angles to the flow of air through the equipment. This permits a more gradual transition from the fan to the duct and increases the static regain in the velocity pressure conversion.

To minimize inlet losses, the distance between the casing walls and the fan inlet should be at least the diameter of the fan wheel. With a single-inlet fan, the length of the transition section should be at least half the width or height of the casing, whichever is longer.

If fans blow through the equipment, the air distribution through the downstream components needs analyzing, and baffles should be used to ensure uniform air distribution. See Chapter 18 of the 1996 *ASHRAE Handbook—Systems and Equipment*.

11.11 Air Distribution

11.11.1 Ductwork

Ductwork should deliver conditioned air to an area as directly, quietly, and economically as possible. Structural features of the building generally require some compromise and often limit depth. Chapter 9 describes ductwork design in detail and gives several methods of sizing duct systems.

It is imperative that the designer coordinate duct design with the structure. In commercially developed projects, it is common that great effort is made to reduce floor-to-floor dimensions. The resultant decrease in the available interstitial space left for ductwork is a major design challenge.

11.11.2 Room Terminals

In some instances, such as in single zone, all-air systems, the air may enter from the supply air ductwork directly into the conditioned space through a grille or diffuser.

In multiple zoned air systems, an intermediate device controls air temperature and/or volume. Various devices are available, including: (1) an air-water induction terminal, which includes a coil or coils in the induced airstream to condition the return air before it mixes with the primary air and enters the space; (2) an all-air induction terminal, which controls the volume of primary air, induces ceiling plenum air and distributes the mixture through low-velocity ductwork to the space; (3) a fan-powered mixing box, which uses a fan to accomplish the mixing rather than depending on the induction principle; (4) a VAV box, which varies the amount of air delivered with no induction; (5) a VAV reheat terminal; (6) a double duct mixing box; and (7) a terminal reheat device.

11.11.3 Insulation

In all new construction (except low-rise residential buildings), air-handling ducts and plenums installed as part of an HVAC air distribution system should be thermally insulated in accordance with Section 9.4 of ASHRAE *Standard* 90.1. See Chapter 32 of the 1997 *ASHRAE Handbook—Fundamentals* for further discussion and calculation methodology.

11.11.4 Ceiling Plenums

The space between a hung ceiling and the floor slab above it is used frequently as a return plenum to reduce sheet metal work. Local and national codes should be consulted before using this approach in new design, because most codes prohibit combustible material in a return air ceiling plenum.

Entrance lobby ceilings with lay-in panels do not work well as return plenums where negative pressures from high-rise elevators or stack effects of high-rise buildings may occur. If the plenum leaks to the low-pressure area, the tiles may lift and drop out when the outside door is opened and closed. Return plenums directly below a roof deck have substantially higher return air gain than a ducted return, which has the advantage of reducing the heat gain to or loss from the space.

11.11.5 Controls

Controls should be automatic and *simple* for best operating and maintenance effectiveness. Operations should follow a natural sequence—depending on the space need, one controlling thermostat closes a normally open heating valve, opens the outdoor air mixing dampers, or opens the cooling valve. In certain applications, an enthalpy controller, which compares the heat content of outdoor air to that of return air, may override the temperature controller. This control opens the outdoor air damper when enthalpy is less than return air or space enthalpy and thus reduces the refrigeration load. On smaller systems, a dry-bulb control saves the cost of the enthalpy control and approaches these savings when an optimum changeover temperature, above the design dew point, is established.

A minimum outdoor air damper with separate motor, selected for a velocity of 1500 fpm, is preferred to one large outdoor air damper with minimum stops. A separate damper simplifies air balancing.

11.11.6 Equipment Isolation

Vibration and sound isolation equipment is required for most central system fan installations. Standard mountings of fiberglass, ribbed rubber, neoprene mounts, and springs are available for both fans and prefabricated units. If the fan manufacturer supplies the vibration isolators, it is common practice to supply neoprene pads for speeds above 1200 rpm, rubber-in-shear isolators (0.5 in. deflection) for speeds between 700 and 1200 rpm and springs with 1 in. deflection for speeds below 700 rpm.

11.11.7 Vibration Isolation

Special consideration is required in the isolation of rotating machinery such as fans and pumps when they are equipped with variable speed drives because of the relationship between frequency (i.e., rotational speed) and the effectiveness of vibration isolation devices.

The transmissibility of vibration isolators is defined as the ratio of the transmitted force to the impressed force, or

$$\mathrm{TR} = \frac{\text{Transmitted force}}{\text{Impressed force}} \qquad (11\text{-}10)$$

Thus, the smaller the transmissibility, the more effective is the isolator. It is common practice to select vibration isolators with a transmissibility between 0.10 and 0.05.

The relationship of the transmissibility to the system frequency is

$$\mathrm{TR} = \frac{1}{(f/f_n)^2 - 1} \qquad (11\text{-}11)$$

where

TR = transmissibility
f = frequency of the rotating mass, Hz
f_n = natural frequency of isolator system, Hz

Then, the frequency of the rotating mass in Hz is

$$f = N/60 \qquad (11\text{-}12)$$

where

N = rotational speed, rpm
60 = seconds per minute

and $$f_n = \frac{1}{2\pi}\sqrt{\frac{g}{y}} \qquad (11\text{-}13)$$

where

g = gravitational constant, 386 in/s^2

y = static deflection of isolator, in.

The solution to Equation (11-11) for rotating fan speeds of 0 to 1000 rpm and static deflections of 0 to 3 in. is plotted in Figure 11-2 for transmissibility of 0.05, 0.10, 1, and ∞. The graph demonstrates that for a given static deflection as the speed is decreased the transmissibility increases to the point where the isolator loses all of its effectiveness when $f/f_n = \sqrt{2}$, below which the isolator becomes an amplifier. Thus, extra care should be taken when selecting and designing isolators for a variable speed device. One method of assuring effective vibration control is to design the isolator at the minimum speed that the system will operate rather than at the design or maximum speed.

Ductwork connections should be made with fireproof fiber cloth sleeves having considerable slack, but without offset between the fan outlet and rigid duct. Misalignment between the duct and fan outlet can cause turbulence, generate noise, and reduce system efficiency. Electrical and piping connections to vibration-isolated equipment should be made with flexible conduit and flexible pipe connections. Special considerations are required in seismic zones.

Equipment noise transmitted through the ductwork can be reduced by sound-absorbing units, acoustical lining, and other means of attenuation. Sound transmitted through the return and relief ducts should not be overlooked. Acoustical

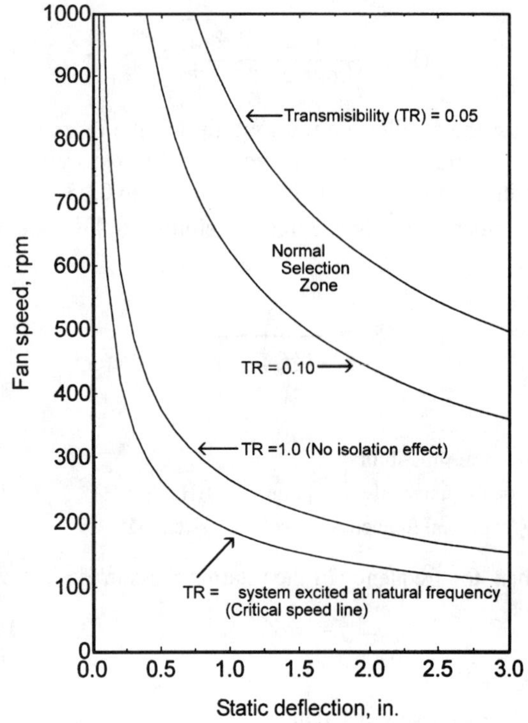

Fig. 11-2 Static Deflection of Isolator Versus Fan Speed

lining sufficient to adequately attenuate any objectionable system noise or locally generated noise should be considered. Chapter 43 of the 1995 *ASHRAE Handbook—Applications*, Chapter 7 of the 1997 *ASHRAE Handbook—Fundamentals*, and ASHRAE *Standard 68* have further information on sound and vibration control.

The designer must account for seismic restraint requirements for the seismic zone in which the particular project is located.

Example 11.3. A fan is selected to be operated at 720 rpm at design conditions and is supplied with a spring vibration isolator with 1 in. static deflection.

(a) What will be the transmissibility of the fan with the selected isolator mount?

Solution:

$$f = N/60 = 720/60 = 12 \text{ Hz}$$

$$f_n = \frac{1}{2\pi}\sqrt{\frac{g}{y}} = \frac{1}{2\pi}\sqrt{\frac{386}{1}} = 3.13 \text{ Hz}$$

$$TR = \frac{1}{(f/f_n)^2 - 1} = \frac{1}{(12/3.13)^2 - 1} = 0.07$$

(b) If the fan is driven by a variable speed drive controlled to reduce the speed to 37% of the design value, what will the transmissibility be at the minimum speed?

$$N_b = 0.37(720) = 266.4 \text{ rpm}$$

$$f = 266.4/60 = 4.44 \text{ Hz}$$

$$TR = \frac{1}{(4.44/3.13)^2 - 1} = 1$$

The isolator would provide no isolation.

11.12 Space Heating

Although steam is an acceptable medium for central system preheat or reheat coils, low-temperature hot water provides a simple and more uniform means of perimeter and general space heating. Individual automatic control of each terminal provides the ideal space comfort. A control system that varies the water temperature inversely with the change in outdoor air temperature provides water temperatures that produce acceptable results without individual room or space control in limited applications. To produce the best results, the most satisfactory ratio of indoor air temperature to that outdoors can be set after the installation is completed and actual operating conditions are ascertained.

Multiple perimeter spaces on one exposure served by a central system may be heated by supplying warm air from the central system. Areas that have heat gain from lights and occupants and no heat loss require cooling in winter as well as in summer, as do perimeter areas in which solar gains in winter combined with internal gains can exceed transmission losses.

In some systems, little or no heating of the return and outdoor air is required when the space is occupied. Local codes dictate the amount of outside air required (see ASHRAE *Standard* 62 for recommended outside air ventilation). For example, with return air at 75°F and outside air at 0°F, the temperature of a 25% outdoor/75% return air mixture would be 56°F, which is close to the temperature of the air supplied to cool such a space in summer. In this instance, a preheat coil installed in the minimum outdoor airstream to warm the outdoor air can produce overheating, unless it is sized as previously recommended. Assuming good mixing, a preheat coil located in the mixed airstream, prevents this problem. The outdoor air damper should be kept closed until room temperatures are reached during warm-up. A return air thermostat can terminate the warm-up period.

When a central air-handling unit supplies both perimeter and interior spaces, the supply air must be cool to handle the interior zones. Additional control is needed to heat the perimeter spaces properly. Reheating the air is the simplest solution, but it is not acceptable by some energy codes. An acceptable solution is to vary the volume of air to the perimeter and combine it with a terminal heating coil or a separate perimeter heating system, either baseboard, overhead air heating, or a fan-powered mixing box with supplemental heat. The perimeter heating should be individually controlled and integrated with the cooling control.

11.13 Primary Systems

The type of central heating and cooling equipment used for air-conditioning systems in large buildings depends chiefly on economic factors, once the total required capacity has been determined. Component choice depends on such factors as the type of fuel available, environmental protection required, structural support, and available space.

Rising energy costs have fostered many designs to recover the internal heat from lights, people, and equipment to reduce the size of the heating plant. Chapter 8 in the 1996 *ASHRAE Handbook—Systems and Equipment* describes several heat recovery arrangements.

The search for energy savings has extended to cogeneration or total energy systems, in which on-site power generation has been added to the heating and air-conditioning project. The economics of this function is determined by gas and electric rate differentials, investment cost of the plant, and by the ratio of electric to heat demands for the project. In these systems, waste heat from the generators can be put into the cooling equipment, either to drive the turbines of centrifugal compressors or to serve absorption chillers. Chapter 7 of the 1996 *ASHRAE Handbook—Systems and Equipment* presents further details on cogeneration or total energy systems.

Among the largest installations of central mechanical equipment are the central cooling and heating plants serving groups of large buildings. These plants provide higher diversity and generally operate more efficiently and with lower maintenance and labor costs than individual plants.

The economics of these systems require extensive analysis. Boilers, gas and steam turbine-driven centrifugals, and absorption chillers may be installed in combination in one plant. In large buildings with core areas that require cooling while perimeter areas require heating, one of several heat reclaim systems could heat the perimeter to save energy. Chapter 8 of the 1996 *ASHRAE Handbook—Systems and Equipment* gives details of these combinations, and Chapters 11, 12, and 14 of the 1996 *ASHRAE Handbook—Systems and Equipment* give design details of central plants.

Most large buildings, however, have their own central heating and cooling plant in which the choice of equipment depends on the following:

- Required capacity and type of usage
- Costs and types of energy available
- Location of the equipment room
- Type of air distribution system
- Owning and operating costs

Many electric utilities impose severe penalties for peak summertime power use, or alternatively, offer incentives for off-peak use. This policy has renewed interest in both water and ice thermal storage systems. The storage capacity installed for summertime load leveling may also be available for use in the winter, making heat reclaim a more viable option. With ice-storage, the low-temperature ice water can provide colder air than that available from a conventional system. Use of high water temperature rise and lower temperature air results in lower pumping and fan energy and, in some instances, offsets the energy penalty due to the lower refrigeration temperature required to make ice.

11.13.1 Heating Equipment

Steam and hot water boilers for heating are manufactured for high or low pressure and use gas, oil, or electricity, and sometimes, coal or waste material for fuel. Low-pressure boilers are rated for a working pressure of 15 psig for steam and 160 psig for water, with a maximum temperature limitation of 250°F. Package boilers, with all components and controls assembled as a unit, are available. Electrode or resistance-type electric boilers are available for either hot water or steam generation. For further information, see Chapter 19.

Where steam or hot water is supplied from a central plant, as on university campuses and in downtown areas of large cities, the service entrance to the building must conform to utility standards. The utility should be contacted at the beginning of the project to determine availability, cost, and the specific requirements of the service.

11.13.2 Fuels

Chapter 19 gives fuel types, properties, and proper combustion factors and includes information for the design, selection, and operation of fuel selection and automatic fuel-burning equipment.

11.13.3 Refrigeration Equipment

The major types of refrigeration equipment used in large systems are reciprocating compressors, helical rotary compressors, screw rotary compressors, centrifugal compressors, and absorption chillers. See Chapter 18 for further discussion of refrigeration equipment, including the general size ranges of available equipment.

Reciprocating, helical or screw rotary, and centrifugal compressors are usually driven by electric motors, however they can, and often are driven by gas and diesel engines and gas and steam turbines. The compressors may be purchased as part of a refrigeration chiller consisting of compressor, drive, chiller, condenser, and necessary safety and operating controls.

Reciprocating and helical or screw rotary compressor units are frequently used in packaged as well as in field-assembled systems, with air-cooled or evaporative condensers arranged for remote installation. Centrifugal compressors are used usually only in packaged chillers.

Absorption chillers are water cooled. They use a lithium bromide/water or water/ammonia cycle and are generally available in the following four configurations: (1) direct fired, (2) indirect fired by low-pressure steam or hot water, (3) indirect fired by high-pressure steam or hot water, and (4) fired by hot exhaust gas. Small direct-fired chillers are single-effect machines with capacities of 3.5 to 25 tons. Larger direct-fired, single-effect and double-effect chillers in the 100 to 2000 ton capacity range are available.

Low-pressure steam at 15 psig or hot water heats the generator of single-effect absorption chillers with capacities from 50 to 1600 tons. Double-effect machines use higher pressure steam up to 150 psig or hot water at an equivalent temperature (365°F). Absorption chillers of this type are available from 350 to 2000 tons.

The absorption chiller is sometimes combined with steam turbine-driven centrifugal compressors in large installations. Steam from the noncondensing turbine is piped to the generator of the absorption machine. When a centrifugal chiller is driven by a gas turbine or an engine, an absorption machine generator may be fed with steam or hot water from the jacket and/or an exhaust gas heat exchanger.

11.13.4 Cooling Towers

Water is usually cooled by the atmosphere for use in water-cooled condensers. Either natural draft or mechanical draft cooling towers or spray ponds are used for the cooling. Of these, the mechanical draft tower, which may be of the forced draft, induced draft, or ejector type, is used for most designs because it does not depend on the wind. Air-conditioning systems use towers ranging from small package units of 5 to 500 tons or field-erected towers with multiple cells in virtually unlimited sizes.

The tower must be winterized if required for operation at ambient outdoor dry-bulb temperatures below 35°F. Winterizing includes the capability of bypassing water directly into the tower return line (either automatically or manually, depending on the installation) and of heating the tower pan water to a temperature above freezing. (See Chapter 13 in the 1996 *ASHRAE Handbook—Systems and Equipment.*)

Heat may be added by steam or hot water coils or electric resistance heaters in the tower pan. Also, it is usually necessary to provide an electric heating cable on the condenser water and makeup water pipes and to insulate these heat-traced sections to prevent the pipes from freezing. Special controls are required when it is necessary to operate the cooling tower at or near freezing conditions.

Where the cooling tower will not operate in freezing weather, provisions for draining the tower and piping are necessary. Draining is the most effective way to prevent the tower and piping from freezing.

Careful attention must also be given to water treatment to keep maintenance required in the refrigeration machine absorbers and/or condensers to a minimum.

Cooling towers may also be used as a cooling source for the building in low temperature seasons by filtering and directly circulating the condenser water through the chilled water circuit, by cooling the chilled water in a separate heat exchanger, or by using the heat exchangers in the refrigeration equipment to produce thermal cooling. Towers are usually selected in multiples so that they may be run at reduced capacity and shut down for maintenance in cool weather. Chapter 18 includes further design and application details.

11.13.5 Air-Cooled Condensers

Air-cooled condensers pass outdoor air over a dry coil to condense the refrigerant. This results in a higher condensing temperature and, thus, a larger power input at peak condition; however, over the year this peak time may be relatively short. The air-cooled condenser is popular in small reciprocating systems because of its low maintenance requirements.

11.13.6 Evaporative Condensers

Evaporative condensers pass air over coils sprayed with water, thus taking advantage of adiabatic saturation to lower the condensing temperature. As with the cooling tower, freeze prevention and close control of water treatment are required for successful operation. The lower power consumption of the refrigeration system and the much smaller footprint from the use of the evaporative versus the air-cooled condenser are gained at the expense of the cost of the water used and increased maintenance costs.

11.13.7 Pumps

Pumps used in heating and air-conditioning systems are usually centrifugal pumps. Pumps for large and heavy-duty systems sometimes have a horizontal split case with a double-suction impeller for easier maintenance and higher efficiency. End suction pumps, either close coupled or flexible connected, are usually used for smaller tasks.

Major applications for pumps in the equipment room are as follows:

- Chilled water
- Heating water

- Condenser water
- Steam condensate pumps
- Boiler feed pumps
- Fuel oil

When the pumps handle hot liquids or have high inlet pressure drops, the required net positive suction head (NPSH) must not exceed the NPSH available at the pump. It is common practice to provide spare pumps to maintain system continuity in case of a pump failure. See Chapter 12 and 39 of the *1996 ASHRAE Handbook—Systems and Equipment*, for more design information on pumps and pumping systems. Section 5 in Chapter 9 also discusses pump selection.

11.13.8 Piping

Air-conditioning piping systems can be divided into two parts: the piping in the main equipment room and the piping required to deliver heat or chilled water to the air-handling equipment throughout the building. The air-handling system piping follows procedures detailed in Chapters 9 and 13.

The major piping in the main equipment room includes fuel lines, refrigerant piping, and steam and water connections. Chapter 10 of the 1996 *ASHRAE Handbook—Systems and Equipment* includes more information on piping for steam systems, and Chapter 12 has information on heating, chilled and dual-temperature water systems.

11.13.9 Instrumentation

All equipment must have adequate gages, thermometers, flow-meters, balancing devices, and dampers for effective system testing, balancing, monitoring and commissioning. In addition, capped thermometer wells, gage cocks, plugged duct openings, volume dampers, and access/inspection doors or ports should be installed at strategic points for system balancing. Chapter 34 of 1995 *ASHRAE Handbook—Applications* indicates the locations and types of fittings required.

A central control console to monitor the many system points should be considered for any large, air-conditioning system. A control panel permits a single operator to monitor and perform functions at any point in the building to increase occupant comfort and to free maintenance staff for other duties. Chapter 42 of the 1995 *ASHRAE Handbook—Applications* describes these systems in detail.

11.14 Space Requirements

In the initial phases of building design, the engineer seldom has sufficient information to finalize the designs. Therefore, most experienced engineers have evaluation criteria to estimate the building space needed.

The air-conditioning system selected, the building configuration, and other variables govern the space required for the mechanical system. The final design is usually a compromise between what the engineer recommends and what the architect can accommodate. Where designers cannot negotiate a space large enough to suit the installation, the judgement of the owners should be called upon.

Although few buildings are identical in design and concept, some basic criteria are applicable to most buildings and help allocate space that approximates the final requirements. These space requirements are often expressed as a percentage of the total building floor area.

11.14.1 Mechanical, Electrical, and Plumbing Facilities

The total mechanical and electrical space requirements range from 4 to 9% of the gross building area, the majority of buildings falling within the 6 to 9% range.

Most of the facilities should be centrally located to minimize long duct, pipe, and conduit runs and sizes; simplify shaft layouts; and centralize maintenance and operation. A central location also reduces pump and fan motor power, which may reduce building operating costs. But for many reasons, it is often impossible to centrally locate all the mechanical, electrical, and plumbing facilities within the building. In any case, the equipment should be kept together to minimize space requirements, centralize maintenance and operation, and simplify the electrical system.

Equipment rooms generally require clear ceiling height range from 12 to 20 ft, depending on equipment sizes and the complexity of ductwork, piping, and conduit.

The main electrical transformer and switchgear rooms should be located as close to the incoming electrical service as practical. If there is an emergency generator, it should be located considering (1) proximity to emergency electrical loads and sources of combustion and cooling air, (2) ease of properly venting exhaust gases to the outdoors, and (3) provisions for noise control.

The main plumbing equipment room usually contains gas and domestic water meters, the domestic hot water system, the fire protection system, and various other elements such as compressed air, special gases, and vacuum, ejector, and sump pump systems. Some water and gas utilities require a remote outdoor meter location.

The heating and air-conditioning equipment room houses the boiler or pressure-reducing station, or both; the refrigeration machines, including the chilled water and condensing water pumps; converters for furnishing hot or cold water for air conditioning; control air compressors; vacuum and condensate pumps; and other miscellaneous equipment. Local codes and ASHRAE *Standard 15* should be consulted for special equipment room requirements.

In high-rise buildings, it is often economical to locate the refrigeration plant at the top of intermediate floors, or on the roof. The electrical service and structural costs will rise, but these may be offset by reducing costs for condenser and chilled water piping, energy consumption, and equipment because of the lower operating pressure. The boiler plant may also be placed on the roof, which eliminates the need for a chimney through the building.

Gas fuel may be more desirable because oil storage and pumping present added design and operating problems, and the cost of oil leak detection and prevention may be substantial. However, restrictions on gas as a boiler fuel may preclude this option. Heat recovery systems, in conjunction with the refrigeration equipment, can appreciably reduce the heating plant size in buildings with large core areas. With well-insulated buildings and electric utility rates structured to encourage a high annual load factor, often electric resistance heat can be attractive, reducing space requirements even further.

Additional space may be needed for a telephone terminal room, a pneumatic tube equipment room, an incinerator, or other equipment.

Most buildings, especially larger ones, need cooling towers, which often present problems. If the cooling tower is on the ground, it should be at least 100 ft away from the building for two reasons: (1) to reduce tower noise in the building and (2) to keep cool season discharge air from fogging the building's windows. Towers should be kept the same distance from parking lots to avoid staining car finishes with water treatment chemicals. When the tower is on the roof, its vibration and noise must be isolated from the building. Some towers are less noisy than others, and some have attenuation housings to reduce noise levels. These options should be explored before selecting a tower.

The bottom of roof mounted towers, especially larger ones, must be set on a steel frame 4 to 5 ft above the roof to allow room for piping and proper tower and roof maintenance. Pumps below the tower should be designed for adequate net positive suction head, but they must be installed to prevent draining the piping on shutdown.

11.14.2 Fan Rooms

Fan rooms should preferably be located as close as possible to the space to be conditioned to reduce both installation cost and fan energy.

The number of fan rooms depends largely on the geometry of the buildings and use schedules of the spaces. Buildings with large floor areas often have multiple fan rooms on each floor. Many high-rise buildings, however, may have one fan room serving 10 to 20 floors—one serving the lower floors, one serving the middle of the building, and one at the roof serving the top portion of the building.

Life safety is a very important factor in fan room location. Chapter 48 of the 1995 *ASHRAE Handbook—Applications* discusses principles of fire spread and smoke management.

11.14.3 Interior Shafts

In tall buildings, interior shaft space accommodates return and exhaust air; interior supply air, hot, chilled, and condenser water piping; steam and return piping; electric closets; telephone closets; plumbing piping; and possibly, pneumatic tubes and conveyer systems.

The shafts must be clear of stairs, elevators and structural beams on at least two sides to allow maximum headroom when the pipes and ducts come out at the ceiling. In general, duct shafts having an aspect ratio of 2:1 to 4:1 are easier to develop than large square shafts. The rectangular shape also makes it easier to go from the equipment in the fan rooms to the shafts.

The size, number, and location of shafts is important in multi-story buildings. Vertical duct distribution systems with little horizontal branch ductwork are desirable because they are usually less costly; easier to balance; create less conflict with pipes, beams, and lights, and enable the architect to design lower floor-to-floor heights.

The number of shafts is a function of building geometry, but, in larger buildings, it is usually more economical, in cost and space to have several smaller shafts rather than one large shaft. Separate supply and exhaust duct shafts may be desired to reduce the number of duct crossovers and to operate the exhaust shaft as a plenum. **From 10% to 15% additional shaft space should be allowed for future expansion and modifications.** The additional space also reduces the initial installation cost.

11.14.4 Equipment Access

Properly designed mechanical equipment rooms must allow for the movement of large, heavy equipment in, out, and within the building. Equipment replacement and maintenance can be very costly if access is not planned properly. Many designers (and some machinery codes), require a minimum of 36" clear aisles between all machines and equipment.

Because systems vary greatly, it is difficult to estimate space requirements for refrigeration and boiler rooms without making block layouts of the system selected. Block layouts allow the engineer to develop the most efficient arrangement of the equipment, with adequate access and serviceability. Block layouts can also be used in preliminary discussions with the owner and architect. Only then can the engineer obtain verification of the estimates and provide a workable and economical design.

Example 11.4. A new law office building is being designed for St. Louis, Missouri, to use the HVAC system shown in the sketch below. Minimum outside air of 15 cfm/person for meeting the ventilation requirements of the anticipated 125 occupants will be maintained throughout the year. During summer operation, the cooling coil supplies air to the conditioned space at 55°F, 90% relative humidity. The space summer design loads and design conditions are:

323,000 Btu/h sensible (gain);
89,000 Btu/h latent (gain)
Outdoor: 94°F db, 75°F wb; Indoor: 78°F

The 55% efficient fan must produce a 3 in. w.g. pressure increase to overcome the friction in the duct system. Determine:

(a) Size of cooling coil, ft² of face area
(b) Rating of chiller unit, Btu/h
(c) Fan motor size, horsepower
(d) Outside air damper face area, ft²

Solution:

$$m_w = 89000/1100 = 80.9 \text{ lb/h}$$

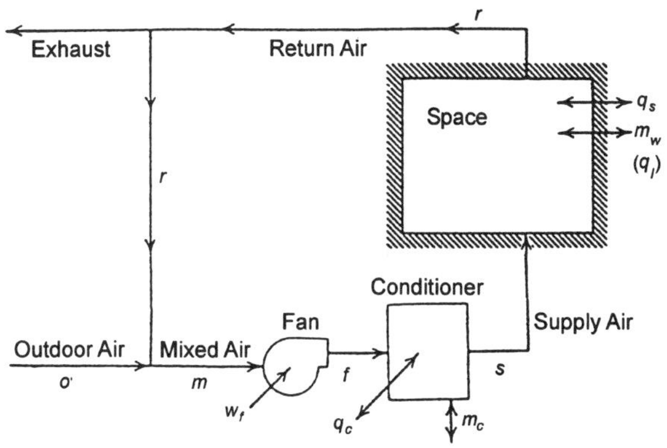

$$m_a = \frac{323000}{0.244(78 - 55)} = 57555 \text{ lb/h}$$

$$m_o = \frac{125 \times 15 \times 60}{13.33} = 8440 \text{ lb/h}$$

$$m_r = 57555 - 8440 = 49115 \text{ lb/h}$$

$$W_r = W_s + \frac{m_w}{m_s} = 0.0083 + \frac{80.9}{57555} = 0.00971$$

$$W_m = \frac{8440(0.0144) + 49115(0.00971)}{57555} = 0.0104 \text{ lb/lb}$$

$$h_m = \frac{8440(38.5) + 49115(29.4)}{57555} = 30.7 \text{ Btu/lb}$$

$$t_m = 80.4\text{°F};\ \phi = 48\%$$

$$h_f = h_m + w_f = 30.7 + 0.49 = 31.2 \text{ Btu/lb}$$

$$W_f = 0.0104 \text{ lb/lb}$$

$$Q = \frac{57555(13.33)}{60} = 12800 \text{ cfm at std. conditions}$$

Coil Size (select 400 fpm face velocity)

$$A_F = 12800/400 = 32 \text{ ft}^2$$

Chiller Size

$$m_a[h_f - h_s - (W_f - W_s)h_c] + Q_c = 0$$

$$57555[31.2 - 22.3 - (0.0104 - 0.0083)23] + Q_c = 0$$

$$Q_c = -509{,}000 \text{ Btu/h}$$

$$Q_{chiller} \approx Q_{coil} = 509{,}000 \text{ Btu/h}$$

Fan Motor Size

$$P_f = \frac{12800(3)}{6350(0.55)} = 11 \text{ hp}$$

Motor size = 15 hp

Outside Air Damper Size

$$\text{OA} = 125 \times 15 = 1875 \text{ cfm}$$

If the recommended face velocity is 1500 fpm:

$$A_D = 1875/1500 = 1.25 \text{ ft}^2$$

11.15 Problems

11.1 A room is to be cooled to a temperature of 75°F and a relative humidity of 50%. If there is negligible latent load within the space, what is the highest dew-point temperature at which the conditioned air can be supplied (t_s)? Why?

11.2 A room has a total space cooling load of 20 tons and a sensible heat ratio of 0.90. If the conditioned air is to be supplied at 20°F less than the room temperature, how much air must be circulated?

11.3 What are the four generic types of air systems expressed by thermodynamic methods?

11.4 What are the 18 fundamental parameters that must be addressed in the selection and design of an HVAC system?

11.5 Before designing a system, the cooling and heating load for each room in a building must be calculated? Why?

11.6 If outdoor air at 95°F dry bulb and 78°F wet bulb is cooled to 75°F dry bulb without any dehumidification, what will the relative humidity be?

11.7 In the air handling unit of Figure 11-1, under design conditions the outdoor air temperature is 95°F dry bulb and 78°F wet bulb and the space temperature is 75°F and 50% rh. The supply fan handles 60,000 cfm of air at 55°F saturated (entering the fan).

(a) If the minimum outdoor air dampers are sized for 6000 cfm of ventilation air, what is the state point (dry bulb and wet bulb temperatures) of the mixed air?
(b) If the maximum outdoor air dampers have 5% leakage (i.e., 5% of full open flow), what is the added refrigeration load?

11.8 An air handling system is designed to circulate 60,000 cfm of air at a total fan pressure rise of 6 in. w.g. The system is a constant flow system and designed to operate constantly. The fan efficiency is 70% and the motor efficiency is 90%.
(a) What size motor (hp) is required to drive the fan?
(b) What will be the annual fan energy consumption?

11.9 If, in the above problem, the sensible space load were reduced by 25% by using a more energy effective building envelope and improved lighting system, and this change were accommodated by reducing the air flow rate at the same fan efficiencies, what would be the reduction in annual fan energy?

11.10 It is desired to transfer a given quantity of heat energy from one location to another location in a building. Two methods being considered are either by an air system operating at 4 in. w.g. total pressure or by a water system with a pump head of 40 feet. Calculate the ratio of fan power required for an air system, to pump power required for a water system with the following system variables:

Fan efficiency	70%
Pump efficiency	80%
Air Δt	20°F
Water Δt	40°F

11.11 A fan with a variable speed drive is selected to operate at 900 rpm, and it is installed on a spring isolator mount with 1 in. static deflection.

(a) What is the transmissibility of the isolator?
(b) What is the minimum speed that the unit can be operated at before the transmissibility is 0.50?

11.12 Specify typical temperatures for the following:

(a) Air leaving a gas-fired warm air furnace
(b) Air leaving a heat pump condenser
(c) Air leaving the cooling coil of a residential air conditioner
(d) Air leaving the cooling coil of a commercial air conditioner
(e) Hot water entering the convectors (radiators) of a hydronic system
(f) Hot water returning to the boiler from the convectors

11.13 An air-conditioned room has a sensible heat load of 200,000 Btu/h, a latent heat load of 50,000 Btu/h, an occupancy of 20 people, and is maintained at 76°F dry bulb and 64°F wet bulb. Twenty-five percent of the air entering the room is vented through cracks and hoods. Outside air is assumed to be at design conditions of 95°F dry bulb and 76°F wet bulb. Conditioned air leaves the apparatus and enters the room at 60°F dry bulb.

Use the following letters to designate state points:

A Outside design conditions
B Inside design conditions
C Air entering apparatus
D Air entering room

(a) Complete the following table:

Point	Dry Bulb	Wet Bulb	*h*	*W*
A				
B				
C				
D				

(b) Calculate the room SHR.
(c) What air quantity must enter the room in
(d) What is the apparatus load in tons?
(e) What is the load of the outside air? In lb per hour? in cfm?
(f) Does the room load plus the outside air load equal the coil load?

11.14 A space has a sensible heat loss of 17.6 kW and a latent loss of 5.86 kW. The space is to be maintained at 21.1°C and 40% rh. The air that passes through the conditioner is 90% recirculated and 10% outdoor air at 4.4°C and 20% rh. The conditioner consists of an adiabatic saturator and a heating coil. Estimate the temperature and humidity ratio of the air entering the conditioned space. What is the flow rate in kg/h and L/s? How much heat is added by the coil to the air in kW? How much water is added to the air by the adiabatic saturator (kg/h)?

11.15 Air at the 800 ft^3/min leaves a residential air conditioner at 65°F with 40% rh. The return air from the rooms has average dry- and wet-bulb temperatures of 75°F and 65°F, respectively. Determine:

(a) Size of the unit in tons (12,000 Btu/h = 1 ton)
(b) Rate of dehumidification

[Ans: 2.58 tons, 20.16 lb/h (9.1 kW, 2.54 g/s)]

11.16 In an air-conditioning unit 2832 L/s (6000 cfm) at 26.7°C (80°F) dry bulb, 50% rh, and standard atmospheric pressure, enter the unit. The leaving condition of the air is 13.9°C (57°F) dry bulb and 90% rh. Calculate:

(a) Cooling capacity of the air-conditioning unit, kW (tons)
(b) Rate of water removal from the unit, kg/h (lb/h)
(c) Sensible heat load on the conditioner, kW (Btu/h)
(d) Latent heat load on the conditioner, kW (Btu/h)
(e) Dew point of the air leaving the conditioner, °C (°F)

11.17 A space in an industrial building has a winter sensible heat loss of 200,000 Btu/h and a negligible latent heat load (latent losses to outside are made up by latent gains within the space). The space is to be maintained at 75°F and 50% rh. Due to the nature of the process, 100% outdoor air is required for ventilation. The outdoor air conditions can be taken as saturated air at 20°F. The amount of ventilation air required is 7000 cfm and the air is to be preheated, humidified with an adiabatic saturator, and then reheated. The temperature out of the adiabatic saturator is to be maintained at 60°F dry bulb. Calculate the following:

(a) Temperature of the air entering the preheater
(b) Temperature of the air entering the space to be heated
(c) Heat supplied to preheat coil, Btu/h
(d) Heat supplied to reheat coil, Btu/h
(e) Quantity of make-up water added to adiabatic saturator, gpm
(f) Temperature of the spray water
(g) Show the processes and label points on the psychrometric diagram

11.18 In winter, a meeting room with a large window is to be maintained at comfort conditions. The inside glass temperature on the design day is 40°F. Condensation on the window is highly undesirable. The room is to accommodate 18 adult males [250 Btu/h (sensible) and 200 Btu/h (latent) per person]. The heat loss through the walls, ceiling, and floor is 33,600 Btu/h. There are 640 watts of lights in the room.

(a) Determine the sensible heat loss or gain.
(b) Specify the desired interior dry-bulb temperature and relative humidity.
(c) If the heating system provides air at 95°F, determine the required airflow (cfm) and the maximum relative humidity permissible in the incoming air.

[Ans: 26,916 Btu/h; 75°F, 28%; 1246 cfm, 14%]

11.19 A zone in a building has a sensible load of 20.5 kW (70,000 Btu/h) and a latent load of 8.8 kW (30,000 Btu/h). The zone is to be maintained at 25°C (77°F) and 50% rh.

(a) Calculate the conditions (t and W) of the entering air to the zone if the air leaves the coil saturated.
(b) What flow rate is required in order to maintain the space temperatures?
(c) If a mixture of 50% return air and 50% outdoor air at 36.1°C (97°F) and 60% rh enters the air conditioner, what is the refrigeration load?

11.20 An Indianapolis, Indiana, plant has a chilled water air-handling unit serving one section of the factory. The unit takes in 2360 L/s (5000 cfm) of outside air at summer design conditions and has the outside air conditioned by a chilled water coil to 17.8°C (64°F) dry bulb and 90% rh. The inside design conditions in the plant are 26.7°C (80°F) dry bulb and 50% rh. The total air supply is 9440 L/s (20,000 cfm).

Mixed air enters a chilled water coil with face and bypass dampers and leaves the coil at 15°C (59°F) db, 50% rh.

Part A. Assume the bypass dampers are closed.
1. What sensible and latent heat quantities does the air-conditioning unit pick up from the plant? What room SHR does the unit exactly satisfy?
2. What refrigeration load does the air-conditioning unit impose on the chilled water distribution system in the plant?

Part B. Assume one-third of the air bypasses the coil.
1. What sensible and latent heat quantities does the air-conditioning unit pick up from the plant?
2. What SHR is satisfied exactly?

11.21 Same plant is the same as in *Problem* 11.20, except the operator now has air at 6.1°C (43°F) dry bulb, 90% rh leaving the coil. The unit takes in 2360 L/s (5000 cfm) of outside air at summer design conditions and has the outside air conditioned by a chilled water coil to 17.8°C (64°F) dry bulb and 90% rh. The inside design conditions in the plant are 26.7°C (80°F) dry bulb and 50% rh. The total air supply is 9440 L/s (20,000 cfm).

Part A. Assume the bypass dampers are closed.
1. What sensible and latent heat quantities does the air-conditioning unit pick up from the plant? What room SHR does the unit satisfy exactly?
2. What refrigeration load does the air-conditioning unit impose on the chilled water distribution system in the plant?

Part B. Assume one-third of the air bypasses the coil.
1. What sensible and latent heat quantities does the air-conditioning unit pick up from the plant?
2. What room SHR does the unit satisfy exactly for this damper setting?

11.22 Sketch (with line diagrams) and list the advantages, disadvantages, and typical uses of the following systems:
(a) Fan-coil units
(b) Terminal reheat system
(c) Multizone system
(d) Double-duct system
(e) Variable volume system
(f) Induction system

11.23 A general office building in Rolla, Missouri, has a winter sensible space heating load of 337 kW (1,150,000 Btu/h) for design conditions of 24 and –20.6°C (75 and –5°F). The heating system operates with 25% outside air mixed with return air.
(a) Schematically draw the flow diagram and label, including temperatures and flow rates at each location.
(b) Specify the necessary furnace size.

11.24 For the building of *Problem* 11.23, determine:
(a) Annual energy requirements for heating, Btu
(b) Annual fuel cost using No. 2 fuel oil at 39.9 cents/liter
(c) Percentage savings in fuel if a 15.6°C (60°F) setback is used between 6 p.m. and 6 a.m., Monday through Thursday, and over the weekend

11.25 To provide comfort conditions for a general office building, 38 ft by 80 ft by 8 ft, an air-treating unit consisting of cooling coil, heating coil, and humidifier is provided for this space with the flow diagram as shown.

Ninety people are normally employed doing light work while seated. The building is in Kansas City, Missouri. Fan operation is constant all year long.

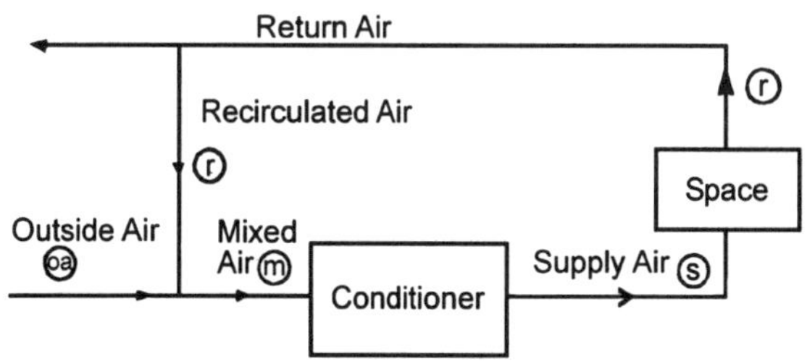

Winter: Sensible space heat loss is 189,000 Btu/h at design conditions, latent load is negligible. Maximum supply air temperature space is 155°F.

Summer: Sensible space heat gain is 101,200 Btu/h at design conditions. Latent load is due entirely to the occupancy. The minimum supply air temperature from the cooling coil is 58°F.
(a) Determine the fan size (scfm) needed to provide sufficient air
(b) Size the heating unit needed, Btu/h
(c) Size the cooling coil needed, Btu/h
(d) Size the humidifier, gal/h

11.26 The air-conditioning unit for the general office building shown in *Problem* 11.25 consists of a cooling coil, heating coil, and humidifier. Ninety people are normally employed doing light work while seated. The building is in Kansas City, Missouri. Fan operation is constant all year long.

Winter: Sensible space heat loss is 60 kW at design conditions; latent load is negligible. Maximum supply air temperature is 68°C.

Summer: Sensible space heat gain is 30 kW at design conditions; latent load is due entirely to the occupancy. Minimum supply air temperature is 14°C.

(a) Determine the fan size needed, L/s
(b) Size the heating unit, kW
(c) Size the cooling coil, kW

11.27 An office building in Jefferson City, Missouri, with the HVAC system shown, has space design loads as follows:

Summer: 314,000 Btu/h sensible (gain); 81,000 Btu/h latent (gain).
Winter: 407,000 Btu/h sensible (loss); negligible latent.

Minimum outside air for meeting the ventilation requirements of the 410 occupants is used.
Specify:

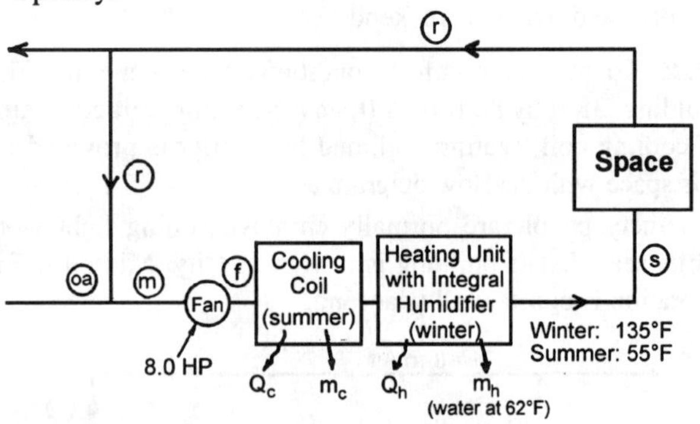

(a) Summer airflow to space, scfm
(b) Cooling coil rating, Btu/h
(c) Sensible cooling coil load, Btu/h
(d) Latent cooling coil load, Btu/h
(e) Actual relative humidity of air leaving space, %
(f) Winter air flow to space, scfm
(g) Heating unit rating, Btu/h
(h) Humidifier rating, gal/h
(i) Latent load on heating/humidifying unit, Btu/h

Plot: All summer points and the summer cycle, with complete labeling, on a psychrometric chart.

11.28 A view of the air-conditioning system for a building in Denver, Colorado (elevation = 5000 ft; barometric pressure = 12.23 psi), is given. Outside air at the rate of 2500 cfm is required for ventilation. Other conditions at summer design are:

Space Loads:
Sensible = 410,000 Btu/h
Latent = 220,000 Btu/h

Outside Air: 91°F, 30% rh

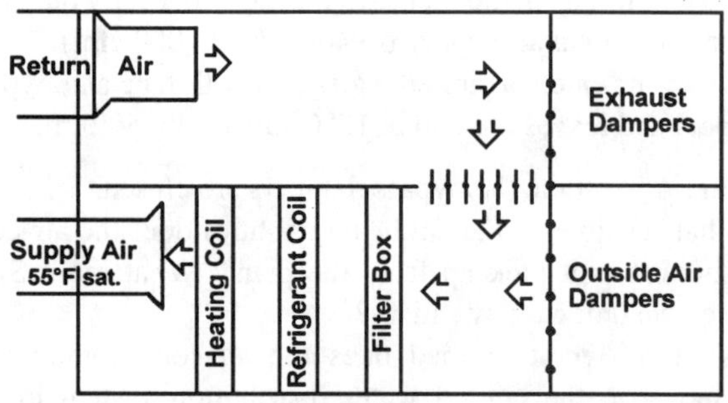

For an indoor design temperature of 78°F, determine:

1. Supply airflow, lb/h
2. Supply airflow, scfm
3. relative humidity at return, %
4. Size of cooling unit, Btu/h
5. Latent component of (4)
6. Sensible component of (4)
7. Sensible cooling load due to outside air, Btu/h

11.16 BIBLIOGRAPHY

ASHRAE. Chapter 1, 1996 *ASHRAE Handbook—Systems and Equipment.*

Wheeler, A.E. 1997. Air Handling Unit Design for Energy Conservation. *ASHRAE Journal* 39(June).

Chapter 12

ALL AIR, AIR-WATER, AND ALL WATER SYSTEMS

In this chapter the various types of HVAC Systems that provide cooling, dehumidifying, heating and humidifying are described. The way the systems are identified with regard to the fluid used for carrying the energy and/or moisture is presented. Details about these various systems are given in Chapters 1, 2, 3, and 4 in the 1996 *Handbook—Systems and Equipment.*

12.1 Introduction

Systems are often classified by the method which they utilize to convey energy to or from the space to be occupied. In this regard, if the unit which provides the psychrometric control of the air is located within the space, and energy is conveyed to or from that unit by water as an intermediate transport fluid, the unit is considered an all water system. If, on the other hand, an air handling system psychometrically conditions the space air at a location remote from the room, then conveys conditioned air to and from the space by an air distribution duct system, that is considered an "all air" system.

However, in addition to thermal conditioning of the space air (heating/humidifying and cooling/dehumidifying) the system must also provide ventilation air. And when the space conditioning is accomplished with a device in the space and the ventilation air is conditioned remotely and the conditioned ventilation air conveyed to the space, the "system" falls into the category of an air-water system because "energy" is essentially conveyed to and from the space by both transport mediums.

For practical purposes, the only commonly used device which qualifies as an all-water system under this definition is the unit ventilator or packaged terminal air conditioning unit, neither of which is commonly used in commercial applications because of the inability to supply known and controlled quantities of outdoor air under controlled psychrometric conditions.

This chapter discusses the most commonly used systems and system combinations in three categories: All-air, air-water and all-water systems.

12.2 All-Air Systems

An all-air system provides complete sensible and latent cooling, preheating, and humidification capacity in the air supplied by the system. No additional cooling or humidification is required at the zone, except in the case of certain industrial systems. Heating may be accomplished by the same airstream, either in the central system or at a particular zone.

In some applications, heating is accomplished by a separate heater. The term zone implies the provision or the need for separate thermostatic control, while the term room implies a partitioned area that may or may not have a separate control.

All-air systems are classified in two basic categories:

- **Single-duct systems**, which contain the main heating and cooling coils in a series flow air path; a common duct distribution system at a common air temperature feeds all terminal apparatus.
- **Dual-stream systems**, which contain the main heating and cooling coils in parallel flow or series-parallel flow air paths with either (1) separate cold and warm air duct distribution systems that blend the air at the terminal apparatus (dual-duct systems), or (2) a separate supply air duct to each zone with the supply air blended to the required temperature at the main unit mixing dampers (multizone).

These classifications may be further divided as follows:

Single duct
Constant volume
  Single zone
  Multiple-zone reheat
  Bypass
Variable air volume (VAV)
  Variable volume only
  Reheat
  Induction
  Fan powered
  Dual conduit
  Variable diffusers

Dual stream
Dual duct
  Constant volume
  Variable air volume
Multizone
  Constant volume
  Variable air volume
  Three-deck or "Texas" multizone

All-air systems may be adapted to many applications for comfort or process work. They are used in buildings that require individual control of multiple zones, such as office buildings; schools and universities; laboratories; hospitals; stores; hotels; and even ships. All-air systems are also used virtually exclusively in special applications for close control of temperature and humidity, including clean rooms, computer rooms, hospital operating rooms, research and development facilities, as well as many industrial/manufacturing facilities.

All-air systems have the following advantages:

- The location of the central mechanical room for major equipment allows operation and the majority of the maintenance to be performed in unoccupied areas. In addition, it allows the maximum range of choices of filtration equipment, vibration and noise control, and the selection of high quality and durable equipment.
- Keeping piping, electrical equipment, wiring, filters, and vibration and noise-producing equipment away from the conditioned area minimizes service needs and reduces potential harm to occupants, furnishings and processes.
- These systems offer the option for use of outside air instead of mechanical refrigeration for cooling.
- Seasonal changeover is simple and adapts readily to automatic control.
- A wide choice of zoning, flexibility, and humidity control under many operating conditions is possible, with the availability of simultaneous heating and cooling even during off-season periods.
- Air-to-air and other heat recovery may be readily incorporated.
- They permit good design flexibility for optimum air distribution, draft control, and adaptability to varying local requirements.
- The systems are well suited to applications requiring unusual exhaust or makeup air quantities (negative or positive pressurization, etc.).
- All-air systems adapt well to winter humidification.

All-air systems have the following disadvantages:

- They require additional duct space, which reduces usable floor space and increases the height of the building.
- Depending on the layout, larger floor plans could be necessary to allow enough space for the vertical shafts required for air distribution.
- Ensuring accessible terminal devices requires close cooperation between architectural, mechanical, and structural designers.
- Air balancing, particularly on large systems, can be more difficult.
- Perimeter heating is not always available to provide temporary heat during construction.

12.3 Single-Duct Systems

12.3.1 Constant Volume

While maintaining constant airflow, single-duct constant volume systems change the supply air temperature in response to the space load (Figure 12-1).

Single-Zone Systems. The simplest all-air system is a supply unit serving a single-temperature control zone. The unit can be installed either within or remote from the space it serves and may operate with or without distribution ductwork. Ideally, this system responds completely to the space needs, and well-designed control systems maintain temperature closely and efficiently. Single-zone systems can be shut down when not required without affecting the operation of adjacent areas.

A return or relief fan may be needed, depending on the capacity of the system and whether 100% outdoor air is used for cooling at some time during the year. Relief fans can be eliminated if provisions are made to relieve overpressurization by other means, such as gravity dampers.

Multiple-Zone Reheat. This system provides (1) zone or space control for areas of unequal loading; (2) simultaneous heating or cooling of perimeter areas with different exposures; and (3) close tolerance of control for process or comfort applications. As the word reheat implies, heat is added as a secondary simultaneous process to either preconditioned (cooled, humidified, etc.) primary air or recirculated room air.

Relatively small low-pressure systems place reheat coils in the ductwork at each zone. More complex designs include higher pressure primary distribution ducts to reduce their size and cost and pressure reduction devices to maintain a constant volume for each reheat zone.

The system uses conditioned air from a central unit generally at a fixed cold air temperature. The temperature can be varied, however, with proper control to reduce both the amount of reheat required and the associated energy consumption. Care must be taken to avoid high internal humid-

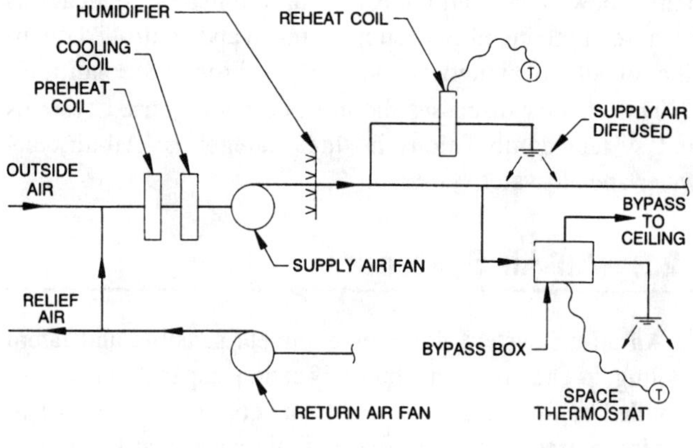

Fig. 12-1 Constant Volume with Reheat and Bypass Terminal Devices

ity if the temperature of air leaving the cooling coil is permitted to rise during the spring and fall.

Bypass. A variation of the constant volume reheat system is the use of a bypass box in lieu of reheat. This system is essentially a constant volume primary system, with a VAV secondary system.

The quantity of room supply air is varied to match the space load by dumping excess supply air into the return ceiling plenum or return air duct, i.e., by bypassing the room. While this reduces the air volume supplied to the space, the system air volume remains constant. Refrigeration or heating at the air-handling unit is reduced due to the lower return air temperature.

A bypass system is seldom used except for small installations where a simple method of temperature control is desired, a modest initial cost is desired, and energy conservation is given less consideration.

12.3.2 Variable Air Volume

A VAV system, as shown in Figure 12-2 controls temperature in a space by varying the quantity of supply air rather than varying the supply air temperature. A VAV terminal device at the zone varies the quantity of supply air to the space. The supply air temperature is held relatively constant, depending on the season.

Variable air volume systems can be applied to interior or perimeter zones, with common or separate fans, with common or separate air temperature control, and with or without auxiliary heating devices. The greatest energy saving associated with VAV occurs at the perimeter zones, where variations in solar load and outside temperature allow the supply air quantity to be reduced.

Humidity control is a potential problem with VAV. If humidity is critical, as in certain research and development laboratories, process work, etc., systems may have to be limited to constant volume airflow or humidity can be controlled with an outdoor air ventilation unit separate from the room temperature control system. If this technique is not used, particular care should be taken in areas where the sensible heat ratio (ratio of sensible heat to sensible plus latent heat to be removed) is low, such as in conference rooms. In these situations, the VAV box minimum set point is usually limited to about 50%, and reheat is added as necessary to prevent overcooling and keep humidity low during part loads.

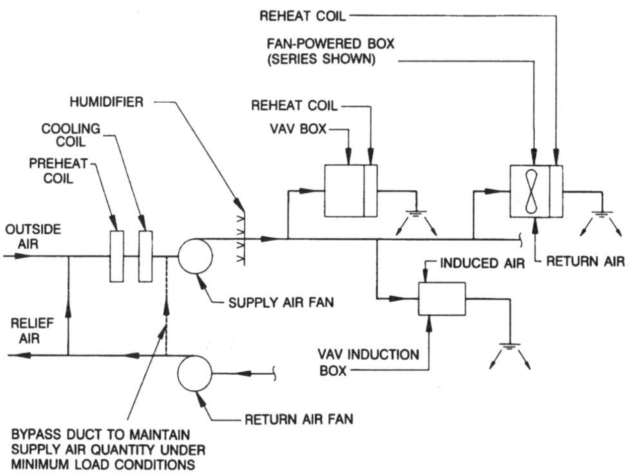

Fig. 12-2 Variable Air Volume with Reheat, Induction, and Fan-Powered Devices

VAV terminal devices are available in many configurations, including the following.

VAV Reheat. This simple VAV system integrates heating at the terminal unit. It is applied to systems requiring full heating and cooling flexibility in interior and exterior zones. The terminal units are set to maintain a predetermined minimum throttling ratio, which is established as the lowest air quantity necessary to (1) offset the heating load, (2) limit the maximum humidity, (3) provide reasonable air movement within the space, and (4) provide required ventilation air. Note, (2) and (4) do not apply if a separate ventilation system is employed.

Variable air volume with reheat permits airflow to be reduced as the first step in control; heat is then initiated as the second step. Compared to constant volume reheat, this procedure reduces operating cost appreciably because the amount of primary air to be cooled and secondary air to be heated is reduced.

A feature can be provided to isolate the availability of reheat during the summer, except in situations where low airflow should be avoided or where an increase in humidity causes discomfort (e.g., in conference rooms when the lights are turned off).

VAV Induction. The VAV induction system uses a terminal unit to reduce cooling capacity by simultaneously reducing primary air and inducing room or ceiling air (replaces the reheat coil) to maintain a relatively constant supply air volume to the room. This operation is the reverse of the bypass box described earlier. The primary air quantity decreases with load, retaining the savings of VAV, while the air supplied to the space is kept relatively constant to avoid the effect of low velocity dumping or low air movement.

The terminal device is usually located in the ceiling cavity to recover heat from lights. This allows the induction box to be used without reheat coils in internal spaces. Provisions must be made for morning warm-up and night heating. Also, interior spaces with a roof load must have heat supplied either separately in the ceiling or at the terminal.

Fan-Powered. Fan-powered systems are available in either parallel or series airflow. In parallel flow units, the fan is located outside the primary airstream to allow intermittent fan operation. In series units, the fan is located within the primary airstream and runs continuously when the zone is occupied. Fan-powered systems, both series and parallel, are often selected because they maintain higher air circulation through a room at low loads while still retaining some of the energy advantages of VAV systems.

As the cold primary air valve modulates from maximum to minimum (or closed), the unit recirculates more plenum air. In a perimeter zone, a hot water heating coil, electric heater, baseboard heater, or remote radiant heater can be sequenced with the cooling to offset external heat losses. Between heating and cooling operations, a dead band in which the fan recirculates ceiling air only is provided. This operation permits heat from lights to be used for space heating for maximum energy saving. During unoccupied periods, the main supply air-handling unit remains off and individual fan-powered heating zone terminals are cycled to maintain required space temperature, thereby reducing operating cost.

Both parallel and series systems use the heat from lights in the ceiling plenum, and both may be provided with filters.

Parallel Arrangement—intermittent Fan. In this device, primary air is modulated in response to cooling demand and energizes an integral fan at a predetermined reduced primary flow to deliver ceiling air to offset heating demand. These devices are primarily used in perimeter zones where auxiliary hot water or electric heating is required. The induction fan operating range normally overlaps the range of the primary air valve. A back-draft damper on the terminal fan prevents conditioned air from backflowing into the return air plenum when the terminal fan is off.

Series Arrangement—Constant Fan. A constant volume (series) fan-powered box mixes primary air with air from the ceiling space using a continuously operating fan; this provides a relatively constant volume to the space. These devices are used for interior or perimeter zones and are supplied with or without an auxiliary heating coil. They can be used to mix primary and return air to raise the temperature of the air supplied to the space such as with low-temperature air systems.

In the series system, since the terminal fan is in series with the main supply fan, the system must be electrically interlocked to assure that all of the terminal fans are running before the supply fan turns on. (If the supply fan turns on before a terminal fan the terminal fan will turn in reverse and then run in that direction when energized.)

Dual Conduit. The dual-conduit system has two air supply paths; one offsets exterior transmission cooling or heating loads, and the other provides cooling throughout the year (Figure 12-3).

The first airstream, the primary air, operates as a constant volume system, and the air temperature is varied to offset transmission only (i.e., it is warm in winter and cool in summer). Often, however, the primary air fan is limited to operating only during peak heating and cooling periods to further save energy. When calculating the heating requirements for this system, the cooling effect of the secondary air must be included., even though the secondary system is operating at minimum flow.

The other airstream, or secondary air, is cool year-round and varies in volume to match the load due to solar heating, lights, power, and occupants. It serves both perimeter and interior spaces.

Variable Diffuser. The discharge aperture of this diffuser is reduced to keep the discharge velocity relatively constant

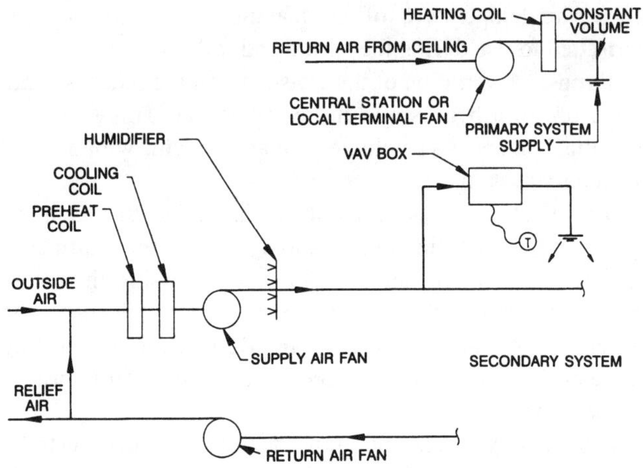

Fig. 12-3 Dual Conduit System

while reducing the conditioned supply airflow. Under these conditions, the induction effect of the diffuser is kept high, and cold air mixes in the space. These devices are of two basic types—one has a flexible bladder that expands to reduce the aperture, and the other has a diffuser plate that physically moves. Both devices are pressure-dependent, which must be considered in the design of the duct distribution system. They are either powered by the system or pneumatically or electrically driven.

12.4 Dual-Duct Systems

A dual-duct system conditions all the air in a central apparatus and distributes it to the conditioned spaces through two parallel mains or ducts. One duct carries cold air and the other carries warm air. In each conditioned space or zone, a valve mixes the warm and cold air in proper proportion to satisfy the load of the space. A dual-duct system uses more energy than a single-duct VAV system, but no pipes that could leak are required in occupied areas.

These systems may be designed as constant volume or variable air volume. As with other VAV systems, certain primary air configurations can cause high relative humidity in the space during the spring and fall unless a separate outdoor ventilation air conditioning system is used.

Constant Volume. Dual-duct constant volume systems are of two types.

Single Fan-No Reheat. This is similar to a single-duct system, except that it contains a face-and-bypass damper at the cooling coil, which is arranged to bypass a mixture of outdoor and recirculated air as the internal heat load fluctuates in response to a zone thermostat (Figure 12-4). A problem occurs during periods of high outdoor humidity, when the internal heat load falls, causing the space humidity to rise rapidly (unless reheat is added). It is identical in concept to face-and-bypass cooling coils.

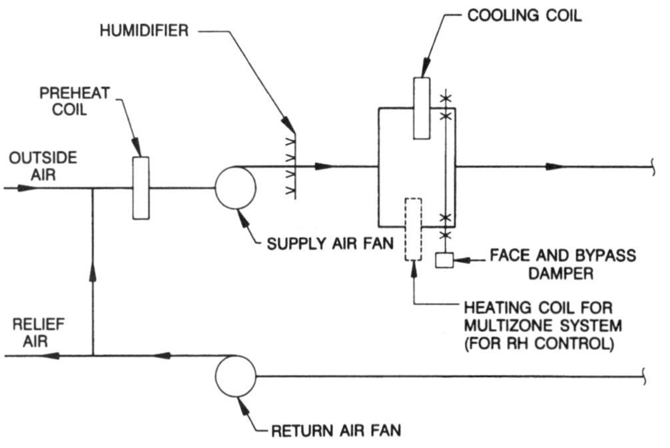

Fig. 12-4 Single Fan-No Reheat

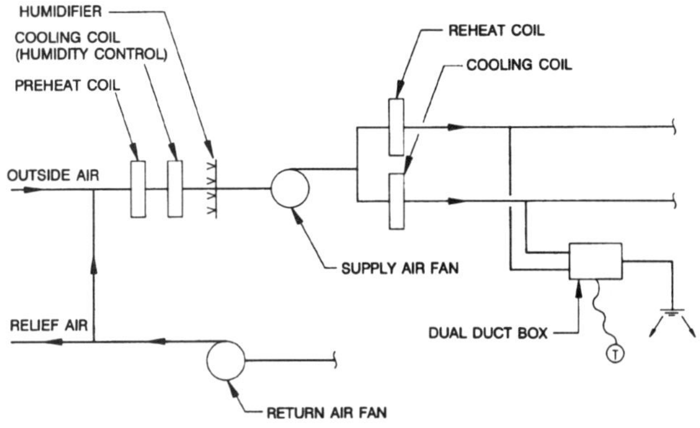

Fig. 12-5 Dual Duct-Single Fan Reheat

This system has limited use in most modern buildings because most occupants demand more consistent temperature and humidity.

Single Fan-Reheat. This method is similar in effect to conventional reheat. The only difference is that reheat is applied at a central point instead of at individual zones (Figure 12-5).

Variable Air Volume. Dual-duct VAV systems blend cold and warm air in various volume combinations. These systems may include single-duct VAV units connected to the cold air chamber of the air handler (cold deck) for cooling only of interior spaces.

Single Fan. In this system, a single supply fan is sized for the coincident peak of the hot and cold decks. Control of the fan is from two static pressure controllers, one located in the hot deck and the other in the cold deck. The duct requiring the highest pressure governs the airflow.

Usually the cold deck is maintained at a fixed temperature, although some central systems permit the temperature to rise during warmer weather to save refrigeration (cold deck reset control). The temperature of the hot deck is often adjusted higher during periods of low outside temperature and high humidity to increase the flow over the cold deck for dehumidification. Other systems, particularly in laboratories,

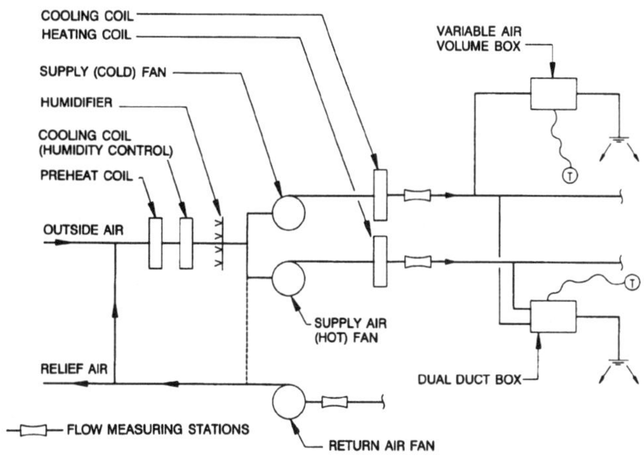

Fig. 12-6 Variable Air Volume, Dual Duct, Dual Fan

use a precooling coil to dehumidify the total airstream or just the outside air to limit humidity in the space.

Return air quantity can be controlled either by flow-measuring devices in the supply and return duct, by holding a fixed negative pressure in the mixing chamber, or by static pressure controls that maintain space static pressure.

Dual Fan. The volume of each supply fan is controlled independently by the static pressure in its respective duct (Figure 12-6). The return fan is controlled based on the sum of the hot and cold fan volumes using flow-measuring stations. Each fan is sized for the anticipated maximum coincident hot or cold volume, not the sum of the instantaneous peaks.

The cold deck can be maintained at a constant temperature either with mechanical refrigeration when minimum fresh air is required or with an economizer when the outside air is below the temperature of the cold deck set point. This operation does not affect the hot deck, which can recover heat from the return air, and the heating coil need operate only when heating requirements cannot be met using return air.

Outdoor air can provide ventilation air via the hot duct when the outdoor air is warmer than the return air. However, controls should be used to prohibit the introduction of excessive amounts of outdoor air beyond the required minimum when that air is more humid than the return air.

12.5 Multizone Systems

The multizone system supplies several zones from a single, centrally located air-handling unit. Different zone requirements are met by mixing cold and warm air through zone dampers at the air handler in response to zone thermostats. The mixed, conditioned air is distributed throughout the building by single-zone ducts. The return air is handled in a conventional manner.

The multizone system is similar to the dual-duct system. In operation, it has the same potential problem with high humidity levels. This system can provide a smaller building with the advantages of a dual-duct system, and it uses packaged equipment, which is less expensive. Multizone packaged equipment is usually limited to about 12 zones, while built-up systems can include as many zones as can be physically incorporated in the layout.

A common variation on the multizone system is called the Texas multizone or three-deck multizone. In this system, the hot deck heating coil is removed from the air handler and replaced with an air resistance plate matching the pressure drop of the cooling coil. Individual heating coils are placed only in each perimeter zone duct. These heating coils are usually located in the equipment room for ease of maintenance. This system is common in humid climates where the cold deck often produces 48 to 52°F air for humidity control. Supply air is then mixed with neutral deck (return) air using the air-handling units' zone dampers to maintain zone conditions. Heat is added only if the zone served cannot be maintained by the delivery of return air alone.

12.6 Special Systems

12.6.1 Primary/Secondary Systems

Some processes use two interconnected all-air systems (Figure 12-7). In these situations, space gains are very high and a large number of air changes are required (e.g., in sterile or clean rooms or where close-tolerance conditions are needed for process work). The primary systems supply the conditioned outside air requirements for the process either to the secondary system or directly to the space. The secondary system provides additional cooling and humidification (and heating, if required) to offset space and fan power gains. Normally, the secondary cooling coil is designed to be dry (i.e., sensible cooling only) which reduces the possibility of bacterial growth, which creates air quality problems. These type systems are finding increasing acceptance because of their ability to provide fixed ventilation air quantities and superior humidity control with a high degree of simplicity in conjunction with variable air volume systems.

12.6.2 Up Air System

In this system, air is supplied from the floor rather than from overhead. Special terminal devices are installed in a raised floor or as part of the furniture to provide individual control for computer workstations, for example. This system is becoming more common, particularly in Europe.

12.6.3 Wetted Duct/Supersaturated System

Some industries spray water into the airstream at central air-handling units in sufficient quantities to create a controlled carryover (Figure 12-8). This supercools the supply air, normally equivalent to an oversaturation of about 10 grains per pound of air and allows less air to be distributed for a given space load. These are used where high humidity is desirable, such as in the textile or tobacco industry, and in climates where adiabatic cooling is sufficient. Extreme care

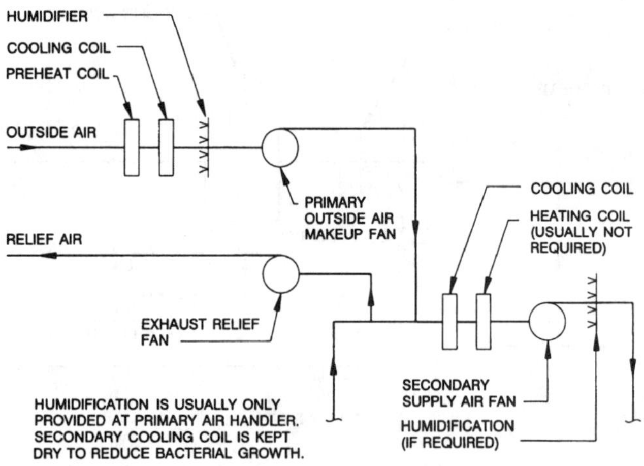

Fig. 12-7 Primary/Secondary System

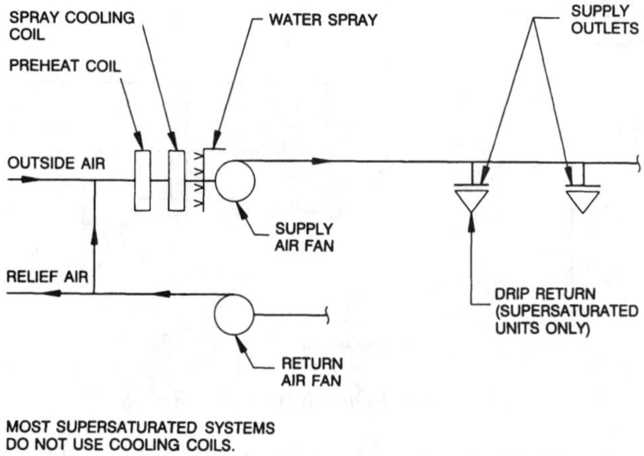

Fig. 12-8 Supersaturated/Wetted Coil

is required in the design of these systems to use non-corrosive hard surface materials and provide for the collection and drainage of moisture and for ease in cleaning.

12.6.4 Low-Temperature Systems

Because ice storage is sometimes used to reduce peak electrical demand, low-temperature systems (where air is supplied at approximately 40°F) are being designed. Because the quantity of air supplied to a zone is so small, special terminal devices ar used to maintain minimum airflow for assurance of ambient air velocity. These high aspiration devices induce return or room air to be mixed with the cold supply air to increase the air circulation rate within the space.

12.7 Air-and-Water Systems

Air-and-water systems condition spaces by distributing air and water sources to terminal units installed in habitable spaces throughout a building. The air and water are cooled or heated in central mechanical equipment rooms. The air supplied is called **primary air**; the water supplied is called **sec-**

ondary water. Sometimes a separate electric heating coil is included in lieu of a hot water coil. This chapter is concerned primarily with air-and-water induction units, fan-coil units, and radiant panels as used in air-water systems.

Air-and-water systems have been applied primarily to exterior spaces of building with high sensible loads and where close control of humidity is not required. They may, however, be applied to interior zones as well. These systems work well in buildings such as office buildings, hospitals, hotels, schools, apartment buildings, and research laboratories. In most climates, these systems are installed in exterior building spaces and are designed to provide (1) all required space heating and cooling needs and (2) simultaneous heating and cooling in different parts of the building.

12.7.1 System Description

An air-and-water system includes central air-conditioning equipment, duct and water distribution systems, and a room terminal. The room terminal may be an induction unit, a fan-coil unit, or a conventional supply air outlet combined with a radiant panel. Larger spaces may be handled by multiple terminals. Generally, the air supply has a constant volume and, as noted in the opening paragraph for the chapter, is called primary air to distinguish it from room air or secondary air that has been recirculated. The primary air provides conditioned outside air for ventilation. In the cooling season, the air is dehumidified sufficiently in the central conditioning unit to achieve comfort humidity conditions throughout the spaces served and to avoid condensation resulting from room latent load on the room cooling coil. In winter, moisture can be added centrally, to limit dryness. As the air is dehumidified, it is also cooled to offset a portion of the room sensible loads. The air may be from outdoors, or may be a mixture of outdoor and return air. Preheating of the primary air is required where low ambient temperatures are found. With induction systems, high efficiency filters must be used to keep the nozzles clean. Whether or not reheat coils are included in the air-handling equipment depends on the type of system.

The quantity of primary air supplied to each space is determined by (1) the ventilation requirement and (2) the required sensible cooling capacity at maximum room cooling load.

In the ideal air-and-water system design, the secondary cooling coil is always dry; this greatly extends terminal unit life eliminates odors and the possibility of bacterial growth. The primary air normally controls the space humidity. Therefore, the moisture content of the supply air must be low enough to offset the room latent heat gain and to maintain a room dew point low enough to preclude condensation on the secondary cooling surface.

Although some systems operate successfully without a secondary coil drain system, a condensate drain is recommended for all air-and-water systems.

In existing induction systems, the energy conservation technique of raising the chilled water temperature on central air-handling cooling coils can damage the terminal cooling coil, causing it to be used constantly as a dehumidifier. Unlike fan-coil units, the induction units are not designed or constructed to handle condensation. Therefore, it is critical that an induction terminal operates dry. It is even more critical that the primary air dehumidification be adequate to prevent condensation on a radiant cooling panel.

The water side, in its basic form, consists of a pump and piping to convey water to the heat transfer surface within each conditioned space. The heat exchange coil may be an integral part of the air terminal (as with induction units), a completely separate component within the conditioned space (as with radiant panels), or a combination (as with fan-coil units). The water can be cooled by direct refrigeration, but it is more commonly cooled by chilled water from the primary cooling system or by heat transfer through a water-to-water exchanger. See Chapter 13. To distinguish it from the primary chilled water circuit, the water side is usually referred to as the secondary water loop or system

Air-and-water systems are categorized as two-pipe, three-pipe, or four-pipe systems. They are basically similar in function and include both cooling and heating capabilities for year-round air conditioning. The numbers are derived from the water distribution system. In two-pipe systems, the water is distributed by one supply and one return pipe for either cold or warm water supply. Two-pipe changeover systems are unsatisfactory during seasonal changeover and should be applied with caution and the owner's full acceptance of their limitations. The three-pipe system has a cold water supply, a warm water supply, and a common return. Because the cold and warm water blends, the three-pipe system has excessive energy waste, is seldom used, and is not recommended. Existing three-pipe systems are ideal candidates for energy conservation retrofit. The four-pipe system distribution of secondary water has cold water supply, cold water return, warm water supply, and warm water return pipes. As discussed in Chapter 13, the arrangements of the secondary water circuits and their control systems differ, depending on the type of secondary water.

12.7.2 Induction Systems

Figure 12-9 shows a basic arrangement for an air-and-water induction terminal. Centrally conditioned primary air is supplied to the unit plenum at medium to high pressure. The acoustically treated plenum attenuate part of the noise generated in the unit and duct system. A balancing damper adjusts the primary air quantity within limits.

The medium-to high-pressure air flows through the induction nozzle and induces secondary air from the room through the secondary coil. The secondary air is either heated or cooled at the coil, depending on the season, the room requirement, or both. Ordinarily, the room coil does no latent cooling, but a drain pan collects condensed moisture from temporary latent loads. Primary and secondary air is mixed and discharged to the room.

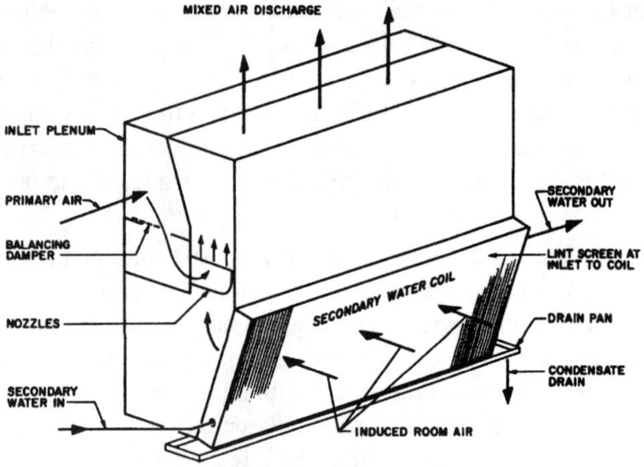

Fig. 12-9 Air-and Water Induction Unit

A lint screen is normally placed across the face of the secondary coil. Induction units are installed in custom enclosures designed for the particular installation or in standard cabinets provided by the unit manufacturer. These enclosures must permit proper flow of secondary air and discharge of mixed air without imposing excessive pressure losses. They must also allow easy servicing.

Induction units are usually installed under a window at a perimeter wall, although units designed for overhead installation are available. During the heating season, the floor-mounted induction unit can function as a convector during off-hours, with hot water to the coil and without a primary air supply. A number of induction unit configurations are available, including units with low overall height or with larger secondary coil face areas to suit particular space or load needs.

Induction systems, like all systems have both advantages and disadvantages. However, improperly applied and designed, some of the disadvantages can become serious problems. The following advantages and disadvantages should be considered when selecting or designing an induction system.

Advantages

1. Individual room temperature control with the capability of adjusting each thermostat for a different temperature.
2. Separate heating and cooling sources in the primary air and secondary water can give the occupant a choice of heating or cooling.
3. Less space is required for the distribution system when the air supply is reduced by using secondary water for cooling and high-velocity air design. The return air duct system is reduced in size and can sometimes be eliminated or combined with the return air system for other building areas, such as the interior spaces.
4. The size of the central air-handling apparatus is smaller than that of other systems because less air must be conditioned.
5. Dehumidification, filtration, and humidification are performed in a central location remote from conditioned spaces.
6. Ventilation air supply is positive and may accommodate recommended outside air quantities.
7. Space can be heated without operating the air system via the secondary water system. Nighttime fan operation is avoided in an unoccupied building. Emergency power for heating, if required, is much lower than for most all-air systems.
8. System components are long-lasting. Room terminals operated dry have an anticipated life of 15 to 25 years. The piping and ductwork longevity should equal that of the building.
9. Individual induction units do not contain fans, motors, or compressors. Routine service is generally limited to temperature controls, cleaning of lint screens, and infrequent cleaning of the induction nozzles.

Disadvantages

1. Relatively low primary air quantities make the two-pipe changeover design for operating during intermediate seasons more critical than in alternate system types.
2. The two-pipe changeover system has operating complexities not present in other systems. The operator must understand the cycles and changeover procedures. The disadvantage, and the need for heating at one time of the day and cooling at another, have effectively ruled out the two-pipe changeover system for many buildings.
3. For most buildings, these systems are limited to perimeter space; separate systems are required for other building areas.
4. Controls tend to be more numerous than for many all-air systems.
5. Secondary airflow can cause the induction or fan-coil unit coils to become dirty enough to affect performance. Lint screens or low-efficiency filters used to protect these terminals require frequent in-room maintenance and reduce unit thermal performance.
6. The primary air supply usually is constant with no provision for shutoff. This is a disadvantage in residential applications, where tenants or hotel room guests may prefer to turn off the air conditioning, or where management may desire to do so to reduce operating expense.
7. A low primary chilled water temperature is needed to control space humidity adequately.
8. The system is not applicable to spaces with high exhaust requirements (e.g., research laboratories), unless supplementary ventilation air is provided.
9. Central dehumidification eliminates condensation on the secondary water heat transfer surface under maximum design latent load. However, abnormal moisture sources (e.g., from open windows, leaky building envelopes, or people congregating) can cause condensation that can have annoying or damaging results.

10. Energy consumption for induction systems is higher than for most other systems due to the increased power required by the primary air pressure drop in the terminal units.
11. The initial cost for four-pipe induction systems is greater than that for most all-air systems.

12.7.3 Fan Coil Units and Panel Systems

In-space fan coil units and panel systems are discussed below under all water systems. However, since neither of those systems have the ability to provide ventilation air, they must be supplemented by a primary air or ventilation air system. Used with fan coil units, room water source heat pumps, panel systems or other types of in-space room temperature control devices, the primary ventilation air system is a 100% outdoor air unit as shown in Figure 12-10.

The unit intake is all outdoor air which is filtered to the extent required by the space air quality requirements and the ambient condition, heated, humidified (it required), cooled, dehumidified, and reheated (if required). The capacity of the ventilation air unit is usually determined by the total design ventilation rate of the spaces served, usually as recommended in ASHRAE *Standard* 62.

The air system component of the total HVAC system is limited in size, not to the capacity of the entire system load, but to the size of only the ventilation load. The control of the ventilation system is generally a simple dewpoint or discharge air temperature control of the heating and cooling coil in sequence, with the option of reheating to reset the supply air temperature up when no cooling is required in humid climates; in most systems reheat is not required.

In applications wherein the humidity control is critical in all seasons in temperate climates (summer and winter), using a sprayed coil in place of the cooling coil will produce supply air, essentially saturated at controlled dewpoint at all times which, in turn, will provide relatively constant space relative humidity unless there are excessive and dynamic space latent gains.

Since the ductwork required for primary air systems is sized for the ventilation load only the air quantities are usually considerably less than for all air systems. This usually allows the designer to size them for low velocities, thus low pressure drops and low power and energy consumption.

In a properly designed system, the entire latent load is handled at the primary air unit, thus significantly reducing the likelihood of condensation on panel cooling surfaces or fan coil unit coils and eliminating the problem of microbial growth at the space cooling coils.

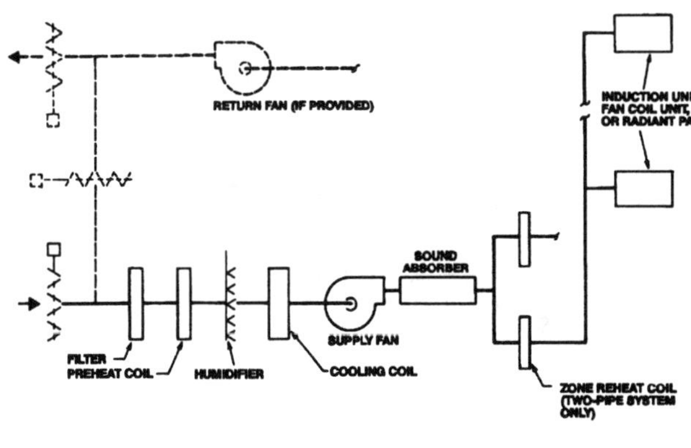

Fig. 12-10 Primary Air System

12.8 All-Water Systems

All-water systems for heating and cooling use either hot or chilled water for space conditioning, with the air in the space heated or cooled by conduction, convection, or radiation. The following are the principal types of all-water systems:

- Baseboard radiation
- Freestanding radiators and convectors
- Wall, floor, or ceiling panels
- Bare pipe (racked on wall)
- Fan-coil units

Additional information on baseboard radiation and freestanding radiators or convectors may be found in Chapters 6 and 32 of the 1996 *ASHRAE Handbook—Systems and Equipment*.

Although fan-coil units rely on fans for the movement of air across the heating or cooling surface, they are included in this section.

12.8.1 Fan-Coil Units

It is common terminology to refer to these systems as all water systems, but since they cannot provide for the ventilation component of the system, they must be used in conjunction with a 100% outdoor air ventilation unit which, in turn, must provide the required amount of ventilation to the space under controlled conditions of temperature and vapor pressure.

Basic elements of fan-coil units are a finned-tube coil, filter, and fan section (Figure 12-11). The fan recirculates air continuously from the space through the coil, which contains

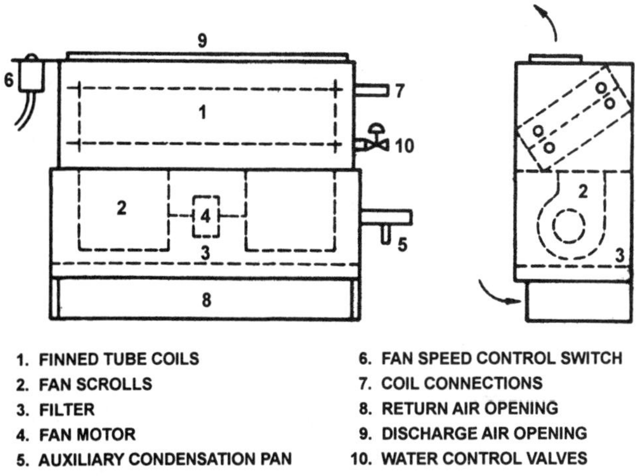

Fig. 12-11 Typical Fan-Coil Unit

either hot or chilled water. The unit may contain an additional electric resistance, steam, or hot water heating coil. The electric heater is often sized for fall and spring to avoid changeover problems in two-pipe systems.

A cleanable or replaceable 35% efficiency filter, located upstream of the fan, prevents clogging the coil with dirt or lint entrained in the recirculated air. It also protects the motor and fan, and reduces the level of airborne contaminants within the conditioned space. The fan-coil unit is equipped with an insulated drain pan. The fan and motor assembly should be arranged for quick removal for servicing. Most manufacturers furnish units with cooling performance that is ARI certified. The prototypes of the units should be tested and labeled by Underwriters' Laboratories (UL), or Engineering Testing Laboratories (ETL), as required by some codes.

Fan coil units, with a dampered opening for connection to apertures in the outside wall, are optional. These units are *not* recommended because wind pressure allows no control over the amount of outside air that is admitted and caution must be exercised for freeze protection in cold climates. Also serious indoor air quality problems and corrosion of cold surfaces could result in humid climates from the excessive condensation.

Room fan coil units are generally available in nominal sizes of 200, 300, 400, 600, 800, and 1200 cfm, often with multispeed fan motors. Means should always be provided to introduce pretreated outside air through a duct system that engages each room or space.

Basic Components. Room fan-coil units are available in may configurations. Figure 12-12 shows several units. Low vertical units are available for use under windows with low sills; however, in some cases, the low silhouette is achieved by compromising such features as filter area, serviceability, and cabinet style.

Floor-to-ceiling, chase-enclosed units are available in which the water and condensate drain risers are part of the factory-furnished unit. Supply and return air systems must be isolated from each other to prevent air and sound interchange between rooms.

Horizontal overhead units may be fitted with ductwork on the discharge to supply several outlets. A single unit may serve several rooms (e.g., in an apartment unit where individual room control is not essential and a common air return is feasible). High static pressure units with larger fan motors handle the higher pressure drops of units with ductwork.

Central ventilation air may be connected to the inlet plenums of the units or introduced directly into the space. If this is done, provisions should be made to ensure that this air is pretreated and held at a temperature equal to the room temperature or to otherwise not cause occupant discomfort when the unit is off. Coil selection must be based on the temperature of the entering mixture of primary and recirculated air, and the air leaving the coil must satisfy the room sensible cooling and heating requirements. Horizontal models conserve floor space and usually cost less, but when located overhead in furred ceilings, they create problems such as condensate collection and disposal, mixing of return air from other rooms, leakage of pans causing damage to ceilings, difficulty of access for maintenance and service, and IAQ concerns.

Vertical models give better results in climates of extremely cold temperatures, since heating is enhanced by under-window or exterior wall locations. Vertical units can be operated as convectors with the fans turned off during winter night setback.

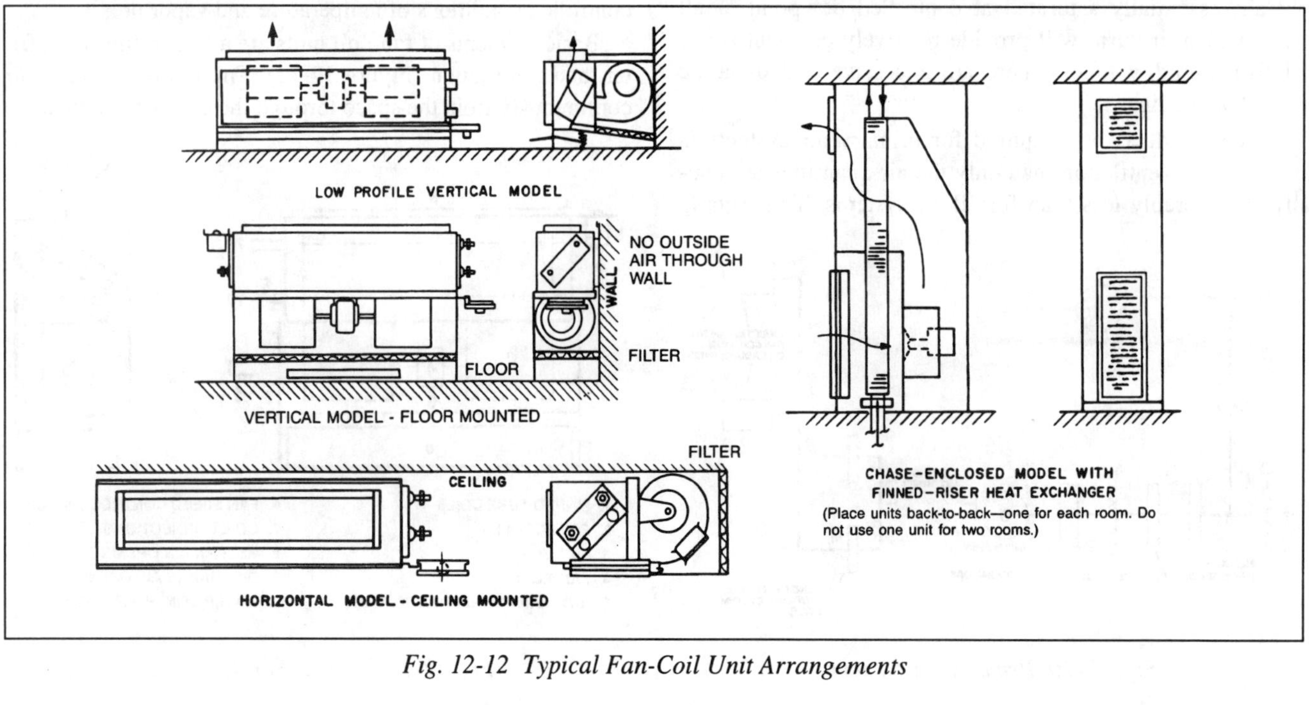

Fig. 12-12 Typical Fan-Coil Unit Arrangements

Selection. Some designers size fan-coil units for nominal cooling at the medium speed setting when a three-speed control switch is provided. This method ensures quieter operation within the space and adds a safety factor, in that capacity can be increased by operating at high speed. Sound power ratings are available from some manufacturers, and as with any in-the-room unit, sound is a very important design parameter.

Only the internal space heating and cooling loads need to be handled by the terminal fan-coil units when outside air is pretreated by a central system to a neutral air temperature of about 70°F. This pretreatment should reduce the size and cost of the terminal units.

Wiring. Fan-coil conditioner fans are driven by small motors generally of the shaded pole or capacitor type, with internal overload protection. Operating wattage of even the largest sizes rarely exceeds 300 W at the high speed setting. Running current rarely exceeds 2.5 A.

Almost all motors on units sold in the United States are wired for 120 V, single-phase, 60 Hz current, and they provide multiple (usually three) fan speeds and an off position or continual speed variation. Other voltages and power characteristics may be encountered, depending on the location, and should be investigated before selecting the fan motor characteristics.

In planning the wiring circuit, local and national electrical codes must be followed. Wiring methods generally provide separate electrical circuits for fan-coil units and do not connect them into the lighting circuit.

Separate electrical circuits connected to a central panel allow the building operator or control system to turn off unit fans from a central point during unoccupied hours. While this panel costs more initially, it can lower operating costs in buildings that do not have 24 hour occupancy.

Piping. Even when outside air is pretreated, a condensate removal system should be installed on the terminal units. This precaution ensures that moisture condensed from air from an unexpected open window that bypasses the ventilation system is carried away. Drain pans should be an integral feature of all units. Condensate drain lines should be oversized to avoid clogging with dirt and other materials, and provision should be made for periodic cleaning of the condensate drain system. Condensation may occur on the outside of the drain piping, which requires that these pipes be insulated. Many building codes have outlawed systems without condensate drain piping due to the damage they could cause.

Capacity Control. Fan-coil unit capacity can be controlled by coil water flow, air bypass, fan speed, or a combination of these. Water flow can be thermostatically controlled by either return air or wall thermostats.

Fan speed control may be automatic or manual. Automatic control is usually on-off with manual speed selection. Units are available with variable-speed motors for modulated speed control. Room thermostats are preferred where fan speed control is used. Return air thermostats do not give a reliable index of room temperature when the fan is off.

On-off speed control is poor because (1) alternating shifts in fan noise level are more obvious than the sound of a constantly running fan, and (2) air circulation patterns (i.e. ambient air circulation) within the room are noticeably affected.

Maintenance. Room fan-coil units are equipped with either cleanable or disposable filters that should be cleaned or replaced when dirty. Good filter maintenance improves sanitation and provides full airflow, ensuring full capacity. The frequency of cleaning varies with the application. Applications in apartments, hotels, and hospitals usually require more frequent filter service because of lint. The condensate drain pan and drain system must be cleaned or flushed periodically to prevent overflow and microbiological buildup.

12.8.2 Water Distribution

Chilled and hot water must run to the fan-coil units. The piping arrangement determines the quality of performance, ease of operation, and initial cost of the system.

Two-Pipe Changeover. This method has low initial cost and supplies either chilled water or hot water through the same piping system (see Chapter 13). The fan-coil unit has a single coil, and room temperature controls reverse their action, depending on whether hot or cold water is available at the unit coil.

This system works well in warm weather when all rooms need cooling and in cold weather when all rooms need heat. The two-pipe system **does not have the simultaneous heating or cooling capability** that is required for most projects during intermediate seasons when some rooms need cooling and others need heat. This problem can be especially troublesome if a single piping zone supplies the entire building. This difficulty may be partly overcome by dividing the piping into zones based on solar exposure. Then each zone may be operated to heat or cool, independent of the others. However, one room may still require cooling while another room on the same solar exposure requires heating—particularly if the building is partially shaded by an adjacent building.

Another difficulty of the two-pipe changeover system is the need for frequent changeover from heating to cooling, which complicates the operation and increases energy consumption to the extent that it may become impractical. For example, two-pipe changeover system hydraulics must consider the water expansion (and relief) that occurs during the cycling from cooling to heating.

Psychrometric principles also show the loss of dehumidification capability throughout the system during the heating cycle.

The designer should consider the disadvantages of the two-pipe system carefully; many installations of this type waste energy and have been unsatisfactory in climates where frequent changeover is required and where interior loads require cooling simultaneously as exterior spaces require heat. Furthermore, most building occupants demand the ability to select either heating or cooling at any time as the thermal conditions *or* their personal metabolism dictates.

Any two-pipe system must be carefully analyzed. In any case, *they are not recommended for commercial buildings.*

Two-pipe changeover with partial electric strip heat. This arrangement provides simultaneous heating and cooling in intermediate seasons by using a small electric strip heater in the fan-coil unit. The unit can handle heating requirements in mild weather, typically down to 40° F, while continuing to circulate chilled water to handle any cooling requirements. When the outdoor temperature drops sufficiently to require heating in excess of the electric strip heater capacity, the water system must be changed over to hot water.

Two-pipe nonchangeover with full electric strip heat. This system is not recommended for energy conservation in temperate or northern climates, but it may be practical in areas with a small heating requirement.

Four-Pipe Distribution. The four-pipe system generally has the highest initial cost, but it has the best fan-coil system performance. It provides (1) all-season availability of heating and cooling at each unit, (2) no summer/winter changeover requirement, (3) simpler operation, and (4) use of any heating fuel, heat recovery, or solar heat. In addition, it can be controlled to maintain a "dead band" between heating and cooling so that there is no possibility of simultaneous heating and cooling.

Central Equipment. Central equipment size is based on the block load of the entire building at the time of building peak load, not on the sum of individual fan-coil unit peak loads. Cooling load should include appropriate diversity factors for lighting and occupant loads. Heating load is based on maintaining the unoccupied building at design temperature, plus an additional allowance for pickup capacity if the building temperature is set back at night.

If water supply temperature or quantities are to be reset at times other than at peak load, the adjusted settings must be adequate for the most heavily loaded space in the building. An analysis of individual room load variations is required.

If the side exposed to the sun or interior zone loads require chilled water in cold weather, the use of condenser water with a water-to-water interchanger should be considered. Varying refrigeration loads require the water chiller to operate satisfactorily under all conditions.

Ventilation requires an outside air pretreatment unit complete with sized heating and cooling coils, filters, and fans, to offset the ventilation load. An additional advantage of the ventilation unit is that, if it is sized for the internal latent load, the terminal cooling coil remains dry.

12.9 Ventilation

Ventilation air is generally the most difficult factor to control and represents a major load component. To save energy, it should be reduced to a minimum. The designer must select the method that meets local codes, performance requirements, cost constraints, and health requirements.

12.9.1 Central Ventilation Systems

A central outside air pretreatment system, which maintains neutral air from 55°F to about 70°F, best controls ventilation air with the greatest freedom from problems related to stack effect and infiltration. Ventilation air may then be introduced to the room through the fan-coil unit or directly to the room as shown in Figure 12-13. Any type of fan-coil unit in any location may be used if the ventilation system has separate air outlets.

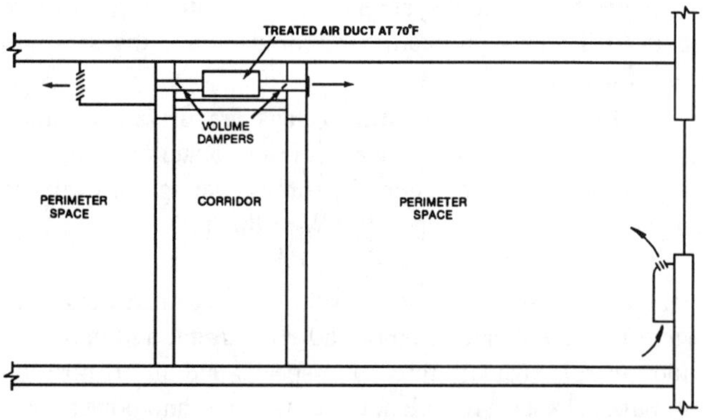

Fig. 12-13 Ventilation from Separate Duct System

Example 12-1. A two-zone building in St. Louis, Missouri has the hourly heating and cooling loads given in the following tables. Assuming that the January day is the coldest for the year, and the August day is the warmest for the year, size the basic components and sketch the equipment arrangement for each of the following types of systems:

1. Separate 4-pipe fan coil units using chilled water supplied at 45°F for cooling and hot water supplied at 190°F for heating.
2. Variable volume with reheat (turndown to 50% of design airflow) with cooling coil discharge at 58°F all year long.
3. Four pipe induction (1:1 induction ratio) with primary air provided at 58°F and 130°F, respectively.
4. Double duct or multizone with design cold and hot deck temperatures of 58°F.

Space Design Conditions:
- Summer: 78°F db
- Winter: 72°F db, 30% rh

Ventilation (Outside) Air Requirements:
- Zone 1: 550 cfm
- Zone 2: 400 cfm

Design Pressure Drop for Duct System:
- 2.8 in. w.g. for Systems 2, 3, 4
- 1.0 in. w.g. for System 1

Solution:

St. Louis

Winter: $t_o = 6°F$, 100% rh $\rightarrow h_o = 2.58$, $W_o = 0.00107$

$t_i = 72°F$, 30% $\rightarrow h_i = 22.9$, $W_i = 0.005$

Summer: $t_o = 94°F/75°F \rightarrow h_o = 38.4$, $W_o = 0.0144$

$t_i = 78°F$

Cold Deck: 58°F (if $\phi = 100\%$); $h_s = 25.2$, $W_s = 0.0103$

JANUARY

Hour	Sensible Load Zone 1 Btu/Hr	Sensible Load Zone 2 Btu/Hr	Latent Load Zone 1 Btu/Hr	Latent Load Zone 2 Btu/Hr
1	-32985.	-32485.	1500.	1800.
2	-33568.	-33068.	1500.	1800.
3	-33918.	-33418.	1500.	1800.
4	-34034.	-33534.	1500.	1800.
5	-34337.	-33837.	1500.	1800.
6	-34477.	-33977.	1500.	1800.
7	-34360.	-33860.	1500.	1800.
8	-26830.	-23173.	1500.	1800.
9	-13237.	-13728.	1500.	1800.
10	- 5232.	-14699.	1500.	1800.
11	2636.	-18162.	1500.	1800.
12	7092.	-21509.	1500.	1800.
13	11608.	-20380.	1500.	1800.
14	16073.	-20729.	1500.	1800.
15	13690.	-21782.	1500.	1800.
16	192.	-23353.	1500.	1800.
17	-27088.	-26588.	1500.	1800.
18	-28183.	-27683.	1500.	1800.
19	-29115.	-28615.	1500.	1800.
20	-30188.	-29688.	1500.	1800.
21	-30980.	-30480.	1500.	1800.
22	-31587.	-31087.	1500.	1800.
23	-32309.	31809.	1500.	1800.
24	-32752.	-32252.	1500.	1800.

AUGUST

Hour	Sensible Load Zone 1 Btu/Hr	Sensible Load Zone 2 Btu/Hr	Latent Load Zone 1 Btu/Hr	Latent Load Zone 2 Btu/Hr
1	1027.	527.	1500.	1800.
2	1820.	1320.	1500.	1800.
3	2426.	1926.	1500.	1800.
4	2659.	2159.	1500.	1800.
5	3195.	2695.	1500.	1800.
6	416.	7621.	1500.	1800.
7	3263.	22148.	1500.	1800.
8	10136.	29670.	1500.	1800.
9	18660.	31112.	1500.	1800.
10	31591.	34088.	1500.	1800.
11	38869.	27952.	1500.	1800.
12	42982.	23170.	1500.	1800.
13	48478.	23717.	1500.	1800.
14	54945.	22592.	1500.	1611.
15	45420.	17379.	1500.	1471.
16	41390.	16062.	1500.	1564.
17	36070.	13277.	1500.	1800.
18	21612.	9042.	1500.	1800.
19	6175.	6675.	1500.	1800.
20	4264.	4764.	1500.	1800.
21	2632.	3132.	1500.	1800.
22	1187.	1687.	1500.	1800.
23	185.	685.	1500.	1800.
24	515.	15.	1500.	1800.

System No. 1: 4-Pipe Fan Coil Units

(Δp = 1.0 in. w.g.)

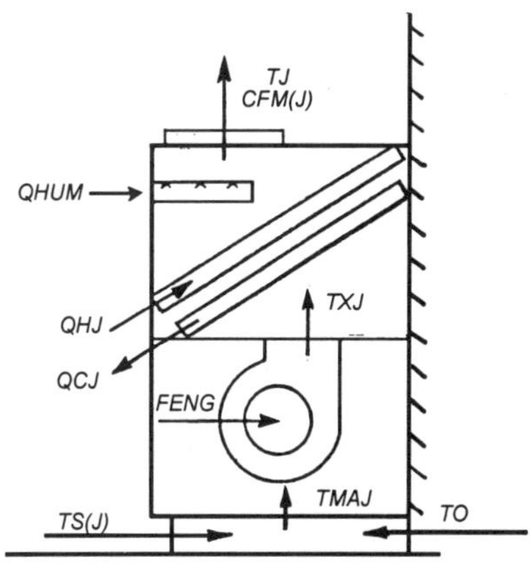

System Sketch

Zone 1

$$Q_1 = \frac{54945}{1.10(78-58)} = 2498 \text{ cfm} \qquad Q_o = 550 \text{ cfm}$$

Summer:

$$W_r = 0.0103 + \frac{1500/1100}{2498 \times 60/13.33} = 0.104$$

$t_r = 78 \quad h_r = 30.2$

$$h_m = \frac{1948(30.2) + 550(38.4)}{2498} = 32.0$$

$$W_m = \frac{1948(0.0104) + 550(0.0144)}{2498} = 0.0133$$

$$W_{fan1} = V\Delta p = \frac{2498(1)(60)(62.4)}{12(778)(2545)} = 0.4 \text{ hp}$$

(2500 cfm, 1 in. w.g.)

$$h_f = 32.0 + \frac{0.4(2545)}{2498 \times 60/13.33} = 32.1$$

$$q_{cc} = \frac{2498(60)}{13.33}[32.1 - 25.2 - (0.0113 - 0.0103)26]$$

$= 76{,}200$ Btu/h

Winter:

$$t_s = 72 + \frac{34477}{1.10(2498)} = 84.5°\text{F}$$

$$W_s = 0.005 - \frac{1500/1100}{2498 \times 60/13.33} = 0.0049$$

$$W_m = \frac{1948(0.005) + 550(0.00107)}{2498} = 0.0041$$

$$t_m = \frac{1948(72) + 550(6)}{2498} = 57.5°\text{F}$$

$$t_f = 57.5 + \frac{0.4(2545)}{11200(0.24)} = 57.9°\text{F}$$

$q_{hc} = 2498(1.1)(84.5 - 57.9) = 73{,}000$ Btu/h heaters

$m_w = 11200(0.0049 - 0.0041) = 9.0$ lb/h humidifiers

Zone 2

$$Q_2 = \frac{34088}{1.10(78-58)} = 1549 \text{ cfm} \quad Q_0 = 400 \text{ cfm}$$

Summer:

$$W_r = 0.0103 + \frac{(1800/1100)}{1549 \times 50/13.33} = 0.0105, \quad h_r = 32.4$$

$$W_m = \frac{1139(0.0105) + 400(0.0144)}{1549} = 0.0115$$

$$W_{fan2} = \frac{1549 \times 60 \times 62.4}{12 \times 778 \times 2545} = 0.244 \text{ hp}, \quad h_f = 32.49$$

$$q_{cc} = \frac{1549 \times 60}{13.33}[32.49 - 25.2 - (0.0115 - 0.0103)26]$$

$$= 50{,}000 \text{ Btu/h}$$

Winter:

$$t_x = 72 + \frac{33977}{1.10(1549)} = 91.9°\text{F}$$

$$W_s = 0.005 - \frac{1800/1100}{1549 \times 60/13.33} = 0.0048$$

$$W_m = \frac{1149(0.005) + 400(0.00107)}{1549} = 0.0040$$

$$t_m = \frac{1149(72) + 400(6)}{1549} = 55.0°\text{F}$$

$$t_f = 55.0 + \frac{0.24(2545)}{6970(0.24)} = 55.4°\text{F}$$

$Q_{Hc} = 1549(1.1)(91.9 - 55.4) = 52{,}200$ Btu/h

$m_w = 6970(0.0048 - 0.0040) = 5.6$ lb/h

System No. 2: VAV with Reheat.

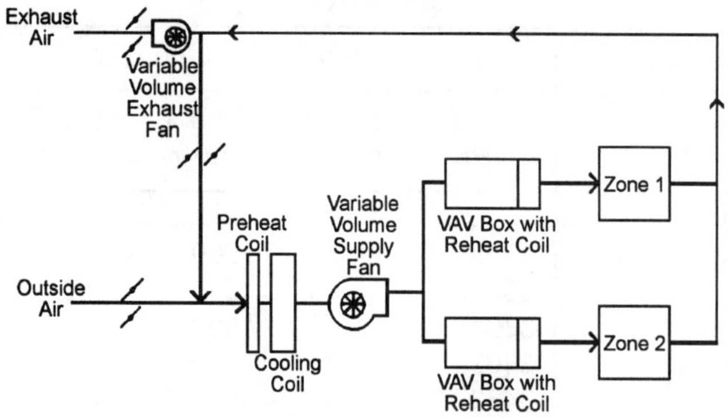

System Sketch

Design Peak Cooling = 77537 = $1.10\, Q_T(78 - 58)$

$Q_T = 3524$ cfm $m = 15860$ lb/h

Space 1 airflow: $54{,}945 = 1.10Q(78 - 58)$
$Q_1 = 2498$ cfm (max), 1249 cfm (min)

Space 2 airflow: $24{,}088 = 1.10Q(78 - 58)$
$Q_2 = 1549$ cfm (max), 775 cfm (min)

$$W_{fan} = \frac{3524(2.8)(62.4)(60)}{12(778)(2545)} = 1.6 \text{ hp}$$

$$\Delta h_f = \frac{1.6(2545)}{15860} = 0.26 \quad \Delta t_f = \frac{\Delta h_f}{c_p} = 1.1°\text{F}$$

Fan: 3500 scfm; $\Delta P = 2.8$ in. w.g.; 1.5 hp motor

$$W_r = W_s + \frac{m_{w1} + m_{w2}}{m_a}$$

$$= 0.0103 + \frac{3111}{15860(1100)} = 0.0105$$

$t_r = 78°\text{F}$ $h_r = 30.3$

$$h_m = \frac{2574(30.3) + 950(38.4)}{3524} = 32.5 \quad h_f = 32.76$$

$$W_m = \frac{2574(0.0105) + 950(0.0144)}{3524} = 0.0116 = W_f$$

$q_{cc} = 15860[32.76 - 25.2 - (0.0116 - 0.0103)26]$
$= 119{,}400$ Btu/h

Winter:

#1 $q_1 = 34477 = 1.10(12490)(t_1 - 72)$ $t_1 = 97°\text{F}$
#2 $q_1 = 33977 = 1.10(775)(t_2 - 72)$ $t_1 = 112°\text{F}$

$q_{rh1} = 1.10(1249)(97 - 58) = 53{,}600$ Btu/h
$q_{rh2} = 1.10(775)(112 - 58) = 46{,}000$ Btu/h

$$W_m = \frac{950(0.00207) + 1074(0.005)}{(950 + 1074)} = 0.0032$$

$$W_s = 0.005 - \frac{3300/1100}{15960/2} = 0.0046$$

$$m_w = \frac{15860}{2}(0.0046 - 0.00232) = 11.3 \text{ lb/h}$$

System No. 3: Four Pipe Induction

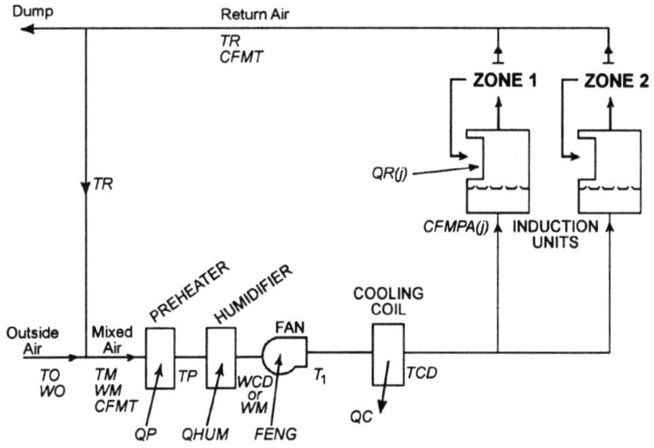

System Sketch

$$Q_1 = \frac{54945}{1.10(78-58)} = 2498 \text{ cfm} \Rightarrow 11240 \text{ lb/h}$$

$$Q_2 = \frac{34088}{1.10(78-58)} = 1549 \text{ cfm} \Rightarrow 6970 \text{ lb/h}$$

$Q_T = 4047$ scfm $\Rightarrow 18200$ lb/h

$Q_p = 1/2(4047) = 2024$ scfm

$$W_r = 0.0103 + \frac{(1500+1611)/1100}{18200} = 0.0105$$

$t_r = 78\,°\text{F} \quad h_r = 30.2$

$$h_m = \frac{1074(30.2)+950(38.4)}{2024} = 34.0$$

$$W_m = \frac{1074(0.0105)+950(0.0144)}{2024} = 0.0123$$

Fan:

$$W_f = \frac{2024(2.8)(62.4)(60)}{12(778)(2545)} = 0.89 \text{ hp}$$

2024 scfm $\quad \Delta P = 2.8$ in. w.g.

$\Delta h_f = 0.89(2545)/(18200/2) = 0.25$

$\Delta t_f = \Delta h_f / c_p = 0.25/0.244 \approx 1\,°\text{F}$

$h_f = 34.0 + 0.25 = 34.25$

Main Coil:

$$q_{cc} = 9100[34.25 - 25.2 - (0.0123 - 0.0103)26]$$
$$= 81{,}900 \text{ Btu/h}$$

Secondary Cooling Coil:

$$q_{c1} = \frac{11240}{2}(30.2 - 25.2)$$
$$= 28{,}100 \text{ Btu/h}$$

Heating Coils:

$$q_{H1} = 34477 + 1.10\left(\frac{2498}{2}\right)(72-58)$$
$$= 53{,}700 \text{ Btu/h}$$

$$q_{H2} = 33977 + 1.10\left(\frac{1549}{2}\right)(72-58)$$
$$= 45{,}900 \text{ Btu/h}$$

Humidifier:

$$m_w = \frac{950(60)}{13.33}(0.005 - 0.00107) - \frac{(1500+1800)}{1100}$$
$$= 14.0 \text{ lb/h}$$

System No. 4: Multizone.

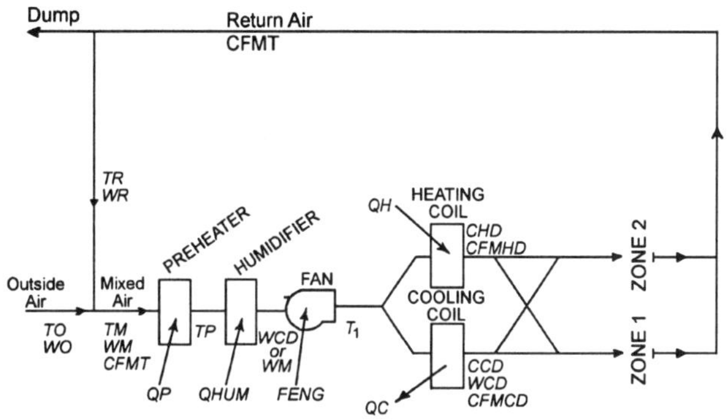

System Sketch

$$q_{1,sMAX} = \frac{54945}{1.10(78-58)} = 2498 \text{ cfm}$$

$$q_{1,wMAX} = \frac{34477}{1.10(130-72)} = 540 \text{ cfm (use 2498 cfm)}$$

$$q_{2,sMAX} = \frac{34088}{1.10(78-58)} = 1549 \text{ cfm}$$

$$q_{2,wMAX} = \frac{33977}{1.10(130-72)} = 533 \text{ cfm (use 1549 cfm)}$$

$m = 4047 \times 60/13.33 = 18200$

Total cfm = 2498 + 1549 = 4047

Fan:

$$\frac{4047 \times 60 \times 2.8 \times 62.4}{12(778)(2545)} = 1.8 \text{ hp}, \quad 4047 \text{ scfm}, \quad 2.8 \text{ in. w.g}$$

$$\Delta h_f = \frac{1.8(2545)}{18200} = 0.25 \quad \Delta t = \frac{0.25}{0.244} \approx 1\,°\text{F}$$

Summer:

$$W_r = 0.0103 + \frac{3111/1100}{18200} = 0.0105 \quad t_r = 78\,°\text{F}$$

$h_r = 30.3$

$$h_m = \frac{3097(30.3)+950(38.4)}{4047} = 32.3$$

$$W_m = \frac{3097(0.0105)+950(0.0144)}{4047} = 0.0114$$

$h_f = 32.2 + 0.25 = 32.45$

$$q_{cc} = 15860[32.45 - 25.2 - (0.0114 - 0.0103)26]$$
$$= 114{,}500 \text{ Btu/h}$$

Winter:

$$m_w = \frac{950(60)}{13.33}(0.005 - 0.00107) - \frac{3300}{1100}$$
$$= 13.8 \text{ lb/h}$$

#1 $1.10Q_{H1}(130 - 72) = 34477 + 1.10(2498 - Q_{H1})(72 - 58)$
$Q_{H1} = 921$ cfm
#2 $1.10Q_{H2}(130 - 72) = 33977 + 1.10(1549 - Q_{H2})(72 - 58)$
$Q_{H2} = 730$ cfm

$Q_H = 921 + 730 = 1652$ cfm

$$t_m = \frac{3097(72) + 950(6)}{4047} = 54.5°\text{F} \quad t_f = 55.5°\text{F}$$

$q_{Hc} = 1.10(1651)(130 - 55.5) = 135{,}300$ Btu/h

12.10 Problems

12.1 From an energy consumption perspective, list the four fundamental psychrometric system types from least consumption to most consumption.

12.2 In a VAV system with series fan powered terminals, why must all of the terminal fans be running prior to turning on the system fan?

12.3 What is the advantage of a parallel fan powered terminal over a series powered terminal?

12.4 What is the purpose of using a fan powered terminal in a variable air volume system?

12.5

(a) Why do some VAV systems also use dual-duct or reheat features?
(b) In your own words, describe the operating sequence of the zone or terminal control of:

(1) A VAV system
(2) A VAV reheat system
(3) A dual-duct VAV system

12.6 What is the primary advantage of a separate outdoor makeup air conditioning unit?

12.7 Why is a high pressure primary system fan required with an induction system?

12.8 Are fan coil units with connections to the outdoors recommended as an acceptable method for providing ventilation air? Why?

12.9 Why are vertical floor mounted fan coil units recommended in some applications in preference to horizontal ceiling mounted units? Explain.

12.10 Size the basic components and sketch the equipment arrangement if the HVAC system now under consideration for the building of Example 12.1 is a triple deck multizone (hot, cold, and neutral decks).

12.11 Size the basic components and sketch the equipment arrangement if the HVAC system now under consideration for the building of *Example* 12.1 is a variable volume, dual fan, dual duct.

12.12 A small single-zone classroom building is being designed for Knoxville, Tennessee, to use the HVAC system shown in the sketch. Minimum outside air for meeting the ventilation requirements of the anticipated 550 occupants will be maintained throughout the year. Fan speed will be changed between summer and winter. The duct system will be designed so that at summer air flow rate the pressure drop does not exceed 3.75 in. of water. At winter design conditions, the air is heated to 130°F at which temperature it is supplied to the conditioned space. The winter conditioning unit includes both a heating coil and a humidifier supplied with city water at 60°F. The humidistat in the return air steam maintains the design relative humidity of 30% in winter. During summer operation, the cooling coil supplied air to the conditioned space at 58°F. The space design loads are:

Summer: 423,000 Btu/h sensible (gain)
139,000 Btu/h latent (gain)

Winter: 645,000 Btu/h sensible (loss)
negligible latent

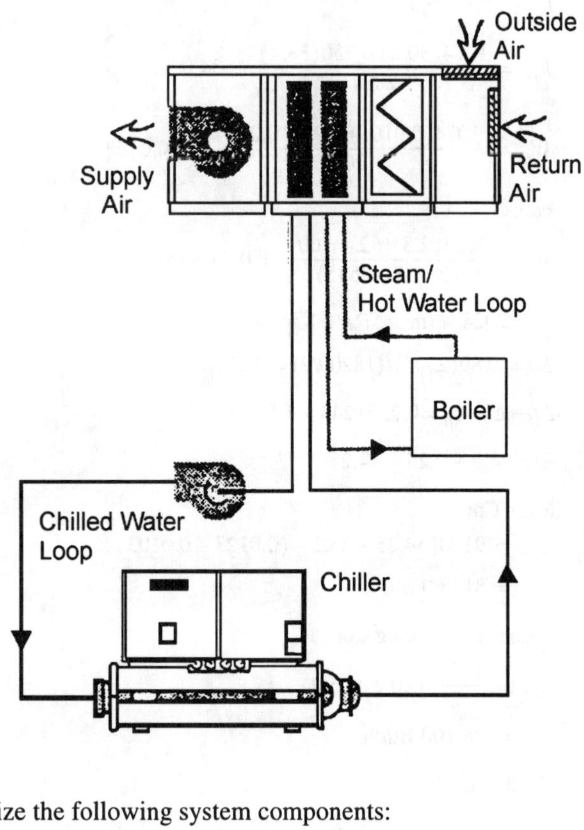

Size the following system components:

(a) Cooling coil, Btu/h and ft^2 of face area
(b) Chiller unit, Btu/h

(c) Heating coil, Btu/h and ft² of face area

(d) Boiler, Btu/h

(e) Humidifier, gph

Select an appropriate air handler from the following data.

Unit Physical Data (Approximate)			
Unit Size	Design cfm	Unit Coil Face Area*, ft²	Max Unit Wt., lb
3	1,660	2.34 – 3.32	
6	2,930	4.31 – 5.86	
8	3,770	5.49 – 7.54	
10	4,820	7.01 – 9.64	
12	6,150	9.46 – 12.3	≤ 3,600
14	7,110	10.2 – 14.2	
17	8,400	12.3 – 16.8	
21	10,390	15.0 – 20.8	
25	12,190	17.8 – 24.4	
30	14,505	21.2 – 29.0	
35	17,050	26.72 – 34.10	
40	19,650	30.78 – 39.30	≤ 4,500
50	24,715	34.22 – 49.43	
66	32,815	48.13 – 65.63	
80	39,375	56.88 – 78.75	≤ 6,000 (all modules)
100	50,180	73.44 – 100.4	

* Actual face area varies with unit coil type.

12.13 A double duct system is to be used for air conditioning of a two-zone building. At winter design outdoor temperature of 0°F, exterior SPACE 1 has a design sensible heat *loss* of 112,000 Btu/h while interior SPACE 2 has a net sensible heat *gain* of 23,500 Btu/h. At summer design outdoor conditions of 95°F db and 75°F wb, SPACE 1 has a design sensible heat gain of 67,000 Btu/h while SPACE 2 experiences a design sensible heat gain of 49,000 Btu/h. Interior design temperatures of both spaces is 75°F, all year long. Duct pressure drop is 3.1 in. water. Outside air requirement is 1400 cfm.

Calculate the size of

(a) Fan (scfm, pressure, motor horsepower)

(b) Heating coil (Btu/h).

12.14 To maintain the necessary close control of humidity as well as temperature required for a computer room, the reheat air-conditioning system shown in the sketch is used. Space loads for the computer room include a heat load of 85,000 Btu/h and a moisture load of 42 lb/h. The return air conditions from the space must be exactly 50% relative humidity and 78°F. After mixing of the outside ventilation air with return air, the mixed air is at 80°F dry bulb with a relative humidity of 0.0114 lb/lb. The air is then cooled to saturation at 50°F by the cooling coil. There is a 2°F temperature rise across the fan. Air flow is controlled by a humidistat in the return air duct. The thermostat controls the temperature leaving the reheater.

Size the reheater (kW) and the cooling coil (Btu/h). From a manufacturer's catalog, select an appropriate electric resistance reheater coil. From a manufacturer's catalog, select an appropriate chilled water cooling coil.

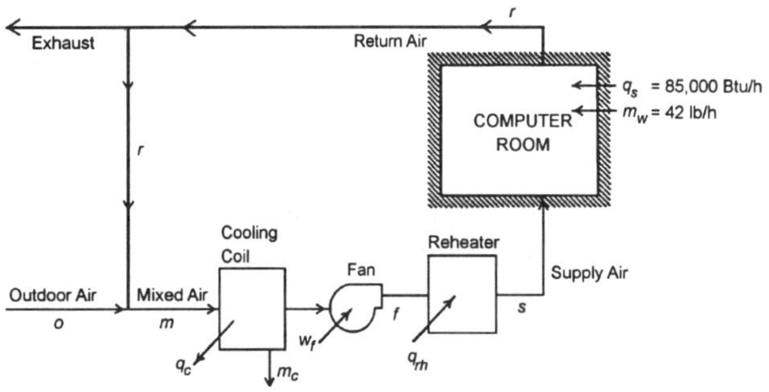

Sketch for Problem 12.14

12.15 A small office building is being designed for St. Louis, Missouri where summer outdoor design conditions are 94°F db and 75°F wb and winter outdoor design conditions are 8°F and 100% rh. The building will be divided into two separate thermostatically controlled zones. A blow-thru induction system will be used with four-pipe induction units in each space. The primary air supply will be 100% outside air with the amount of outside air equal to the minimum ventilation requirement of 15 cfm per person in accordance with ASHRAE *Standard* 62-1989. Design occupancies are 160 people for Space 1 and 110 people for Space 2. The duct system will be designed so that the pressure drop does not exceed 2.5 in. w.g. Fan efficiency is estimated at 63%. In winter, the humidistat in the common return air duct is set at 30% rh and will control the operation of the spray washer (located between the fan and the primary cooling coil) being used as the humidifier. Neglect the effect of the spray washer at summer design. The primary cooling coil is to be selected to provide air at 54°F with a relative humidity of 90% or less throughout the year. At summer design, supply air (primary + induced) to the space is to be provided at 60°F. A closed loop run-around air-to-air energy recovery system having a sensible effectiveness of 79% has been selected for transferring energy between the exhaust air and the incoming outside ventilation air.

The space design loads at indoor design temperatures of 78°F summer and 72°F winter are:

Summer:

Zone 1: 116,000 Btu/h sensible; 43,000 latent (gains)

Zone 2: 190,000 Btu/h sensible; 39,000 latent (gains)

Winter:

Zone 1: –215,000 Btu/h sensible (loss); negligible latent

Zone 2: –71,000 Btu/h sensible (loss); negligible latent

Do a preliminary sizing of the following components:

Fan: _____scfm _____hp

Primary Cooling Coil: _____Btu/h

Spray Washer: _____gallons/hour; _____% Efficiency

Cooling Coil, Space 1: _____Btu/h

Cooling Coil, Space 2: _____Btu/h

Heating Coil, Space 1: _____Btu/h

Heating Coil, Space 2: _____Btu/h

Sketch System And Label Completely.

12.16 A small commercial building located in St. Louis, Missouri is to be conditioned using a variable air volume (VAV) system with reheat, as shown in the following sketch. At this stage of the process, preliminary sizing of the central cooling unit, of the reheaters, and of the fan (scfm) is to take place. There are four zones (separately thermostated spaces) in the building. Supply air from the cooling coil is maintained at 55°F during the summer and 58°F during the winter. Relative humidity off the coil is approximately 90% in both cases. Minimum outside air of 4000 scfm is maintained at all times (just don't ask how). The VAV boxes are not to be cut back beyond 50% of rated flow. The design conditions and calculated design load for each zone are as follow:

Zone 1

Winter inside temperature = 72°F
Winter design heat loss = –55,000 Btu/h (a loss)
Summer inside temperature = 78°F
Summer design heat gains = 124,000 Btu/h (sensible) and 31,000 Btu/h (latent)

Zone 2 (an interior space)

Winter inside temperature = 78°F
Winter design heat loss = 40,000 Btu/h (a gain)
Summer inside temperature = 78°F
Summer design heat gains = 220,000 Btu/h (sensible) and 71,000 Btu/h (latent)

Zone 3 (an interior space)

Winter inside temperature = 78°F
Winter design heat loss = 115,000 Btu/h (a gain)
Summer inside temperature = 78°F
Summer design heat gains = 140,000 Btu/h (sensible) and 42,000 Btu/h (latent)

Zone 4

Winter inside temperature = 72°F
Winter design heat loss = –180,000 Btu/h (a loss)
Summer inside temperature = 78°F
Summer design heat gains = 210,000 Btu/h (sensible) and 52,500 Btu/h (latent)

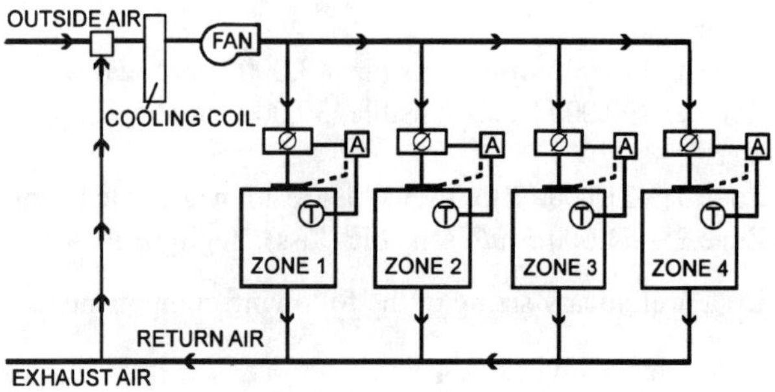

Sketch for Problem 12.16

12.17 A commercial three zone office building is being designed for St. Louis, Missouri where summer outdoor design conditions are 94°F db and 75°F *wb* and winter outdoor design conditions are 3°F and 100% rh. Each zone is to contain 10,000 sq ft of floor space. A blow-thru multizone unit will be used with cold deck temperature maintained at 58°F all year long and with hot deck temperature varying from a maximum of 130°F at winter design to 85°F during the summer. The amount of outside air is to equal the recommended 20 cfm per person in accordance with ASHRAE *Standard* 62-1989. Design occupancy is to be 10 people per 1000 ft^2 of floor area. The duct system will be designed so that the pressure drop does not exceed 2.0 in. w.g. Fan efficiency is estimated at 65%. In winter, the control humidistat in the common return air duct is set at 30% rh. Due to the building orientation and internal zoning, all spaces will experience their peak loads at the same time. The space design loads at indoor design temperatures of 78°F summer and 72°F winter are:

Summer:

Zone 1: 116,000 Btu/h sensible, 43,000 Btu/h latent (gains)
Zone 2: 290,000 Btu/h Sensible, 59,000 Btu/h Latent (gains)
Zone 3: 190,000 Btu/h sensible, 39,000 Btu/h latent (gains)

Winter:

Zone 1: –215,000 Btu/h sensible (loss), negligible latent
Zone 2: 110,000 Btu/h sensible (gain), negligible latent
Zone 3: –171,000 Btu/h sensible (loss), negligible latent

Conduct the preliminary sizing of the fan (scfm and horsepower), cooling coil (scfm and Btu/h), heating coil (scfm and Btu/h), and humidifier (gal/h). Provide a completely labeled sketch of the system.

12.18 An air-conditioning unit takes in 2000 cfm of outside air at 95°F dry bulb and 76°F wet bulb, and 6000 cfm of return air at 78°F dry bulb and 50% rh. The conditioned air leaves the chilled water coil at 52°F dry bulb and 90% rh.

(a) What is the refrigeration load on the chiller in tons?
(b) Assume the conditioned air were reheated to 58.5°F dry bulb with electric heaters. What would be the operating cost of these heaters at 2.5 cents per kWh?

12.19 In *Problem* 12.18, assume 2000 cfm of return air bypasses the chilled water coil and is used for reheat.

(a) How does the final condition of the air compare with the reheated air in part (b) of 12.18? [Ans: 58°F, $W = 0.0081$]

(b) Comment on the ability of the leaving air to absorb latent load in the conditioned space. [Ans: Less than in *Example* 12.1]

12.20 For the building and reheat system shown below, determine:

(a) Fan rating, scfm
(b) Return air relative humidity at summer design conditions, %
(c) Size cooling coil, Btu/h
(d) Size reheat coils, Btu/h and scfm for each

Winter: Outside 6°F, $W = 0.001$; indoor 72°F, no humidity control.

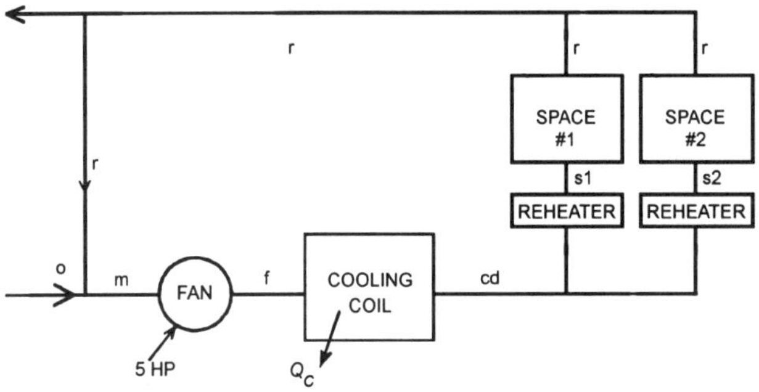

Sensible design heating loads:
Space 1: 162,000 Btu/h
Space 2: 143,000 Btu/h

Summer: Outdoor 95°F dry bulb, 78°F wet bulb; indoor 78°F.
Sensible design cooling loads:
Space 1: 64,500 Btu/h
Space 2: 55,000 Btu/h
Latent design loads (moisture produced):
Space 1: 38 lb/h
Space 2: 26 lb/h

Year-round: 10% by mass outside air required for ventilation.
Conditions of cooling coil: 58°F, 90% rh.

12.21 A two-zone building has the following design loads:
Zone 1: Winter sensible, 320,000 Btu/h; summer sensible, 295,000 Btu/h
Zone 2: Winter sensible, 56,000 Btu/h; summer sensible, 413,000 Btu/h.

If a standard reheat system is used, size the reheaters in Btu/h.

12.22 A basic reheat system has been retrofitted with an improved control system. For the operating conditions shown in the sketch below and with all thermostats set at 78°F, for what cooling coil discharge temperature *T* should the logic system of the controller be calling if there is no humidity override?

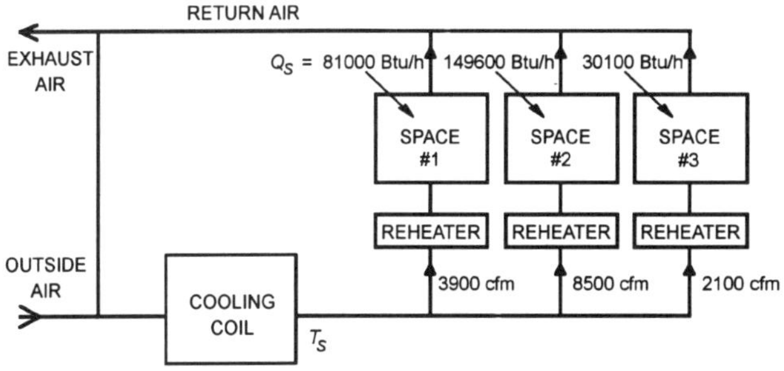

12.23 An office building has the following loads:
Summer: 1,500,000 Btu/h sensible, 830,000 Btu/h latent
Winter: 2,600,000 Btu/h sensible

It is to be conditioned using a double-duct system. Summer inside design conditions are 76°F dry bulb, 68°F wet bulb, maximum. During summer operation, the air temperature in the cold air duct is 53°F; temperature of air in the hot duct is 86°F. During winter operation, cold duct air temperature is 55°F with a hot duct air temperature of 128°F. Based on comfort, air cannot enter the conditioned space at less than 56°F during summer operation. Find suitable design cold duct and hot duct airflows.

12.24 For the office building of *Problem* 12.23, existing summer outside conditions are 98°F dry bulb and 77°F wet bulb. Ventilation requirements call for 12,000 cfm of outside air. Air leaves the cooling coils at 53°F with 95% rh.

(a) Sketch and label (with temperatures and airflows) a line diagram of a possible double duct system with: (i) one return air fan and a simple supply fan; and (ii) one return air fan and separate hot and cold duct supply fans.
(b) Find the mixed air temperature and humidity ratio entering the cooling coils.
(c) Find the final humidity ratio and relative humidity of the return air from the conditioned space.

12.25 The periphery of an office building is air conditioned with a high-pressure induction system. The interior zones are air conditioned with a conventional air distribution arrangement. The primary air component takes in 5000 cfm at 95°F dry bulb and 76°F wet bulb. The air leaves a chilled water coil at 47.5°F dry bulb and 90% rh.

Part A
(a) What is the refrigeration load on the coil?
(b) What should be the chilled water flow for a 20°F rise?
(c) What are the dry- and wet-bulb temperatures and humidity ratio for air at a typical unit if there is a 4°F temperature rise due to fan power and duct heat gain?

Part B
In a typical exterior office, the induction unit is supplied with 70 cfm primary air. The room is maintained at 75°F dry bulb and 50% rh. Secondary water enters the coil at 50°F and leaves at 60°F. The unit has an induction ratio of 5:1. Air is cooled to 68°F dry bulb as it flows through the secondary coil.

(a) Find the condition of the air leaving the induction unit.
(b) What room sensible heat ratio is satisfied exactly by the given operating conditions?

12.26 A perimeter room of an office building is to be maintained at 78°F dry bulb and 50% rh; it has a sensible heat ratio of 0.90. A fan-coil unit with a capacity of 400 cfm is in the room. It cools room air 14°F. The primary air apparatus takes in air at 95°F dry bulb and 76°F wet bulb and it delivers air to the room at 54°F dry bulb and 53°F dew point. What quantity of primary air should be used?

12.11 Bibliography

ASHRAE. 1996 *ASHRAE Handbook—HVAC Systems and Equipment.*

Sauer, H.J., Jr. and R.H. Howell. 1992. Estimating the indoor air quality and energy performance of VAV systems. *ASHRAE Journal* 34(July).

Delp, W.W., H.J. Sauer, Jr., R.H. Howell, and B. Subbarao. 1993. Control of outside air and building pressurization in VAV systems. *ASHRAE Transactions* 99(1).

Chapter 13

HYDRONIC HEATING AND COOLING SYSTEM DESIGN

This chapter provides information useful for the design of hydronic heating and cooling systems. It provides information on the classification of systems, system descriptions and design procedures. Additional information can be obtained from the 1996 *ASHRAE Handbook—Systems and Equipment* and the 1995 *ASHRAE Handbook—Applications.*

13.1 Introduction

Water systems that convey heat to or from a conditioned space or process with hot or chilled water are frequently called hydronic systems. The water flows through piping that connects a boiler, water heater, or chiller to suitable terminal heat transfer units located at the space or process.

Water systems can be classified by (1) operating temperature, (2) flow generation, (3) pressurization, (4) piping arrangement, and (5) pumping arrangement.

Classified by flow generation, hydronic heating systems may be (1) gravity systems, which use the difference in density between the supply and return water columns of a circuit or system to circulate water; or (2) forced systems, in which a pump, usually driven by an electric motor, maintains the flow. Gravity systems are seldom used today.

Water systems can be either once-through or recirculating systems. This chapter describes forced recirculating systems.

13.1.1 Principles

The design of effective and economical water systems is affected by complex relationships between the various system components. The design water temperature, flow rate, piping layout, pump selection, terminal unit selection, and control method are all interrelated. The size and complexity of the system determine the importance of these relationships to the total system operating success. In the United States, present hydronic heating system design practice originated in residential heating applications, where a temperature drop Δt of 20°F was used to determine flow rate. Besides producing satisfactory operation and economy in small systems, this Δt enabled simple calculations because 1 gpm conveys 10,000 Btu/h. However, almost universal use of hydronic systems for both heating and cooling of large buildings and building complexes has rendered this simplified approach obsolete.

13.1.2 Temperature Classifications

Water systems can be classified by operating temperature as follows.

Low temperature water (LTW) system. This hydronic heating system operates within the pressure and temperature limits of the ASME *Boiler and Pressure Vessel Code* for low-pressure boilers. The maximum allowable working pressure for low-pressure boilers is 160 psig, with a maximum temperature limitation of 250°F. The usual maximum working pressure for boilers for LTW systems is 30 psi, although boilers specifically designed, tested, and stamped for higher pressures are frequently used. Steam-to-water or water-to-water heat exchangers are also used for heating low-temperature water. Low temperature water systems are used in buildings ranging from small, single dwellings to very large and complex structures.

Medium-temperature water (MTW) system. This hydronic heating system operates at temperatures between 250 and 350°F, with pressures not exceeding 160 psi. The usual design supply temperature is approximately 250 to 325°F, with a usual pressure rating of 150 psi for boilers and equipment.

High-temperature water (HTW) system. This hydronic heating system operates at temperatures over 350°F and usual pressures of about 300 psi. The maximum design supply water temperature is usually about 400°F, with a pressure rating for boilers and equipment of about 300 psi. The pressure-temperature rating of each component must be checked against the system's design characteristics.

Chilled water (CW) system. This hydronic cooling system normally operates with a design supply water temperature of 40 to 55°F, usually 44 or 45°F, and at a pressure of up to 120 psi. Anti-freeze or brine solutions may be used for applications (usually process applications) that require temperatures below 40°F or for coil freeze protection. Well water systems can use supply temperatures of 60°F or higher.

Dual-temperature water (DTW) system. This hydronic combination heating and cooling system circulates hot and/or chilled water through common piping and terminal heat transfer apparatus. These systems operate within the pressure and temperature limits of LTW systems, with usual winter design supply water temperatures of about 100 to 150°F and summer supply water temperatures of 40 to 45°F.

Terminal heat transfer units include convectors, cast-iron radiators, baseboard and commercial finned-tube units, fan-coil units, radiant panels, and snow-melting panels. A large storage tank may be included in the system to store energy to use when such heat input devices as the boiler or a solar energy collector are not supplying energy.

13.2 Closed Water Systems

Because most hot and chilled water systems are closed, this chapter addresses only closed systems. The fundamental difference between a closed and an open water system is the interface of the water with a compressible gas (such as air) or an elastic surface (such as a diaphragm). A closed water system is defined as one with no more than one point of interface with a compressible gas or surface. This definition is fundamental to understanding the hydraulic dynamics of these systems. Earlier literature referred to a system with an open or vented expansion tank as an "open" system, but such a system is actually a closed system; the atmospheric interface of the tank simply establishes the system pressure.

An open system, on the other hand, has more than one such interface. For example, a cooling tower system has at least two points of interface: the tower basin and the discharge pipe or nozzles entering the tower. One of the major differences in hydraulics between open and closed systems is that certain hydraulic characteristics of open systems cannot occur in closed systems. For example, in contrast to the hydraulics of an open system, in a closed system (1) flow cannot be motivated by static head differences, (2) pumps do not provide static lift, and (3) the entire piping system is always filled with water.

13.2.1 Basic System

Figure 13-1 shows the fundamental components of a closed hydronic system. Actual systems generally have additional components such as valves, vents, regulators, etc., but they are not essential to the basic principles underlying the system.

These fundamental components are

- Loads
- Source
- Expansion chamber
- Pump
- Distribution system

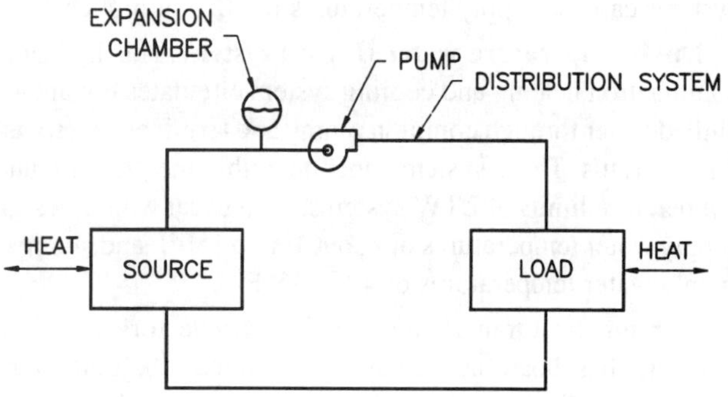

Fig. 13-1 Hydronic System—Fundamental Components

Theoretically, a hydronic system could operate with only these five components.

The components are subdivided into two groups-thermal components and hydraulic components. The thermal components consist of the load, the source, and the expansion chamber. The hydraulic components consist of the distribution system, the pump, and the expansion chamber. The expansion chamber is the only component that serves both a thermal and a hydraulic function.

13.2.2 Thermal Components

Loads. The load is the point where heat flows out of or into the system to or from the space or process; it is the independent variable to which the remainder of the system must respond. Outward heat flow characterizes a heating system, and inward heat flow characterizes a cooling system. The quantity of heating or cooling is calculated by one of the following means.

Sensible Heating or Cooling. The rate of heat entering or leaving an airstream is expressed as follows:

$$q = 60 Q_a \rho_a c_p \Delta t \qquad (13\text{-}1)$$

where

q = heat transfer rate to or from air, Btu/h
Q_a = airflow rate, cfm
ρ_a = density of air, lb/ft^3
c_p = specific heat of air, Btu/lb·°F
Δt = temperature increase or decrease of air, °F

For standard air with a density of 0.075 lb/ft^3 and a specific heat of 0.244 Btu/lb·°F, Equation (13-1) becomes

$$q = 1.1 Q_a \Delta t \qquad (13\text{-}2)$$

The heat exchanger or coil must then transfer this heat from or to the water. The rate of sensible heat transfer to or from the heated or cooled medium in a specific heat exchanger is a function of the heat transfer surface area; the mean temperature difference between the water and the medium; and the overall heat transfer coefficient, which itself is a function of the fluid velocities, properties of the medium, geometry of the heat transfer surfaces, and other factors. The rate of heat transfer may be expressed by

$$q = UA(\text{LMTD}) \qquad (13\text{-}3)$$

where

q = heat transfer rate through heat exchanger, Btu/h
U = overall coefficient of heat transfer, Btu/h·ft^2·°F
A = heat transfer surface area, ft^2
LMTD = logarithmic mean temperature difference, heated or cooled medium to water, °F

Cooling and Dehumidification. The rate of heat removal from the cooled medium when both sensible cooling and dehumidification are present is expressed by

$$q_t = w\Delta h \quad (13\text{-}4)$$

where

q_t = total heat transfer rate from cooled medium, Btu/h
w = mass flow rate of cooled medium, lb/h
Δh = enthalpy difference between entering and leaving conditions of cooled medium, Btu/lb

Expressed for an air-cooling coil, this equation becomes

$$q_t = 60\, Q_a \rho_a \Delta h \quad (13\text{-}5)$$

which, for standard air with a density of 0.075 lb/ft³, reduces to

$$q_t = 4.5 Q_a \Delta h \quad (13\text{-}6)$$

Heat Transferred to or from Water. The rate of heat transfer to or from the water is a function of the flow rate, the specific heat, and the temperature rise or drop of the water as it passes through the heat exchanger. The heat transferred to or from the water is expressed by

$$q_w = mc_p \Delta t \quad (13\text{-}7)$$

where

q_w = heat transfer rate to or from water, Btu/h
m = mass flow rate of water, lb/h
c_p = specific heat of water, Btu/lb·°F
Δt = water temperature increase or decrease across unit, °F

With water systems, it is common to express the flow rate as volumetric flow, in which case Equation (13-7) becomes

$$q_w = 8.02 \rho_w c_p Q_w \Delta h \quad (13\text{-}8)$$

where

Q_w = water flow rate, gpm
ρ_w = density of water, lb/ft³

For standard conditions in which the density is 62.4 lb/ft³ and the specific heat is 1 Btu/lb·°F, Equation (13-8) becomes

$$q_w = 500 Q_W \Delta t \quad (13\text{-}9)$$

Equation (13-8) or (13-9) can be used to express the heat transfer across a single load or source device, or any quantity of such devices connected across a piping system. In the design or diagnosis of a system, the load side may be balanced with the source side using these equations.

Heat Carrying Capacity of Piping. Equations (13-8) and (13-9) are also used to express the heat carrying capacity of the piping or distribution system or any portion thereof. When the existing temperature differential Δt, sometimes called the temperature range, is identified for any flow rate Q_w through the piping, q_w is called the **heat carrying capacity**.

Load systems can be any system in which heat is conveyed to or from the water for heating or cooling the space or process. Most load systems are basically a water-to-air finned-coil heat exchanger or a water-to-water exchanger. The specific configuration is usually used to describe the load device. The most common configurations include the following:

Heating load devices

- Preheat coils in central units
- Heating coils in central units
- Zone or central reheat coils
- Finned-tube radiators
- Baseboard radiators
- Convectors
- Unit heaters
- Fan-coil units
- Water-to-water heat exchangers
- Radiant heating panels
- Snow-melting panels

Cooling load devices

- Coils in central units
- Fan-coil units
- Induction unit coils
- Radiant cooling panels
- Water-to-water heat exchangers

Source. The source is the point where heat is added to (heating) or removed from (cooling) the system. Except for the pump energy, the amount of energy entering or leaving the source equals the amount entering or leaving through the load system(s). Under steady-state conditions, the load energy and source energy are equal and opposite. Also, when properly measured or calculated, temperature differentials and flow rates across the source and loads are all equal. Equations (8) and (9) are used to express the source capacities as well as the load capacities.

Any device that can be used to heat or cool water under controlled conditions can be used as a source device. The most common source devices for heating and cooling systems are the following:

Heating source devices

- Hot water generator or boiler
- Steam-to-water heat exchanger
- Water-to-water heat exchanger
- Solar heating panels
- Heat recovery or salvage heat device, (e.g., water jacket of an internal combustion engine)
- Exhaust gas heat exchanger
- Incinerator heat exchanger
- Heat pump condenser
- Air-to-water heat exchanger

Cooling source devices

- Electric compression chiller
- Thermal absorption chiller
- Heat pump evaporator
- Air-to-water heat exchanger
- Water-to-water heat exchanger

The two primary considerations in selecting a source device are the design capacity and the part-load capability, sometimes called the turndown ratio. The turndown ratio, expressed in percent of design capacity, is

$$\text{Turndown ratio} = 100\,\frac{\text{Minimum capacity}}{\text{Design capacity}} \qquad (13\text{-}10)$$

The reciprocal of the turndown ratio is sometimes used (for example, a turndown ratio of 25% may also be expressed as a turndown ratio of 4).

The turndown ratio has a significant effect on performance; not considering the source system's part-load capability has been responsible for many systems that either do not function properly or do so at the expense of excess energy consumption. The turndown ratio has a significant impact on the ultimate equipment and/or system design selection.

System Temperatures. Design temperatures and temperature ranges are selected by considering the performance requirements and the economics of the components. For a cooling system that must maintain 50% rh at 75°F, the dew-point temperature is 55°F, which sets the maximum return water temperature at about 55°F (60°F maximum); on the other hand, the lowest reasonable temperature for refrigeration, considering the freezing point and economics, is about 40°F. This temperature spread then sets constraints for a chilled water system.

For a heating system, the maximum hot water temperature is normally established by the ASME Low-Pressure Code as 250°F, and with space temperature requirements of little over 75°F, the actual operating supply temperatures and the temperature ranges are set by the design of the load devices. The most economical systems related to distribution and pumping favor the use of the maximum possible temperature range Δt.

Expansion Chamber. The expansion chamber (also called an expansion or compression tank) serves both a thermal function and a hydraulic function. In its thermal function the tank provides a space into which the noncompressible liquid can expand or from which it can contract as the liquid undergoes volumetric changes with changes in temperature. To allow for this expansion or contraction, the expansion tank provides an interface point between the system fluid and a compressible gas. *Note:* By definition, a closed system can have only one such interface; thus, a system designed to function as a closed system can have only one expansion chamber.

Expansion tanks are of three basic configurations: (1) a closed tank, which contains a captured volume of compressed air and water, with an air water interface (sometimes called a plain steel tank); (2) an open tank (i.e., a tank open to the atmosphere); and (3) a diaphragm tank, in which a flexible membrane is inserted between the air and the water (another configuration of a diaphragm tank is the bladder tank).

In the plain steel tank and the open tank, gases can enter the water through the interface and can adversely affect performance. Thus, current design practice normally uses diaphragm tanks.

Sizing the tank is the primary thermal concern in including a tank in a system. However, prior to sizing the tank, the control or elimination of air must be considered. The amount of air that will be absorbed and can be held in solution with the water is expressed by Henry's equation (Pompei 1981):

$$x = p/H \qquad (13\text{-}11)$$

where

x = solubility of air in water (% by volume)
p = absolute pressure
H = Henry's constant

Henry's constant, however, is constant only for a given temperature (Figure 13-2). Combining the data of Figure 13-2 (Himmelblau 1960) with Equation (13-11) results in the solubility diagram of Figure 13-3. With that diagram, the solubility can be determined if the temperature and pressure are known.

If the water is not saturated with air, it will absorb air at the air/water interface until the point of saturation has been reached. Once absorbed, the air moves through the water either by mass migration or by molecular diffusion until the water is uniformly saturated.

If the air/water solution changes to a state that reduces solubility, the excess air will be released as a gas. For example, if the air/water interface is at a high pressure, the water will absorb air to its limit of solubility at that point; if at another point the pressure is less, some of the dissolved air will be released. In the design of systems with open or plain steel expansion tanks, the tank is commonly used as the major air control or release point in the system.

The following equations are used to size the three common configurations of expansion tanks (Coad 1980b):

For closed tanks with air/water interface,

$$V_t = V_s\,\frac{[(v_2/v_1)-1]-3\alpha\Delta t}{(P_a/P_1)-(P_a/P_2)} \qquad (13\text{-}12)$$

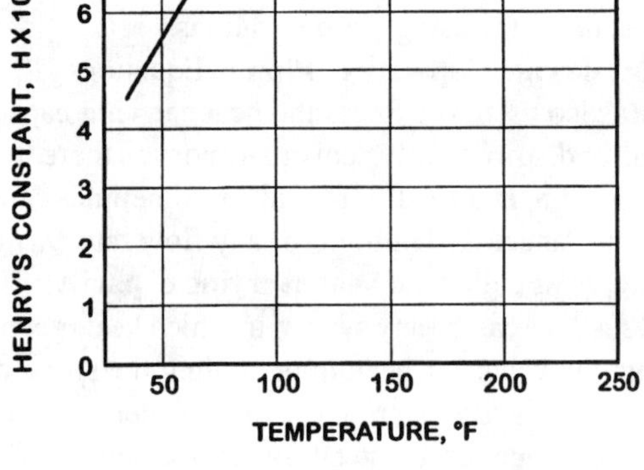

Fig. 13-2 Henry's Constant Versus Temperature for Air and Water

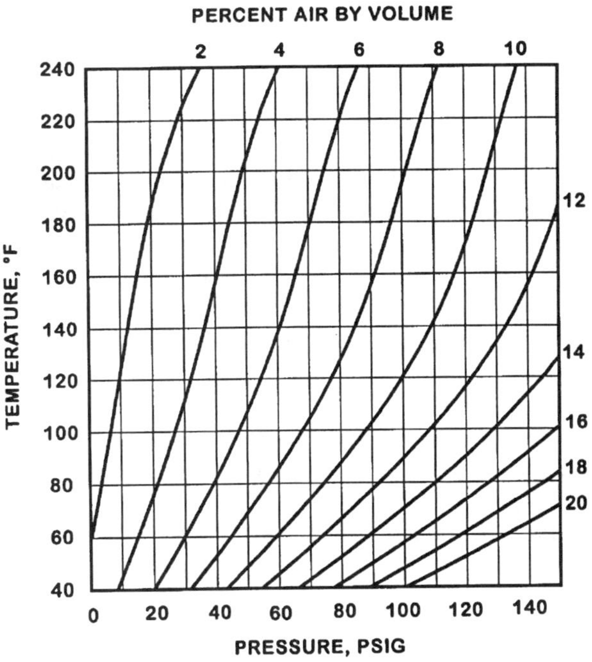

Fig. 13-3 Solubility Versus Temperature and Pressure for Air/Water Solutions

For open tanks with air/water interface,

$$V_t = 2\{V_s[(v_2/v_1) - 1] - 3\alpha\Delta t\} \qquad (13\text{-}13)$$

For diaphragm tanks,

$$V_t = V_s\frac{[(v_2/v_1) - 1] - 3\alpha\Delta t}{1 - (P_1/P_2)} \qquad (13\text{-}14)$$

where

V_t = volume of expansion tank, gal
V_s = volume of water in system, gal
t_1 = lower temperature, °F
t_2 = higher temperature, °F
P_a = atmospheric pressure, psia
P_1 = pressure at lower temperature, psia
P_2 = pressure at higher temperature, psia
v_1 = specific volume of water at lower temperature, ft^3/lb
v_2 = specific volume of water at higher temperature, ft^3/lb
α = linear coefficient of thermal expansion, in/in °F
= 6.5×10^{-6} in/in °F for steel
= 9.5×10^{-6} in/in °F for copper
$\Delta t = (t_2 - t_1)$, °F

As an example, the lower temperature for a heating system is usually normal ambient temperature at fill conditions (e.g., 50°F) and the higher temperature is the operating supply water temperature for the system. For a chilled water system, the lower temperature is the design chilled water supply temperature, and the higher temperature is ambient temperature (e.g., 95°F). For a dual-temperature hot/chilled system, the lower temperature is the chilled water design supply temperature, and the higher temperature is the heating water design supply temperature.

For specific volume and saturation pressure of water at various temperatures, see Table 3 in Chapter 6 of the 1997 *ASHRAE Handbook—Fundamentals.*

At the tank connection point, the pressure in closed tank systems increases as the water temperature increases. Pressures at the expansion tank are generally set by the following parameters:

- The lower pressure is usually selected to hold a positive pressure at the highest point in the system (usually about 10 psig).
- The higher pressure is normally set by the maximum pressure allowable at the location of the safety relief valve(s) without opening them.

Other considerations are to ensure that (1) the pressure at no point in the system will ever drop below the saturation pressure at the operating system temperature and (2) all pumps have sufficient net positive suction head (NPSH) available to prevent cavitation.

Example 13-1. Size an expansion tank for a water heating system that will operate at 180 to 220°F. The minimum pressure at the tank is 10 psig (24.7 psia) and the maximum pressure is 25 psig (39.7 psia). (Atmospheric pressure is 14.7 psia.) The volume of water is 3000 gal. The piping is steel.

1. Calculate the required size for a closed tank with an air/ water interface.

Solution: For lower temperature t_1, use 40°F.

From Table 3 in Chapter 6 of the 1997 *ASHRAE Handbook—Fundamentals,*

v_1 (at 40°F) = 0.01602 ft^3/lb and v_2 (at 220°F) = 0.01677 ft^3/lb

Using Equation (13-12),

$$V_t = 3000\frac{[(0.01677/0.01602) - 1] - 3(6.5 \times 10^{-6})(220 - 40)}{(14.7/24.7) - (14.7/39.7)}$$

$$= 578 \text{ gal}$$

If a diaphragm tank were to be used in lieu of the plain steel tank, what tank size would be required?

Solution: Using Equation (13-14),

$$V_t = 3000\frac{[(0.01677/0.01602) - 1] - 3(6.5 \times 10^{-6})(220 - 40)}{1 - (14.7/39.7)}$$

$$= 206 \text{ gal}$$

13.2.3 Hydraulic Components

Distribution System. The distribution system is the piping system connecting the various other components of the system. The primary considerations in designing this system are (1) sizing the piping to handle the heating or cooling capacity required and (2) arranging the piping to ensure flow in the quantities required at design conditions and at all other loads.

The flow requirement of the pipe is determined by Equation (13-8) or (13-9). After Δt is established based on the thermal requirements, either of these equations (as applicable) can be used to determine the flow rate. First-cost economics and energy consumption make it advisable to design for the greatest practical Δt because the flow rate is inversely proportional to Δt; that is, if Δt doubles, the flow rate is reduced by half.

The three related variables in sizing the pipe are flow rate, pipe size, and pressure drop. The primary consideration in selecting a design pressure drop is the relationship between the economics of first cost and energy costs.

Once the distribution system is designed, the pressure loss at design flow is calculated by the methods discussed in Chapter 9 in this book or in Chapter 33 of the 1997 *ASHRAE Handbook—Fundamentals.* The relationship between flow rate and pressure loss can be expressed by

$$Q = C_v\sqrt{\Delta p} \qquad (13\text{-}15)$$

where

Q = system flow rate, gpm
Δp = pressure drop in system, psi
C_v = system constant (sometimes called valve coefficient, which is discussed in Chapter 41 in 1996 *ASHRAE Handbook—Systems and Equipment*)

Equation (13-15) may be modified as follows:

$$Q = C_s\sqrt{\Delta h} \qquad (13\text{-}16)$$

where

Δh = system head loss, ft of fluid [$\Delta h = \Delta p/\rho$]
C_s = system constant
[$C_s = 0.67\ C_v$ for water with a density = 62.4 lb/ft^3]

Equations (13-15) and (13-16) are the system constant form of the Darcy-Weisbach equation. If the flow rate and head loss are known for a system, Equation (13-16) may be used to calculate the system constant C_s. From this calculation, the pressure loss can be determined at any other flow rate. Equation (13-16) can be graphed as a system curve (Figure 13-4).

The system curve changes if anything occurs that changes the flow/pressure drop characteristics. Examples of this are a strainer that starts to block or a control valve closing, either of which increases the head loss at any given flow rate, thus changing the system curve in a direction from curve A to curve B in Figure 13-4.

Pump or Pumping System. Centrifugal pumps are the type most commonly used in hydronic systems (see Chapter 38 in 1996 *ASHRAE Handbook—Systems and Equipment* or Chapter 9 in this book). Circulating pumps used in water systems can vary in size from small in-line circulators delivering 5 gpm at 6 or 7 ft head to base-mounted or vertical pumps handling hundreds or thousands of gallons per minute, with pressures limited only by the characteristics of the system. Pump operating characteristics must be carefully matched to system operating requirements.

Pump Curves and Water Temperature. Performance characteristics of centrifugal pumps are described by pump curves, which plot flow versus head or pressure, as well as by efficiency and power information. The point at which a pump operates is the point at which the pump curve intersects the system curve (Figure 13-5).

A complete piping system follows the same water flow/pressure drop relationships as any component of the system [see Equation (13-16)]. Thus, the pressure required for any proposed flow rate through the system may be determined and a system curve constructed. A pump may be selected by using the calculated system pressure at the design flow rate as the base point value.

Figure 13-6 illustrates how a shift of the system curve to the right affects system flow rate. This shift can be caused by incorrectly calculating the system pressure drop by using arbitrary safety factors or overstated pressure drop charts. Variable system flow caused by control valve operation or improperly balanced systems (subcircuits having substantially lower pressure drops than the longest circuit) can also cause a shift to the right.

Pumps for closed-loop piping systems should have a flat pressure characteristic and should operate slightly to the left of the peak efficiency point on their curves. This characteristic permits the system curve to shift to the right without causing undesirable pump operation, overloading, or reduction in available pressure across circuits with large pressure drops.

Many dual-temperature systems are designed so that the chillers are bypassed during the winter months. The chiller

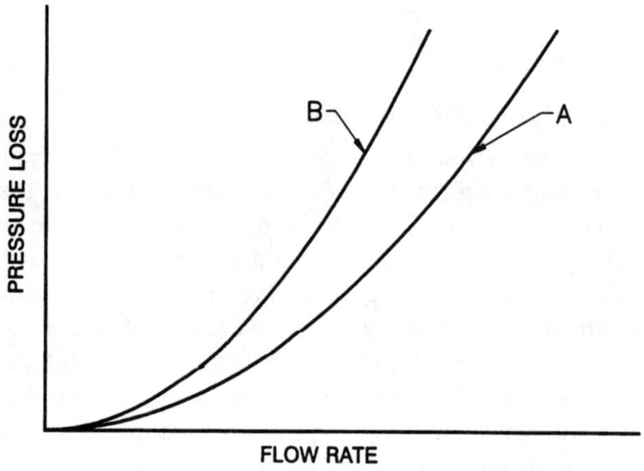

Fig. 13-4 Typical System Curves for Closed System

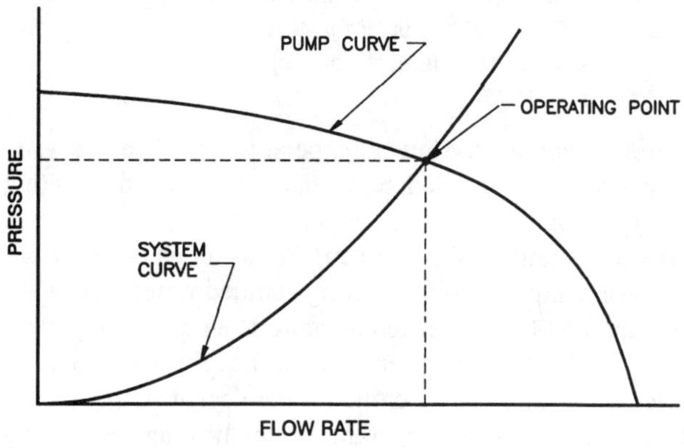

Fig. 13-5 Pump Curve and System Curve

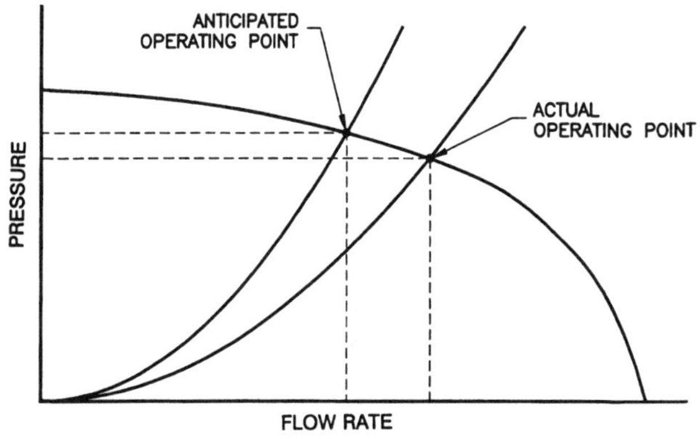

Fig. 13-6 Shift of System Curve due to Circuit Unbalance

pressure drop, which may be quite high, is thus eliminated from the system pressure drop, and the pump operating point shift to the right may be quite large. For such systems, system curve analysis should be used to check winter operating points.

Operating points may be highly variable, depending on (1) load conditions, (2) the types of control valves used, and (3) the piping circuitry and heat transfer elements. In general, the best selection will be

- For design flow rates calculated using pressure drop charts that illustrate actual closed-loop hydronic system piping pressure drops
- To the left of the maximum efficiency point of the pump curve to allow shifts to the right caused by system circuit unbalance, direct-return circuitry applications, and modulating three-way valve applications
- A pump with a flat curve to compensate for unbalanced circuitry and to provide a minimum pressure differential increase across two-way control valves

Parallel Pumping. When pumps are applied in parallel, each pump operates at the same head, and provides its share of the system flow at that pressure (Figure 13-7). Generally, pumps of equal size are used, and the parallel pump curve is established by doubling the flow of the single pump curve (with identical pumps).

Plotting a system curve across the parallel pump curve shows the operating points for both single and parallel pump operation (Figure 13-7). Note that single pump operation does not yield 50% flow. The system curve crosses the single pump curve considerably to the right of its operating point when both pumps are running. This leads to two important concerns: (1) the pumps must be powered to prevent overloading during single-pump operation, and (2) a single pump can provide standby service of up to 80% of design flow; the actual amount depends on the specific pump curve and system curve.

Series Pumping. When pumps are operated in series, each pump operates at the same flow rate and provides its share of the total pressure at that flow. A system curve plotted across the series pump curve shows the operating points for both single and series pump operation (Figure 13-8). Note that the single pump can provide up to 80% flow for standby and at a lower power requirement.

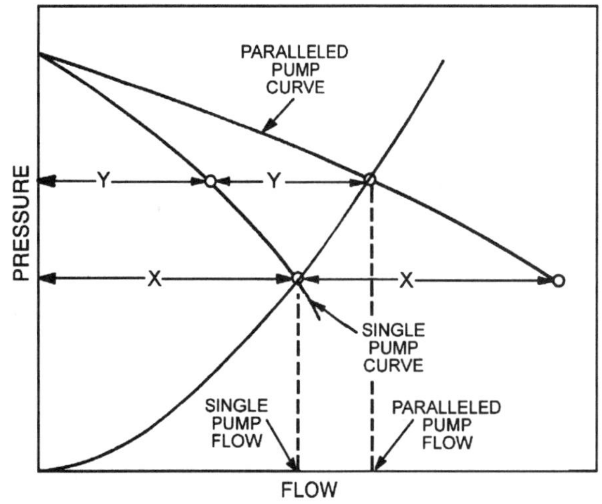

Fig. 13-7 Operating Conditions for Parallel Pump Installation

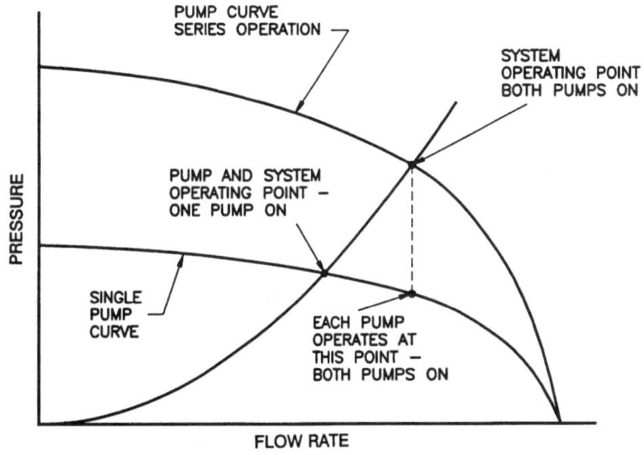

Fig. 13-8 Operating Conditions for Series Pump Installation

Series pump installations are often used in heating and cooling systems so that both pumps operate during the cooling season to provide maximum flow and head, while only a single pump operates during the heating season. Note that both parallel and series pump applications require that the actual pump operating points be used to accurately determine the pumping point. Adding artificial safety factor head, using improper pressure drop charts, or incorrectly calculating pressure drops may lead to an unwise selection.

Multiple-Pump Systems. Care must be taken in designing systems with multiple pumps to ensure that if pumps ever operate in either parallel or series, such operation is fully understood and considered by the designer. Pumps performing unexpectedly in series or parallel have been the cause of performance problems in hydronic systems. Typical problems resulting from pumps functioning in parallel and series when not anticipated by the designer are the following.

Parallel. With pumps of unequal pressures, one pump may create a pressure across the other pump in excess of its cutoff pressure, causing flow through the second pump to diminish significantly or to cease. This phenomenon can cause flow problems or pump damage.

Series. With pumps of different flow capacities, the pump of greater capacity may overflow the pump of lesser capacity, which could cause damaging cavitation in the smaller pump and could actually cause a pressure drop rather than a pressure rise across that pump. In other circumstances, unexpected series operation can cause excessively high or low pressures that can damage system components.

Standby Pump Provision. If total flow standby capacity is required, a properly valved standby pump of equal capacity is installed to operate when the normal pump is inoperable. A single standby may be provided for several similarly sized pumps. Parallel or series pump installation can provide up to 80% standby, which is often sufficient.

Compound Pumping. In larger systems, compound pumping, also known as primary-secondary pumping, is often employed to provide system advantages that would not be available with a single pumping system. The concept of compound pumping is illustrated in Figure 13-9.

In Figure 13-9, Pump No. 1 can be referred to as the source or primary pump and Pump No. 2 as the load or secondary pump. The short section of pipe between A and B is called the common pipe because it is common to both the source and load circuits. Other terms used for the common pipe are the decoupling line and the neutral bridge. In the design of compound systems, the common pipe should be kept as short and as large in diameter as practical to minimize the pressure loss between those two points. Care must be taken, however, to ensure adequate length in the common pipe to prevent recirculation from entry or exit turbulence. There should never be a valve or check valve in the common pipe. If these conditions are met and the pressure loss in the common pipe can be assumed to be zero, then neither pump will affect the other. Then, except for the system static pressure at any given point, the circuits can be designed and analyzed and will function dynamically independently of one another.

In Figure 13-9, if Pump No. 1 has the same flow capacity in its circuit as Pump No. 2 has in its circuit, all of the flow

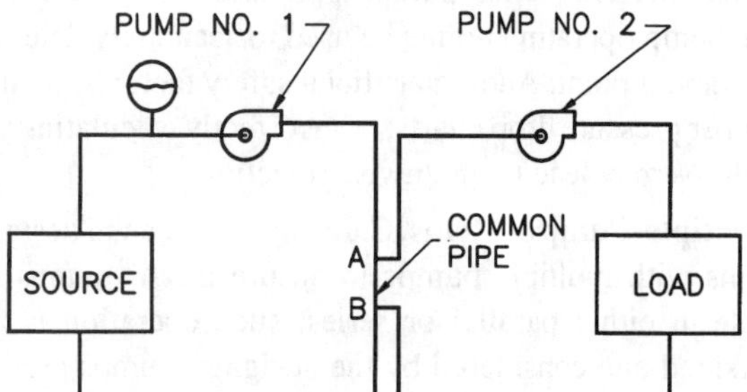

Fig. 13-9 Compound Pumping (Primary-Secondary Pumping)

entering Point A from Pump No. 1 will leave in the branch supplying Pump No. 2, and no water will flow in the common pipe. Under this condition, the water entering the load will be at the same temperature as that leaving the source.

If the flow capacity of Pump No. 1 exceeds that of Pump No. 2, some water will flow downward in the common pipe. Under this condition, Tee A is a diverting tee, and Tee B becomes a mixing tee. Again, the temperature of the fluid entering the load is the same as that leaving the source. However, because of the mixing taking place at Point B, the temperature of the water returning to the source is between the source supply temperature and the load return temperature.

On the other hand, if the flow capacity of Pump No. 1 is less than that of Pump No. 2, then Point A becomes a mixing point because some water must recirculate upward in the common pipe from Point B. Under this condition, the temperature of the water entering the load is between the supply water temperature from the source and the return water temperature from the load.

For example, if Pump No. 1 circulates 25 gpm of water leaving the source at 200°F, and Pump No. 2 circulates 50 gpm of water leaving the load at 100°F, then the water temperature entering the load is

$$t_{load} = 200 - (25/50)(200 - 100) = 150°F$$

The following are some advantages of compound circuits:

1. They enable the designer to achieve different water temperatures and temperature ranges in different elements of the system.
2. They decouple the circuits hydraulically, thereby making the control, operation, and analysis of large systems much less complex. Hydraulic decoupling also prevents unwanted series or parallel operation.
3. Circuits can be designed for different flow characteristics. For example, a chilled water load system can be designed with two way valves for better control and energy conservation while the source system operates at constant flow to protect the chiller from freezing.

Expansion Chamber. As a hydraulic device, the expansion tank serves as the reference pressure point in the system, analogous to a ground in an electrical system (Lockhart and Carlson 1953). Where the tank connects to the piping, the pressure equals the pressure of the air in the tank plus or minus any fluid pressure due to the elevation difference between the tank liquid surface and the pipe (Figure 13-10).

As previously stated, a closed system should have only one expansion chamber. The presence of more than one chamber or of excessive amounts of undissolved air in a piping system can cause the closed system to behave in unexpected (but understandable) ways, causing extensive damage from shock waves or water hammer.

With a single chamber on a system, assuming isothermal conditions for the air, the air pressure can change only as a result of displacement by the water. The only thing that can cause the water to move into or out of the tank (assuming no

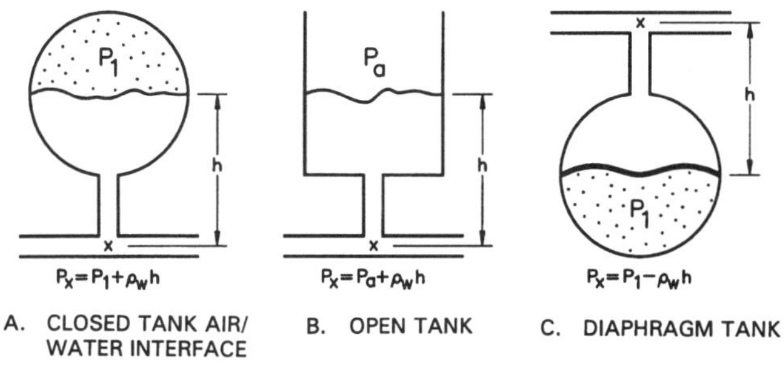

Fig. 13-10 Tank Pressure Related to "System" Pressure

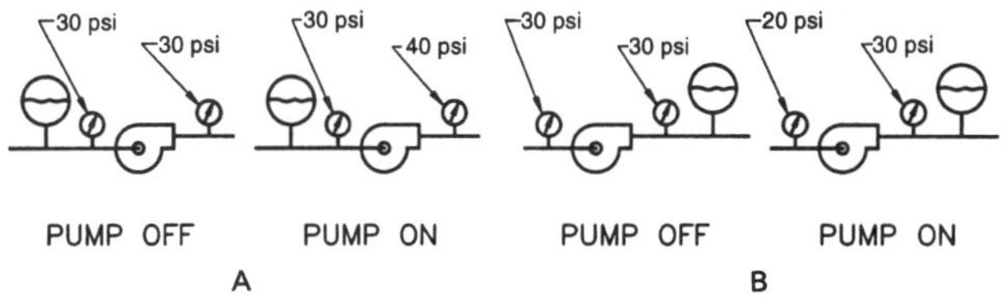

Fig. 13-11 Effect of Expansion Tank Location with Respect to Pump Pressure

water is being added to or removed from the system) is expansion or shrinkage of the water in the system. Thus, in sizing the tank, thermal expansion is related to the pressure extremes of the air in the tank [Equations (13-12), (13-13), and (13-14)].

The point of connection of the tank should be based on the pressure requirements of the system, remembering that the pressure at the tank connection will not change as the pump is turned on or off. For example, consider a system containing an expansion tank at 30 psig and a pump with a pump head of 23.1 ft (10 psig). Figure 13-11 shows alternative locations for connecting the expansion tank; in either case, with the pump off, the pressure will be 30 psig on both the pump suction and discharge. With the tank on the pump suction side, when the pump is turned on, the pressure increases on the discharge side by an amount equal to the pump pressure (Figure 13-11A). With the tank connected on the discharge side of the pump, the pressure decreases on the suction side by the same amount (Figure 13-11B).

Other considerations relating to the tank connection include the following:

- A tank open to the atmosphere must be located above the highest point in the system.
- A tank with an air/water interface is generally used with an air control system that continually revents the air into the tank. For this reason, it should be connected at a point where air can best be released.
- Within reason, the lower the pressure in a tank, the smaller is the tank [see Equations (13-12) and (13-14)]. Thus, in a vertical system, the higher the tank is placed, the smaller it can be.

13.3 Design Considerations

13.3.1 Piping Circuits

Hydronic systems are designed with many different configurations of piping circuits. In addition to simple preference by the design engineer, the method of arranging the circuiting can be dictated by such factors as the shape or configuration of the building, the economics of installation, energy economics, the nature of the load, part-load capabilities or requirements, and others.

Each piping system is a network; the more extensive the net work, the more complex it is to understand, analyze, or control. Thus, a major design objective is to maintain the highest degree of simplicity.

Load distribution circuits are of four general types:

- Full series
- Diverting series
- Parallel direct return
- Parallel reverse return

Series Circuit. A simple series circuit is shown in Figure 13-12. Series loads generally have the advantage of both lower piping costs and higher temperature drops that result in smaller pipe sizes and lower energy consumption. A disadvantage is that the different circuits cannot be controlled separately. Simple series circuits are generally limited to residential and small commercial standing radiation systems. Figure 13-13 shows a typical layout of such a system with two zones for residential or small commercial heating.

Diverting Series. The simplest diverting series circuit diverts some of the flow from the main piping circuit through a special diverting tee to a load device (usually standing radiation) that has a low pressure drop. This system is generally limited to heating systems in residential or small commercial applications.

Figure 13-14 illustrates a typical one-pipe diverting tee circuit. For each terminal unit, a supply and a return tee are installed on the main. One of the two tees is a special diverting tee that creates a pressure drop in the main flow to divert part of the flow to the unit. One (return) diverting tee is usually sufficient for upfeed (units above the main) systems. Two special fittings (supply and return tees) are usually required to overcome thermal pressure in down feed units. Special tees

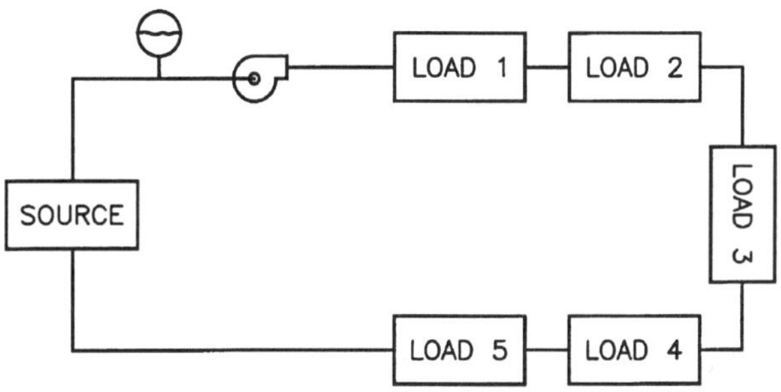

Fig. 13-12 Flow Diagram of Simple Series Circuit

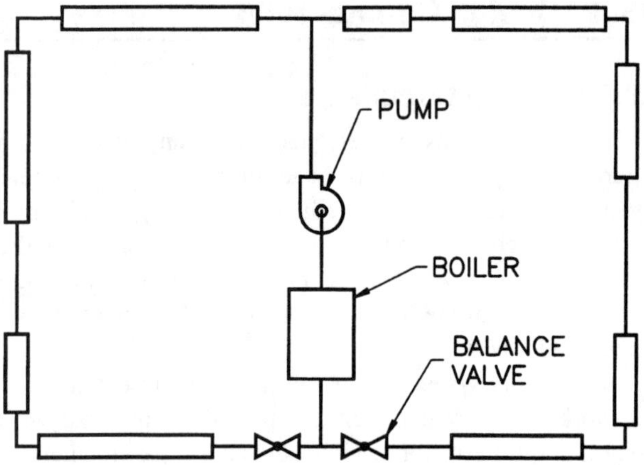

Fig. 13-13 Series Loop System

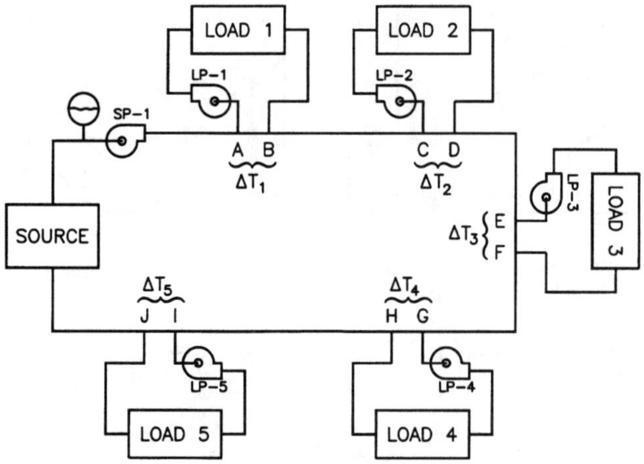

Fig. 13-15 Series Circuit with Load Pumps

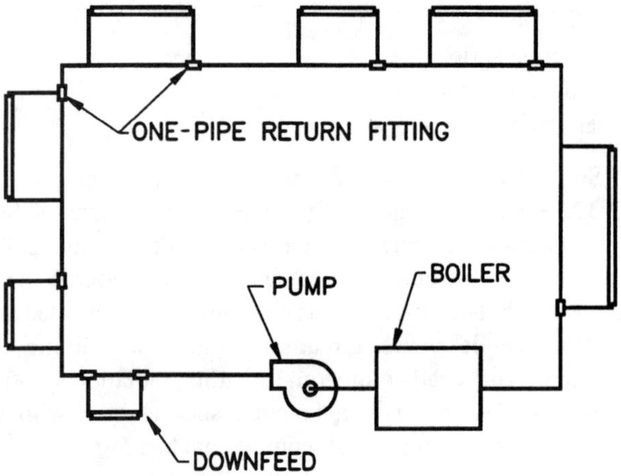

Fig. 13-14 One-Pipe Diverting Tee System

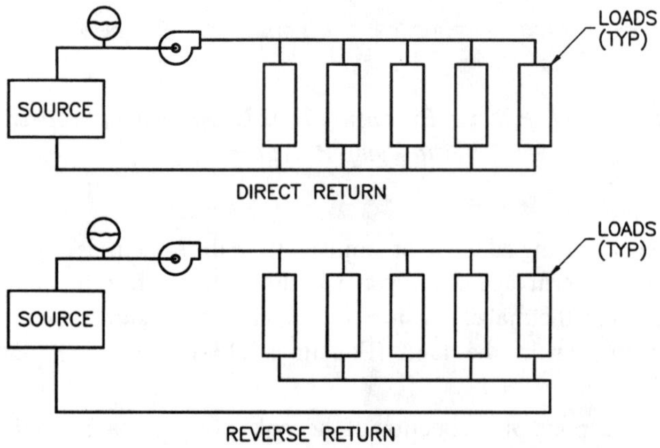

Fig. 13-16 Direct- and Reverse-Return Two-Pipe Systems

are proprietary; consult manufacturer's literature for flow rates and pressure drop data on these devices. Unit selection can be only approximate without these data.

One-pipe diverting series circuits allow manual or automatic control of flow to individual heating units. On-off rather than flow modulation control is preferred because of the relatively low pressure drop allowable through the control valve in the diverted flow circuit. This system is likely to cost more than the series loop because extra branch pipe and fittings, including special tees, are required. Each unit usually requires a manual air vent because of the low water velocity through the unit. The length and load imposed on a one-pipe circuit are usually small because of these limitations.

Because only a fraction of the main flow is diverted in a one-pipe circuit, the flow rate and pressure drop are less variable. When two or more one-pipe circuits are connected to the same two-pipe mains the circuit flow may need to be mechanically balanced. After balancing, sufficient flow must be maintained in each one-pipe circuit to ensure adequate flow diversion to the loads.

When coupled with compound pumping systems, series circuits can be applied to multiple control zones on larger commercial or institutional systems (Figure 13-15). Note that in the series circuit with compound pumping, the load pumps need not be equal in capacity to the system pump. If, for example, load pump LP-1 circulates less flow (Q_{LP1}) than system pump SP-1 (Q_{SP1}), the temperature difference across Load 1 would be greater than the circuit temperature difference between A and B (i.e., water would flow in the common pipe from A to B). If, on the other hand, the load pump LP-2 is equal in flow capacity to the system pump SP-1, the temperature differentials across Load 2 and across the system from C to D would be equal and no water would flow in the common pipe. If Q_{LP3} exceeds Q_{SP1}, mixing occurs at Point E and, in a heating system, the temperature entering pump LP-3 would be lower than that available from the system leaving load connection D.

Thus, a series circuit using compound or load pumps offers many design options. Each of the loads shown in Figure 13-15 could also be a complete piping circuit or network.

Parallel Piping. These networks are the most commonly used in hydronic systems because they allow the same temperature water to be available to all loads. The two types of parallel networks are direct return and reverse return (Figure 13-16).

In the direct-return system, the length of supply and return piping through the subcircuits is unequal, which may cause unbalanced flow rates and require careful balancing to provide each subcircuit with design flow. Ideally, the reverse-return system provides nearly equal total lengths for all terminal circuits.

Direct-return piping has been successfully applied where the designer has guarded against major flow unbalance by

1. Providing for pressure drops in the subcircuits or terminals that are significant percentages of the total, usually establishing pressure drops for close subcircuits at higher values than those for the far subcircuits
2. Minimizing distribution piping pressure drop (In the limit, if the distribution piping loss is zero and the loads are of equal flow resistance, the system is inherently balanced.)
3. Including balancing devices and some means of measuring flow at each terminal or branch circuit
4. Using control valves with a high head loss at the terminals

13.3.2 Capacity Control of Load System

The two alternatives for controlling the capacity of hydronic systems are on-off control and variable-capacity or modulating control. The on-off option is generally limited to smaller systems (e.g., residential or small commercial) and individual components of larger systems. In smaller systems where the entire building is a single zone, control is accomplished by cycling the source device (the boiler or chiller) on and off. Usually a space thermostat allows the chiller or boiler to run, then a water temperature thermostat (aquastat) controls the capacity of the chiller(s) or boiler(s) as a function of supply or return water temperature. The pump can be either cycled with the load device (usually the case in a residential heating system) or left running (usually done in commercial hot or chilled water systems).

In these single-zone applications, the piping design requires no special consideration for control. Where multiple zones of control are required, the various load devices are controlled first; then the source system capacity is controlled to follow the capacity requirement of the loads.

Control valves are commonly used to control loads. These valves control the capacity of each load by varying the amount of water flow through the load device when load pumps are not used. Control valves for hydronic systems are straight-through (two-way) valves and three-way valves (Figure 13-17). The effect of either valve is to vary the amount of water flowing through the load device.

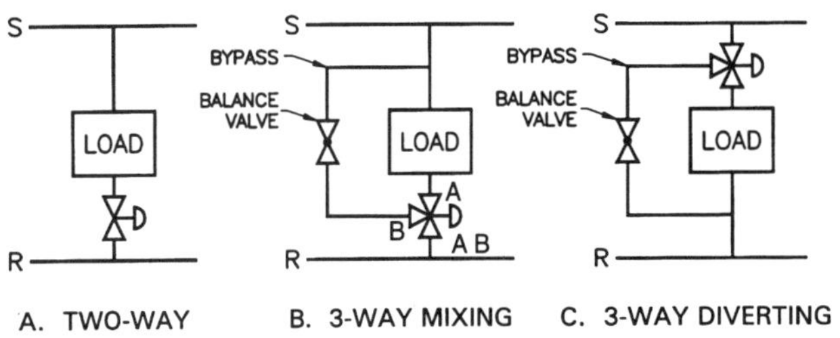

Fig. 13-17 Load Control Valves

With a two-way valve (Figure 13-17A), as the valve strokes from full-open to full-closed, the quantity of water flowing through the load gradually decreases from design flow to no flow. With a three way mixing valve (Figure 13-17B) in one position, the valve is open from Port A to AB, with Port B closed off. In that position, all the flow is through the load. As the valve moves from the A-AB position to the B-AB position, some of the water bypasses the load by flowing through the bypass line, thus decreasing flow through the load. At the end of the stroke, Port A is closed, and all of the fluid will flow from B to AB with no flow through the load. Thus, the three-way mixing valve has the same effect on the load as the two way valve-as the load reduces, the quantity of water flowing through the load decreases.

The effect on load control with the three-way diverting valve (Figure 13-17C) is the same as with the mixing valve in a closed system-the flow is either directed through the load or through the bypass in proportion to the load. Because of the dynamics of valve operation, diverting valves are more complex in design and are thus more expensive than mixing valves; because they accomplish the same function as the simpler mixing valve, they are seldom used in closed hydronic systems.

In terms of load control, a two-way valve and a three-way valve perform identical functions-they both vary the flow through the load as the load changes. The fundamental difference between the two-way valve and the three-way valve is that as the source or distribution system sees the load, the two-way valve provides a variable flow load response and the three-way valve provides a constant flow load response.

According to Equation (13-9), the load q is proportional to the product of Q and Δt. Ideally, as the load changes, Q changes, while Δt remains fixed. However, as the system sees it, as the load changes with the two-way valve, Q varies and Δt is fixed, whereas with a three-way valve, Δt varies and Q is fixed. This principle is illustrated in Figure 13-18. An understanding of this concept is fundamental to the design or analysis of hydronic systems.

The flow characteristics of two-way and three-way valve ports are described in Chapter 42, Automatic Control, of the 1995 *ASHRAE Handbook—Applications* and must be understood. The equal percentage characteristic is recommended for proportional control of the load flow for two-way and

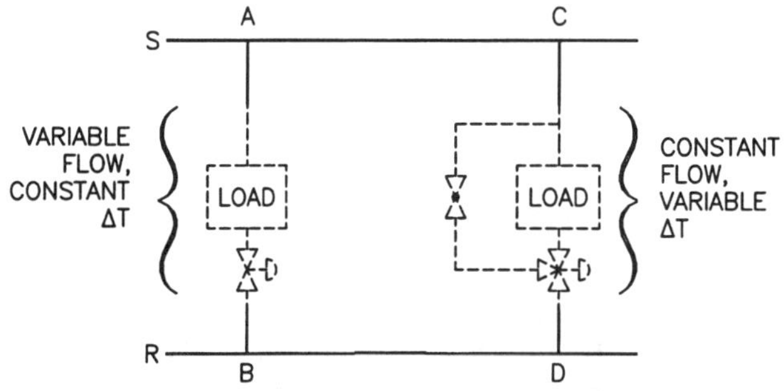

Fig. 13-18 System Flow with Two-Way and Three-Way Valves

three-way valves; the bypass flow port of three-way valves should have the linear characteristic to maintain a uniform flow during part-load operation.

13.3.3 Sizing Control Valves

For stable control, the pressure drop in the control valve at the full-open position should be no less than one-half the pressure drop in the branch. For example, in Figure 13-18 the pressure drop at full open position for the two-way valve should equal one-half the pressure drop from A to B, and for the three-way valve, the full-open pressure drop should be half that from C to D. The pressure drop in the bypass balancing valve in the three-way valve circuit should be set to equal that in the coil (load).

Control valves should be sized on the basis of the valve coefficient C_V. For more information, see the section on Control Valve Sizing in Chapter 41 in 1996 *ASHRAE Handbook—Systems and Equipment*.

If a system is to be designed with multiple zones of control such that load response is to be by constant flow through the load and variable Δt, control cannot be achieved by valve control alone; a load pump is required.

Several control arrangements of load pump and control valve configurations are shown in Figure 13-19. Note that in all three configurations the common pipe has no restriction or check valve. In all configurations there is no difference in control as seen by the load. However, the basic differences in control are

1. With the two-way valve configuration (Figure 13- 19A), the distribution system sees a variable flow and a constant Δt, whereas with both three-way configurations, the distribution system sees a constant flow and a variable Δt.
2. Configuration B differs from C in that the pressure required through the three-way valve in Figure 13-19B is provided by the load pump, while in Figure 13-19C it is provided by the distribution pump(s).

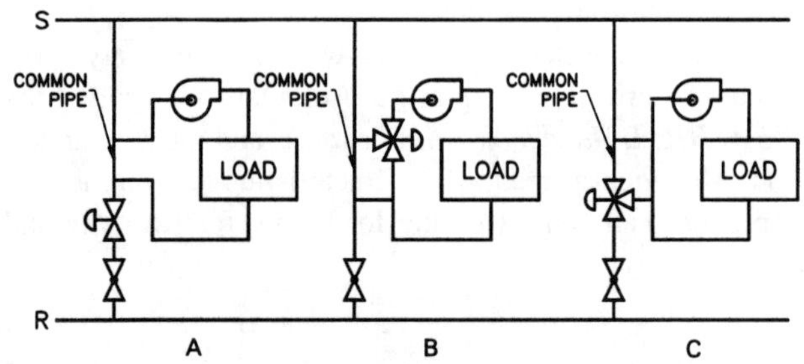

Fig. 13-19 Load Pumps with Valve Control

13.3.4 Low-Temperature Heating Systems

These systems are used for heating spaces or processes directly, as with standing radiation and process heat exchangers, or indirectly, through air-handling unit coils for preheating, for reheating, or in hot water unit heaters. These systems are generally designed with supply water temperatures from 180 to 240°F and temperature drops from 20 to 100°F.

In the United States, hot water heating systems were historically designed for a 200°F supply water temperature and a 20°F temperature drop. This practice evolved from earlier gravity system designs and provides convenient design relationships for heat transfer coefficients related to coil tubing and finned-tube radiation and for calculations (one gallon per minute conveys 10,000 Btu/h at 20°F Δt). Because many terminal devices still require these flow rates, it is important to recognize this relationship in selecting devices and designing systems.

However, the greater the temperature range (and related lower flow rate) that can be applied, the less costly the system is to install and operate. A lower flow rate requires smaller and less expensive piping, less secondary building space, and smaller pumps. Also, smaller pumps require less energy, so operating costs are lower.

Nonresidential Heating Systems. Possible approaches to enhancing the economics of large heating systems include (1) higher supply temperatures, (2) primary-secondary pumping, and (3) terminal equipment designed for smaller flow rates. The three techniques may be used either singly or in combination.

Using higher supply water temperatures achieves higher temperature drops and smaller flow rates. Terminal units with a reduced heating surface can be used. These smaller terminals are not necessarily less expensive, however, because their required operating temperatures and pressures may increase manufacturing costs and the problems of pressurization, corrosion, expansion, and control. System components may not increase in cost uniformly with temperature, but rather in steps conforming to the three major temperature classifications. Within each classification, the most economical design uses the highest temperature in that classification.

Primary-secondary or compound pumping reduces the size and cost of the distribution system and also may use larger flows and lower temperatures in the terminal or secondary circuits. A primary pump circulates water in the primary distribution system while one or more secondary pumps circulate the terminal circuits. The connection between primary and secondary circuits provides complete hydraulic isolation of both circuits and permits a controlled interchange of water between the two. Thus, a high supply water temperature can be used in the primary circuit at a low flow rate and high temperature drop, while a lower temperature and conventional temperature drop can be used in the secondary circuit(s).

For example, a system could be designed with primary-secondary pumping in which the supply temperature from the boiler was 240°F, the supply temperature in the secondary was 200°F, and the return temperature was 180°F. This design results in a conventional 20°F Δt in the secondary zones, but permits the primary circuit to be sized on the basis of a 60°F drop. This primary-secondary pumping arrangement is most advantageous with terminal units such as convectors and finned radiation, which are generally unsuited for small flow rate design.

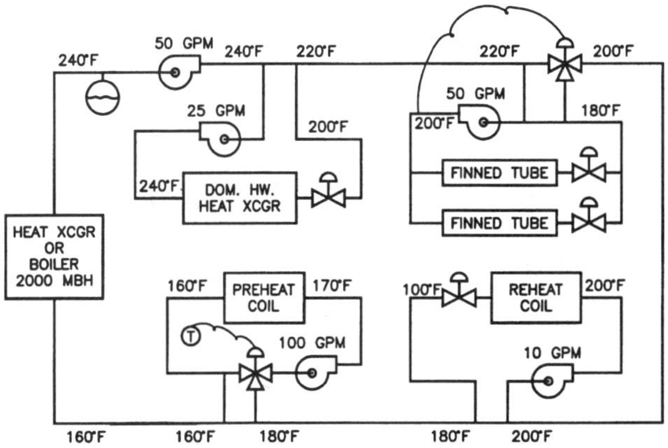

Fig. 13-20 Example of Series-Connected Loads

Many types of terminal heat transfer units are being designed to use smaller flow rates with temperature drops up to 100°F in low-temperature systems and up to 150°F in medium-temperature systems. Fan apparatus, the heat transfer surface used for air heating in fan systems, and water-to-water heat exchangers are most adaptable to such design.

A fourth technique is to put certain loads in series utilizing a combination of control valves and compound pumping (Figure 13-20). In the system illustrated, the capacity of the boiler or heat exchanger is 2×10^6 Btu/h, and each of the four loads is 0.5×10^6 Btu/h. Under design conditions, the system is designated for an 80°F water temperature drop, and the loads each provide 20°F of the total Δt. The loads in these systems, as well as the smaller or simpler systems in residential or commercial applications, can be connected in a direct-return or a reverse-return piping system. The different features of each load are as follows:

1. The domestic hot water heat exchanger has a two-way valve and is thus arranged for variable flow (while the main distribution circuit provides constant flow for the boiler circuit).
2. The finned-tube radiation circuit is a 20°F Δt circuit with the design entering water temperature reduced to and controlled at 200°F.
3. The reheat coil circuit takes a 100°F temperature drop for a very low flow rate.
4. The preheat coil circuit provides constant flow through the coil to keep it from freezing.

When loads such as water-to-air heating coils in LTW systems are valve controlled (flow varies), they have a heating characteristic of flow versus capacity as shown in Figure 13-21 for 20°F and 60°F temperature drops. For a 20°F Δt coil, 50% flow provides approximately 90% capacity; valve control will tend to be unstable. For this reason, proportional temperature control is required, and equal percentage characteristic two-way valves should be selected such that 10% flow is achieved with 50% valve lift. This combination of the valve characteristic and the heat transfer characteristic of the coil makes the control linear with respect to the control signal.

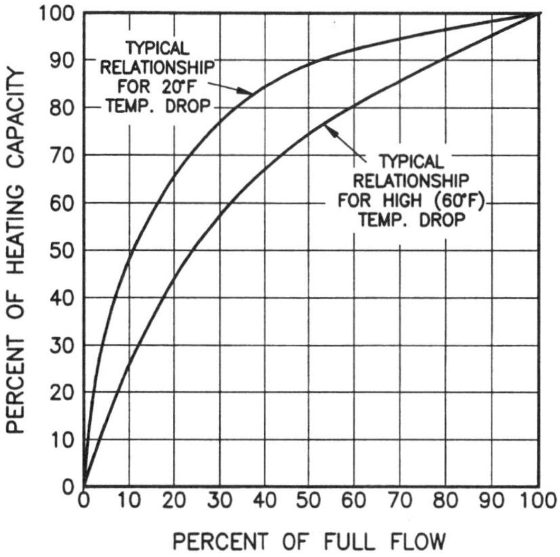

Fig. 13-21 Heat Emission Versus Flow Characteristic of Typical Hot Water Heating Coil

This type of control can be obtained only with equal percentage two-way valves and can be further enhanced if piped with a secondary pump arrangement as shown in Figure 13-19A. See Chapter 42 of the 1995 *ASHRAE Handbook—Applications* for further information on automatic controls.

13.3.5 Chilled Water Systems

Designers have less latitude in selecting supply water temperatures for cooling applications because there is only a narrow range of water temperatures low enough to provide adequate dehumidification and high enough to avoid chiller freeze-up. circulated water quantities can be reduced by selecting proper air quantities and heat transfer surface at the terminals. Terminals suited for a 12°F rise rather than an 8°F rise reduce circulated water quantity and pump power by one-third and increase chiller efficiency.

A proposed system should be evaluated for the desired balance between installation cost and operating cost. Table 13-1 shows the effect of coil circuiting and chilled water temperature on water flow and temperature rise. The coil rows, fin spacing, air-side performance, and cost are identical for all selections. Morabito (1960) showed how such changes in coil circuiting affect the overall system. Considering the investment cost of piping and insulation versus the operating cost of refrigeration and pumping motors, higher temperature rises, (i.e., 16 to 24°F temperature rise at about 1.0 to 1.5 gpm per ton of cooling) can be applied on chilled water systems with long distribution piping runs; larger flow rates should be used only where reasonable in close-coupled systems.

For the most economical design, the minimum flow rate to each terminal heat exchanger is calculated. For example, if one terminal can be designed for an 18°F rise, another for 14°F, and others for 12°F, the highest rise to each terminal should be used, rather than designing the system for an overall temperature rise based on the smallest capability.

Table 13-1 Chilled Water Coil Performance

Coil Circuiting	Chilled Water Inlet Temp., °F	Coil Pressure Drop, psi	Chilled Water Flow gpm/ton	Chilled Water Temp. Rise, °F
Full[a]	45	1.0	2.2	10.9
Half[b]	45	5.5	1.7	14.9
Full[a]	40	0.5	1.4	17.1
Half[b]	40	2.5	1.1	21.8

Note: Table is based on cooling air from 81°F dry bulb, 67°F wet bulb to 58°F dry bulb, 56°F wet bulb.

[a]Full circuiting (also called single circuit). Water at the inlet temperature flows simultaneously through all tubes in a plane transverse to airflow; it then flows simultaneously through all tubes, in unison, in successive planes (i.e., rows) of the coil.

[b]Half circuiting. Tube connections are arranged so there are half as many circuits as there are tubes in each plane (row) thereby using higher water velocities through the tubes. This circuiting is used with small water quantities.

The control system selected also influences the design water flow. For systems using multiple terminal units, diversity factors can be applied to flow quantities before sizing pump and piping mains if exposure or use prevents the unit design loads from occurring simultaneously and if two-way valves are used for water flow control. If air-side control (e.g., face-and-bypass or fan cycling) or three-way valves on the water side are used, diversity should not be a consideration in pump and piping design, although it should be considered in the chiller selection.

A primary consideration with chilled water system design is the control of the source systems at reduced loads. the constraints on the temperature parameters are (1) a water freezing temperature of 32°F, (2) economics of the refrigeration system in generating chilled water, and (3) the dew-point temperature of the air at nominal indoor comfort conditions (55°F dew point at 75°F and 50% rh). These parameters have led to the common practice of designing for a supply chilled water temperature of 44 to 45°F and a return water temperature between 55 and 64°F.

Historically, most chilled water systems have used three-way control valves to achieve constant water flow through the chillers. However, as systems have become larger, as designers have turned to multiple chillers for reliability and controllability, and as energy economics have become an increasing concern, the use of two-way valves and source pumps for the chillers has greatly increased.

A typical configuration of a small chilled water system using two parallel chillers and loads with three-way valves is illustrated in Figure 13-22. Note that the flow is essentially constant. A simple energy balance [Equation (13-9)] dictates that with a constant flow rate, at one-half of design load, the water temperature differential drops to one-half of design. At this load, if one of the chillers is turned off, the return water circulating through the off chiller mixes with the supply water. This mixing raises the temperature of the supply chilled water and can cause a loss of control if the designer does not consider this operating mode.

A typical configuration of a large chilled water system with multiple chillers and loads and compound piping is shown in Figure 13-23. This system provides variable flow, essentially constant supply temperature chilled water, multiple chillers, more stable two-way control valves, and the advantage of adding chilled water storage with little additional complexity.

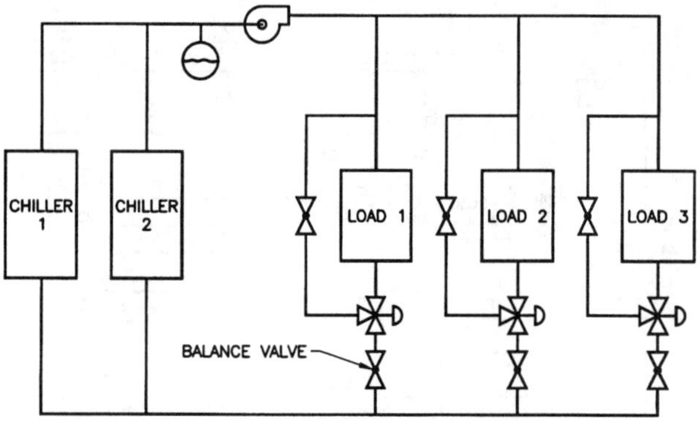

Fig. 13-22 Constant Flow Chilled Water System

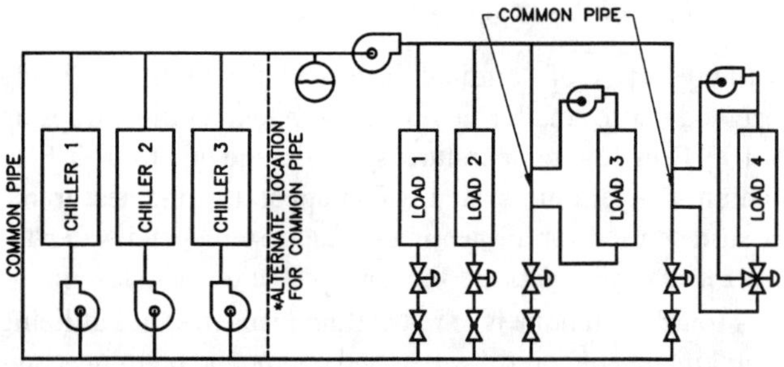

Fig. 13-23 Variable Flow Chilled Water System

One design issue illustrated in Figure 13-23 is the placement of the common pipe for the chillers. With the common pipe as shown, the chillers will unload from left to right. With the common pipe in the alternate location shown, the chillers will unload equally in proportion to their capacity (i.e., equal percentage).

13.3.6 Dual-Temperature Systems

Dual-temperature systems are used when the same load devices and distribution systems are used for both heating and cooling (e.g., fan-coil units and central station air-handling unit coils). In the design of dual-temperature systems, the cooling cycle design usually dictates the requirements of the load heat exchangers and distribution systems. Dual-temperature systems are basically of three different configurations, each requiring different design techniques:

1. Two-pipe systems
2. Four-pipe common load systems
3. Four-pipe independent load systems

Two-Pipe Systems. In a two-pipe system, the load devices and the distribution system circulate chilled water when cooling is required and hot water when heating is required (Figure 13-24). Design considerations for these systems include the following:

- Loads must all require cooling or heating coincidentally; that is, if cooling is required for some loads and heating for

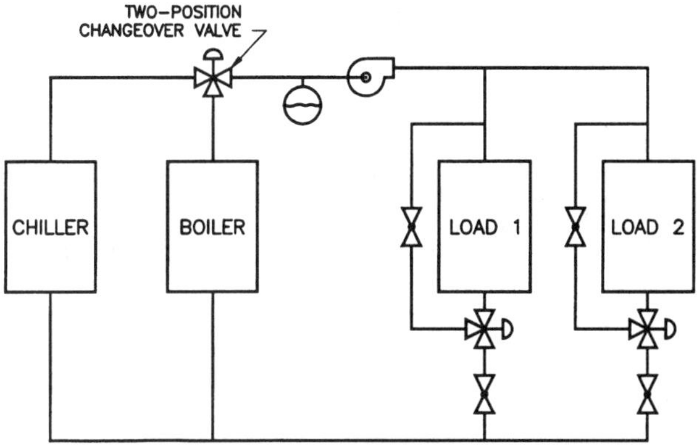

Fig. 13-24 Simplified Diagram of Two-Pipe System

other loads at a given time, this type of system should not be used.

- When designing the system, the flow and temperature requirements for both the cooling and the heating media must be calculated first. The load and distribution system should be designed for the more stringent, and the water temperatures and temperature differential should be dictated by the other mode.
- The changeover procedure should be designed such that the chiller evaporator is not exposed to damaging high water temperatures and the boiler is not subjected to damaging low water temperatures. To accommodate these limiting requirements, the changeover of a system from one mode to the other requires considerable time. If rapid load swings are anticipated, a two-pipe system should not be selected, although it is the least costly of the three options.

Four-Pipe Common Load Systems. In the four-pipe common load system, load devices are used for both heating and cooling as in the two-pipe system. The four-pipe common load system differs from the two-pipe system in that both heating and cooling are available to each load device, and the changeover from one mode to the other takes place at each individual load device, or grouping of load devices, rather than at the source. Thus, some of the load systems can be in the cooling mode while others are in the heating mode. Figure 13-25 is a flow diagram of a four-pipe common load system, with multiple loads and a single boiler and chiller.

Although many of these systems have been installed, many have not performed successfully due to problems in implementing the design concepts.

One problem that must be addressed is the expansion tank connection(s). Many four-pipe systems were designed with two expansion tanks-one for the cooling circuit and one for the heating circuit. However, with multiple loads, these circuits become hydraulically interconnected, thus creating a system with two expansion chambers. The preferred method of handling the expansion tank connection sets the point of reference pressure equal in both circuits (Figure 13-25).

Another potential problem is the mixing of hot and chilled water. At each load connection, two three-way valves are required-a mixing valve on the inlet and a diverting valve on

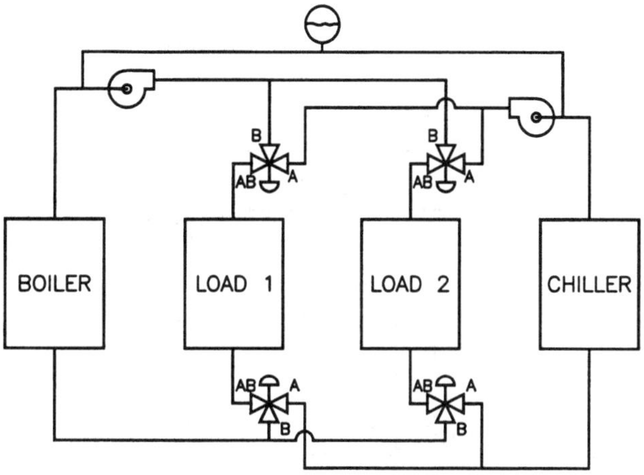

Fig. 13-25 Four-Pipe Common Load System

the outlet. These valves operate in unison in just two positions-opening either Port B to AB or Port A to AB. If, for example, the valve on the outlet does not seat tightly and Load 1 is indexed to cooling and Load 2 is indexed to heating, return heating water from Load 2 will flow into the chilled water circuit, and return chilled water from Load 1 will flow into the heating water circuit. The probability of this occurring increases as the number of loads increases because the number of control valves increases.

Another disadvantage of this system is that the loads have no individual capacity control as far as the water system is concerned. That is, each valve must be positioned to either full heating or full cooling with no control in between.

Because of these disadvantages, four-pipe common load systems should be limited to those applications in which there are no independent load circuits (i.e., radiant ceiling panels or induction unit coils).

Four-Pipe Independent Load Systems. The four-pipe independent load system is preferred for those hydronic applications in which some of the loads are in the heating mode while others are in the cooling mode. Control is simpler and more reliable than for the common load systems, and in many applications, the four-pipe independent load system is less costly to install. Also, the flow through the individual loads can be modulated, providing both the control capability for variable capacity and the opportunity for variable flow in either or both circuits.

A simplified example of a four-pipe independent load system with two loads, one boiler, and two chillers is shown in Figure 13-26. Note that both hydronic circuits are essentially independent, so that each can be designed with disregard for the other system. Although both circuits in the figure are shown as variable flow distribution systems, they could be constant flow (three-way valves) or one variable flow and one constant flow. Generally, the control modulates the two load valves in sequence with a dead band at the control midpoint.

This type of system offers additional flexibility when some selective loads are arranged for heating only or cooling only, such as unit heaters or preheat coils. Then, central station sys-

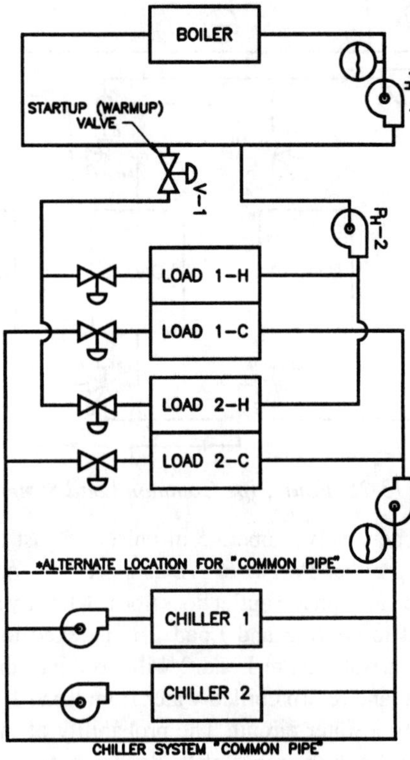

Fig. 13-26 Four-Pipe Independent Load System

tems can be designed for humidity control with reheat through configuration at the coil locations and with proper control sequences.

13.3.7 Other Design Considerations

Makeup and Fill Water Systems. Generally, a hydronic system is filled with water through a valved connection to a domestic water source, with a service valve, a back flow preventer, and a pressure gage. (The domestic water source pressure must exceed the system fill pressure.)

Because the expansion chamber is the reference pressure point in the system, the water makeup point is usually located at or near the expansion chamber.

Many designers prefer to install automatic makeup valves, which consist of a pressure-regulating valve in the makeup line. However, the quantity of water being made up must be monitored to avoid scaling and oxygen corrosion in the system.

Safety Relief Valves. Safety relief valves should be installed at any point at which pressures can be expected to exceed the safe limits of the system components. Causes of excessive pressures include

- Overpressurization from fill system
- Pressure increases due to thermal expansion
- Surges caused by momentum changes (shock or water hammer)

Overpressurization from the fill system could occur due to an accident in filling the system or due to the failure of an automatic fill regulator. To prevent this, a safety relief valve

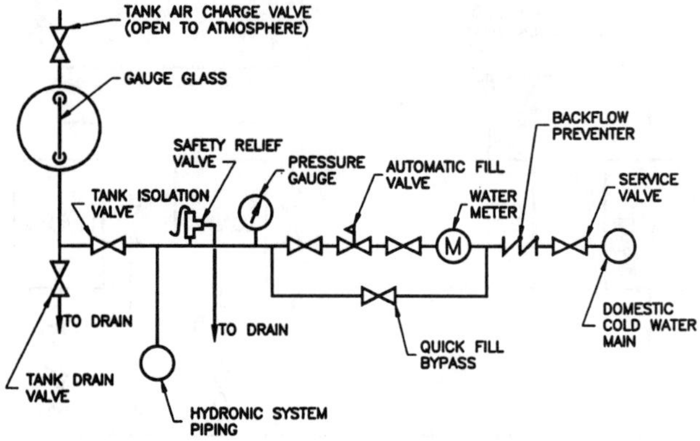

Fig. 13-27 Typical Makeup Water and Expansion Tank Piping Configuration for Plain Steel Expansion Tank

is usually installed at the fill location. Figure 13-27 shows a typical piping configuration for a system with a plain steel or air/water interface expansion tank. Note that no valves are installed between the hydronic system piping and the safety relief valve. This is a mandatory design requirement if the valve in this location is also to serve as a protection against pressure increases due to thermal expansion.

An expansion chamber is installed in a hydronic system, to allow for the volumetric changes that accompany water temperature changes. However, if any part of the system is configured such that it can be isolated from the expansion tank and its temperature can increase while it is isolated, then overpressure relief should be provided.

The relationship between pressure change due to temperature change and the temperature change in a piping system is expressed by the following equation:

$$\Delta p = \frac{(\beta - 3\alpha)\Delta t}{(5/4)(D/E\Delta r) + \gamma} \qquad (13\text{-}17)$$

where

Δp = pressure increase, psi

β = volumetric coefficient of thermal expansion of water, 1/°F (for standard water, approximately 1×10^{-4}/°F)

α = linear coefficient of thermal expansion for piping, 1/°F (for steel, approximately 6.5×10^{-6}/°F; for copper, approximately 9.0×10^{-6}/°F)

Δt = water temperature increase, °F

D = mean diameter of pipe, in.

E = modulus of elasticity of piping material, psi

γ = volumetric compressibility of water, in²/lb (for standard water, approximately 3.1×10^{-6}/°F)

Δr = thickness of pipe wall, in.

Figure 13-28 shows a solution to Equation (13-17) demonstrating the pressure increase caused by any given temperature increase for 1 in. and 10 in. steel piping. If the temperature in a chilled water system with piping spanning sizes between 1 and 10 in. were to increase by 15°F, the pressure would increase between 340 and 420 psi, depending on the average pipe size in the system.

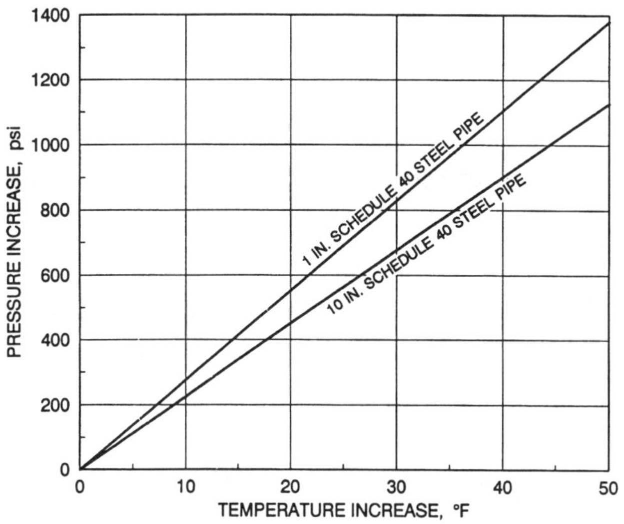

Fig. 13-28 Pressure Increase Resulting from Thermal Expansion as Function of Temperature Increase

Safety relief should be provided to protect boilers, heat exchangers, cooling coils, chillers, and the entire system when the expansion tank is isolated for air charging or other service. As a minimum, the ASME Boiler Code requires that a dedicated safety relief valve be installed on each boiler and that isolating or service valves be provided on the supply and return connections to each boiler.

Potential forces caused by shock waves or water hammer should also be considered in design. Chapter 33 of the 1997 *ASHRAE Handbook—Fundamentals* discusses the causes of shock forces and the methodology for calculating the magnitude of these forces.

Air Elimination. If air and other gases are not eliminated from the flow circuit, they may cause binding in the terminal heat transfer elements, corrosion, noise, reduced pumping capacity, and loss of hydraulic stability. A closed tank without a diaphragm can be installed at the point of the lowest solubility of air in water. When a diaphragm tank is used, air in the system can be removed by an air separator and air elimination valve installed at the point of lowest solubility. Manual vents should be installed at high points to remove all trapped air during initial operation and to ensure that the system is tight. Shutoff valves should be installed on any automatic air removal device to permit servicing without draining the system.

Drain and Shutoff. All low points should have drains. Separate shutoff and draining of individual equipment and circuits should be possible so that the entire system does not have to be drained to service a particular item. Whenever a device or section of the system is isolated, and the water in that section or device could increase in temperature following isolation, overpressure safety relief protection must be provided.

Balance Fittings. Balance fittings or valves and a means of measuring flow quantity should be applied as needed to permit balancing of individual terminals and subcircuits.

Pitch. Piping need not pitch but can run level, providing that flow velocities exceeding 1.5 fps are maintained or a diaphragm tank is used.

Strainers. Strainers should be used where necessary to protect system elements. Strainers in the pump suction must be checked carefully to avoid cavitation. Large separating chambers can serve as main air venting points and dirt strainers ahead of pumps. Automatic control valves or other devices operating with small clearances require protection from pipe scale, gravel, and welding slag, which may readily pass through the pump and its protective separator. Individual fine mesh strainers may therefore be required ahead of each control valve.

Thermometers. Thermometers or thermometer wells should be installed to assist the system operator in routine operation and troubleshooting. Permanent thermometers, with the correct scale range and separate sockets should be used at all points where temperature readings are regularly needed. Thermometer wells should be installed where readings will be needed only during start-up and infrequent trouble-shooting. If a central monitoring system is provided, a calibration well should be installed adjacent to each sensing point in insulated piping systems.

Flexible Connectors and Expansion Compensation. Flexible connectors are sometimes installed at pumps and machinery to reduce pipe stress. See Chapter 43 of the 1995 *ASHRAE Handbook—Applications* for vibration isolation information. Expansion, flexibility, and hanger and support information is in Chapter 40 of the 1996 *ASHRAE Handbook—Systems and Equipment Handbook.*

Gage Cocks. Gage cocks or quick-disconnect test ports should be installed at points requiring pressure readings. Gages permanently installed in the system will deteriorate because of vibration and pulsation and will, therefore, be unreliable. It is good practice to install gage cocks and provide the operator with several quality gages for diagnostic purposes.

Insulation. Insulation should be applied to minimize pipe thermal loss and to prevent condensation during chilled water operation (see Chapter 22 of the 1997 *Handbook—Fundamentals*). On chilled water systems, special rigid metal sleeves or shields should be installed at all hanger and support points, and all valves should be provided with extended bonnets to allow for the full insulation thickness without interference with the valve operators.

Condensate Drains. Condensate drains from dehumidifying coils should be trapped and piped to an open-sight plumbing drain. Traps should be deep enough to overcome the air pressure differential between drain inlet and room, which ordinarily will not exceed 2 in. of water. Pipe should be noncorrosive and insulated to prevent moisture condensation. Depending on the quantity and temperature of condensate, plumbing drain lines may require insulation to prevent sweating.

Common Pipe. In compound (primary-secondary) pumping systems, the common pipe is used to dynamically decouple the two pumping circuits. Ideally, there is no pressure drop in this section of piping; however, in actual systems, it is recommended that this section of piping be a minimum of 10 diameters in length to reduce the likelihood of unwanted mixing resulting from velocity (kinetic) energy or turbulence.

13.4 Design Procedures

13.4.1 Preliminary Equipment Layout

Flows in Mains and Laterals. Regardless of the method used to determine the flow through each item of terminal equipment, the desired result should be listed in terms of mass flow on the preliminary plans or in a schedule of flow rates for the piping system. (In the design of small systems and chilled water systems, the determination may be made in terms of volumetric flow).

In an equipment schedule or on the plans, starting from the most remote terminal and working toward the pump, progressively list the cumulative flow in each of the mains and branch circuits in the distribution system.

Preliminary Pipe Sizing. For each portion of the piping circuit, select a tentative pipe size from the unified flow chart in Chapter 33 of the 1997 *ASHRAE Handbook—Fundamentals*, using a value of pipe friction loss ranging from 0.75 to 4 ft per 100 ft (approximately 0.1 to 0.5 in/ft).

Residential piping size is often based on pump preselection using pipe sizing tables, which are available from the Hydronics Institute or from manufacturers.

Preliminary Pressure Drop. Using the preliminary pipe sizing indicated above, determine the pressure drop through each portion of the piping. The total pressure drop in the highest pressure drop circuit (usually the longest circuit) determines the maximum pressure drop through the piping (including terminals and control valves) that must be made available by the pump.

Preliminary Pump Selection. The preliminary selection should be based on the pump's ability to fulfill the determined capacity requirements. It should be selected at a point left of center on the pump curve and should not overload the motor. Because pressure drop in a flow system varies as the square of the flow rate, the flow variation between the nearest size of stock pump and an exact point selection will be relatively minor.

13.4.2 Final Pipe Sizing and Pressure Drop Determination

Final Piping Layout. Examine the overall piping layout to determine whether pipe sizes in some areas need to be readjusted. Several principal circuits should have approximately equal pressure drops so that excessive pressures are not needed to serve a small portion of the building.

Consider both the initial costs of the pump and piping system and the pump's operating cost when determining final system friction loss. Generally, lower heads and larger piping are more economical when longer amortization periods are considered, especially in larger systems. However, in small systems such as in residences, it may be most economical to select the pump first and design the piping system to meet the available pressure. In all cases, adjust the piping system design and pump selection until the optimum design is found.

Final Pressure Drop. When the final piping layout has been established, determine the friction loss for each section of the piping system from the pressure drop charts (Chapter 33 of the 1997 *ASHRAE Handbook—Fundamentals)* for the mass flow rate in each portion of the piping system.

After calculating the friction loss at design flow for all sections of the piping system and all fittings, terminal units, and control valves, sum them for several of the longest piping circuits to determine the pressure against which the pump must operate at design flow.

Final Pump Selection. After completing the final pressure drop calculations, select the pump by plotting a system curve and pump curve and selecting the pump or pump assembly that operates closest to the calculated design point.

13.4.3 Freeze Prevention

All circulating water systems require precautions to prevent freezing, particularly in makeup air applications in temperate climates (1) where coils are exposed to outdoor air at below-freezing temperatures, (2) where undrained chilled water coils are in the winter airstream, or (3) where piping passes through unheated spaces. Freezing will not occur as long as flow is maintained and the water is at least warm. Unfortunately, during extremely cold weather or in the event of a power failure, water flow and temperature cannot be guaranteed. Additionally, continuous pumping can be energy-intensive and cause system wear. The following are precautions to avoid flow stoppage or damage from freezing:

1. Select all load devices (such as preheat coils) that are subjected to outdoor air temperatures for constant flow, variable Δt control.
2. Position the coil valves of all cooling coils with valve control that are dormant in winter months to the full-open position at those times.
3. If intermittent pump operation is used as an economy measure, use an automatic override to operate both chilled water and heating water pumps in below-freezing weather.
4. Select pump starters that automatically restart after power failure (i.e., maintain contact control).
5. Select nonoverloading pumps.
6. Instruct operating personnel never to shut down pumps in sub freezing weather.
7. Do not use aquastats, which can stop a pump, in boiler circuits.
8. Avoid sluggish circulation, which may cause air binding or dirt deposit. Properly balance and clean systems. Provide proper air control or means to eliminate air.
9. Install low temperature detection thermostats that have phase change capillaries wound in a serpentine pattern across the leaving face of the upstream coil.

In fan equipment handling outdoor air, take precautions to avoid stratification of air entering the coil. The best methods for proper mixing of indoor and outdoor air are the following:

1. Select dampers for pressure drops adequate to provide stable control of mixing, preferably with dampers installed several equivalent diameters upstream of the air-handling unit.
2. Design intake and approach duct systems to promote natural mixing.
3. Select coils with circuiting to allow parallel flow of air and water.

Freeze-up may still occur with any of these precautions. If an antifreeze solution is not used, water should circulate at all times. Valve-controlled elements should have low-limit thermostats, and sensing elements should be located to ensure accurate air temperature readings. Primary-secondary pumping of coils as in Figure 13-19 is advantageous. Use outdoor reset of water temperature wherever possible.

13.4.4 Antifreeze Solutions

In systems in danger of freeze-up, water solutions of ethylene glycol and propylene glycol are commonly used. Freeze protection may be needed (1) in snow-melting applications (see Chapter 46 of the 1995 *ASHRAE Handbook—Applications);* (2) in systems subjected to 100% outdoor air, where the methods outlined above may not provide absolute antifreeze protection; (3) in isolated parts or zones of a heating system where intermittent operation or long runs of exposed piping increase the danger of freezing; and (4) in process cooling applications requiring temperatures below 40°F. Although using ethylene glycol or propylene glycol is comparatively expensive and tends to create corrosion problems unless suitable inhibitors are used, it may be the only practical solution in many cases.

Solutions of triethylene glycol, as well as certain other heat transfer fluids, may also be used. However, ethylene glycol and propylene glycol are the most common substances used in hydronic systems because they are less costly and provide the most effective heat transfer.

Heat Transfer and Flow. Chapter 20 of the 1997 *ASHRAE Handbook—Fundamentals* presents density, specific heat, thermal conductivity, and viscosity of various aqueous solutions of ethylene glycol and propylene glycol.

System heat transfer rate is affected by relative density and specific heat according to the following equation:

$$q_w = 500\, Q(\rho/\rho_w)c_p\Delta t \qquad (13\text{-}18)$$

where

q_w = total heat transfer rate, Btu/h
Q = flow rate, gpm
ρ = fluid density, lb/ft^3
ρ_w = density of water at 60°F, lb/ft^3
c_p = specific heat of fluid, Btu/lb·°F
Δt = temperature increase or decrease, °F

Effect on Heat Source or Chiller. Generally, ethylene glycol solutions should not be used directly in a boiler because of the danger of chemical corrosion caused by glycol breakdown on direct heating surfaces. However, properly inhibited glycol solutions can be used in low-temperature water systems directly in the heating boiler if proper operation can be ensured. Automobile antifreeze solutions are not recommended because the silicate inhibitor can cause fouling, pump seal wear, fluid gelation, and reduced heat transfer. The area or zone requiring the antifreeze protection can be isolated with a separate heat exchanger or converter. Glycol solutions are used directly in water chillers in many cases.

Glycol solutions affect the output of a heat exchanger by changing the film coefficient of the surface contacting the solution. This change in film coefficient is caused primarily by viscosity changes. Figure 13-29 illustrates typical changes in output for two types of heat exchangers, Curve A for a steam-to-liquid converter and Curve B for a refrigerant-to-liquid chiller. The curves are plotted for one set of operating conditions only and reflect the change in ethylene glycol concentration as the only variable. Propylene glycol has a similar effect on heat exchanger output.

Because many other variables, such as liquid velocity, steam or refrigerant loading, temperature difference, and unit construction affect the overall coefficient of a heat exchanger, designers should consult manufacturers' ratings when selecting such equipment. The curves indicate only the magnitude of these output changes.

Effect on Terminal Units. Because the effect of glycol on the capacity of terminal units may vary widely with temperature, the manufacturer's rating data should be consulted when selecting heating or cooling units in glycol systems.

Effect on Pump Performance. Centrifugal pump characteristics are affected to some degree by glycol solutions because of viscosity changes. Figure 13-30 shows these effects on pump capacity, head, and efficiency. Figures in Chapter 20 of the 1997 *ASHRAE Handbook—Fundamentals* plot the viscosity of aqueous ethylene glycol and propylene glycol. Centrifugal pump performance is normally cataloged

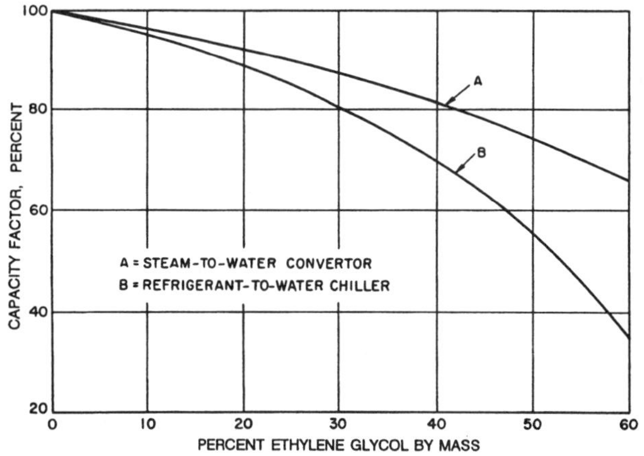

Fig. 13-29 Example of Effect of Acqueous Ethylene Glycol Solutions on Heat Exchanger Output

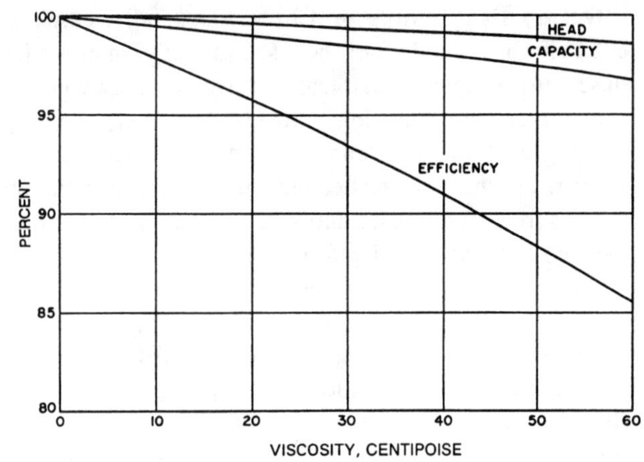

Fig. 13-30 Effect of Viscosity on Pump Characteristics

for water at 60 to 80°F. Hence, absolute viscosity effects below 1.1 centipoise can safely be ignored as far as pump performance is concerned. In intermittently operated systems, such as snow-melting applications, viscosity effects at start-up may decrease flow enough to slow pickup.

Effect on Piping Pressure Loss. The friction loss in piping also varies with viscosity changes. Figure 13-31 gives correction factors for various ethylene glycol and propylene glycol solutions. These factors are applied to the calculated pressure loss for water [Equation (13-17)]. No correction is needed for ethylene glycol and propylene glycol solutions above 160°F.

Installation and Maintenance. Because glycol solutions are comparatively expensive, the smallest possible concentrations to produce the desired antifreeze properties should be used. The total water content of the system should be calculated carefully to determine the required amount of glycol (Craig et al. 1993). The solution can be mixed outside the system in drums or barrels and then pumped in. Air vents should be watched during filling to prevent loss of solution. The system and the cold water supply should not be permanently connected, so automatic fill valves are usually not used.

Ethylene glycol and propylene glycol normally include an inhibitor to help prevent corrosion. Solutions should be checked each year using a suitable refractometer to determine glycol concentration. Certain precautions regarding the use of inhibited ethylene glycol solutions should be taken to extend their service life and to preserve equipment:

1. Before injecting the glycol solution, thoroughly clean and flush the system.
2. Use waters that are soft and low in chloride and sulfate ions to prepare the solution whenever possible.
3. Limit the maximum operating temperature to 250°F in a closed hydronic system. In a heat exchanger, limit glycol film temperatures to 300 to 350°F (steam pressures 120 psi or less) to prevent deterioration of the solution.
4. Check the concentration of inhibitor periodically, following procedures recommended by the glycol manufacturer.

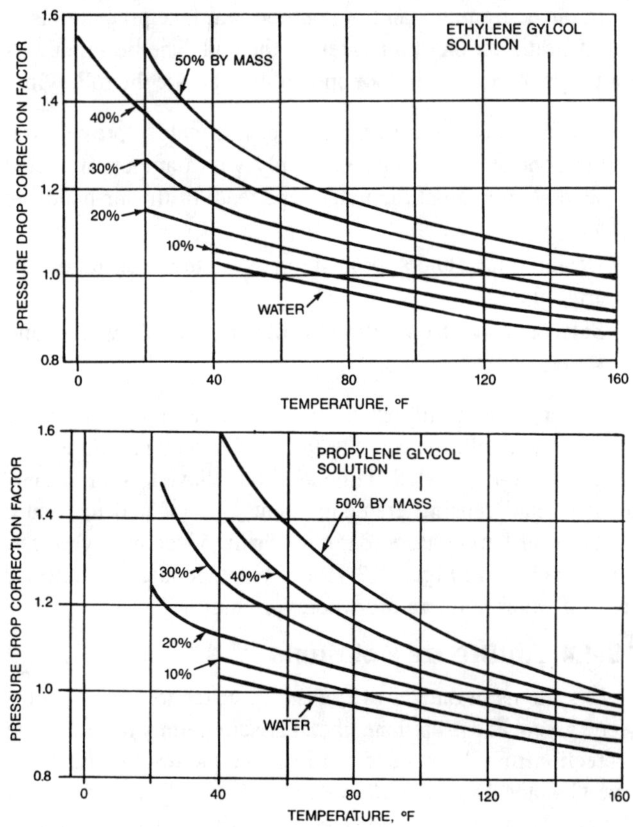

Fig. 13-31 Pressure Drop Correction for Glycol Solutions

13.5 Problems

13.1 What is the maximum temperature at which a heating water system can be operated if the boiler (hot water generator) is rated as low pressure by the ASME *Boiler and Pressure Vessel Code*?

13.2 Sketch the fundamental components for a chilled water system with a single load and source, and a capacity of 100 tons of cooling, then:

(a) What is the water circulation rate (GPM) required if the temperature range of the water is 12°F.

(b) If the head loss in the system is 60 feet, and the pump is 80% efficient, what is the pump horsepower? Motor size?

(c) If the motor is 90% efficient and it operates for one-third of the total hours in the year, what is the annual energy consumption of the pump?

13.3 Calculate the size of the expansion tank for a hot water heating system of 1,200,000 Btu/h heating capacity if the tank is a closed tank with an air/water interface and the following system parameters are known:

Supply water temperature	210°F
Ambient temperature	60°F
Fill pressure (at tank)	30 psig
Max. operating pressure (at tank)	35 psig

System water volume	6,000 gallons
Steel piping system material	

13.4 What tank size diaphragm tank would be required for the above system?

13.5 In a given chilled water system, the pump head required at 640 gpm is 80 ft.

(a) What is the system constant, C_s?

(b) Plot the system curve from 0 to 800 gpm.

13.6 In a chilled water system, the pump is located in a basement equipment room with the expansion tank connected to the pump suction. The pump is the lowest point in the system and the highest point is a pipe in the penthouse, which is 115 feet above the pump? The dynamic head losses in the system are:

Piping and fittings	30 ft.
Chiller	20 ft.
Control valve	10 ft.
Cooling coil	10 ft.

When the system is filled (at 95° ambient temperature) it is desired to have a pressure of 10 psig at the highest point in the system which will reduce to 5 psig when the water temperature reduces to 45°F.

(a) What operating pressures (p_1, p_2) should the expansion tank be designed for?

(b) What pump head is required?

(c) With the pump off and a cold (45°F) system, what is the pressure at the pump suction? The pump discharge?

(d) With the pump on and a cold (45°F) system, what is the pressure at the pump suction? The pump discharge?

13.7 In your own words, explain the difference between a three-way control valve and a two-way control valve as they affect the hydraulics of the system.

13.8 A control valve is to be sized for a cooling coil with a capacity of 30 tons of cooling. The water temperature entering the coil is at 44°F with a 12°F Δt. It is determined that the valve should have a pressure drop of 5 psi. What is the required C_v of the valve?

13.9 A section of 1 in. steel pipe in a 45° chilled water system at 50 psig is in a pipe chase and is isolated between two service valves. With a cold system (45°) the section is isolated by closing off the two service valves. If the chase is at a temperature of 95°F and the pipe reaches thermal equilibrium with the chase, what will the final pressure be?

13.6 References

ASME. 1995. *Boiler and Pressure Vessel Codes.* American Society of Mechanical Engineers, New York.

Carlson, G.F. 1981. The design influence of air on hydronic systems. *ASHRAE Transactions* 87(1):1293-1300.

Coad, W.J. 1980a. Air in hydronic systems. *Heating/Piping/Air Conditioning* (July).

Coad, W.J. 1980b. Expansion tanks. *Heating/Piping/Air Conditioning* (May).

Coad, W.J. 1985. Variable flow in hydronic systems for improved stability, simplicity, and energy economics. *ASHRAE Transactions* 91 (1B): 224-37.

Craig, N.C., B.W. Jones, and D.L. Fenton. 1993. Glycol concentration requirements for freeze burst protection. *ASHRAE Transactions* 99(2):200-09

Himmelblau, D.M. 1960. Solubilities of inert gases in water *Journal of Chemical and Engineering Data* 5(1).

Hull, R.E 1981. Effect of air on hydraulic performance of the HVAC system. *ASHRAE Transactions* 87(1):1301-25.

Lockhart, H.A. and G.E Carlson. 1953. Compression tank selection for hot water heating systems. *ASHVE Journal* 25(4):132-39. Also in *ASHVE Transactions* 59:55-76.

Morabito, B.R 1960. How higher cooling coil differentials affect system economics. *ASHRAE Journal* 2(8):60.

Pierce, J.D. 1963. Application of fin tube radiation to modern hot water heating systems. *ASHRAE Journal* 5(2):72.

Pompei, E 1981. Air in hydronic systems: How Henry's law tells us what happens. *ASHRAE Transactions* 87(1):1326-42.

Stewart, W.E. and C.L. Dona. 1987. Water flow rate limitations. *ASHRAE Transactions* 93(2):811-25.

Chapter 14

UNITARY AND ROOM AIR CONDITIONERS

This chapter discusses the availability of the various types of unitary units and room air conditioners. Additional details on this equipment can be found in Chapters 43 and 44 in the 1996 *ASHRAE Handbook—Systems and Equipment*.

14.1 Unitary Air Conditioners

Unitary air-conditioning equipment is an assembly of factory-matched refrigerant cycle components for inclusion in field designed air-conditioning systems. Some of the many types of unitary air conditioners available include the following characteristics:

Arrangement: Single or split.
Heat rejection: Air cooled, water cooled, evaporative condenser.
Unit exterior: Decorative for in-space applications, functional for equipment room and ducts, weatherproofed for outdoors.
Placement: Floor standing, wall mounted, ceiling suspended, roof mounted.
Indoor air: Vertical upflow or downflow, horizontal flow, 90° and 180° turns, with fan, or for use with forced-air furnaces.
Locations: *Indoor*—exposed with plenums or furred in ductwork concealed in closets, attic, crawl spaces, basements, garages, utility rooms, or equipment rooms. Wall, window or transom mounted.
Outdoor—rooftop, wall mounted, or on ground
Heat: May be combined with electric heat, gas heat, hot water, or steam coil.

Unitary air-conditioners, in contrast to room air-conditioners, include fans capable of operating with ductwork, although some units may be applied with plenums. Heat pumps are also offered in many of the same types and capacities as unitary air conditioners. Packaged reciprocating and centrifugal water chillers are considered to be unitary air conditioners, particularly when applied with unitary chilled-water blower coil units.

Single-package air conditioners are depicted in Figures 14-1 through 14-4. Split systems, condensing units with coils and with blower coil units are shown in Figures 14-5 through 14-7.

The many combinations of coil configurations, evaporator temperatures, air handling arrangements, refrigerating capacities, and variations thereof that are available in central systems are seldom possible with unitary systems. Consequently, a higher level of design ingenuity and performance is required to develop superior system performance from unitary equipment.

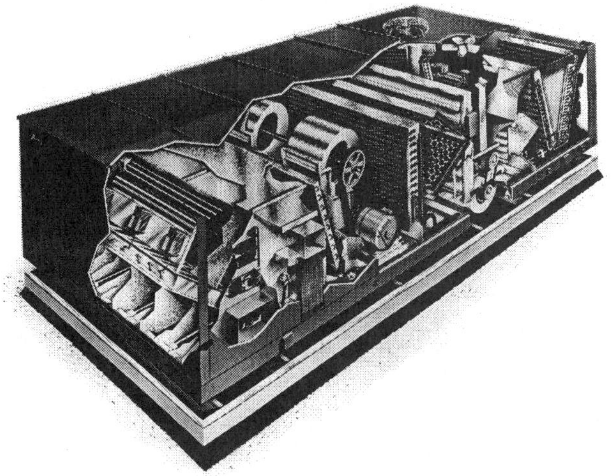

Fig. 14-1 Typical Rooftop Air-Cooled Single Package Air Conditioner

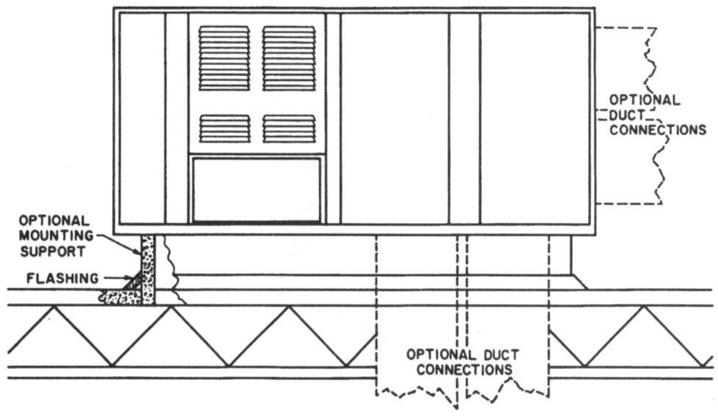

Fig. 14-2 Rooftop Installation of a Single-Package Unit

Unitary equipment tends to serve zoned systems, with each zone served by its own unit. The room conditioner carries this concept to relatively small rooms.

For large single spaces where central systems are at their best advantage, multiple central systems are often advantageous because as load sources move within the larger space, the many smaller interlocked and independent systems have more flexibility than one central system.

However, rooms with less than 0.5-ton (2-kW) or over 25-tons (100-kW) cooling load are seldom conditioned by their own single unit in multiple-unit systems. Multiple-unit systems generally provide the following advantages over central system alternatives:

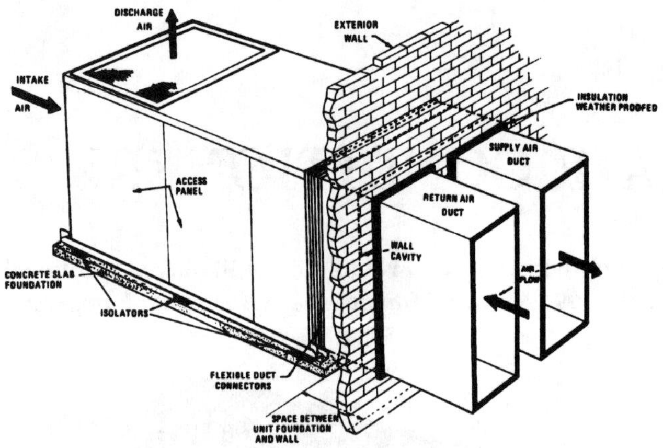

Fig. 14-3 Typical Through-the-Wall Air-Cooled Single-Package Unit

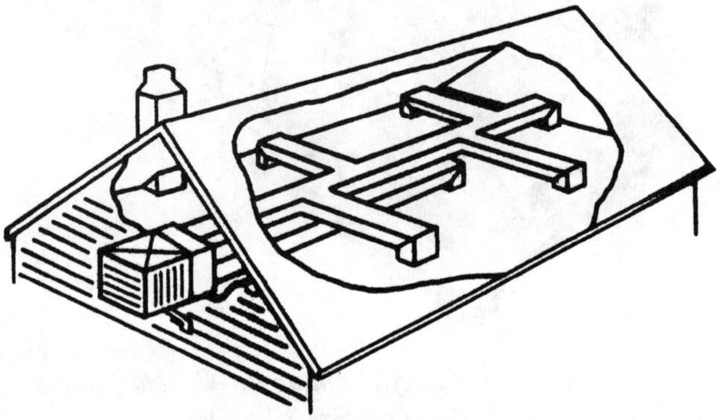

Fig. 14-4 Through-the-Wall Installation of a Single-Package Unit

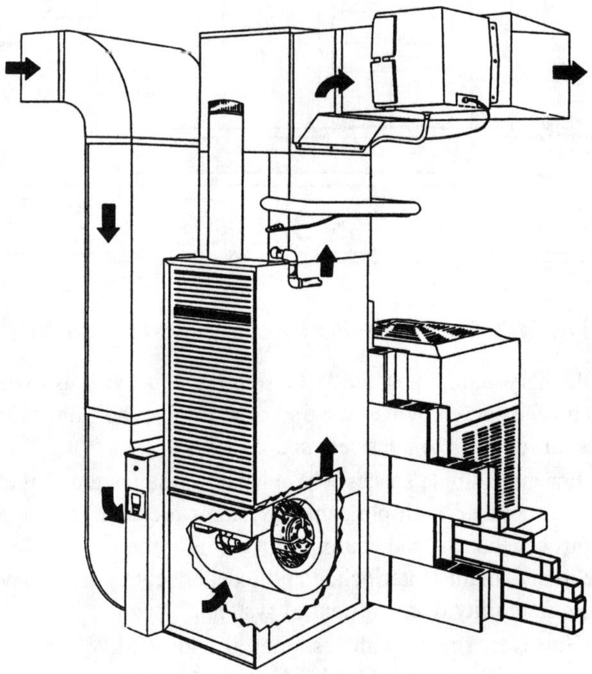

Fig. 14-5 Residential Installation of Split-System Air-Cooled Condensing Unit with Indoor Coil and Upflow Furnace

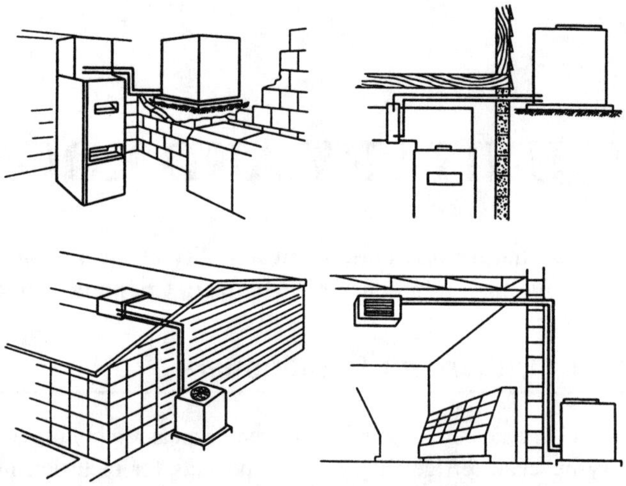

Fig. 14-6 Outdoor Installations of Split-System Air-Cooled Condensing Units with Coil and Upflow Furnace or with Indoor Blower Coils

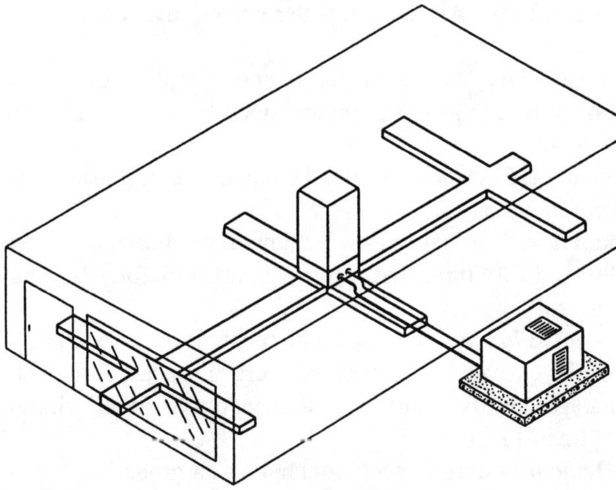

Fig. 14-7 Outdoor Installation of Split-System Air-Cooled Condensing Unit with Indoor Coil and Downflow Furnace

- Simple and inexpensive individual room control
- Individual air-distribution for each room, usually with convenient and simple adjustment
- Heating and cooling capability at all times, independent of the mode of operation of other spaces in the building
- Individual ventilation air, normally operating whenever (and only when) the conditioner operates
- Consistent performance assured by manufacturer-matched components
- Generally has published certified ratings and performance data
- Single source of accountability because manufacturer assembles components
- Manufacturer instructions and multiple-unit nature simplify and systematize installation through repetition of tasks
- Only one terminal zone or conditioner is affected in the event of equipment malfunction
- Usually saves some space

- Usually quick availability and installation are possible
- Usually lower initial cost
- Responsibility for performance of complete package(s) rests with one manufacturer and its agents who provide information on application, installation, maintenance, and service
- Equipment serving spaces that become vacant can be turned off locally or from a central point, without affecting occupied spaces

Multiple-unit systems may have the following disadvantages:

- Limited performance options are available because airflow and cooling coil and condenser sizing is fixed.
- Not generally suited for close humidity control, except when using special purpose equipment such as packaged units for a computer room.
- Energy use may be greater than for central systems if efficiency of the unitary equipment is less than that of the combined central system components.
- Low cost cooling by outdoor air economizers is not always available.
- Air distribution control may be limited.
- Operating sound levels can be high.
- Ventilation capabilities are fixed by equipment design.
- Overall appearance can be unappealing.
- Air filtration options are limited.
- Maintenance may be difficult because of the many pieces of equipment and their locations.

14.2 Window Air Conditioners

A window air conditioner is an encased assembly designed as a unit primarily for mounting in a window. These units are designed for comfort cooling and provide delivery of conditioned air to the room either without ducts or with very short ducts up to a maximum of about 48 in. (1.2 m).

A window air conditioner cools, dehumidifies, filters or cleans, and circulates room air. Ventilation may also be provided by introducing outdoor air into the room, and/or by exhausting room air to the outside. Some conditioners provide heating by reverse cycle (heat pump) operation, by steam or hot water coils, or by electric resistance elements.

A typical window air conditioner is shown in Figure 14-8. Warm room air passes over the cooling coil, giving up its sensible and latent heat. The conditioned air is then circulated in the room by a fan or blower.

The cooling and heating capacities of window air conditioners are always measured and stated in terms of Btu/h (W). A wide range of capacities is available [from approximately 4000 to 36,000 Btu/h (1.2 to 10.5 kW)].

The design of a window air conditioner is usually based on one or more of the following criteria, any one of which automatically limits the freedom of the designer in overall system design:

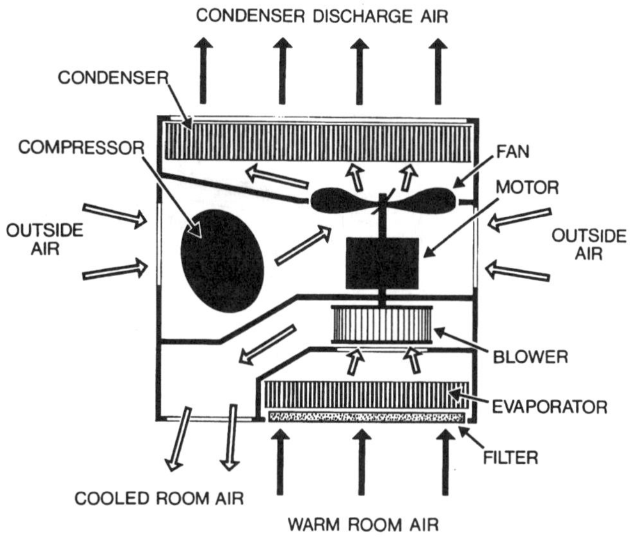

Fig. 14-8 Schematic View of Window Air Conditioner

- Lowest initial cost
- Lowest operating cost (highest efficiency)
- Low sound level
- Physical chassis size
- An unusual chassis shape (minimal depth, height, etc.)
- An amperage limitation (7.5 A, 12 A, etc.)
- Weight

The basic design is a carefully selected group of components consisting of an evaporator, a condenser, a compressor, one or more fan motors, air impellers for evaporator and condenser airflow, and a restrictor device, usually consisting of one or more capillary tubes.

14.3 Through-the-Wall Conditioner System

A through-the-wall system is an air-cooled room air conditioner designed for mounting through the wall and normally capable of providing both heating and cooling. Design and manufacturing specifications range from appliance grade to heavy-duty commercial grade. The latter is called **packaged terminal air conditioner**, and is defined as such by ARI in the "Packaged Terminal Air Conditioners" subsection of the *Air Conditioning Heat Transfer Products*; all others are covered by AHAM *Standard* CN-1.

System Concept and Description. The through-the- wall concept incorporates a complete air-cooled refrigeration and air-handling system in an individual package, using space normally occupied by the building wall for equipment, with the remainder projecting inside the room.

Each packaged terminal air conditioner has a self-contained, direct-expansion cooling system, heating coil (electric, hot water, or steam), and packaged controls. Two

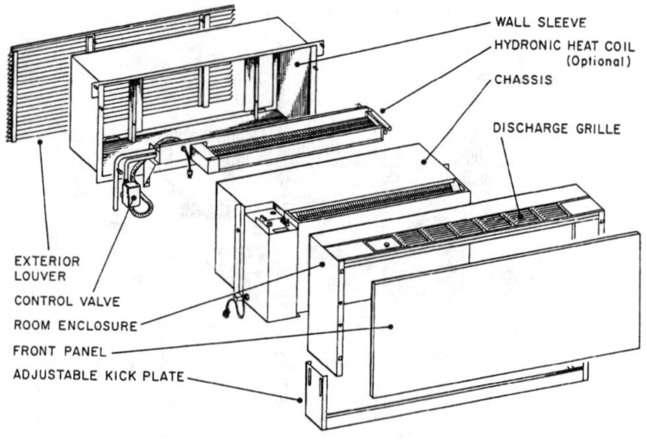

Fig. 14-9 Packaged Terminal Air Conditioner with Separate Heat Section and Cooling Chassis

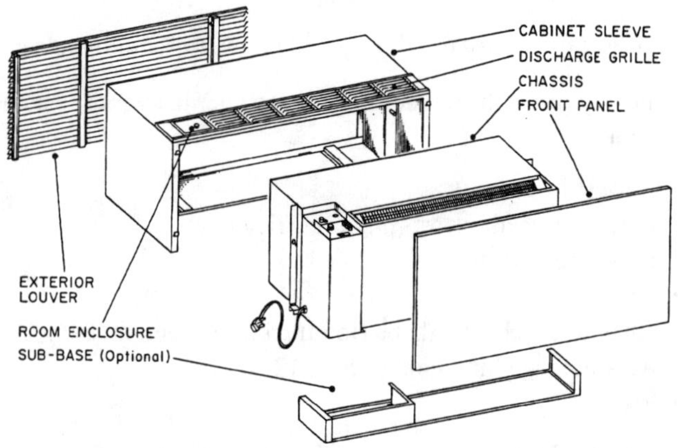

Fig. 14-10 Packaged Terminal Air Conditioner with Combination Heating and Cooling Chassis

general configurations used consist of (1) wall box, heat section, room cabinet, outdoor louver, and cooling chassis (Figure 14-9); and (2) a combination wall sleeve and room cabinet, combination heating and cooling chassis, and outdoor louver (Figure 14-10).

The exterior louver is installed flush (or nearly so) with the outside wall of the building and receives a variety of architectural treatments, such as emphasizing the existing louvers and using them as aesthetic highlights, hiding them completely with solid or pierced wall coverings, or designing the building so that the louvers blend into the overall exterior.

Advantages. The initial cost of the through-the-wall system in multiroom applications is considerably less than central systems adapted to simultaneously heat or cool each room under control of the room occupants. The cost differences may run as high as 20 to 50%, depending on the design and components.

Because a through-the-wall system has no system auxiliaries, the energy consumption may be lower than for central systems. For this reason, economical comparisons between central systems and through-the-wall conditioners should include all system components, including fans, pumps and heat rejection devices. Keep in mind that fan and motor efficiencies will be significantly lower for the through-the-wall air-conditioner.

A through-the-wall system requires less space because it requires no ductwork nor equipment rooms. This space savings can range from 5 to 15% of the total building space when the savings are considered on a floor-by-floor basis.

Limitations. The through-the-wall system is limited to multizone systems and generally cannot be used economically in large spaces requiring more than three units per zone. However, where the packaged terminal air-conditioner system is coordinated with a well-designed core system, it can be economically used for large office areas while allowing for maximum flexibility in moving partitions. Through-the-wall units are more likely to be limited by their ability to throw air across the room.

Current products do not include individual conditioner humidifier systems. Humidification and reheat can be achieved with a through-the-wall system but must be done through a separate core system or a central fresh air supply with zone humidistat control. However, the higher initial cost associated with humidity control generally restricts its use for most comfort heating and cooling applications. The through-the-wall system should not be used where there are high sensible load requirements coming from a concentration of heat-producing equipment, such as is used in telephone equipment rooms or radio and television stations.

Applications. Through-the-wall systems are best applied in multizone applications. The system lends itself to both low- and high-rise buildings. The system is most generally applied in

- Office buildings
- Motels and hotels
- Apartments and dormitories
- Schools and other educational buildings
- Nursing homes

This system is also applicable for renovating existing buildings because all or part of the existing heating system can be used. This equipment causes less disruption and construction-forced sacrifice of rentable space than alternative systems. The result is an automatically controlled heating system and a completely self-contained cooling system with pressure ventilation air.

14.4 Typical Performance

Specially constructed equipment cannot be justified for small commercial and residential applications. Furthermore, these applications generally have a higher sensible heat factor (SHF), so dehumidification is not as critical as in large commercial buildings. Therefore, the equipment is manufactured to operate at or near one set of conditions.

For example, typical residential and light commercial cooling equipment operates with a coil SHF of 0.75 to 0.8

with the air entering the coil at about 80°F (27°C) dry-bulb and 67°F (19°C) wet-bulb temperature. This equipment usually has a capacity of less than 10 tons (35 kW). When the peak cooling load and latent heat requirements are appropriate, this less expensive type of equipment is used.

Selected equipment should be within the range of 95 to 115% of the peak cooling load. The air quantity is specified by the manufacturer for each unit, and is about 400 cfm/ton (50 L/s per kW). The total air quantity is then divided among the various rooms according to the cooling load of each room. Typical performance data for residential and light commercial cooling equipment are listed in Table 14-1.

Table 14-1 Typical Residential or Light Commercial Cooling Coil Performance Data (Split System)

Capacity		Airflow		Coil Pressure Loss	
Btu/h	kW	cfm	m^3/s	in. of water	Pa
18,000	5.3	600	0.28	0.18	45
24,000	7.0	800	0.38	0.30	75
30,000	8.8	1050	0.50	0.13	32
41,000	10.3	1270	0.60	0.20	50
48,000	14.1	1750	0.83	0.25	62
59,000	17.3	2140	1.01	0.30	75

Example 14.1 An air-conditioning unit selected for a residence has a rated total cooling capacity of 36,000 Btu/h and a sensible cooling capacity of 27,000 Btu/h. The manufacturer also lists a SEER of 13 for this unit. The unit is expected to operate for 1900 hours during each cooling season.

a) Determine the latent cooling capacity.
b) What is the sensible heat ratio for the unit?
c) What is the expected energy use per cooling season?

Solution:

a) $Q_{latent} = Q_{Total} - Q_{sensible}$

$Q_{latent} = 36{,}000 - 27{,}000 = 9000$ Btu/h

b) Sensible Heat Ratio (SHR) $= \dfrac{Q_{sensible}}{Q_{Total}}$

$$\text{SHR} = \frac{27{,}000}{36{,}000} = 0.75$$

c) $$\frac{36{,}000\ \text{Btu/h} \times 1900\ \text{h}}{13\ \text{Btu/h}\cdot\text{W} \times 1000\ \text{W/kW}} = 5262\ \text{kWh}$$

14.5 Problems

14.1 For the residence shown below and located in Cedar Rapids, Iowa, size and select the heating and cooling equipment.

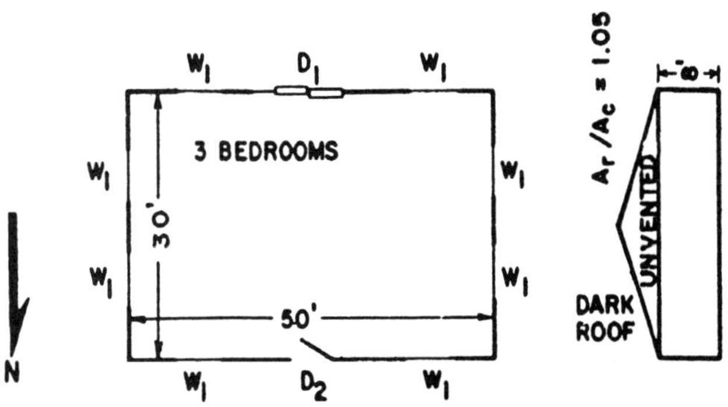

Ceiling/Roof: $U = 0.05$ Btu/h·ft^2·°F

Wall Construction: Face brick, 25/32-in. insulating board sheathing, 2 by 6 studs on 24-in. centers, 1/4-in. paneling. Neglect effect of studs. Full wall insulation (glass-fiber type) is used.

Floor: Concrete slab, 24 in. width of $R = 5.0$ insulation

Window type:

W1 = 4 ft by 5 ft single-glazed windows, wood sash, and storm window. No interior shading.

Door types:

D1 = 6 ft by 7 ft sliding glass patio door, double-glazed, 1/2-in. airspace, aluminum frame

D2 = wood door with storm door

Humidifier: None

14.2 For the residence shown below, located in Cleveland, Ohio, size and select the heating and cooling equipment and estimate the annual energy requirements.

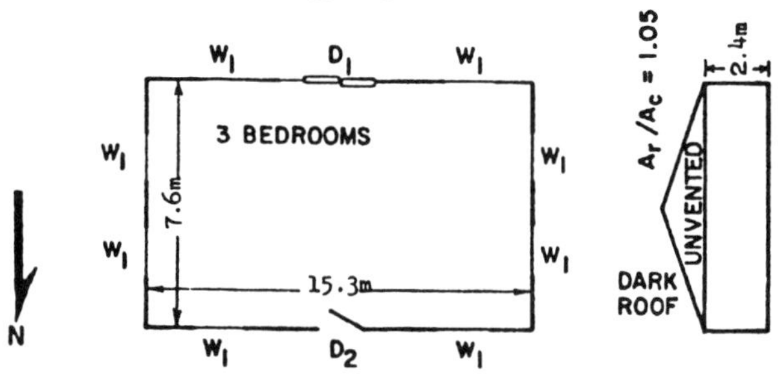

Ceiling/Roof: $U = 0.34$ W/m^2·K

Wall construction: Face brick, 20-mm insulating board sheathing, 38 mm by 140 mm studs on 0.61-m centers, 6.4-mm paneling. Neglect effect of studs. Full wall insulation (glass-fiber type) is used.

Floor: Concrete slab, 0.61 m width of $R = 0.88$ m^2·K/W insulation

Window:

W_1 = 1.2 m by 1.5 m single-glazed windows, wood sash, and storm window. *No interior shading.*

Door:

D_1 = 1.8 m by 2.1 m sliding glass patio door, double-glazed, 13-mm airspace, aluminum frame

D_2 = wood door with storm door

Humidifier: Yes

14.3 For the light commercial building shown below, located in Cleveland, Ohio, size and select the heating and cooling equipment and estimate the annual energy requirements.

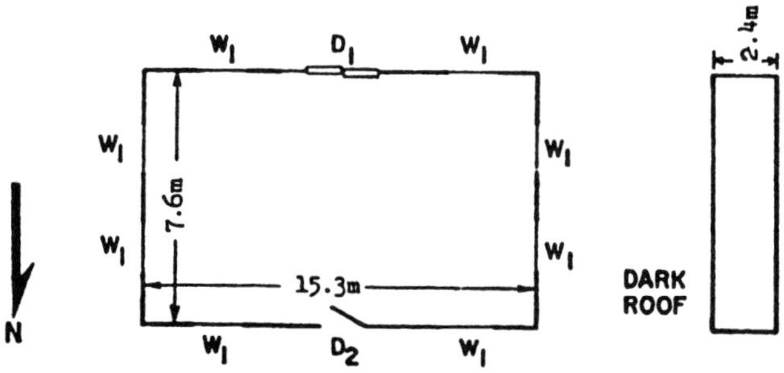

Roof: $U = 0.34$ W/m^2·K; suspended ceiling; 25.4-mm wood with 76.2-mm glass-fiber insulation

Wall construction: Face brick; 20-mm insulating board sheathing; 38 mm by 140 mm studs on 0.61-m centers; 6.4-mm paneling. Full wall insulation (glass-fiber type) is used. Neglect effect of studs.

Floor: Concrete slab with 0.61 m wide, $R = 0.88$ m^2·K/W insulation

Window:

$W_1 = 1.2$ m by 1.5 m single-glazed windows, wood sash, and storm window. *No interior shading.*

Doors:

$D_1 = 1.8$ m by 2.1 m sliding glass patio door, double-glazed, 13-mm airspace, aluminum frame

D_2 = wood door with storm door

Humidifier: Yes

Lights: 1 W/ft^2

People: Six doing light office work between 9 A.M. and 5 P.M. Air conditioning is on only when building is occupied.

14.6 Bibliography

ASHRAE. Chapter 43, Room Air Conditioners and Dehumidifiers. 1996 *ASHRAE Handbook—HVAC Systems and Equipment.*

ASHRAE. Chapter 44, Unitary Air Conditioners and Unitary Heat Pumps. 1996 *ASHRAE Handbook—HVAC Systems and Equipment.*

ASHRAE. Chapter 5, Unitary Refrigerant Based Systems for Air Conditioning. 1996 *ASHRAE Handbook—HVAC Systems and Equipment.*

Chapter 15

PANEL HEATING AND COOLING SYSTEMS

This chapter discusses the principles and equipment available for panel heating and cooling systems. Additional details can be found in Chapter 6, Panel Heating and Cooling in the 1996 *ASHRAE Handbook—Systems and Equipment*.

15.1 General

Radiant panel systems combine temperature control of room surfaces with central air conditioning. Radiant surfaces may be located in the floor, walls, or ceiling, and the temperature is maintained by circulating water or air, or by electric resistance. The central air system can be a basic, one zone, constant-temperature, constant-volume system; or it can include some or all of the features used in properly designed dual-duct, reheat, multizone, or variable volume systems. A controlled temperature surface is called a **radiant panel** if 50% or more of the heat transfer is by radiation to other surfaces.

Residential heating applications usually consist of pipe coils embedded in masonry floors or plaster ceilings. This construction serves well where loads are relatively stable and where solar effects are minimized by building design. However, in buildings with large glass areas and rapid load changes, the slow response, lag, and override effect of masonry panels is unsatisfactory. Lightweight metal panel ceiling systems quickly respond to load changes and can be used for cooling as well as heating.

Warm air and electric heating elements are used where local factors influence such use. In the warm air system, air is supplied to a cavity behind or under the panel surface. The air may leave the cavity through a normal diffuser and flow into the room. These systems are used as floor radiant panels in schools and in floors subject to extreme cold, such as in an overhang. Electric heating elements embedded in the floor or ceiling construction and unitized electric ceiling panels are used in residences, apartments, and various applications for local spot heating. Two factors to consider when using electric radiant panels are local electric codes and the relative difference between electric and fossil fuel heating costs.

The radiant panel is most often located in the ceiling of a room. A ceiling is used because it sees all other surfaces and objects in the room; it is not subject to unpredictable coverings, as are floors; higher surface temperatures can be used; it is of smaller mass and therefore has quicker response to load changes; radiant cooling can be incorporated, and, in the case of the metal ceiling system, the piping is accessible for servicing.

Ceiling panel systems commonly used are an outgrowth of the perforated metal, suspended, acoustical ceiling. These radiant ceiling systems are usually designed into buildings where the features of the suspended acoustical ceiling can be combined with panel heating and cooling. The panels can be designed as small units to fit the building module and provide extensive flexibility for zoning and control; or, for maximum economy, the panels can be arranged as large continuous areas. Two types of metal ceiling systems are available. One type consists of lightweight aluminum panels, usually 12 in. by 24 in. (305 mm by 610 mm), that are attached in the field to 0.5-in. (15-mm) galvanized pipe coils. The second type consists of a copper coil metallurgically bonded to the aluminum face sheet forming a modular panel. Modular panels are available in sizes up to approximately 36 in. by 60 in. (910 mm by 1520 mm) and are held in position by various ceiling suspension systems.

The arrangement of components in radiant panel systems are similar to other air-water systems. Room thermal conditions are primarily maintained by direct transfer of radiant energy, rather than by convective heating and cooling. The room heating and cooling loads are calculated in the conventional manner. Manufacturers' generally rate their equipment in the form of total performance, which can be applied directly to the calculated room load.

These are the principal advantages of panel heating and cooling systems:

1. Comfort levels are better than those experienced in any other conditioning system because radiant loads are treated directly and air motion in the space is at normal ventilation levels.
2. Panel systems do not require any mechanical equipment at the outside walls, thus simplifying the wall, floor, and structural systems.
3. All pumps, fans, filters, and so forth, are centrally located, thereby simplifying maintenance and operation.
4. Cooling or heating may be obtained during any season, without central zoning or seasonal changeover, when three- and four-pipe systems are used.
5. Supply air quantities usually do not exceed those required for ventilation and dehumidification.
6. No mechanical equipment requiring maintenance or repair is placed within the occupied space.
7. Draperies and curtains can be installed at the outside wall without interfering with heating and cooling systems.
8. The modular panel provides flexibility to meet changes in partitioning.
9. No space is required within the air-conditioned room for the mechanical equipment. This feature is especially

valuable when compared to other conditioning methods for applications in existing buildings, hospital patient rooms, and other applications where space is at a premium, where maximum cleanliness is essential, or where dictated by legal requirements.

10. A common central air system can serve both the interior and perimeter zones.
11. Wet surface cooling coils are eliminated from the occupied space, thus reducing the potential for septic contamination.

Other essential factors when considering the use of panel systems are as follows:

1. Evaluate early to plan an optimum physical arrangement of the building to take full advantage of the panel system.
2. Select recessed lighting fixtures, air diffusers, hung ceiling, and other ceiling devices to provide the maximum ceiling area possible for use as radiant panels.
3. The air-side design must maintain humidity levels at or below design conditions at all times to eliminate any possibility of condensation on the panels.
4. Do not use cooling panels in, or adjacent to, high humidity areas.
5. As with any hydronic system, design the piping system to avoid noises from entrained air, high velocity or high-pressure drop devices, or from pump and pipe vibrations.
6. Anticipate thermal expansion of the ceiling and other devices in or adjacent to the ceiling.

15.2 Types

The most common forms of panels applied in panel heating and cooling systems are:

- metal ceiling panels
- embedded piping in ceilings, walls, or floors
- air-heated floors
- electrically heated ceilings or floors

Metal Ceiling Panels. Metal ceiling panels are normally integrated into a system that both heats and cools. In such a system, a source of dehumidified ventilation air is required in summer, and the system is classed as one of the combination air-water systems. In such a system, various amounts of forced air are supplied year-round. When metal panels are applied for heating purposes only, a ventilation system may or may not be required, depending on local codes.

A metal ceiling panel system using copper tubing metallurgically bonded to an aluminum panel is shown in Figure 15-1. This panel can be mounted into various ceiling suspension systems.

Two-pipe, three-pipe, and four-pipe distribution systems have been used successfully with metal ceiling panels. Common design practice calls for a 20°F (11°C) drop for heating across a given grid and a 5°F (3°C) rise for cooling, but higher temperature differentials may apply in some cases.

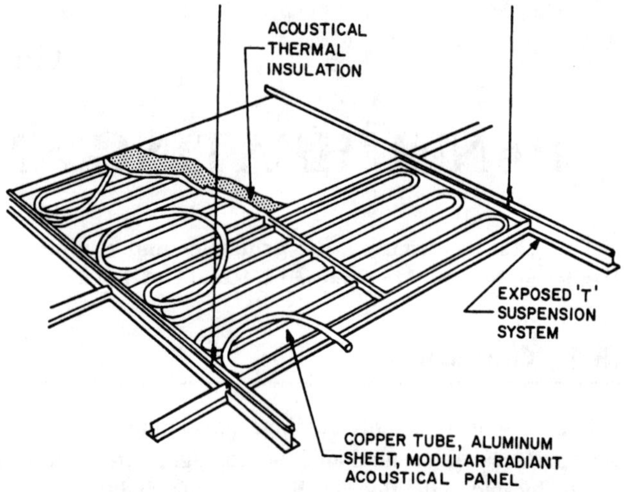

Fig. 15-1 Metal Ceiling Panels Metallurgically Bonded to Copper Tubing

Some ceiling installations require that active grids cover only a part of the room, and consequently, compatible matching standard acoustical panels are normally used for the remaining ceiling area.

Embedded Piping in Ceilings, Walls, and Floors. When piping is embedded in ceilings, the construction used is generally one of the following:

1. Pipe or tube is embedded in the lower portion of a concrete slab, generally within an inch of its lower surface. If plaster is to be applied to the concrete, the piping may be placed directly on the wood forms. If the slab is to be used without plaster finish, then the piping should be installed not less than 0.75 in. (19 mm) above the undersurface of the slab. This method of construction is shown in Figure 15-2. The minimum coverage must be in compliance with the local building code requirements.
2. Pipe or tube is embedded in a metal lath and plaster ceiling. If the lath is suspended to form a hung ceiling, both the lath and the heating coils are securely wired to the supporting members in such a way that the lath is below, but in good contact with, the coils. Plaster is then applied to the metal lath, with care being taken to embed the coil.
3. Copper tube of the smaller diameters is attached to the underside of a wire lath or gypsum lath. Plaster is then applied to the lath to embed the tube (Figure 15-3).

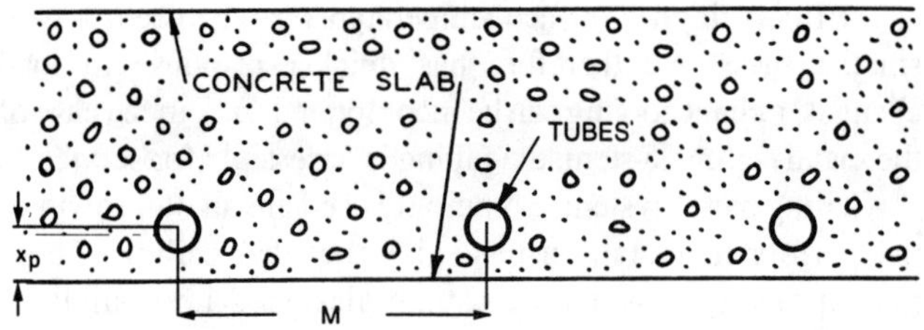

Fig. 15-2 Coils in Structural Concrete Slab

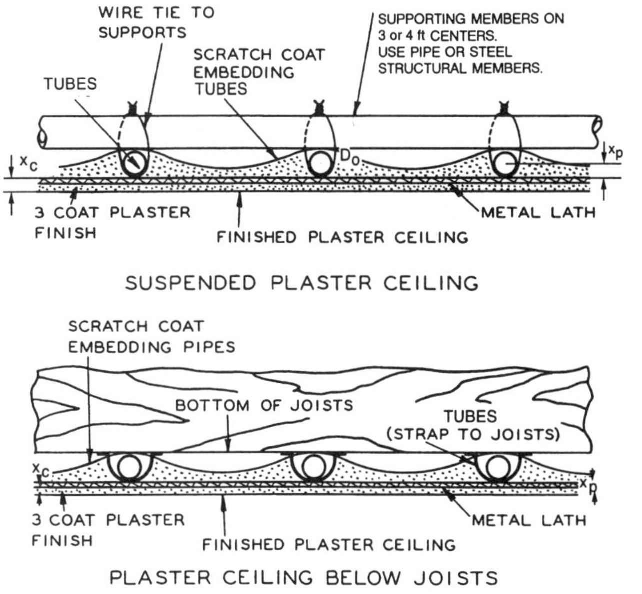

Fig. 15-3 Coils in Plaster above Lath

4. Other forms of ceiling construction are composition board, wood paneling, etc., with warm water piping, tube, or channels built into the panel sections.

Coils are usually of the sinuous type, although some header or grid-type coils have been used in ceilings. Coils may be of plastic, ferrous or nonferrous pipe or tube, with coil pipes spaced from 4.5 to 9 in. (115 to 230 mm) on centers, depending on the required output, pipe or tube size, and other factors.

Although not so universally used as ceiling panels, wall panels may be constructed by any of the methods described for ceilings.

The construction for piping embedded in floors depends on whether (1) the floor is laid on grade, or (2) the floor is above grade.

On-Grade Floor. Plastic, ferrous, and nonferrous pipe and tube are used in floor slabs which rest on grade. The coils are constructed as either sinuous, continuous pipe coils, or arranged as heater coils with the pipes spaced from 6 to 18 in. (150 to 460 mm) on centers. The coils are generally installed with 1.5 to 4 in. (40 to 100 mm) of cover above the coils. Insulation should be used to reduce the perimeter and reverse side losses. Illustrated in Figure 15-4 is the application of pipe coils in slabs resting on grade. Coils should be embedded completely and should not rest on an interface. Any supports used for positioning the heating coils should be nonabsorbent and inorganic.

Above-Grade Floor. Where the coils are embedded in structural load-supporting slabs above grade, construction codes may affect their position. Otherwise, the coil piping is installed in the same manner as described for slabs resting on grade.

Air-Heated Floors. Several methods have been devised to warm interior room surfaces by circulating heated air through

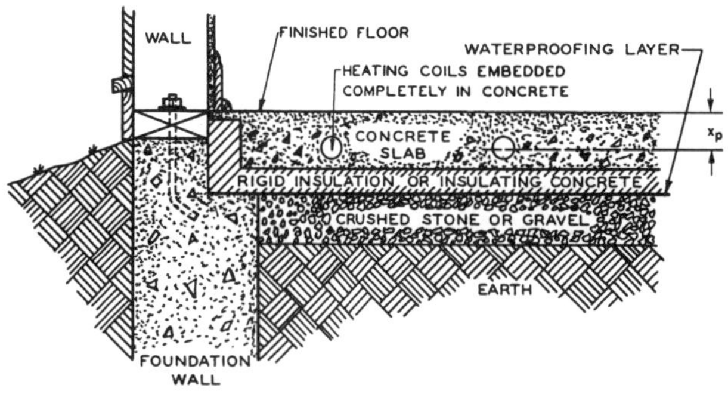

Fig. 15-4 Coils in Floor Slab on Grade

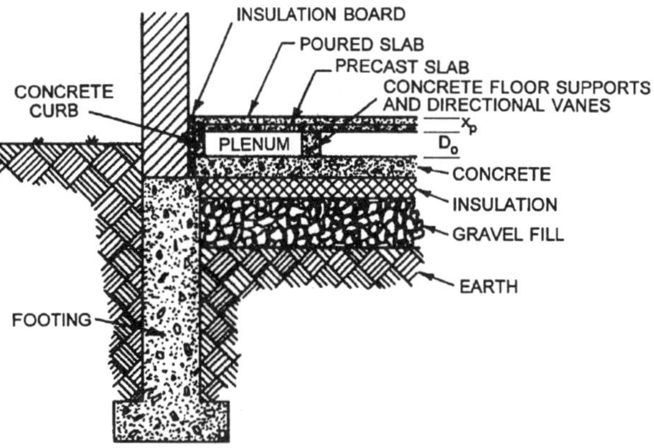

Fig. 15-5 Warm Air Floor Panel Construction

passages in the floor. In some cases, the heated air is recirculated in a closed system. In others, all or part of the air is passed through the room on its way back to the furnace to provide supplementary heating and ventilation (Figure 15-5). Any building codes that might apply must be followed.

Electrically Heated Ceilings. Several types of electric resistance units are available for heating interior room surfaces. These include: (1) electric heating cables that may be embedded in concrete or plaster, or laminated in drywall ceiling construction; (2) prefabricated electric heating panels to be attached to room surfaces; and (3) electrically heated fabrics or other materials for application to, or incorporation into, finished room surfaces.

Ceiling Cables. The details of ceiling cable installation for plastered and drywall construction is shown in shown in Figure 15-6.

Electric Heating Panels. A variety of prefabricated electric heating panels are used for either supplemental or full room heating. These panels are available in sizes for 2 ft by 4 ft to 6 ft by 12 ft (0.6 m by 1.2 m to 1.8 m by 3.6 m). They are constructed from a variety of materials such as gypsum board, glass, steel, and vinyl. Different panels have rated inputs varying from 10 to 95 W/ft^2 (108 to 1023 W/m^2) for 120, 208, and 240 V service. Maximum operating temperatures vary from about 100 to about 300°F (38 to 149°C) depending on watt density.

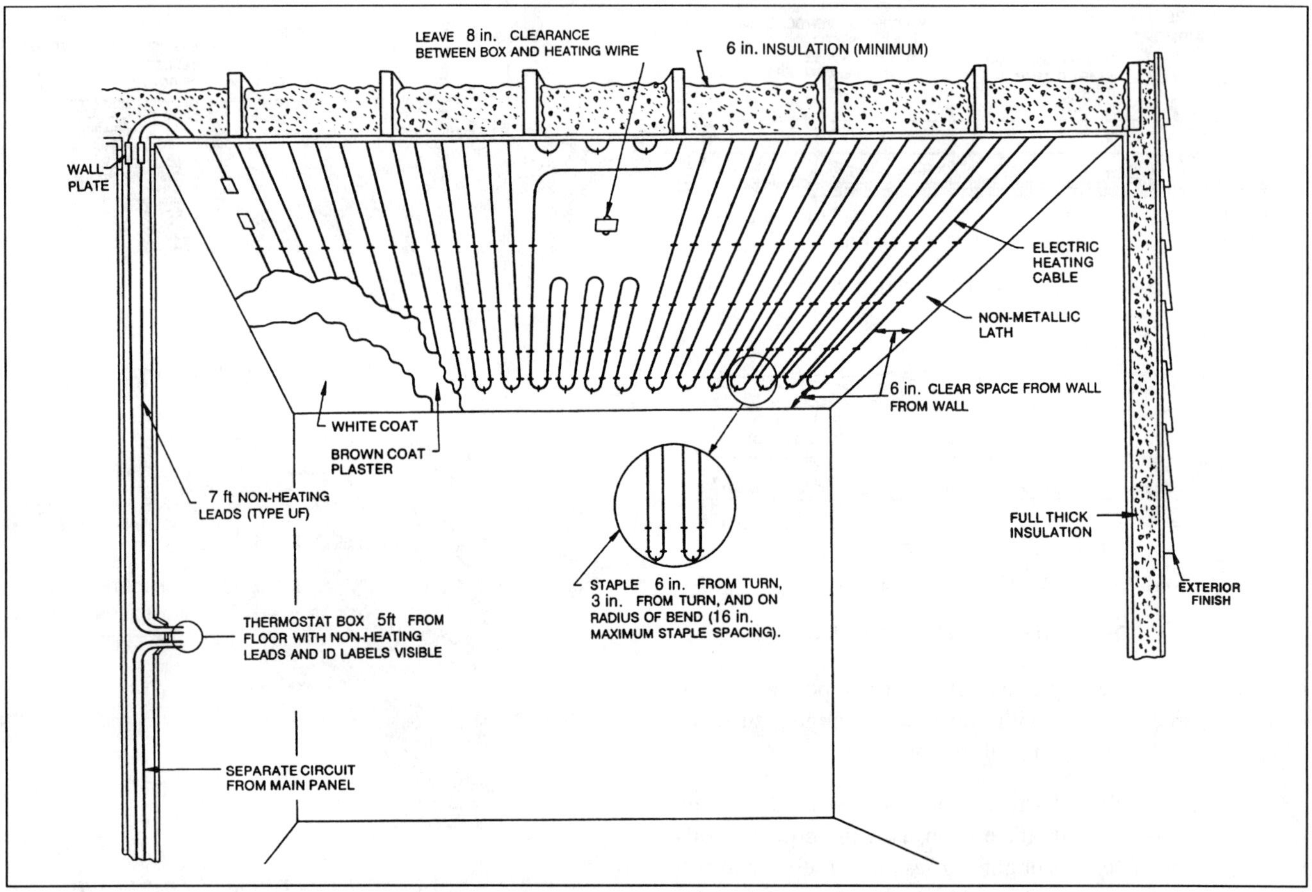

Fig. 15-6 Electric Heating Panel for Wet Plastered Ceiling

Panel heating elements may be embedded conductors, laminated conductive coatings, or printed circuits. Nonheating leads are connected and furnished as part of the panel.

Some panels may be cut to fit available space; others must be installed as received. Panels may be either flush or surface mounted. In some cases, they are finished as part of the ceiling. Rigid panels that are about 1 in. (25 mm) thick and weigh about 25 lb (11 kg) each are available to fit standard 2 ft by 4 ft (0.6 m by 1.2 m) modular tee-bar ceilings.

Cable embedded in walls, similar to ceiling construction, is occasionally found in Europe. Because of possible damage due to nails driven for hanging pictures or because of building alteration, most codes prohibit such panels in the United States.

Some of the prefabricated panels described in the preceding section are also used for wall panel heating.

Electric heating cable assemblies, such as those used for ceiling panels, are sometimes used for concrete floor heating systems.

15.3 Design Steps

Panel design requires specification of the following: panel area, size and location of the heating elements in the panel, insulation on the reverse side and edge of the panel, required input to panel, and temperature of the heating elements. Specific procedures are given in Chapter 6 in 1992 *ASHRAE Handbook—Systems and Equipment*. The procedure is summarized as follows:

1. Calculate heat loss for each room.
2. Determine the available area for panels in each room.
3. Calculate the required unit panel output.
4. Determine the required panel surface temperature.
5. Select the means of heating the panel and the size and location of the heating elements.
6. Select insulation for the reverse side and edge of panel.
7. Determine panel heat loss and required input to the panel.
8. Determine the other temperatures that are required or developed.
9. Design the system for heating the panels in accordance with conventional practice and manufacturers recommendations.

In the steps outlined for design, the effect of each assumption or choice on comfort should be considered carefully. The following general rules may be followed:

1. Place panels near cold areas where heat losses occur.
2. Do not use high-temperature ceiling panels in very low ceilings.
3. Keep floor temperatures at or below 85°F (30°C).

Example 15-1 The living room in a home is occupied by adults in light clothing and engaged in sedentary activity. The room has a net outside wall area of 275 ft^2 with a surface temperature of 540℉, 45 ft^2 of glass with a surface temperature of 200℉; 540 ft^2 of ceiling with a surface temperature of 600℉; 670 ft^2 of partitions with a surface temperature of 700℉; and 540 ft^2 of floor with a surface temperature of 700℉. If the air movement is 20 fpm, determine the air temperature necessary for comfort.

Solution:

Mean radiant temperature = MRT =

$$\text{MRT} = \frac{275(54) + 45(20) + 540(60) + 670(70) + 540(70)}{275 + 45 + 540 + 670 + 540}$$

$$\text{MRT} = 64.1°\text{F}$$

for sedentary activity with light clothing at 20 fpm from Figure 4-3:

$$t_{dry\ bulb} = 90℉ \text{ for comfort}$$

15.4 Problems

15.1 A room has a net outside wall area of 300 ft^2 that has a surface temperature of 55°F; 50 ft^2 of glass with a surface temperature of 30°F; 560 ft^2 of ceiling with a surface temperature of 70°F; and 560 ft^2 with a surface temperature of 70°F. Estimate the average unheated surface temperature or the area-weighted mean radiant temperature. [Ans: 65.6°F]

15.2 For the room in *Problem* 15.1, estimate the following:

(a) radiant output for a 100 ft^2 heating panel with a panel surface temperature of 120°F

(b) natural convection output for the ceiling panel when the air temperature is 70°F

15.3 A room has 1500 ft^2 of surface area and 320 ft^2 is to be heated. The average unheated surface temperature in the room is 67°F. The air temperature in the room is 75°F. The room is occupied by adults in light clothing at a sedentary activity. Determine the surface temperature of the heated panel necessary to produce comfort if the air velocity is 20 fpm. [Ans: 131°F]

15.4 For *Problem* 15.3, determine the total heat transferred by the ceiling heating panel.

15.5 Bibliography

ASHRAE, 1996. Chapter 6—*Panel Heating and Cooling, HVAC Systems and Equipment Handbook*, ASHRAE, Atlanta, GA.

Chapter 16

HEAT PUMP, TOTAL ENERGY, AND HEAT RECOVERY SYSTEMS

This chapter discusses applied heat pump systems, heat recovery systems, and cogeneration (total energy) systems. Specific details on these subjects can be found in Chapters 7 and 8 of the 1996 *ASHRAE Handbook—HVAC Systems and Equipment*.

16.1 General

The thermal cycle of a heat pump is the same as that for refrigeration, but controls allow heat to be either added to the conditioned space from the condenser or removed by the evaporator as desired. Sometimes both the heating and cooling effects are used.

A heat pump extracts heat from a source and transfers it to a sink at a higher temperature. According to this definition, all pieces of refrigeration equipment, including air conditioners and chillers with refrigeration cycles, are heat pumps. In engineering, however, the term heat pump is generally reserved for equipment that heats for beneficial purposes, rather than that which removes heat for cooling only. Dual-mode heat pumps alternately provide heating or cooling. Heat reclaim heat pumps provide heating only, or simultaneous heating and cooling.

An applied heat pump requires competent field engineering for the specific application, in contrast to the use of a manufacturer-designed unitary product. Applied heat pumps include built-up heat pumps (field-, custom-assembled from components) and industrial process heat pumps. Although most heat pump compressors are powered by electric motors, limited use is also made of engine and turbine drives. Applied heat pumps having capacities ranging from 24,000 to 150,000,000 Btu/h operate in many facilities. Decentralized systems with water loop heat pumps are common, using multiple water-source heat pumps connected to a common circulating water loop. They can also include ground coupling, heat rejectors (cooling towers and dry coolers), supplementary heaters (boilers and steam heat exchangers), loop reclaim heat pumps, solar collection devices, and thermal storage. Community and district heating and cooling systems based on both centralized and distributed heat pump systems are feasible.

Unitary heat pumps (as opposed to applied heat pumps) consist of one or more factory-made assemblies that include an outdoor conditioning coil, compressor(s), and chiller-condenser or outdoor coil, and means to both heat and cool. The units are shipped from the factory as a complete preassembled unit, including internal wiring controls and piping. Only the ductwork, external power wiring, and condensate piping are required to complete the installation. Such equipment may be provided in more than one assembly, which requires connecting the refrigerant piping between the indoor and outdoor sections. Unitary heat pump casings closely resemble those of conventional air-conditioning units of equal capacity. Capacities of typical unitary heat pumps range from about 1.5 to 20 tons (5 to 70 kW), although larger capacities are possible. This equipment is used in residential and smaller commercial and industrial installations. The multiunit installation (with a number of individual units) is particularly advantageous because it provides the opportunity for heating or cooling in each zone on demand.

Compressor-type heat pumps used in large central systems vary from one large, centrifugal unit to as many as eight multicylinder reciprocating units. A single or central system is generally used throughout the building, but in some instances the total capacity is divided among several separate heat pump systems to facilitate zoning. Well water, air, and internal building heat are used as heat sources. The refrigerant is compressed in two stages for some projects. Frequently, heating service and cooling service are supplied simultaneously to separate zones of the building.

16.2 Types of Heat Pumps

Heat pumps for air-conditioning service may be classified according to (a) the type of heat source and sink; (b) the heating and cooling distribution fluid; (c) the type of thermodynamic cycle; (d) the type of building structure; and (e) the size and configuration. The more common types are shown in Table 16-1.

The air-to-air heat pump is the most widely used type for residential and commercial applications. It is particularly suited for factory-built unitary heat pumps. The first diagram in Table 16-1 is typical of the refrigeration circuit used. In some installations, the forced convection indoor heat transfer surface has been replaced by a radiant panel.

In air-to-air heat pump systems, as shown in the second diagram of Table 16-1, the air circuits may be interchanged by dampers (motor-driven or manually operated) to obtain either heated or cooled air. With this system, one heat-exchanger coil is always the evaporator and the other is always the con-

Table 16-1 Common Types of Heat Pumps

(Figure 5, Chapter 8, 1996 *ASHRAE Handbook—Systems and Equipment*)

Heat Source and Sink	Distribution Fluid	Thermal Cycle	Diagram (Heating / Cooling / Heating and Cooling)
Air	Air	Refrigerant changeover	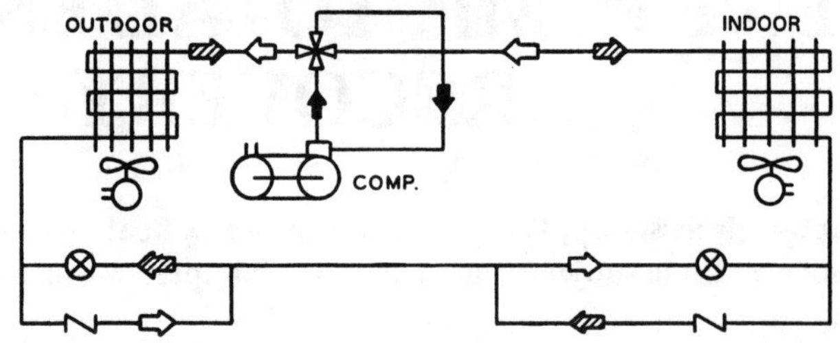
Water	Air	Refrigerant changeover	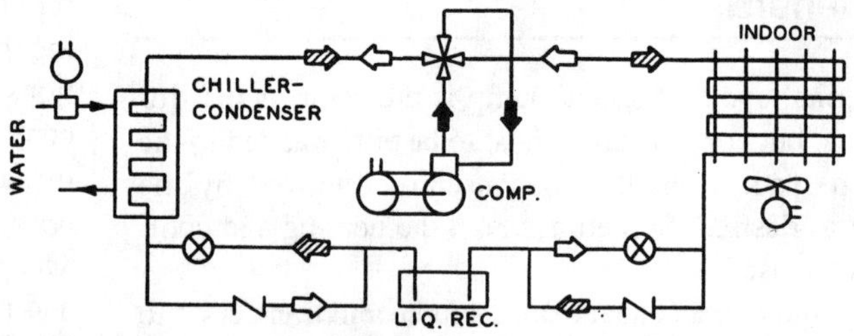
Water	Water	Water changeover	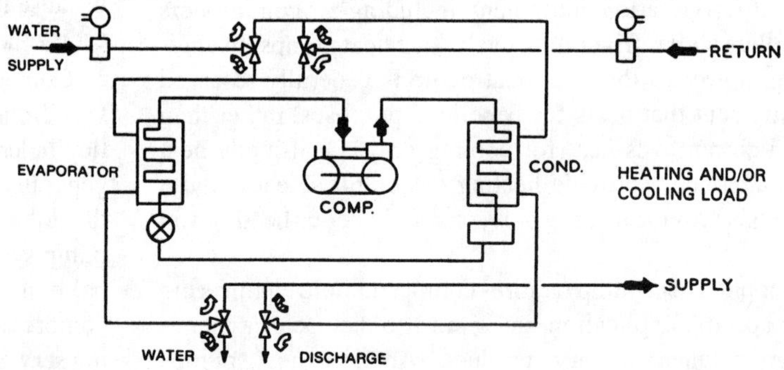
Ground-coupled (or Closed-loop ground-source)	Air	Refrigerant changeover	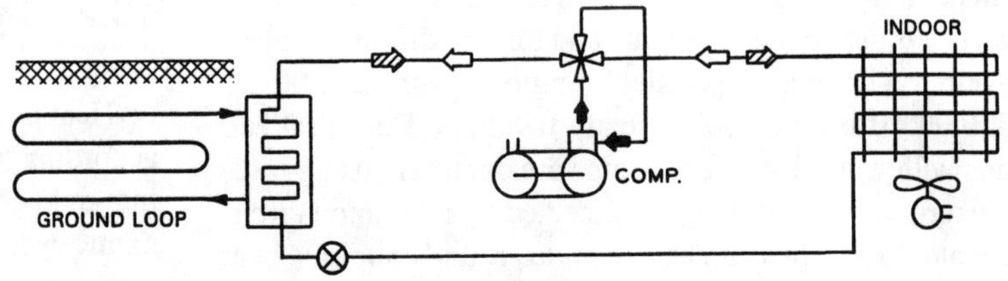
Ground-source, Direct-expansion	Air	Refrigerant changeover	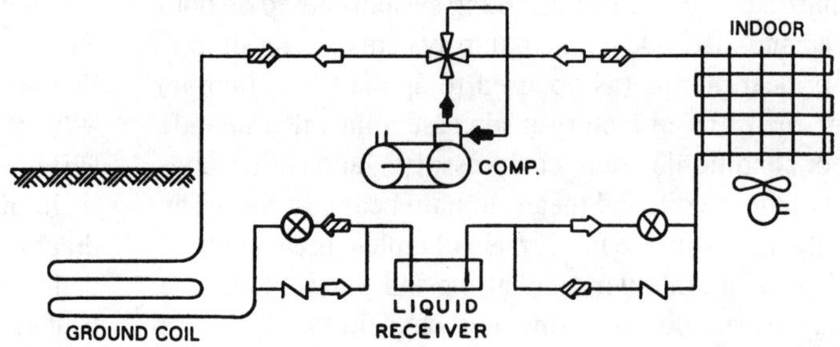

denser. The conditioned air passes over the evaporator during the cooling cycle and the outdoor air passes over the condenser. The change from cooling to heating is accomplished by positioning the dampers.

A water-to-air heat pump uses water as a heat source and sink, and air transfers heat to or from the conditioned space (Table 16-1). Air-to-water heat pumps are commonly used in large buildings where zone control is necessary. They are also sometimes used in industrial applications to produce hot or cold water.

Earth-to-air heat pumps may use direct expansion of the refrigerant in an embedded coil (Table 16-1), or they may be of the indirect type.

A water-to-water heat pump uses water as the heat source and sink for both cooling and heating operation. Heating and cooling may be changed over in the refrigerant circuit, but, in many cases, it is more convenient to perform the switching in the water circuits (Table 16-1).

An earth-to-water heat pump is similar to the earth-to-air heat pump, except a refrigerant-water heat exchanger is substituted for the finned coil. It may also be similar to the water-to-water system when a secondary-fluid ground coil is used.

Internal source heat pumps use the heat generated from the cooling load in modern buildings directly for heating or store it for later use.

Some heat pumps that use earth as the heat source and sink are essentially of the water-to-air type. An antifreeze solution is pumped through a circuit consisting of the chiller-condenser and a pipe coil embedded in the earth. Earth source and sink systems are seldom used today.

Other types of heat pumps are possible. An example is one that uses solar energy as a source of heat; its refrigerant circuit may resemble the water-to-air, air-to-air, or other types.

Another variation is the use of more than one heat source. Some heat pumps use air as the primary heat source, but are changed over to extract heat from water (e.g., from a well or storage tank) during periods of peak load. Heat pumps that use solar energy require another heat source during periods of insufficient solar radiation.

Theoretically, any thermodynamic cycle capable of producing a cooling effect may be used as a heat pump. Other than the ordinary vapor-compression cycle, possible cycles include (a) the heat-operated absorption cycle; (b) the ejector cycle; (c) gas cycles— both open and closed; and (d) the thermoelectric cycle.

16.3 Heat Sources and Sinks

The principal media used with heat pumps as a heat source for heating and as a heat sink for cooling are shown in Table 16-1. The choice for a particular application is primarily influenced by geographic location, climatic conditions, initial cost, availability, and the type of structure. Factors to consider for each source are given in Table 16-2.

Air. Outdoor air may be used as a universal heat source or heat sink for the heat pump. Extended-surface, forced convection heat-transfer coils normally transfer heat between the air and the refrigerant. Typically, these surfaces are 50 to 100% larger than the corresponding surface on the indoor side of heat pumps using air as the distributive medium. The volume of outdoor air handled is usually greater in about the same proportions. When operated as a heater, the temperature difference between the outdoor air and the evaporating refrigerant is generally about 10 to 25°F (5 to 15°C).

When selecting or designing an air-source heat pump, two factors must be considered: (1) temperature variation experienced in a given locality and (2) frost formation.

As the outdoor temperature decreases, the heating capacity of an air-source heat pump decreases. Therefore, selecting equipment for a given outdoor heating design temperature is more critical than for a fuel-fired system. Consequently, the equipment must be sized for as low a balance temperature as is practicable for heating without having excess cooling capacity during the summer periods.

Early air-source heat pumps had wide fin spacing of 4 to 5 fins/in. (5 to 6 mm between fins). However, 8 to 13 fins/in. (2 to 3 mm between fins) is now used.

Water. Water may be a satisfactory, and in many cases an ideal, heat source, subject to the considerations listed in Table 16-2. Well water is particularly attractive because of its relatively high and nearly constant temperature [generally about 50°F (10°C) in northern areas and 60°F (15°C) and higher in the south]. However, sources of suitable water are becoming increasingly scarce and the application of this type of system is rather limited. Frequently, sufficient water may be available from wells, but the condition of the water often causes either corrosion in heat exchangers or induces scale formation. Other considerations are a means for disposal of used water, and the drilling, piping, and pumping costs.

Surface or stream water may be used, but under reduced winter temperatures, the cooling spread between inlet and outlet must be limited to prevent freeze-up in the water chiller that is absorbing the heat. Some large heat pump systems in Europe operate in areas where winter stream temperatures of about 35°F (2°C) permit inlet-outlet temperature spreads of only 1 or 2°F (0.5 or 1°C).

Under certain industrial circumstances, waste process water, such as spent warm water in laundries and warm condenser water, may be a source for special heat pump operations.

Water use for cooling generally follows conventional practice with water-cooled condensers.

Water-refrigerant heat exchangers are usually direct-expansion water coolers, either of the shell-and-coil type or of the shell-and-tube type. They are circuited for use as a refrigerant condenser during the heating cycle and as a refrigerant evaporator during the cooling cycle.

Earth. Earth as a heat source and sink, by heat transfer through buried coils, has not been used extensively, possibly due to high installation expense, ground area requirements, and the difficulty and uncertainty of predicting performance.

Table 16-2 Heat Pump Sources and Sinks

(Table 1, Chapter 8, 1996 *ASHRAE Handbook—Systems and Equipment*)

		Suitability		Availability		Cost		Temperature		Common Practice	
Medium	**Examples**	**Heat Source**	**Heat Sink**	**Location Relative to Need**	**Coincidence with Need**	**Installed**	**Operation and Maintenance**	**Level**	**Variation**	**Use**	**Limitations**
AIR											
Outdoor	Ambient air	Good, but efficiency and capacity in heating mode decrease with decreasing outdoor air temperature	Good, but efficiency and capacity in cooling mode decrease with increasing outdoor air temperature	Universal	Continuous	Low	Moderate	Variable	Generally extreme	Most common, many standard products	Defrosting and supplemental heat usually required
Exhaust	Building ventilation	Excellent	Fair	Excellent if planned for in building design	Excellent	Low to moderate	Low unless exhaust is laden with dirt or grease	Excellent	Very low	Excellent as energy-conservation measure	Insufficient for typical loads
WATER											
Well[a]	Ground-water well may also provide a potable water source	Excellent	Excellent	Poor to excellent, practical depth varies by location	Continuous	Low if existing well used or shallow wells suitable; can be high otherwise	Low, but periodic maintenance required	Generally excellent, varies by location	Extremely stable	Common	Water disposal and required permits may limit; may require double-wall exchangers; may foul or scale
Surface	Lakes, rivers, oceans	Excellent for large water bodies or high flow rates	Excellent for large water bodies or high flow rates	Limited, depends on proximity	Usually continuous	Depends on proximity and water quality	Depends on proximity and water quality	Usually satisfactory	Depends on source	Available, particularly for fresh water	Often regulated or prohibited; may clog, foul, or scale
Tap (city)	Municipal water supply	Excellent	Excellent	Excellent	Continuous	Low	Low energy cost, but water use and disposal may be costly	Excellent	Usually very low	Use is decreasing due to regulations	Use or disposal may be regulated or prohibited; may corrode or scale
Condens-ing	Cooling towers, re-frigeration systems	Excellent	Poor to good	Varies	Varies with cooling loads	Usually low	Moderate	Favorable as heat source	Depends on source	Available	Suitable only if heating need is coincident with heat rejection
Closed loops	Building water-loop heat pump systems	Good, loop may need supplemental heat	Favorable, may need loop heat rejection	Excellent if designed as such	As needed	Low	Low to moderate	As designed	As designed	Very common	Most suitable for medium or large buildings
Waste	Raw or treated sewage, gray water	Fair to excellent	Fair, varies with source	Varies	Varies, may be adequate	Depends on proximity, high for raw sewage	Varies, may be high for raw sewage	Excellent	Usually low	Uncommon, practical only in large systems	Usually regulated; may clog, foul, scale, or corrode
GROUND[a]											
Ground-coupled	Buried or submerged fluid loops	Good if ground is moist, other-wise poor	Fair to good if ground is moist, other-wise poor	Depends on soil suitability	Continuous	High to moderate	Low	Usually good	Low, particularly for vertical systems	Rapidly increasing	High initial costs for ground loop
Direct-expan-sion	Refrig-erant circulated in ground coil	Varies with soil conditions	Varies with soil conditions	Varies with soil conditions	Continuous	High	High	Varies by design	Generally low	Extremely limited	Leak repair very expensive; requires large refrigerant quantities
SOLAR ENERGY											
Direct or heated water	Solar collectors and panels	Fair	Poor, usually un-acceptable	Universal	Highly intermittent, night use requires storage	Extremely high	Moderate to high	Varies	Extreme	Very limited	Supplemental source or storage required
INDUSTRIAL PROCESS											
Process heat or exhaust	Distilla-tion, molding, refining, washing, drying	Fair to excellent	Varies, often impractical	Varies	Varies	Varies	Generally low	Varies	Varies	Varies	May be costly unless heat need is near rejected source

[a]Groundwater-source heat pumps are also considered ground-source heat pump systems.

Soil composition, which varies from wet clay to sandy soil, has a predominant effect on thermal properties and attendant overall performance. Heat transfers through the soil primarily by bulk temperature change with time (e.g., transient heat flow). Thermal diffusivity—the ratio of thermal conductivity to the product of unit density and specific heat—is a dominant factor and is difficult to determine at different building sites. Likewise, moisture content has an influence, since moisture movement may transport energy through the soil.

Earth coils are usually horizontally spaced 3 to 6 ft (0.9 to 1.8 m) apart and are submerged 3 to 6 ft (0.9 to 1.8 m) below the surface. Though a lower depth might be preferred, excavation cost requires a compromise. Mean undisturbed ground temperatures generally follow the mean annual climatic temperature for any location.

Solar. Although still largely in the research stage, solar energy as a heat source, either on a primary basis or in combination with other sources, attracts interest. The principal advantage of solar radiation is that, when available, it provides heat at a higher temperature level than other sources, thus giving an increased coefficient of performance. As compared to a solar heating system without a heat pump, the collector efficiency and capacity are materially increased due to the lower collector temperature required.

Research and development in the use of solar energy for heat pump operation has been concerned with both direct and indirect systems. In the **direct system**, refrigerant evaporator tubes are incorporated in a solar collector, usually of the flat-plate type. When the collector has no glass cover plates, the same collector surface extracts heat from the outdoor air. The same surface may act as a condenser using outdoor air as a heat sink for cooling. The refrigeration circuit may resemble that shown in Table 16-1 for an earth-to-air heat pump.

An **indirect system** uses either water or air, which is circulated through the solar collector. The first system shown in Table 16-1 for an air-to-air heat pump is an example of an indirect system. The collector is added such that (1) it can serve as an outdoor-air preheater, (2) the outdoor-air loop can be closed so that all source heat is derived from the sun, or (3) the collector may be disconnected and the outdoor air used as the source or sink. When water is circulated through the collector, the heat pump circuit may be of either the water-to-air or water-to-water type illustrated in Table 16-1.

All heat pump systems that use solar energy as the only heat source require an alternate heating system or a means of storing heat during periods of insufficient solar radiation.

16.4 Total Energy Concept

Total energy designates on-site electrical generating systems that salvage byproduct or waste heat from the generating process. The magnitude, duration, and coincidence of electrical and thermal loads must be analyzed, and prime movers and waste heat recovery systems must be selected to determine system feasibility and design. The basic components of the total energy plant are (1) prime movers, (2) generators, (3) waste heat recovery systems, (4) control systems, and (5) connections to building mechanical and electrical services.

The normal prime movers are reciprocating internal combustion engines, combustion gas turbines, expansion turbines, and steam boiler-turbine combinations. These units transfer fuel (liquid, solid, gaseous, or nuclear) into rotating shaft energy.

Use of the prime mover heat determines overall system efficiency and is one of the critical factors of economic feasibility. Two kinds of energy are available from the prime mover: (1) mechanical energy from the shaft and (2) unused heat energy remaining after the fuel or steam has acted on the shaft.

Shaft loads (generators, centrifugal chillers, compressors, process equipment) require a given amount of rotating mechanical energy. Once the prime mover has been selected to provide the required shaft output, it has a fixed relationship to system efficiency, that is dependent upon the prime mover fuel versus load and the load versus heat balance curves.

Steam turbine drives can be arranged to extract steam at intermediate turbine stages. The waste heat value of a steam turbine is the enthalpy of the steam at the point it is extracted from the turbine or at the turbine's exhaust outlet. This steam, reduced in pressure and temperature by the amount of shaft work, is fed to heat exchange equipment, absorption chillers, and steam turbine driven centrifugal chillers.

The gas turbine cycle has a thermal efficiency of approximately 20 to 30%, with the remainder of the fuel energy exhausted or radiated. A minimum exhaust temperature of approximately 300°F (150°C) is required to prevent condensation. The recoverable heat per unit of power is greater for a gas turbine than for a reciprocating engine because of the larger exhaust flow. The net result is an increase in overall thermal efficiency to approximately 60% and up. Because gas turbine exhaust contains a large percentage of excess air, afterburners or boost burners may be installed in the exhaust to create a supplementary boiler system. This system can provide additional steam or level the steam production during reduced turbine loads. Boost burning can further increase cycle efficiency to a maximum of 93%. Figure 16-1 illustrates a gas turbine heat recovery system.

In all reciprocating internal combustion engines except small air-cooled units, heat can be reclaimed from the lubricating system, jacket cooling water system, and the exhaust.

Coolant fluids and lubricating oil are generally circulated to remove excess heat conducted into the power train during combustion and heat from friction. Some engines are constructed to convert cooling water to steam within the engine.

The approximate distribution of input fuel energy is as follows:

Useful work	33%
Friction and radiation	7%
Rejected in jacket water	30%
Rejected in exhaust	30%

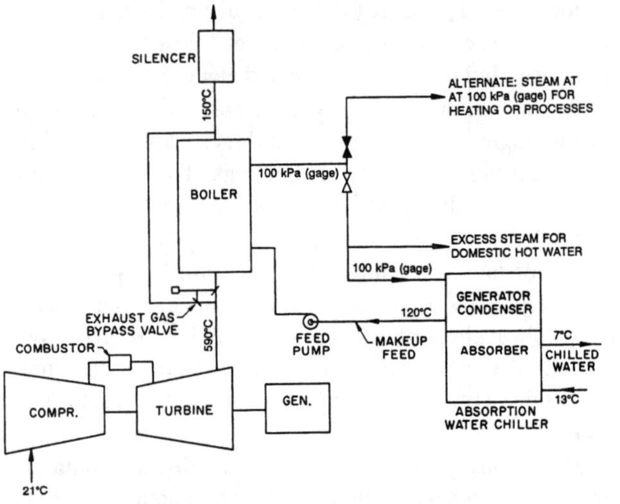

Fig. 16-1 Typical Heat Recovery Cycle for Gas Turbine

Depending on engine design, these amounts vary. However, they do indicate that overall cycle thermal efficiency can be greatly improved by waste heat recovery systems.

Example 16.1. A 200 kW internal combustion engine power unit produces 2570 lb/h of exhaust gas at 950°F. The exhaust gas mixture has a specific heat of 0.252 Btu/lb·°F. Energy in the exhaust gas is to be used in a waste heat boiler to produce dry saturated steam at 280°F from water supplied at 60°F. The exhaust gas is cooled during the process from 950°F to 400°F. Determine the quantity of steam that can be produced, lb/h.

Solution:

From Table 2.1, Thermodynamic Properties of Water:

$$h_g \text{ (at 280°F)} = 1173.94 \text{ Btu/lb}$$

$$h_f \text{ (at 60°F)} = 28.07 \text{ Btu/lb}$$

Equating the heat transfer rate from the exhaust gas to that for the water/steam, yields:

$$m_g c_p (t_{g,in} - t_{g,out}) = m_s(h_g - h_f)$$

$$2570(0.252)(950 - 400) = m_s(1173.4 - 28.07)$$

$$m_s = 311 \text{ lb/h}$$

16.5 Heat Recovery Terminology and Concepts

The following definitions serve as an introduction to heat recovery systems.

Internal heat is the total heat generated in a conditioned space from any normal source plus heat added by mechanical work done in the system (such as fan and pump gains and heat of compression).

External heat is heat added from sources outside the system (such as boilers, electric heaters, and gas heaters) to supplement the internal heat in the conditioned space to maintain space temperature.

Breakeven temperature t_{be} is the outdoor temperature at which heat losses from the conditioned space equal the internal heat.

Artificial breakeven temperature is the outdoor temperature at which heat losses from the conditioned space equal the internal heat plus any external heat added above t_{be}.

Recovered heat is that portion of internal heat used to overcome heat losses from the conditioned space to the extent of the recovery capacity of the system.

A **wide range coil** is a coil where the water range for both heating and cooling is substantially more than the 10 to 15°F (5 to 8°C) normally used and is about 20 to 30°F (11 to 17°C) in the cooling cycle.

Balanced heat recovery pertains to the functions of reclaiming internal building heat, raising the temperature to a usable level, and redistributing this energy to the required locations in the proper amounts. Heat shall be generated only if there is an insufficient amount of reclaimed heat to serve those areas needing heat. Each of these functions warrants detailed consideration to determine the overall effect of the entire system.

A **balanced system** is one in which all of the components work together year-round to use all internal heat before adding additional heat. When internal heat exceeds the project requirements, the excess heat is automatically rejected.

When the outdoor temperature drops sufficiently, the internal heat may be insufficient to supply the project requirements. Also, on nights and weekends, the building may be shut down with little or no internal heat available. Under these circumstances, a balanced system must provide heat from an external source.

When, for any reason, the internal heat recurs, the external source heat must be automatically reduced to equal only the instantaneous difference between the total required and the recovered internal heat.

An **unbalanced heat recovery system** is one in which part or all of the excess internal heat is transferred by the equipment without providing instantaneous balance.

It is relatively easy to transfer excess heat within a project. For example, air heated or cooled by exhaust air from parts of the system may produce economies at certain times of the year and cause penalties at other times. Heat recovered from exhaust air may add heat to a project that already has more heat than can be used at an outdoor temperature higher than the breakeven temperature t_{be}. At a lower outdoor temperature, the added heat from exhaust air provides all or part of the supplementary heat required.

In large internal space projects, a substantial amount of heat is available for recovery and must be removed year-round. This heat can be a source of heat for the perimeter conduction losses and can be used to heat the outdoor ventilating air at low outdoor temperatures. But, as the outdoor temperature drops, more heat is needed for the perimeter conduction losses.

The usable temperature range for heat recovery from the centrifugal compressor condensers and absorption equipment is limited for presently offered standard equipment. A system should use standard equipment for heat recovery because it is less costly to use the same equipment that supplies cooling during the summer without expensive additional equipment.

Heat recovery must be properly analyzed to avoid pitfalls. For example, if the quantity of recovered heat must be supplemented by using external high-temperature heat for the periphery or for reheat, the total recovered heat plus the necessarily added external heat may exceed the instantaneous project requirements. When this happens, part of the surplus heat, including the recovered heat, must be rejected, or some part of the building will overheat. It is uneconomical to remove heat while supplying heat from an external source.

Generally, recovered and external heat are mixed in the return air. An unbalanced heat recovery system can waste heat intended for recovery, the end result being that more and more external heat must be added. For example, raising temperatures by adding perimeter external heat in the conditioned spaces, may cause an economizer control to extend itself to its limit of 100% outdoor air, causing more external heat to be added to overcooled interior spaces and internal heat to be exhausted.

Unbalanced heat recovery systems can defeat the purpose they are intended to correct. Their performance may be no better than conventional systems that do not attempt to transfer internally recovered heat.

16.6 Balanced Heat Recovery Analysis

Heat balance involves the amount of heat either added to or removed from the overall project at any ambient temperature and building condition. The benefits of balanced heat recovery often exceed the operating economies of reduced heating costs. Possibly the greatest advantage is the ability to solve between-season problems. Additionally, properly applying heat recovery fundamentals may save valuable space in the building and, in many cases, capital costs may also be reduced. Savings in heating equipment and between-season cooling apparatus and controls may offset the initial costs of any additional equipment required to reclaim and redistribute otherwise wasted heat.

Regardless of the system being considered, a heat balance analysis establishes the relative merits of balanced heat recovery at various outdoor temperatures. Penalties can also be determined if heat recovery is omitted.

Outdoor air is often used for low-cost cooling when the outdoor temperature is low enough, notably about 55°F (13°C). However, if this cooling is controlled from a local room or duct thermostat, excess outdoor air may automatically enter and may remove internal heat, and heat introduced elsewhere to satisfy another thermostat. Under these circumstances, any system, whether or not it is intended to include heat recovery, can be very expensive to operate.

Heat Redistribution Within a Project. Many air-conditioned buildings, especially those with large interior areas, have more heat generated within the overall project than can be used for most of the year. The outdoor temperature at which the internal heat is equal to the various heat losses is the breakeven temperature t_{be}. The t_{be} may be calculated as soon as heat loads can be estimated.

In practice, the actual t_{be} and the calculated t_{be} may not be the same. The t_{be} shifts if heat is added to or is rejected from the overall system. Minimum operating cost can be obtained when the system is operating under natural t_{be} conditions, for example, if gains equal losses, the cost of energy for heating or cooling can reach the lowest value. A much higher operating cost can result if an artificial t_{be} is created by adding or removing heat unnecessarily. The operating costs are increased by simultaneously incurring greater heating costs, which create a need for greater cooling costs.

Optimum equipment and system selections are frequently discovered only after analysis of heat balance and its effect on system operation. Fuel or electric power costs may, in themselves, not be the dominant factor regarding operating costs until a choice is made at the proper t_{be}. Equipment that substantially lowers the t_{be} may result in higher operating costs than equipment that has higher fuel or power costs.

Heat Balance Concept. An overall building project or single space must adhere to the heat balance concept, which requires that one of the following takes place on demand: (1) heat must be removed; (2) heat must be added; or (3) heat generated must exactly balance the heat required, in which case, no heat should be either added or removed.

Small air-conditioning projects serving only one space must supply either cooling or heating to satisfy thermostat demands. If humidity control is not needed, the problem is simple. Assuming that heating and cooling are both available, the thermostat may call for the automatic controls to furnish either. A system should not furnish both heating and cooling simultaneously to the same space.

Multiroom buildings often require heating in some rooms and cooling in others. Good design considers the building as a whole and transfers excess internal heat from one area to another area as required. The heat balance concept is violated when this occurs.

A system must maintain the desired temperature and humidity without adding or removing more heat than necessary. Large amounts of outdoor air with high wet-bulb temperatures, as well as certain types of humidity control, may require adding reheat, which could upset the desirable heat balance. In general, humidity control can be obtained without upsetting the balance. When reheat is completely unavoidable, internally transferred heat can always be used to the extent available from the refrigeration plant before using heat from an externally generated source, such as a boiler. As it affects the heat balance and may have to be treated as a variable internal load, the effect of the added reheat must be analyzed.

In general, when a building needs heat and the refrigeration plant is not in use, the outdoor air is sufficiently dry so that the ventilating air can handle internal moisture requirements and dehumidification is not required. This situation is often true for occupancies of a maximum of one person per 75 ft^2 (7 m^2) and without other internal latent loads, but it should be reviewed for each design. Various types of air distribution and distributing equipment, including variable air volume systems, can be used to satisfy temperature and humidity requirements of different projects with normal outdoor air proportions and without using reheat.

The methods of analysis that follow are intended to predict and correct the undesirable situations that sometimes occur in nonrecovery and unbalanced heat recovery systems.

Heat Balance Studies. Three graphs of the major components comprising the total air-conditioning load of a building are shown in Figure 16-2. These components are plotted above and below a zero line and indicate how they vary in response to outdoor temperature. Values above the zero line are cooling loads; values below the zero line are heating loads.

Note that on an individual basis, the ventilation and conduction loads cross the zero line. This indicates that, depending on the outdoor temperature, these loads can be a heating or a cooling load. The solar load and internal loads comprising lights, people, and equipment are always a cooling load and are, therefore, plotted above the zero line.

Figure 16-3 is a graph that combines all of the loads shown in Figure 16-2. The graph is obtained by plotting the conduction load of a building at various outdoor temperatures and then adding or subtracting the various other loads at each temperature. The project load lines with and without solar effect cross the zero line at 16 and 30°F (−9 and −1°C), respectively. These are the outdoor temperatures for the plotted conditions when the naturally created internal load exactly balances the losses.

As plotted, this heat balance diagram includes only the building loads; no allowance has been made for additional external heat from a boiler or from other components. If, because of system design, external heat is necessary, the heat balance diagram should be changed to include the additional heat.

A case when heat recovery is not considered is illustrated in Figure 16-4. Here, it is assumed that at some temperature, shown as 70°F (21°C) in this case, heat is added from an external source to balance the perimeter loss in increasing amounts down to the minimum outdoor temperature winter design condition.

Also shown in Figure 16-4 is the heat required for the peripheral zone ventilation. The outdoor air that makes up part or all of the supply air must be heated to room temperature. Thus, only the temperature range above the room temperature is effective for heating to balance the perimeter conduction loss.

At the minimum outdoor winter design temperature, these two loads are plotted in a new line ADE. When the solar effect is not considered, this line crosses the zero line at −35°F (−37°C), which becomes the artificially created breakeven temperature rather than +30°F. When the sun shines, the added solar heat at the minimum design temperature further lowers the −35°F (−37°C) breakeven temperature.

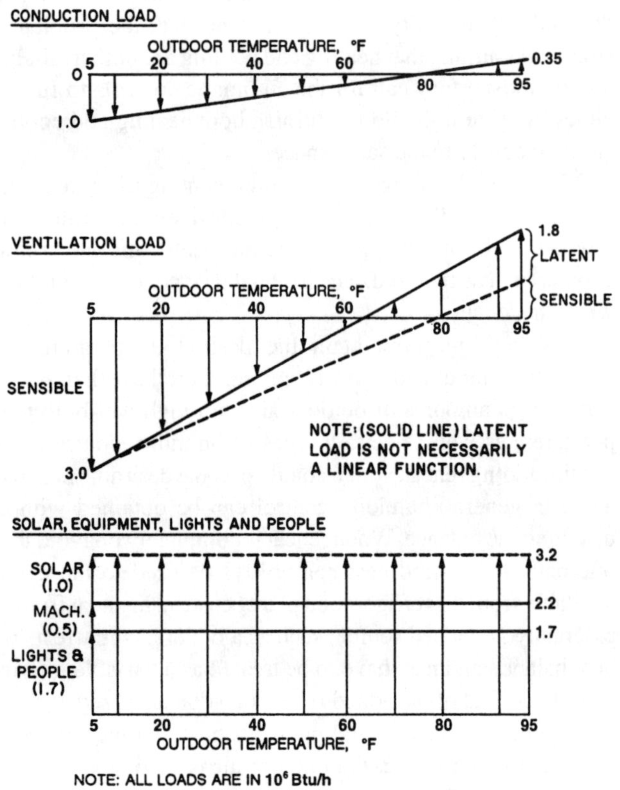

Fig. 16-2 Major Load Components

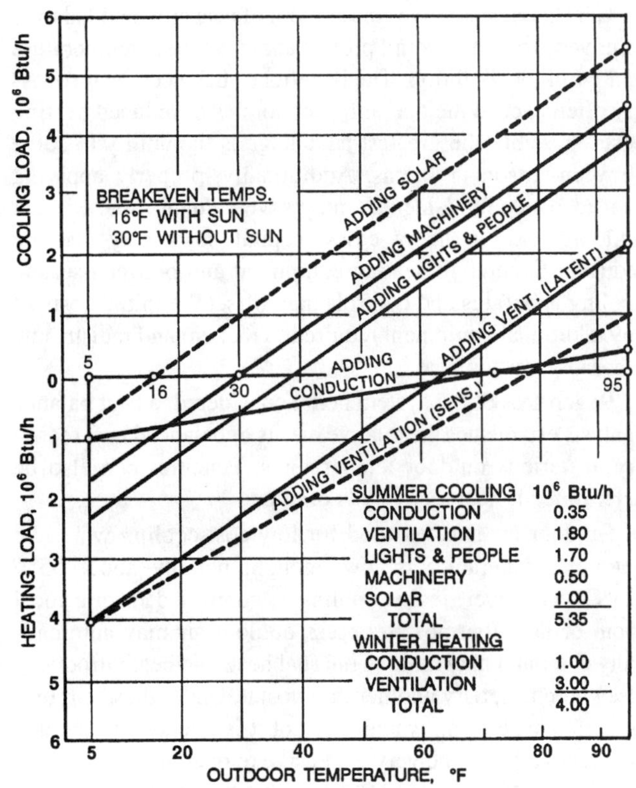

Fig. 16-3 Composite Plot of Loads in Fig. 16-2

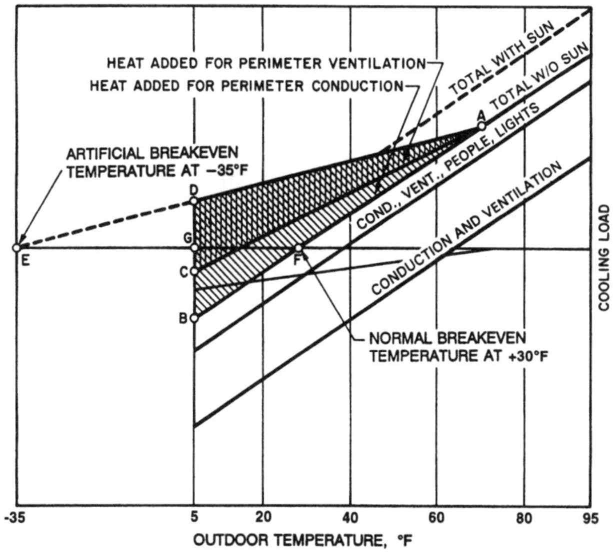

Fig. 16-4 Nonheat Recovery System

Such a design adds more heat than the overall project requires and does not use a balanced heat recovery system to use the available internal heat. This problem is most evident during mild weather with systems not designed for year-round operation.

16.7 Heat Recovery Systems

Figures 16-5 through 16-9 show several possible heat recovery/simultaneous heating cooling systems. Figure 16-5 illustrates one method of using water as the heat source or sink and as the heating and cooling medium. The compressor, evaporator, condenser, refrigerant piping, and accessories are essentially standard and are available as a factory-packaged water-to-water heat pump.

The cycle is flexible, and the heating or cooling medium is instantly available at all times. Heating can be provided exclusively to the zone conditioners by closing valves 2 and 3 and opening valves 1 and 4. With the valves in these positions, the water is divided into two separate circuits. The warm water circuit consists of the condenser (where the heat is supplied by the high-temperature refrigerant), valve 1, zone conditioners, and a circulating pump. The cold water circuit consists of the evaporator (where heat is taken from the water by the low-temperature refrigerant), valve 4, a heat exchanger (where heat is taken from the source water), valve 1, and a circulating pump. The refrigerating compressor operates to maintain the desired leaving water temperature from the condenser.

Similarly, cooling can be exclusively obtained in the cycle of Figure 16-5 by opening valves 2 and 3 and closing valves 1 and 4. With this arrangement, the cold water circuit consists of the evaporator (where heat is removed from the water by the low-temperature refrigerant), valve 2, zone conditioners, and a circulating pump. The warm water circuit consists of the condenser (which receives the heat from the refrigerant), valve 3, a heat exchanger (where heat is rejected to the source

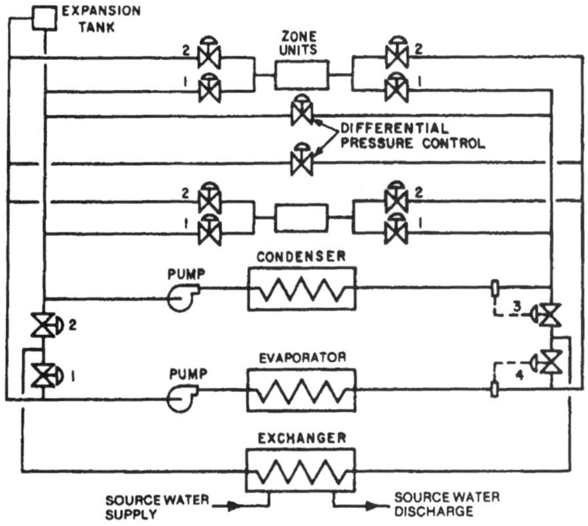

Fig. 16-5 Water-to-Water Heat Pump Cycle

water), valve 2, and a circulating pump. The refrigerating compressor operates to maintain the desired water temperature leaving the evaporator.

During the intermediate season, simultaneous heating and cooling can be provided by the cycle shown in Figure 16-5. Valves 3 and 4 are modulated when valves 1 and 2 are open. Valve 3 is adjusted to maintain 85 to 140°F (29° to 60°C) water in the condenser circuit and valve 4 to maintain 45 to 50°F (7° to 10°C) in the evaporator circuit. The excess heating or cooling effect is discharged to the exchanger, which passes it on to the source water.

The source or sink water, if of suitable quality, can be supplied directly to the condenser and evaporator instead of using an exchanger (Figure 16-5). This eliminates one heat transfer surface and its performance penalty.

A water loop heat pump (WLHP) cycle that combines load transfer characteristics with water-to-air heat pump units is illustrated in Figure 16-6. Each module or space has one or more water-to-air heat pumps. The units in both the building core and perimeter areas are connected hydronically with a common two-pipe system. Each unit cools conventionally, supplying air to the individual module and rejecting the heat removed to the two-pipe system through its integral condenser. The total heat gathered by the two-pipe system is expelled through a common heat rejection device. This device often includes a closed circuit evaporative cooler with an integral spray pump. If and when some of the modules, particularly on the northern side, require heat, the individual units switch (by means of four-way refrigerant valves) into the heating cycle. The units derive their heat source from the two-pipe water loop, basically obtaining heat from a relatively high source, that is, the condenser water of the other units. When only heating is required, all units are in the heating cycle and, consequently, an external heat input source is needed to provide 100% heating capability. The heat of compression should be considered in heat source sizing. The water loop is usually 60 to 90°F (15° to 32°C) and, therefore, seldom requires piping insulation.

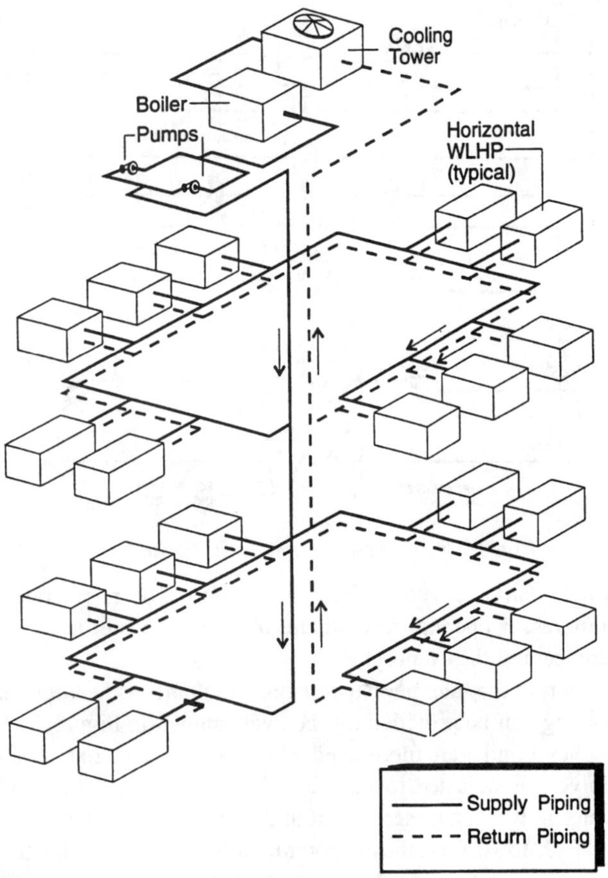

Fig. 16-6 Heat Recovery System Using Water-to-Air Heat Pump in Closed Loop

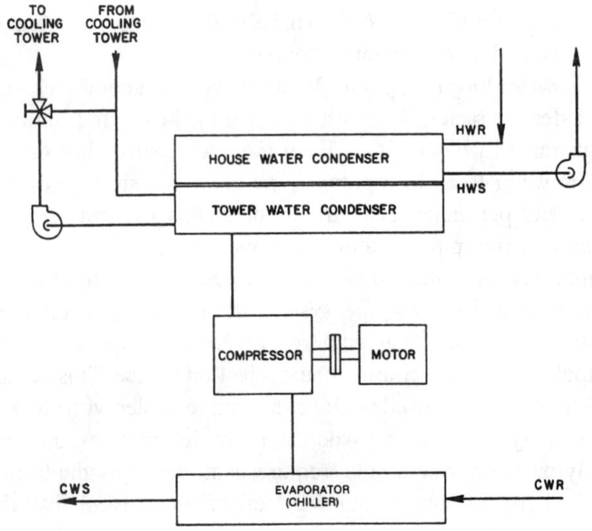

Fig. 16-7 Heat Transfer Heat Pump with Double Bundle Condenser

A water-to-water heat pump can be added in the closed water loop before the heat rejection device for further heat reclaim. This heat pump reuses the heat and provides domestic hot water or elevates water temperatures in a storage tank to be bled back into the loop.

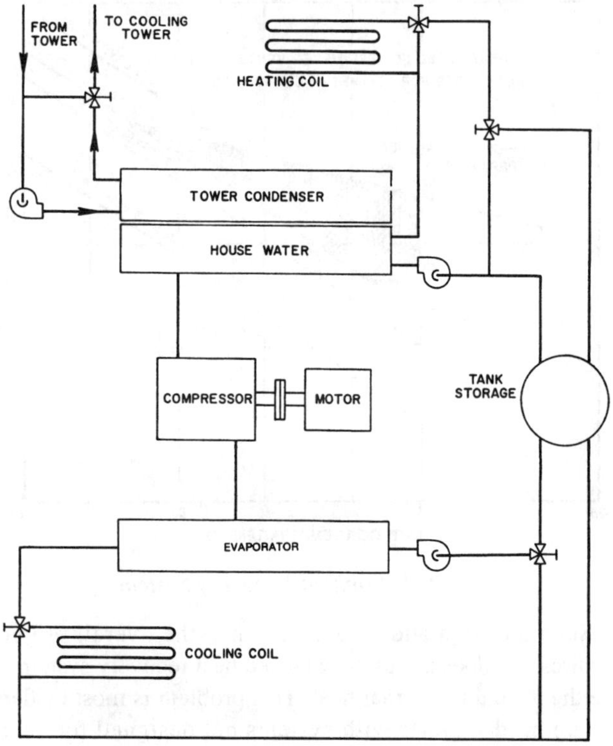

Fig. 16-8 Heat Transfer System with Storage Tank

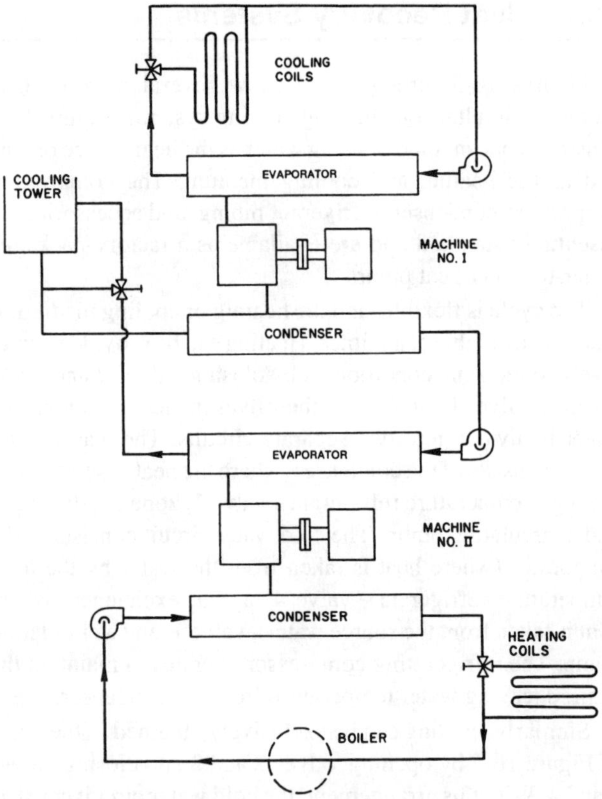

Fig. 16-9 Multistage (Cascade) Heat Transfer System

In many large buildings, internal heat gains require year-round chiller operation. This internal heat is often discharged through a cooling tower. Prudent design may dictate cascade systems with chillers in parallel or series. Manufacturers can assist with custom components to meet a wide range of load and temperature requirements. The double-bundle condenser working with a reciprocating or centrifugal compressor is most often used in this application. Figure 16-7 shows the basic configuration of this system, which makes heat available in the range of 100 to 130°F (38° to 54°C). The warm water is supplied as a secondary function of the heat pump and represents recovered heat.

Figure 16-8 shows a similar cycle, except that a storage tank has been added, enabling the system to store heat during occupied hours by raising the temperature of the water in the tank. During unoccupied hours, water from the tank is gradually fed to the evaporator providing load for the compressor and condenser that heats the building during off hours.

Figure 16-9 is another transfer system capable of generating 130 to 140°F (54° to 60°C) or warmer water whenever there is a cooling load by cascading two compressors hydronically. In this configuration, one chiller can be considered as a chiller only and the second unit as a heating. only heat pump.

16.8 Problems

16.1 A heat pump is used in place of a furnace for heating a house. In winter, when the outside air temperature is −10°C, the heat loss from the house is 200 kW if the inside is maintained at 21°C. Determine the minimum electric power required to operate the heat pump.

16.2 A solar powered heat pump is designed to operate as shown in the accompany diagram. Solar energy is used as the heat source for the boiler in a Rankine power system operating with R-22 as the working fluid. The turbine output drives the compressor in a regular R-12 heat pump system. For the conditions shown, find the minimum square footage of solar collectors if the heat loss from the house is 45,000 Btu/h.

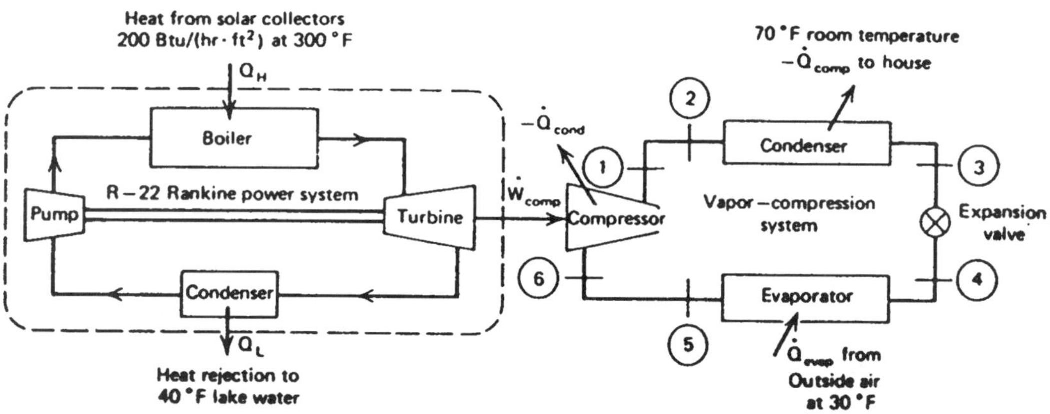

Diagram for Problem 16.2

16.3 A heat pump is to be used for both air conditioning and heating a small office building, maintaining the interior at 75°F all year long. In summer, when the outside air temperature is 96°F, the heat gain by the building is 360,000 Btu/h. In winter, when the outside air temperature is 4°F, the heat loss by the office building is 520,000 Btu/h. If the heat pump is sized for cooling, determine the minimum amount of auxiliary heating (Btu/h and kW) needed for the 4°F winter condition.

16.4 A building located in Rochester, New York is shown in the accompanying sketch. Size the heat pump and estimate the annual energy requirements for heating and cooling. There is no humidifier.

Walls and roof: 3 in. of glass fiberboard, organically bonded, sandwiched between metal sheets

Floor: Concrete slab on ground with edge-only insulation, R = 2.50 °F· ft^2· h/Btu

Doors: 2-in. thick, solid wood

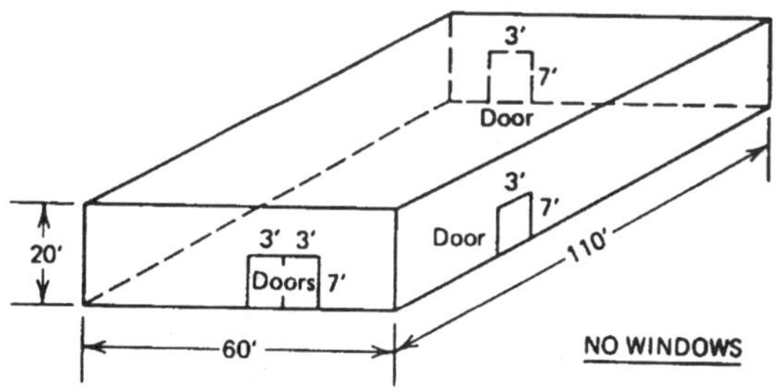

Sketch for Problem 16.4

16.9 Bibliography

Anantapantula, V. S. and H. J. Sauer, Jr. 1994. "Heat Recovery and the Economizer for HVAC Systems," *ASHRAE Journal*, pp. 48-53, November.

ASHRAE. 1996. *Practical Guide to Cool Storage Projects*, ASHRAE, Atlanta, GA

ASHRAE. 1995. Commercial/Institutional Ground-Source Heat Pump Engineering Manual, ASHRAE, Atlanta, GA

Dorgan, C. E. and J. S. Elleson. 1993. *Design Guide for Cool Thermal Storage*, ASHRAE, Atlanta, GA

Orlando, J. 1996. *Cogeneration Design Guide*, ASHRAE, Atlanta, GA

Sauer, H. J., Jr. and R. H. Howell. 1988. "Design Guidelines for Use of an Economizer with Heat Recovery," *ASHRAE Transactions*, V. 94, Pt. 2.

SI Figures

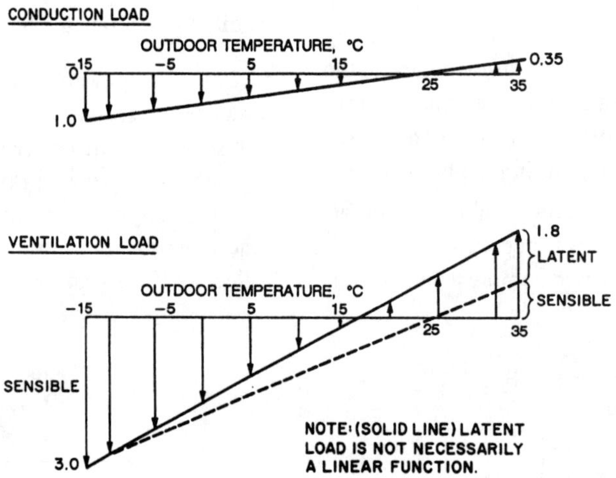

Fig. 16-2 SI Major Load Components

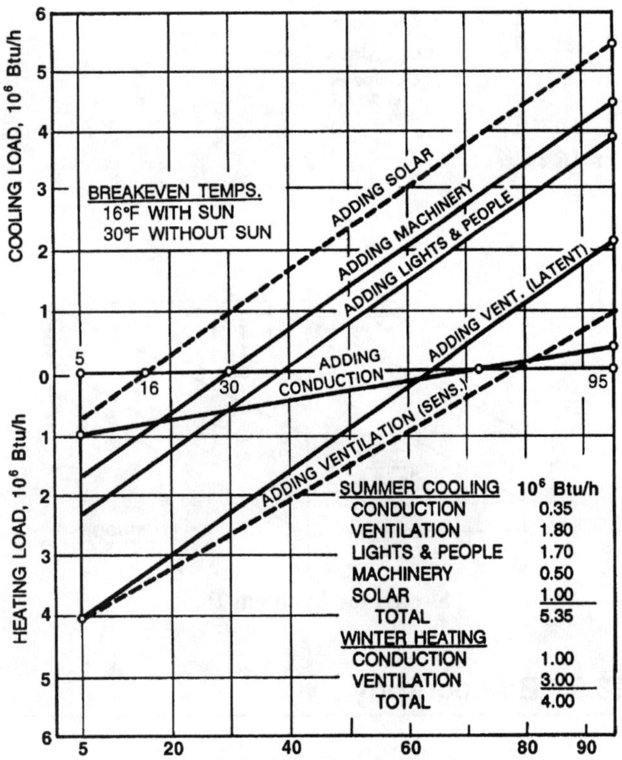

Fig. 16-3 SI Composite Plot of Loads in Fig. 16-2

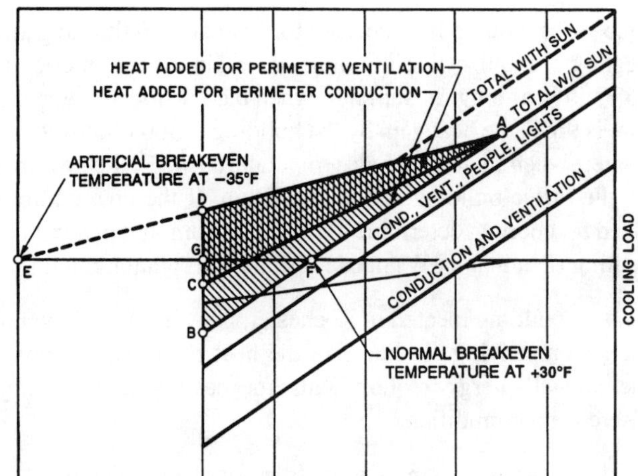

Fig. 16-4 SI Nonheat Recovery-System

Chapter 17

AIR-PROCESSING EQUIPMENT

Cooling, heating, humidifying, dehumidifying, and cleaning of air are some of the processes for which mechanical equipment is needed in HVAC systems. These kinds of air-processing equipment are examined in this chapter, along with air-to-air energy recovery equipment. For additional information of these topics, the reader is referred to Chapters 19 through 24 of the 1996 *ASHRAE Handbook—Systems and Equipment*. Chapters 2 and 3 of the 1997 *ASHRAE Handbook—Fundamentals* provide the heat transfer background for much of this equipment.

17.1 Air Handling Equipment

Air handling units consist of the equipment that filter, heat, humidify, cool, dehumidify, and move the air. The three major types of air handlers are:

- factory fabricated units
- built-up units
- customized units

Each category contains both single zone and multizone units.

Factory fabricated units usually contain the fan and cooling coil assembled in a cabinet, usually of sheet metal. Filters, mixing boxes, and heating coils are also assembled in sheet metal enclosures that are attached as desired. Standard arrangements and options available with factory assembled units include:

- draw-through or blow-through
- horizontal or vertical assembly
- chilled water or DX cooling coils
- hot water, steam, or electric heating coils
- forward-curved, backward-curved, or airfoil fans
- flat or "V" bank filter boxes
- mixing boxes with damper assemblies

Factory fabricated units are less expensive than field erected built-up systems and the delivery time is usually shorter than for the purchase and assembly of a built-up unit.

Rooftop units may be considered a special type of factory fabricated unit, being similar to such indoor units, except that they are located on the roof, saving valuable space that would otherwise be needed for the mechanical equipment room. Packaged rooftop units are completely self-contained including the condensing unit and usually either a gas-fired or electric heating section. On the negative side, rooftop units generally require higher maintenance and have a shorter service life than units protected in mechanical equipment rooms.

Built-up air handling units consist of separate casings enclosing fans, coils, filters, mixing boxes, and plenums. Built-up unit casings may be factory made or fabricated by a local sheet metal shop. Dimensions of built-up units can often be varied for the floor area available, being limited only by the coil and fan selections. There is almost no limit to the capacity of built-up units.

Customized air handling units are normally selected to provide either a higher level of quality or special component configurations for a special application.

17.2 Cooling Coils

Coils are used to cool an airstream under forced convection. Such equipment may consist of a single coil section or several individual coil sections built into banks. Coils are also used extensively as components in central station air-handling units, room terminals, and in factory-assembled, self-contained air conditioners.

Chilled water, brines, or volatile refrigerants are the usual cooling media. Cooling coils that use relatively high- temperature water usually do not dehumidify the air; however, most coil equipment is designed to remove sensible heat and dehumidify simultaneously. The coil assembly usually includes a means to protect the coil from dirt accumulation and to keep dust and foreign matter out of the conditioned space.

17.2.1 Coil Construction and Arrangement

Coils include bare tubes or pipe, and those with extended or finned surfaces. The design of coils with extended surfaces on the air side considers the materials, fin size and spacing, ratio of extended surface area to that of the tube area, tube nesting center dimensions, staggered or in-line tube arrangement, and use of turbulators.

Staggered tubes increase the total heat transfer over that of the in-line arrangement, and turbulators may also increase total heat transfer. The surface arrangement has a great effect on the air-film heat transfer resistance and associated air-side pressure drop. Several arrangements are illustrated in Figure 17-1.

In fin or extended surface coils, the external surface of the tubes is **primary**, and the fin surface is **secondary**. The primary surface consists of rows of round tubes or pipes, which may be staggered or placed in line with respect to the airflow. Some tubes are flattened or have nonround internal passageways. The inside surface of the tubes is usually smooth and plain, but some designs have internal fins or turbulence promoters (either fabricated or extruded) to provide additional

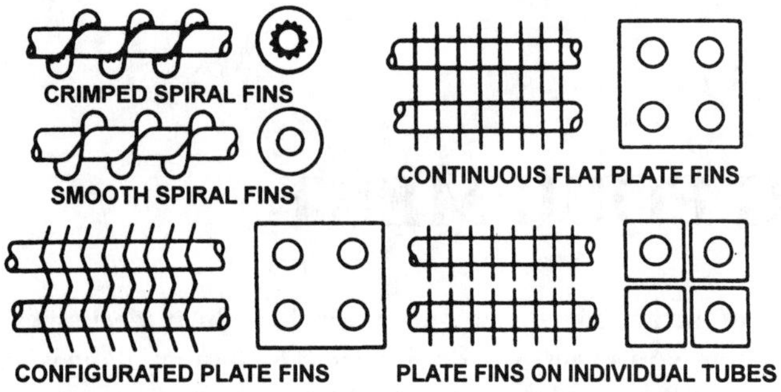

Fig. 17-1 Types of Fin-Coil Arrangements

inside surface area for enhancing performance. Individual tubes are generally interconnected by return bends, sometimes together with hairpin tubes to form the required serpentine arrangement of multipass tube circuits. Some flattened tubes are folded into continuous serpentine circuits with fins metallurgically bonded between adjacent tube passes. Numerous fin arrangements are used; the most common are smooth spiral, crimped spiral, flat plate, and configurated plate. A good thermal bond between the tube and the fin must be maintained permanently to assure low resistance to heat transfer from fin to tube.

In some coils, fins are wound under pressure onto the tubes in order to upset the metal slightly at the fin root. They are then coated with solder while the fin and tube are still revolving, to assure a uniform solder coating. In other types of coils, the spiral fin may be knurled into a shallow groove on the exterior of the tube. The tube may be expanded after the fins are assembled, or the tube-hole flanges of a flat or configurated fin may be made to override those in the preceding fin and so compress them on the tube. Some construction techniques even form the fin from the material of the tube itself.

Cooling coils for water or for volatile refrigerants frequently have aluminum fins and copper tubes, although copper fins on copper tubes are also used and the combination of aluminum fins on aluminum tubes is finding use. Adhesive bonding is sometimes used in making header connections, return bends, and fin-tube joints, particularly for aluminum-to-aluminum joints. Many types of lightweight, extended-surface cooling coils are made for both heating and cooling. Tube outside diameters are commonly 1/4, 3/16, 3/8, 5/8, 3/4, and 1 in. (6.4, 9.5, 12.7, 15.9, 19.1 and 25 mm), and fins are fins spaced from 3 to 14 per inch (1.8 to 8.5 mm apart). The tube spacing varies from about 5/8 to 2-1/2 in. (16 to 64 mm) on centers, depending on the width of individual fins and other performance considerations. Fin spacing should be chosen for the duty to be performed, with special attention paid to air friction, possible lint accumulation, and, especially at lower temperatures, frost accumulation.

17.2.2 Water Coils

Water coil performance depends on eliminating air from the water circuit and properly distributing the water. Unless the system is vented, air may accumulate in the coil circuits, which reduces thermal performance and may cause noise or vibration. Air vent connections are usually provided on the coil water headers. Depending on performance requirements, the water velocity inside tubes usually ranges from approximately 1 to 8 ft/s (0.3 to 2.4 m/s), and the design water pressure drop across coils varies from about 5 to 50 ft of water (15 to 150 kPa).

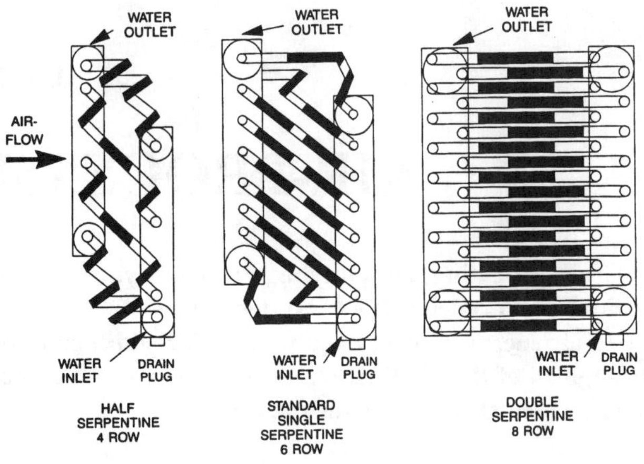

Fig. 17-2 Typical Water Circuit Arrangements

A variety of circuit arrangements, and combinations thereof, for varying the number of parallel water flow passes within the tube core are usually available. Some typical arrangements are shown in Figure 17-2.

17.2.3 Direct-Expansion Coils

Direct-expansion coils present more complex problems of cooling fluid distribution than water or brine coils. The coil should be effectively and uniformly cooled throughout, and the compressor must be protected from entrained, unevaporated refrigerant. Direct-expansion coils are used on both flooded and dry-expansion refrigeration systems.

The **flooded system** is mainly used for low-temperature applications where a small temperature difference between the air and refrigerant is advantageous. However, a relatively large volume of refrigerant is required, together with extra components such as a surge tank and interconnecting piping. Other applications of direct-expansion coils generally use dry expansion. For **dry-expansion systems**, the most commonly used refrigerant liquid metering devices are the capillary tube and the thermostatic expansion valve.

The **capillary tube system** is applied on evaporator coils in factory-assembled, self-contained air conditioners up to approximately 10 tons (35 kW) capacity and is used extensively on the smaller capacity models such as window or room units. In this system, the bore and length of a capillary tube are sized so that at full load, just enough refrigerant liquid is metered from the condenser to the evaporator coil to be completely evaporated.

The **thermostatic expansion valve system** is common for all dry-expansion coil applications, particularly for field assembled coil sections in central air-handling units, as well as for the larger factory-assembled hermetic air conditioners. A schematic typical of a coil and thermostatic expansion valve assembly is shown as Figure 17-3. The thermostatic expansion valve automatically regulates the rate of refrigerant liquid flow to the coil in direct proportion to the rate of evaporation of refrigerant liquid in the coil, thereby maintaining the superheat at the coil suction outlet within the usual predetermined limits of 6 to 10°F (3 to 6°C).

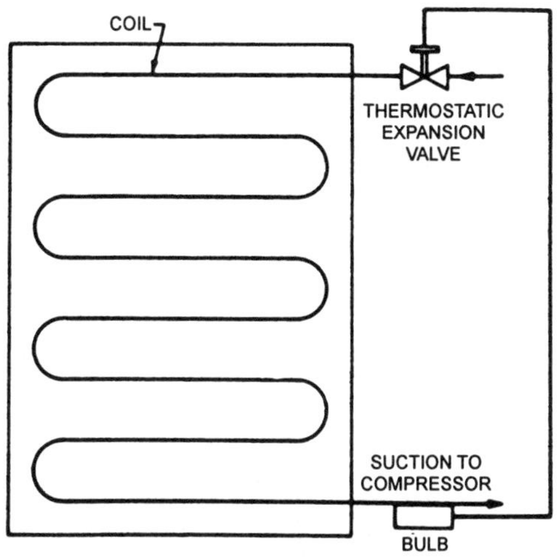

Fig. 17-3 Dry Expansion Coil with Thermostatic Expansion Valve

17.2.4 Coil Selection

When selecting a coil, the following factors must be considered:

- Job requirements: Cooling, dehumidifying, and the capacity required to maintain balance with other system components, for example, compressor equipment in the case of direct-expansion coils.
- Temperature of entering air: Dry bulb only if there is no dehumidification; dry and wet bulb if moisture is to be removed.
- Available cooling media and its operating temperature and quantity.
- Space and dimensional limitations.
- Air quantity limitations.
- Allowable frictional resistances in cooling media piping system (including coils).
- Allowable frictional resistances in air circuit (including coils).
- Characteristics of individual coil designs.
- Individual installation requirements, such as the type of automatic control to be used or the presence of a corrosive atmosphere.
- Coil air face velocity.

Coil ratings and selection procedures are usually presented in one of two ways:

Basic Data Method. Coil performance parameters are published in the form of tables or charts from which the coil row depth is calculated, after determining the required coil sensible and total heat capacities and other design variables from the job conditions. The initial selection generally indicates a nonintegral row depth requirement. It is frequently necessary to recheck and reselect the coil to match more closely the required air and refrigerant conditions with the integral row depth actually installed, particularly for dehumidifying coils. The method is generally used in selecting coils or coil banks for field assembly, since there is a vast number of size and row depth combinations available.

Unit Rating Method. Performance for specific combinations of coil face area and row depth are presented in tables or charts. This method provides a direct selection of specific coils to match the required capacity under the job conditions. This method is frequently used in selecting coils for central station air-handling units and also in determining performance for factory-assembled, self-contained air conditioners.

With either method, various combinations of coil face area, row depth, air velocity, and air quantity may be chosen to do the same job. Coil selection requires understanding each case, and selection should be based on an economic analysis of the plant as a whole.

Table 17-1 provides an illustration of coil performance data as may be found in a typical cooling coil catalog.

17.2.5 Application Range

Based on information in ARI *Standard* 410-91, dry surface (sensible cooling) coils and dehumidifying coils (which both cool and dehumidify), particularly for field assembled coil banks, factory-assembled coil banks, or factory-assembled central station air conditioners using different combinations of coils, are usually rated within the following limits:

Entering air temperature	65 to 100°F (18 to 38°C)
Entering air wet bulb	60 to 85°F (15 to 30°C)
Air face velocity	300 to 800 fpm (1.5 to 4.0 m/s) (sometimes as low as 200 and as high as 1500 fpm)
Refrigerant saturated temperature	30 to 55°F (−1 to 13°C) at coil suction outlet [refrigerant vapor superheat at coil suction outlet is 6°F (3.3°C) or higher]
Entering liquid	35 to 65°F (2 to 18°C) temperature
Water quantity	1.2 to 6 gpm per ton (0.02 to 0.1 L/s per kW) [equivalent to a water temperature rise of from 4 to 20°F (2 to 11°C)]
Water velocity	1 to 8 fps (0.3 to 2.4 m/s)

17.2.6 Determining Refrigeration Load

The following method of calculating refrigeration load shows a division of the true sensible and latent heat loss of the air, which is accurate within the limitations of the data. This division does not correspond to load determination obtained from approximate factors or constants.

Table 17-1 Typical Cooling Coil Catalog Data

EDB/EWB=80/67

WTR=8

FPS	ROW	FPF	400 FPM MBH	400 FPM LDB	400 FPM LWB	500 FPM MBH	500 FPM LDB	500 FPM LWB	600 FPM MBH	600 FPM LDB	600 FPM LWB	700 FPM MBH	700 FPM LDB	700 FPM LWB
2	2	80	6.5	67.8	62.1	7.1	68.8	62.8	7.5	69.7	63.3	8.0	70.3	63.6
		100	7.4	66.0	61.4	8.1	67.2	62.2	8.6	68.1	62.7	9.1	68.8	63.1
		120	8.1	64.5	60.8	8.9	65.7	61.6	9.5	66.6	62.2	10.1	67.4	62.7
		140	8.8	63.2	60.3	9.6	64.5	61.2	10.3	65.5	61.8	10.9	66.0	62.3
		160	9.3	62.3	59.8	10.2	63.6	60.8	10.9	64.6	61.5	11.5	65.1	62.0
	4	80	11.3	60.6	58.2	12.5	62.1	59.3	13.5	63.2	60.1	14.4	64.2	60.7
		100	12.6	58.7	57.1	14.0	60.2	58.3	15.2	61.3	59.2	16.2	62.3	59.9
		120	13.6	57.2	56.2	15.2	58.7	57.4	16.6	59.9	58.4	17.7	60.9	59.2
		140	14.5	56.0	55.4	16.2	57.6	56.7	17.7	58.8	57.8	18.8	59.8	58.6
		160	15.2	55.2	54.8	17.0	56.8	56.2	18.5	58.0	57.3	19.8	59.1	58.2
	6	80	14.9	56.1	55.0	16.7	57.6	56.4	18.3	58.9	57.4	19.7	60.0	58.2
		100	16.3	54.3	53.8	18.4	55.9	55.1	20.3	57.1	56.3	21.9	58.2	57.1
		120	17.3	53.0	52.7	19.8	54.5	54.2	21.8	55.8	55.3	23.5	56.9	56.3
		140	18.2	52.1	51.9	20.8	53.6	53.4	23.0	54.9	54.6	24.9	56.0	55.6
		160	18.9	51.4	51.3	21.6	52.9	52.8	23.9	54.2	54.0	25.9	55.3	55.1
	8	80	17.5	53.0	52.6	20.0	54.6	54.0	22.1	55.9	55.1	24.0	57.0	56.1
		100	18.9	51.5	51.3	21.8	52.9	52.7	24.2	54.2	53.9	26.3	55.3	54.9
		120	19.9	50.4	50.3	23.1	51.8	51.7	25.8	53.0	52.9	28.1	54.1	53.9
		140	20.7	49.6	49.5	24.1	51.0	50.9	27.0	52.2	52.1	29.5	53.3	53.2
		160	21.3	49.0	48.9	24.8	50.4	50.3	27.9	51.6	51.5	30.5	52.7	52.6
4	2	80	7.4	67.0	61.4	8.0	68.2	62.2	8.6	69.1	62.7	9.1	69.8	63.1
		100	8.5	65.1	60.6	9.3	66.3	61.3	10.1	67.3	62.0	10.7	68.0	62.4
		120	9.5	63.3	59.7	10.5	64.6	60.6	11.3	65.7	61.3	12.0	66.5	61.8
		140	10.3	61.9	59.0	11.4	63.2	60.0	12.3	64.3	60.7	13.1	65.3	61.3
		160	11.1	60.7	58.4	12.2	62.2	59.5	13.2	63.3	60.3	14.0	64.3	60.9
	4	80	12.6	59.5	57.1	14.0	61.0	58.3	15.3	62.2	59.1	16.3	63.2	59.8
		100	14.1	57.3	55.8	15.9	58.8	57.0	17.4	60.0	57.9	18.7	61.1	58.7
		120	15.4	55.6	54.6	17.4	57.1	55.9	19.2	58.3	56.9	20.7	59.4	57.7
		140	16.4	54.2	53.6	18.7	55.8	55.0	20.6	57.0	56.1	22.2	58.1	57.0
		160	17.3	53.2	52.8	19.7	54.8	54.2	21.7	56.1	55.4	23.4	57.2	56.4
	6	80	16.2	54.8	53.8	18.4	56.4	55.1	20.4	57.7	56.2	22.1	58.8	57.1
		100	17.8	52.9	52.3	20.5	54.3	53.6	22.8	55.6	54.7	24.8	56.7	55.7
		120	19.1	51.4	51.1	22.1	52.8	52.4	24.7	54.0	53.6	27.0	55.1	54.5
		140	20.0	50.3	50.1	23.3	51.7	51.5	26.2	52.9	52.6	28.7	54.0	53.7
		160	20.8	49.5	49.4	24.3	50.8	50.7	27.3	52.1	51.9	30.0	53.2	53.0
	8	80	18.8	51.7	51.3	21.8	53.2	52.7	24.3	54.5	53.8	26.6	55.6	54.7
		100	20.3	50.1	49.9	23.8	51.4	51.1	26.8	52.6	52.3	29.4	53.7	53.2
		120	21.4	48.8	48.7	25.2	50.1	50.0	28.6	51.2	51.1	31.6	52.3	52.1
		140	22.2	48.0	47.9	26.3	49.2	49.1	30.0	50.3	50.2	33.2	51.3	51.2
		160	22.8	47.4	47.3	27.2	48.5	48.4	31.0	49.6	49.5	34.5	50.6	50.5
6	2	80	7.8	66.7	61.1	8.5	67.8	61.9	9.2	68.7	62.4	9.7	69.5	62.9
		100	9.0	64.6	60.1	10.0	65.9	61.0	10.8	66.8	61.6	11.4	67.7	62.1
		120	10.1	62.8	59.2	11.2	64.1	60.1	12.2	65.2	60.8	13.0	66.1	61.4
		140	11.1	61.2	58.4	12.3	62.6	59.4	13.4	63.7	60.2	14.2	64.7	60.8
		160	11.9	60.0	57.6	13.3	61.4	58.8	14.4	62.6	59.6	15.3	63.6	60.3
	4	80	13.1	59.0	56.6	14.7	60.5	57.8	16.1	61.7	58.7	17.2	62.8	59.4
		100	14.7	56.7	55.2	16.7	58.2	56.4	18.4	59.4	57.3	19.9	60.5	58.1
		120	16.1	54.9	53.9	18.4	56.3	55.1	20.4	57.6	56.2	22.1	58.7	57.0
		140	17.3	53.4	52.8	19.8	54.9	54.1	22.0	56.2	55.2	23.8	57.3	56.2
		160	18.2	52.3	51.9	21.0	53.8	53.3	23.3	55.1	54.4	25.3	56.3	55.4
	6	80	16.8	54.2	53.3	19.2	55.8	54.6	21.3	57.1	55.7	23.1	58.2	56.5
		100	18.5	52.2	51.7	21.4	53.7	53.0	23.9	54.9	54.0	26.1	56.0	55.0
		120	19.7	50.7	50.4	23.1	52.0	51.7	26.0	53.2	52.8	28.5	54.3	53.7
		140	20.8	49.5	49.4	24.4	50.8	50.6	27.6	52.0	51.7	30.4	53.1	52.7
		160	21.6	48.7	48.6	25.4	49.9	49.8	28.8	51.1	50.9	31.8	52.2	51.9
	8	80	19.4	51.2	50.8	22.5	52.6	52.1	25.3	53.9	53.2	27.7	55.0	54.2
		100	20.9	49.4	49.3	24.6	50.7	50.5	27.9	51.9	51.6	30.8	52.9	52.5
		120	22.0	48.3	48.2	26.1	49.4	49.2	29.8	50.4	50.3	33.1	51.4	51.2
		140	22.8	47.4	47.3	27.2	48.4	48.3	31.2	49.4	49.3	34.8	50.4	50.3
		160	23.4	46.8	46.7	28.1	47.8	47.7	32.3	48.7	48.6	36.1	49.6	49.5
8	2	80	8.0	66.5	60.9	8.8	67.6	61.7	9.5	68.6	62.3	10.1	69.3	62.7
		100	9.3	64.3	59.9	10.3	65.6	60.7	11.2	66.6	61.4	11.9	67.4	61.9
		120	10.5	62.4	58.9	11.7	63.8	59.8	12.7	64.8	60.5	13.6	65.8	61.1
		140	11.5	60.8	58.0	12.9	62.2	59.0	14.0	63.4	59.8	15.0	64.4	60.5
		160	12.5	59.5	57.2	13.9	61.0	58.3	15.1	62.2	59.2	16.2	63.2	59.9
	4	80	13.4	58.7	56.3	15.1	60.2	57.5	16.6	61.4	58.4	17.8	62.5	59.1
		100	15.1	56.3	54.8	17.3	57.8	56.0	19.0	59.1	57.0	20.6	60.1	57.8
		120	16.6	54.4	53.5	19.0	55.9	54.7	21.1	57.1	55.7	22.9	58.2	56.6
		140	17.7	53.0	52.4	20.5	54.4	53.6	22.8	55.7	54.7	24.8	56.8	55.7
		160	18.7	51.8	51.4	21.7	53.3	52.7	24.2	54.5	53.9	26.4	55.7	54.9
	6	80	17.1	53.9	52.9	19.7	55.5	54.3	21.8	56.8	55.3	23.7	57.9	56.2
		100	18.8	51.8	51.3	21.9	53.2	52.6	24.5	54.5	53.7	26.9	55.6	54.6
		120	20.2	50.3	50.0	23.6	51.6	51.2	26.7	52.7	52.3	29.4	53.8	53.2
		140	21.2	49.1	49.0	25.0	50.3	50.1	28.4	51.5	51.2	31.4	52.5	52.2
		160	22.0	48.2	48.1	26.1	49.4	49.3	29.7	50.5	50.4	32.9	51.6	51.3
	8	80	19.7	50.9	50.5	23.0	52.3	51.8	25.8	53.6	52.9	28.4	54.7	53.8
		100	21.2	49.1	48.9	25.1	50.4	50.1	28.5	51.5	51.2	31.5	52.5	52.1
		120	22.3	47.9	47.8	26.6	49.0	48.9	30.5	50.0	49.8	34.0	51.0	50.8
		140	23.1	47.1	47.0	27.7	48.0	47.9	31.9	48.9	48.8	35.7	49.8	49.7
		160	23.7	46.4	46.3	28.6	47.3	47.2	33.0	48.2	48.1	37.1	49.1	49.0

WTR=10

400 FPM MBH	400 FPM LDB	400 FPM LWB	500 FPM MBH	500 FPM LDB	500 FPM LWB	600 FPM MBH	600 FPM LDB	600 FPM LWB	700 FPM MBH	700 FPM LDB	700 FPM LWB	FPF	ROW	FPS
6.2	68.0	62.3	6.8	69.0	62.9	7.3	69.8	63.4	7.7	70.5	63.7	80	2	2
7.1	66.3	61.7	7.7	67.4	62.3	8.3	68.2	62.9	8.8	68.6	63.3	100		
7.8	64.8	61.1	8.6	65.9	61.8	9.2	66.8	62.4	9.7	67.4	62.8	120		
8.5	63.5	60.5	9.3	64.7	61.4	9.9	65.7	62.0	10.5	66.4	62.5	140		
9.0	62.5	60.1	9.8	63.8	61.0	10.5	64.8	61.7	11.1	65.6	62.2	160		
10.9	61.0	58.6	12.0	62.4	59.6	13.0	63.5	60.4	13.9	64.4	61.0	80	4	
12.1	59.1	57.5	13.5	60.5	58.6	14.6	61.7	59.5	15.6	62.6	60.1	100		
13.1	57.6	56.6	14.7	59.1	57.8	16.0	60.2	58.7	17.1	61.2	59.5	120		
14.0	56.5	55.9	15.7	57.9	57.1	17.0	59.1	58.1	18.2	60.1	58.9	140		
14.6	55.7	55.2	16.4	57.2	56.6	17.9	58.4	57.6	19.1	59.4	58.5	160		
14.3	56.6	55.5	16.1	58.1	56.8	17.6	59.3	57.8	19.0	60.3	58.6	80	6	
15.7	54.9	54.3	17.8	56.3	55.6	19.5	57.6	56.7	21.1	58.6	57.5	100		
16.8	53.6	53.3	19.1	55.0	54.6	21.1	56.3	55.8	22.7	57.3	56.7	120		
17.6	52.6	52.5	20.2	54.1	53.9	22.3	55.3	55.1	24.1	56.4	56.0	140		
18.3	51.9	51.8	21.0	53.4	53.3	23.2	54.7	54.5	25.1	55.8	55.5	160		
16.9	53.6	53.1	19.3	55.1	54.5	21.4	56.3	55.6	23.1	57.4	56.5	80	8	
18.3	52.0	51.8	21.1	53.5	53.2	23.4	54.7	54.4	25.5	55.8	55.3	100		
19.3	50.9	50.8	22.4	52.3	52.2	25.0	53.5	53.4	27.2	54.6	54.4	120		
20.1	50.1	50.0	23.4	51.5	51.4	26.2	52.7	52.6	28.6	53.8	53.7	140		
20.7	49.5	49.4	24.2	50.9	50.8	27.1	52.2	52.1	29.6	53.2	53.1	160		
7.0	67.3	61.7	7.7	68.4	62.4	8.3	69.3	62.9	8.8	70.0	63.3	80	2	4
8.1	65.4	60.9	8.9	66.6	61.6	9.6	67.5	62.2	10.2	68.3	62.6	100		
9.1	63.7	60.1	10.0	64.9	60.9	10.8	65.9	61.5	11.5	66.8	62.1	120		
9.9	62.3	59.4	11.0	63.5	60.3	11.8	64.6	61.0	12.6	65.5	61.6	140		
10.6	61.1	58.8	11.8	62.5	59.8	12.7	63.6	60.5	13.5	64.5	61.2	160		
12.0	60.0	57.6	13.4	61.4	58.7	14.6	62.6	59.5	15.7	63.5	60.1	80	4	
13.5	57.9	56.3	15.3	59.3	57.4	16.7	60.5	58.3	18.0	61.5	59.0	100		
14.8	56.1	55.1	16.8	57.6	56.3	18.4	58.8	57.3	19.9	59.8	58.1	120		
15.8	54.8	54.2	18.0	56.3	55.5	19.8	57.5	56.5	21.4	58.6	57.4	140		
16.7	53.8	53.4	19.0	55.3	54.7	21.0	56.6	55.8	22.6	57.6	56.8	160		
15.6	55.4	54.4	17.7	56.9	55.6	19.6	58.2	56.7	21.2	59.2	57.5	80	6	
17.2	53.4	52.9	19.8	54.9	54.2	22.0	56.1	55.2	23.9	57.2	56.1	100		
18.5	51.9	51.7	21.4	53.4	53.0	23.9	54.6	54.1	26.0	55.6	55.0	120		
19.4	50.8	50.7	22.6	52.2	52.0	25.3	53.4	53.2	27.7	54.5	54.2	140		
20.2	50.0	49.9	23.6	51.4	51.3	26.5	52.6	52.4	29.0	53.7	53.5	160		
18.2	52.3	51.9	21.0	53.8	53.2	23.5	55.1	54.3	25.6	56.1	55.2	80	8	
19.7	50.6	50.4	23.0	52.0	51.7	25.9	53.2	52.8	28.4	54.2	53.8	100		
20.8	49.4	49.3	24.5	50.6	50.5	27.8	51.8	51.6	30.6	52.8	52.6	120		
21.7	48.5	48.4	25.7	49.7	49.6	29.2	50.8	50.7	32.2	51.8	51.7	140		
22.3	47.9	47.8	26.5	49.0	48.9	30.2	50.1	50.0	33.5	51.1	51.0	160		
7.4	67.0	61.4	8.1	68.1	62.1	8.7	69.0	62.7	9.3	69.7	63.1	80	2	6
8.6	65.0	60.5	9.5	66.2	61.2	10.3	67.1	61.8	10.9	67.9	62.3	100		
9.6	63.2	59.6	10.7	64.4	60.4	11.6	65.5	61.1	12.4	66.3	61.6	120		
10.6	61.6	58.8	11.8	63.0	59.7	12.8	64.1	60.5	13.7	65.0	61.1	140		
11.4	60.4	58.1	12.7	61.8	59.1	13.8	63.0	59.9	14.7	63.9	60.6	160		
12.5	59.5	57.1	14.1	61.0	58.2	15.4	62.1	59.1	16.5	63.1	59.7	80	4	
14.1	57.3	55.7	16.1	58.7	56.8	17.7	59.9	57.8	19.1	60.9	58.5	100		
15.5	55.4	54.5	17.7	56.9	55.7	19.6	58.1	56.7	21.2	59.1	57.5	120		
16.7	54.0	53.4	19.1	55.5	54.7	21.2	56.7	55.7	22.9	57.8	56.6	140		
17.6	52.9	52.5	20.2	54.4	53.8	22.4	55.6	55.0	24.3	56.7	55.9	160		
16.1	54.9	53.9	18.5	56.4	55.1	20.4	57.6	56.2	22.2	58.7	57.0	80	6	
17.8	52.8	52.3	20.6	54.2	53.5	23.0	55.4	54.6	25.2	56.5	55.5	100		
19.2	51.3	51.0	22.3	52.6	52.2	25.1	53.8	53.3	27.5	54.8	54.3	120		
20.2	50.1	50.0	23.7	51.4	51.2	26.7	52.6	52.3	29.4	53.6	53.3	140		
21.0	49.2	49.1	24.7	50.5	50.4	28.0	51.7	51.5	30.8	52.7	52.5	160		
18.7	51.8	51.4	21.7	53.3	52.7	24.4	54.5	53.8	26.7	55.6	54.7	80	8	
20.3	50.1	49.9	23.8	51.3	51.1	27.0	52.5	52.1	29.7	53.5	53.1	100		
21.5	48.8	48.7	25.4	49.9	49.8	28.9	51.0	50.9	32.1	52.0	51.8	120		
22.3	47.9	47.8	26.6	49.0	48.9	30.4	50.0	49.9	33.8	50.9	50.8	140		
23.0	47.2	47.1	27.5	48.3	48.2	31.5	49.2	49.1	35.2	50.2	50.1	160		
7.6	66.8	61.3	8.3	68.0	62.0	9.0	68.8	62.5	9.6	69.6	62.9	80	2	8
8.8	64.8	60.2	9.8	65.9	61.0	10.7	66.9	61.6	11.4	67.7	62.1	100		
10.0	62.9	59.3	11.2	64.1	60.2	12.2	65.2	60.8	13.0	66.0	61.4	120		
11.0	61.3	58.4	12.3	62.6	59.4	13.4	63.7	60.1	14.3	64.7	60.8	140		
11.9	60.0	57.7	13.3	61.4	58.7	14.5	62.6	59.6	15.5	63.5	60.2	160		
12.8	59.2	56.9	14.4	60.7	58.0	15.8	61.9	58.8	17.0	62.9	59.5	80	4	
14.5	56.9	55.4	16.5	58.4	56.5	18.3	59.5	57.4	19.7	60.6	58.2	100		
15.9	55.0	54.1	18.3	56.4	55.3	20.3	57.7	56.2	22.0	58.7	57.1	120		
17.1	53.5	52.9	19.7	55.0	54.2	22.0	56.2	55.2	23.9	57.3	56.1	140		
18.1	52.4	52.0	20.9	53.8	53.3	23.3	55.1	54.4	25.4	56.2	55.4	160		
16.5	54.6	53.6	18.9	56.1	54.8	20.9	57.3	55.9	22.8	58.4	56.7	80	6	
18.2	52.5	51.9	21.1	53.9	53.2	23.7	55.1	54.2	25.9	56.1	55.1	100		
19.6	50.9	50.6	22.9	52.2	51.8	25.8	53.3	52.9	28.4	54.4	53.8	120		
20.6	49.7	49.5	24.3	50.9	50.7	27.5	52.1	51.8	30.3	53.1	52.8	140		
21.5	48.8	48.7	25.4	50.0	49.9	28.8	51.1	51.0	31.9	52.1	51.9	160		
19.0	51.5	51.1	22.1	53.0	52.4	24.9	54.2	53.5	27.3	55.2	54.4	80	8	
20.6	49.7	49.5	24.3	51.0	50.7	27.6	52.1	51.8	30.5	53.1	52.7	100		
21.8	48.4	48.3	25.9	49.5	49.4	29.6	50.6	50.4	32.9	51.5	51.3	120		
22.6	47.6	47.5	27.1	48.6	48.5	31.1	49.5	49.4	34.7	50.4	50.3	140		
23.3	46.9	46.8	28.0	47.8	47.7	32.2	48.7	48.6	36.1	49.6	49.5	160		

MBH = 1000 Btu/h per square foot of coil face area
WTR = water temperature rise, °F
FPS = water velocity, ft/s
FPM = air velocity, ft/min
LDB = leaving dry bulb, °F
LWB = leaving wet bulb, °F
EWT = entering water temp., °F
FPF = fins per foot

Note: When using turbulators make selection based on double the actual water velocity.

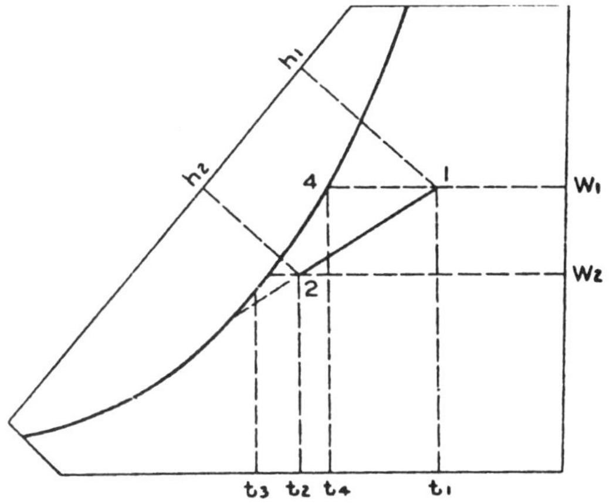

Fig. 17-4 Psychrometric Performance of Cooling and Dehumidifying Coil

The total refrigeration load q_t of a cooling and dehumidifying coil (or air washer) per unit of dry air is indicated in Figure 17-4 and consists of the following components:

1. The sensible heat q_s removed from the dry air and moisture in cooling from entering temperature t_1 to leaving temperature t_2.
2. The latent heat q_1 removed to condense the moisture at the dew point t_4 of the entering air.
3. The heat of subcooling qw removed from the condensate in cooling it from the condensing temperature t_4 to the leaving condensate temperature t_3.

Items 1, 2, and 3 may be related by:

$$q_t = q_s + q_l + q_w \tag{17-1}$$

If only the total heat value is desired, it may be computed by

$$q_t = (h_1 - h_2) - (W_1 - W_2)\, h_{f3} \tag{17-2}$$

where

h_1 and h_2 = enthalpy of air at points 1 and 2, respectively
W_1 and W_2 = humidity ratio at Points 1 and 2, respectively
h_{f3} = enthalpy of saturated liquid at final temperature t_3

If a breakdown into latent and sensible heat components is desired, the following relations may be used. The latent heat may be found from

$$q_1 = (W_1 - W_2)\, h_{fg4} \tag{17-3}$$

where

h_{fg4} = latent heat of water vapor at condensing temperature t_4

The sensible heat may be shown to be

$$q_s + q_w = (h_1 - h_2) - (W_1 - W_2)h_{g4} + (W_1 - W_2)(h_{f4} - h_{f3}) \tag{17-4}$$

or

$$q_s + q_w = (h_1 - h_2) - (W_1 - W_2)(h_{fg4} - h_{f3}) \tag{17-5}$$

where

$h_{g4} = h_{fg4} + h_{f4}$ = enthalpy of saturated liquid at the condensing temperature t_4

The last term in Equation (17-4) is the heat of subcooling the condensate from the condensing temperature t_4 to its final temperature t_3. Then

$$q_w = (W_1 - W_2)(h_{f4} - h_{f3}) \tag{17-6}$$

The final condensate temperature t_3 leaving the system is subject to substantial variations, depending on the method of coil installation, as affected by such factors as coil face orientation, airflow direction, and air duct insulation. In practice, t_3 is frequently the same as the leaving wet-bulb temperature. Within the normal air-conditioning range, precise values of t_3 are not necessary since energy in the condensate $(W_1 - W_2)h_{f3}$ removed from the air usually represents about 0.5 to 1.5% of the total refrigeration load. All values for solving the foregoing equations may be found on the ASHRAE Psychrometric Chart (Chart 1) and Tables 1 and 2 of Chapter 6 of the 1997 *ASHRAE Handbook—Fundamentals.*

Example 17-1 Air enters a coil at 32.2°C dry bulb, 23.9°C wet bulb; it leaves at 16.1°C dry bulb, 14.4°C wet bulb; leaving water is at 12.2°C. Find the total, latent, and sensible cooling loads on the coil with the air at standard barometric pressure.

Solution:

From the ASHRAE Psychrometric Chart, find the following variables:

h_1 = 89.52 kJ/kg of dry air
h_2 = 58.48 kJ/kg of dry air
t_4 = 20.6°C dew point of entering air
W_1 = 15.25 g/kg of dry air
W_2 = 9.6 g/kg of dry air

From Table 2, Chapter 6 of the 1997 Fundamentals, find the following:

h_{f4} = 86.37 kJ/kg
h_{f3} = 51.45 kJ/kg
h_{fg4} = 2456.45 kJ/kg
h_{g4} = 2542.82 kJ/kg

From Equation (17-2), the total heat is

$$q_t = (89.52 - 58.48) - 51.45[(15.25 - 9.6)/(1000 \text{ g/kg})]$$
$$= 31.04 - 0.29 = 30.75 \text{ kJ/kg (of dry air) (13.2 Btu/lb)}$$

From Equation (17-3), the latent heat is

$$q_l = 0.00565 \times 2456.45$$
$$= 13.88 \text{ kJ/kg (of dry air) (5.96 Btu/lb of dry air)}$$

The sensible heat, by difference, is

$$qs + qw = qt - q_l = 30.75 - 13.88$$
$$= 16.87 \text{ kJ/kg (of dry air) (7.24 Btu/lb of dry air)}$$

Or the sensible heat may be computed from Equation (17-4) as

$$q_s + q_w = (89.52 - 58.48) - (0.00565 \times 2542.82)$$
$$+ 0.00565(86.37 - 51.45)$$
$$= 31.04 - 14.37 + 0.20$$
$$= 16.87 \text{ kJ/kg (of dry air) (7.24 Btu/lb of dry air)}$$

The subcooling of the condensate as a part of the sensible heat is the last term of the equation, or 0.20 kJ/kg.

17.3 Heating Coils

Generally, extended-surface coils are used for heating air with steam or hot water.

17.3.1 Steam Coils

For proper performance of steam heating coils, condensate and air or other noncondensables must be rapidly eliminated and the steam must be uniformly distributed to the individual tubes. Noncondensable gases (such as carbon dioxide) that remain in the coil cause chemical corrosion and result in early coil failure.

Steam is distributed uniformly by methods such as:

- individual orifices in the tubes
- distributing plates in the steam headers
- perforated, small-diameter, inner steam-distributing tubes extending to the larger tubes of the primary surface

Coils with perforated inner tubes are constructed with different arrangements such as:

- supply and return on one end, with the incoming steam used to heat the leaving condensate (nonfreeze type)
- supply and return on opposite ends
- supply and return on one end and a supply on the opposite end (nonfreeze type)

Properly designed and selected steam distribution coils distribute steam throughout the full length of all primary tubes, even when the leaving air temperature is controlled by modulating the steam supply through a steam-metering valve. Thus, more uniform leaving air temperatures are produced over the entire length and face of the coil than from a single-tube coil.

Piping, controls, and installation must be designed to protect the coils from freeze-up due to incomplete draining of condensate. When the entering air temperature is 32°F (0°C) or below, the steam supply to the coil should not be modulated. A series of coils in the airstream, with each coil sized to be on or completely off in a specific sequence depending on the entering air temperature, has little likelihood for a freeze-up. Bypass dampers are also common. When less than full load conditions occur, air is bypassed around the steam coil with full steam being kept on the coil. In this system, the high-velocity jets of low-temperature air must not impinge on the coil when the face dampers are in a partially closed position.

17.3.2 Water Coils

In order to produce the desired heating capacity, hot water comfort heating systems usually require no more than one or two rows of tubes in the direction of airflow. Various circuits are used to produce the most efficient capacity without excessive water pressure drop through the coil. The relative directions of fluid flows influence the performance of heat transfer surfaces. In air-heating coils with only one row of tubes, the air flows at right angles relative to the heating medium. In coils with more than one row of tubes in the direction of the airflow, the heating medium in the tubes may be circuited in various ways.

Although crossflow is common in steam-heating coils, parallel flow and counterflow arrangements are common in water coils. Counterflow is the preferred arrangement to obtain the highest possible mean temperature difference.

A single-tube serpentine circuit on small-size booster heaters requires small water quantities up to a maximum of approximately 4 or 5 gpm (0.25 or 0.32 L/s). With this arrangement, a single tube handles the entire water quantity, provided the tube is circuited such that it makes a number of passes across the airstream.

Commonly selected water circuits are illustrated in Figure 17-5. When entering air temperatures are below freezing (an antifreeze brine would be preferable to water), piping the coil for parallel flow rather than counterflow should be considered, placing the highest water temperature on the entering air side. Coils piped for counterflow have water enter the coil in the tube row on the exit air side of the coil. Coils piped for parallel flow have water enter the tube row on the entering air side of the coil.

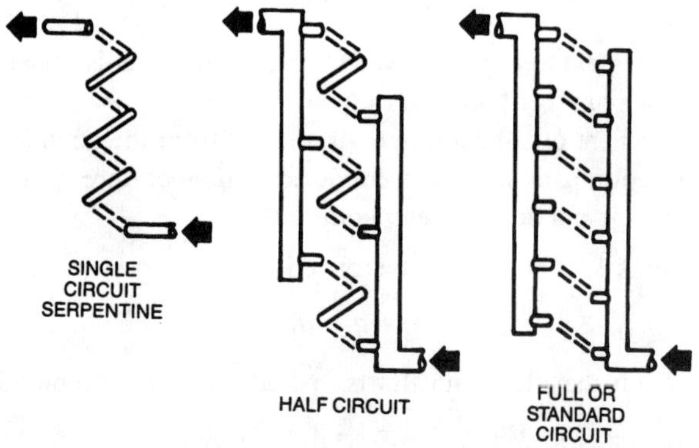

Fig. 17-5 Water Circuit Arrangements for Heating Coils

17.3.3 Electric Heating Coils

An electric heating coil consists of a length of resistance wire (commonly nickel/chromium) to which a voltage is applied. The resistance wire may be bare or sheathed. The sheathed coil is a resistance wire encased by an electrically insulating layer such as magnesium oxide, which is encased in a finned steel tube. The sheathed coils are more expensive, have a higher air-side pressure drop, and require more space. The outer surface temperature of sheathed coils is lower, the coils are mechanically stronger, and contact with body or housing is not dangerous.

17.3.4 Coil Ratings

Steam and hot water coils are usually rated within these limits, which may be exceeded for special applications:

Air face velocity — Between 200 and 1500 fpm (1 to 8 m/s), based on air at standard density of 0.075 lb/ft^3 (1.2 kg/m^3)

Entering air temperature	−20° to 100°F (−30 to 38°C) for steam coils; 0 to 100°F (−20 to 38°C) for hot water coils
Steam pressures	From 2 to 250 psia (14 to 1700 kPa) at the coil steam supply connection (pressure drop through the steam control valve must be considered)
Hot water	Between 120 and 250°F (50 and 120°C) temperature
Water velocities	From 0.5 to 8 fps (0.2 to 2.5 m/s)

Individual installations vary widely, but the following values can be used as a guide. The most common air face velocities used are between 500 and 1000 fpm. Delivered air temperatures vary from about 72°F for ventilation only to about 150°F for complete heating. Steam pressures vary from 2 to 15 psig, with 5 psig being the most common. A minimum steam pressure of 5 psig is recommended for systems with entering air temperatures below freezing. Water temperatures for comfort heating are commonly between 180 and 200°F, with water velocities between 4 and 6 fps. Water quantity is usually based on about 20°F temperature drop through the coil. Air resistance is usually limited to 0.4 to 0.6 in. of water for commercial buildings and to about 1 in. for industrial buildings. High-temperature water systems have water temperatures commonly between 300 and 400°F, with up to 100°F drops through the coil.

17.4 Evaporative Air-Cooling Equipment

In its broadest sense, the evaporative cooling principle applies to all equipment that exchanges sensible heat for latent heat. Cooling towers, evaporative condensers, vacuum cooling apparatus, air washers, and packaged evaporative coolers cool air by evaporation. This equipment falls into two general categories: (1) apparatus for air cooling and (2) apparatus for heat rejection.

Evaporative air cooling evaporates water into an airstream. Illustrated in Figure 17-6 are thermodynamic changes that take place between air and water that are in direct contact in the moving airstream. The continuously recirculated water has reached an equilibrium temperature that equals the entering air wet-bulb temperature. The heat and mass transfer process between the air and water lowers the air dry-bulb temperature and increases the humidity ratio at constant wet-bulb temperature.

The extent to which the leaving air temperature approaches the thermodynamic wet-bulb temperature of the entering air, or the extent to which complete saturation is approached, is conveniently expressed as cooling or saturation efficiency and is defined as:

$$e_c = (t_1 - t_2)/(t_1 - t')$$

where

e_c = cooling or saturation efficiency
t_1 = dry-bulb temperature of the entering air
t_2 = dry-bulb temperature of the leaving air
t' = thermodynamic wet-bulb temperature of entering air

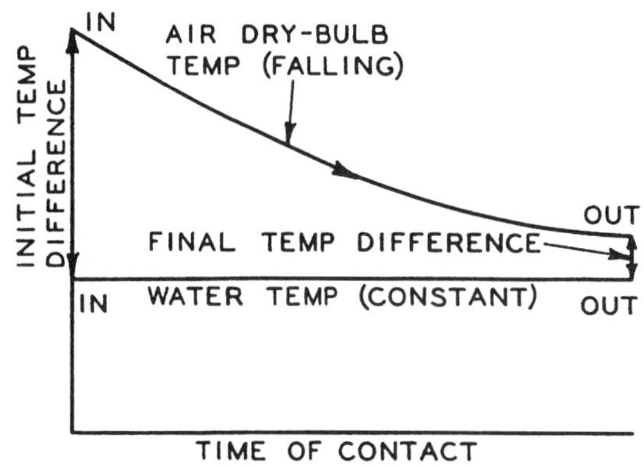

Fig. 17-6 Interaction of Air and Water in Evaporative Air Coolers

If warm or cold unrecirculated water is used, the air can be heated and humidified or cooled and dehumidified.

Evaporative air-cooling equipment can be placed in two general classes, direct and indirect. In the direct system, air is cooled by direct contact with the water, either from the wetted surface of an extended-surface material (as in packaged air coolers) or with a series of sprays (as in an air washer). In the indirect system, air is cooled in a heat exchanger by a secondary stream of air and water that has been evaporatively cooled, such as by a cooling tower and cooling coil.

By applying recirculating, regenerating principles, temperatures below the initial wet bulb may be produced. However, the cost of these more complex devices has restricted their use.

The random media air coolers contains an evaporative pad made of aspen wood (or other) fibers and a water circulating pump to lift water from a sump to a distributing system. The water then runs down through the pads and back into the sump (Figure 17-7). A fan within the cooler pulls the air through the evaporative pads and delivers it to the space to be cooled. The fan discharges either through the side of the cooler cabinet when the cabinet is mounted on the outside wall of a building, or through the sump bottom when installed on the roof. Wetted-pad packaged air coolers are made in sizes from 2000 to 20,000 cfm (1 to 10 m^3/s).

The slinger cooler contains a slinger that throws a spray of water into the air and onto the evaporative pad (Figure 17-8). An eliminator on the downstream side of the pad removes the entrained moisture. The air-handling part of the cooler is similar to that of the wetted-pad cooler. Slinger coolers are built in capacities from 3000 to 30,000 cfm (1.4 to 14 m^3/s), typically with 80% cooling efficiencies.

The rotary cooler wets and washes the evaporative pad by rotating it through a water bath (Figure 17-9). The evaporative pad and other parts in contact with the water are usually made with corrosion resistant copper alloy. Like the slinger cooler, this cooler has a cooling section and a blower compartment. The air-handling part of the cooler is similar to that

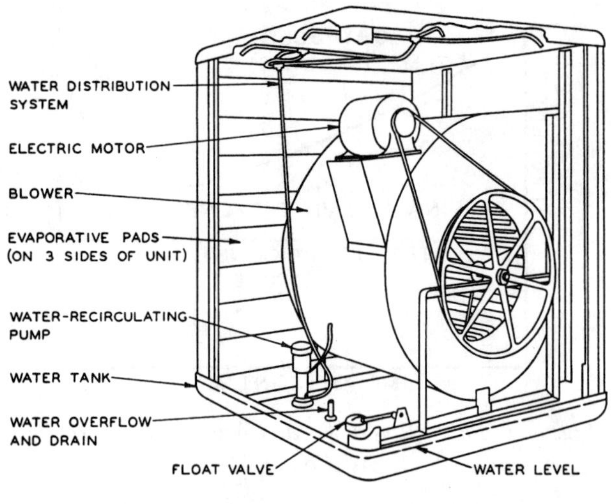

Fig. 17-7 Wetted-Pad Evaporative Cooler

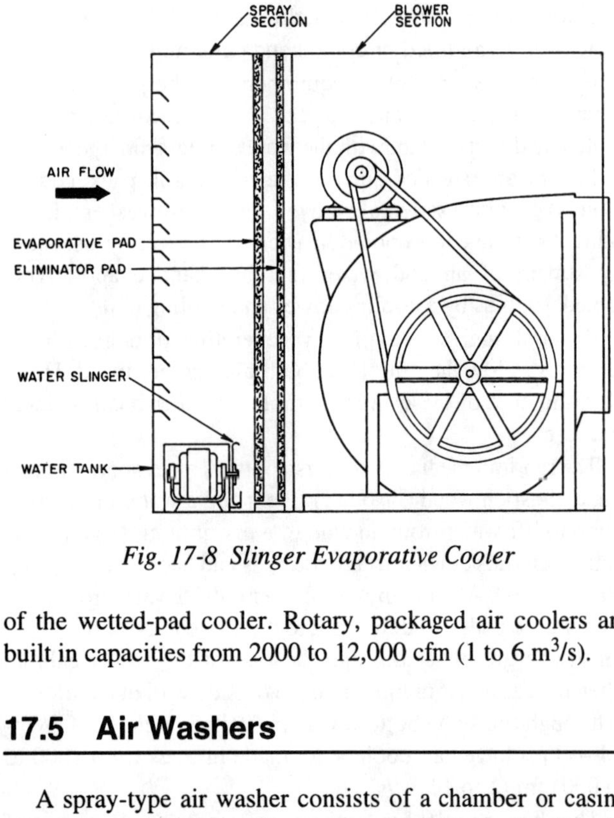

Fig. 17-8 Slinger Evaporative Cooler

of the wetted-pad cooler. Rotary, packaged air coolers are built in capacities from 2000 to 12,000 cfm (1 to 6 m^3/s).

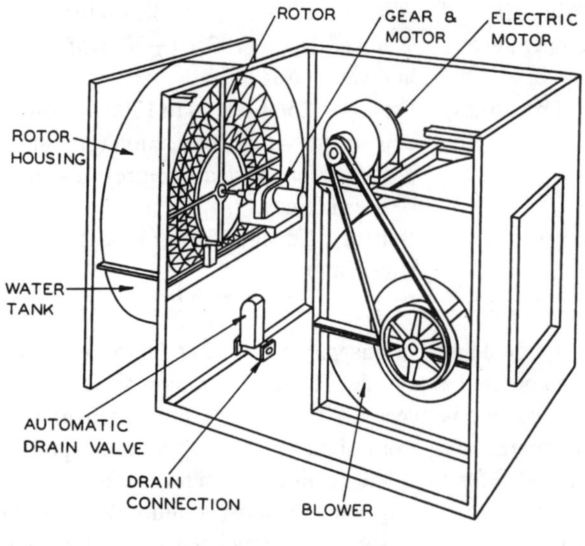

Fig. 17-9 Rotary Evaporative Cooler

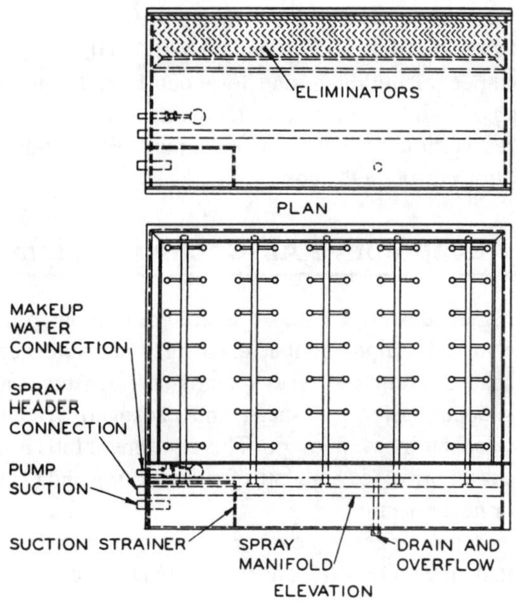

Fig. 17-10 Single-Bank Air Washer

17.5 Air Washers

A spray-type air washer consists of a chamber or casing containing a spray nozzle system, a tank for collecting the spray water as it falls, and an eliminator section at the discharge to remove the entrained drops of water from the air. A pump recirculates water at a rate in excess of the evaporation rate. Heat and mass transfer between the air and the water cools the water.

Construction features of conventional spray-type air washers are shown in Figure 17-10. Requirements of air washer operation are

- uniform distribution of air across the spray chamber
- air velocities from 300 to 700 fpm (1.5 to 3.5 m/s) in the washer chamber
- adequate spray water broken up into fine droplets at pressures from 20 to 40 psig [140 to 280 kPa (gage)]
- good spray distribution across the airstream
- sufficient length of travel through the spray and wetted surfaces
- elimination of free moisture from the outlet air

Spray water requirements for spray-type air washers used for washing or evaporative cooling vary from 4 gpm per 1000 cfm with a single bank to 10 gpm per 1000 cfm for double banks (0.5 to 1.3 L/s per m^3/s). Pumping heads usually range from 55 to 150 ft of water (160 to 450 kPa), depending on such factors as spray pressure, height of apparatus, and pressure losses in pipe and strainers.

17.6 Dehumidification

Dehumidification is the reduction of the water content of air, gases, or other fluids. Dehumidification is normally limited to equipment operating at essentially atmospheric pressures, built to standards similar to other types of air-handling equipment.

Drying of gases has become an increasingly important operation. Some commercial applications include the following:

1. lowering the relative humidity to facilitate manufacturing and handling of hygroscopic materials
2. air conditioning for comfort (in combination with cooling, under certain design conditions, such as high moisture load in comparison to sensible heat load)
3. providing protective atmospheres for the heat treatment of metals
4. maintaining controlled humidity conditions in warehouses and caves for storage
5. preserving ships and other surplus equipment, which would otherwise deteriorate
6. condensation and corrosion control
7. drying air for wind tunnels
8. drying natural gas
9. drying instrument air and plant air
10. drying of process and industrial gases
11. dehydration of liquids

17.6.1 Methods of Dehumidification

Dehumidification can be accomplished by compression, refrigeration, liquid sorption, solid sorption, or combinations of these systems.

Three methods by which sorbent materials or sorbent equipment dehumidify air are illustrated in the psychrometric chart shown in Figure 17-11. Air at point A can be dehumidified and cooled to point B by a liquid sorption system with intercooling directly. Alternatively, it may be dehumidified in a solid sorption unit by precooling and dehumidifying from point A to point C, desiccating from point C to point E, and finally cooling to point B. Air could also be dehumidified with solid sorption equipment by desiccating from point A to point D and then by refrigeration from point D to point B.

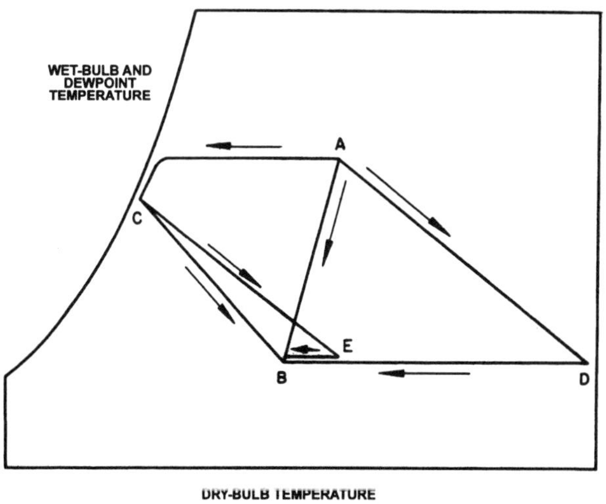

Fig. 17-11 Methods of Dehumidification

Compression Dehumidification. Compressing a gas to be dehumidified reduces its absolute moisture content, but it generally produces a saturated condition at the elevated pressure. This method is uneconomical, but is of value for pressure systems since part of the moisture is removed by compression of the gas; the remaining moisture may be removed by cooling alone, with sorption, or both, depending on the final dew point required. Expansion of high-pressure gas also lowers the dew point.

Refrigeration Dehumidification. Refrigerating gas below its dew point is the most common method of dehumidification. This method is advantageous when the gas (1) is comparatively warm, (2) has a high moisture content, and (3) requires an outlet dew point above 40°F (5°C). Frequently, refrigeration is used in combination with sorption dehumidifiers to obtain an extremely low dew point at minimum cost.

Direct Sorption Dehumidification. Sorbent materials used in dehumidification equipment may either be liquids or solids. The performance of the different sorption dehumidification machines is, to some extent, a function of the sorbent used. Sorbents either retain water on their surface (adsorption) or chemically combine with water (absorption). In regenerative equipment, the water must be removed from the sorbent to regenerate it for further use.

Nonregenerative equipment uses hygroscopic salts such as calcium chloride, urea, or sodium chloride. In regenerative systems, the sorbent is usually a form of silica, alumina gel, activated alumina, molecular sieves, lithium chloride salt, lithium chloride solution, or glycol solution.

In liquid sorption dehumidification systems, the gas passes through sprays of a liquid sorbent such as lithium chloride or a glycol solution. The sorbent in active state has a vapor pressure below that of the gas to be dehumidified and absorbs moisture from the gas stream. The sorbent solution during the process of absorption becomes diluted with moisture, which during regeneration is given up to an outdoor airstream in which the solution is heated. A partial bleed-off of the solution is used for continuous reconcentration of the sorbent in a closed circuit between the spraying or contactor unit and the regenerator unit.

In solid sorption, the gas stream passes through or over granular beds of fixed desiccant structures. A number of commercially available desiccants may be used, depending on such factors as the character of the gas to be dried, inlet temperature, moisture levels, and required final dew point. Outdoor air is passed through beds or layers of the sorbent, which in its active state has a vapor pressure below that of the gas to be dehumidified and absorbs moisture from the gas stream. After becoming saturated with moisture, the desiccant is periodically reactivated to give up previously absorbed moisture to an outdoor air or gas stream.

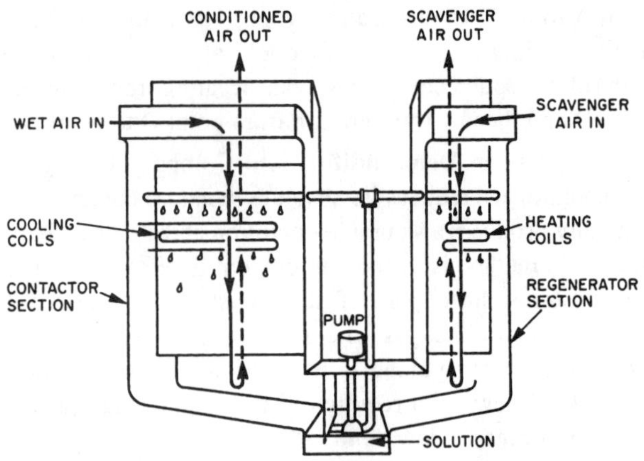

Fig. 17-12 Flow Diagram for Liquid-Absorbent Dehumidifier

17.6.2 Liquid Absorption Equipment

The flow diagram for a typical liquid absorption system with extended-surface contactor coils is shown in Figure 17-12. For dehumidifying operation, the strong absorbent solution is pumped from the sump of the unit and sprayed over the contactor coils.

Air to be conditioned passes over the contactor coils and comes in contact with the hygroscopic solution. Airflow can be either parallel with or counter to the sprayed solution flow, depending on the space and application requirements.

The degree of dehumidification depends on the concentration, temperature, and characteristics of the hygroscopic solution. Moisture is absorbed from the air by the solution due to the vapor pressure difference between the air and the liquid absorbent. The moisture content of the outlet air can be precisely maintained by varying the coolant flow in the coil to control the absorbent solution contact temperature. The absorbent solution is maintained at the proper concentration by continuous regeneration.

The heat generated in absorbing moisture from the air consists of the latent heat of condensation of water vapor and the heat of solution, or the heat of mixing, of the water and the absorbent. The heat of mixing varies with the liquid absorbent used and with the concentration and temperature of the absorbent. The total heat removal required by the conditioner coil consists of the heat of absorption, sensible heat removed from the air, and the residual heat load added by the regeneration process.

17.6.3 Solid Sorption

Dehumidification by use of a solid desiccant, such as silica gel, molecular sieves, activated alumina, or hygroscopic salts, may be performed under either static or dynamic conditions. In the static method, the air or gas is not forced through the desiccant. Instead, the air immediately surrounding the desiccant dries, and through convection and vapor diffusion, water vapor from surrounding areas reaches the desiccant where it is absorbed. In dynamic dehumidification, the air or gas being dried flows through the desiccant bed or structure. In the air-conditioning industry, which is primarily concerned with operation at atmospheric pressure, an air-moving device such as a fan forces the gas through the desiccant bed and a heater or other means periodically reactivates the desiccant.

17.6.4 Solid Absorption Equipment

The arrangement of major components of a typical solid absorption system is shown in Figure 17-13. To achieve dehumidification, moist air is passed through a desiccant structure, where the water vapor in the air is absorbed by the desiccant. The systems employ a desiccant structure that may be a disc, drum, or wheel, filled or saturated with an absorbent, such as lithium chloride. The desiccant structure rotates slowly through a heated stream of air where the desiccant is desorbed or reactivated. By continuous rotation, freshly reactivated portions of the desiccant are always available for drying.

The amount of drying depends on the temperature and absolute humidity of the air and the useful concentration of desiccant. The useful concentration of the desiccant is affected by

- quantity of desiccant in relation to the mass flow of air and water vapor
- energy (amount of heat and temperature) for reactivation
- frequency of reactivation (speed of rotation)

Performance typical of a solid absorption dehumidifier using a fixed desiccant structure is shown in Figure 17-14.

17.7 Humidification

When selecting humidification equipment, both the environmental conditions of the occupancy or process and the characteristics of the building enclosure must be considered.

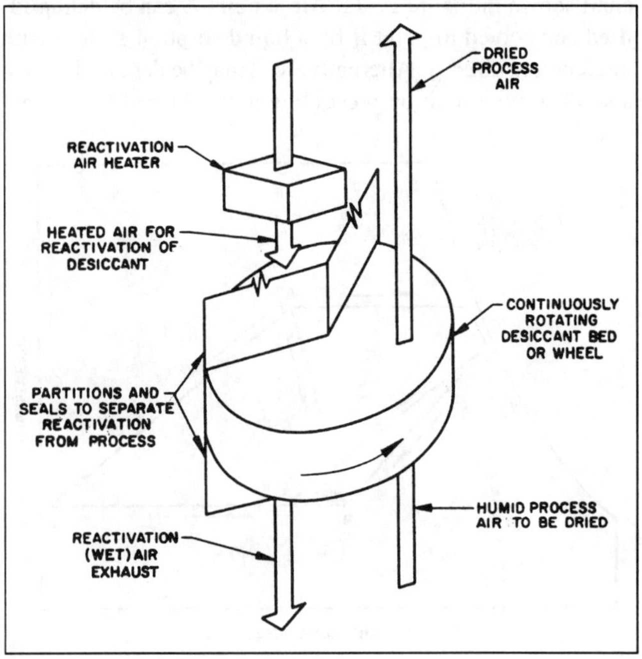

Fig. 17-13 Rotary Dehumidification Unit

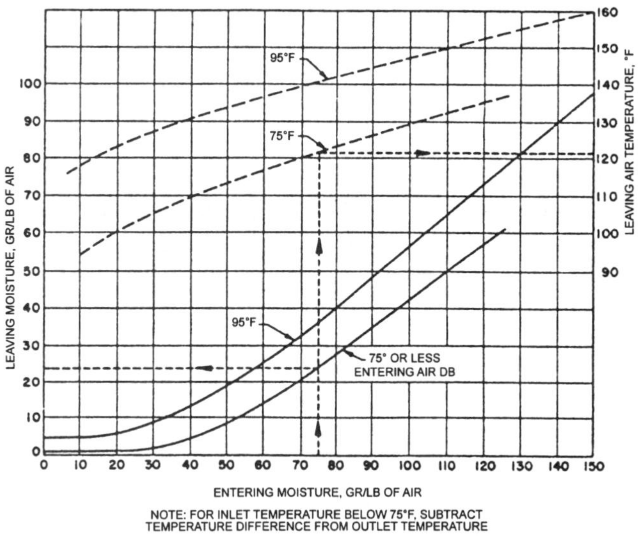

Fig. 17-14 Performance Data for Rotary Solid Absorption Dehumidifier

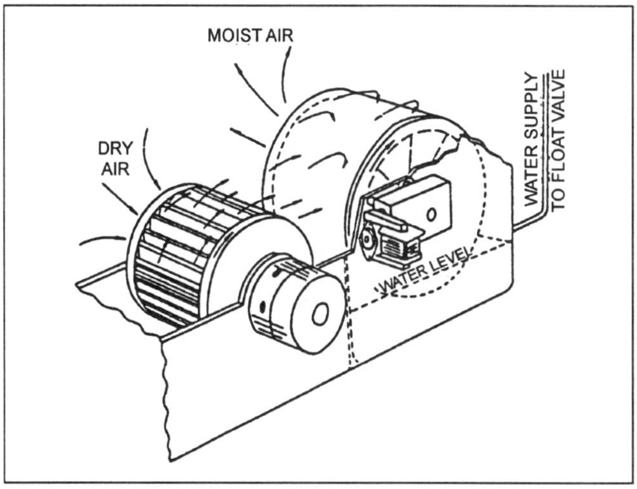

Fig. 17-16 Wetted-Drum Humidifier

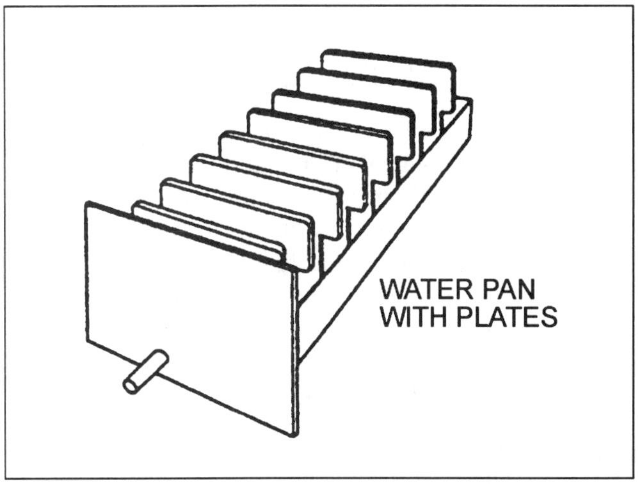

Fig. 17-15 Pan-Type Humidifier

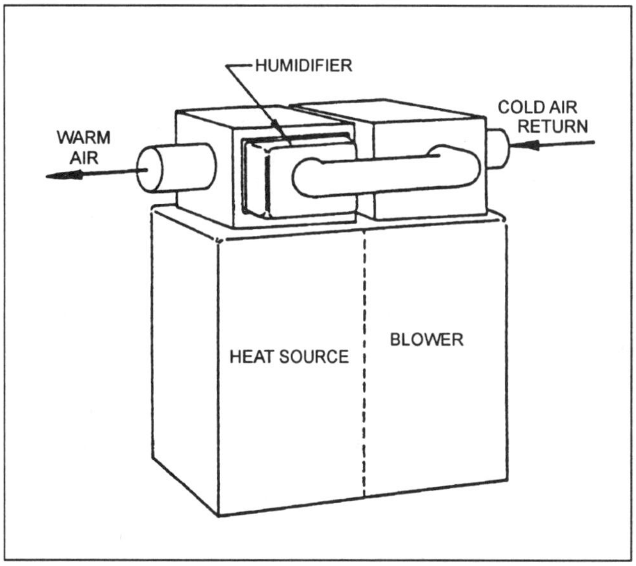

Fig. 17-17 Bypass Wetted-Element Humidifier

These may not always be compatible and a compromise solution may be necessary.

Air washers and evaporative coolers may be used as humidifiers, but are usually selected to provide some additional function, such as air cooling or air cleaning, as discussed in the section on air washers.

Residential Humidifiers for Central Air Systems. This type of unit depends on airflow in the heating system for evaporation and distribution. General principles of operation and description of equipment are as follows:

Pan Type. The humidification rate varies with temperature, humidity, and velocity of the air in the system (Figure 17-15).

Wetted Elements. These units use an open textured, wetted media, through or over which air is circulated. The evaporating surface may take the form of a fixed pad, wetted by sprays or by water flowing through by gravity from a header at the top, or the pad may be a paddle wheel, drum, or belt rotating through a water reservoir. Figures 17-16 and 17-17 are examples of this type of humidifier.

Residential Humidifiers for Nonducted Applications. Many portable or room humidifiers are available for use in residences and apartments heated by nonducted systems, such as hydronic or electric, or where the occupant is prevented from making a permanent installation. An example of this type of humidifier is shown in Figure 17-18.

Industrial/Commercial Humidifiers for Central Air Systems. Humidification equipment commonly used in central air-handling systems incorporates a heated water pan, direct steam injection, or atomizers. Specific types are shown in Figure 17-19 and discussed briefly in the following paragraphs.

Heated Pan. These units offer a broad range of capacity and may be heated by an electric element, steam, or hot water coil (see Figure 17-19A). Some units are designed to be attached directly to the underside of a system duct. Others are

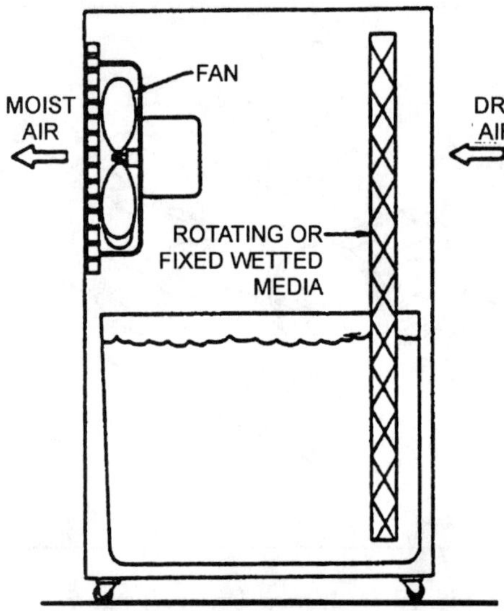

Fig. 17-18 Portable Humidifier

provided with a fan or a steam hose, which allows them to be installed remote from the ductwork.

Steam. Direct steam injection humidifiers cover a wide range of designs and capacities. Since water vapor is steam at low pressure and temperature, the whole process can be simplified by introducing steam directly into the air to be humidified. This method is essentially an isothermal process because the temperature of the air remains constant as the moisture is added in vapor form. The steam control valve may be modulating or two-position in response to a humidity controller. The steam may be either used from an external source with enclosed grid, cup, or jacketed dry steam humidifiers or produced within the humidifier, as in the self-contained type.

- *Enclosed steam grid humidifiers* (Figure 17-19B) should be used on low steam pressures to prevent splashing of condensate in the duct.
- A *cup* or *pot-type humidifier* (Figure 17-19C) is usually attached under a system duct. Steam is attached tangentially to the inner periphery of the cup by one or more steam inlets, depending on the capability of the unit. The steam supply line should have a suitable steam trap.
- A *jacketed steam humidifier* uses an integral steam valve with a steam-jacketed duct-traversing dispersing tube and condensate separator to prevent condensate from being introduced into the airstream (Figure 17-19D). An inverted bucket-type steam trap is required to drain the separating chamber.

The aforementioned humidifiers inject steam directly from the boiler into the space or duct system. Some boiler treatment chemicals can be discharges, which can affect indoor air quality.

- A *self-contained steam humidifier* converts tap water to steam by electrical energy using either the electrode boiler principle or resistance heating. This steam is injected into the duct system through a dispersion manifold (Figure 17-19E), or the humidifier may be freestanding for nonducted applications.

Atomizing humidifiers with optional filter eliminator (Figure 17-19F). Centrifugal atomizers use a high-speed disc, that slings water through a fine comb to create a fine mist that is introduced directly into the air where it is evaporated. The ability of the air to absorb the moisture depends on temperature, air velocity, and moisture content. Where mineral fallout from hard water is a problem, optional filter eliminators may be added to remove mineral dust from humidified air, or water demineralizers may be installed. Additional atomizing methods use nozzles; one uses water pressure and the other uses both air and water, as shown in Figure 17-19G. Mixing air and water streams at combined pressures atomizes water into a fine mist, which is evaporated in the room or air duct.

Wetted-element humidifier. Wetted-element humidifiers have a wetted media, sometimes in modular configurations, through or over which air is circulated to evaporate water. This unit depends on airflow for evaporation; the rate varies with temperature, humidity, and velocity of the air.

17.8 Air Cleaners

In buildings, dust content seldom exceeds 2 mg/m^3 and is usually less than 0.2 mg/m^3 of air. This concentration is in contrast to exhaust gases from processes and flue gases where dust concentration typically ranges from 200 to 40 000 mg/m^3.

With certain exceptions, the air cleaners described in this section are not applicable to the cleaning of exhaust gases. Atmospheric dust is a complex mixture of smokes, mists, fumes, dry granular particles, and fibers (such particles, when suspended in a gas, are called aerosols). A sample of atmospheric dust gathered at any point generally contains materials common to that locality, together with other components that originated at a distance but have been transported by air currents or diffusion.

These components vary with the geography of the locality in question, the season of the year, the direction and strength of the wind, and the proximity of dust sources. A sample of atmospheric dust usually contains soot and smoke, silica, clay, decayed animal and vegetable matter, organic materials in the form of lint and plant fibers, and metallic fragments. It may also contain living organisms, such as mold spores, bacteria, and plant pollens, which may cause diseases or allergic responses. Chapter 11 of the 1993 *Handbook—Fundamentals* contains further information on atmospheric contaminants.

The particles in the atmosphere can range in size from less than 0.01 mm to dimensions of lint, leaves, and insects. Almost all conceivable shapes and sizes are represented. This wide variety makes it impossible to design one cleaner that is best for all applications. For example, in industrial ventilation, only the coarser dust particles may need to be removed from the airstream for cleanliness of the structure and protection of mechanical equipment. In other applications, surface discoloration must be prevented. Unfortunately, the smaller

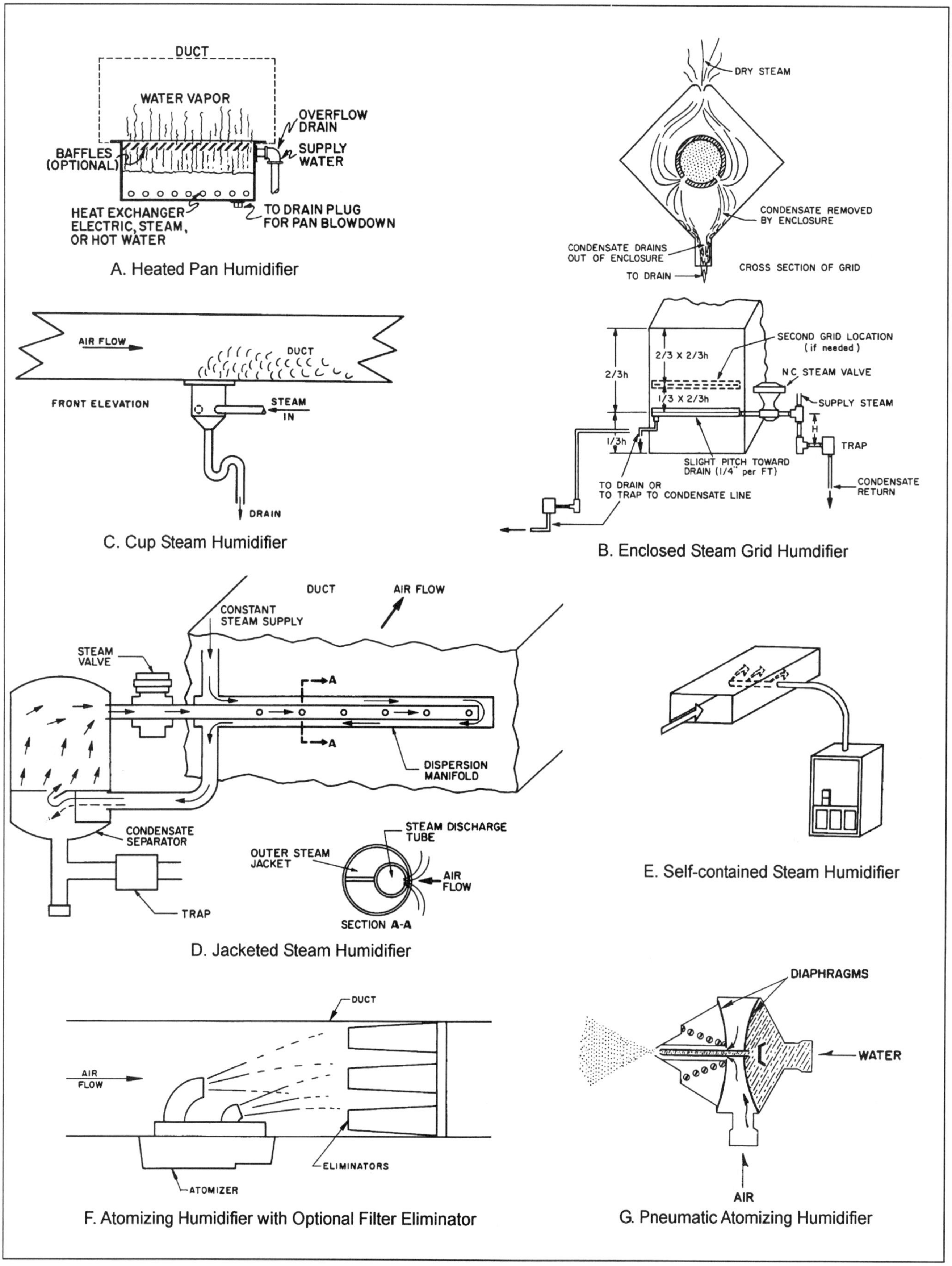

Fig. 17-19 Commercial Humidifiers

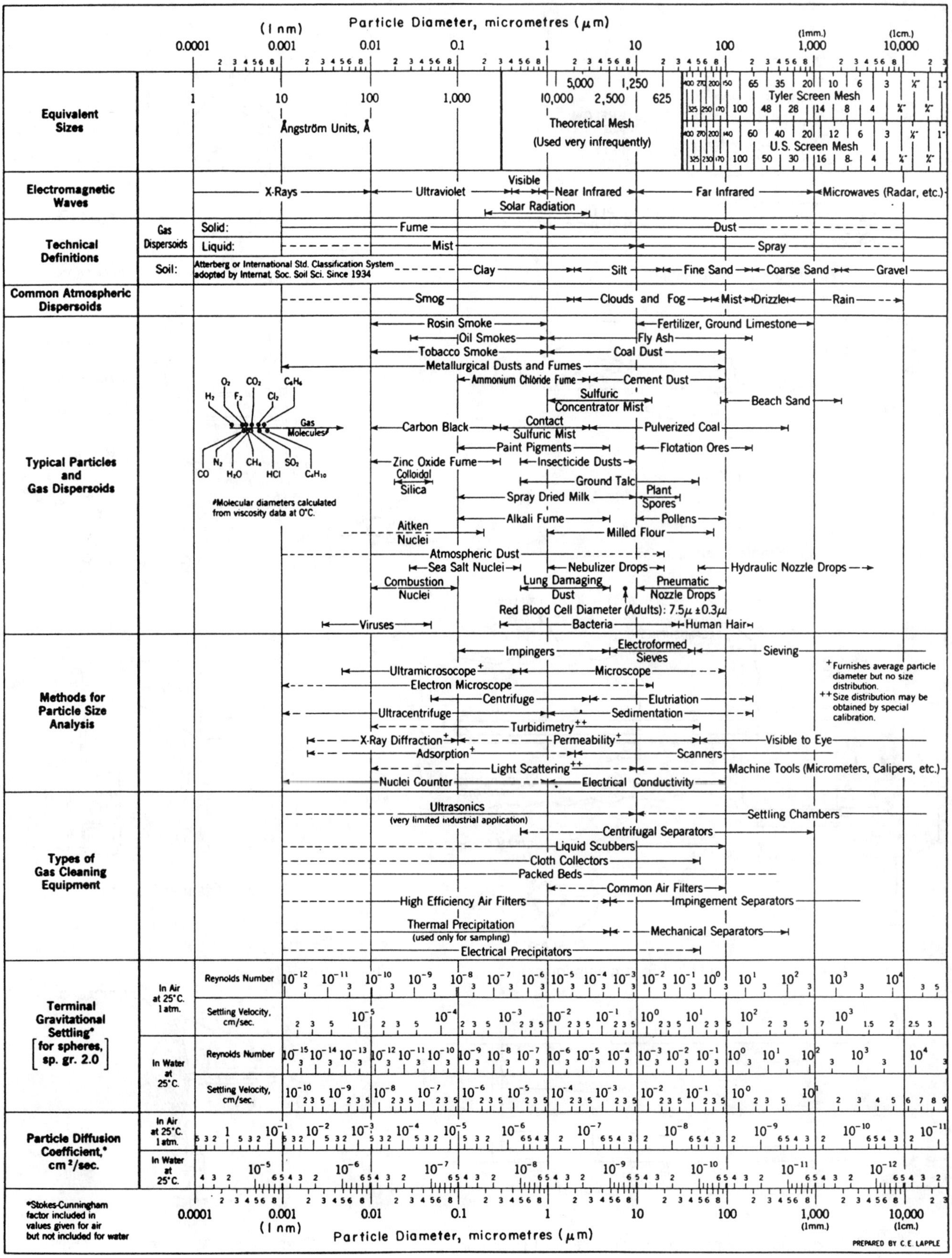

Fig. 17-20 Characteristics of Particles

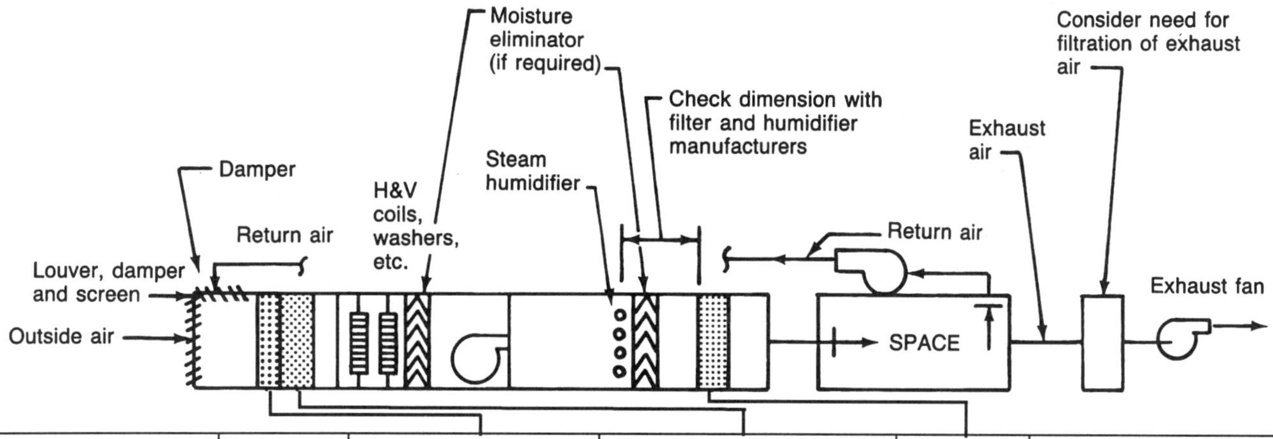

Application	System Designator[b]	Prefilter		Prefilter/Filter		Final Filter	Application Notes
Warehouse, storage, shop and process areas, mechanical equipment rooms, electrical control rooms, protection for heating and cooling coils	A1	None	None	50 to 85% arrestance	Panel-type or automatic roll	None	Reduce larger particle settling. Protect coils from dirt and lint.
	A2	None	None	25 to 30% dust spot	Pleated panel or extended surface	None	
Special process areas, electrical shops, paint shops, average general offices and laboratories	B1	None	None	75 to 90% arrestance, 35 to 60% dust spot	Extended surface, cartridge, bag-type, or electronic (manually cleaned or replaceable media)	None	Average housecleaning. Reduces lint in airstream. Reduces ragweed pollen >85% at 35%. Removes all pollens at 60%, somewhat effective on particles causing smudge and stain.
Analytical laboratories, electronics shops, drafting areas, conference rooms, above-average general offices	C1	75 to 85% arrestance, 25 to 40% dust spot	Extended surface, cartridge, or bag-type	>98% arrestance, 80 to 85% dust spot	Bag-type, cartridge, or electronic (semi-automatic cleaning)	None	Above average housecleaning. No settling particles of dust. Cartridge and bag-types very effective on particles causing smudge and stain, partially effective on tobacco smoke. Electronic types quite effective on smoke.
	C2	None	None	>98% arrestance, 80 to 85% dust spot	Electronic (agglomerator) with bag or cartridge section	None	
Hospitals, pharmaceutical R&D and manufacturing (non-aseptic areas only), some clean ("gray") rooms	D1	75 to 85% arrestance, 25 to 40% dust spot	Extended surface, cartridge, or bag-type	>98% arrestance, 80 to 85% dust spot	Bag-type, cartridge, electronic (semi-automatic cleaning)	95% DOP disposable cell	Excellent housecleaning. Very effective on particles causing smudge and stain, smoke and fumes. Highly effective on bacteria.
	D2	None	None	>98% arrestance, 80 to 95% dust spot	Electronic (agglomerator) with bag or cartridge section	None	
Aseptic areas in hospital and pharmaceutical R&D and manufacturing. Clean rooms in film and electronics manufacturing, radioactive areas, etc.[c]	E1	75 to 85% arrestance, 25 to 40% dust spot	Extended surface, cartridge, or bag-type	>98% arrestance, 80 to 85% dust spot	Bag-type, cartridge, electronic (semi-automatic cleaning)	≥99.97% DOP disposable cell	Protects against bacteria, radioactive dusts, toxic dusts, smoke, and fumes.

[a] Adapted from a similar table courtesy of E.I. du Pont de Nemours & Company.
[b] System designators have no significance other than their use in this table.
[c] Electronic agglomerators and air cleaners are not usually recommended for clean room applications.

Fig. 17-21 Typical Filter Applications

components of atmospheric dust are the worst offenders in smudging and discoloring building interiors. Electronic air cleaners or high-efficiency dry filters are required for small particle removal. In clean room applications or when radioactive or other dangerous particles are present, extremely high-efficiency mechanical filters should be used.

The most important characteristics of aerosols affecting the performance of an air filter include particle size and shape, density, and concentration. The most important of these is particle size. Data on the sizes and characteristics of airborne particulate matter and the wide range of particle size encountered are given in Figure 17-20. Cleaning efficiency is also affected by the velocity of the airstream. The degree of air cleanliness required is a major factor influencing filter design and selection. Removal of particles becomes progressively more difficult as particle size decreases.

Cost considerations (both in initial investment and maintenance), space requirements, and airflow resistance, in addition to wide-ranging criteria as to degree of air cleanliness, have resulted in a wide variety of commercial air cleaners.

To evaluate filters and air cleaners properly for a particular application, the following factors should be considered:

- Degree of air cleanliness required
- Disposal of dust after it is removed from the air
- Amount and type of dust in the air filtered
- Operating resistance to airflow (pressure drop)
- Space available for filtration equipment
- Cost of maintaining or replacing filters
- Initial cost of the system

Figure 17-21 lists some applications of filters classified according to their efficiencies and type.

17.8.1 Types of Air Cleaners

Air cleaners fall into the following three categories:

1. *Fibrous media unit filters* in which accumulating dust load causes pressure drop to increase up to some maximum permissible value. During this period, efficiency normally increases; however, at high dust loads, dust may adhere poorly to filter fibers, and efficiency drops. Filters in such condition should be replaced or reconditioned, as should filters that have reached their terminal (maximum permissible) pressure drop. This category includes both viscous impingement and dry air filters.
2. *Renewable media filters* in which fresh media is introduced into the airstream as needed to maintain essentially constant resistance. This also maintains essentially constant efficiency.
3. *Electronic air cleaners*, which have essentially constant pressure drop and efficiency unless their precipitating elements become severely dust-loaded.

17.8.2 Fibrous Media Unit Filters

Viscous Impingement Filters. These flat panel filters consist of coarse fibers and have a high porosity. The filter media is coated with a viscous substance, such as oil, which acts as an adhesive for particles that impinge on the fibers. Design air velocity through the media is usually in the range of 250 to 700 fpm (1 to 4 m/s). These filters are characterized by low pressure drop, low cost, and good efficiency on lint, but low efficiency on normal atmospheric dust. They are commonly 1/2 to 4 in. (13 to 100 mm) thick; 1- to 2- in. (25- to 50-mm) nominal thickness is most popular. The thicker configurations have a high dust-holding capacity. Unit panels are available in standard and special sizes up to about 24 in. by 24 in. (610 mm by 610 mm). This type of filter is often used as a prefilter to higher efficiency filters.

Many different materials have been used as the filtering medium, including coarse (15 to 60 μm diameter) glass fibers, animal hair, vegetable fibers, synthetic fibers, metallic wools, expanded metals and foils, crimped screens, random-matted wire, and synthetic open-cell foams.

Although viscous impingement filters usually operate in the range of 300 to 600 fpm (1.5 to 3 m/s), they may operate at higher velocities. The limiting factor other than increased flow resistance is the danger of blowing off agglomerates of collected dust and the viscous coating on the filter.

The rate of filter loading depends on the type and concentration of the dirt being handled and on the operating cycle of the system. Manometers or draft gages are often installed to measure the pressure drop across the filter bank and thereby indicate when the filter needs servicing. The final allowable pressure drop may vary from one installation to another; but, in general, unit filters are serviced when their operating resistance reaches 0.5 in. of water (120 Pa). The decline in filter efficiency that occurs when all the viscous coating has been absorbed by the collected dust, rather than the increased resistance due to dust load, may be the limiting factor in operating life.

Dry Air Filters. The media used in dry air filters are random fiber mats or blankets of varying thicknesses, fiber sizes, and densities. Media of bonded glass fiber, cellulose fibers, wool felt, asbestos, synthetics, and other materials have been used commercially. The medium in filters of this class is frequently supported by a wire frame in the form of pockets or V-shaped pleats. In other designs, the media may be self-supporting because of inherent rigidity or because airflow inflates it into extended form. Pleating of the media provides a high ratio of media area to face area, thus allowing reasonable pressure drop despite the density and fineness of the media.

The efficiency of dry air filters is usually higher than that of viscous impingement filters, and the variety of media available makes it possible to furnish almost any degree of cleaning efficiency desired. Modern dry filter media and filter configurations also have higher dust-holding capacities than viscous impingement filters. Coarse prefilters placed ahead of high-efficiency dry filters may be economically justified by the even longer life they give the main filters.

Electronic Air Cleaners. These ionizing filters are efficient, low pressure drop devices for removing fine dust and smoke particles. Collector plates are often coated with a special oil as an adhesive. Cleaning is generally accomplished by washing the cells in place with hot water from a water hose or by a fixed or moving nozzle system.

Electrical forces drive most particles to the collecting surface but cannot hold them there. In fact, after a particle touches the collecting surface, the electrical force reverses and tends to pull it off, and the dust is held only by intermolecular adhesion forces. It is, therefore, very important with the washed type of electronic air cleaner to ensure that either the dust is naturally adherent or that the plates are always covered with adhesive.

Electronic air cleaners, however, are often used without any adhesive treatment on the plates. Under such conditions, the precipitator forms agglomerates that eventually blow off the plates. They must be followed downstream by a secondary filter or storage section. The dry agglomerates produced in the precipitator are allowed to blow off and be caught by the downstream filter. An automatic replaceable media filter for catching these agglomerates gives a combination with a high degree of cleaning efficiency and also the convenient maintenance associated with an automatic filter. A schematic diagram of an ionizing electronic air cleaner is shown in Figure 17-22.

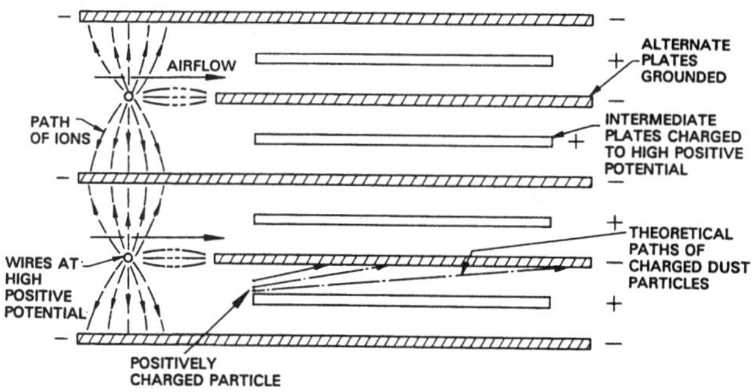

Fig. 17-22 Cross-Section of Ionizing Electronic Air Cleaner

17.9 Air-to-Air Energy Recovery Equipment

Energy can be recovered from exhaust air, as well as transferred from one location to another. This can be done using rotary devices, heat pipe heat exchangers, coil heat recovery loops, twin tower heat recovery loops, fixed plate exchangers, and thermosiphon heat exchangers.

Table 17-1 provides comparative data for common types of air-to-air energy recovery devices. The following sections describe the construction, operation, and unique features of the various devices.

17.9.1 Performance Rating of Equipment

Performance of air-to-air heat exchangers is usually expressed in terms of their effectiveness in transferring (1) sensible energy (dry-bulb temperature), (2) latent energy (humidity ratio), or (3) total energy (enthalpy). The effectiveness e of a heat exchanger is defined as follows:

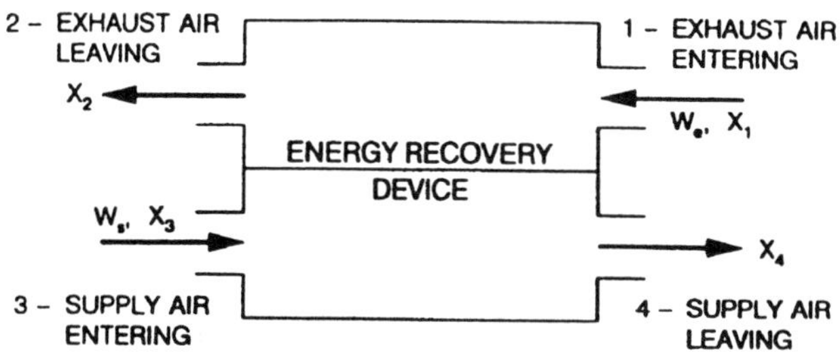

Fig. 17-23 Nomenclature for Effectiveness Evaluation

$$\varepsilon = \frac{\text{Actual transfer for given device}}{\text{Maximum possible transfer between airstreams}}$$

Referring to Figure 17-23,

$$\varepsilon = \frac{W_e(X_1 - X_2)}{W_{min}(X_1 - X_3)} = \frac{W_s(X_4 - X_3)}{W_{min}(X_1 - X_3)} \qquad (17\text{-}7)$$

where

ε = sensible, latent, or total heat effectiveness
X = dry-bulb temperature, humidity ratio, or enthalpy at locations indicated in Figure 17-23

For the latent and total heat effectiveness,

W_s = mass flow rate of supply
W_e = mass flow rate of exhaust

For the sensible heat effectiveness,

W_s = (specific heat)(mass flow rate) for the supply
W_e = (specific heat)(mass flow rate) for the exhaust
W_{min} = smaller of W_s and W_e

The leaving supply air condition is then

$$X_2 = X_1 - \varepsilon(X_1 - X_3)(W_{min}/W_s) \qquad (17\text{-}8a)$$

The leaving exhaust air condition is:

$$X_4 = X_3 + \varepsilon(X_1 - X_3)(W_{min}/W_3) \qquad (17\text{-}8b)$$

The effectiveness of a particular air-to-air energy recovery device is a function of several variables, including the supply and exhaust mass flow rates and the energy transfer characteristics of the device. Because of this combination, performance data must be established for each device.

17.9.2 Economics of Air-to-Air Energy Recovery

In analyzing any air-to-air energy recovery application, consider both first and operating costs.

First Cost

- Energy recovery device
- Installing energy recovery device
- Additional ductwork to accommodate device, or cost of piping for energy transfer liquid
- Larger fans and/or motors to overcome static pressure loss of energy recovery device
- Additional air filtration required, if any

Table 17-2 Comparison of Air-to-Air Energy Recovery Devices

	Fixed Plate	Rotary Wheel	Heat Pipe	Runaround Coil Loop	Thermosiphon	Twin Towers
Airflow arrangements	Counterflow Crossflow Parallel flow	Counterflow Parallel flow	Counterflow Parallel flow	Counterflow Parallel flow	Counterflow Parallel flow	
Equipment size range, cfm	50 and up	50 to 70,000	100 and up	100 and up	100 and up	
Type of heat transfer (typical effectiveness)	Sensible (50 to 80%)	Sensible (50 to 80%) Total (55 to 85%)	Sensible (45 to 65%)	Sensible (55 to 65%)	Sensible (40 to 60%)	Sensible (40 to 60%)
Face velocity, fpm (most common design velocity)	100 to 1000 (200 to 1000)	500 to 1000	400 to 800 (450 to 550)	300 to 600	400 to 800 (450 to 550)	300 to 450
Pressure drop, in. of water (most likely pressure)	0.02 to 1.8 (0.1 to 1.5)	(0.4 to 0.7)	(0.4 to 2.0)	(0.4 to 2.0)	(0.4 to 2.0)	0.7 to 1.2
Temperature range	–70 to 1500°F	–70 to 1500°F	–40 to 95°F	–50 to 900°F	–40 to 104°F	–40 to 115°F
Typical mode of purchase	Exchanger only Exchanger in case Exchanger and blowers Complete system	Exchanger only Exchanger in case Exchanger and blowers Complete system	Exchanger only Exchanger in case	Coil only Complete system	Exchanger only Exchanger in case	Complete system
Unique advantages	No moving parts Low pressure drop Easily cleaned	Latent transfer Compact large sizes Low pressure drop	No moving parts except tilt Fan location not critical Allowable pressure differential up to 60 in. of water	Exhaust airstream can be separated from supply air Fan location not critical	No moving parts Exhaust airstream can be separated from supply air Fan location not critical	Latent transfer from remote airstreams Multiple units in a single system Efficient microbiological cleaning of both supply and exhaust airstreams
Limitations	Latent available in hygroscopic units only	Cold climates may increase service Cross-air contamination possible	Effectiveness limited by pressure drop and cost Few suppliers	High effectiveness requires accurate simulation model	Effectiveness may be limited by pressure drop and cost Few suppliers	Few suppliers
Cross-leakage	0 to 5%	1 to 10%	0%	0%	0%	0.025%
Heat rate control (HRC) schemes	Bypass dampers and ducting	Wheel speed control over full range	Tilt angle down to 10% of maximum heat rate	Bypass valve or pump speed control over full range	Control valve over full range	Control valve or pump speed control over full range

- Capacity controls
- Any auxiliary heaters required for frost control
- Savings of boiler or heating equipment due to reduced design load
- Savings of heating coils and associated piping and pumps due to reduced design capacity
- Savings of chiller or cooling plant due to reduced design load
- Savings of cooling coils and associated piping and pumps due to reduced design capacity
- Savings of electric supply equipment

Operating Cost

- Maintaining the energy recovery device
- Operating fans to overcome additional static pressure
- Maintaining additional filtration, if any
- Operating energy recovery device drive, pumps, controls, and defrost heaters
- Savings of annual heating energy, based on weather data for the system location
- Savings of annual cooling energy, based on weather data for the system location

17.9.3 Rotary Air-to-Air Energy Exchangers

A rotary air-to-air energy exchanger, often called a heat wheel, is a revolving cylinder filled with an air permeable medium with a large internal surface area for contact with the air passing through it. Adjacent supply and exhaust airstreams each flow through half the exchanger in a counterflow pattern (Figure 17-24). Media material may be selected to recover either sensible heat only or total heat (sensible heat plus latent heat).

Sensible heat is recovered (transferred) as the medium picks up and stores heat from the hot airstream and gives it up to the cold one. Latent heat is transferred as the medium (1) condenses moisture from the airstream having the higher humidity ratio (by means of absorption for liquid desiccants and adsorption for solid desiccants), with a simultaneous release of heat and (2) then releases the moisture through evaporation (and heat pick-up) into the airstream with the lower humidity ratio. Thus, more moist air is dried while drier air is humidified. In total heat transfer, both sensible and latent heat recovery processes take place simultaneously.

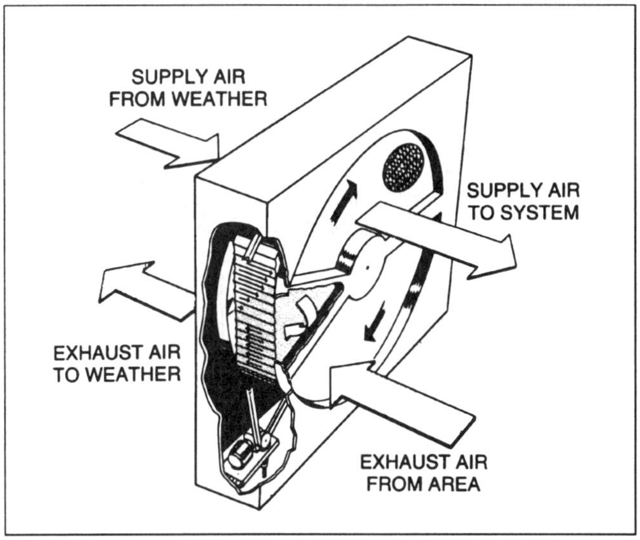

Fig. 17-24 Rotary Energy Exchanger

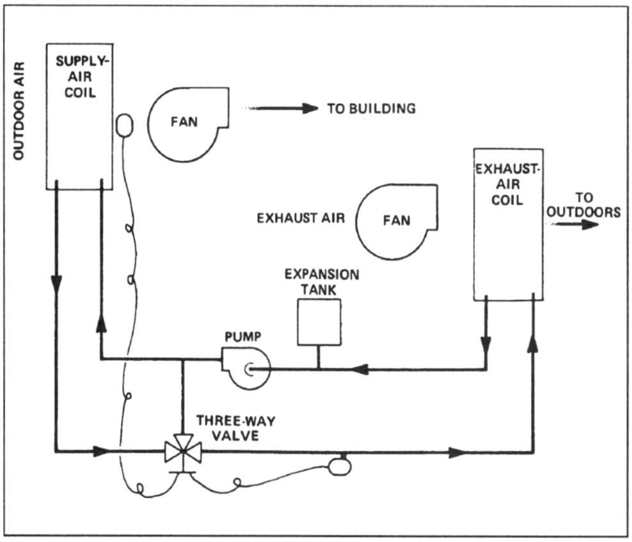

Fig. 17-25 Arrangement of Coil Energy Recovery Loop

Choice of structural material for the casing, rotor structure, and medium of a rotary energy exchanger is influenced by the contaminants, dew point, and temperature of the exhaust air, as well as by the properties of the supply air. Aluminum and steel are the usual casing and rotor materials for normal comfort ventilating systems. Exchanger media are fabricated from metal, mineral, or man-made materials and classified as providing either random flow or directionally-oriented flow through their structures.

The performance of a rotary energy exchanger is defined by the exchanger's effectiveness and the media pressure drops. Face velocities for most energy recovery applications range from 500 to 800 fpm (2.5 to 4.0 m/s). Low face velocities give lower pressure drop, higher effectiveness, and lower operating costs, but require larger size units with higher capital costs and more installation space.

Typical pressure drops for various types of media at 500 fpm (2.5 m/s) vary from 0.4 to 0.7 in. of water (100 to 170 Pa). (Consult the manufacturer's catalog in each case for actual data.) Average effectiveness values for sensible and total heat exchangers lie in the 70 to 85% range for equal supply and exhaust air mass flow rates and usual exchanger face velocities.

Rotary energy exchangers are available in single units to 68,000 cfm (32 m^3/s) capacity; they are usually not larger than 14 ft (4.25 m) in diameter due to difficulty in shipping, erecting, and fitting into buildings. Multiple units may be used to provide greater single-system capacities. Units are available for temperatures −70 to 1500°F (−60 to 800°C). When installed horizontally (vertical airflow), units greater than 8 ft (2.4 m) in diameter may require special structural considerations due to their size and weight.

17.9.4 Coil Energy Recovery Loops

The coil energy recovery loop system uses extended- surface, finned-tube water coils placed in the supply, and exhaust airstreams of a building or process. The coils are connected in a closed loop via counterflow piping and an intermediate heat transfer fluid of water (typically) or a freeze-protected solution is pumped through the coils.

This system allows energy to transfer from the warmer to the cooler airstream. In a typical comfort-to-comfort application, the system is seasonally reversible—the supply air preheats when outdoor air is cooler than the exhaust air and precools when the outdoor air is warmer. This system operates generally for sensible heat recovery.

As with other air-to-air energy recovery equipment, measures must be taken to prevent potential freezing of exhaust air condensate. A dual purpose, three-way temperature control valve is used to prevent exhaust coil freeze-up. The valve is controlled to maintain an entering solution temperature to the exhaust coil of not less than 30°F (−1°C). This is accomplished by bypassing some of the warmer solution from the supply air coil. The valve can also ensure that a prescribed leaving air temperature from the supply air coil is not exceeded for those applications where the energy recovered must be limited.

This system affords a high degree of flexibility, which makes it well-suited for renovation and industrial applications. The system accommodates remotely located supply and exhaust ducts. It also allows simultaneous energy recovery from multiple supply and exhausts. A basic arrangement of the coil energy recovery loop is depicted in Figure 17-25.

17.9.5 Twin-Tower Enthalpy Recovery Loop

This system is an air-to-liquid, liquid-to-air enthalpy recovery system. It consists of one or more contactor towers to handle the building or process supply air and also one or more contactor towers to handle the building or process exhaust air. A sorbent liquid is continuously recirculated between the supply and exhaust air contactor towers; alternately, it contacts both supply and exhaust airstreams (Figure 17-26). The sorbent acts as a vehicle for transporting humidity, as well as heat, between the two airstreams. In a typical comfort-conditioning application, building supply air is

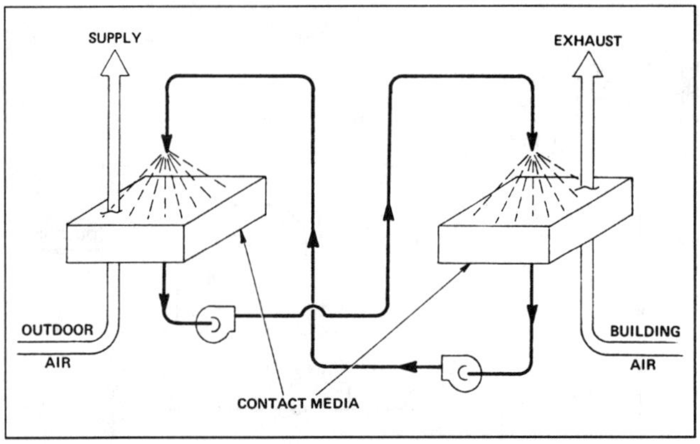

Fig. 17-26 Twin-Tower Enthalpy Recovery Loop

cooled and dehumidified during summer operation and heated and humidified during winter operation.

The sorbent solution is usually a halogen salt solution, such as lithium chloride in water. Pumps are used to circulate the solution between supply and exhaust towers.

Contactor towers are manufactured in both vertical and horizontal airflow configurations. In the vertical airflow tower, the supply or exhaust airstream passes vertically through the contact surface in a counterflow relationship to the sorbent liquid to achieve high contact efficiency. In the horizontal airflow contactor, the airstream passes horizontally through the contact surface in a crossflow relationship to the sorbent liquid, yielding a contact efficiency that is slightly lower. Vertical and horizontal contactor towers can be combined in a common system. Contactor towers of both configurations are supplied with airflow capacities of up to 100,000 scfm (47 m^3/s).

The contactor surface is usually made of nonmetallic materials, while the tower casing is made of steel with protective coatings. Air leaving the contactor tower passes through demister pads that remove any entrained droplets of the sorbent solution.

17.9.6 Heat Pipe Heat Exchangers

A heat pipe heat exchanger has no moving parts; it is a passive energy recovery device. Although it appears similar to a standard steam or chilled water coil, it differs in two major aspects. As shown schematically in Figure 17-27, each tube is an individual heat pipe, that operates independently and acts as a superconductor of heat. Secondly, the heat pipe heat exchanger is divided into two airflow paths. Hot air passes through one side of the exchanger and cold air through the other side in the opposite direction, that is, in a counterflow arrangement. Sensible energy from the hot air is transferred by the heat pipes to the other side of the exchanger, where it is captured by the cold air, thereby warming it. Although the heat pipes span the width of the unit, a sealed partition separates the two airstreams, preventing any cross contamination between them.

Figure 17-28 is a schematic of a heat pipe. A heat pipe is a tube that is fabricated with a capillary wick structure, filled

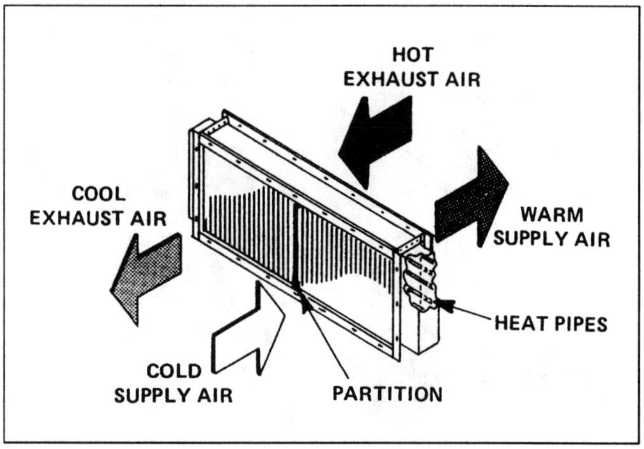

Fig. 17-27 Heat Pipe Heat Exchanger

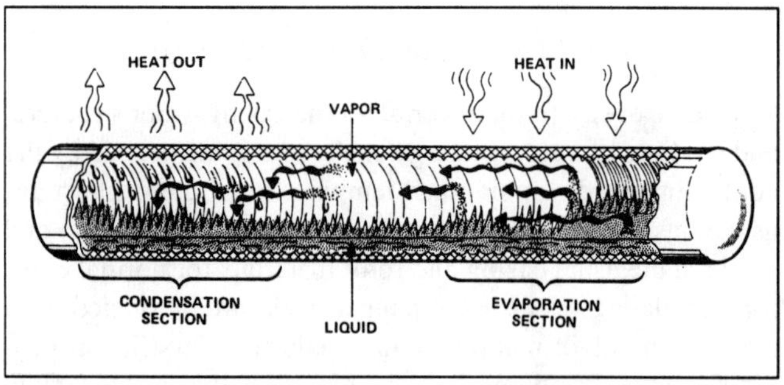

Fig. 17-28 Heat Pipe

with a refrigerant or suitable heat transfer fluid, and permanently sealed.

Basically, the heat pipe operates on a condensation/evaporation cycle that is continuous as long as there is a temperature difference to drive the process. Energy transfer within a heat pipe is accomplished with a very small temperature drop; a heat pipe is essentially an isothermal device.

Thermal energy applied to either end of the pipe causes the fluid at the end to vaporize. The vapor then travels to the other end of the pipe where the removal of thermal energy causes the vapor to condense into liquid again, thus giving up the latent heat of condensation. The condensed liquid then flows back to the evaporator section (i.e., the hot end) to be reused, completing the cycle.

Heat pipes have a finite heat transfer capacity affected by such factors as wick design, tube diameter, working fluid, and tube orientation relative to horizontal. Design face velocities for heat pipe heat exchangers range from 400 to 800 fpm (2.0 to 4.1 m/s), with 450 to 550 fpm (2.3 to 2.8 m/s) most common. Design face velocities are generally established on allowable pressure drop rather than recovery performance.

Pressure drops at 60% effectiveness range from 0.4 to 0.7 in. of water (100 to 170 Pa) at 400 fpm (2.0 m/s) up to 1.5 to 2.0 in. of water (370 to 500 Pa) at 800 fpm (4.1 m/s). Recovery performance, or effectiveness, decreases with increasing velocity, but the effect is not as pronounced as with pressure drop.

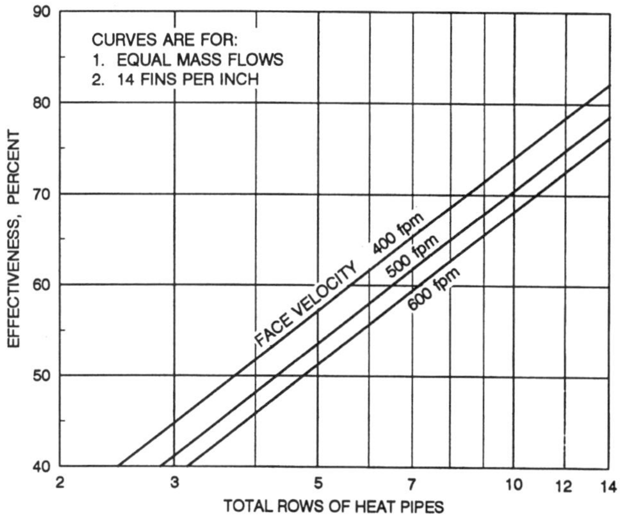

Fig. 17-29 Heat Pipe Exchanger Effectiveness

Available fin designs include continuous corrugated plate fins, continuous plain plate fins, and spiral fins. These fin designs and tube spacing cause the variation in pressure drop, noted previously, at a given face velocity.

Figure 17-29 presents a typical effectiveness curve for various face velocities and rows of tubes. As the number of rows increases, effectiveness increases at a decreasing rate. For example, doubling the rows of tubes in a 60% effective heat exchanger increases the effectiveness to 75%.

17.9.7 Fixed Plate Exchangers

The plate heat exchanger is a static device that has no leakage between airstreams. Since it uses no secondary heat transfer medium, such as water or refrigerant, its temperature range is the broadest of all air-to-air energy recovery equipment.

A fixed surface plate exchanger can be classified as (1) a **pure-plate heat exchanger**, consisting of only a primary heat transfer surface or (2) a **plate-fin heat exchanger**, which is made up of alternate layers of separate plates and interconnecting fins. The pure-plate exchanger is usually a counterflow design, whereas the basic plate-fin exchanger is a crossflow design with combinations sometimes arranged to approach a counterflow unit. Counterflow provides the greatest temperature difference for maximum heat transfer, but crossflow can sometimes give more convenient air connections.

Fixed surface plate exchangers have no moving parts. Alternate layers of plates, separated and sealed (referred to as the heat exchanger core) form the exhaust and supply airstream passages (Figure 17-30). Plate spacings range from 0.1 to 0.5 in. (2.5 to 13 mm), depending on the design and application. Heat transfers directly from the warm airstreams through the separating plates into the cool airstreams.

Normally, both latent heat of condensation, from moisture condensed as the temperature of the warm (exhaust) airstream drops below its dew point, and sensible heat are conducted through the separating plates into the cool (supply) airstream. Thus, latent energy but not actual moisture may be transferred. Recovering upward of 80% of the available waste exhaust heat is not uncommon.

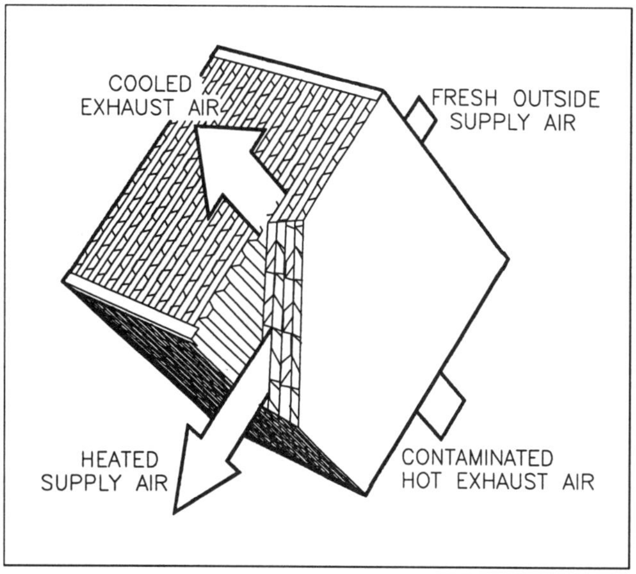

Fig. 17-30 Fixed Plate Heat Exchanger

Plate exchangers are of many proprietary designs, with weights, sizes, and flow patterns depending on the manufacturer (Figure 17-31). Most manufacturers of plate exchangers offer the equipment in modular design.

17.9.8 Thermosiphon Heat Exchangers

Thermosiphon heat exchangers use the natural gravity circulation of a boiling and condensing intermediate fluid to transfer energy between exhaust and supply airstreams. They may be classified as sealed tube thermosiphons and coil loop thermosiphons.

The sealed tube type is essentially the same as a heat pipe and is often given that name. The only distinction made between the two is that heat pipes are usually considered to use, if not solely rely on, capillary forces to cause the intermediate liquid to flow from the cold to the hot end of the tubes, whereas the thermosiphon tubes rely only on gravity. The coil loop type is similar in appearance to the coil energy recovery loop discussed previously. The most obvious difference is the absence of a circulating pump in the thermosiphon loop and the need for evaporator and condenser coils rather than single-phase liquid coils.

Example 17-2 Determine the leaving conditions for a hygroscopic rotary exchanger with the following conditions:

Cooling:

1. Design conditions: outdoor air = 94°F (34.4°C) dry bulb, 77°F (25°C) wet bulb
2. Design conditions: space = 75°F (23.9°C) dry bulb, 62.5°F (16.9°C) wet bulb

Heating:

1. Design conditions: outdoor air = 0°F (−17.8°C) dry bulb, −3°F (−19.4°C) wet bulb
2. Design conditions: space = 75°F (23.9°C) dry bulb, 59.5°F (15.3°C) wet bulb

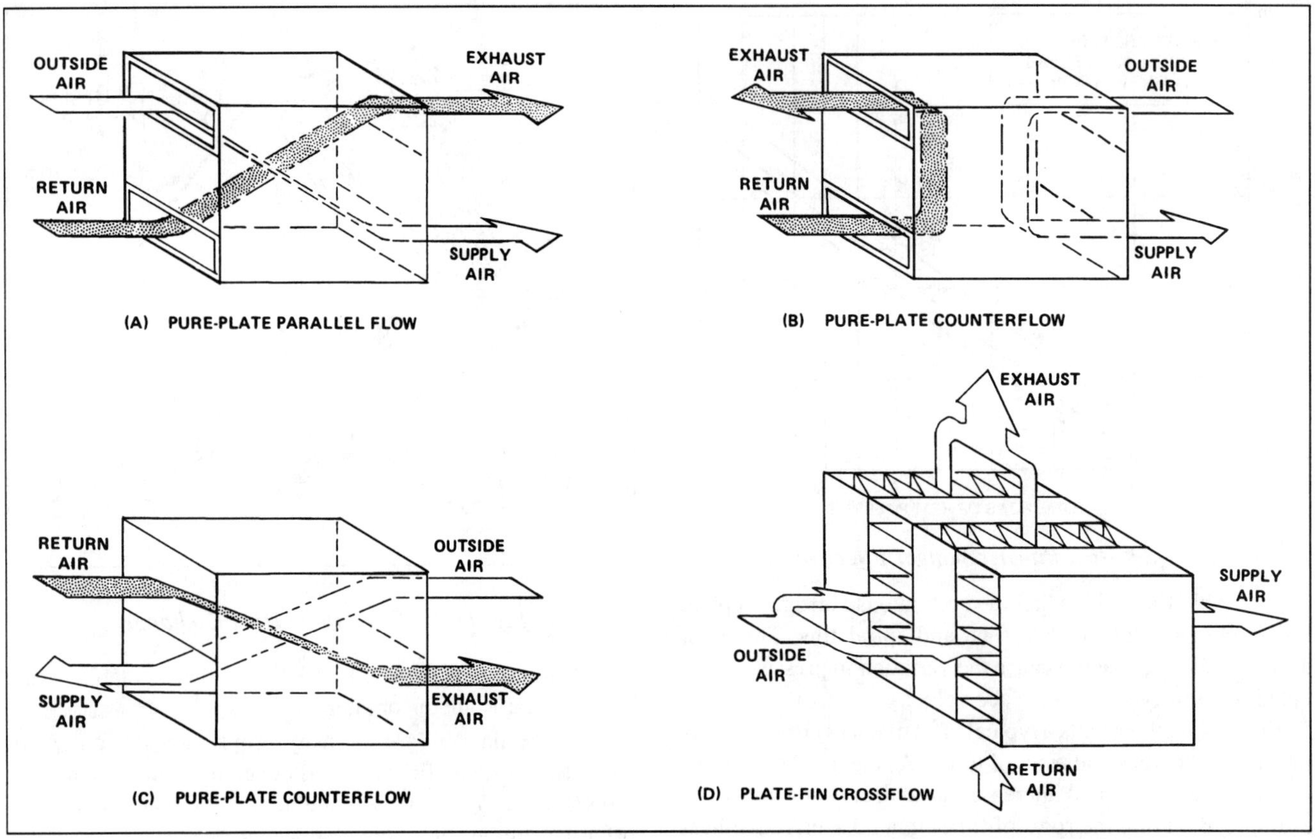

Fig. 17-31 Pure-Plate and Plate-Fin Models

Cooling and Heating:

Exchanger effectiveness = 80% on sensible heat and 80% on latent heat. Equal mass flow rates.

Solution:

Dry-bulb temperature and humidity ratio are calculated from Equation (17-8).

Summer dry-bulb temperature

$$X_2 = X_1 - \varepsilon(X_1 - X_2) = 94 - 0.8(94 - 75)$$
$$= 78.8°F\ (26.0°C)$$

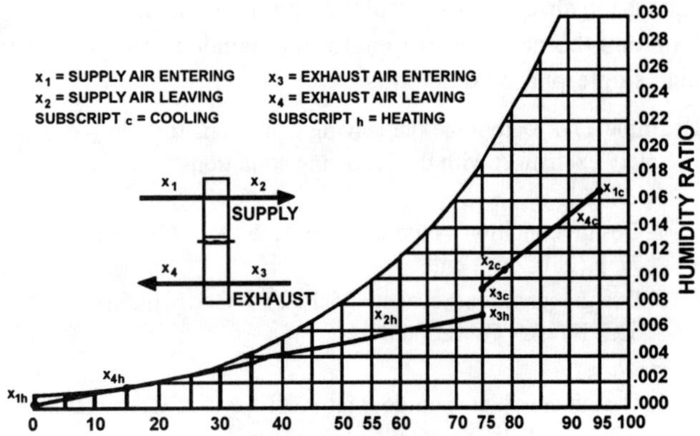

Conditions for Example 17-2

Summer humidity ratio

$$X_2 = X_1 - \varepsilon(X_1 - X_2) = 0.0162 - 0.8(0.0162 - 0.0092)$$
$$= 0.0106\ lb/lb\ (0.0106\ kg/kg)$$

Winter dry-bulb temperature

$$X_2 = X_1 - \varepsilon(X_1 - X_2) = 0 - 0.8(0 - 75)$$
$$= 60°F\ dry\ bulb\ (15.5°C)$$

Winter humidity ratio

$$X_2 = X_1 - \varepsilon(X_1 - X_2) = 0.0001 - 0.8(0.0001 - 0.0074)$$
$$= 0.0059\ lb/lb\ (0.0059\ kg/kg)$$

Example 17-3 Determine the leaving conditions for a hygroscopic exchanger with the following comfort conditions:

Cooling:

1. Design conditions. Outdoor air = 95°F (35°C) dry bulb, 78°F (25.6°C) wet bulb and 41.3 Btu/lb (96.1 kJ/kg).
2. Design conditions. Space = 75°F (23.9°C) dry bulb, 62.5°F (17°C) wet bulb and 28.3 Btu/lb (65.8 kJ/kg) of dry air).

Heating:

1. Design conditions. Outdoor air = 20°F (−6.7°C) dry bulb and 5.0 Btu/lb (11.6 kJ/kg) of dry air.
2. Design conditions. Space = 75°F (23.9°C) dry bulb and 22.4 Btu/lb (52.1 kJ/kg) of dry air.

Cooling and Heating:

Exchanger effectiveness = 80% on sensible heat and 65% on total heat. Equal mass flow rates.

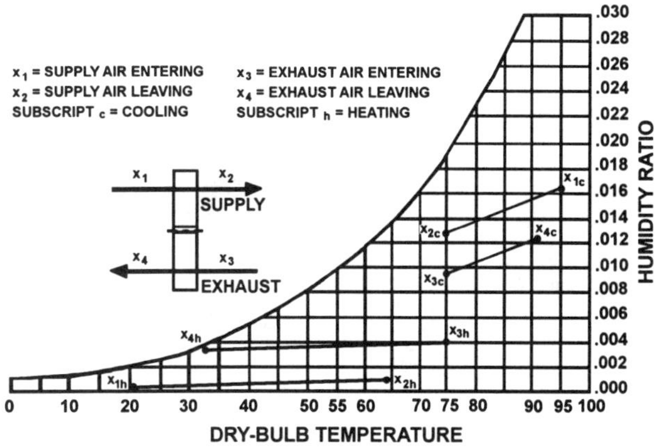

Conditions for Example 17-3

Solution:

Dry-bulb temperature and enthalpy are calculated from Equation (17-8).

Summer dry-bulb temperature

$$X_2 = X_1 - \varepsilon(X_1 - X_3) = 95 - 0.8(95 - 75)$$
$$= 79°F\ (26.1°C)$$

Summer enthalpy

$$X_2 = X_1 - \varepsilon(X_1 - X_3) = 41.3 - 0.65(41.3 - 28.3)$$
$$= 32.9\ \text{Btu/lb}\ (76.5\ \text{kJ/kg})$$

Winter dry-bulb temperature

$$X_2 = X_1 - \varepsilon(X_1 - X_3) = 20 - 0.8(20 - 75)$$
$$= 64°F\ (17.8°C)$$

Heating enthalpy

$$X_2 = X_1 - \varepsilon(X_1 - X_3) = 0.5 - 0.65(5.0 - 22.4)$$
$$= 16.3\ \text{Btu/lb}\ (37.9\ \text{kJ/kg})$$

Example 17-4 Calculate recovered temperatures and volumes (measured at point 2), as well as energy savings, for a metallic exchanger handling 8000 cfm (3.8 m^3/s) of process exhaust at 300°F (149°C) measured at point 3, considered dry air. Assume an equal mass of makeup air at winter design conditions of 0°F (−17.8°C). Exchanger effectiveness is 80% at equal mass flows. Neglect cross leakage and purge volume.

Solution:

1. For conditions at 300°F (149°C)

$$8000\ \text{ft}^3/\text{min}/19.13\ \text{ft}^3/\text{lb} = 418\ \text{lb/min}\ (189.3\ \text{kg/min})$$

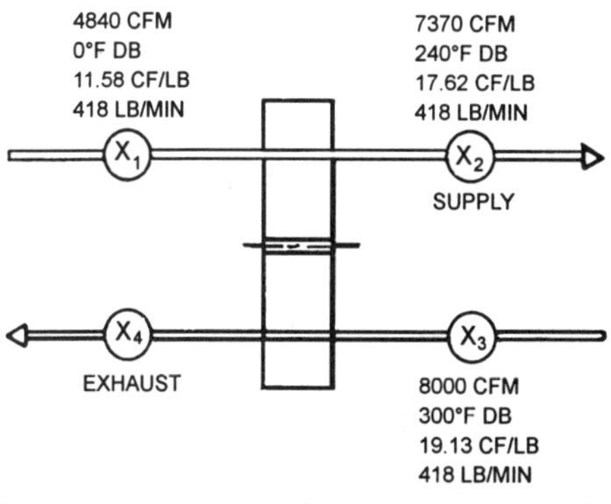

Schematic and Conditions for Example 17-4

2. For conditions of 0°F (-17.8°C)

$$v_1 = 11.58\ \text{ft}^3/\text{lb}$$

418 lb/min × 11.58 ft^3/lb = 4840 cfm at Point 1 (2.28 m^3/s)

3. Temperature at Point 2 from Equation (17-8):

$$X_2 = X_1 - \varepsilon(X_1 - X_3) = 0 - 0.8(0 - 300)$$
$$= 240°F\ \text{dry bulb}\ (115.5°C)$$

4. Specific volume at 240°F dry bulb (115.5°C)

$$v_2 = 17.62\ \text{ft}^3/\text{lb}$$

418 lb/min × 17.62 ft^3/lb = 7370 cfm (3.5 m^3/s)

5. Savings at winter design conditions
[specific heat = 0.242 Btu/(lb·°F)]

$$418\ \text{lb/min} \times 60\ \text{min/h} \times 0.242\ \text{Btu/(lb·°F)} \times (240 - 0)$$
$$= 1{,}460{,}000\ \text{Btu/h}\ (428\ \text{kW})$$

Example 17-5 Determine the leaving conditions for a heat pipe exchanger with the following comfort conditions:

Cooling:

1. Design conditions, outdoor air = 95°F dry bulb (35°C)
2. Design conditions, space = 75°F dry bulb (23.9°C)

Heating:

1. Design conditions, outdoors = 10°F dry bulb (-12.2°C)
2. Design conditions, space = 75°F dry bulb (23.9°C)

Cooling and Heating:

Exchanger effectiveness = 65% on sensible heat at equal mass flows.

Solution:

Dry-bulb temperature is calculated from Equation (17-8).

Cooling dry-bulb temperature

$$X_2 = X_1 - \varepsilon(X_1 - X_3) = 95 - 0.65(95 - 75)$$
$$= 82°F\ (27.8°C)$$

Heating dry-bulb temperature

$$X_2 = X_1 - \varepsilon(X_1 - X_3) = 10 - 0.65(10 - 75)$$
$$= 52.3°F\ (11.3°C)$$

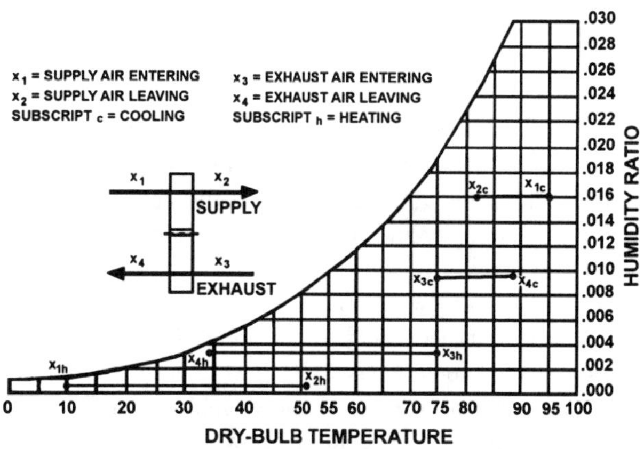

Conditions for Example 17-5

17.10 Economizers

An economizer uses outside air to reduce the refrigeration required to provide cooling for the building. Either the air-side or the water-side economizer is an attractive option for reducing energy costs with self-contained HVAC systems. Although climate often dictates which economizer type is selected, either one can provide advantages.

The air-side economizer is usually a field-installed accessory that includes an outdoor air damper, relief damper, return air damper, filters, actuator, and linkage. Economizer controls are usually a factory-installed option. The air-side economizer takes advantage of cool outdoor air to either assist mechanical cooling or, if the outdoor air is sufficiently cool, provide total system cooling. However, if the building has significant simultaneous heating and cooling requirements, the interaction of the economizer with an installed heat recovery system must be thoroughly investigated.

Self-contained units do not include return air fans. It is necessary to include a variable volume relief fan unit when air-side economizers are employed. The relief fan volume is generally controlled with discharge dampers in response to building space pressure. The relief fan is off and discharge dampers are closed when the air-side economizer is inactive. Advantages of air-side economizers include:

- substantially reduced compressor, cooling tower, and condenser water pump energy requirement
- lower air-side pressure drop than a water-side economizer

However, the installed cost is generally higher than that for a water-side economizer due to exhaust system requirements.

Typically, in an air-side economizer, an enthalpy sensor or dry bulb temperature probe energizes the unit to bring in outside air as the first stage of cooling. An outside air damper modulated the flow to meet a design temperature, and when outside air can no longer provide enough cooling, compressors are energized.

The water-side economizer consists of a water coil located upstream of the main cooling coil. All economizer control valves, piping between the economizer coil and the condenser, and economizer control wiring can be factory installed. The water-side economizer takes advantage of low cooling tower water temperature (approaching ambient wet bulb temperature) to either precool the entering air, assist mechanical cooling, or, if the cooling water is cold enough, to provide total system cooling. If the economizer is unable to maintain the supply air set point for VAV units or zone set point for constant volume units, factory-mounted controls integrate economizer and compressor operation to meet cooling requirements.

Cooling water flow rate is controlled by two valves (Figure 17-32), one at the economizer coil inlet (A) and one in the bypass loop to the condenser (B). Two control methods are common - constant water flow and variable water flow.

Standard modulating control allows constant condenser water flow during operation. The two control valves are wired

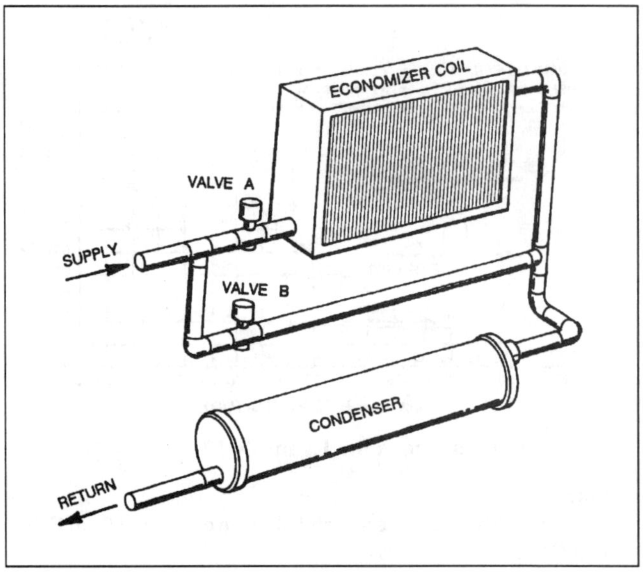

Fig. 17-32 Water-Side Economizer

for complementary operation, where one valve is drive open while the other is driven closed. Energy saving modulating valve control allows variable condenser water flow during operation. The valve in the bypass loop (B) is an on-off valve and is closed when the economizer is enabled. Water flow through the economizer coil is modulated by valve A. As the cooling load increases, valve A open, increasing water flow through the economizer coil. If the economizer is unable to completely satisfy the cooling requirements, the control system integrate economizer and compressor operation. When the system is not in the cooling mode, both valves are closed.

17.11 Problems

17.1 Air enters a coil at 95°F dry-bulb and 78°F wet-bulb temperature and leaves at 62°F dry-bulb and 60°F wet-bulb temperature. The condensate is assumed to be at a temperature of 56°F. Find the total, latent, and sensible cooling loads on the coil with air at 14.7 psia.

17.2 Air enters a direct expansion coil at 29.4°C dry bulb (21.1°C wet bulb) and leaves at 16.7°C d.b. and 90% rh.

(a) How much sensible heat and how much latent heat is removed from the air by the coil?
(b) What is the dew point of the apparatus?
(c) How much condensate drains off the coil?

17.3 Air enters a direct-expansion coil at 90°F dry bulb (32.2°C) 60% rh and leaves the coil at 60°F dry bulb (15.6°C), 95% rh. Find:

(a) heat removed from air
(b) moisture condensed from air
(c) SHR for the condition line

[Ans: (a) 19.2 Btu/lb (44.6 kJ/kg), (b) 0.008 lb/lb (0.008 kg/kg), (c) 0.45]

17.4 Water flowing at 60 lb/min and at 51°F is chilled in an evaporator to 40°F. The heat transfer area is 20 ft^2 and the heat exchanger has an overall heat transfer coefficient of 60 Btu/h· ft^2 ·°F. The direct-expansion evaporator uses R-12 and operates at 35°F. Find the evaporator effectiveness.

17.5 Outside air at 35°F and 70% rh is supplied to an air-conditioning apparatus. Recirculated air is returned from the plant at 69°F dry bulb and 40% rh; 8100 cfm of outside air mixes with 18,900 cfm of recirculated air. The mixture is heated by a steam coil and humidified by a pan humidifier to final conditions of 115°F d.b. and 20% rh.

(a) What steam flow, in pounds per hour, should be supplied to the heating coil?

(b) Estimate the steam consumption of the humidifier.

17.6 Outdoor air (8000 cfm) at 10°F dry bulb and 50% rh enters the central apparatus of a split heating system. It is tempered to 55°F dry bulb. Then, it flows through a spray humidifier where the leaving sump water is maintained at 50°F. The spray humidifier has a performance factor of 0.80. After leaving the humidifier, the air flows through a steam heating coil and is heated to 70°F dry bulb.

(a) What is the final relative humidity and humidity ratio of the air as it leaves the heating coil?

(b) Assume steam at 2 psig and 90% quality is supplied to the tempering coil, the sump water heat exchanger, and the heating coil. How many pounds of steam per hour should be supplied to each?

17.7 The heat exchanger for the spray water in *Problem* 17.6 is out of service for maintenance. The split heating system is operating as specified except that the sump water is recirculated. Assume make-up water to the sump is 37°F and saturating effectiveness equals the performance factor.

(a) What is the final relative humidity and humidity ratio of the air leaving the heating coil?

(b) What is the steam rate (lb/h) for the tempering coils and for the heating coil?

17.8 Air at 105°F dry bulb (40.6°C) and 75% rh passes through a chilled water spray. Air leaves the spray chamber at 45°F dry bulb (7.2°C) saturated. How many grains of moisture per pound of entering air are condensed?

17.9 Air enters a coil at 35°C dry-bulb and 26°C wet-bulb temperatures and leaves at 17°C dry-bulb and 16°C wet-bulb temperatures. The condensate is assumed to be at a temperature of 13.5°C. Find the total, latent, and sensible cooling loads on the coil with air at 101 kPa.

17.10 A building space is to be maintained at 70°F and 35 percent relative humidity when outdoor design temperature is 10°F. Design heat losses from the space are 250,000 Btu/h, sensible, and 45,000 Btu/h, latent. Ventilation requires that 1500 cfm of outdoor air be used. Supply air is to be at 120°F. Determine:

(a) the amount of supply air required, lb/h, and cfm;

(b) the capacity of the heating coil, Btu/h, if

1) the humidifier is a spray washer using recirculated spray water with makeup water provided at 60°F;

2) the humidifier is a steam humidifier using dry, saturated steam at 17.2 psia;

(c) the capacity of the humidifier, lb/h.

The conditioning equipment and nomenclature are shown in the following sketch.

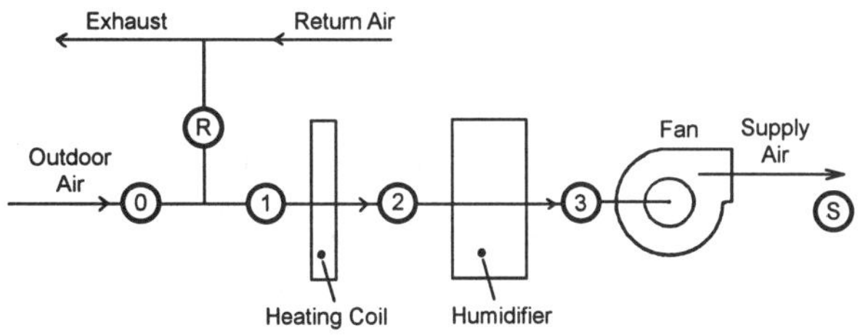

17.11 A spray-type air washer is to be used for humidification as well as cleaning of 9000 SCFM of air. Inlet conditions to the washer are 75°F db and 48 F wb. Desired humidity ratio at outlet is 0.005 lb_w/lb_a. Determine: (a) the necessary humidification efficiency of the washer, %, and (b) the make-up water requirements (humidifying capacity) of the unit, lb_w/h.

17.12 A heat pipe air-to-air energy recovery device is being considered for a system requiring 9000 SCFM of outside air. Initially, a separate preheater was planned for bringing the outside aire from its −2°F design ambient outdoor temperature to 40°F. Determine: (a) the rating (Btu/h) and (b) the sensible effectiveness (%) to specify for the heat pipe unit if it is to eliminate the need for the air preheater.

17.13 The HVAC system for a hospital operating room which requires 100% outside air is shown in the following figure and includes an air-to-air heat pipe energy recovery unit having a sensible effectiveness of 73%. The air leaving the cooling coil is maintained at 58°F, 90% rh, all year long. During winter operation, air leaves the heater at 130°F. Fan speed is changed between summer and winter operation. Design duct system pressure drop (summer) is 3.25 in. water.

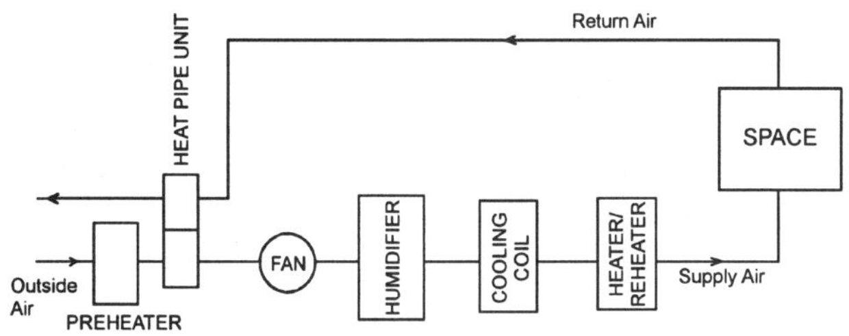

1. At winter design conditions (Indoor: 72°F & 30% rh; Outdoor: 5°F & 100% rh) the space load is 235,000 Btu/h (sensible) with negligible latent. Determine: (a) the necessary

size of heating unit (Btu/h) both with and without the energy recovery unit and (b) the humidifier size (gallons/day). Neglect fan effects.

2. At summer design conditions (Indoor: 78 °F; Outdoor: 95 °F db/76 °F wb), the space cooling loads are 146,000 Btu/h (sensible) and 79,000 Btu/h (latent). Determine: (a) fan size (HP & SCFM), (b) sensible coil load, Btu/h, (c) latent coil load, Btu/h, and (d) necessary size of cooling unit, Btu/h, both with and without the energy recovery unit. Include fan effects.

17.12 Bibliography

ASHRAE. 1991. Method of testing air-to-air heat exchangers. ASHRAE *Standard* 84-91.

ASHRAE. 1996. *Handbook—Systems and Equipment.*

Gudac, G.J., M.A. Mueller, J.J. Bosch, R.H. Howell, and H.J. Sauer, Jr. 1981. "Effectiveness and Pressure Drop Characteristics of Various Types of Air-to-Air Energy Recovery Systems," *ASHRAE Transactions*, V. 87, Pt. 1.

Sauer, H. J., Jr. and R. H. Howell. 1981. "Promise and Potential of Air-to-Air Energy Recovery Systems," *ASHRAE Transactions*, V. 87, Pt. 1.

SI Table

Table 17-2 SI Comparison of Air-to-Air Energy Recovery Devices

(Table 2, Chapter 42, 1996 *Handbook—Systems and Equipment*, SI Version)

	Fixed Plate	Rotary Wheel	Heat Pipe	Runaround Coil Loop	Thermosiphon	Twin Towers
Airflow arrangements	Counterflow Crossflow Parallel flow	Counterflow Parallel flow	Counterflow Parallel flow	Counterflow Parallel flow	Counterflow Parallel flow	
Equipment size range, L/s	25 and up	25 to 35 000 and up	50 and up	50 and up	50 and up	
Type of heat transfer (typical effectiveness)	Sensible (50 to 80%)	Sensible (50 to 80%) Total (55 to 85%)	Sensible (45 to 65%)	Sensible (55 to 65%)	Sensible (40 to 60%)	Sensible (40 to 60%)
Face velocity, m/s (most common design velocity)	0.5 to 5 (1 to 5)	2.5 to 5	2 to 4 (2.2 to 2.7)	1.5 to 3	2 to 4 (2.2 to 2.7)	1.5 to 2.2
Pressure drop, Pa (most likely pressure)	5 to 450 (25 to 370)	(100 to 170)	(100 to 500)	(100 to 500)	(100 to 500)	170 to 300
Temperature range	–60 to 800°C	–60 to 800°C	–40 to 35°C	–45 to 500°C	–40 to 40°C	–40 to 46°C
Typical mode of purchase	Exchanger only Exchanger in case Exchanger and blowers Complete system	Exchanger only Exchanger in case Exchanger and blowers Complete system	Exchanger only Exchanger in case	Coil only Complete system	Exchanger only Exchanger in case	Complete system
Unique advantages	No moving parts Low pressure drop Easily cleaned	Latent transfer Compact large sizes Low pressure drop	No moving parts except tilt Fan location not critical Allowable pressure differential up to 15 kPa	Exhaust airstream can be separated from supply air Fan location not critical	No moving parts Exhaust airstream can be separated from supply air Fan location not critical	Latent transfer from remote airstreams Multiple units in a single system Efficient microbiological cleaning of both supply and exhaust airstreams
Limitations	Latent available in hygroscopic units only	Cold climates may increase service Cross-air contamination possible	Effectiveness limited by pressure drop and cost Few suppliers	High effectiveness requires accurate simulation model	Effectiveness may be limited by pressure drop and cost Few suppliers	Few suppliers
Cross-leakage	0 to 5%	1 to 10%	0%	0%	0%	0.025%
Heat rate control (HRC) schemes	Bypass dampers and ducting	Wheel speed control over full range	Tilt angle down to 10% of maximum heat rate	Bypass valve or pump speed control over full range	Control valve over full range	Control valve or pump speed control over full range

Chapter 18

REFRIGERATION EQUIPMENT

This chapter provides a relatively brief treatment of the systems and components used for providing the cooling requirements of building HVAC systems. Primary topics are vapor compression refrigeration, absorption refrigeration, and cooling towers. Additional information can be obtained from 1994 *ASHRAE Handbook—Refrigeration* and the 1996 *ASHRAE Handbook—Systems and Equipment.*

18.1 Mechanical Vapor Compression

The basic components of the mechanical vapor compression cycle are the compressor, condenser, expansion valve, and evaporator (Figure 18-1). The basic principles of the vapor compression cycle are detailed in Chapter 2 of this book. Additional information is also provided in Chapter 1 of the 1997 *ASHRAE Handbook—Fundamentals.*

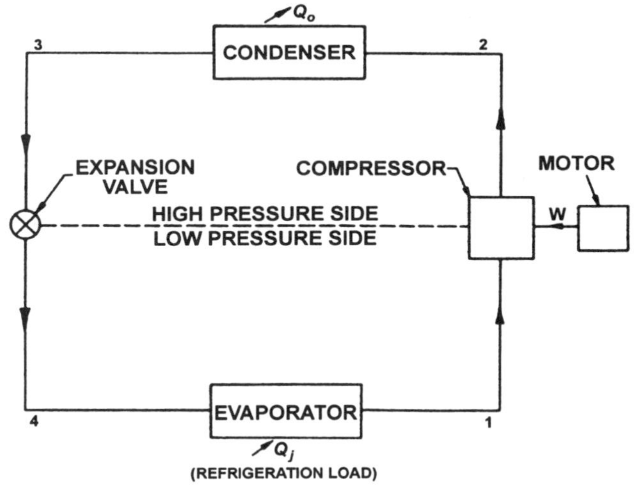

Fig. 18-1 Equipment Diagram for the BasicVapor-Compression Cycle

18.1.1 Compressors

The compressor is one of the essential parts of the compression refrigeration system and serves both to provide the necessary increase in pressure of the refrigerant vapor and as a refrigerant pump to circulate the refrigerant through the system in a continuous cycle.

There are two basic types of compressors: positive displacement and dynamic. Positive-displacement compressors increase the pressure of refrigerant vapor by reducing the volume of the compressor chamber through work applied to the compressor's mechanism. This class of compressor includes reciprocating, rolling piston, rotary vane, single screw, double screw, and scroll. Dynamic compressors increase the pressure of refrigerant vapor by a continuous transfer of angular momentum from the rotating member to the vapor followed by the conversion of this momentum into a pressure rise. Centrifugal compressors function based on these principles.

Compressor performance is the result of design compromises involving physical limitations of the refrigerant, compressor, and motor, while attempting to provide the following:

- Greatest trouble-free life expectancy
- Most refrigeration effect for the least power input
- Lowest applied cost
- Wide range of operating conditions
- Acceptable vibration and sound level

Two useful measures of compressor performance are capacity (which is related to compressor volume displacement) and efficiency. Compressor refrigerating capacity is the rate of heat removal by the refrigerant pumped by the compressor in a refrigerating system at the evaporator. Capacity equals the product of the mass flow rate of refrigerant pumped by the compressor and the difference in specific enthalpies of the refrigerant when it leaves the evaporator and when it enters the evaporator.

Reciprocating Compressors. Most reciprocating compressors are single acting, using pistons driven directly through a pin and connecting rod from the crankshaft. Double-acting compressors are not extensively used.

The halocarbon compressor is the most widely used and is manufactured in three designs: (1) open, (2) semihermetic or bolted hermetic, and (3) welded-shell hermetic. Ammonia

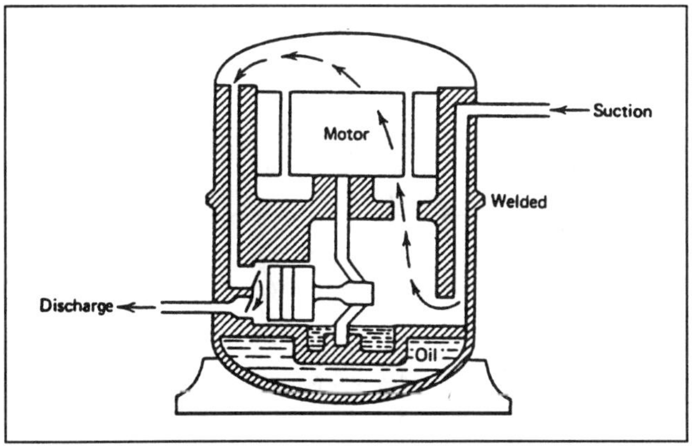

Fig. 18-2 Hermetic Compressor

Table 18-1 Typical Design Features of Reciprocating Compressors

Item	Halocarbon Compressor Open	Halocarbon Compressor Semi-hermetic	Halocarbon Compressor Welded Hermetic	Ammonia Compressor Open
1. Number of cylinders—one to:	16	12	6	16
2. Power range*	0.17 hp and up	0.5 to 150 hp	0.17 to 25 hp	10 hp and up
3. Cylinder arrangement				
a. Vertical, V or W, radial	X	X		
b. Radial, horizontal opposed			X	
c. Horizontal, vertical V or W				X
4. Drive				
a. Hermetic compressors, induction electric motor		X	X	
b. Open compressors—direct drive, V belt chain, gear, by electric motor or engine	X			X
5. Lubrication—splash or force feed, flooded	X	X	X	X
6. Suction and discharge valves—ring plate or ring or reed flexing	X	X	X	X
7. Suction and discharge valve arrangement				
a. Suction and discharge valves in head	X	X	X	X
b. Uniflow—suction valves in top of piston, suction gas entering through cylinder walls; discharge valves in head	X			X
8. Cylinder cooling				
a. Suction gas cooled	X	X	X	X
b. Water jacket cylinder wall, head, or cylinder wall and head	X			X
c. Air cooled	X	X	X	X
d. Refrigerant cooled heads	X			X
9. Cylinder head				
a. Spring loaded	X	X	X	X
b. Bolted head	X	X	X	X
10. Bearings				
a. Sleeve, antifriction	X	X	X	X
b. Tapered roller	X			X
11. Capacity control, if provided—manual or automatic				
a. Suction valve lifting	X	X	X	X
b. Bypass-cylinder heads to suction	X	X	X	X
c. Closing inlet	X	X		X
d. Adjustable clearance	X	X		X
e. Variable speed	X	X	X	X
12. Materials				
Motor insulations and rubber materials must be compatible with refrigerant and lubricant mixtures; otherwise, no restrictions		X	X	
No copper or brass				X
13. Lubricant return				
a. Crankcase separated from suction manifolds, oil return check valves, equalizers, spinners, foam breakers	X	X		X
b. Crankcase common with suction manifold			X	
14. Synchronous speeds (50 to 60 Hz)	250 to 3600	1500 to 3600	1500 to 3600	250 to 1500
15. Pistons				
a. Aluminum or cast iron	X	X	X	X
b. Ringless	X	X	X	X
c. Compression and oil control rings	X	X	X	X
16. Connecting rod				
Split rod with removable cap or solid eccentric strap	X	X	X	X
17. Mounting				
Internal spring mount		X	X	
External spring mount		X	X	
Rigidly mounted on base	X	X		X

* 1 hp = 0.746 kW

Table 18-2 Typical Performance Values

Compressor Size and Type	R-404a: Evap. Temp. = −40°F, Cond. Temp. = 105°F, Suction Gas = 65°F, Subcooling = 0°F	R-134a: Evap. Temp. = 0°F, Cond. Temp. = 110°F, Suction Gas = 65°F, Subcooling = 0°F	R-22: Evap. Temp. = 40°F, Cond. Temp. = 105°F, Suction Gas = 55°F, Subcooling = 0°F	R-22: Evap. Temp. = 45°F, Cond. Temp. = 130°F, Suction Gas = 65°F, Subcooling = 0°F
Large, over 25 hp				
Open	0.21 tons/hp	0.40 tons/hp	1.05 tons/hp	1.07 tons/hp
Hermetic	3.15 Btu/h per W	6.00 Btu/h per W	14.2 Btu/h per W	10.4 Btu/h per W
Medium, 5 to 25 hp				
Open	0.19 tons/hp	0.37 tons/hp	1.00 ton/hp	1.00 tons/hp
Hermetic	2.89 Btu/h per W	5.60 Btu/h per W	14.0 Btu/h per W	10.2 Btu/h per W
Small, under 5 hp				
Open	—	—	—	—
Hermetic	—	3.80 Btu/h per W	13.8 Btu/h per W	10.0 Btu/h per W

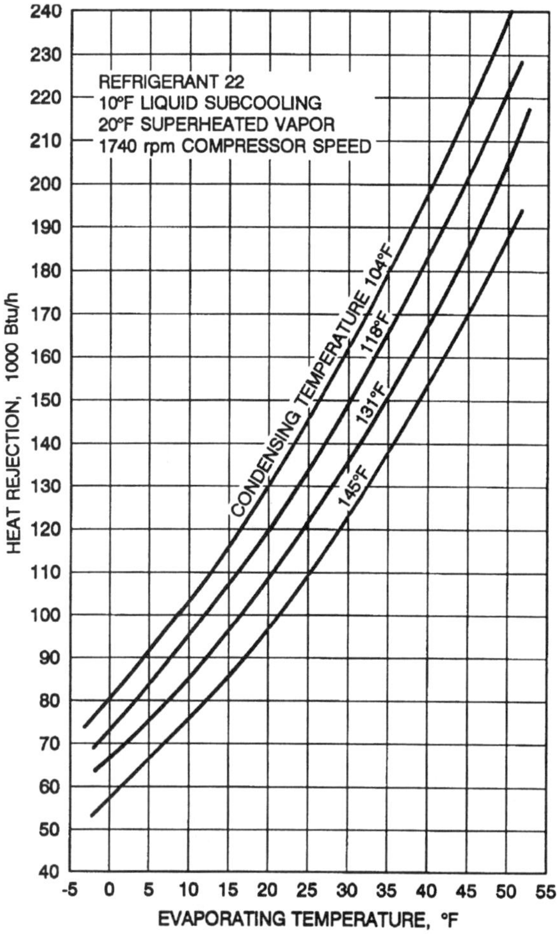

Fig. 18-3 Heat Rejection Curve for Reciprocating Compressor

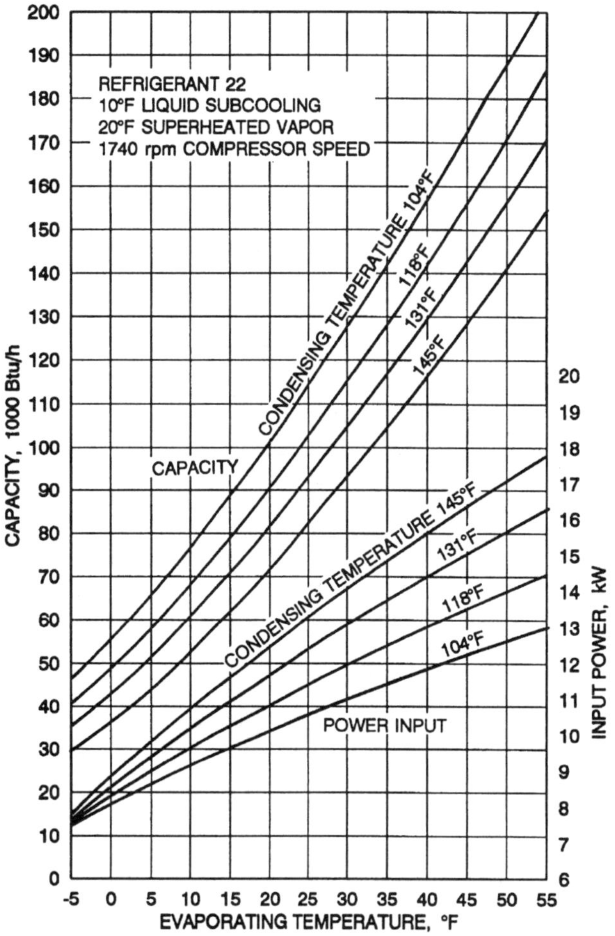

Fig. 18-4 Typical Capacity and Power for Reciprocating Compressor

compressors are manufactured only in the open design, in which the driveshaft extends through a seal in the crankcase for an external drive.

In hermetic compressors, the motor and compressor are contained within the same pressure vessel; the motor shaft is integral with the compressor crankshaft, and the motor is in contact with the refrigerant. A hermetic compressor is shown in Figure 18-2. A semi-, bolted, accessible, or serviceable hermetic compressor is bolted together and may be repaired in the field. The motor compressor in a welded shell (sealed) hermetic compressor is mounted inside a steel shell, which in turn is sealed by welding. Table 18-1 shows combinations of common design features and Table 18-2 gives typical performance values for halocarbon compressors.

Capacity data is given in Figure 18-3, which is a typical set of curves for a four-cylinder semi-hermetic compressor, 2 3/8 in. (60 mm) bore, 1 3/4-in. (44 mm) stroke, 1720 rpm, operating with R-22. A set of power curves for the same compressor is also shown. The heat rejection curves for the same compressor are shown in Figure 18-4.

Reciprocating compressors are most commonly used for systems in the range of 0.5 to 100 tons (2 to 350 kW) and larger. They are used in unitary heat pumps and, in most cases, are either fully or accessibly hermetic.

One of the important thermodynamic considerations for this compressor is the effect of the clearance volume (i.e., the volume occupied by the refrigerant within the compressor that is not displaced by the moving member). The effect is illustrated, in the case of the piston-type compressor, by considering the clearance volume between the piston and the cylinder head when the piston is at top dead-center position. The clearance gas remaining in this space after the compressed gas is discharged from the cylinder re-expands as the piston moves downward, preventing a fresh charge into the cylinder until the pressure falls to the inlet (suction) pressure (see Figure 18-5). As a consequence, the volume (and mass) of refrigerant entering the cylinder is less than the volume swept by the piston. This effect is quantitatively expressed by the volumetric efficiency e_v as:

$$e_v/100 = m_a/m_i$$

where

m_a = actual mass of new gas entering the compressor

m_i = theoretical mass, equal to piston displacement divided by specific volume of refrigerant vapor at suction conditions

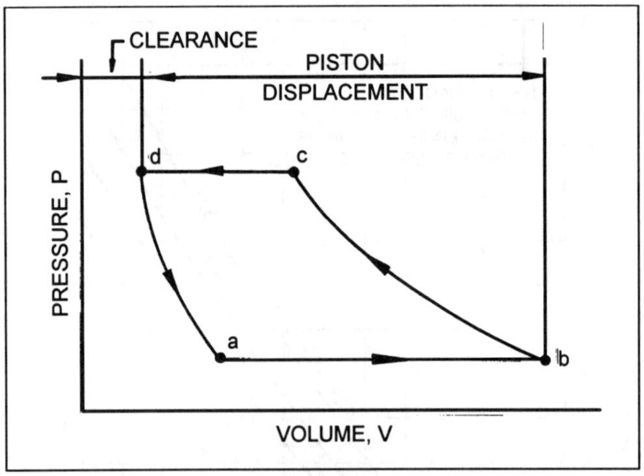

Fig. 18-5 Cycle for Idealized Piston Compressor

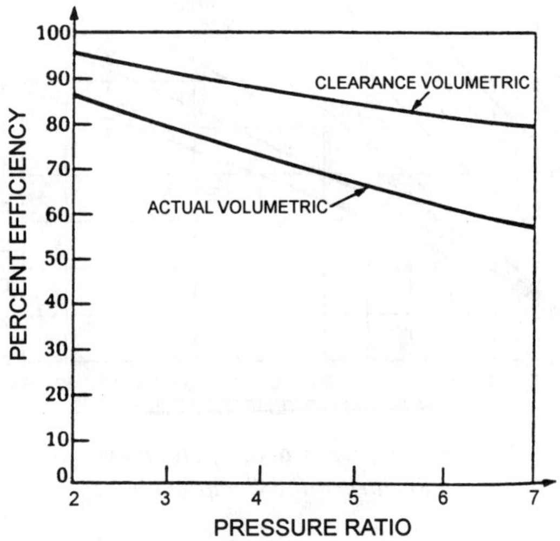

Fig. 18-6 Volumetric Efficiency

The volumetric efficiency due only to reexpansion of the clearance volume gas can be calculated as follows:

$$\frac{e_v}{100} = 1 + C\left(\frac{v_s}{v_d}\right)$$

where

C = clearance ratio = $(V_b - V_a)/(V_b - V_d)$

v_s = specific volume of refrigerant at suction conditions

v_d = specific volume of refrigerant at discharge conditions

V_a, V_b and V_d = the volumes at the locations given in Figure 18-5

The actual volumetric efficiency is affected by other factors such as cylinder wall heating due to friction and pressure drops through the inlet and discharge valves and is best obtained by actual laboratory measurements of the amount of refrigerant compressed and delivered by the compressor. The difference between actual and predicted volumetric efficiency, considering only clearance volume effects, is illustrated in Figure 18-6.

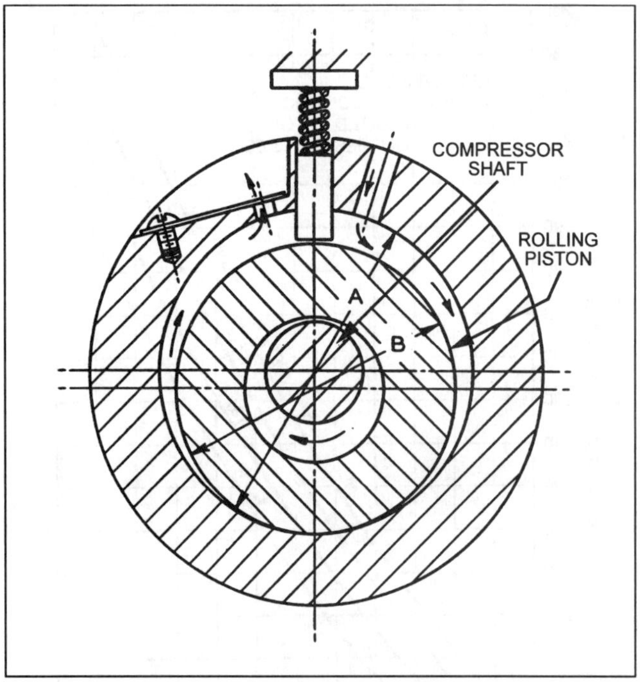

Fig. 18-7 Rolling Piston Compressor

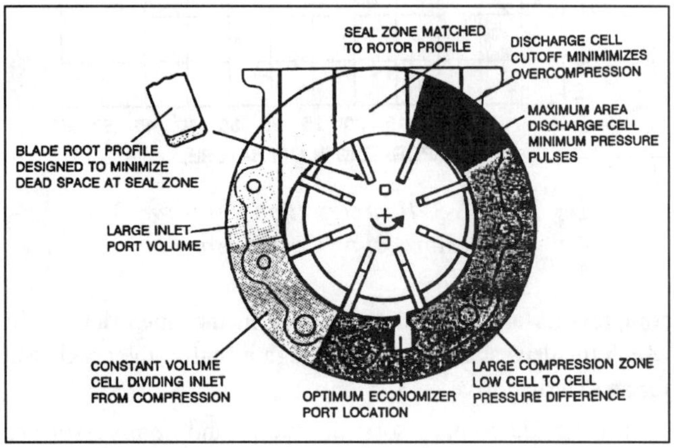

Fig. 18-8 Rotary Vane Compressor

Rotary Compressors. Rotary compressors operate with a circular, or rotary, motion instead of reciprocating motion. Their positive-displacement compression process is nonreversing and either continuous or cyclical, depending on the type of mechanism. Most are direct drive machines.

The rolling piston rotary compressor is shown in Figure 18-7; the rotary vane type is shown in Figure 18-8. These two machines are similar in size, weight, thermodynamic performance, field of applications, range of capacities, durability, and sound level.

Internal leakage is controlled in rotary compressors through hydrodynamic sealing; thus, precision fits and optimum clearance are design requirements. The hydrodynamic sealing depends on clearances, surface speed, oil viscosity, and surface finish of the parts. Smoother finishes and closer clearances are used with low-viscosity oil in small machines.

Larger machines have greater clearances and usually use a higher viscosity oil.

Rotary compressor performance is characterized by high volumetric efficiency due to the small clearance volume and by correspondingly low reexpansion loss.

The **rolling piston compressor** uses a roller mounted on an eccentric shaft. A single vane or blade positioned in the nonrotating cylindrical housing reciprocates as the eccentrically moving roller turns. Rolling piston compressors are used in household refrigerators and air-conditioning units in sizes up to about 3 hp (2 kW).

Displacement for this compressor can be calculated from the following equation:

$$V_d = \frac{\pi H(A^2 - B^2)}{4}$$

where

V_d = displacement
H = cylinder block height
A = cylinder diameter
B = roller diameter

Suction gas is directly piped into the suction port of the compressor, and the compressed gas is discharged into the compressor housing shell. This high-side shell design is used because of the simplicity of its lubrication system and the absence of oiling and compressor cooling problems. Compressor performance is also improved because this arrangement minimizes heat transfer to the suction gas and reduces gas leakage areas.

The performance typical of rolling piston compressors is illustrated in Figure 18-9.

The **rotating vane compressor** has a rotor concentric with the shaft, with vanes in the rotor; this assembly is off center with respect to the cylindrical housing. An oval shaped bore produces a double lobe or a two-cylinder compressor. Rotary vane compressors have a low weight-to-displacement ratio, which, in combination with their compact size, makes them suitable for transport applications. Small compressors in the 3 to 50 hp (2 to 40 kW) range are single staged, for a saturated suction temperature range of –40 to 45°F (–40 to 7°C) at saturated condensing temperatures of up to 140°F (60°C). By employing a second stage, low-temperature applications down to –60°F (–50°C) are possible. Currently, R-22, R-502, and R-717 refrigerants are used.

Screw Compressors. The helical rotary compressor, or the screw compressor, belongs to the class of positive-displacement compressors. Screw compressors currently in production for refrigeration and air-conditioning applications comprise two distinct types: single screw and twin screw. Both are conventionally used in the fluid injection mode where sufficient fluid cools and seals the compressor. Single-screw compressors have the capability to operate at pressure ratios above 20:1 single stage. The capacity range currently available is from 20 to 1300 tons (70 to 4600 kW).

The single-screw compressor consists of a single cylindrical main rotor that works with a pair of gaterotors. Both the main rotor and gaterotors can vary widely in terms of form and mutual geometry. Figure 18-10 shows the design normally encountered in refrigeration.

The main rotor has six helical grooves, with a cylindrical periphery and a globoid (or hourglass shape) root profile. The two identical gaterotors each have 11 teeth and are located on opposite sides of the main rotor. The casing

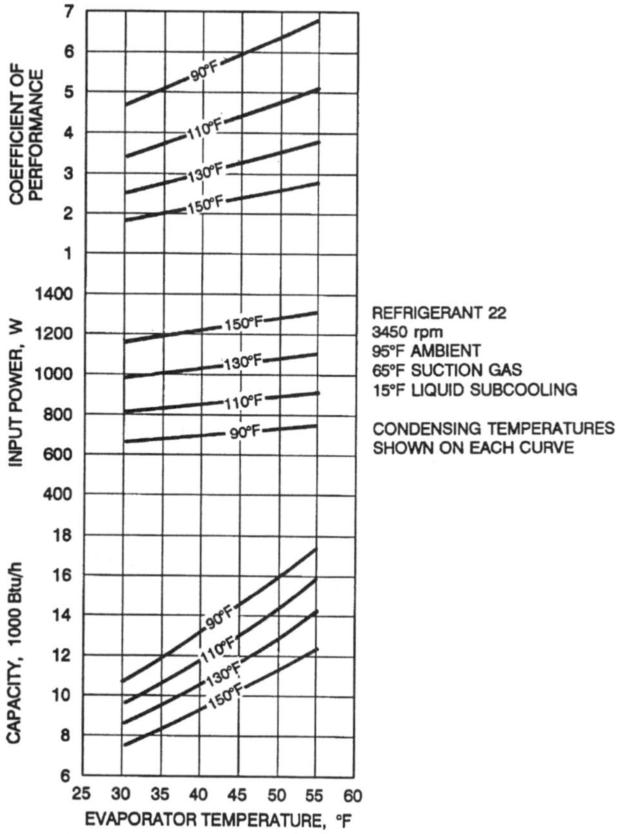

Fig. 18-9 Typical Rolling Piston Compressor Performance

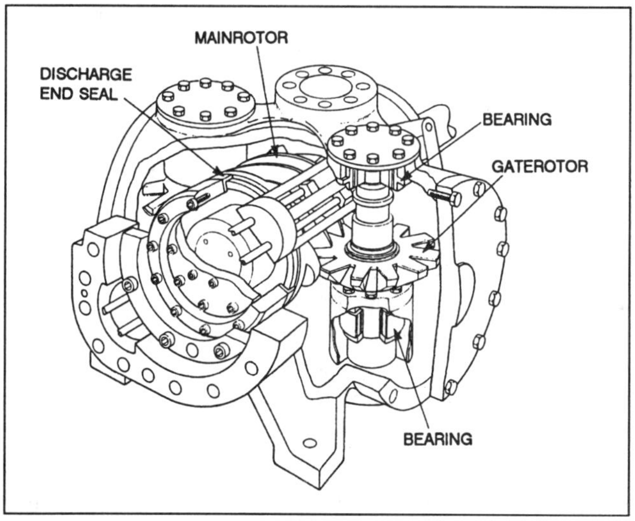

Fig. 18-10 Section of Single-Screw Compressor

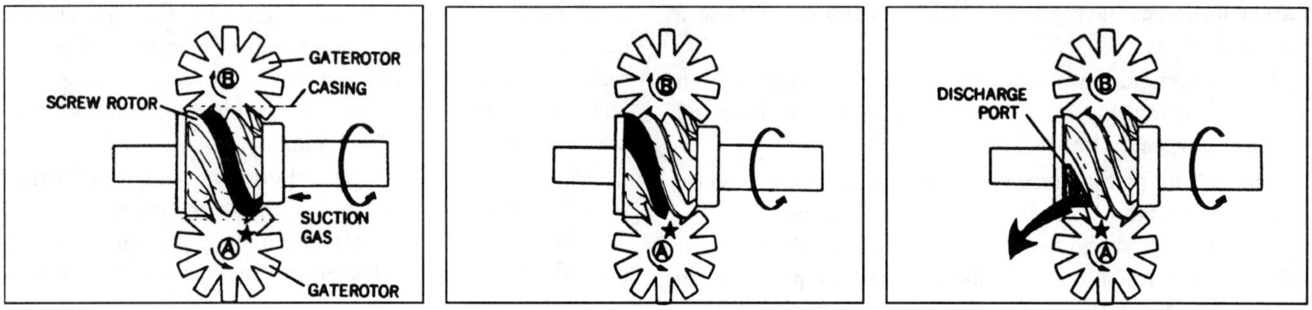

Suction. During rotation of the main rotor, a typical groove in open communication with the suction chamber gradually fills with suction gas. The tooth of the gaterotor in mesh with the groove acts as an aspirating piston.

Compression. As the main rotor turns, the groove engages a tooth on the gaterotor and is covered simultaneously by the cylindrical main rotor casing. The gas is trapped in the space formed by the three sides of the groove, the casing, and the gaterotor tooth. As rotation continues, the groove volume decreases and compression occurs.

Discharge. At the geometrically fixed point where the leading edge of the groove and the edge of the discharge port coincide, compression ceases, and the gas discharges into the delivery line until the groove volume has been reduced to zero.

Fig. 18-11 Sequence of Compression Process in Single-Screw Compressor

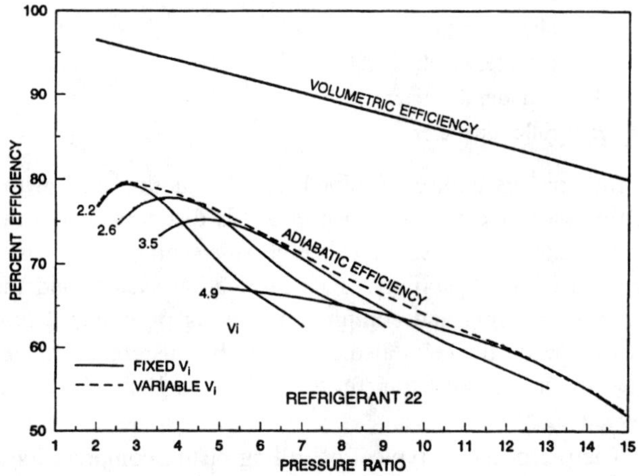

Fig. 18-12 Typical Screw Compressor Performance with R-22

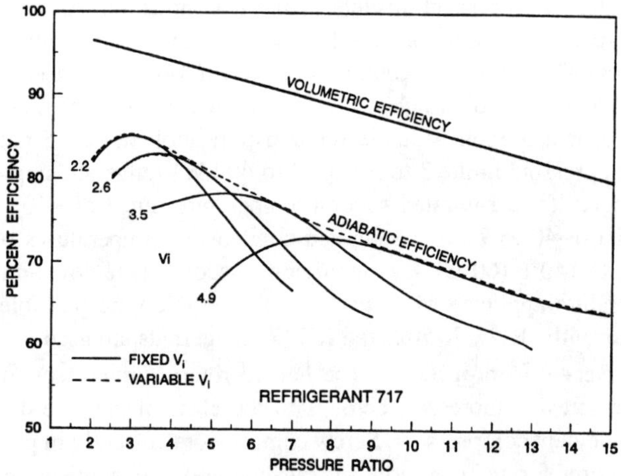

Fig. 18-13 Typical Screw Compressor Performance with R-717 (Ammonia)

enclosing the main rotor has two slots, which allow the teeth of the gaterotors to pass through them. Two diametrically opposed discharge ports use a common discharge manifold located in the casting. The compressor is driven through the main rotor shaft, and the gaterotors follow by direct meshing action at 6:11 ratio of the main rotor speed. The geometry of the single-screw compressor is such that 100% of the gas compression power is transferred directly from the main rotor to the gas. No power (other than small frictional losses) is transferred across the meshing points to the gaterotors.

Compression is obtained by direct volume reduction with pure rotary motion as illustrated in Figure 18-11.

The four basic continuous phases of the working cycle are as follows:

Suction. As a lobe of the male rotor begins to unmesh from an interlobe space in the female rotor, a void is created and gas is drawn in through the inlet port. As the rotors continue to turn, the interlobe space increases in size and gas flows continuously into the compressor. Prior to the point at which the interlobe space leaves the inlet port, the entire length of the interlobe space is completely filled with gas.

Transfer. As rotation continues, the trapped gas pocket in the interlobe space is moved circumferentially around the compressor housing at constant suction pressure.

Compression. Further rotation starts meshing of another male lobe with the female interlobe space on the suction end and progressively squeezes (compresses) the gas in the direction of the discharge port. Thus, the occupied volume of the trapped gas within the interlobe space is decreased and the gas pressure consequently increased.

Discharge. At a point determined by the design built-in volume ratio, the discharge port is uncovered and the compressed gas is discharged by further meshing of the lobe and interlobe space.

During the remeshing period of compression and discharge, a fresh charge is drawn through the inlet on the opposite side of the meshing point. With four male lobes rotating at 3600 rpm, four interlobe volumes are filled and discharged per revolution, providing 14,400 discharges per minute or 240 per second. Since the intake and discharge cycles overlap effectively, a smooth, continuous flow of gas results.

Figures 18-12 and 18-13 show typical efficiencies of all single-screw compressor designs. High isentropic and volumetric efficiencies are the result of internal compression, the absence of suction and discharge valves and their losses, and extremely small clearance volumes. The curves show the importance of selecting the correct volume ratio in fixed volume ratio compressors.

Twin screw is a common designation for double helical rotary screw compressors. A twin-screw compressor consists of two mating helically grooved rotors–male (lobes) and female (flutes or gullies) in a stationary housing with inlet and outlet gas ports (Figure 18-14).

While operating, some twin-screw compressors adjust the volume ratio of the compressor to the most efficient ratio for whatever system pressures are encountered. The comparative efficiencies of fixed and variable volume ratio screw compressors are shown in Figure 18-15 for full-load operation on ammonia and R-22 refrigerants. The greater the change in either suction or condensing pressure a given system experiences, the more benefits are possible with a variable volume ratio. Efficiency improvements as high as 30% are possible, depending on the application, refrigerant, and system operating range. Hermetic screw compressors are commercially available through 400 tons (1.4 MW) of refrigeration using R-22.

Scroll compressors are rotary motion, positive-displacement machines that compress with two interfitting, spiral-shaped scroll members. They are currently used in residential and commercial air-conditioning and heat pump applications as well as in automotive air-conditioning systems. Capacities range from 10,000 to 170,000 Btu/h (3 to 50 kW). To function effectively, the scroll compressor requires close tolerance machining of the scroll members, which has become possible only recently due to current advances in manufacturing technology. This positive-displacement, rotary motion compressor includes performance features, such as high efficiency and low noise.

Scroll members are typically a geometrically matched pair, assembled 180° out of phase. Each scroll member is open on one end of the vane and bound by a base plate on the other. The two scrolls are fitted to form pockets between their respective base plate and various lines of contact between their vane walls. One scroll is held fixed, while the other moves in an orbital path with respect to the first. The flanks of the scrolls remain in contact, although the contact locations move progressively inward. Relative rotation between the pair is prevented by a coupling. An alternate approach creates relative orbital motion via two scrolls synchronously rotating about noncoincident axes.

Compression is accomplished be sealing suction gas in pockets of a given volume at the outer periphery of the scrolls and progressively reducing the size of these pockets as the scroll relative motion moves then inwards toward the discharge port. Figure 18-16 shows the sequence of suction, compression, and discharge phases.

As the outermost pockets are sealed off (Figure 18-16a), the trapped gas is at suction pressure and has just entered the compression process. At stages (b) through (f), orbiting motion moves the gas toward the center of the scroll pair, and pressure rises as pocket volumes are reduced. At stage

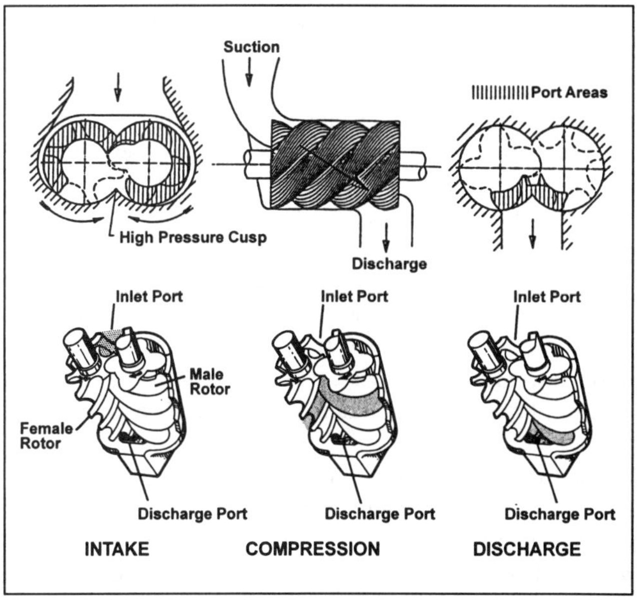

Fig. 18-14 Twin-Screw Compressor

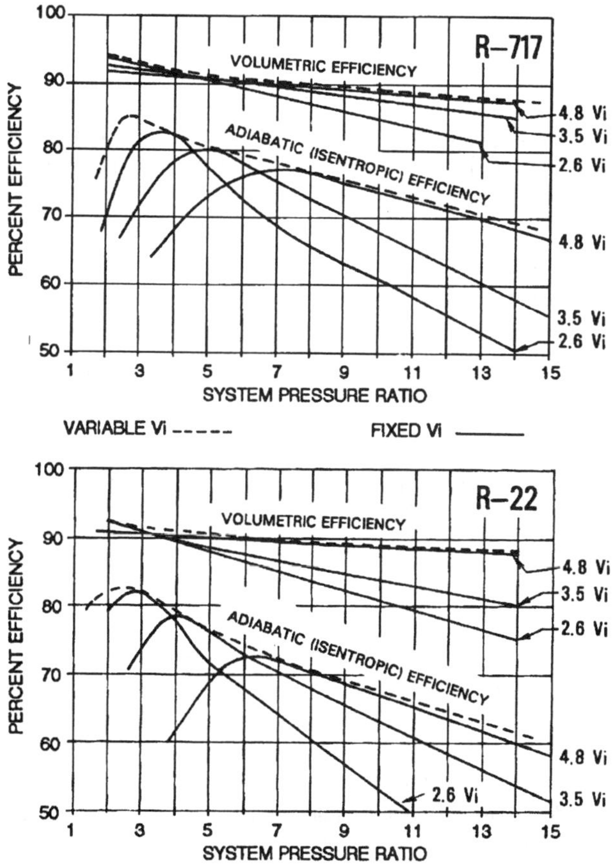

Fig. 18-15 Twin-Screw Compressor Efficiency Curves

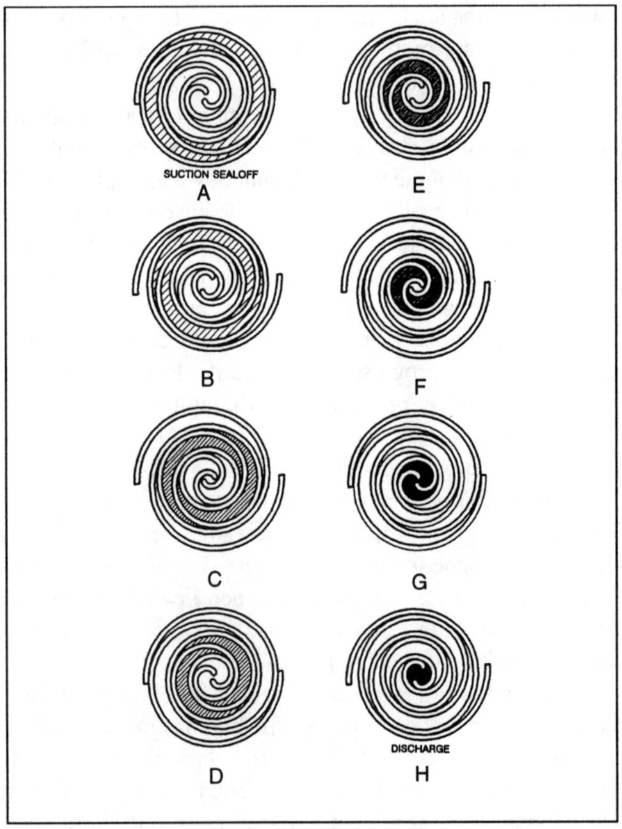

Fig. 18-16 Scroll Compression Process

(g), the gas reaches the central discharge port and begins to exit the scrolls. Stages (a) through (h) show that two distinct compression paths operate simultaneously in a scroll set. The discharge process is nearly continuous, since new pockets reach the discharge stage very shortly after the previous discharge pockets have been evacuated.

Both high-side and low-side shells are available. In the former, the entire compressor is at discharge pressure, except for the outer areas of the scroll set. Suction gas is introduced into the suction port of the scrolls through piping, which keeps it discrete from the rest of the compressor. Discharge gas is directed into the compressor shell, which acts as a plenum. In the low-side type, most of the shell is at suction pressure, and the discharge gas exiting the scrolls is routed outside the shell, sometimes through a discrete or integral plenum.

Scroll technology offers an advantage in performance for a number of reasons. Large suction and discharge ports reduce pressure losses incurred in the suction and discharge processes. Physical separation of these processes also reduces heat transfer to the suction gas. The absence of valves and reexpansion volumes and the continuous flow process results in high volumetric efficiency over a wide range of operation conditions. Figure 18-17 illustrates this effect.

The built-in volume ratio can be designed for lowest over- or undercompression at typical demand conditions (2.5 to 3.5 pressure ratio for air conditioning). Isentropic efficiency in the range of 70% is possible at such pressure ratios, and it remains quite close to the efficiency of other compressor types at high

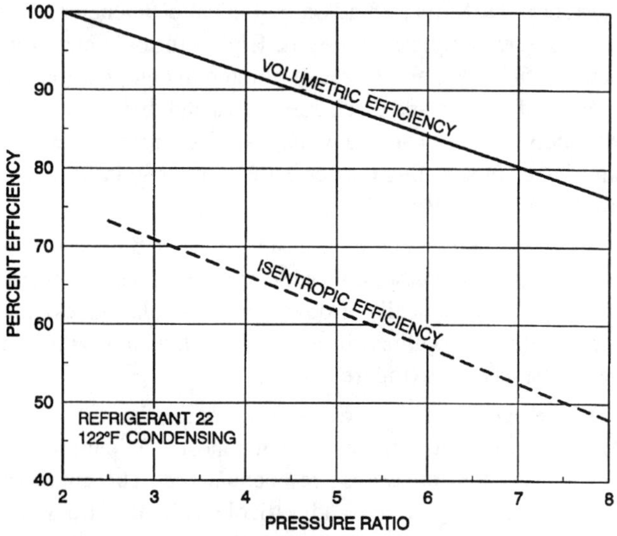

Fig. 18-17 Volumetric and Isentropic Efficiency for Scroll Compressor

pressure ratios. Scroll compressors offer a flatter capacity versus outdoor ambient curve than reciprocating products, which means that they can more closely approach indoor requirements at high demand conditions. As a result, the heat pump mode requires less supplemental heating; the cooling mode is more comfortable, because cycling is less as demand decreases. Scroll compressors available in the United States are typically specified as producing ARI operating efficiencies (COP) in the range of 3.10 to 3.34.

Centrifugal Compressors. Centrifugal compressors, or turbocompressors, are characterized by a continuous exchange of angular momentum between a rotating mechanical element and a steadily flowing fluid. Because their flows are continuous, turbomachines have greater volumetric capacities, size-for-size, than do positive-displacement devices. For effective momentum exchange, their rotative speeds must be higher, but little vibration or wear results because of the steadiness of the motion and the absence of contacting parts.

Centrifugal compressors are well suited for air-conditioning and refrigeration applications because of their ability to produce high pressure ratios (as compared to other turbocompressors). The suction flow enters the rotating element, or impeller, in the axial direction and is discharged radially at a higher velocity. The change in diameter through the impeller increases the velocity of the gas flow. This dynamic head is then converted to static head, or pressure, through a diffusion process, which generally begins within the impeller and ends in a radial diffuser and scroll outboard of the impeller.

Centrifugal compressors are used in a variety of refrigeration and air-conditioning installations. Suction flow rates range between 60 and 30,000 cfm (0.03 and 14 m^3/s), with rotational speeds between 1800 and 90,000 rpm. However, the high angular velocity associated with a low volumetric flow establishes a minimum practical capacity for most centrifugal applications. The upper capacity limit is determined by physical size, a 30,000 cfm (14 m^3/s) compressor being about 6 or 7 ft (2 m) in diameter.

A centrifugal compressor can be single stage, having only one impeller, or it can be multistage, having two or more impellers mounted in the same casing as shown in Figure 18-18. For process refrigeration applications, a compressor can have as many as ten stages.

The suction gas generally passes through a set of adjustable inlet guide vanes or an external suction damper before entering the impeller. The vanes (or suction damper) are used for capacity control.

Suction temperatures are usually between 50 and −150°F (10 and −100°C), with suction pressures between 2 and 100 psia (14 and 700 kPa) and discharge pressures up to 300 psia (2100 kPa). Pressure ratios range between 2 and 30. Almost any refrigerant can be used; R-123 is currently replacing R-11 as the most common.

The momentum exchange, or energy transfer, between a centrifugal impeller and a flowing refrigerant is expressed by the following equation:

$$W_i = u_i\, c_u/g$$

where

W_i = impeller work input per unit mass of refrigerant

u_i = impeller blade tip speed

c_u = tangential component of refrigerant velocity leaving impeller blades

g = gravitational constant

These velocities are shown in Figure 18-19, where refrigerant flows out from between impeller blades with relative velocity *b* and absolute velocity *c*. The relative angle β is a few degrees smaller than the blade angle because of a phenomenon known as slip. This equation assumes that the refrigerant enters the impeller without any tangential velocity component or swirl. This is generally the case at design flow conditions.

At least at low refrigerant flow rates, the tip speed of the impeller and the tangential velocity of the refrigerant are nearly identical. Thus, for a mass flow rate *m*, the ideal power can be estimated by

$$P = mc_u^2 = mu_i^2$$

Another expression for the ideal power input comes from the first law of thermodynamics:

$$P = m\Delta h_i$$

where Δh_i is the isentropic change in enthalpy across the compressor.

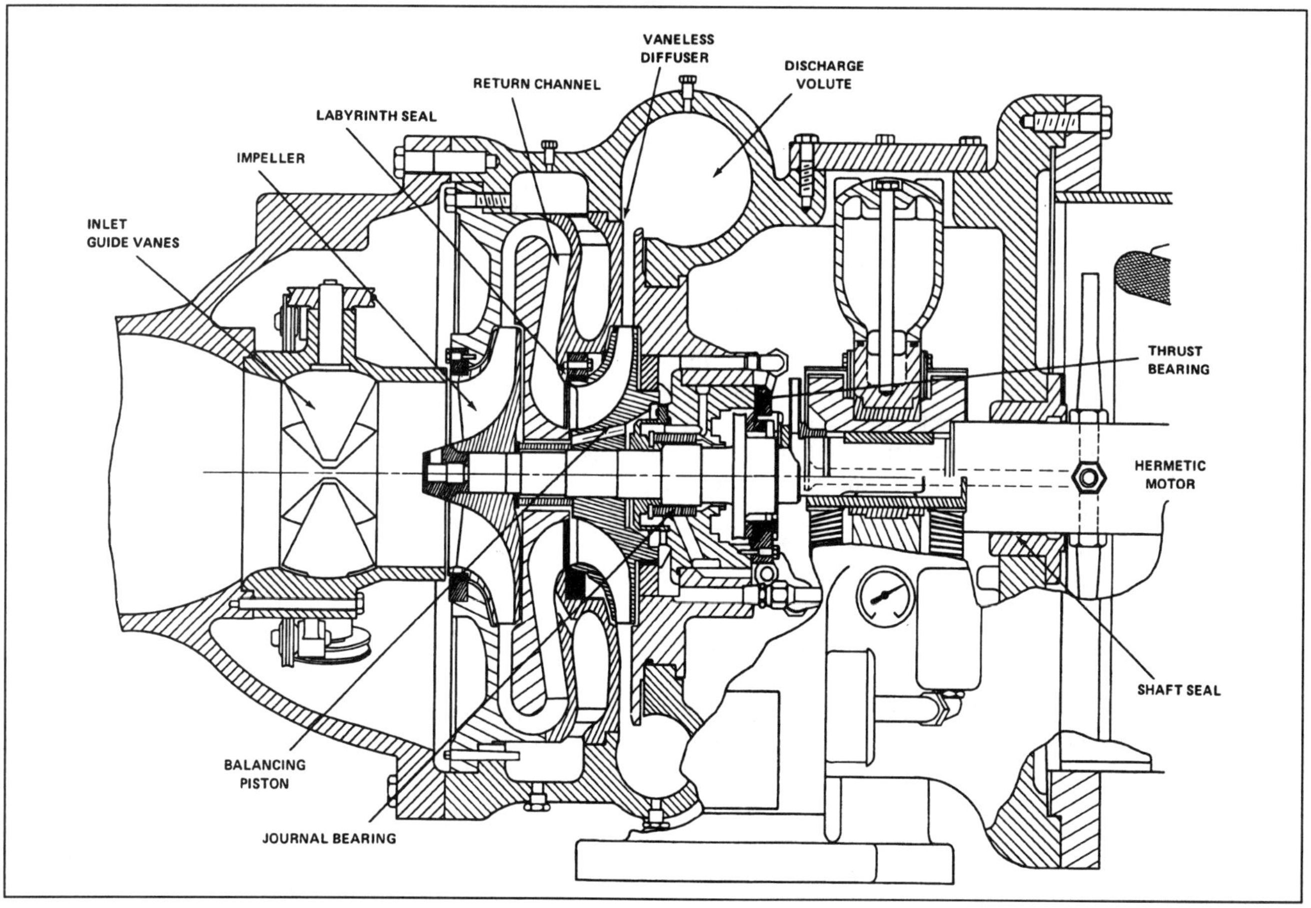

Fig. 18-18 Centrifugal Refrigeration Compressor

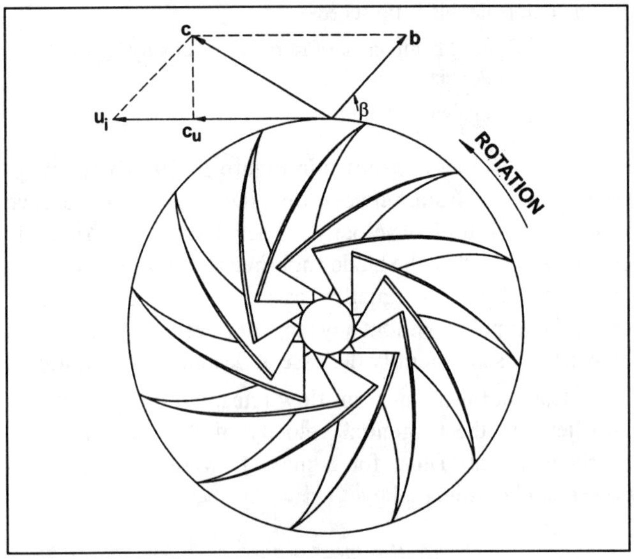

Fig. 18-19 Impeller Exit Velocity Diagram

Equating the two expressions for power yields an order-of-magnitude estimate of the tip speed:

$$u_i^2 = \Delta h_i(g)$$

Example 18-1 Estimate the impeller tip speed needed to compress R-717 (ammonia) from saturated vapor at 20°F to a pressure corresponding to a condensing temperature of 100°F.

Solution:

From Figure 21, Chapter 19, 1997 *ASHRAE Handbook—Fundamentals*:

$$\Delta h_i = 320 - 210 = 110 \text{ Btu/lb}$$

The tip speed is

$$u_i = [(32.2)(110)(778)]^{1/2} = 1660 \text{ ft/s}$$

Note: $g = 32.2$ ft/s^2 and 778 ft-lb/Btu is a conversion factor.

Some of the work done by the impeller increases the refrigerant pressure, while the remainder only increases its kinetic energy. The ratio of pressure-producing work to total work is known as the impeller reaction. Since this varies from about 0.4 to 0.7, an appreciable amount of kinetic energy leaves the impeller with magnitude $c^2/2g$. To convert this kinetic energy into additional pressure, a diffuser is located after the impeller. Radial vaneless diffusers are most common, but vaned, scroll, and conical diffusers are also used. In a multistage compressor, the flow leaving the first diffuser is guided to the inlet of the second impeller and so on through the machine. The total compression work input is the sum of the individual stage inputs provided that the mass flow rate is constant throughout the compressor:

$$W = \Delta W_i$$

18.1.2 Condensers

The condenser removes (from the refrigerant gas) the heat of compression and the heat absorbed by the refrigerant in the evaporator. The refrigerant is thereby converted back into the liquid phase at the condenser pressure and is available for reexpansion into the evaporator. The common forms of condensers may be classified on the basis of the cooling medium as (1) water-cooled, (2) air-cooled, and (3) evaporative (air and water) cooled.

Water-cooled condensers consist of the following types:

- shell-and-tube (vertical)
- shell-and-tube (horizontal)
- shell-and-coil (horizontal and vertical)
- double pipe
- atmospheric

The selection of a water-cooled condenser depends on the cooling load, the refrigerant used, the source and temperature of the available cooling water, the amount of water that can be circulated, the condenser location, the required operating pressures, and maintainability.

The heat rejection rate of the condenser for each unit of refrigeration produced in the evaporator may be estimated from Figure 18-20. Similar plots can be prepared for other refrigerants from tables of thermodynamic properties. In practice, the heat removed is 5 to 10% higher than the theoretical values because of losses during compression.

An accurate determination of the heat rejection requirement q_o can usually be made from known values of evaporator load q_i and the heat equivalent of the actual power required q_w for compression:

$$q_o = q_i + q_w \quad (18\text{-}1)$$

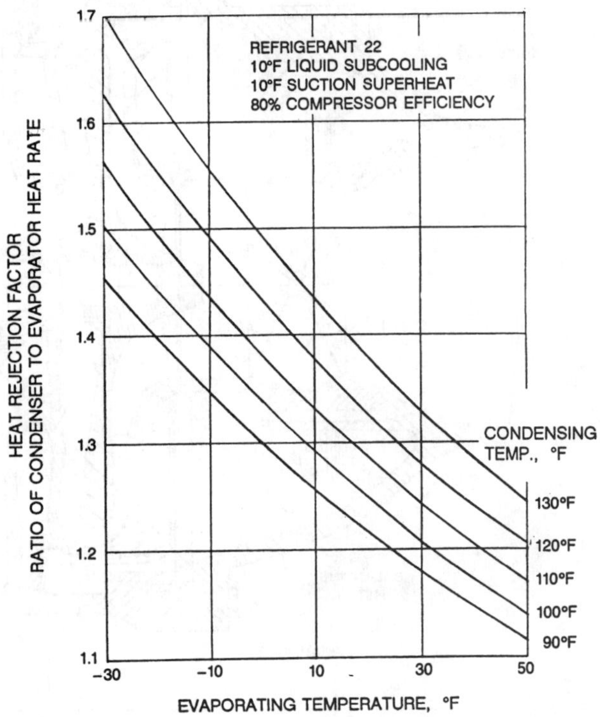

Fig. 18-20 Heat Rejection Rate for R-22 Condenser

Note: q_w is reduced by any independent heat rejection processes such as oil cooling and motor cooling.

The volumetric flow rate Q of condensing water required may be found from the following equation:

$$Q = \frac{q_o}{\rho c_p(t_2 - t_1)} \tag{18-2}$$

where

q_o = heat rejection rate
ρ = density of water
t_1 = temperature of water entering condenser
t_2 = temperature of water leaving condenser
c_p = specific heat of water

The heat rejection rate may also be determined as:

$$q_o = UA\Delta t_m \tag{18-3}$$

where

U = overall heat transfer coefficient
A = surface area associated with U
Δt_m = mean temperature difference

The computation of overall heat transfer in a water-cooled condenser with water inside the tubes may be made from calculated or test-derived heat transfer coefficients of the water and refrigerant sides, from physical measurements of the condenser tubes, and from a fouling factor on the water side, by using

$$U_o = \frac{1}{(S_r/h_w) + S_R r_{fw} + (X/k)(A_o/A_m) + 1/h_r\phi_w} \tag{18-4}$$

where

U_o = overall heat transfer coefficient, based on the external surface and the log mean temperature difference, between the external and internal fluids, Btu/h · ft^2 °F [(W/(m^2 · K)]
S_R = ratio of external to internal surface area
h_w = internal or water side film coefficient, Btu/h· ft^2· °F [W/(m^2· K)]
r_{fw} = fouling resistance on water side, ft^2·°F· h/Btu (m^2· K/W)
X = thickness of tube wall, ft (m)
k = thermal conductivity of tube material, Btu/h· ft· °F [W/(m · K)]
A_o/A_m = ratio of external surface to mean heat transfer area of metal wall
h_r = external, or refrigerant side coefficient, Btu/h· ft^2· °F [W/(m^2 · K)]
ϕ_w = weighted fin efficiency (100% for bare tubes)

Values of the water-side coefficient may be calculated from equations in Chapter 3 of the 1997 *ASHRAE Handbook—Fundamentals*. For turbulent flow, at Reynolds numbers exceeding 10,000 in horizontal tubes and using average water temperatures, the general equation is

$$\frac{h_w D}{k} = 0.023\left(\frac{DG}{\mu}\right)^{0.8}\left(\frac{c_p\mu}{k}\right)^{0.4} \tag{18-5}$$

where

D = inside tube diameter, ft (m)
k = thermal conductivity of water, Btu/h· ft· °F [W/(m · K)]
G = mass velocity of water, lb/s · ft^2 (kg/s · m^2)
μ = viscosity of water, lb/ft · h (mPa · s)
c_p = specific heat of water at constant pressure, Btu/lb· °F [kJ/(kg· K)]

Note: The constant (0.023) in this equation applies only to tubes with plain inside diameters.

Because of its strong influence on the value of h_w, water velocity should be maintained as high as permitted by water pressure drop considerations. Maximum velocities with clean water of 6 to 10 ft/s (1.8 to 3 m/s) are commonly used. A minimum velocity of 3 ft/s (1 m/s) is considered good practice when the water quality is such that noticeable fouling or corrosion could result. With clean water, the velocity may be lower if dictated by conservation or low supply temperature considerations.

Factors that influence the value of h_r are

- Type of refrigerant being condensed
- Geometry of condensing surface (plain tube, outside diameter, finned tube, fin spacing, height, and cross-section profile)
- Condensing temperature
- Condensing rate, in terms of mass velocity or rate of heat transferred
- Arrangement of tubes in bundle
- Vapor distribution and flow rate
- Condensate drainage

Values of the refrigerant side coefficients may be estimated from correlations shown in Chapters 3 or 4 of the 1997 *ASHRAE Handbook—Fundamentals*.

Example 18-2 Estimate the volumetric flow rate of condensing water required for the condenser of an R-22 water chilling unit assumed to be operating at a condensing temperature of 100°F, and evaporating temperature of 40°F, an entering condensing water temperature of 86°F, a leaving condensing water temperature of 95°F, and a refrigeration load of 100 tons.

Solution:

From Figure 18-20, the heat rejection factor is found to be 1.17.

$$q_o = 100 \times 1.17 = 117 \text{ tons} = 1{,}404{,}000 \text{ Btu/h}$$

ρ = 62.2 lb/ft^3 at 90.5°F
c_p = 1 Btu/lb·°F

From Equation (18-2),

$$Q = 1{,}404{,}000/[62.2 \times 1(95 - 86)] = 2500 \text{ ft}^3\text{/h} = 310 \text{ gpm}$$

A typical horizontal closed shell-and-tube ammonia condenser is shown in Figure 18-21.

Air-Cooled Condensers. The heat transfer process in an air-cooled condenser has three main phases: (1) desuperheating, (2) condensing, and (3) subcooling. The changes of state of R-134a passing through the condenser coil and the corre-

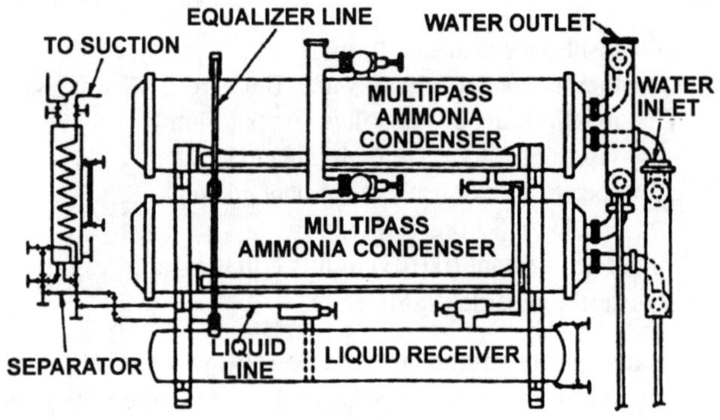

Fig. 18-21 Horizontal Shell-and-Tube Ammonia Condenser and Receiver

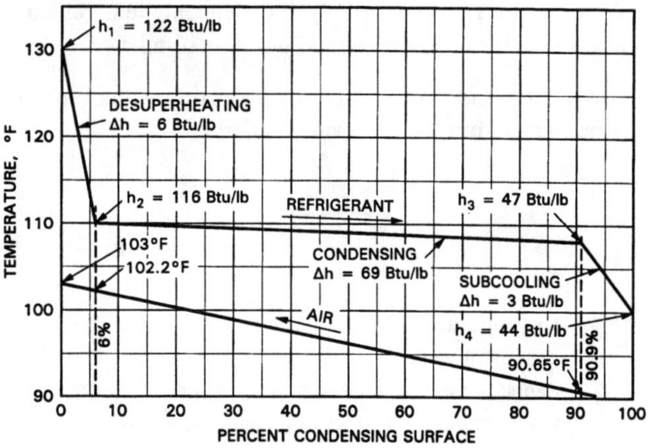

Fig. 18-22 Temperature and Enthalpy Changes in Air-Cooled Condenser with R 134a

sponding temperature change of the cooling air as it passes through the coil are shown in Figure 18-22. Desuperheating, condensing, and subcooling zones vary 5 to 10%, depending on the entering gas temperature and the leaving liquid temperature, but Figure 18-22 is typical for most of the commonly used refrigerants.

Condensing occurs in approximately 85% of the condenser area at a substantially constant temperature. The drop in condensing temperature is due to the friction loss through the condenser coil.

Coils in air-cooled condensers are commonly constructed of copper, aluminum, or steel tubes, ranging from 1/4 to 3/4 in. (8 to 20 mm) diameter. Copper is easy to use in manufacturing and requires no protection against corrosion. Aluminum requires exact manufacturing methods, and special protection must be provided if aluminum to copper joints are made. Steel tubing is used, but weather protection must be provided.

Fins are used to improve the air-side heat transfer. Fins are usually made of aluminum, but copper and steel are also used. The most common forms are plate fins making a coil bank, plate fins individually fastened to the tube, or a fin spirally wound onto the tube. Other forms such as plain tube-fin extrusions or tube extrusions with accordion type fins are also used. The number of fins per inch varies from 4 to 30 (0.8 to 6.4 mm fin spacing). The most common range is 8 to 18 (1.4 to 3.2 mm spacing).

Evaporative Condensers. As with water-cooled and air-cooled condensers, evaporative condensers reject heat

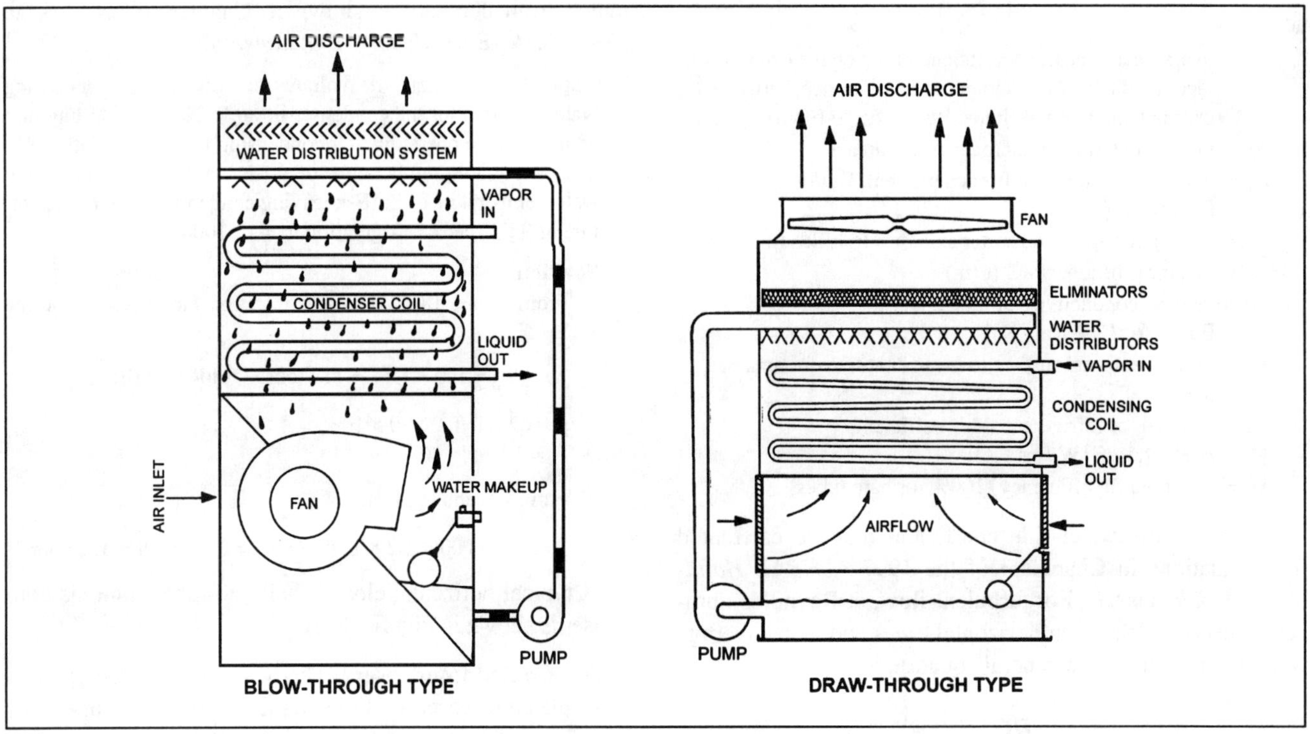

Fig. 18-23 Functional View of Evaporative Condenser

from a condensing vapor into the environment. In an evaporative condenser, hot high-pressure vapor from the compressor discharge circulates through a condensing coil that is continually wetted on the outside by a recirculating water system. As seen in Figure 18-23, air is simultaneously directed over the coil, causing a small portion of the recirculated water to evaporate. This evaporation removes heat from the coil, thus cooling and condensing the vapor.

Evaporative condensers reduce the water pumping and chemical treatment requirements associated with cooling tower/refrigerant condenser systems. In comparison with an air-cooled condenser, an evaporative condenser requires less coil surface and airflow to reject the same heat, or alternately, greater operating efficiencies can be achieved by operating at a lower condensing temperature.

The evaporative condenser can operate at a lower condensing temperature than an air-cooled condenser because the air-cooled condenser is limited by the ambient dry-bulb temperature. In the evaporative condenser, heat rejection is limited by the ambient wet-bulb temperature, which is normally 14 to 24°F (8 to 13°C) lower than the ambient dry bulb. The evaporative condenser also provides lower condensing temperatures than the cooling tower/water-cooled condenser because the heat transfer/mass transfer steps are reduced from two (between the refrigerant and the cooling water and between the water and ambient air) to one step (refrigerant directly to ambient air). While both the water-cooled condenser/cooling tower combination and the evaporative condenser use evaporative heat rejection, the former has added a second step of nonevaporative heat transfer from the condensing refrigerant to the circulating water, requiring more surface area. Evaporative condensers are, therefore, the most compact for a given capacity.

18.1.3 Expansion and Control Devices

Any refrigeration system requires that the flow of refrigerant be controlled. Valves are used to start, stop, direct, and modulate the flow of refrigerant to satisfy load requirements. To assure satisfactory performance, valves should be adequately protected from foreign material, excessive moisture, and corrosion. Such protection is accomplished by installing properly sized strainers and driers.

Thermostatic Expansion Valves. The thermostatic expansion valve controls the flow rate of liquid refrigerant entering the evaporator in response to the superheat of the refrigerant gas leaving the evaporator. It keeps the entire evaporator active, without permitting unevaporated refrigerant liquid to be returned through the suction line to the compressor. The thermostatic expansion valve does so by controlling the mass flow rate of refrigerant entering the evaporator so that it equals the rate at which the refrigerant can be completely vaporized in the evaporator by heat absorption. Since the thermostatic expansion valve is opera-ted by the superheated refrigerant gas leaving the evaporator and is responsive to changes in superheat of this gas, a portion of the evaporator must be devoted to superheating the refrigerant gas.

Unlike the constant pressure expansion valve, the thermostatic expansion valve is not limited to constant load applications. It is used to control refrigerant flow to all types of direct-expansion evaporators in air-conditioning, commercial, low-temperature, and ultralow temperature refrigeration systems.

A schematic cross section of the thermostatic expansion valve, with the principal components identified, is shown in Figure 18-24. Three forces are shown that govern thermostatic expansion valve operation:

p_1 = vapor pressure of the thermostatic element (a function of the bulb temperature), which is applied to the top of the diaphragm and acts to open valve

p_2 = evaporator pressure, which is applied underneath the diaphragm through the equalizer passage, and acts in a closing direction

p_3 = pressure equivalent of the superheat spring force, which is applied underneath the diaphragm, and is also a closing force

At any constant operating condition, these forces are balanced and $p_1 = p_2 + p_3$.

An additional force is that arising from the unbalanced pressure across the valve port. It can affect thermostatic expansion valve operation to a degree. For the configuration shown in Figure 18-24, the force due to port unbalance is the product of the pressure drop across the port and the difference in area of the port and the stem, and it would be an opening force. In other designs, depending on the direction of flow through the valve, the port unbalance might result in a closing force.

The principal effect of port unbalance is on valve control stability. As with any modulating control, if the ratio of power element area to port area is kept large, the unbalanced port effect is minor. Large capacity valves are made with

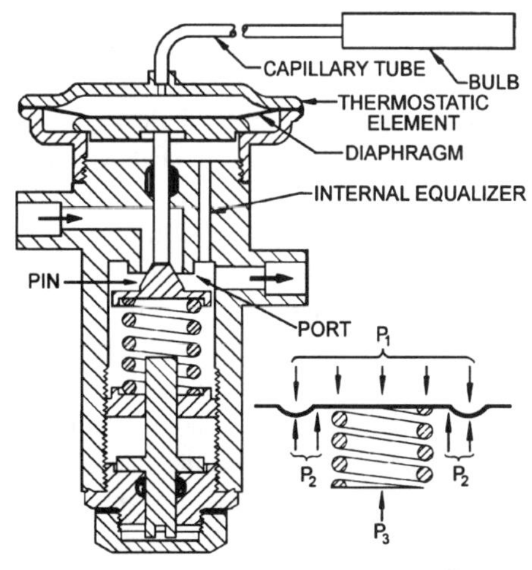

Fig. 18-24 Typical Thermostatic Expansion Valve

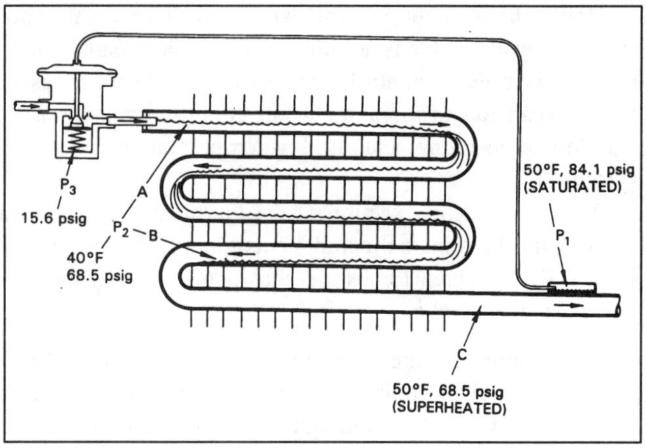

Fig. 18-25 Thermostatic Expansion Valve Controlling Flow of Liquid R-12 Entering Evaporator (Assuming R-12 Charge in Bulb)

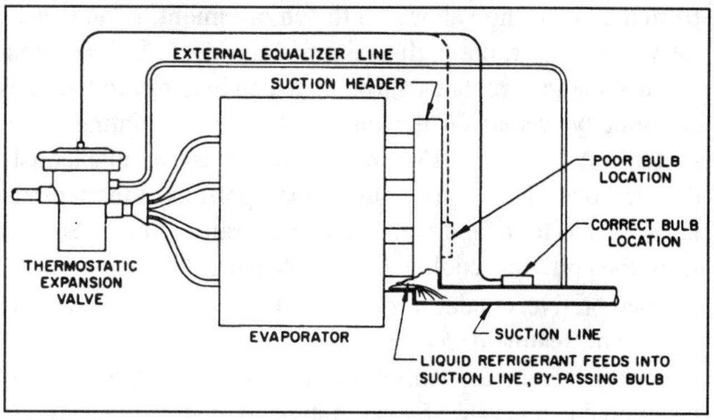

Fig. 18-26 Bulb Location for Thermostatic Expansion Valve

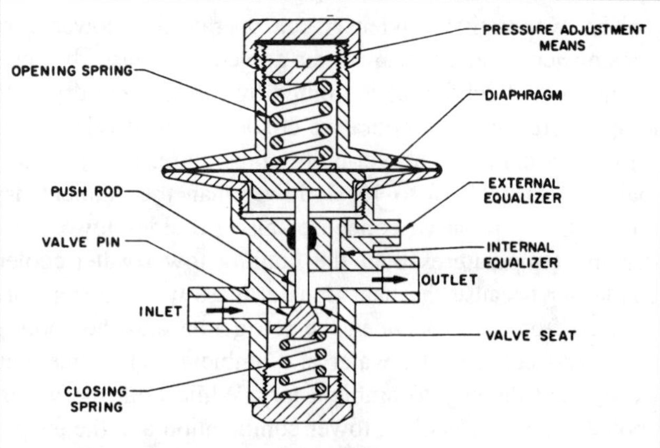

Valve is used with either internal or external equalizer, but not with both.

Fig. 18-27 Constant Pressure Expansion Valve

double-ported, or semibalanced, construction to minimize the effect of unbalanced pressure.

An evaporator using R-12 and operating at a saturation temperature of 40°F (4.4°C), and a pressure of 37 psig (255 kPa) is shown in Figure 18-25. Liquid refrigerant enters the expansion valve, is reduced in pressure and temperature at the valve port, and enters the evaporator at point A as a mixture of saturated liquid and vapor. As flow continues through the evaporator, more and more of the boiling refrigerant is evaporated. The refrigerant temperature remains at 40°F (4.4°C) until the liquid portion is completely evaporated by the absorption of heat at point B. From this point, additional heat absorption increases the temperature and superheats the refrigerant gas, while the pressure remains constant at 37 psig (255 kPa), until at point C (the outlet of the evaporator), the refrigerant gas temperature is 50°F (10°C). At this point, the superheat is 10°F (from 40 to 50°F) [5.6°C (from 4.4 to 10°C)].

An increase in the heat load on the evaporator increases the temperature of the refrigerant gas leaving the evaporator. The bulb of the thermostatic expansion valve senses this increase; the thermostatic charge pressure (p_1) increases and causes the valve to open wider. The increased flow rate results in a higher evaporator pressure (p_2) and a balanced control point is established again. Conversely, a decrease in the heat load on the evaporator decreases the temperature of the refrigerant gas leaving the evaporator and causes the thermostatic expansion valve pin to move in a closing direction.

External pressure equalizing thermostatic expansion valves are also used. A pressure line is connected between the valve and the suction side of the evaporator. This connection compensates for the frictional pressure loss in the evaporator. A common technique for this type of valve installation is illustrated in Figure 18-26.

Constant Pressure Expansion Valves. The constant pressure expansion valve is operated by the evaporator or valve outlet pressure to regulate the mass flow rate of liquid refrigerant entering the evaporator and thereby maintain this pressure at a constant value.

Figure 18-27 shows a schematic cross section of a constant pressure expansion valve. The valve has an adjustable spring that exerts its force on top of the diaphragm in an opening direction, and a spring beneath the diaphragm that exerts its force in a closing direction. Evaporator pressure admitted beneath the diaphragm, through either the internal or external equalizer passage, combines with the closing spring to counterbalance the opening spring pressure.

With the valve set and feeding refrigerant at a given pressure, a small increase in the evaporator pressure forces the diaphragm upward and causes the valve pin to move in a closing direction, thereby restricting refrigerant flow and limiting evaporator pressure. When the evaporator pressure, because of a decrease in load, drops below the valve setting, the top spring pressure moves the valve pin in an opening direction, thereby increasing the refrigerant flow in an effort to raise the evaporator pressure to the balanced valve setting. This valve controls the evaporation of the liquid refrigerant in the evaporator at a constant temperature.

Evaporator Pressure Regulators. The evaporator pressure regulator (back pressure regulator) regulates the evaporator pressure (pressure entering the regulator) at a constant value. It is used in the evaporator outlet or suction line to prevent frosting on the coil or to keep the leaving air temper-

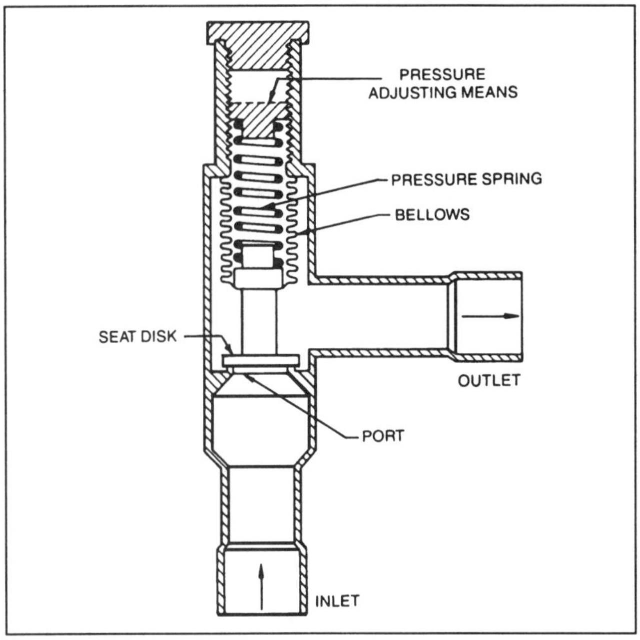

Fig. 18-28 Direct-Acting Evaporator Pressure Regulator

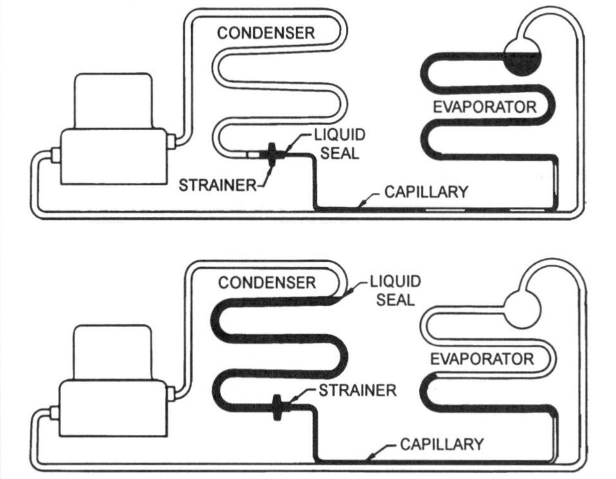

Notes:

1. Capillary selected for capacity balance conditions. Liquid seal at capillary inlet but no excess liquid in condenser. Compressor discharge and suction pressure normal. Evaporator properly charged.
2. too much capillary resistance—liquid refrigerant backs up in condenser and causes evaporator to be undercharged. Compressor discharge pressure may be abnormally high. Suction pressure below normal. Bottom of condenser subcooled.

Fig. 18-29 Effect of Capillary Tube Selection of Refrigerant Distribution

ature from lowering under light load conditions. These pressure regulators are commonly used on multiple evaporators served by a single compressor or when different suction pressures are required by multiple evaporator coils.

As illustrated in Figure 18-28, the inlet pressure acts on the bottom of the seat disk and is opposed by the adjusting spring. The outlet pressure acts on the underside of the bellows and the top of the seating disk, and, since the effective areas of the bellows and the port are equal, the two forces cancel and the valve is responsive to inlet pressure only. When the evaporator pressure rises above the force exerted by the spring, the valve moves in the opening direction. When the evaporator pressure drops below the force exerted by the spring, the valve moves in the closing direction. In actual operation, the valve assumes a throttling position to balance system load.

Capillary Tubes. Every refrigerating unit requires a pressure-reducing device to meter the refrigerant flow to the low side in accordance with the system demands. The capillary tube is popular for smaller unitary hermetic equipment, such as household refrigerators and freezers, dehumidifiers, and room air conditioners. It is also used in larger units such as unitary air conditioners in sizes up to 10 tons (35 kW) capacity. The capillary operates on the principle that liquid passes through it more readily than does gas. It consists of a small diameter line that connects the outlet of the condenser to the inlet of the evaporator. It is sometimes soldered to the outer surface of the suction line for heat exchange purposes.

Assume that a condenser-to-evaporator capillary has been sized to permit the desired flow of refrigerant with a liquid seal at its inlet. If a system unbalance occurs so that some gas (uncondensed refrigerant) enters the capillary, this gas tends to considerably reduce the mass flow of refrigerant with little or no change in the system pressures. If the opposite type of unbalance occurs, liquid refrigerant backs up in the condenser. This condition tends to cause subcooling and increases the mass flow of refrigerant. Thus, a capillary properly sized for the application tends to automatically compensate for load and system variations and gives acceptable performance over a wide range of operating conditions.

A refrigerating system is operating at the **condition of capacity balance** when the resistance of the capillary is sufficient to maintain a liquid seal at its entrance without excess liquid accumulating in the high side of the system (Figure 18-29). Only one such capacity balance point exists for any given compressor discharge pressure.

18.1.4 Evaporators for Liquid Chillers

A liquid cooler (hereafter called a cooler) is a component of a refrigeration system in which the refrigerant is evaporated to produce a cooling effect on a fluid (usually water or brine). Various types of water and brine coolers, as well as refrigerant flow control, capacity range, and refrigerants commonly used, are listed in Table 18-3.

In the **direct-expansion cooler**, the refrigerant is expanded into the inside of the tubes and vaporizes completely before leaving. The fluid being cooled is circulated on the outside of the tube surface within an enclosing shell. These coolers are usually used with positive-displacement compressors, such as reciprocating, rotary, or rotary screw compressors, to cool water or brine. Shell-and-tube is the most common arrangement, although tube-in-tube and brazed plate cooler are also available.

Figure 18-30 shows a typical shell-and-tube cooler. A series of baffles channels the fluid throughout the shell side.

Table 18-3 Types of Liquid Coolers

Type of Cooler	Usual Refrigerant Feed Device	Usual Capacity Range, tons (kW)	Commonly Used Refrigerants
Flooded shell-and-tube	Low-pressure float High-pressure float Fixed orifice(s) Weir	25 to 2000 (90 to 7000)	11, 12, 22, 113, 114, 123, 134a, 500, 502, 717
Spray-type shell-and-tube[a]	Low-pressure float High-pressure float	50 to 10,000 (180 to 35 000)	11, 12, 13B1, 22, 113, 114, 123, 134a
Direct-expansion shell-and-tube	Thermal expansion valve Electronic modulation valve	2 to 1000 (7 to 3500)	12, 22, 134a, 500, 502, 717
Baudelot (flooded)	Low-pressure float	10 to 100 (35 to 350)	22, 717
Baudelot (direct-expansion)	Thermal expansion valve	5 to 25 (18 to 90)	12, 22, 134a, 717
Tube-in-tube	Thermal expansion valve	5 to 25 (18 to 90)	12, 22, 134a, 717
Shell-and-coil	Thermal expansion valve	2 to 10 (7 to 35)	12, 22, 134a, 717
Brazed or semiwelded plate[b]	Thermal expansion valve Fixed orifice	0.5 to 2000 (2 to 7000)	12, 22, 134a, 500, 502, 717

[a]See the section on Flooded Shell-and-Tube. [b]See the section on Direct-Expansion.

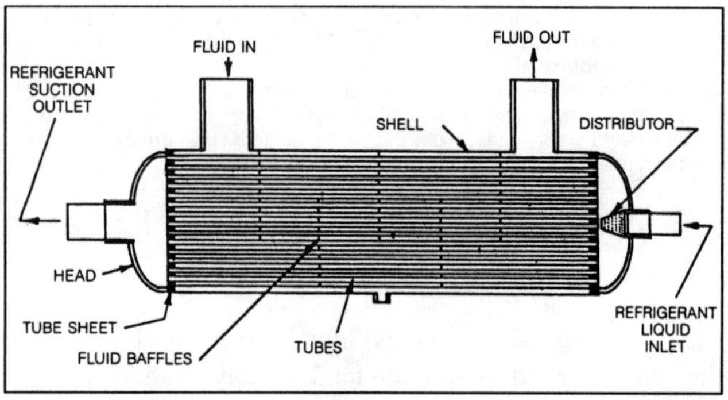

Fig. 18-30 Direct-Expansion Shell-and-Tube Cooler

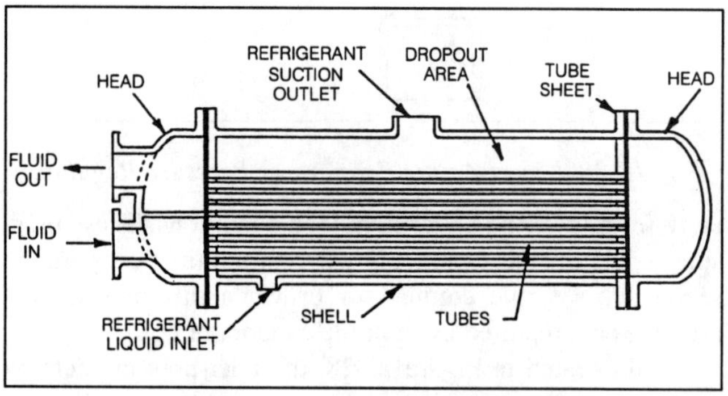

Fig. 18-31 Flooded Shell-and-Tube Cooler

The baffles increase the velocity of the fluid, thereby increasing its heat transfer coefficient. The velocity of the fluid flowing perpendicular to the tubes should be at least 2 ft/s (0.6 m/s) to clean the tubes and less than 10 ft/s (3 m/s) to prevent erosion.

Distribution is critical in direct-expansion coolers. If some tubes are fed more refrigerant than others, they tend to bleed liquid refrigerant into the suction line. Since most direct-expansion coolers are controlled to a given suction super-heat, the remaining tubes must produce a higher super-heat to evaporate the liquid bleeding through. This unbalance causes poor heat transfer. Uniform distribution is often achieved by a spray distributor. Most direct-expansion coolers are designed for horizontal mounting.

In a **flooded cooler**, the refrigerant vaporizes on the outside of tubes, which are submerged in liquid refrigerant within a closed shell. The fluid flows through the tubes as shown in Figure 18-31. Flooded coolers are usually used with rotary screw or centrifugal compressors to cool water or brine.

Refrigerant liquid/vapor mixture usually feeds into the bottom of the shell through a distributor that distributes the refrigerant vapor equally under the tubes. The relatively warm fluid in the tubes heats the refrigerant liquid surrounding the tubes, causing it to boil. As bubbles rise up through the space between tubes, the liquid surrounding the tubes becomes increasingly bubbly (or foamy, if much oil is present). The refrigerant vapor must be separated from the separation method is provided by a dropout area between the top row of tubes and the suction connections. If this dropout area is insufficient, a coalescing filter may be required between the tubes and connectors.

The size of tubes, number of tubes, and number of passes should be determined to maintain the fluid velocity typically between 3 and 10 ft/s (1 and 3 m/s). In some cases, the minimum velocity may be determined by a lower Reynolds number limit to ensure turbulent flow. Flooded shell-and-tube coolers are generally unsuitable for other than horizontal orientation.

A **spray cooler** is similar to a flooded shell-and-tube cooler except that the refrigerant liquid is recirculated through spray nozzles located above the top tubes. None of the tubes are submerged in liquid.

A simple **shell-and-coil cooler** is used in small capacitiesfor cooling water for drinking purposes, bakeries, and mist generated by the boiling refrigerant. The simplest photographic laboratories (Figure 18-32). It consists of a steel or alloy tank containing a helical coil through which refrigerant is circulated. The water is contained in the tank surrounding the coil. This type of cooler has the advantage of having cold water storage capacity, which is useful where peak loads occur at intervals.

Table 18-4 Overall Heat Transfer Coefficients for Liquid Coolers

Type of Evaporator	Overall U, Btu/h·ft^2·°F (W/(m^2·K)) Minimum	Maximum	Surface Side Basis for U
Flooded shell-and-plain-tube (water to Refrigerants 12, 22, and 717)	130 (740)	190 (1080)	Refrigerant
Flooded shell-and-finned-tube (water to Refrigerants 12, 22, or 500)	90 (510)	170 (970)	Refrigerant
Flooded shell-and-plain-tube (brine to Refrigerant 717)	45 (260)	100 (570)	Refrigerant
Flooded shell-and-plain-tube (brine to Refrigerants 12, 22, or 502)	30 (170)	90 (510)	Refrigerant
Direct-expansion, shell-and-plain-tube (water to Refrigerants 12, 22, and 717) (Refrigerant in Tubes)	80 (450)	220 (1250)	Liquid
Direct-expansion, shell-and-internal-finned-tubes (water to Refrigerants 12 or 22) (Refrigerant in Tubes)	160 (910)	250 (1420)	Liquid
Direct-expansion, shell-and-plain-tube (brine to Refrigerants 12, 22, 717, or 502) (Refrigerant in Tubes)	60 (340)	140 (790)	Liquid
Direct-expansion, shell-and-internal-finned-tubes (nonsalt brines to Refrigerants 12, 22, or 502)	60 (340)	170 (970)	Liquid
Shell-and-plain-tube coil (water in shell)(Refrigerant 12, 22, or 717 in coil)	10 (57)	25 (140)	Liquid
Baudelot cooler, flooded (Refrigerant 12 or 22 to water)	100 (570)	200 (1130)	Liquid
Baudelot cooler, direct expansion (Refrigerant 717 to water)	60 (340)	150 (850)	Liquid
Baudelot cooler, direct expansion (Refrigerant 12 or 22 to water)	60 (340)	120 (680)	Liquid
Double-pipe cooler (Refrigerant 717 to water)	50 (280)	150 (850)	Liquid
Double-pipe cooler (Refrigerant 717 to water)	50 (280)	125 (710)	Liquid
Tank-and-agitator, coil type water cooler (flooded, Refrigerant 717)	80 (450)	125 (710)	Liquid
Tank-and-agitator, coil type water cooler (flooded, Refrigerant 12, 22, or 500)	60 (340)	100 (570)	Liquid
Tank, ammonia (Refrigerant 717) to brine cooling, coils between cans in ice	15 (85)	40 (230)	Liquid
Tank-and-agitator, coil type water cooler (flooded, Refrigerant 717)	80 (450)	110 (620)	Liquid

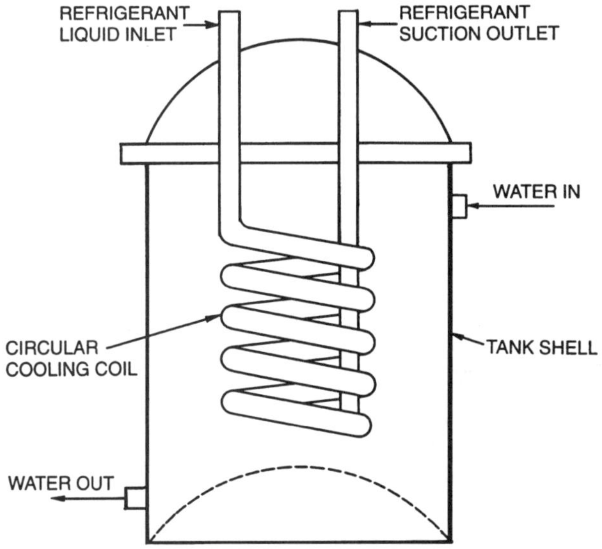

Fig. 18-32 Shell-and-Coil Cooler

The rate at which heat is transferred in the evaporator is given by the following equation:

$$q = U_o A_o \Delta t_m \quad (18\text{-}6)$$

where

q = heat transfer rate, Btu/h (W)
U_o = overall heat transfer coefficient based on outside surface, Btu/h·ft^2·°F [W/(m^2·K)]
A_o = outside surface area, ft^2 (m^2)
Δt_m = logarithmic mean temperature difference, °F (°C)

Details on determining these quantities are given in Chapter 2 of the 1993 *ASHRAE Handbook—Fundamentals.*

Listed in Table 18-4 are approximate minimum and maximum values for U_o.

18.1.5 Refrigerants

The choice of a refrigerant for a particular application often depends on properties not directly related to its ability to remove heat. Such properties are flammability, toxicity,density, viscosity, and availability. As a rule, the selection of a refrigerant is a compromise between conflicting desirable properties. For example, the pressure in the evaporator should be as high as possible, and at the same time, a low condensing pressure is desirable.

Table 18-5 provides the ASHRAE standard designation of refrigerants given in ANSI/ASHRAE *Standard* 34. Table 18-6 lists the basic physical properties of these refrigerants. Table 18-7 gives the comparative refrigerant performance per unit (ton or kW) of refrigeration.

A discussion of the properties of various refrigerants, as well as their relative performance characteristics, is presented in Chapter 18 of the 1997 *ASHRAE Handbook—Fundamentals.* Complete thermodynamic and thermophysical properties for the refrigerants may be found in Chapter 19 of the 1997 *ASHRAE Handbook—Fundamentals.*

18.2 Absorption Air-Conditioning and Refrigeration Equipment

Absorption refrigeration cycles are heat-operated cycles in which a secondary fluid, the **absorbent**, is used to absorb the **primary fluid**, a gaseous refrigerant, which has been vaporized in the evaporator. The basic absorption cycle is shown in Figure 18-33.

Table 18-5 Standard Designation of Refrigerants (ASHRAE *Standard* 34)

Refrigerant Number	Chemical Name or Composition (% by mass)	Chemical Formula
Methane Series		
10	tetrachloromethane (carbon tetrachloride)	CCl_4
11	trichlorofluoromethane	CCl_3F
12	dichlorodifluoromethane	CCl_2F_2
12B1	bromochlorodifluoromethane	$CBrClF_2$
12B2	dibromodifluoromethane	CBr_2F_2
13	chlorotrifluoromethane	$CClF_3$
13B1	bromotrifluoromethane	$CBrF_3$
14	tetrafluoromethane (carbon tetrafluoride)	CF_4
20	trichloromethane (chloroform)	$CHCl_3$
21	dichlorofluoromethane	$CHCl_2F$
22	chlorodifluoromethane	$CHClF_2$
22B1	bromodifluoromethane	$CHBrF_2$
23	trifluoromethane	CHF_3
30	dichloromethane (methylene chloride)	CH_2Cl_2
31	chlorofluoromethane	CH_2ClF
32	difluoromethane (methylene fluoride)	CH_2F_2
40	chloromethane (methyl chloride)	CH_3Cl
41	fluoromethane (methyl fluoride)	CH_3F
50	methane	CH_4
Ethane Series		
110	hexachloroethane	CCl_3CCl_3
111	pentachlorofluoroethane	CCl_3CCl_2F
112	1,1,2,2-tetrachloro-1,2-difluoroethane	CCl_2FCCl_2F
112a	1,1,1,2-tetrachloro-2,2-difluoroethane	CCl_3CClF_2
113	1,1,2-trichloro-1,2,2-trifluoroethane	CCl_2FCClF_2
113a	1,1,1-trichloro-2,2,2-trifluoroethane	CCl_3CF_3
114	1,2-dichloro-1,1,2,2-tetrafluoroethane	$CClF_2CClF_2$
114a	1,1-dichloro-1,2,2,2-tetrafluoroethane	CCl_2FCF_3
114B2	1,2-dibromo-1,1,2,2-tetrafluoroethane	$CBrF_2CBrF_2$
115	chloropentafluoroethane	$CClF_2CF_3$
116	hexafluoroethane	CF_3CF_3
120	pentachloroethane	$CHCl_2CCl_3$
123	2,2-dichloro-1,1,1-trifluoroethane	$CHCl_2CF_3$
123a	1,2-dichloro-1,1,2-trifluoroethane	$CHClFCClF_2$
124	2-chloro-1,1,1,2-tetrafluoroethane	$CHClFCF_3$
124a	1-chloro-1,1,2,2-tetrafluoroethane	CHF_2CClF_2
125	pentafluoroethane	CHF_2CF_3
133a	2-chloro-1,1,1-trifluoroethane	CH_2ClCF_3
134a	1,1,1,2-tetrafluoroethane	CH_2FCF_3
140a	1,1,1-trichloroethane (methyl chloroform)	CH_3CCl_3
141b	1,1-dichloro-1-fluoroethane	CCl_2FCH_3
142b	1-chloro-1,1-difluoroethane	$CClF_2CH_3$
143a	1,1,1-trifluoroethane	CF_3CH_3
150a	1,1-dichloroethane	$CHCl_2CH_3$
152a	1,1-difluoroethane	CHF_2CH_3
160	chloroethane (ethyl chloride)	CH_3CH_2Cl
170	ethane	CH_3CH_3
Propane Series		
216ca	1,3-dichloro-1,1,2,2,3,3-hexafluoropropane	$CClF_2CF_2CClF_2$
218	octafluoropropane	$CF_3CF_2CF_3$
245cb	1,1,1,2,2-pentafluoropropane	$CF_3CF_2CH_3$
290	propane	$CH_3CH_2CH_3$
Cyclic Organic Compounds		
C316	1,2-dichloro-1,2,3,3,4,4-hexafluorocyclobutane	$C_4Cl_2F_6$
C317	chloroheptafluorocyclobutane	C_4ClF_7
C318	octafluorocyclobutane	C_4F_8
Zeotropic Blends (% by mass)		
400	R-12/114 (must be specified)	
401A	R-22/152a/124 (53/13/34)	
401B	R-22/152a/124 (61/11/28)	
401C	R-22/152a/124 (33/15/52)	
402A	R-125/290/22 (60/2/38)	
402B	R-125/290/22 (38/2/60)	
Zeotropes (*Continued*)		
403A	R-290/22/218 (5/75/20)	
403B	R-290/22/218 (5/56/39)	
404A	R-125/143a/134a (44/52/4)	
405A	R-22/152a/142b/C318 (45/7/5.5/42.5)	
406A	R-22/600a/142b (55/4/41)	
407A	R-32/125/134a (20/40/40)	
407B	R-32/125/134a (10/70/20)	
407C	R-32/125/134a (23/25/52)	
407D	R-32/125/134a (15/15/70)	
408A	R-125/143a/22 (7/46/47)	
409A	R-22/124/142b (60/25/15)	
409B	R-22/124/142b (65/25/10)	
410A	R-32/125 (50/50)	
410B	R-32/125 (45/55)	
411A	R-1270/22/152a (1.5/87.5/11.0)	
411B	R-1270/22/152a (3/94/3)	
412A	R-22/218/142b (70/5/25)	
Azeotropic Blends (% by mass)		
500	R-12/152a (73.8/26.2)	
501	R-22/12 (75.0/25.0)*	
502	R-22/115 (48.8/51.2)	
503	R-23/13 (40.1/59.9)	
504	R-32/115 (48.2/51.8)	
505	R-12/31 (78.0/22.0)*	
506	R-31/114 (55.1/44.9)	
507A	R-125/143a (50/50)	
508A	R-23/116 (39/61)	
508B	R-23/116 (46/54)	
509A	R-22/218 (44/56)	
Miscellaneous Organic Compounds		
Hydrocarbons		
600	butane	$CH_3CH_2CH_2CH_3$
600a	2-methyl propane (isobutane)	$CH(CH_3)_3$
Oxygen Compounds		
610	ethyl ether	$C_2H_5OC_2H_5$
611	methyl formate	$HCOOCH_3$
Sulfur Compounds		
620	(Reserved for future assignment)	
Nitrogen Compounds		
630	methyl amine	CH_3NH_2
631	ethyl amine	$C_2H_5NH_2$
Inorganic Compounds		
702	hydrogen	H_2
704	helium	He
717	ammonia	NH_3
718	water	H_2O
720	neon	Ne
728	nitrogen	N_2
732	oxygen	O_2
740	argon	Ar
744	carbon dioxide	CO_2
744A	nitrous oxide	N_2O
764	sulfur dioxide	SO_2
Unsaturated Organic Compounds		
1112a	1,1-dichloro-2,2-difluoroethene	$CCl_2{=}CF_2$
1113	1-chloro-1,2,2-trifluoroethene	$CClF{=}CF_2$
1114	tetrafluoroethene	$CF_2{=}CF_2$
1120	trichloroethene	$CHCl{=}CCl_2$
1130	1,2-dichloroethene (trans)	$CHCl{=}CHCl$
1132a	1,1 difluoroethene (vinylidene fluoride)	$CF_2{=}CH_2$
1140	1-chloroethene (vinyl chloride)	$CHCl{=}CH_2$
1141	1-fluoroethene (vinyl fluoride)	$CHF{=}CH_2$
1150	ethene (ethylene)	$CH_2{=}CH_2$
1270	propene (propylene)	$CH_3CH{=}CH_2$

*The exact composition of this azeotrope is in question.

Table 18-6 Physical Properties of Selected Refrigerants[a]

Refrigerant No.	Refrigerant Chemical Name or Composition (% by mass)	Chemical Formula	Molecular Mass	Boiling Pt. (NBP) at 14.696 psia, °F	Freezing Point, °F	Critical Temperature, °F	Critical Pressure, psia	Critical Volume, ft^3/lb	Refractive Index of Liquid[b,c]
704	Helium	He	4.0026	−452.1	None	−450.3	33.21	0.2311	1.021 (NBP) 5461 Å
702p	Hydrogen, para	H_2	2.0159	−423.2	−434.8	−400.3	187.5	0.5097	1.09 (NBP)[f]
702n	Hydrogen, normal	H_2	2.0159	−423.0	−434.5	−399.9	190.8	0.5320	1.097 (NBP) 5791 Å
720	Neon	Ne	20.183	−410.9	−415.5	−379.7	493.1	0.03316	—
728	Nitrogen	N_2	28.013	−320.4	−346.0	−232.4	492.9	0.05092	1.205 (83 K) 5893 Å
729	Air	—	28.97	−317.8	—	−220.95	548.9	0.0530	
						−221.1	546.3	0.05007	
740	Argon	Ar	39.948	−302.55	−308.7	−188.48	704.9	0.0301	1.233 (84 K) 5893 Å
732	Oxygen	O_2	31.9988	−297.332	−361.8	−181.424	731.4	0.03673	1.221 (92 K) 5893 Å
50	Methane	CH_4	16.04	−258.7	−296	−116.5	673.1	0.099	
14	Tetrafluoromethane	CF_4	88.01	−198.3	−299	−50.2	543	0.0256	
1150	Ethylene	C_2H_4	28.05	−154.7	−272	48.8	742.2	0.070	1.363(−148)[1]
744A[2]	Nitrous oxide	N_2O	44.02	−129.1	−152	97.7	1048	0.0355	
170	Ethane	C_2H_6	30.07	−127.85	−297	90.0	709.8	0.0830	
503	R-23/13 (40.1/59.9)	—	87.5	−127.6	—	67.1	607	0.0326	
23	Trifluoromethane	CHF_3	70.02	−115.7	−247	78.1	701.4	0.0311	
13	Chlorotrifluoromethane	$CClF_3$	104.47	−114.6	−294	83.9	561	0.0277	1.146 (77)[4]
744	Carbon dioxide	CO_2	44.01	−109.2[d]	−69.9[e]	87.9	1070.0	0.0342	1.195 (59)
13B1	Bromotrifluoromethane	$CBrF_3$	148.93	−71.95	−270	152.6	575	0.0215	1.239 (77)[4]
504	R-32/115 (48.2/51.8)	—	79.2	−71.0	—	151.5	690.5	0.0324	
32	Difluoromethane	CH_2F_2	52.02	−61.1	−213	173.14	845.6	0.03726	
125	Pentafluoroethane	C_2HF_5	120.03	−55.43	−153.67	151.34	526.57	—	—
1270	Propylene	C_3H_6	42.09	−53.86	−301	197.2	670.3	0.0720	1.3640 (−58)[1]
502[5]	R-22/115 (48.8/51.2)	—	111.63	−49.8	—	179.9	591.0	0.0286	
290	Propane	C_3H_8	44.10	−43.76	−305.8	206.1	616.1	0.0726	1.3397 (−43)
22	Chlorodifluoromethane	$CHClF_2$	86.48	−41.36	−256	204.8	721.9	0.0305	1.234 (77)[4]
115	Chloropentafluoroethane	$CClF_2CF_3$	154.48	−38.4	−159	175.9	457.6	0.0261	1.221 (77)[4]
500	R-12/152a (73.8/26.2)	—	99.31	−28.3	−254	221.9	641.9	0.0323	
717	Ammonia	NH_3	17.03	−28.0	−107.9	271.4	1657	0.068[d]	1.325 (61.7)
12	Dichlorodifluoromethane	CCl_2F_2	120.93	−21.62	−252	233.6	596.9	0.0287	1.288 (77)[4]
134a	Tetrafluoroethane	CF_3CH_2F	102.03	−15.08	−141.9	214.0	589.8	0.029	—
152a	Difluoroethane	CHF_2CH_3	66.05	−13.0	−178.6	236.3	652	0.0439	
40[2]	Methyl chloride	CH_3Cl	50.49	−11.6	−144	289.6	968.7	0.0454	
124	Chlorotetrafluoroethane	$CHClFCF_3$	136.47	8.26	−326.47	252.5	530.84	—	—
600a	Isobutane	C_4H_{10}	58.13	10.89	−255.5	275.0	529.1	0.0725	1.3514 (−13)[1]
764[6]	Sulfur dioxide	SO_2	64.07	14.0	−103.9	315.5	1143	0.0306	
142b	Chlorodifluoroethane	$CClF_2CH_3$	100.5	14.4	−204	278.8	598	0.0368	
630[6]	Methyl amine	CH_3NH_2	31.06	19.9	−134.5	314.4	1082		1.432 (63.5)
C318	Octafluorocyclobutane	C_4F_8	200.04	21.5	−42.5	239.6	403.6	0.0258	
600	Butane	C_4H_{10}	58.13	31.1	−217.3	305.6	550.7	0.0702	1.3562 (5)[1]
114	Dichlorotetrafluoroethane	$CClF_2CClF_2$	170.94	38.8	−137	294.3	473	0.0275	1.294 (77)
21[7]	Dichlorofluoromethane	$CHCl_2F$	102.92	47.8	−211	353.3	750	0.0307	1.332 (77)[4]
160[2]	Ethyl chloride	C_2H_5Cl	64.52	54.32	−216.9	369.0	764.4	0.0485	
631[6]	Ethyl amine	$C_2H_5NH_2$	45.08	61.88	−113	361.4	815.6		
11	Trichlorofluoromethane	CCl_3F	137.38	74.87	−168	388.4	639.5	0.0289	1.362 (77)[4]
123	Dichlorotrifluoroethane	$CHCl_2CF_3$	152.93	82.17	−160.87	362.82	532.87	—	—
611[6]	Methyl formate	$C_2H_4O_2$	60.05	89.2	−146	417.2	870	0.0459	
141b	Dichlorofluoroethane	CCl_2FCH_3	116.95	89.6	—	399.6	616.4	—	
610[6]	Ethyl ether	$C_4H_{10}O$	74.12	94.3	−177.3	381.2	523	0.0607	1.3526 (68)
216ca	Dichlorohexafluoropropane	$C_3Cl_2F_6$	220.93	96.24	−193.7	356.0	399.5	0.0279	
30[6]	Methylene chloride	CH_2Cl_2	84.93	104.4	−142	458.6	882		1.4244 (68)[3]
113	Trichlorotrifluoroethane	CCl_2FCClF_2	187.39	117.63	−31	417.4	498.9	0.0278	1.357 (77)[4]
1130[8]	Dichloroethylene	$CHCl{=}CHCl$	96.95	118	−58	470	795		
1120[6]	Trichloroethylene	$CHCl{=}CCl_2$	131.39	189.0	−99	520	728		1.4782(68)[3]
718[6]	Water	H_2O	18.02	212	32	705.18	3200	0.0498	

Notes:

[a]Data from ASHRAE *Thermodynamic Properties of Refrigerants* (Stewart et al. 1986) or from McLinden (1990), unless otherwise noted.

[b]Temperature of measurement (°F, unless kelvin is noted) shown in parentheses. Data from CRC *Handbook of Chemistry and Physics* (CRC 1987), unless otherwise noted.

[c]For the sodium D line.

[d]Sublimes.

[e]At 76.4 psia.

[f]Dielectric constant data.

References:

[1]Kirk and Othmer (1956).

[2]*Matheson Gas Data Book* (1966).

[3]Electrochemicals Department, E.I. duPont de Nemours & Co.

[4]*Bulletin* B-32A (duPont).

[5]*Bulletin* T-502 (duPont 1980).

[6]*Handbook of Chemistry* (1967).

[7]*Bulletin* G-1 (duPont).

[8]CRC *Handbook of Chemistry and Physics* (CRC 1987).

Table 18-7 Comparative Refrigerant Performance per Ton of Refrigeration[a]

Refrigerant No.	Refrigerant Chemical Name or Composition (% by mass)	Evaporator Pressure, psia	Condenser Pressure, psia	Compression Ratio	Net Refrigerating Effect, Btu/lb_m	Refrigerant Circulated, lb_m/min	Liquid Circulated, in^3/min	Specific Volume of Suction Gas, ft^3/lb_m	Compressor Displacement, cfm	Power Consumption, hp	Coefficient of Performance	Comp. Discharge Temp., °F
170	Ethane	236.410	674.710	2.85	69.27	2.88704	289.1266	0.5344	1.543	1.733	2.72	123
744	Carbon dioxide	332.375	1045.360	3.15	57.75	3.46320	158.5272	0.2639	0.914	1.678	2.81	156
13B1	Bromotrifluoromethane	77.820	264.128	3.39	28.45	7.02901	129.7814	0.3798	2.669	1.134	4.16	104
125	Pentafluoroethane	58.870	228.110	3.87	37.69	5.30645	126.8148	0.6281	3.333	1.283	3.67	108
1270	Propylene	52.704	189.440	3.59	123.15	1.62401	90.7048	2.0487	3.327	1.035	4.56	108
290	Propane	42.37	156.820	3.70	120.30	1.66251	95.0386	2.4589	4.088	1.031	4.57	98
502	R-22/115 (48.8/51.2)	50.561	191.290	3.78	44.91	4.45305	103.3499	0.8015	3.569	1.067	4.42	98
22	Chlorodifluoromethane	42.963	172.899	4.02	69.90	2.86144	67.6465	1.2394	3.546	1.011	4.67	128
717	Ammonia	34.170	168.795	4.94	474.20	0.42177	19.6087	8.1790	3.450	0.989	4.77	210
500	R-12/152a (73.8/26.2)	31.064	127.504	4.10	60.64	3.29834	80.1925	1.5022	4.955	1.005	4.69	105
12	Dichlorodifluoromethane	26.505	107.991	4.07	50.25	3.97981	85.2280	1.4649	5.830	0.992	4.75	100
134a	Tetrafluoroethane	23.790	111.630	4.69	64.77	3.08785	71.8199	1.9500	6.021	1.070	4.41	108
124	Chlorotetrafluoroethane	12.960	64.590	4.98	50.93	3.92696	81.1580	2.7140	10.658	1.054	4.47	90
600a	Isobutane	12.924	59.286	4.59	113.00	1.76991	90.0059	6.4189	11.361	1.070	4.41	80
600	Butane	8.176	41.191	5.04	125.55	1.59299	77.7772	10.2058	16.258	0.952	4.95	88
114	Dichlorotetrafluoroethane[b]	6.747	36.493	5.41	43.02	4.64889	89.5631	4.3400	20.176	1.015	4.65	86
11	Trichlorofluoromethane	2.937	18.318	6.24	67.21	2.97592	56.2578	12.2400	36.425	0.939	5.02	110
123	Dichlorotrifluoroethane	2.290	15.900	6.94	61.19	3.26829	62.3495	14.0800	46.018	0.974	4.84	94
113	Trichlorotrifluoroethane[b]	1.006	7.884	7.83	52.08	3.84047	68.5997	26.2845	100.945	1.105	4.27	86

Notes: [a]Based on 5°F evaporation and 86°F condensation. [b]Saturated suction except R-113 and R-114. Enough superheat was added to give saturated discharge.

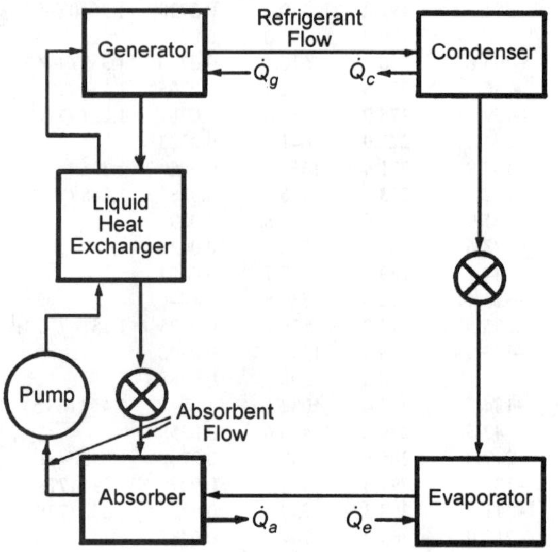

Fig. 18-33 Basic Absorption Refrigeration Cycle

Chapter 1 of the 1997 *ASHRAE Handbook—Fundamentals* discusses operating principles and thermodynamics of the basic absorption cycle and other information on the thermodynamics of workable absorbent-refrigerant combinations. A complete thermodynamic analysis of the absorption cycle is complex. However, a detailed analysis is not necessary to understanding the operating principles of the cycle.

The absorption cycle and the mechanical compression cycle have in common the evaporation and condensation of a refrigerant liquid; these processes occur at two pressure levels within the unit. The two cycles differ in that the absorption cycle uses a pump and a heat-operated generator to produce the pressure differential, whereas the mechanical compression cycle uses a compressor; the absorption cycle substitutes physiochemical processes for the purely mechanical processes of the compression cycle. Both cycles require energy for operation: heat in the absorption cycle, mechanical energy in the compression cycle.

Of the many combinations that have been tried, only the lithium bromide-water and the ammonia-water cycles remain in common use for air-conditioning. In addition, ammonia-water absorption equipment has been used in large industrial applications requiring low temperatures for process work.

Figure 18-34 is a typical schematic diagram of machines available in the form of indirect-fired liquid chillers in capacities of 50 to 1500 tons (180 to 5300 kW). Figure 18-35 is a similar machine with components arranged in a single shell.

Generators (concentrators) are tube bundles submerged in the solution, heated by steam or hot liquids.

Condensers are tube bundles located in the vapor space over the generator and shielded from carryover of salt by eliminators. Cooling water to the condenser first passes through the absorber.

Absorbers are tube bundles over which strong absorbent is sprayed. Refrigerant vapor is condensed into the absorbent, releasing heat to the cooling water passing through.

Evaporators (coolers) are tube bundles over which the refrigerant water is sprayed and evaporated. The liquid to be cooled passes inside the tubes.

Solution heat exchangers are of all steel shell-and-tube construction.

Solution and evaporator pumps are generally electric-motor-driven centrifugal pumps of hermetic design that use the cycle fluids for cooling and lubrication.

Purgers are used to remove noncondensable gases. Noncondensable gases present in small quantities can raise the total pressure in the absorber sufficiently to significantly

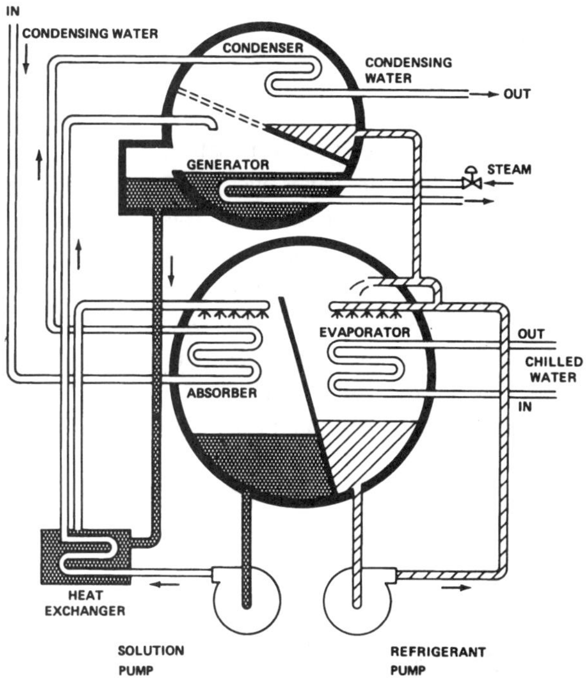

Fig. 18-34 Diagram of Two-Shell Lithium Bromide Cycle Water Chiller

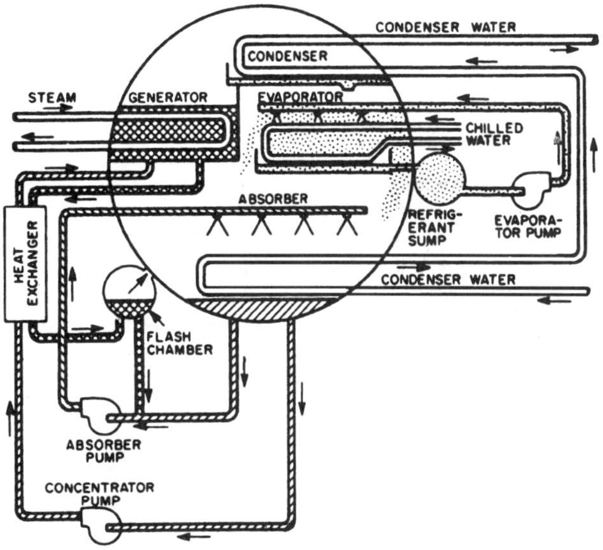

Fig. 18-35 Diagram of One-Shell Lithium Bromide Cycle Water Chiller

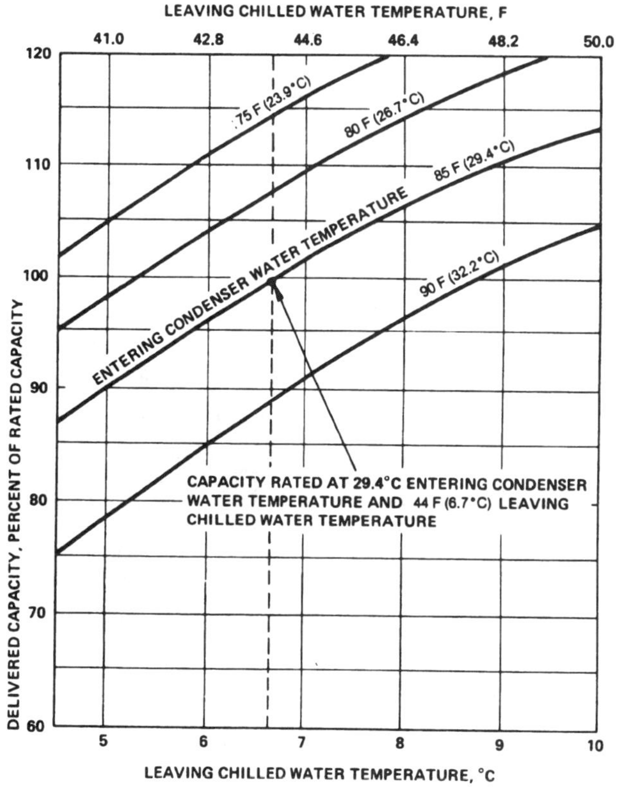

Fig. 18-36 Performance Characteristics of Lithium Bromide Cycle Water Chiller

change the evaporator pressure. Small pressure increases cause appreciable change in the refrigerant evaporating temperature.

Expansion devices commonly used in absorption machines are usually an orifice or fixed restriction, which controls the flow of refrigerant liquid between the condenser and the evaporator.

Lithium bromide-water cycle absorption machines meet load variations and maintain chilled water temperature control by varying the rate of reconcentration of the absorbent solution. At any given constant load, the chilled water temperature is maintained by a temperature difference between refrigerant and chilled water. In turn, the refrigerant temperature is maintained by the absorber being supplied with a flow rate and concentration of solution, and by the absorber cooling water temperature.

Load changes are reflected by corresponding changes in chilled water temperature. A load reduction, for example, results in less temperature difference needed in the evaporator and a reduced requirement for solution flow or concentration. The resultant chilled water temperature drop is met by adjusting the rate of reconcentration to match the reduced requirements of the absorber. The typical performance characteristics of a lithium bromide-water cycle absorption machine with an indirect heat source generator are shown in Figure 18-36.

The coefficient of performance (COP) of a lithium bromide-water cycle absorption machine operating at the nominal conditions shown in Table 18-8 is typically in the range of 0.65 to 0.70. Whenever chilled water temperatures are above the nominal, or condensing water temperatures are

Table 18-8 Nominal Rating Conditions for Heat-Operated Units

Leaving chilled water temperature	44°F	6.7°C
Chilled water temperature differential	10°F	5.5°C
Entering condenser water temperature	85°F	30°C
Steam pressure at control valve inlet, gage pressure dry and saturated	9–12 psi	60–80 kPa
Scale factor for evaporator, condenser, and absorber	0.0005 $h \cdot ft^2 \cdot °F/Btu$	0.09 $(m^2 \cdot K)/kW$

below the nominal, a COP as high as 0.70 can be reached. Reversing the temperature conditions cited reduces the COP to below 0.60. A coefficient of performance of 0.68 corresponds approximately to a steam rate of 18 lb/h per ton of refrigeration (1.45 kW/kW).

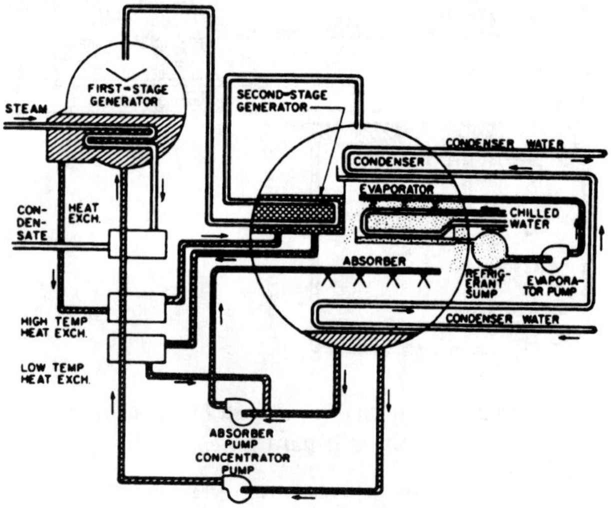

Fig. 18-37 Diagram of One-Shell Lithium Bromide Cycle-Water Chiller with Two-Stage Generator

Absorption machines can be made with a two-stage generator. Such a unit may be called **dual effect**. Figure 18-37 is a schematic diagram of a nominally single-shell design with a two-stage generator. The first-effect generator receives the external heat, which boils refrigerant from the weak absorbent. This hot refrigerant vapor then goes to a second generator and supplies heat for further refrigerant vaporization from the absorbent of intermediate concentration, which flows from the first generator and is cooled by passing through a first-stage heat economizer. Other than the generator, all components of the single-stage lithium bromide-water absorption units are common to the two-stage units. The advantage of the dual-effect unit is higher performance, with steam rates approximately two-thirds those of single-stage machines. Heat source temperature for the dual-effect unit is over 120°F (67°C) higher than for the single-effect unit, requiring higher steam pressures.

18.3 Cooling Towers

A cooling tower, through a combination of mass and energy transfer, cools water by exposing it as an extended sur-

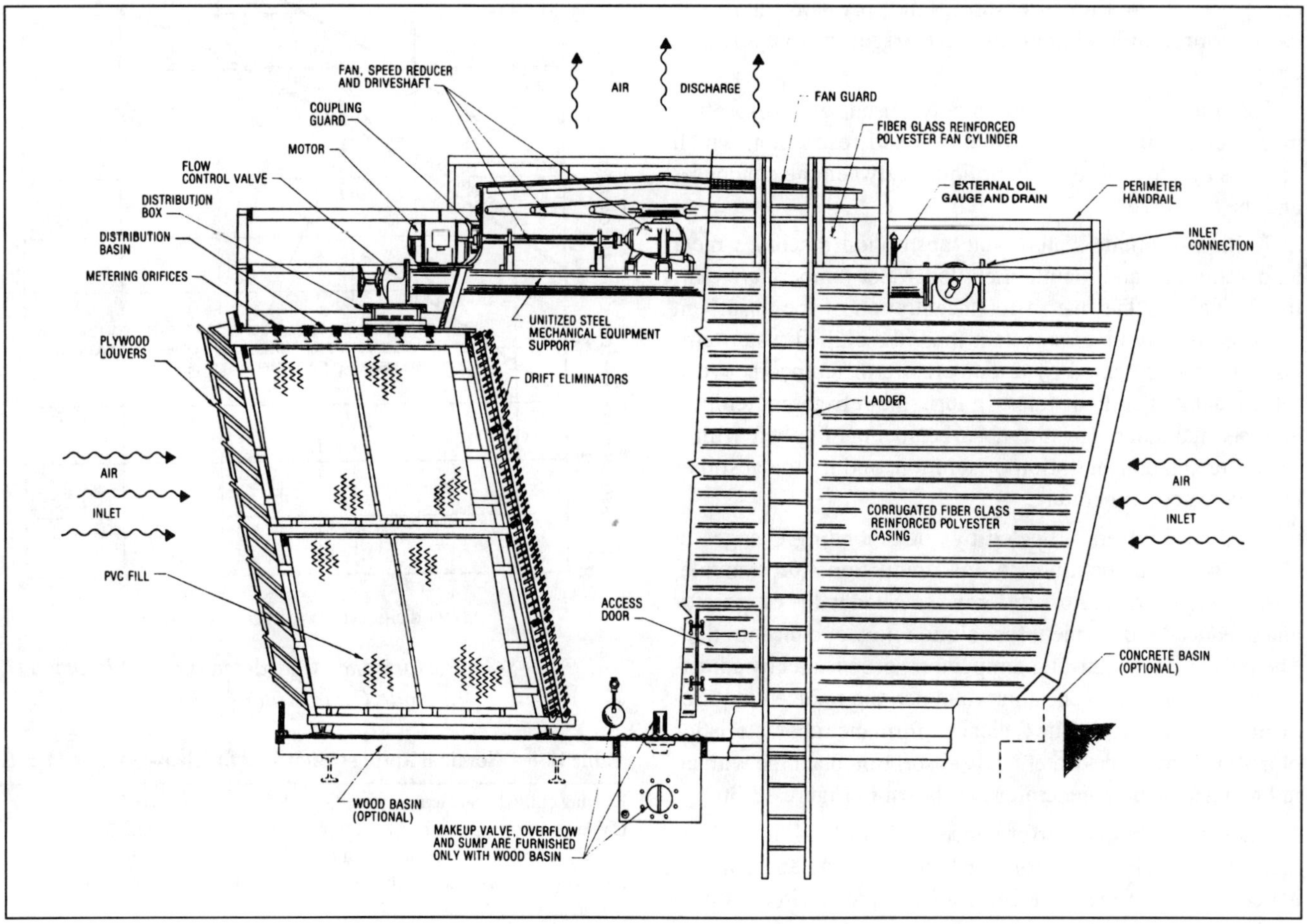

Fig. 18-38 Crossflow Mechanical-Draft Tower

face to the atmosphere. The water fills the tower to present a wetted surface or create drops due to splashing, or is sprayed, producing droplets. The airflow may be caused by mechanical means, by convection currents due to variation in density, or by natural wind currents. The airflow may be crossflow or counterflow. Crossflow describes air flowing horizontally in the filled portion of the tower or normal to the water flow, whereas counterflow implies the airstream rises vertically or countercurrent to the falling stream of water.

Counterflow mechanical-draft towers are principally found in air-conditioning applications. The main advantage of counterflow is its adaptability to restrictive space limitations. Factory-assembled towers often use centrifugal blowers in forced-draft configurations. The field-erected designs are usually induced-draft units with axial flow fans.

Crossflow towers are widely used in air-conditioning, process, and industrial applications. Crossflow towers have: (1) low air-side pressure drop in relation to high transfer surface areas and (2) the inherent capability to obtain uniform distributional characteristics of both the air and water streams.

The thermal capability of any cooling tower may be defined by the following parameters:

- entering and leaving water temperatures
- entering air wet-bulb temperature
- water flow rate

The variations in tower performance associated with changes in these parameters are discussed in Chapter 36 of the 1996 *ASHRAE Handbook—Systems and Equipment.*

The thermal capability of cooling towers for air-conditioning applications is usually stated in terms of nominal refrigeration tonnage based on heat dissipation of 15,000 Btu/h per ton (1.25 kW/kW) and a water circulation rate of 3 gpm per ton (0.054 L/s per kW) cooled from 95 to 85°F (35 to 29.4°C) at 78°F (25.6°C) wet-bulb temperature. For industrial applications, nominal tonnage ratings are not used and the performance capability of the cooling tower is usually stated in terms of flow rate at specified operating conditions (entering and leaving water temperature and entering air wet-bulb temperature).

Fans in the mechanical-draft tower provide a positive and constant airflow. Since performance does not depend on the wind, mechanical-draft towers may be designed for exacting conditions. The fans may operate to provide forced or induced draft, depending on their location at the inlet or outlet of the tower. The tower may be crossflow (Figure 18-38) or counterflow (Figure 18-39). The addition of the fan makes it possible to design wider towers that are more compact than the long, narrow atmospheric towers.

Factory-assembled cooling towers in both crossflow and counterflow designs are available. Water distribution is by gravity or low-pressure flume with crossflow design, and spray nozzles are used on counterflow units.

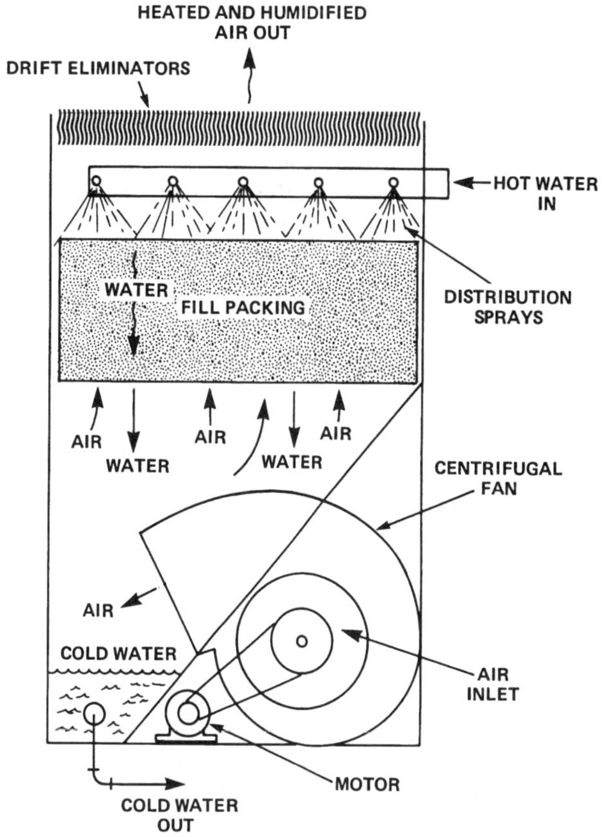

Fig. 18-39 Conterflow Forced-Draft Cooling Tower

18.3.1 Spray Ponds

Heat dissipates from the surface of a body of water by evaporation, radiation, and convection. A spray pond divides the water into small droplets, greatly extending the water surface and bringing it into contact with the air. Heat transfer is largely due to evaporative cooling. Temperature control, large space requirements, limited ability to approach the wet-bulb temperature, and winter operational difficulties have generally ruled out the spray pond in favor of more compact and more controllable mechanical-draft or hyperbolic towers.

18.4 Problems

18.1 A condenser used in a refrigeration system has a capacity of 10 tons at a 40°F evaporating temperature. When 20 gpm of cooling water enters at 75°F, the condensing temperature is 90°F. The manufacturer claims a U-value of 95 Btu/h·ft^2·°F, with a heat transfer area of 83 ft^2. Are these claims reasonable? Why? [Ans: No, inconsistent LMTD]

18.2 Saturated water vapor at 40°F is mixed in a steady-flow chamber with a saturated lithium bromide-water solution having a concentration of 0.30 lb LiBr/lb mixture. The mass of the liquid solution mixed is four times the mass of the water vapor mixed. The mixing process occurs at constant pressure. Determine:

(a) Concentration of the resulting mixture
(b) Heat that must be removed from the final mixture to produce a saturated liquid solution
[Ans: (a) 0.24, (b) 216.5 Btu/lb]

18.3 Given a compressor using R-22 condensing at 80°F (26.7°C) and evaporating at 20°F (−6.7°C), find the enthalpy of the refrigerant when it enters the
(a) compressor
(b) condenser
(c) evaporator
Find the power required for the compressor.
[Ans: (a) 0.24, (b) 216.5 Btu/lb]

18.4 Given a compressor that uses R-11, which condenses at 100°F (37.8°C) and evaporates at –10°F (-23.3°C), calculate the compressor displacement, mass flow rate, and power required for the compressor under regular assumptions.

18.5 What is the maximum theoretical COP of a refrigeration device operating between 0°F and 75°F (–17.8°C and 23.9°C). Why is this theoretical limit difficult to obtain?[Ans: 6.14]

18.6 A reference book on refrigeration indicates that a compressor using R-22 requires a displacement of 40.59 cfm per ton for evaporation at –100°F and condensing at –30°F. Is this correct? Substantiate your answer with calculations based on knowledge of R-22 for these conditions. Also, verify the mass flow rate in lb per min.

18.7 An R-134a refrigerating system develops 10 tons of refrigeration when operating at 100°F condensing and +10°F evaporating, with no liquid cooling or vapor superheating. Determine the volume of the refrigerant leaving the expansion valve in cubic feet per minute.

18.8 An expansion device has a mass flow rate for R-134a given by

$$m = 60 + 0.25\Delta p$$

where m = flow rate in lb/min and Δp = pressure drop across valve in psi.

For an evaporator temperature of 0°F and a condenser temperature of 100°F, estimate the piston displacement required for a compressor if C = 0.04 and the polytropic compression coefficient n = 1.1 for the compression process. [Ans: 236 cfm]

18.9 A liquid-to-suction heat exchanger is installed in an R-134a system to cool liquid that comes from the condenser with vapor that flows from the evaporator. The evaporator generates 10 tons (35.17 kW) of refrigeration at 30°F (–1.1°C). Liquid leaves the condenser saturated at 100°F (37.8°C), vapor leaves the evaporator saturated, and vapor leaves the heat exchanger at a temperature of 50°F (10°C). What is the flow rate of the refrigerant?

18.10 An eight-cylinder ammonia compressor is designed to operate at 800 rpm and deliver 30 tons of refrigeration. The evaporator is to operate at 10°F with a condensing temperature of 100°F. The vapor enters the compressor at 30°F. The ammonia leaves the condenser as saturated liquid. If the average piston speed is to be 600 ft/min and the actual volumetric efficiency at this condition is 83%, find the bore of the compressor.

18.11 Find the coefficient of performance for the ideal compound system shown in the figure. [Ans: 4.18]

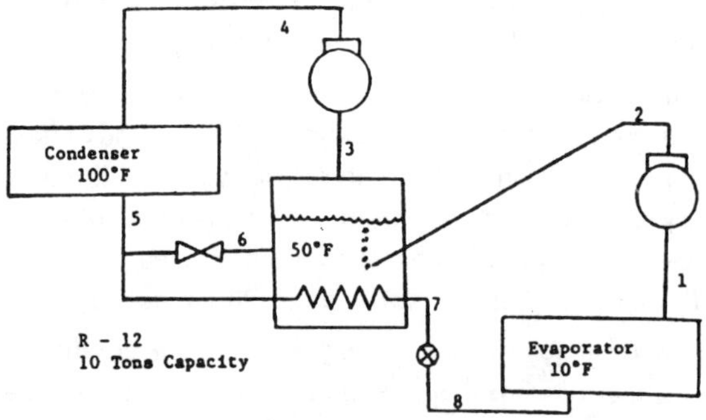

18.12 A condenser is to be selected for a system that generates 30 tons (105.5 kW) of refrigeration at 10°F (–12.2°C). The condenser is to operate at 110°F (43.3°C) and is cooled with 90 gpm (5.68 L/s) of water at 85°F (29.4°C). If the expected U-value of the condenser is 130 Btu/h· ft^2·°F [738 W/(m^2·K)], calculate the condensing area required.

18.13 A food storage plant requires a refrigeration system of 12-ton capacity at an evaporator temperature of 20°F and a condenser temperature of 90°F. The refrigerant R-134a is subcooled 9°F before entering the expansion valve, and the vapor is superheated 9°F before leaving the evaporator. Compression of the refrigerant is isentropic. The volumetric efficiency is 70%. A two-cylinder vertical compressor with stroke equal 1.5 times the bore is used and operates at 900 rpm. Find the bore and stroke of the compressor.

18.14 A lithium bromide-water absorption refrigeration system operates at the pressure and temperature shown in the figure. Calculate the flow at point 1 per lb/min at point 2. [Ans: 5.4 lb/min]

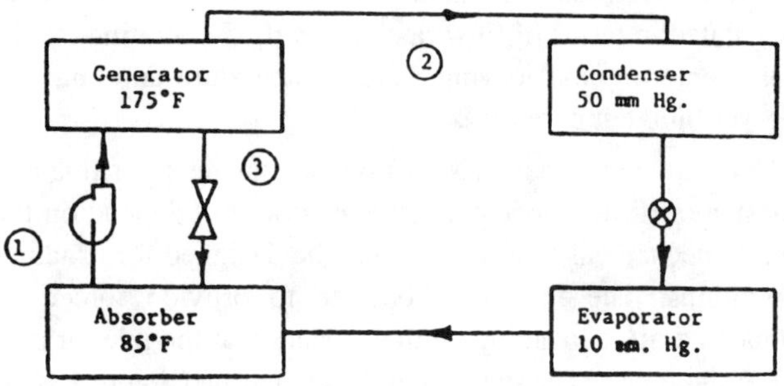

18.15 A closed air-cycle refrigeration system produces 10 tons of refrigeration. Air enters the compressor at 65 psia and 20°F and is compressed polytropically ($Pv^{1.35} = C$) to 225 psia. The temperature of the air leaving the air cooler is 80°F. Expansion is polytropic with n = 1.30. Assume frictionless flow. Calculate the mass rate of airflow and the power required to drive the unit, assuming the expander helps drive the compressor.

18.16 A 30 ft by 84 ft cooling tower cools 7650 gpm through a 15°F range and a 10°F approach. For 70°F wet bulb, what is the rating factor and rated area for the tower?

18.17 Green beans are to be brought in from a field located at 40°N latitude for cooling and storage. Two tons of beans are to be picked and cooled per day. The beans are to be stored at 45°F and are brought in at 75°F. It is desired to cool the beans to 45°F in three hours, and then store them for the remainder of the day. The heat lost through the walls of the cooler is 400 Btu/h and the volume of the room is 2000 ft^3. Four 100-watt light bulbs are left burning. The outdoor temperature is 75°F. How much heat is removed from the cooler for a 24-h day? [Ans: 157,500 Btu]

18.18 The tower in *Problem 18-16* is still supplied with 7650 gpm, but the wet-bulb temperature is now 80°F. If the cooling range is to remain at 15°F, what approach must be used? At what temperature does water leave the tower?

18.19 A cooling tower cools water by passing it through a stream of air. If 1000 cfm of air at 95°F dry bulb and 78°F wet bulb enters the tower and leaves saturated at 84°F, to what temperature can this air cool water that enters at 110°F with a flow of 80 lb/min? What is the makeup water rate?

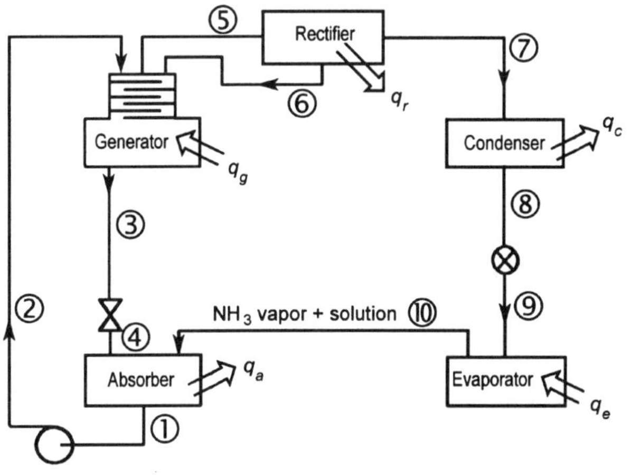

Pt.	Temp., °C	Pressure, kPa	Concentration, kg/kg	Enthalpy, kJ/kg	Flow Rate, kg/s
1	30				
2					
3					
4					
5	120	1300			
6					
7			0.98		
8					
9					
10	0	125			

18.20 Water flowing at 28 kg/min at 11°C is chilled in an evaporator to 4.5°C. The heat transfer area is 1.9 m^2 and the heat exchanger has an overall heat transfer coefficient of 341 W/(m^2· K). The direct-expansion evaporator uses R-12 and operates at 2°C. Find the evaporator effectiveness.

18.21 An eight-cylinder ammonia compressor is designed to operate at 800 rpm and deliver 30 tons of refrigeration. The evaporator is to operate at –12°C with a condensing temperature of 38°C. The vapor enters the compressor at –1°C. The ammonia leaves the condenser as saturated liquid. If the average piston speed is to be 3.1 m/s and the actual volumetric efficiency at this condition is 83%, find the bore of the compressor.

18.22 A cooling tower cools water by passing it through a stream of air. If 475 L/s of air at 35°C dry bulb and 26°C wet bulb enter the tower and leaves saturated at 29°C, to what temperature can this air cool water that enters at 43°C with a flow of 37 kg/min? What is the make-up water rate?

18.23 For the aqua-ammonia absorption system shown in the sketch to the left, complete the table and determine the energy quantities q_g, q_c, q_a, q_r per kW of refrigeration. [Ans: 6.83, –1.19, –6.03, –0.61]

18.24 A large Li-Br absorption refrigeration system is rated at 700 kW of cooling. The unit operates with hot water from solar collectors and with a cooling tower that provides the cooling water for the absorber and condenser. The unit and operating conditions are shown in the figure below. Determine all energy quantities (Q_c, Q_a, Q_g) and the COP$_c$.

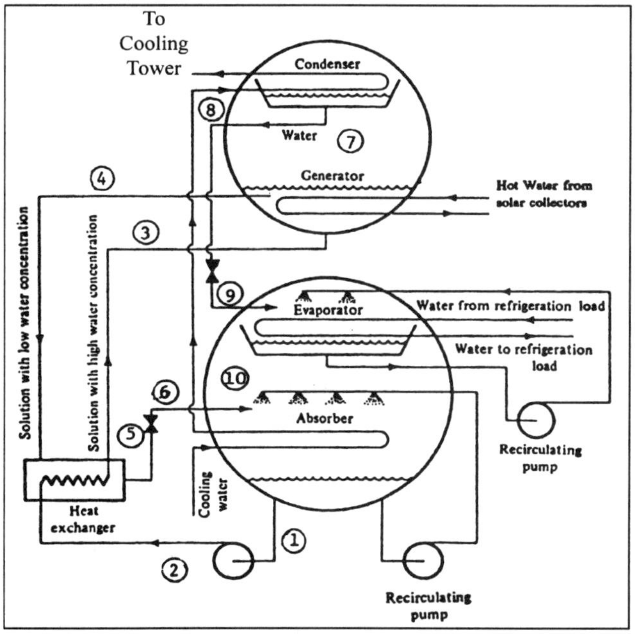

Pt.	Temp., °C	Pt.	Temp., °C
1	25	6	—
2	—	7	80
3		8	30
4	80	9	5
5	*	10	5

* Minimum without crystallization

18.5 Bibliography

ASHRAE. 1996 *ASHRAE Handbook—Systems and Equipment.*

ASHRAE. 1997 *ASHRAE Handbook—Fundamentals.*

Sauer, H.J., Jr. and Howell, R.H. 1983. *Heat Pump Systems.* Wiley Interscience, New York.

Stoecker, W. and Jones, J. 1987. *Refrigeration and Air Conditioning*, 3rd ed. McGraw-Hill, New York.

SI Figures and Tables

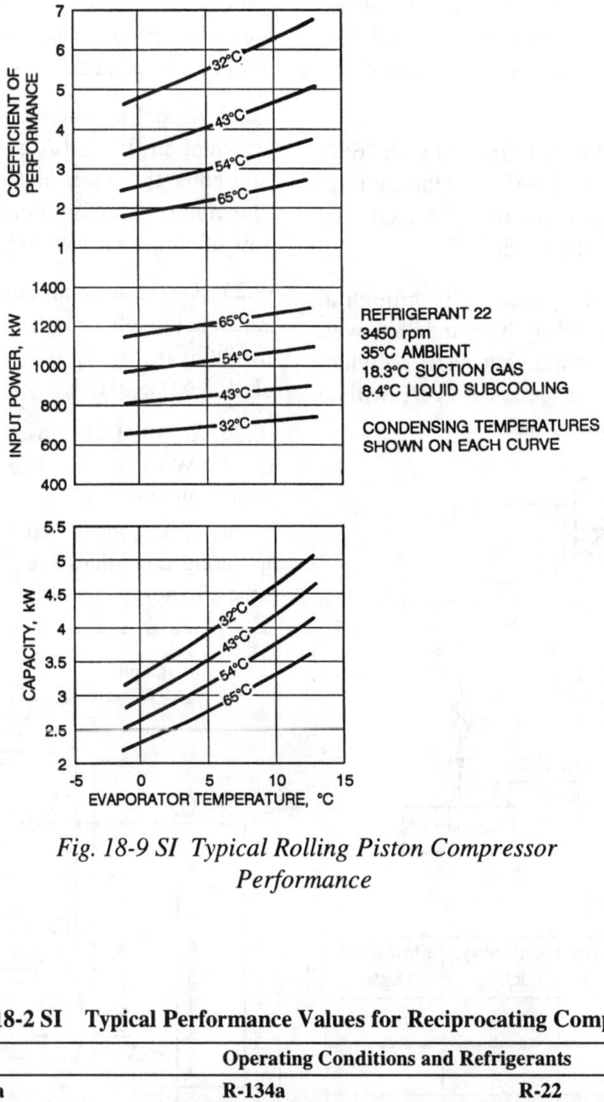

Fig. 18-9 SI Typical Rolling Piston Compressor Performance

Table 18-2 SI Typical Performance Values for Reciprocating Compressors

	Operating Conditions and Refrigerants			
	R-404a	R-134a	R-22	R-22
Compressor Size and Type	Evap. Temp. = −40°C Cond. Temp. = 41°C Suction Gas = 18.3°C Subcooling = 0 K	Evap. Temp. = −17.8°C Cond. Temp. = 43°C Suction Gas = 18.3°C Subcooling = 0 K	Evap. Temp. = 4.4°C Cond. Temp. = 41°C Suction Gas = 12.8°C Subcooling = 0 K	Evap. Temp. = 7.2°C Cond. Temp. = 54.4°C Suction Gas = °18.3C Subcooling = 0 K
Large, over 19 kW	Refrigerant Output/Power Input, W/W			
Open	0.99	1.89	4.95	5.04
Hermetic	0.92	1.76	4.16	3.05
Medium, 4 to 19 kW				
Open	0.90	1.74	4.71	4.71
Hermetic	0.85	1.64	4.10	3.02
Small, 4 kW				
Open	—	—	—	—
Hermetic	—	1.11	4.04	2.93

Table 18-6 SI Physical Properties of Selected Refrigerants[a]

Refrigerant No.	Refrigerant Chemical Name or Composition (% by mass)	Chemical Formula	Molecular Mass	Boiling Pt. (NBP) at 101.325 kPa, °C	Freezing Point, °C	Critical Temperature, °C	Critical Pressure, kPa	Critical Volume, L/kg	Refractive Index of Liquid[b,c]
704	Helium	He	4.0026	−268.9	None	−267.9	228.8	14.43	1.021 (NBP) 546.1 nm
702p	Hydrogen, para	H_2	2.0159	−252.9	−259.3	−240.2	1292	31.82	1.09 (NBP)[f]
702n	Hydrogen, normal	H_2	2.0159	−252.8	−259.2	−239.9	1315	33.21	1.097 (NBP) 579.1 nm
720	Neon	Ne	20.183	−246.1	−248.6	−228.7	3397	2.070	—
728	Nitrogen	N_2	28.013	−198.8	−210	−146.9	3396	3.179	1.205 (83 K) 589.3 nm
729	Air	—	28.97	−194.3	—	−140.53	3785	3.31	
						−140.6	3764	3.126	
740	Argon	Ar	39.948	−185.86	−189.3	−122.49	4860	1.88	1.233 (84 K) 589.3 nm
732	Oxygen	O_2	31.9988	−182.962	−218.8	−118.569	5042.9	2.293	1.221 (92 K) 589.3 nm
50	Methane	CH_4	16.04	−161.5	−182.2	−82.5	4638	6.181	
14	Tetrafluoromethane	CF_4	88.01	−127.9	−184.9	−45.7	3741	1.598	
1150	Ethylene	C_2H_4	28.05	−103.7	−169	9.3	5114	4.37	1.363 (−100)[1]
744A[2]	Nitrous oxide	N_2O	44.02	−89.5	−102	36.5	7221	2.216	
170	Ethane	C_2H_6	30.07	−88.8	−183	32.2	4891	5.182	
503	R-23/13 (40.1/59.9)	—	87.5	−88.7	—	19.5	4182	2.035	
23	Trifluoromethane	CHF_3	70.02	−82.1	−155	25.6	4833	1.942	
13	Chlorotrifluoromethane	$CClF_3$	104.47	−81.4	−181	28.8	3865	1.729	1.146 (25)[4]
744	Carbon dioxide	CO_2	44.01	−78.4[d]	−56.6[e]	31.1	7372	2.135	1.195 (15)
13B1	Bromotrifluoromethane	$CBrF_3$	148.93	−57.75	−168	67.0	3962	1.342	1.239 (25)[4]
504	R-32/115 (48.2/51.8)	—	79.2	−57.2	—	66.4	4758	2.023	
32	Difluoromethane	CH_2F_2	52.02	−51.8	−136	78.4	5830	2.326	
125	Pentafluoroethane	C_2HF_5	120.03	−48.57	−103.15	66.3	3630.6	—	—
1270	Propylene	C_3H_6	42.09	−47.7	−185	91.8	4618	4.495	1.3640 (−50)[1]
502[5]	R-22/115 (48.8/51.2)	—	111.63	−45.4	—	82.2	4075	1.785	
290	Propane	C_3H_8	44.10	−42.09	−187.7	96.70	4248	4.53	1.3397 (−42)
22	Chlorodifluoromethane	$CHClF_2$	86.48	−40.76	−160	96.0	4974	1.904	1.234 (25)[4]
115	Chloropentafluoroethane	$CClF_2CF_3$	154.48	−39.1	−106	79.9	3153	1.629	1.221 (25)[4]
500	R-12/152a (73.8/26.2)	—	99.31	−33.5	−159	105.5	4423	2.016	
717	Ammonia	NH_3	17.03	−33.3	−77.7	133.0	11417	4.245[d]	1.325 (16.5)
12	Dichlorodifluoromethane	CCl_2F_2	120.93	−29.79	−158	112.0	4113	1.792	1.288 (25)[4]
134a	Tetrafluoroethane	CF_3CH_2F	102.03	−26.16	−96.6	101.1	4067	1.81	—
152a	Difluoroethane	CHF_2CH_3	66.05	−25.0	−117	113.5	4492	2.741	
40[2]	Methyl chloride	CH_3Cl	50.49	−12.4	−97.8	143.1	6674	2.834	
124	Chlorotetrafluoroethane	$CHClFCF_3$	136.47	−13.19	−199.15	122.5	3660	—	—
600a	Isobutane	C_4H_{10}	58.13	−11.73	−160	135.0	3645	4.526	1.3514 (−25)[1]
764[6]	Sulfur dioxide	SO_2	64.07	−10.0	−75.5	157.5	7875	1.910	
142b	Chlorodifluoroethane	$CClF_2CH_3$	100.5	−9.8	−131	137.1	4120	2.297	
630[6]	Methyl amine	CH_3NH_2	31.06	−6.7	−92.5	156.9	7455		1.432 (17.5)
C318	Octafluorocyclobutane	C_4F_8	200.04	−5.8	−41.4	115.3	2781	1.611	
600	Butane	C_4H_{10}	58.13	−0.5	−138.5	152.0	3794	4.383	1.3562 (−15)[1]
114	Dichlorotetrafluoroethane	$CClF_2CClF_2$	170.94	3.8	−94	145.7	3259	1.717	1.294 (25)
21[7]	Dichlorofluoromethane	$CHCl_2F$	102.92	8.9	−135	178.5	5168	1.917	1.332 (25)[4]
160[2]	Ethyl chloride	C_2H_5Cl	64.52	12.4	−138.3	187.2	5267	3.028	
631[6]	Ethyl amine	$C_2H_5NH_2$	45.08	16.6	−80.6	183.0	5619		
11	Trichlorofluoromethane	CCl_3F	137.38	23.82	−111	198.0	4406	1.804	1.362 (25)[4]
123	Dichlorotrifluoroethane	$CHCl_2CF_3$	152.93	27.87	−107.15	183.79	3674	—	—
611[6]	Methyl formate	$C_2H_4O_2$	60.05	31.8	−99	214.0	5994	2.866	
141b	Dichlorofluoroethane	CCl_2FCH_3	116.95	32	—	204.2	4250	—	
610[6]	Ethyl ether	$C_4H_{10}O$	74.12	34.6	−116.3	194.0	3603	3.790	1.3526 (20)
216ca	Dichlorohexafluoropropane	$C_3Cl_2F_6$	220.93	35.69	−125.4	180.0	2753	1.742	
30[6]	Methylene chloride	CH_2Cl_2	84.93	40.2	−97	237.0	6077		1.4244 (20)[3]
113	Trichlorotrifluoroethane	CCl_2FCClF_2	187.39	47.57	−35	214.1	3437	1.736	1.357 (25)[4]
1130[8]	Dichloroethylene	$CHCl{=}CHCl$	96.95	47.8	−50	243.3	5478		
1120[6]	Trichloroethylene	$CHCl{=}CCl_2$	131.39	87.2	−73	271.1	5016		1.4782 (20)[3]
718[6]	Water	H_2O	18.02	100	0	373.99	22064	3.11	

Notes:

[a]Data from ASHRAE *Thermodynamic Properties of Refrigerants* (Stewart et al. 1986) or from McLinden (1990), unless otherwise noted.

[b]Temperature of measurement (Celsius, unless kelvin is noted) is shown in parentheses. Data from CRC *Handbook of Chemistry and Physics* (CRC 1987), unless otherwise noted.

[c]For the sodium D line.

[d]Sublimes.

[e]At 527 kPa.

[f]Dielectric constant data.

References:

[1]Kirk and Othmer (1956).

[2]*Matheson Gas Data Book* (1966).

[3]Electrochemicals Department, E.I. duPont de Nemours & Co.

[4]*Bulletin* B-32A (duPont).

[5]*Bulletin* T-502 (duPont 1980).

[6]*Handbook of Chemistry* (1967).

[7]*Bulletin* G-1 (duPont).

[8]CRC *Handbook of Chemistry and Physics* (CRC 1987).

Table 18-7 SI Comparative Refrigerant Performance per Kilowatt of Refrigeration[a]

Refrigerant No.	Refrigerant Chemical Name or Composition (% by mass)	Evaporator Pressure, MPa	Condenser Pressure, MPa	Compression Ratio	Net Refrigerating Effect, kJ/kg	Refrigerant Circulated, kg/s	Liquid Circulated, L/s	Specific Volume of Suction Gas, m^3/kg	Compressor Displacement, L/s	Power Consumption, kW	Coefficient of Performance	Comp. Discharge Temp., K
170	Ethane	1.623	4.637	2.86	162.44	0.00616	0.0232	0.0335	0.206	0.364	2.74	324
744	Carbon dioxide	2.291	7.208	3.15	134.24	0.00745	0.0123	0.0087	0.065	0.338	2.96	343
13B1	Bromotrifluoromethane	0.536	1.821	3.39	66.14	0.01512	0.0101	0.0237	0.358	0.274	3.65	313
125	Pentafluoroethane	0.400	1.570	3.93	87.76	0.01139	0.0098	0.0394	0.449	0.272	3.68	315
1270	Propylene	0.362	1.304	3.60	286.48	0.00349	0.0070	0.1285	0.449	0.197	5.07	354
290	Propane	0.291	1.077	3.71	279.88	0.00357	0.0074	0.1542	0.551	0.211	4.74	320
502	R-22/115 (48.8/51.2)	0.349	1.319	3.78	104.39	0.00958	0.0080	0.0500	0.479	0.226	4.43	310
22	Chlorodifluoromethane	0.296	1.192	4.03	162.46	0.00616	0.0053	0.0774	0.476	0.210	4.75	326
717	Ammonia	0.236	1.164	4.94	1102.23	0.00091	0.0015	0.5106	0.463	0.207	4.84	371
500	R-12/152a (73.8/26.2)	0.214	0.879	4.11	140.95	0.00709	0.0062	0.0938	0.665	0.213	4.69	314
12	Dichlorodifluoromethane	0.183	0.745	4.07	116.58	0.00858	0.0066	0.0914	0.784	0.213	4.69	311
134a	Tetrafluoroethane	0.160	0.770	4.81	150.71	0.00664	0.0056	0.1224	0.812	0.226	4.42	316
124	Chlorotetrafluoroethane	0.090	0.440	4.89	118.49	0.00844	0.0063	0.1705	1.439	0.224	4.47	305
600a	Isobutane	0.089	0.407	4.60	262.84	0.00380	0.0070	0.4029	1.533	0.220	4.55	318
600	Butane	0.056	0.283	5.05	292.01	0.00342	0.0060	0.6641	2.274	0.214	4.68	318
114	Dichlorotetrafluoroethane[b]	0.047	0.252	5.41	99.19	0.01008	0.0070	0.2700	2.722	0.225	4.44	303
11	Trichlorofluoromethane	0.020	0.126	6.24	156.22	0.00640	0.0044	0.7641	4.891	0.196	5.09	313
123	Dichlorotrifluoroethane	0.016	0.110	5.50	142.30	0.00703	0.0045	0.8853	6.221	0.229	4.36	301
113	Trichlorotrifluoroethane[b]	0.007	0.054	7.84	127.34	0.00785	0.0051	1.6793	13.187	0.173	5.77	303

Notes: [a]Based on 258 K evaporation and 303 K condensation. [b]Saturated suction except R-113 and R-114. Enough superheat was added to give saturated discharge.

Chapter 19

HEATING EQUIPMENT

In this chapter the principles of combustion and data concerning various types of fuels common to HVAC systems are discussed. The information in this chapter has been extracted from Chapter 17 in the 1997 *ASHRAE Handbook—Fundamentals* and Chapters 26 through 33 in the 1996 *ASHRAE Handbook—Systems and Equipment.*

19.1 Fuels and Combustion

19.1.1 Principles of Combustion

Combustion is the chemical process in which an oxidant reacts rapidly with a fuel to liberate stored energy as thermal energy, generally in the form of high-temperature gases. The oxidant is usually oxygen in the air.

Conventional hydrocarbon fuels contain primarily hydrogen and carbon, in either elemental form or in various compounds. Their complete combustion produces mainly carbon dioxide and water; however, small quantities of carbon monoxide and partially reacted flue gas constituents may form. Most conventional fuels also contain small amounts of sulfur, oxidized to SO_2 or SO_3 during combustion, and non-combustible substances, i.e., mineral matter (ash), water, and inert gases. Flue gas is the product of complete or incomplete combustion including excess air (if present), but not dilution air.

The rate of fuel combustion depends on: (1) the chemical reaction rate of combustible fuel constituents with oxygen; (2) the rate at which oxygen is supplied to fuel (mixing of air and fuel); and (3) the temperature in the combustion region. The reaction rate is fixed by fuel selection. Increasing the mixing rate or temperature increases the combustion rate. In complete combustion of hydrocarbon fuels, all hydrogen and carbon in the fuel are oxidized to H_2O and CO_2.

For complete combustion, excess oxygen or excess air must generally be supplied beyond the amount theoretically required to oxidize the fuel; this is usually expressed as a percentage of the air required to completely oxidize the fuel. Incomplete combustion occurs when a fuel element is not completely oxidized in the combustion process. For example, a hydrocarbon may not completely oxidize to carbon dioxide and water, but may form partially oxidized compounds such as carbon monoxide, aldehydes, and ketones. Conditions that promote incomplete combustion include:

- Insufficient air and fuel mixing causing local fuel-rich and fuel-lean zones.
- Insufficient air supply to the flame providing less than the required quantity of oxygen.
- Insufficient reactant residence time in the flame preventing completion of combustion reactions.
- Flame impingement on a cold surface quenching combustion reactions.
- Too-low flame temperature slowing combustion reactions.

Incomplete combustion uses fuel inefficiently, contributes to air pollution, and can be hazardous because of carbon monoxide production.

Combustion of oxygen with the combustible elements and compounds in fuels occurs according to fixed chemical principles, including:

- Chemical reaction equations.
- Law of matter conservation. The mass of each element in the reaction products must equal the mass of that element in the reactants.
- Law of combining mass. Chemical compounds are formed by elements combining in fixed mass relationships.
- Chemical reaction rates.

Oxygen for combustion is normally obtained from air, which is a physical mixture of nitrogen, oxygen, small amounts of water vapor, carbon dioxide, and inert gases. For practical combustion calculations, dry air consists of 20.95% oxygen and 79.05% inert gases, primarily nitrogen, by volume, or 23.15% oxygen and 76.85% inert gases by mass. For calculation purposes, nitrogen is assumed to pass through the combustion process unchanged (although small quantities of nitrogen oxides are known to form).

The quantity of heat generated by complete combustion of a unit of specific fuel is constant and is called the **heating value**, **heat of combustion**, or **caloric value** of that fuel. The heating value of a fuel can be determined by measuring the heat evolved during combustion of a known quantity of the fuel in a calorimeter, or it can be estimated from chemical analysis of the fuel and the heating value of the several chemical elements in the fuel.

Higher heating value, gross heating value, or total heating value is determined when water vapor in fuel combustion products is condensed and the latent heat of vaporization is included in the fuel's heating value. Conversely, lower heating value or net heating value is obtained when latent heat of vaporization is not included. When the heating value of a fuel is specified without designating higher or lower, it generally means the higher heating value in the United States. (lower heating value is mainly used for internal combustion engine fuels.)

Table 19-1 Heating Values of Selected Fuels
(Table 4, Chapter 17, 1997 *ASHRAE Handbook—Fundamentals*)

Substance	Molecular Symbol	Higher Heating Values,[a] Btu/lb	Lower Heating Values,[a] Btu/lb	Specific Volume,[b] ft³/lb	Higher Heating Values,[c] MJ/kg	Lower Heating Values,[c] MJ/kg	Density,[d] kg/m³
Carbon (to CO)	C	3950	3950		9.188	9.188	
Carbon (to CO_2)	C	14,093	14,093		32.788	32.780	
Carbon Monoxide	CO	4347	4347	13.5	10.111	10.111	1.187
Hydrogen	H_2	61,095	51,623	188.0	142.107	118.680	0.085
Methane	CH_4	23,875	21,495	23.6	55.533	49.997	0.679
Ethane	C_2H_6	22,323	20,418	12.5	51.922	47.492	1.28
Propane	C_3H_8	21,669	19,937	8.36	50.402	46.373	1.92
Butane	C_4H_{10}	21,321	19,678	6.32	49.593	45.771	2.53
Ethylene	C_2H_4	21,636	20,275		50.325	47.160	
Propylene	C_3H_6	21,048	19,687	9.01	48.958	45.792	1.78
Acetylene	C_2H_2	21,502	20,769	14.3	50.028	48.309	1.120
Sulfur (to SO_2)	S	3980	3980		9.257	9.257	
Sulfur (to SO_3)	S	5940	5940		13.816	13.816	
Hydrogen Sulfide	H_2S	7097	6537	11.0	16.508	15.205	1.456

a All values corrected to 60 °F, 30 in. Hg dry. For gases saturated with water vapor at 60°F, deduct 1.74% of the value to adjust for gas volume displaced by water vapor.
b At 32 °F and 29.92 in. Hg
c All values corrected to 16 °C, 101.4 kPa dry. For gases saturated with water vapor at 16°F, deduct 1.74% of the value to adjust for gas volume displaced by water vapor.
d At 32 °F and 29.92 in. Hg

Heating values are usually expressed in Btu/ft³ (kJ/m³) for gaseous fuels, Btu/gal (kJ/m³) for liquid fuels, and Btu/lb (kJ/kg) for solid fuels. Heating values are always given in relation to a certain reference temperature and pressure, usually 60, 68, or 77°F and 14.696 psia (15, 20, or 25°C and 103.325 kPa), depending on the particular industry practice. Heating values of several substances and common fuels are listed in Table 19-1.

When combustion is incomplete, not all fuel is completely oxidized, and the heat released is less than the heating value of the fuel. Therefore, the quantity of heat produced per unit of fuel consumed decreases, implying lower combustion efficiency.

Not all heat released during combustion can be used effectively. The greatest heat loss is in the form of increased temperature (thermal energy) of hot exhaust gases above the temperature of incoming air and fuel. Other heat losses include radiation and convection heat transfer from outer walls of combustion equipment to the environment.

19.1.2 Fuels

Generally, hydrocarbon fuels are classified according to physical state (gaseous, liquid, or solid). Different types of combustion equipment are usually needed to burn fuels in different physical states. Gaseous fuels can be burned in premix or diffusion burners that take advantage of the gaseous state. Liquid fuel burners must include a means of atomizing or vaporizing fuel into small droplets or to a vapor for burning, and must provide adequate mixing of fuel and air. Solid fuel combustion equipment must: (1) heat fuel to vaporize sufficient volatiles to initiate and sustain combustion; (2) provide residence time to complete combustion; and (3) provide space for ash containment.

Principal uses of fuel include space heating and cooling of residential, commercial, industrial, and institutional buildings; service water heating; steam generation; and refrigeration. Fuels for these applications are natural and liquefied petroleum gases, fuel oils, diesel and gas turbine fuels (for total energy applications), and coal.

Gaseous Fuels. Heating and cooling applications are presently limited to natural and liquefied petroleum gases. Natural gas is a nearly odorless and colorless gas that accumulates in the upper parts of oil and gas wells. Raw natural gas is a mixture of methane (55 to 98%), higher hydrocarbons (primarily ethane), and noncombustible gases. Some constituents, principally water vapor, hydrogen sulfide, helium, liquefied petroleum gases, and gasoline are removed prior to distribution.

Heating values of natural gases vary from 900 to 1200 Btu/ft³ (34 to 45 MJ/m³); the usual range is 1000 to 1050 Btu/ft³ (37 to 39 MJ/m³) at sea level. Three liquefied petroleum gases—butane, propane, and a mixture of the two—are commercially available.

Commercial propane consists primarily of propane, but generally contains about 5 to 10% propylene. It has a heating value of about 21,560 Btu/lb (50.15 MJ/kg) or about 2500 Btu/ft³ (93 MJ/m³) of gas. At atmospheric pressure, commercial propane has a boiling point of about –40°F (–40°C). The low boiling point of propane makes it usable during winter in cold climates such as the northern United States. It is available in cylinders, bottles, tank trucks, or tank cars.

Commercial butane consists primarily of butane, but may contain up to 5% butylene. It has a heating value of about 21,180 Btu/lb (49.26 MJ/kg) or 3200 Btu/ft3 (119 MJ/m³).

Commercial propane-butane mixtures with varying ratios of propane and butane are available. Their properties generally fall between those of the unmixed fuels. Propane air and butane-air mixtures are used in place of natural gas in small communities and by natural gas companies at peak loads. Typical heating values are listed in Table 19-2.

Liquid Fuels. Liquid fuels, with few exceptions, are mixtures of hydrocarbons refined from crude petroleum. Fuel oils for heating are broadly classified as distillate fuel oils

Table 19-2 Heating Values of Gaseous Fuels

Gas	Btu/ft^3	MJ/m^3	Specific Gravity Air = 1.0
Natural	1030	38.4	0.60
Propane	2500	93.1	1.53
Butane	3175	118.3	2.00

Table 19-3 Typical API Gravity, Density, and Heating Value of Standard Grades of Fuel Oil

Grade No.	API Gravity	Density, lb/gal[a]	Heating Value, Btu/gal[b]
1	38 to 45	6.950 to 6.675	137,000 to 132,900
2	30 to 38	7.296 to 6.960	141,800 to 137,000
4	20 to 28	7.787 to 7.396	148,100 to 143,100
5L	17 to 22	7.940 to 7.686	150,000 to 146,800
5H	14 to 18	8.080 to 7.890	152,000 to 149,400
6	8 to 15	8.448 to 8.053	155,900 to 151,300

[a] 1 lb/gal = 120 kg/m^3
[b] 1 Btu/gal = 279 kJ/m^3

(lighter oils) or residual fuel oils (heavier oils). ASTM has established specifications for fuel oil properties which subdivide the oils into various grades. Grades No. 1 and 2 are distillate fuel oils. Grades 4,5 (Light), 5 (Heavy), and 6 are residual fuel oils. Specifications for the grades are based on required characteristics of fuel oils for use in different types of burners. Typical gravity and heating values of standard grades of fuel oil are shown in Table 19-3.

Solid Fuels. Solid fuels include coal, coke, wood, and waste products of industrial and agricultural operations. Of these, only coal is widely used. Chemically, coal consists of carbon, hydrogen, oxygen, nitrogen, sulfur, and a mineral residue, ash. Heating values may be reported on an as received, dry, dry and mineral-matter-free, or moist and mineral-matter-free basis. Higher heating values of coals are frequently reported with their proximate analysis. When more specific data are lacking, the higher heating value of higher quality coals can be calculated by the Dulong Formula:

$$\text{Higher Heating Value (Btu/lb)} = 14{,}54C + 62{,}028\,[H - (O/8)] + 4050S \quad (19\text{-}1a)$$

or

$$\text{Higher Heating Value (MJ/kg)} = 33.829C + 194.28\,[H - (O/8)] + 9.42S \quad (19\text{-}1b)$$

where C, H, O, and S are the mass fractions of carbon, hydrogen, oxygen, and sulfur in the coal. Typical values for coal are listed in Table 19-4.

19.1.3 Combustion Calculations

Calculations of the quantity of air required for combustion and quantity of flue gas products generated during combustion are frequently needed for sizing system components and as input to efficiency calculations. Other calculations, such as values for excess air and theoretical CO_2, are useful in estimating combustion system performance. Details on combustion calculations are given in Chapter 17 of the 1997 *ASHRAE Handbook—Fundamentals*.

Table 19-4 Heating Value of Coal

Rank	Heating Value As Received Btu/lb	MJ/kg
Anthracite	12,700	29.5
Semianthracite	13,600	31.6
Low-volatile bituminous	14,350	33.4
Medium-volatile bituminous	14,000	32.6
High-volatile bituminous A	13,800	32.1
High-volatile bituminous B	12,500	29.1
High-volatile bituminous C	11,000	25.6
Subbituminous B	9000	20.9
Subbituminous C	8500	19.8
Lignite	6900	16.0

Example 19-1. Carbon burns with 160% theoretical air. Combustion goes to completion. Determine: (a) the air/fuel ratio by mass, and (b) the Orsat gas analysis and dew point of the products.

Solution:

Theoretical:

$$C + O_2 + 3.76N_2 \rightarrow CO_2 + 3.76N_2$$

Actual:

(a) $A/F = [1.6(32) + 1.6(3.76)28]/12 = 18.3\ lb_{air}/lb_{fuel}$

(b)

CO_2	1.0 moles/7.62	=	13.1%
O_2	0.6 moles/7.62	=	7.9% ORSAT
N_2	6.02 moles/7.6	=	79.0%
	7.62 moles	=	100.0%

No water in products → *No dew point*

Note: Assuming air is 79% N_2, 21% O_2 by volume:

$$1\ \text{mol}\ O_2 + 3.76\ \text{mol}\ N_2 = 4.76\ \text{mol air}$$

Example 19-2. The flue gas analysis of a hydrocarbon fuel on a percent by volume dry basis shows: CO_2 = 12.4%, O_2 = 3.2%, CO = 0.1%, H_2 = 0.2%, and N_2 = 84.1%. Determine the air/fuel ratio by volume.

Solution:

$$C_xH_y + (84.1/3.76)\ O_2 + 84.1\ N_2 \rightarrow 12.4\ CO_2 + 3.2\ O_2 + 0.1\ CO + 0.2\ H_2 + 84.1\ N_2 + z\ H_2O$$

$x = 12.4 + 0.1 = 12.5$ — Carbon balance

$22.4 = 12.4 + 3.2 + 0.05 + z/2$ — O_2 balance

$z = 13.5$

$y = 0.4 + 27 = 27.4$ — Hydrogen balance

$$C_{12.5}H_{27.4} + 22.4O_2 + 84.1N_2 \rightarrow 12.4CO_2 + 3.2O_2 + 0.1CO + 0.2H_2 + 84.1N_2 + 13.5H_2O$$

$$A/F = (22.4\ \text{moles}\ O_2 + 84.1\ \text{moles}\ N_2)/\text{mole fuel}$$

$$A/F = 106.5/1\ \text{by volume}$$

19.2 Burners

When heating is required within a controlled environment, it is normally done using hot water, warm air, steam, radiant heat, or electric heat. Water, air, and steam can be heated using gas, oil, coal, or electric energy. In some instances, energy for heating can be provided by heat recovery techniques or solar energy.

19.2.1 Domestic Gas Burning Equipment

A gas burner is used to convey gas, or a mixture of gas and air to the combustion zone. Burners are of the atmospheric injection, luminous flame, or power burner types.

Domestic gas burners may be classified as either those types designed for central heating plants or those designed for unit application. Gas-designed units and conversion burners are available for the several kinds of central systems and for other applications where the units are installed in the heated space. Central heating appliances include warm air furnaces and steam or hot water boilers.

Warm air furnaces are of two types, gravity and forced air. Forced warm-air furnaces use a motor-driven blower to circulate air over the heat exchanger and through the ducts. A draft hood is attached to the outlet of the furnace and replaces the barometric damper.

Gas-designed boilers for hot water or steam heating are available in cast-iron, steel, and non-ferrous metals. Burners are located beneath the sections; the flue gases pass upwards between the sections to the flue collector. Some boilers are designed to provide domestic hot water, using tankless or instantaneous heaters.

Some gas furnaces and boilers are available with sealed combustion chambers. These units have no draft hood and are called **direct vent appliances**. Combustion air is piped, usually through a side wall from outdoors, directly to the combustion chamber.

The air intake pipe terminates in the same location as the flue gas vent, sometimes as concentric pipes, with an appropriate terminal covering or cowl. No chimney or vertical flue is needed with such units.

Floor furnaces are used in mild climates for auxiliary heating, heating of single rooms, and in some cases, heating of several rooms. Floor furnaces are not usually considered central heating systems. However, some are furnished with a circulating fan and as many as eight takeoff ducts. This type floor furnace is a central heating system. In such a system, piping is below the floor as in other central warm air systems.

Space heaters are generally used for heating a single room or limited area. They differ from central heating equipment in the extent of distribution systems used. Both natural convection and forced-circulation systems distribute the warm air; however, no ductwork distributes heat beyond the immediate area occupied by the heater. Domestic, gas-fired space heaters include: floor furnaces (without ductwork), vented wall-furnaces, vented and unvented room heaters, radiant heaters, baseboard-sealed combustion system wall furnace, wall heaters and unit heaters. Some small room heaters are operated without vents, but they must be used with caution. Both manual and automatic controls are used. An automatic pilot or ignition system must be a part of any control system.

Under controlled conditions, an oil burner combines fuel oil and air for combustion. Fuel oil may be either **atomized** or **vaporized** for the combustion process. Air for combustion is supplied by natural or mechanical draft. Ignition is generally accomplished by an electric spark, gas pilot flame, oil pilot flame, or combination of these. Burners of different types operate with luminous or nonluminous flame. Operation may be continuous, modulating, or intermittent with high-low flame.

Residential oil burners are ordinarily used in the range of 0.5 to 3.5 gph (0.5 to 3.7 mL/s) fuel consumption rate. However, burners up to 7.0 gph (7.2 mL/s) sometimes fall in the residential classification because of similarities in controls and standards. Burner capacity of 7.0 gph (7.35 mL/s) and above is classified as commercial-industrial. Generally, No. 2 fuel oil is used, although burners in the residential size range can also operate on No. 1 fuel oil. In addition to boilers and furnaces for space heating, burners in the 0.5 to 1.0 gph (0.5 to 1.0 mL/s) size range are also used for separate tank type residential hot water heaters, infrared heaters, space heaters, and other commercial equipment.

Most burners manufactured (over 95%) are high-pressure, atomizing gun burners. While other types of burners are still in operation, only a few of these types are currently in production.

The high-pressure, atomizing gun burner illustrated in Figure 19-1 supplies oil to the atomizing nozzle at 100 to 300 psi (700 to 2100 kPa). A blower supplies air for combustion, and a damper or other device regulates the air supply at the burner. Ignition is usually accomplished by a high voltage electric spark, which may be intermittent, sometimes called either **constant ignition** ("on" when the burner motor is on) or **interrupted** (on only to start combustion). Typically, these burners fire into a combustion chamber in which negative draft is maintained.

Present high-pressure atomizing gun burner design includes retention heads and residential burner motors operating at 3450 rpm instead of 1725 rpm. The retention head assists combustion by providing better air-oil mixing, turbulence, and shear. Using the higher speed 3450 rpm motors (often combined with a retention head design) results in a

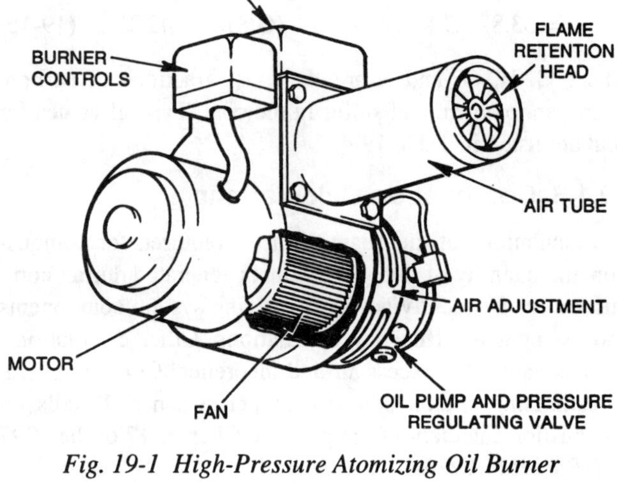

Fig. 19-1 High-Pressure Atomizing Oil Burner

more compact burner having equal capacity to one operating at 1725 rpm, and one that has a wide tolerance for varying combustion chamber and draft conditions.

Vaporizing burners are designed for use with No. 1 fuel oil. Fuel is ignited by manual pilot or electric spark. The combustion process usually provides enough heat for oil vaporization.

Oil-designated boiler-burner units for hydronic (hot water or steam) heating are constructed of cast iron, steel, and non-ferrous metals. The oil burner is usually located at, or near, the base of the boiler; the flue gases pass upward and around the heat transfer sections and then out the chimney connector. Most oil-powered boiler burner units provide domestic hot water by incorporating a water heating coil (tankless heater) within the boiler.

Warm air furnaces with oil burner units are normally of forced-air design. A blower circulates air over the heat exchanger and through the duct. Upflow, counterflow, horizontal, or downflow furnaces are available. Most forced warm-air furnaces make provisions for installing direct expansion air conditioning directly in the unit.

Additional details concerning commercial and industrial gas and/or oil burning equipment, as well as solid fuel burning equipment, can be found in Chapter 26 of the 1996 *ASHRAE Handbook—Systems and Equipment*. Details about various types of steam and hot water boilers are in Chapter 27 of the above reference.

19.3 Residential Furnaces

19.3.1 Equipment Variations

Residential furnaces provide heated air through a system of ductwork into the space being heated. They are of two basic types:

Fuel-Burning Furnaces. Combustion takes place within a combustion chamber. Circulating air passes over the outside surfaces of the heat exchanger so that it does not contact the fuel or the products of combustion. The products of combustion are passed to the outside atmosphere through a vent.

Electric Furnaces. A resistance-type heating element heats the circulating air either directly or through a metal sheath enclosing the resistance element.

Residential furnaces may be further categorized by:

- Fuel type
- Mounting arrangement
- Airflow direction
- Combustion system
- Installation location

A forced air furnace is a self-enclosed appliance used to heat air that is circulated through the enclosure and discharged directly into the space being heated, or air that is conveyed through ducts to the space to be heated. An induced draft gas-fired unit is illustrated in Figure 19-2.

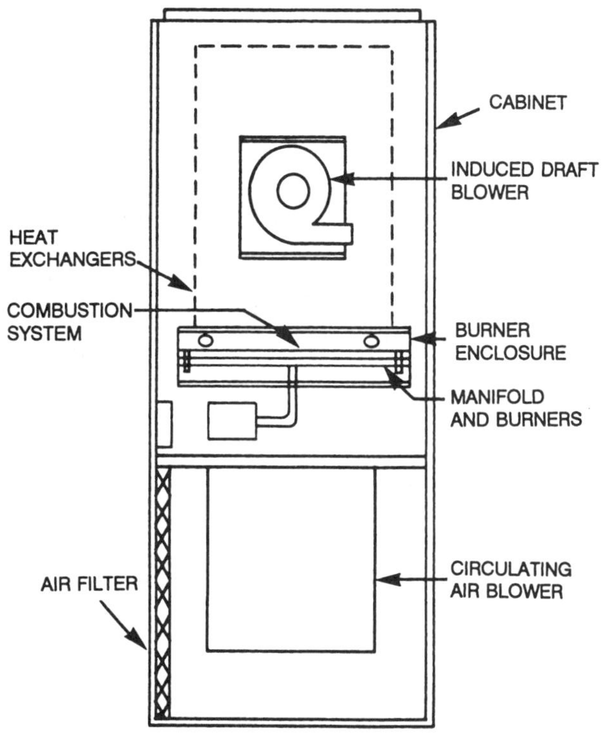

Fig. 19-2 Induced Draft Gas Furnace

In fuel-burning furnaces, combustion occurs within a metal-walled heat exchanger. Air passes over the outside surfaces of the heat exchanger and the heat is transferred through the heat exchanger walls; the circulating air does not come in contact with the fuel or the products of combustion. The products of combustion are conveyed to the outside atmosphere through a flue or vent.

In an electric furnace, the heating element, heated by its electric resistance, heats the circulating air either directly or through a metal sheath enclosing the resistance element.

Residential forced air furnaces usually have a capacity under 250,000 Btu/h (74 kW) output. Residential furnaces are often used in commercial installations. The reverse is usually not true since more than one residential furnace would usually be used in an extremely large home rather than a furnace intended for commercial use.

The furnace may be designed and manufactured to combine components in a variety of ways. The relative positions of the components in the different types of furnaces are described below:

1. In a **horizontal furnace**, the blower is located beside the heat exchanger (Figure 19-3). The air enters one end and travels horizontally through the blower, over the heat exchanger, and discharges out of the opposite end. Such furnaces are used for locations with limited head room (*e.g.*, attics and crawl spaces). These units are often designed to allow for component rearrangement so that airflow may be from left to right or from right to left.
2. The blower in an **upflow furnace** is beneath the heat exchanger and discharges vertically upward (Figure 19-4).

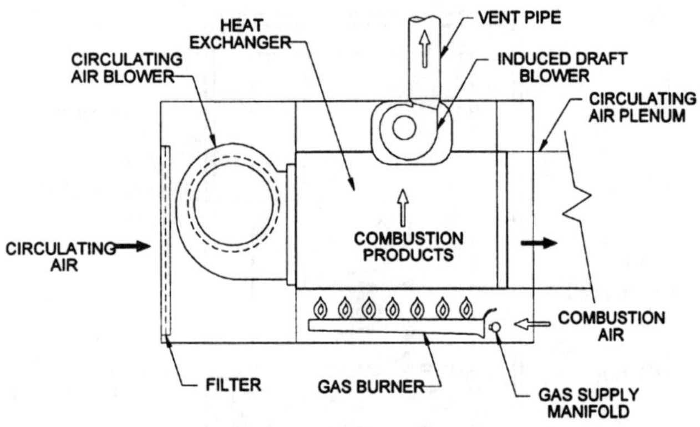

Fig. 19-3 Horizontal Forced Warm-Air Furnace

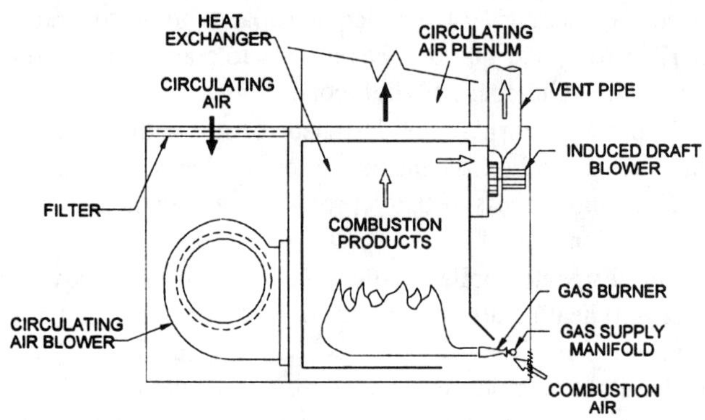

Fig. 19-5 Basement Forced Warm-Air Furnace

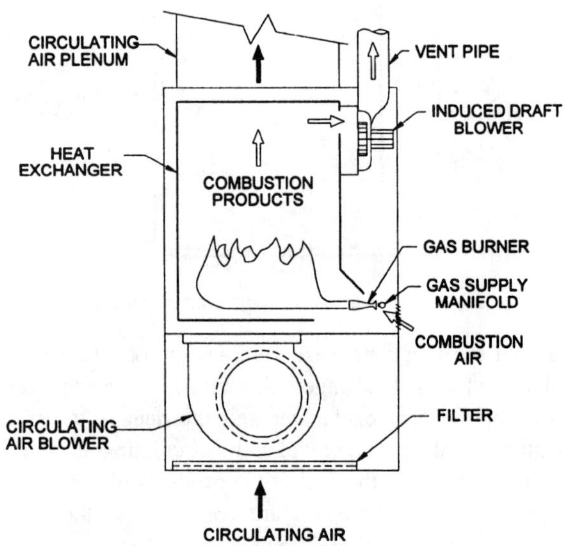

Fig. 19-4 Upflow Forced Warm-Air Furnace

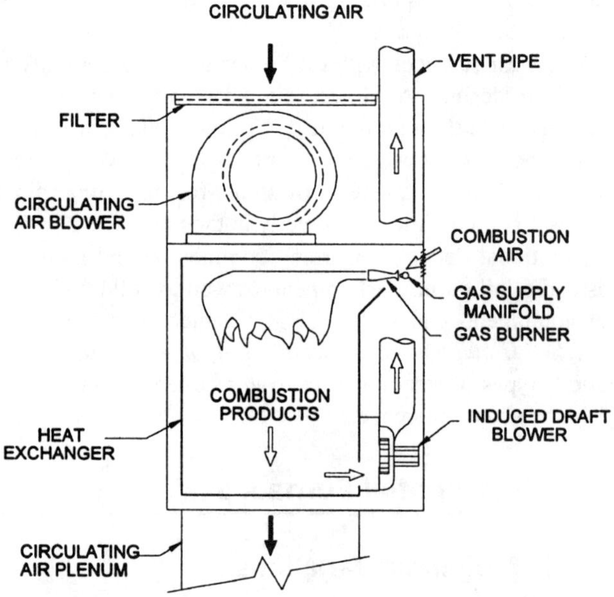

Fig. 19-6 Downflow (Counterflow) Warm-Air Furnace

Air enters through the bottom or the side of the blower compartment and leaves at the top. Such furnaces may be used in utility rooms on the first floor of homes without basements or in basements with the return air ducted down to the blower compartment entrance.

3. The **basement furnace**, which is a variation of the upflow furnace, requires less head room (Figure 19-5). The blower is located at the bottom beside the heat exchanger. Air enters the top of the cabinet, flows down through the blower, discharges over the heat exchanger, and leaves vertically at the top.
4. The blower in the **downflow** or **counterflow furnace** is located above the heat exchanger and discharges downward (Figure 19-6). Air enters at the top and discharges vertically at the bottom. This style furnace is used in a house without a basement that has a perimeter heating system.

Further discussion about furnaces and space heaters can be found in Chapter 28 of the 1996 *ASHRAE Handbook—Systems and Equipment*.

19.3.2 Capacity Selection

Heating capacity depends on several variables that may operate alone or in combination.

Design heating requirement of building. The heat loss of the structure can be calculated by using the procedures in Chapters 6 or 7.

Additional heating required if furnace is operating on night setback cycle. During the morning recovery period, additional capacity is required to bring the conditioned space temperature up to the desired level.

Internal loads. Normally, the heat gain from internal loads is neglected when selecting a furnace, but if the internal loads are constant, they should be used to reduce the required capacity of the furnace. This is particularly applicable in nonresidential applications.

Energy required for humidification. Humidification energy depends on the desired level of relative humidity and the rate at which moisture must be supplied to maintain the specified level. Net moisture requirements must take into account internal gains as the result of people, equipment, and appliances, and losses through migration in exterior surfaces, plus air infiltration.

Influence of off-peak storage devices. A storage device, when used in conjunction with a furnace, decreases the required capacity of the furnace. The storage device can supply the additional capacity required during the morning recovery of a night setback cycle, or reduce the daily peak loads to assist in load shedding.

Influence of backup systems. A furnace can exist as a backup to a solar system, a heat recovery system, or a structure requiring multiple units for uninterrupted service. Oversizing results in higher initial costs, possible increased operating costs, and decreased comfort control. Undersizing produces unacceptable comfort control near the design conditions.

Capacity to accommodate air conditioning. Even if air conditioning is not initially planned, the cabinet should be large enough to accept a cooling coil that satisfies the design cooling load. The blower and motor should have sufficient capacity to provide increased airflow rates typically required in air-conditioning applications.

19.3.3 Performance Criteria

Some typical efficiencies encountered in performance criteria of a furnace are: (1) steady-state efficiency, (2) use efficiency, and (3) annual fuel use efficiency.

These efficiencies are generally used by the furnace industry in the following manner:

Steady-state efficiency is the efficiency of a furnace when it is operated under equilibrium conditions. It is calculated by measuring the energy input, subtracting the losses for exhaust gases, and then dividing by the fuel input (cabinet loss not included), i.e.,

$$SS\ (\%) = 100(\text{Fuel input} - \text{Flue loss} - \text{Condensate loss})/\text{Fuel input}$$

For furnaces tested under the isolated combustion system (ICS) method, cabinet heat loss must also be deducted from the energy input.

$$SS\ (\%)(ICS) = 100(\text{Fuel input} - \text{Flue loss} - \text{Condensate loss} - \text{Jacket loss})/\text{Fuel input}$$

Utilization efficiency is obtained from an empirical equation developed by the National Institute of Standards and Technology (NTIS Order No. PB 289484) by starting with 100% efficiency and deducting losses for exhausted latent and sensible heat, cyclic effects, infiltration, and pilot-burner effect.

Annual fuel utilization efficiency (AFUE) is the same as **utilization efficiency**, except that losses from a standing pilot during nonheating season time are deducted. The equation for AFUE can also be found in NTIS *Order No.* PB 289484 or ANSI/ASHRAE *Standard* 103.

Federal law requires manufacturers of furnaces to use AFUE to rate efficiency. Typical values of AFUE for various types of furnaces are listed in Table 19-5.

Table 19-5 AFUE Values of Various Furnaces Located in Conditioned Space

	AFUE, %	
Type of Gas Furnace	**Indoor**	**ICS[a]**
1. Natural-draft with standing pilot	64.5	63.9
2. Natural-draft with intermittent ignition	69.0	68.5
3. Natural-draft with intermittent ignition and auto vent damper	78.0	68.5
4. Fan-assisted combustion with standing pilot or intermittent ignition	80.0	78.0
5. Same as 4, except with improved heat transfer	82.0	80.0
6. Direct vent with standing pilot, preheat	66.0	64.5
7. Direct vent, fan-assisted combustion, and intermittent ignition	80.0	78.0
8. Fan-assisted combustion (induced-draft)	80.0	78.0
9. Condensing	93.0+	91.0+
Type of Oil Furnace	Indoor	ICS[a]
1. Standard	71.0	69.0
2. Same as 1, with improved heat transfer	76.0	74.0
3. Same as 2, with auto vent damper	83.0	74.0
4. Condensing	91.0	89.0

[a]Isolated combustion system.

19.4 Commercial Furnaces

19.4.1 Equipment Variations

The basic difference between residential and commercial furnaces is the size and heating capacity of the equipment. The heating capacity of a commercial furnace may range from 150,000 Btu/h (44 kW) to over 2,000,000 Btu/h (600 kW). Generally, furnaces with output capacities less than 320,000 Btu/h (93 kW) are classified as light commercial, and those above 320,000 Btu/h (93 kW) are large commercial equipment. In addition to the difference in capacity, commercial equipment is constructed from material having increased structural strength and more sophisticated control systems.

Light commercial heating equipment comes in many flow arrangements and design variations. Some are identical to residential equipment, while others are unique to commercial applications. Some commercial units function as a part of a ducted system; others operate as unducted space heaters.

Ducted Equipment. Upflow gas-fired commercial furnaces are available up to 300,000 Btu/h (88 kW) and supply enough airflow to handle up to 10 tons (35 kW) of air conditioning. These furnaces may develop high static pressure, have belt-driven blowers, and frequently consist of two standard upflow furnaces tied together in a side-by-side arrangement.

Horizontal gas-fired duct furnaces are also available for built-in light commercial systems. This furnace is not equipped with its own blower, but is designed for uniform airflow across the entire furnace.

Duct furnaces are normally certified for operation either upstream or downstream of an air-conditioner cooling coil. Electric duct furnaces are available in a great range of sizes and are suitable for operation in upflow, downflow, or horizontal positions. These units are also used to supply auxiliary heat with the indoor section of a split-heat pump.

The most common commercial furnace is the combination package unit, which is sometimes called a combination rooftop unit. They are available as air-conditioning units with liquified petroleum gas (LPG) and natural gas furnaces, electric resistance heaters, or heat pumps. Combination oil-heat-electric cool units are not commonly available. Combination units come in a full range of sizes covering air-conditioning ratings from 5 to 50 tons (18 to 176 kW) with matched furnaces supplying heat-to-cool ratios of approximately 1.5:1.

Combination units of 15 tons (53 kW) and under are available as single-zone units. The entire unit must be in either the heating or cooling mode. All air delivered by the unit is at the same temperature. Large combination units in the 15- to 50-ton (50- to 180-kW) range are available as single-zoned units, as are small units; however, they are also available as multizoned units. A multizone unit supplies conditioned air at several different zones of a building in response to individual thermostats controlling those zones. These units are capable of supplying heating to one or more zones at the same time cooling is being supplied to other zones.

Large combination units are normally available only in a curbed configuration; *i.e.*, the units are mounted on a rooftop over a curbed opening in the roof. The supply and return air enter through the bottom of the unit. Smaller units may be available for either curbed or uncurbed mounting. In either case, the unit is always connected to ductwork within the building to distribute the conditioned air.

Unducted Heaters. Three types of commercial heating equipment used as unducted space heaters are unit heaters, infrared heaters, and floor furnaces.

Unit heaters are available from about 25,000 to 320,000 Btu/h (7 to 94 kW). Normally, they are mounted from ceiling hangers and blow air across the heat exchanger into the heated space. Natural gas, LPG, and electric heat units are available.

Infrared heaters are mounted from ceiling hangers and transmit heat downward by radiation. Low- and medium intensity infrared heaters are compact, self-contained, direct-heating devices. They are used in hangars, factories, warehouses, foundries, greenhouses, and gymnasiums, and for areas such as loading docks, racetrack stands, under marquees, outdoor restaurants, and around swimming pools. Low-temperature radiant heaters are used in office buildings and other commercial buildings.

These heaters can be used with variable-air-volume systems. Infrared heating units may be electric, gas fired, or oil fired. They consist of an infrared source or generator operating in a temperature range of 350 to 5000°F (180 to 2800°C), with the specific temperature determined by the energy source, size, and application. Reflectors can be used to distribute radiation in specific patterns. Common configurations for gas-fired and electric infrared heaters are shown in Figures 19-7 and 19-8, respectively.

Radiant heaters transfer energy directly to solid objects. As floor and objects are warmed by the infrared energy, they, in turn, reradiate heat to solid objects, as well as transfer heat to the air by convection. Dry-bulb temperatures can be maintained slightly less than the mean radiant temperature. With convective heat, the converse is true. Since human comfort is determined by the average of mean radiant and dry-bulb temperatures, dry-bulb temperature may be lowered when heating with radiation. Heat loss to ventilating air and by transmission is correspondingly lower, as is energy consumption. Because buildings heated by infrared require less heating fuel for a given application, equipment that handles only 80 to 85% of the design heat loss calculated by ASHRAE methodology is typically installed.

Floor furnaces are used as large area unducted heaters. They are available in capacities ranging from 200,000 to 2,000,000 Btu/h (60 to 590 kW). Floor furnaces direct heated air through nozzles for task heating or use air circulators to heat large industrial spaces.

19.4.2 System Design and Equipment Selection

The procedure for design and selection of a commercial furnace is similar to that for a residential furnace. First, the design capacity of the heating system must be determined, considering structure heat loss, recovery load, internal load, humidification, off-peak storage, waste heat recovery, and backup capacity. Since most commercial buildings use setback periods during weekends, evenings, or other long periods of inactivity, the recovery load is important, as are internal loads and waste heat recovery.

Commercial sizing criteria are essentially the same as for residential furnaces. The furnace should be oversized 30% above the total load if setback is anticipated. Since combination units must be sized accurately for the cooling load, it is possible that the smallest gas-fired capacity available is larger than the 30% oversize value. This is especially true for the warmer climates of the United States.

Commercial units have about the same efficiency as residential units. Two-stage gas valves are frequently used with commercial furnaces, but the efficiency of a two-stage system may be lower than that of a single-stage system. At a reduced firing rate, the excess combustion airflow through the burners increases, which decreases the steady-state operating efficiency of the furnace. Multistage furnaces with multistage thermostats and controls provide more uniform distribution of heat within the building.

The useful life of commercial heating and cooling equipment is about 20 years.

19.5 Boilers

A boiler is a pressure vessel designed to transfer heat produced by combustion to a fluid. Heat is normally produced by combustion, but electrical resistance elements or electrodes acting directly on the fluid are also used. In boilers of

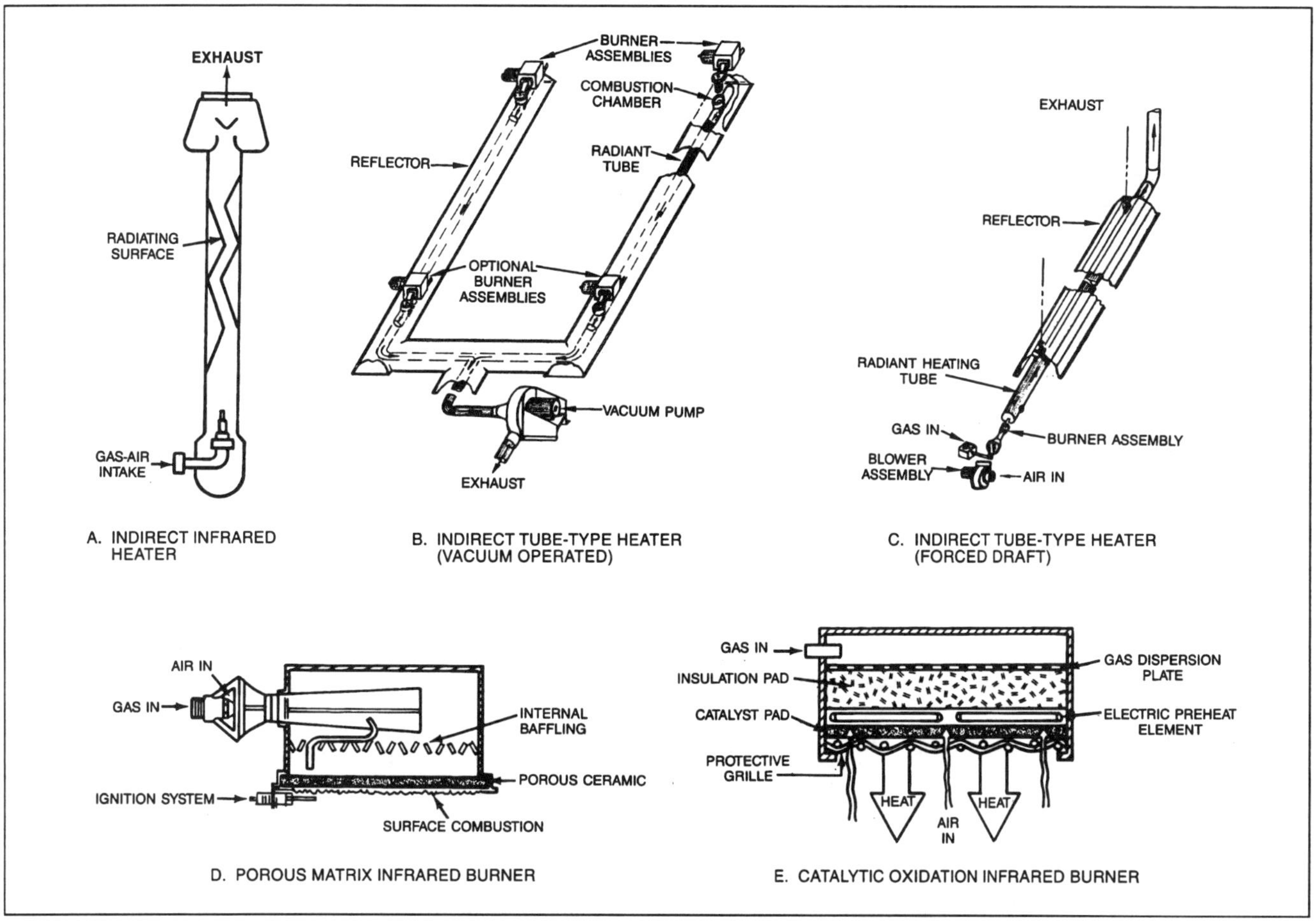

Fig. 19-7 Gas-Fired Infrared Heaters

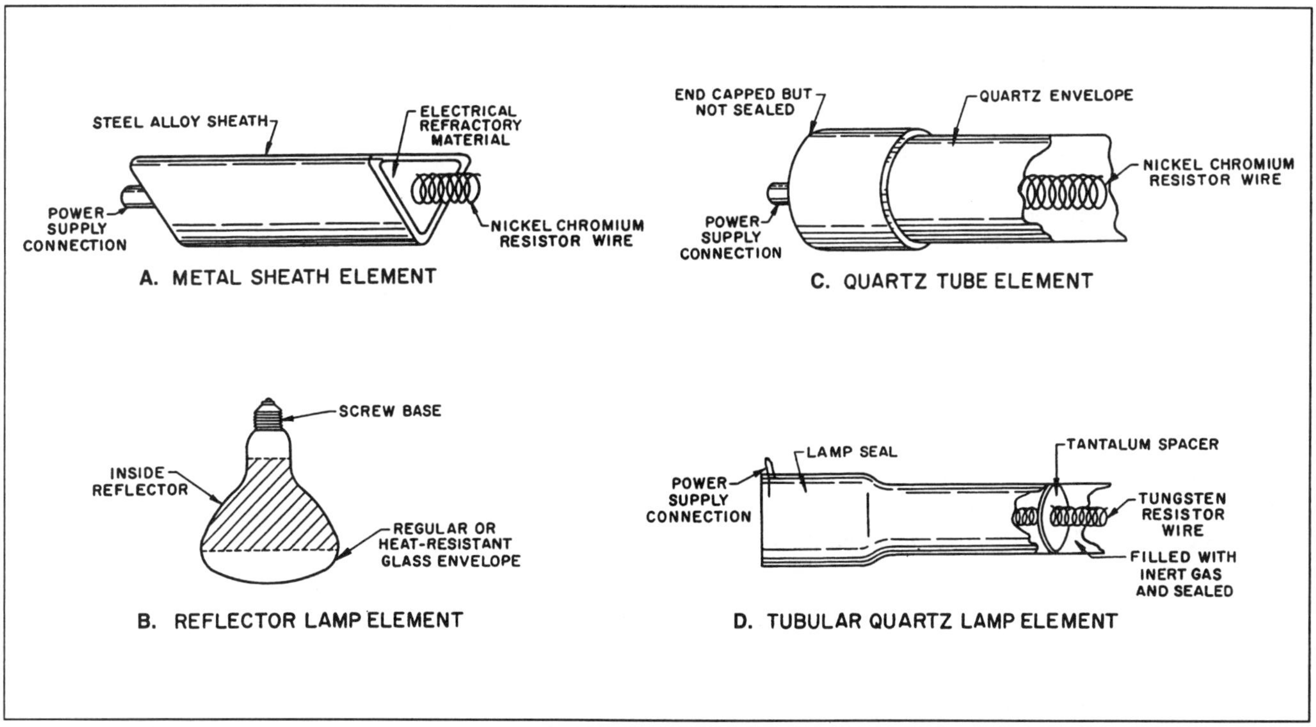

Fig. 19-8 Electric Infrared Heaters

interest to ASHRAE, the fluid is usually water, in the form of liquid or steam. If the fluid being heated is air, the heat-exchange device is called a furnace. The firebox, or combustion space, of some boilers is also called the furnace.

Excluding special and unusual fluids, materials, and methods, a boiler is a cast-iron, steel, or copper pressure vessel heat exchanger, designed with and for fuel-burning devices and other equipment (1) to burn fossil fuels (or use electric current) and (2) to transfer the released heat to water (in water boilers) or to water and steam (in steam boilers). Boiler heating surface is the area of fluid-backed surface exposed to the products of combustion, or the fire-side surface. Various codes and standards define allowable heat transfer rates in terms of heating surface. Boiler design provides for connections to a piping system, which delivers heated fluid to the point of use and returns the cooled fluid to the boiler.

19.5.1 Boiler Classifications

Boilers may be grouped into classes based on such criteria as working pressure and temperature, fuel used, shape and size, use (such as heating or process), and steam or water.

Working Pressure/Temperature. With few exceptions, all boilers are constructed to meet the ASME *Boiler and Pressure Vessel Code.*

Low-pressure boilers are constructed for maximum working pressures of 15 psi (103 kPa) steam and up to 160 psi (1100 kPa) hot water. Hot water boilers are limited to 250°F (120°C) operating temperature.

Medium- and high-pressure boilers are designed to operate at above 15 psi (103 kPa) steam or above 160 psi (1100 kPa) water or 250°F (120°C) water boilers.

Steam boilers are available in standard sizes of up to 50,000 lb steam/h (60,000 to 50,000,000 Btu/h or 17 to 15 000 kW), many of which are used for space heating in both new and existing systems. On larger installations, they may also provide steam for auxiliary uses, such as hot-water heat exchangers, absorption cooling, laundry, and sterilizers. In addition, many steam boilers provide steam at various temperatures and pressures for a wide variety of industrial processes.

Water boilers are available in standard sizes of up to 50,000,000 Btu/h (15 MW) from 50,000 Btu/h (15 kW), many of which are in the low-pressure class and are used for space heating in both new and existing systems. Some water boilers may be equipped with either internal or external heat exchangers to supply domestic (service) hot water.

Every steam or water boiler is rated at the maximum working pressure determined by the ASME *Boiler Code Section* (or other code) under which it is constructed and tested. When installed, it must also be equipped with safety controls and pressure relief devices mandated by such code provisions.

Fuel Used. Boilers may be designed to burn coal, wood, various grades of fuel oil, various types of fuel gas, or to operate as electric boilers. A boiler designed for one specific fuel type may not be convertible to another type of fuel. Some boiler designs can be adapted to burn coal, oil, or gas. Several designs allow firing with oil or gas by burner conversion or by using a dual fuel burner.

Construction Materials. Most boilers, other than special or unusual models, are made of cast iron or steel. Some small boilers are made of copper or copper-clad steel.

Cast iron boilers are constructed of individually cast sections, assembled into blocks (assemblies) or sections. Push or screw nipples, gaskets, or an external header join the sections pressure-tight and provide passages for the water, steam, and products of combustion. The number of sections assembled determines boiler size and energy rating. Sections may be vertical or horizontal, the vertical design being the most common. The boiler may be dry-base (the firebox is beneath the fluid-backed sections), wet-leg (the firebox top and sides are enclosed by fluid-backed sections), or wet-base (the firebox is surrounded by fluid-backed sections, except for necessary openings).

Steel boilers are fabricated into one assembly of a given size and rating, usually by welding. The heat-exchange surface past the firebox usually is an assembly of vertical, horizontal, or slanted tubes. The tubes may be firetube (flue gas inside, heated fluid outside) or watertube (fluid inside, hot gas outside). The tubes may be in one or more passes. Dry-base, wet-leg, or wet-base design may be used. Most small steel heating boilers are of dry-base, vertical firetube design. Larger boilers usually have horizontal or slanted tubes; both firetube and watertube designs are used. A popular design for medium and large steel boilers is the Scotch, or Scotch Marine, which is characterized by a central fluid-backed cylindrical firebox, surrounded by firetubes in one or more passes, all within the outer shell.

Cast iron boilers range in size from 35,000 to 10,000,000 Btu/h (10 to 2900 kW) gross output. Steel boilers range in size from 50,000 Btu/h (15 kW) to the largest boilers made.

Condensing or Non-Condensing Boilers. Because higher boiler efficiencies can be achieved with lower water temperatures, condensing boilers purposely allow the flue gas water vapor in the boiler to condense and drain. Illustrated in Figure 19-9 is a typical relationship of overall boiler efficiency to return water temperature. The dew point of 130°F (55°C) shown varies with the percent of hydrogen in the fuel and the CO_2 (or excess air) in the flue gas.

Low return water temperatures and condensing boilers are particularly important because they are so efficient at part-load operation when high water temperatures are not required. For example, a hot water heating system that operates under light load conditions at 80°F (27°C) return water temperature has a potential overall boiler efficiency of 97% when operated with natural gas of the specifications applicable for Figure 19-9.

19.5.2 Selection Parameters

Boiler selection should be based on a competent review of the following parameters:

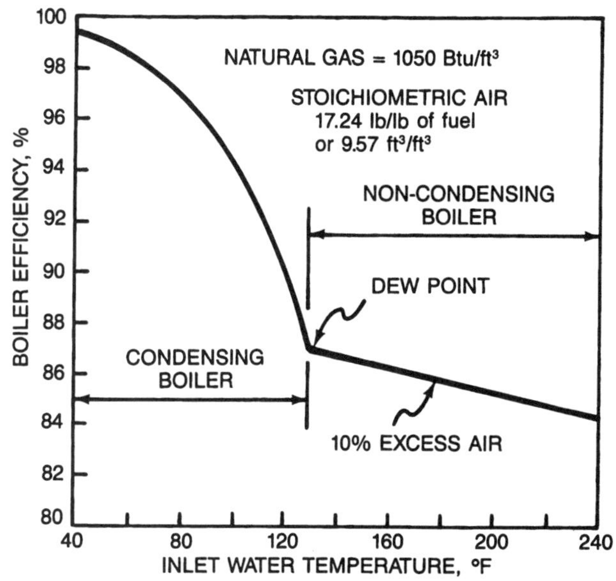

Fig. 19-9 Boiler Efficiency

All Boilers

- ASME Code Section, under which the boiler is constructed and tested
- Net boiler output capacity, Btu/h (kW)
- Total heat transfer surface, ft^2 (m^2)
- Water content, lb (kg)
- Auxiliary power requirements, kWh
- Internal water-flow patterns
- Cleaning provisions for all heat transfer surfaces
- Operational efficiency
- Space requirements and piping arrangement
- Water treatment requirements

Fuel-Fired Boilers

- Combustion space (furnace volume), ft^2 (m^2)
- Internal flow patterns of combustion products
- Combustion air and venting requirements
- Steam Boilers
- Steam space, ft^3 (m^3)

Electric Boilers

Electric boilers are in a separate class. Since no combustion occurs, no boiler heating surface and no flue openings are necessary. Heating surface is the surface of the electric elements or electrodes immersed in the boiler water. The design of electric boilers is largely determined by the shape and heat release of the electric heating elements used.

19.5.3 Efficiency: Input and Output Ratings

Efficiency of fuel-burning boilers is defined by combustion efficiency and overall efficiency. Overall efficiency of electric boilers is in the 92 to 96% range.

Combustion efficiency is input minus stack (chimney) loss, divided by input, and ranges from 75 to 86% for most non-condensing, mechanically fired boilers. Condensing boilers operate in the range of 88% to over 95% efficiency.

Overall efficiency is gross output divided by input. Gross output is measured in the steam or water leaving the boiler and depends on individual installation characteristics. Overall efficiency is lower than combustion efficiency by the percentage of heat lost from the outside surface of the boiler (this loss is usually termed **radiation loss**). Overall efficiency can be determined only by testing under fixed conditions. Approximate combustion efficiency can be determined under any operating condition by measuring operating flue-gas temperature and percentage CO_2 or O_2 and by consulting a chart or table for the fuel being used.

Heating boilers are usually rated according to standards developed by (1) The Hydronics Institute [formerly the Institute of Boiler and Radiator Manufacturers (IBR) and The Steel Boiler Institute (SBI)], (2) The American Gas Association (AGA), and (3) The American Boiler Manufacturers Association (ABMA).

19.5.4 Boiler Sizing

Boiler sizing is the selection of boiler output capacity to meet connected load. The boiler gross output is the rate of heat delivered by the boiler to the system under continuous firing at rated input. Net rating (IBR rating) is gross output minus a fixed percentage to allow for an estimated average piping heat loss plus an added load for initially heating the water in a system (sometimes called pickup).

Piping loss is variable. If all piping is run within the space defined as load, loss is zero. If piping runs through unheated spaces, heat loss from the piping may be higher than accounted for by the fixed net rating factor. Pickup is also variable. Pickup factor may be unnecessary when actual connected load is less than design load. On the design's coldest day, extra system output (boiler and radiation) is needed to pick up the load from a shutdown or low night setback. If night setback is not used, or if no extended shutdown occurs, no pickup load exists. Standby system capacity for pickup, if needed, can be in the form of excess capacity in base-load boilers, or in a standby boiler.

19.5.5 Control of Boiler Input and Output

Boiler controls regulate the rate of fuel input (on-off, step-firing, or modulating) in response to a control signal representing load change, so that average boiler output equals load within some accepted control tolerance. Boiler controls include safety controls that shut off fuel flow when unsafe conditions develop.

Steam boilers are operated by boiler-mounted, pressure actuated controls, which vary the input of fuel to the boiler. Common examples of controls are on-off, high-low-off, and modulating. Modulating controls continuously vary the fuel input from 100% down to a selected minimum point. The ratio of maximum to minimum is called the **turndown ratio**. The minimum input is usually between 5% and 25%, *i.e.*, 20:1 to 4:1, and depends on the size and type of fuel-burning apparatus.

19.5.6 Hydronic Systems

Hot water heating systems are frequently called **hydronic systems**. Water systems can be classified by: (1) temperature, (2) flow generation, (3) pressurization, (4) piping arrangement, and (5) pumping arrangement. Water systems are either once-through or recirculating systems.

The two types of hot water heating systems classified by flow generation are: (1) the **gravity system**, which uses the difference in density between the supply and return water columns of a circuit or system to circulate water; and (2) the **forced system**, in which a pump, usually driven by an electric motor, maintains the flow.

Low-temperature hot water systems (LTHW) are the most widely used heating systems for residential, commercial, and institutional systems where loads consist primarily of space heating and domestic water heating and do not exceed 5,000,000 Btu/h (1.5 MW) total. The maximum allowable working pressure for low-pressure heating boilers is 160 psia (1100 kPa), with a maximum temperature limitation of 250°F (120°C). The usual maximum working pressure for boilers for LTHW systems is 30 psia (200 kPa), although boilers specifically designed, tested, and stamped for higher pressures may frequently be used with working pressures to 160 psia (1100 kPa). Steam-to-water or water-to-water heat exchangers are also often used.

Medium-temperature hot water systems (MTHW) (350°F [175°C] or less) are most commonly used for space heating in large commercial and institutional buildings or in industrial applications with process loads, and where total loads range from 5×10^6 to 20×10^9 Btu/h (1.5 to 6 MW). In a medium-temperature system, the usual design supply temperature is above 250°F (120°C) and below 350°F (175°C) with a usual pressure rating for boilers and equipment of 150 psia (1030 kPa).

High-temperature hot water systems (HTHW) are generally limited to campus-type district heating installations and to applications requiring process heating temperatures of 350°F (175°C) or higher.

The design of water systems is affected by complex relationships between the various system components. The design water temperature, flow rate, piping layout, pump selection, terminal unit selection, and control method are all interrelated. The size and complexity of the system determines the importance of these relationships in affecting the total operating success. Present hot water heating system design practice originated in residential heating applications where a 20°F (11°C) temperature drop (TD) was used to determine flow rate. Besides producing satisfactory operation and economy in small systems, this TD enabled simple calculations because 1 gpm conveys 10,000 Btu/h (1 L/s conveys 41 kW with a 10°C TD).

Boiler piping connections and components for a multizone hot water system are illustrated in Figure 19-10. Requirements for such a system include a high limit control, a safety relief valve, and other safety controls and devices on the boiler, and a boiler efficiency with an accepted test rating.

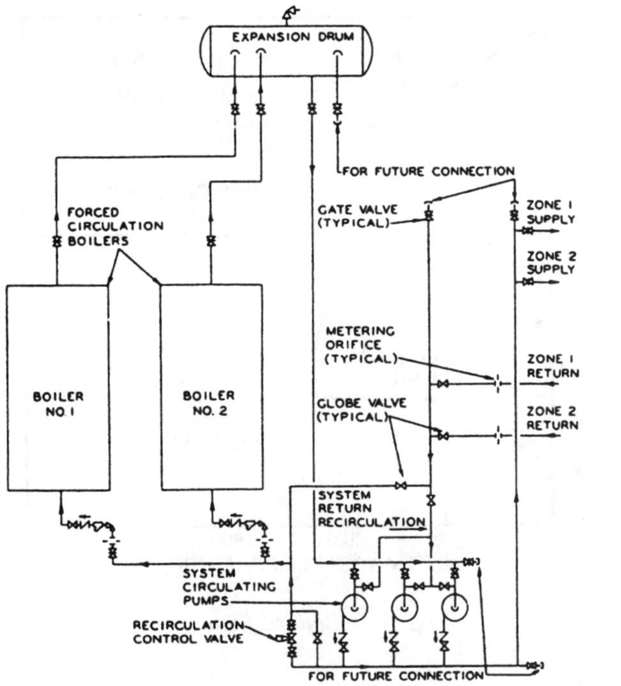

Fig. 19-10 HTHW Piping for Combined One Pump System

19.6 Terminal Units

Radiators, convectors, baseboard, and finned tube units are commonly used to distribute heat to the space provided by the steam or LTHW systems. They supply heat through a combination of radiation and convection. In general, these units are placed at the points of greatest heat loss of the space such as under windows, along exposed walls, and at door openings.

A **radiator** is generally considered a sectional cast-iron unit of columns, large tube, or small tube type (Fig. 19-11).

A **convector** is a heat-distributing unit that operates with gravity circulated air. The heating element contains two or more tubes with headers at both ends. The heating element is surrounded by an enclosure with an air inlet below and an air outlet above (Fig. 19-11).

Baseboard and **baseboard radiation heat distributing units** are installed at the base of walls in place of the conventional baseboard. They may be made of cast iron, with a substantial portion of the front face directly exposed to the room, or with a finned-tube element in a sheet metal enclosure (Fig. 19-11).

Finned tube or **fin-tube** refers to heat-distributing units fabricated from metallic tubing with metallic fins bonded to the tube. They operate with gravity-circulated room air, and may be installed bare, with an expanded metal grille, a cover, or an enclosure having top, front, or inclined outlets.

19.6.1 Radiators

The small-tube type radiators, with a length of only 1 3/4 in. (44 mm) per section, occupy less space than the older column and large-tube units, and are particularly suited to installation in recesses. Shown in Fig. 19-12 are the types of units now being manufactured.

19.6.2 Convectors

Convectors are made in a wide variety of depths, sizes, and lengths in both cabinet and enclosure style. The heating elements are fabricated in ferrous and non-ferrous metals. The air enters the enclosure below the heating element, is heated as it passes through the element, and leaves the enclosure through the outlet grille located above the heating element. Factory assembled units comprised of a heating element and enclosure are widely used. These may be free standing, wall hung, or recessed, and may have outlet grilles and arched inlets or inlet grilles (Figure 19-11).

19.6.3 Baseboard Units

Baseboard heat-distributing units are divided into two types: (1) radiant-convector, and (2) finned tube.

A **radiant-convector baseboard heating unit** is made of cast iron or steel. The units have air openings at the top and bottom to permit circulation of room air over the wall side of the unit. The wall side of the unit has an extended surface to provide increased heat output. A large portion of the heat is transferred by convection (Fig. 19-11).

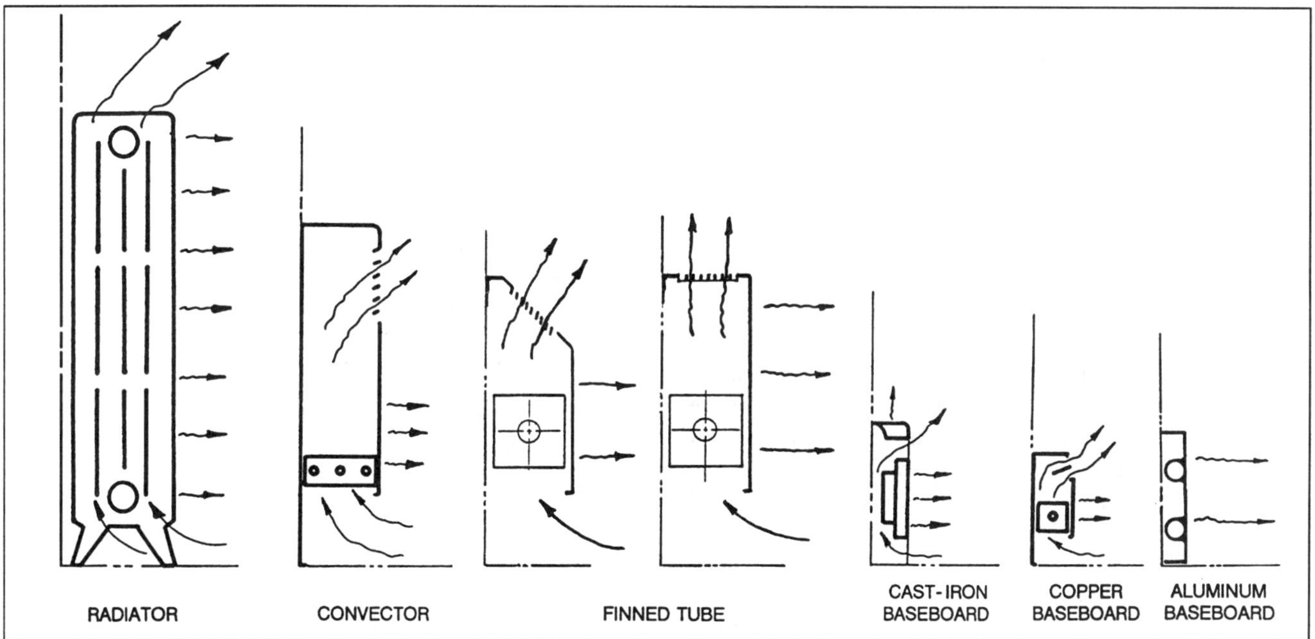

Fig. 19-11 Terminal Units

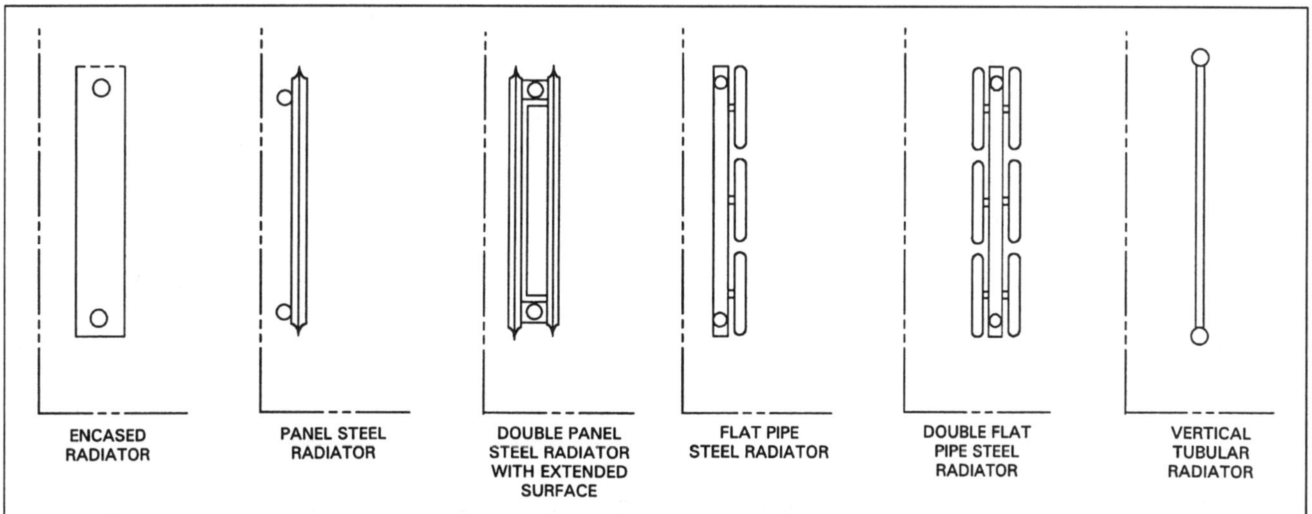

Fig. 19-12 Typical Radiators

A **finned tube baseboard heating unit** has a finned-tube heating element that is concealed by a long, low sheet-metal enclosure or cover. Most of the heat is transferred to the room by convection. Optimum comfort for room occupants is obtained when units are installed along as much of the exposed wall as possible.

The baseboard unit has the following advantages: (1) it is normally placed along the cold walls and under areas where the greatest heat loss occurs, (2) it is inconspicuous, (3) it offers minimum interference with furniture placement, and (4) it distributes heat near the floor. This last characteristic reduces the floor-to-ceiling temperature gradient to about 2 to 4°F (1 to 2°C) and helps produce uniform temperatures throughout the room. It also makes baseboard heat-distributing units adaptable to homes without basements, where cold floors are prevalent.

19.7 Electric Heating

For many applications, the compactness, simplicity, responsiveness, accuracy of control, safety, and cleanliness of electric heating may outweigh its disadvantages. Electric space heating is often used where minimum initial cost is the dominating factor.

19.7.1 Electric Heating Elements

Electric heating elements usually are composed of metal-alloy wire or ribbons, non-metallic carbon compounds in rod or other shapes, or printed circuits. Heating elements may have exposed resistor coils mounted on insulators, metallic resistors embedded within refractory insulation encased in a protective metal sheath, or a printed circuit on glass sheets or vitrified panels. Fins or extended surfaces may be used to increase heat dissipation. Elements are made in many forms. Metal or oxide conductive films on glass and ceramics have been used, usually in panel form. Tubular elements may be immersed in liquids, used bare, formed into coils, or cast into metal.

Cloth fabrics, incorporating flexible resistor wires, are used for low-temperature purposes such as heating pads, sheets, blankets, aviators' clothing, window draperies, and some radiant panel heating installations. Paper or fabric incorporating a surface resistor on the back is applied for ceiling panel heating installations.

19.7.2 Electric Space Heating Systems

Types of electric heating equipment and complete heating systems in use are listed in Table 19-6. The sequence shown is for convenient reference only, and does not indicate the relative performance or extent of use. Installations of all types listed are in successful operation, but operating characteristics depend largely on proper application.

Table 19-6 Types of Electric Space-Heating Equipment

Decentralized Systems
Natural Convection Units
Floor drop-in units
Wall insert and surface-mounted heaters
Baseboard convectors
Hydronic baseboard convectors with immersion elements
Forced Air units
Unit ventilators
Unit heaters
Wall insert heaters
Baseboard heaters
Floor drop-in heaters
Radiant Units (High Intensity)
Radiant wall, insert, or surface mounted (open ribbon or wire element)
Metal-sheathed element with focusing reflector
Quartz tube element with focusing reflector
Quartz lamp with focusing reflector
Heat lamps
Valance (cove) heaters
Radiant Panel Systems (Low Intensity)
Radiant ceiling with embedded conductors
Prefabricated panels
Radiant floor with embedded conductors
Radiant-convector panel heaters
Centralized Systems
Heated Water Systems
Electric boiler
Electric boiler with hydronic off-peak storage
Heat pumps
Integrated heat recovery systems
Steam Systems
Electric boiler with immersion element or electrode
Heated-Air Systems
Duct heaters
Electric furnaces
Heat pumps
Integrated heat recovery systems
Unit ventilators
Self contained heating and cooling units
Storage units (ceramic, water)

19.7.3 Calculating Capacities

The procedure outlined in Chapters 27 and 28 of the 1997 *ASHRAE Handbook—Fundamentals* for calculating heating load of residential and non-residential buildings may be used for electric systems. The NEMA Manual for Electric Comfort Conditioning published by the National Electrical Manufacturers Association, gives heat loss factors and describes methods for calculating load directly in kilowatts.

The most economical electric heating systems from an operating standpoint are decentralized, with the thermostat provided on each unit or for each room. This permits each room to compensate for heat contributed by auxiliary sources such as sunshine, lighting, and appliances. Such an arrangement also gives a better diversity of the power demand because the electric load from all units of an installation does not coincide. Manual switches allow the heat to be turned off or allow for reduced temperatures in rooms that are not in use. When manual switches are used, adequate capacity for warmup should be provided.

Residences and other buildings designed for electric heat should be well insulated. Depending on the climate, storm or multiple-glazed windows and storm doors are generally recommended to reduce heat loss and further increase comfort. Weather stripping doors and windows effectively reduces air infiltration.

19.8 Problems

In all problems, assume air is 79% N_2 and 21% O_2.

19.1 Set up the necessary combustion equations and determine the mass of air required to burn 0.45 kg (lb) of pure carbon to equal masses of CO and CO_2.

19.2 The gravimetric analysis of a gaseous mixture is: CO_2 = 32%, O_2= 54.5%, and N_2 = 11.5%. The mixture is at a pressure of 20.7 kPa (3 psia). Determine: (a) the volumetric analysis and (b) the partial pressure of each component.

19.3 A liquid petroleum fuel, C_2H_6OH is burned in a space heater at atmospheric pressure.

(a) For combustion with 20% excess air, determine the air/fuel ratio by mass, the mass of water formed by combustion per pound of fuel, and the dew point of the combustion products. [Ans: 14.5, 1.34, 133.9°F]
(b) For combustion with 80% theoretical air, determine the dry analysis of the exhaust gases in percentage by volume. [Ans: 5.94% CO_2, 11.04% CO, 83.02% N_2]

19.4 19.4 Find the air/fuel ratio by mass when benzene (C_6H_6) burns with theoretical air and determine the dew point at atmospheric pressure of the combustion products if an air/fuel ratio of 20:1 by mass is used.

19.5 A diesel engine uses 30 lb_m of fuel per hour (3.8 g/s) when the brake output is 75 hp. If the heating value of the fuel is 19,600 Btu/lb (45,600 kJ/kg), what is the brake thermal efficiency of the engine?

19.6 Methane (CH_4) is burned with air at atmospheric pressure. The Orsat analysis of the flue gas gives: CO_2 = 10.00%, O_2 = 2.41%, CO = 0.52%, and N_2 = 87.07%. Balance the combustion equation and determine the air-fuel ratio, the percent theoretical air, and the percent excess air. [Ans: 10.48 (vol.), 18.89 (mass), 110.1%, 10.1%]

19.7 Fuel oil composed of $C_{16}H_{32}$ is burned with the chemically correct air-fuel ratio. Find:

(a) Moisture formed per kg of fuel; moisture formed per lb of fuel
(b) Partial pressure of the water vapor, kPa; water vapor psia
(c) Percentage of CO_2 in the stack gases on an Orsat basis
(d) Volume of exhaust gases per unit mass of oil, if the gas is at 260°C (500°F) and 102 kPa (14.8 psia).

19.8 Determine the composition of a hydrocarbon fuel if the Orsat analysis gives: CO_2 = 8.0%, CO = 1.0%, O_2 = 8.7%, and N_2 = 82.3%.

19.9 Determine the air/fuel ratio by mass when a liquid fuel of 16% hydrogen and 84% carbon by mass is burned with 15% excess air. [Ans: 17.49]

19.10 Compute the compositions of the flue gases on a percent by volume on dry basis (same as Orsat) resulting from the combustion of C_8H_{18} with 84% theoretical air.

19.11 A liquid petroleum fuel having a hydrogen to carbon ratio of 0.169 by mass is burned in a heater with an air/fuel ratio of 17 by mass. Determine: (a) the volumetric analysis on both wet and dry bases of the exhaust gases; and (b) the dew point of the exhaust gas.

19.12 Compare the heating value for semianthracite coal as given in Table 9, Chapter 17, 1997 *ASHRAE Handbook—Fundamentals* with the value predicted using the Dulong Formula. [Ans: 1.24% difference]

19.13 Natural gas with a volumetric composition of 93.32% methane, 4.17% ethane, 0.69% propane, 0.19% butane, 0.05% pentane, 0.98% carbon dioxide and 0.61% nitrogen burns with 30% excess air. Calculate the volume of dry air at 60°F, 30 in. Hg (15.6°C, 101.5 kPa) used to burn 1000 ft^3 (28.3 mL) of gas at 68°F and 29.92 in. Hg (20°C and 101.4 kPa) and find the dew point of the combustion products.

19.14 The proximate analysis of a coal is: moisture = 4.33%, volatile matter = 40.21%, fixed carbon = 45.07%, and ash = 10.39%. The heating value was determined as 29 000 kJ/kg (12,490 Btu/lb). Find the ASTM rank of the coal.

19.15 A fuel oil shows an API gravity of 36. Calculate the specific gravity at 60°F and the pounds per gallon of fuel. Estimate the ASTM Grade. [Ans: 0.845, 7.05, No. 2]

19.16 A representative No. 4 fuel oil has a gravity of 25 degrees API and the following composition: carbon = 87.4%, hydrogen = 10.7%, sulfur = 1.2%, nitrogen = 0.2, moisture = 0, and solids = 0.5%.

(a) Estimate its higher heating value.
(b) Compute the mass of air required to burn, theoretically, one gallon of the fuel.

19.17 The following data was taken from a test on an oil-fired furnace:

Fuel rate = 20 gal oil/h
Specific gravity of fuel oil = 0.89% by mass
Hydrogen in fuel = 14.7%
Temperature of fuel for combustion = 80°F
Temperature of entering combustion air = 80°F
Relative humidity of entering air = 45%
Temperature of flue gases leaving furnace = 550°F

(a) Calculate the heat loss in water vapor in products formed by combustion.
(b) Calculate the heat loss in water vapor in the combustion air.

[Ans: 1672.5 Btu/lb (3888 kJ/kg), 29.4 Btu/lb (68.3 kJ/kg)]

19.18 An office building requires 2901 MJ (2.75×10^9 Btu) of heat for the winter season. Compute the seasonal heating costs, if the following fuel is used:

(a) Bituminous coal; 31 380 kJ/kg (13,500 Btu/lb); $36.00 per ton

(b) No. 2 fuel oil, 38 500 kJ/L (138,000 Btu/gal); 99 cents per gallon.

Assume that the conversion efficiency is 75% for the oil and 61% for the coal.

19.19 Saturated air at 41°F dry bulb (5°C) enters a furnace; it leaves the furnace at 110°F dry bulb (43.3°C) and 0.00543 lb_v/lb_a (0.00543 kg/kg) and circulates through a factory. Air leaves the factory at 65°F dry bulb (18.3°C) and 63°F wet bulb (17.2°C).

(a) What is the sensible and latent heat change for the air passing through the factory?
(b) State whether the air gains or loses sensible and latent heat during each process. [Ans: q_s = +6 Btu/lb (14.0 kJ/kg), q_l = +7 Btu/lb (16.3 kJ/kg)]

19.20 A plant is maintained at 70°F dry bulb, 60% rh, and has a low-pressure steam heating system. A makeup air system is being added to the plant and it has been decided that the input air should be 10,127 cfm. Outside design conditions are –1°F dry bulb, 50% rh. The plant is 250 ft by 560 ft and normally has 325 people working per shift.

(a) What are the total steam requirements for the heating coil and the humidifier?
(b) What capacity should the humidifier have in pounds of water per hour?

19.21 A residence with a design heating load of 26 kW (89,000 Btu/h) is to use an oil-fired warm air system with forced circulation. Return air to the furnace is at 22.2°C (72°F). Specify the following:

(a) Supply air temperature
(b) Airflow rate
(c) Make and catalog number of suitable furnace

19.22 A residence with a design heating load of 16 kW (55,000 Btu/h) is to use a forced circulation hot-water baseboard radiator system. The baseboard units house copper tubing with aluminum fins and operate with the inlet air temperature at 18.3°C (65°F). Specify the following:

This problem requires catalog data.

(a) Hot water inlet temperature and outlet temperature
(b) Total water flow rate
(c) Total length of radiator panel for house
(d) Location of panels
(e) Make and catalog number of suitable hot water heater

19.23 For the residence of *Problem 19-22*, electric baseboard units replace the hot water system. Specify:

This problem requires catalog data.

(a) Total rating of electric system, kW
(b) Total length of baseboard units

19.24 A large classroom has a winter design heat loss of 19.9 kW (68,000 Btu/h) with installed forced circulation hot-water baseboard radiators. The baseboard units house copper tubing with aluminum fins and operate with the inlet air temperature at 18.3°C (65°F). Specify the following:

(a) Hot water inlet temperature and outlet temperature
(b) Water flow rate
(c) Length of radiator panel

19.25 A large classroom has a winter design load of 26 kW (89,000 Btu/h). A forced circulation warm air system is to be used with return air at 23.3°C (74°F). Specify:

(a) Supply air temperature
(b) Airflow rate

19.26 For a heat loss from the space to be conditioned of Q, write the expression for determining:

(a) Amount of air L/s (cfm), which must be supplied if a hot air system is used
(b) Amount of hot water L/s (gpm), which must be supplied if a hydronic system is used
(c) Amount of steam kg/h (lb/h), which must be supplied if a steam heating system is used
(d) Size, in watts, of electric heaters required if electric heat is used

19.27 List the steps taken when designing a forced-circulation hot water heating system.

19.28 Compute the increase in length of 28.3 m (93 ft) of steel steam pipe when the average steam temperature is 113°C (235°F) and the air is 21°C (70°F). The pipe was installed during a period when the temperature was 15.6°C (60°F).

19.29 The total mass of steel in the boiler and piping of a school's heating system is 9080 kg (20,000 lb). The piping and boiler also contain 6810 kg (15,000 lb) of water. After a weekend shut-down, the temperature of the system is 10°C (50°F). The operating temperature is 93°C (200°F).

(a) Assuming the system should be warmed up in one hour, determine the required furnace size.
[Ans: 764 kW (2,610,000 Btu/h)]
(b) For a furnace size of 146 kW (500,000 Btu/h) output, when should the furnace be started to be up to the operating temperature of 93°C (200°F) by 7:30 a.m. Monday morning? [Ans: 2:16 a.m. Sunday]

19.9 Bibliography

ASHRAE. Chapter 17, 1997 *ASHRAE Handbook—Fundamentals*.

ASHRAE. Chapters 26 through 33, 1996 *ASHRAE Handbook—HVAC Systems and Equipment*.

Strehlow, R.A. 1984. *Combustion Fundamentals*. McGraw Hill, New York.

NFPA. 1992. Chimneys, Fireplaces, Vents and Solid Fuel-Burning Appliances. *Standard* 211-92. National Fire Protection Association, Quincy, MA.

Appendix A

SI FOR HVAC&R

This guide conforms to ANSI SI 10-1997, *Standard for Use of the International System of Units* (SI): *The Modern Metric System*. See ANSI SI 10 for more information and a complete list of conversion factors with more significant digits.

ASHRAE METRIC POLICY

The metric unit use or application policy shall include, as a minimum, time-dated directions on the use of SI and I-P units in all ASHRAE publications.

1. The Technical Committee on terminology, TC 1.6, shall serve as the authority on SI and I-P usage and application.
2. Research projects, Standards and Guidelines, Special Publications, Insights articles, Journal articles, and Handbooks shall be prepared using inch-pound (I-P) units and/or the International System of Units (SI) in formats approved by the Publishing Council.
3. The Publishing Council shall review annually the approved formats to be used in ASHRAE publications—considering suggestions from members, Technical Committees/Task Groups/Technical Resource Groups, Standards Project Committees, Research and Technical Committee, Journal, Handbook, and other General Committees, and shall establish any changes in the approved formats.
4. The Publishing Council shall consider this policy annually and shall recommend to the Board of Directors the formats to be used in ASHRAE publications.
   a. The format for ASHRAE publications shall be dual units, except in cases determined by the Publishing Council, where two separate versions are to be published, one rational I-P and the other rational SI. For selected ASHRAE Standards and Guidelines, the Standards Committee may approve use of SI units only.
   b. In dual unit publications, the units used in calculating the work being reported shall be listed first. The alternate system of units should follow in parenthesis. Authors shall round off equivalents in the alternate system of units so that they imply the same accuracy as is implied with primary units.
   c. Exceptions require the approval of the Director of Communications and Publications.
   d. All Handbook volumes are published in separate I-P and SI editions.

SI PRACTICE

1 General

1.1 The International System of Units (SI) consists of seven base units listed in Table 1 and numerous derived units, which are combinations of base units (Table 2).

Table 1 SI Base Units

Quantity	Name	Symbol
length	metre	m
mass	kilogram	kg
time	second	s
electric current	ampere	A
thermodynamic temperature	kelvin	K
amount of substance	mole	mol
luminous intensity	candela	cd

2 Units

2.1 In SI each physical quantity has only one unit. The base and derived units may be modified by prefixes as indicated in Section 4. All derived units are defined by simple formulas using the base units. The basic simplicity of the system can only be kept by adhering to the approved units.

2.2 **Angle.** The unit of plane angle is the radian. The degree and its decimal fractions may be used, but the minute and second should not be used.

2.3 **Area.** The unit of area is the square metre. Large areas are expressed in hectares (ha) or square kilometres (km^2). The hectare is restricted to land or sea areas and equals 10 000 m^2.

2.4 **Energy.** The unit of energy, work, and quantity of heat is the joule (J). The kilowatthour (kWh) is presently permitted as an alternative in electrical applications, but should not be introduced in new applications.

1 kilowatthour (kWh) = 3.6 megajoules (MJ)

The unit of power and heat flow rate is the watt (W).

1 watt (W) = 1 joule per second (J/s)

2.5 **Force.** The unit of force is the newton (N). The newton is also used in derived units which include force.

Examples: pressure or stress = N/m^2 = Pa (pascal)
work = N·m = J (joule)
power = N·m/s = W (watt)

2.6 **Length.** The unit of length is the metre. The millimetre is used on architectural or construction drawings and mechanical or shop drawings. The symbol mm does not need to be placed after each dimension; a note, "All dimensions in mm" is sufficient.

The centimetre is used only for cloth, clothing sizes, and anatomical measurements.

The metre is used for topographical and plot plans. It is always written with a decimal and three figures following the decimal, i.e., 38.560.

2.7 **Mass.** The unit of mass is the kilogram (kg). The unit of mass is the only unit whose name, for historical reasons, contains a prefix. Names of multiples of the unit mass are formed

Table 2 Some SI Derived Units

Quantity	Expression in Other SI Units	Name	Symbol
acceleration			
angular	rad/s²		
linear	m/s²		
angle			
plane	dimensionless	radian	rad
solid	dimensionless	steradian	sr
area	m²		
Celsius temperature	K	degree Celsius	°C
conductivity, thermal	W/(m·K)		
density			
heat flux	W/m²		
mass	kg/m³		
energy, enthalpy			
work, heat	N·m	joule	J
specific	J/kg		
entropy			
heat capacity	J/K		
specific	J/(kg·K)		
flow, mass	kg/s		
flow, volume	m³/s		
force	kg·m/s²	newton	N
frequency			
periodic	1/s	hertz	Hz
rotating	rev/s		
inductance	Wb/A	henry	H
magnetic flux	V·s	weber	
moment of a force	N·m		
potential, electric	W/A	volt	V
power, radiant flux	J/s	watt	W
pressure, stress	N/m²	pascal	Pa
resistance, electric	V/a	ohm	Ω
velocity			
angular	rad/s		
linear	m/s		
viscosity			
dynamic (absolute)(m)	Pa·s		
kinematic (n)	m²/s		
volume	m³		
volume, specific	m³/kg		

by attaching prefixes to the word gram. The megagram, Mg, (1000 kg, metric ton or tonne, t) is the appropriate unit for describing large masses. Do not use the term *weight* when *mass* is intended.

2.8 **Pressure.** The unit of stress or pressure, force per unit area, is the newton per square metre. This unit is called the *pascal* (Pa). SI has no equivalent symbol for psig or psia. If a misinterpretation is likely, spell out Pa (absolute) or Pa (gage).

2.9 **Volume.** The unit of volume is the cubic metre. Smaller units are the litre, L (m³/1000); millilitre, mL; and microlitre, μL. No prefix other than m or μ is used with litre.

2.10 **Temperature.** The unit of thermodynamic (absolute) temperature is the Kelvin. Celsius temperature is measured in degrees Celsius. Temperature intervals may be measured in kelvins or degrees Celsius and are the same in either scale. Thermodynamic temperature is related to Celsius temperature as follows:

$$t_c = T - T_0$$

where

t_c = Celsius temperature, °C
T = thermodynamic temperature, kelvins (K)
T_0 = 273.15 K by definition

2.11 **Time.** The unit of time is the second, which should be used in technical calculations. However, where time relates to life customs or calendar cycles, the minute, hour, day, and other calendar units may be necessary.

Exception: Revolutions per minute may be used, but revolutions per second is preferred.

3 Symbols

3.1 The correct use of symbols is important because an incorrect symbol may change the meaning of a quantity. Some SI symbols are listed in Table 3.

3.2 SI has no abbreviations—only symbols. Therefore, no periods follow a symbol except at the end of a sentence.

Examples: SI, *not* S.I.; s, *not* sec; A, *not* amp

3.3 Symbols appear in lower case unless the unit name has been taken from a proper name. In this case the first letter of the symbol is capitalized.

Examples: m, metre; W, watt; Pa, pascal

Exception: L, litre

3.4 Symbols and prefixes are printed in upright (roman) type regardless of the type style in surrounding text.

Example: . . . *a distance of* 56 km *between* . . .

3.5 Unit symbols are the same whether singular or plural.

Examples: 1 kg, 14 kg; 1 mm, 25 mm

3.6 Leave a space between the value and the symbol.

Examples: 55 mm, *not* 55mm; 100 W, *not* 100W

Table 3 SI Symbols

Symbol	Name	Quantity	Formula
A	ampere	electric current	base unit
a	atto	prefix	10^{-18}
Bq	becquerel	activity (of a radio nuclide)	1/s
C	coulomb	quantity of electricity	A·s
°C	degree Celsius	temperature	°C = K
c	centi	prefix	10^{-2}
cd	candela	luminous intensity	base unit
d	deci	prefix	10^{-1}
da	deka	prefix	10^{1}
E	exa	prefix	10^{18}
F	farad	electric capacitance	C/V
f	femto	prefix	10^{-15}
G	giga	prefix	10^{9}
Gy	gray	absorbed dose	J/kg
g	gram	mass	kg/1000
H	henry	inductance	Wb/A
Hz	hertz	frequency	1/s
h	hecto	prefix	10^{2}
ha	hectare	area	10 000 m²
J	joule	energy, work, heat	N·m
K	kelvin	temperature	base unit
k	kilo	prefix	10^{3}

Table 3 SI Symbols (*Continued*)

Symbol	Name	Quantity	Formula
kg	kilogram	mass	base unit
L	litre	volume	$m^3/1000$
lm	lumen	luminous flux	cd·sr
lx	lux	illuminance	lm/m^2
M	mega	prefix	10^6
m	metre	length	base unit
m	milli	prefix	10^{-3}
mol	mole	amount of substance	base unit
μ	micro	prefix	10^{-6}
N	newton	force	$kg \cdot m/s^2$
n	nano	prefix	10^{-9}
Ω	ohm	electric resistance	V/A
P	peta	prefix	10^{15}
Pa	pascal	pressure, stress	N/m^2
p	pico	prefix	10^{-12}
rad	radian	plane angle	dimensionless
S	siemens	electric conductance	A/V
Sv	sievert	dose equivalent	J/kg
s	second	time	base unit
sr	steradian	solid angle	dimensionless
T	tera	prefix	10^{12}
T	tesla	magnetic flux density	Wb/m^2
t	tonne, metric ton	mass	1000 kg; Mg
V	volt	electric potential	W/A
W	watt	power, radiant flux	J/s
Wb	weber	magnetic flux	V·s

Exception: No space is left between the numerical value and symbol for degree Celsius and degree of plane angle.

Note: Symbol for degree Celsius is °C; for coulomb, C.

Examples: 20°C, not 20 °C or 20° C; 45°, not 45 °

3.7 Do not mix symbols and names in the same expression.

Examples: m/s or metres per second,
not metres/second; *not* metres/s

J/kg or joules per kilogram,
not joules/kilogram; *not* joules/kg

3.8 Symbol for product—use the raised dot (·)

Examples: N·m; mPa·s; $W/(m^2 \cdot K)$

3.9 Symbol for quotient—use one of the following forms:

Examples: m/s or $\frac{m}{s}$ or use negative exponent

Note: Use only one solidus (/) per expression.

3.10 Place modifying terms such as electrical, alternating current, etc. parenthetically after the symbol with a space in between.

Examples: MW (e); *not* MWe; *not* MW(e)
V (ac); *not* Vac; *not* V(ac)
kPa (gage); *not* kPa(gage); *not* KPa gage

4 Prefixes

4.1 Most prefixes indicate orders of magnitude in steps of 1000. Prefixes provide a convenient way to express large and small numbers and to eliminate nonsignificant digits and leading zeros in decimal fractions. Some prefixes are listed in Table 4.

Examples: 126 000 watts is the same as 126 kilowatts
0.045 metre is the same as 45 millimetres
65 000 metres is the same as 65 kilometres

4.2 To realize the full benefit of the prefixes when expressing a quantity by numerical value, choose a prefix so that the number lies between 0.1 and 1000. For simplicity, give preference to prefixes representing 1000 raised to an integral power (i.e., μm, mm, km).

Exceptions:

1. In expressing area and volume, the prefixes hecto, deka, deci, and centi are sometimes used; for example, cubic decimetre (L), square hectometre (hectare), cubic centimetre.
2. Tables of values of the same quantity.
3. Comparison of values.

Table 4 SI Prefixes

Prefix	Pronunciation	Symbol	Represents	
exa	ex'a (a as in about)	E	10^{18}	
peta	pet'a (e as in pet, a as in about)	P	10^{15}	
tera	as in *terra* firma	T	10^{12}	
giga	jig' (i as in jig, a as in about)	G	10^9	
mega	as in *mega*phone	M	10^6	
kilo	kill'oh	k	10^3	= 1000
hecto	heck' toe	h*	10^2	= 100
deka	deck'a (a as in about)	da*	10^1	= 10
deci	as in *deci*mal	d*	10^{-1}	= 0.1
centi	as in *centi*pede	c*	10^{-2}	= 0.01
milli	as in *mili*tary	m	10^{-3}	= 0.001
micro	as in *micro*phone	μ	10^{-6}	
nano	nan'oh (an as in ant)	n	10^{-9}	
pico	peek'oh	p	10^{-12}	

*See paragraph 4.2 regarding use of this prefix.

4. For certain quantities in particular applications. For example, the millimetre is used for linear dimensions in engineering drawings even when the values lie far outside the range of 0.1 mm to 1000 mm; the centimetre is usually used for body measurements and clothing sizes.

4.3 **Compound units.** A compound unit is a derived unit expressed with two or more units. The prefix is attached to a unit in the numerator.

Examples: V/m *not* mV/mm
mN·m *not* N·mm (torque)
MJ/kg not kJ/g

4.4 Compound prefixes formed by a combination of two or more prefixes are not used. Use only one prefix.

Examples: 2 nm *not* 2 mμm
$6\ m^3$ *not* 6 kL
6 MPa *not* 6 kkPa

4.5 **Exponential Powers.** An exponent attached to a symbol containing a prefix indicates that the multiple (of the unit with its prefix) is raised to the power of 10 expressed by the exponent.

Examples: $1\ mm^3 = (10^{-3}\ m)^3 = 10^{-9}\ m^3$

$$1\ \text{ns}^{-1} = (10^{-9}\ \text{s})^{-1} = 10^{9}\ \text{s}^{-1}$$
$$1\ \text{mm}^2/\text{s} = (10^{-3}\ \text{m})^2/\text{s} = 10^{-6}\ \text{m}^2/\text{s}$$

5 Numbers

5.1 **Large Numbers.** International practice separates the digits of large numbers into groups of three, counting from the decimal to the left and to the right, and inserts a space to separate the groups. In numbers of four digits, the space is not necessary except for uniformity in tables.

Examples: 2.345 678; 73 846; 635 041; 600.000; 0.113 501; 7 258

5.2 **Small Numbers.** When writing numbers less than one, always put a zero before the decimal marker.

Example: 0.046

5.3 **Decimal Marker.** The recommended decimal marker is a dot on the line (period). (In some countries, a comma is used as the decimal marker.)

5.4 **Billion.** Because billion means a thousand million in the United States and a million million in most other countries, avoid using the term in technical writing.

5.5 **Roman Numerals.** Do not use M to indicate thousands (MBtu for a thousand Btu), nor MM to indicate millions, nor C to indicate hundreds because they conflict with SI prefixes.

6 Words

6.1 The units in the international system of units are called SI units—not Metric Units and not SI Metric Units.

(Inch-Pound units are called I-P units—not conventional units, not U.S. customary units, not English units, and not Imperial units.)

6.2 Treat all spelled out names as nouns. Therefore, do not capitalize the first letter of a unit except at the beginning of a sentence or in capitalized material such as a title.

Examples: watt; pascal; ampere; volt; newton; kelvin

Exception: Always capitalize the first letter of Celsius.

6.3 Do not begin a sentence with a unit symbol—either rearrange the words or write the unit name in full.

6.4 Use plurals for spelled out words when required by the rules of grammar.

Examples: metre — metres; henry — henries; kilogram — kilograms; kelvin — kelvins

Irregular: hertz — hertz; lux — lux; siemens — siemens

6.5 Do not put a space or hyphen between the prefix and unit name.

Examples: kilometre not kilo metre or kilo-metre; milliwatt not milli watt or milli-watt

6.6 When a prefix ends with a vowel and the unit name begins with a vowel, retain and pronounce both vowels.

Example: kiloampere

Exceptions: hectare; kilohm; megohm

6.7 When compound units are formed by multiplication, leave a space between units that are multiplied.

Examples: newton metre, not newton-metre; volt ampere, not volt-ampere

6.8 Use the modifier squared or cubed after the unit name.

Example: metre per second squared

Exception: For area or volume place the modifier before the units. *Example*: square millimetre; cubic metre

6.9 When compound units are formed by division, use the word *per*, not a solidus (/).

Examples: metre per second, *not* metre/second; watt per square metre, *not* watt/square metre

TEMPERATURE CONVERSION

(exact)

$t_C = (t_F - 32)/1.8$ $\quad$ $t_F = 1.8\,t_C + 32$

$t_C = T - 273.15$ $\quad$ $t_F = T_R - 459.67$

$T = T_R/1.8$ $\quad$ $T_R = 1.8T$

$T = t_C + 273.15$ $\quad$ $T_R = t_F + 459.67$

where

t_C = Celsius temperature, °C
T = thermodynamic (absolute) temperature, kelvins (K)
t_F = Fahrenheit temperature, °F
T_R = thermodynamic (absolute) temperature, degrees Rankine (°R)

and °C = K = 1.8°F $\quad$ °F = °R = °C/1.8

Table 5 SI Units for HVAC&R Catalogs

Quantity	Unit
Boilers	
Heat output	kW
Heat input	kW
Heat release	kW/m^2
Steam generation rate	kg/s
Fuel firing rate:	
solid	kg/s
gaseous	L/s
liquid	kg/s, L/s
Volume flow rate (combust. products)	m^3/s, L/s
Power input (to drives)	kW
Operating pressure	kPa
Hydraulic resistance	kPa
Draft conditions	Pa
Coil, Cooling and Heating	
Heat exchange rate	kW
Primary medium:	
mass flow rate	kg/s
hydraulic resistance	kPa
Air volume flow rate	m^3/s, L/s
Airflow static pressure loss	Pa
Face area	m^2
Fin spacing, center to center	mm
Controls and Instruments	
Flow rate:	
mass	kg/s
volume	m^3/s, L/s, mL/s
Operating pressure	kPa
Hydraulic resistance	kPa
Rotational frequency	rev/s (rpm)*
Cooling Towers	
Heat extraction rate	kW
Volume flow rate:	
air	m^3/s, L/s
water	m^3/s, L/s
Power input (to drive)	kW

Quantity	Unit
Diffusers and Grilles	
Air volume flow rate	m^3/s, L/s
Airflow pressure loss	Pa
Velocity	m/s
Fans	
Air volume flow rate	m^3/s, L/s
Power input (to drive)	kW
Fan static pressure	Pa
Fan total pressure	Pa
Rotational frequency	rev/s (rpm)*
Outlet velocity	m/s
Air Filters	
Air volume flow rate	m^3/s, L/s
Static pressure loss	Pa
Face area	m^2
Fuels	
Heating value:	
solid	MJ/kg
gaseous	MJ/m^3
liquid	MJ/kg
Heat Exchangers	
Heat output	kW
Mass flow rate	kg/s
Hydraulic resistance	kPa
Operating pressure	kPa
Flow velocity	m/s
Heat exchange surface	m^2
Fouling factor	m^2/W
Induction Terminals	
Heating or cooling output	kW
Primary air volume flow rate	m^3/s, L/s
Primary air static pressure loss	Pa
Secondary water mass flow rate	kg/s
Secondary water hydraulic resistance	kPa

Quantity	Unit
Pumps	
Mass flow rate	kg/s
Volume flow rate	L/s
Power input (to drive)	kW
Developed pressure	kPa
Operating pressure	kPa
Rotational frequency	rev/s (rpm)*
Space Heating Apparatus	
Heat output	kW
Airflow volume flow rate	m^3/s, L/s
Power input (to drive)	kW
Primary medium mass flow rate	kg/s
Hydraulic resistance	kPa
Operating pressure	kPa
Airflow static pressure loss	Pa
Vessels	
Operating pressure	kPa
Volumetric capacity	m^3, L
Air Washers	
Volume flow rate:	
air	m^3/s, L/s
water	m^3/s, L/s
Mass flow rate, water	kg/s
Power input (to drive)	kW
Airflow static pressure loss	Pa
Hydraulic resistance	kPa
Water Chillers	
Cooling capacity	kW
Mass flow rate, water	kg/s
Power input (to drive)	kW
Refrigerant pressure	kPa
Hydraulic resistance	kPa

*Acceptable

PHYSICAL PROPERTIES

Atmospheric Pressure

Standard pressure = 101.325 kPa, exact value by definition (approximately 29.921 in. Hg at 32°F; 760 mm Hg at 0°C; 14.696 psi at 32°F).

Gravity

Standard acceleration = 9.806 65 m/s^2, exact value by definition (approximately 32.1740 ft/s^2).

Table 6 Typical Densities (kg/m^3 at 20°C)

Gases (101.325 kPa)		Liquids		Solids	
butane	2.412	mercury	13 550	lead	11 300
propane	1.829	sulphuric acid	1 830	copper	8 900
oxygen	1.330	refrigerant 12	1 329	steel	7 830
air, dry	1.204	glycerine	1 264	cast iron	7 200
carbon dioxide	1.970	battery electr.	1 260	aluminum	2 700
air, 50% rh	1.191	refrigerant 22	1 213	glass	2 500
acetylene	1.173	water	998	concrete	2 300
nitrogen	1.164	mineral oil	900	brick	1 920
natural gas	0.719	kerosene	820	hardwood	750
helium	0.166	ethyl alcohol	791	softwood	540
hydrogen	0.083	gasoline	730	fiberglass board	80
		propane	580	polystyrene	20

Standard Air

Dry air at 101.325 kPa and 20°C (density ≈ 1.204 kg/m^3)

Specific heat (constant pressure), $c_p = 1.006$ kJ/(kg·K)

Heating of Air

Sensible heat $q_s = 1.2\,Q\Delta t$

Latent heat $q_l = 3.0\,Q\Delta w$

Total heat $q_t = 1.2\,Q\Delta h$

where

Δt = temperature difference, K or °C

Δw = moisture content difference, g/kg (dry air)

Δh = enthalpy difference, kJ/kg (dry air)

Q = volume flow rate, m^3/s (standard air)

q_s, q_l, q_t = heat flow, kW

Water

Heat of vaporization

at 101.325 kPa and 100°C = 2257 kJ/kg

Heat of fusion at 0°C = 334 kJ/kg

CONVERSION FACTORS

When making conversions, remember that a converted value is no more precise than the original value. Round off the final value to the same number of significant figures as those in the original value.

CAUTION: The conversion values are rounded to three or four significant figures, which is sufficiently accurate for most applications. See ANSI SI 10 for additional conversions with more significant figures.

Multiply	By	To Obtain
acre	0.4047	ha
atmosphere, standard	*101.325	kPa
bar	*100	kPa
barrel (42 US gal, petroleum)	159	L
Btu, (International Table)	1.055	kJ
Btu/ft^2	11.36	kJ/m^2
Btu·ft/h·ft^2·°F	1.731	W/(m·K)
Btu·in/h·ft^2·°F (thermal conductivity, *k*)	0.1442	W/(m·K)
Btu/h	0.2931	W
Btu/h·ft	0.9615	W/m
Btu/h·ft^2	3.155	W/m^2
Btu/h·ft^2·°F (heat transfer coefficient, *U*)	5.678	W/(m^2·K)
Btu/lb	*2.326	kJ/kg
Btu/lb·°F (specific heat, c_p)	4.184	kJ/(kg·K)
bushel	0.03524	m^3
calorie, (thermochemical)	*4.184	J
calorie, nutrition (kilocalorie)	*4.184	kJ
candle, candlepower	*1.0	cd
centipoise, dynamic vicosity, μ	*1.00	mPa·s
centistokes, kinematic viscosity, ν	*1.00	mm^2/s
clo	0.155	m^2·K/W
dyne/cm^2	*0.100	Pa
EDR hot water (150 Btu/h)	44.0	W
EDR steam (240 Btu/h)	70.3	W
fuel cost comparison at 100% eff.		
cents per gallon (no. 2 fuel oil)	0.0677	\$/GJ
cents per gallon (no. 6 fuel oil)	0.0632	\$/GJ
cents per gallon (propane)	0.113	\$/GJ
cent per kWh	2.78	\$/GJ
cents per therm	0.0948	\$/GJ
ft	*0.3048	m
ft	*304.8	mm
ft/min, fpm	*0.00508	m/s
ft/s, fps	*0.3048	m/s
ft of water	2.99	kPa
ft of water per 100 ft of pipe	0.0981	kPa/m
ft^2	0.09290	m^2
ft^2·h·°F/Btu (thermal resistance, *R*)	0.176	m^2·K/W
ft^2/s, kinematic viscosity, ν	92 900	mm^2/s
ft^3	28.32	L
ft^3	0.02832	m^3
ft^3/h, cfh	7.866	mL/s
ft^3/min, cfm	0.4719	L/s
ft^3/s, cfs	28.32	L/s
footcandle	10.76	lx
ft·lb$_f$ (torque or moment)	1.36	N·m
ft·lb$_f$ (work)	1.36	J
ft·lb$_f$/lb (specific energy)	2.99	J/kg
ft·lb$_f$/min (power)	0.0226	W
gallon, US (*231 in^3)	3.785	L
gph	1.05	mL/s
gpm	0.0631	L/s
gpm/ft^2	0.6791	L/(s·m^2)
gpm/ton refrigeration	0.0179	mL/J
grain (1/7000 lb)	0.0648	g
gr/gal	17.1	g/m^3
horsepower (boiler)(33,470 Btu/h)	9.81	kW
horsepower (550 ft·lb$_f$/s)	0.746	kW
inch	*25.4	mm
inch of mercury (60°F)	3.377	kPa
inch of water (60°F)	248.8	Pa
To Obtain	**By**	**Divide**

Multiply	By	To Obtain
in/100 ft (thermal expansion)	0.833	mm/m
in·lb$_f$ (torque or moment)	113	mN·m
in^2	645	mm^2
in^3 (volume)	16.4	mL
in^3/min (SCIM)	0.273	mL/s
in^3 (section modulus)	16 400	mm^3
in^4 (section moment)	416 200	mm^4
km/h	0.278	m/s
kWh	*3.60	MJ
kW/1000 cfm	2.12	kJ/m^3
kilopond (kg force)	9.81	N
kip (1000 lb$_f$)	4.45	kN
kip/in^2 (ksi)	6.895	MPa
litre	*0.001	m^3
MBtuh (1000 Btu/h)	0.2931	kW
met	58.15	W/m^2
micron (μm) of mercury (60°F)	133	mPa
mil (0.001 in.)	*25.4	mm
mile	1.61	km
mile, nautical	1.85	km
mph	1.61	km/h
mph	0.447	m/s
millibar	*0.100	kPa
mm of mercury (60°F)	0.133	kPa
mm of water (60°F)	9.80	Pa
ounce (mass, avoirdupois)	28.35	g
ounce (force of thrust)	0.278	N
ounce (liquid, US)	29.6	mL
ounce (avoirdupois) per gallon	7.49	kg/m^3
perm (permeance)	57.45	ng/(s·m^2·Pa)
perm inch (permeability)	1.46	ng/(s·m·Pa)
pint (liquid, US)	473	mL
pound		
lb (mass)	0.4536	kg
lb (mass)	453.6	g
lb$_f$ (force or thrust)	4.45	N
lb/ft (uniform load)	1.49	kg/m
lb$_m$/(ft·h) (dynamic viscosity, μ)	0.413	mPa·s
lb$_m$/(ft·s) (dynamic viscosity, μ)	1490	mPa·s
lb$_f$·s/ft^2 (dynamic viscosity, μ)	47 880	mPa·s
lb/min	0.00756	kg/s
lb/h	0.126	g/s
lb/h (steam at 212°F)(970 Btu/h)	0.284	kW
lb$_f$/ft^2	47.9	Pa
lb/ft^2	4.88	kg/m^2
lb/ft^3 (density, ρ)	16.0	kg/m^3
lb/gallon	120	kg/m^3
ppm (by mass)	*1.00	mg/kg
psi	6.895	kPa
quad (10^{15} Btu)	1.06	EJ
quart (liquid, US)	0.946	L
revolutions per minute (rpm)	*1/60	Hz
square (100 ft^2)	9.29	m^2
tablespoon (approx.)	15	mL
teaspoon (approx.)	5	mL
therm (100,000 Btu)	105.5	MJ
ton, short (2000 lb)	0.907	Mg; t (tonne)
ton, refrigeration (12,000 Btu/h)	3.517	kW
torr (1 mm Hg at 0°C)	133	Pa
watt per square foot	10.8	W/m^2
yd	*0.9144	m
yd^2	0.836	m^2
yd^3	0.7646	m^3
To Obtain	**By**	**Divide**

Note: In this list the kelvin (K) expresses temperature intervals. The degree Celsius symbol (°C) is often used for this purpose as well.

*Conversion factor is exact.

Appendix B

SYSTEMS DESIGN PROBLEMS

1 Combination Water Chillers

(Centrifugal and Absorption Machines in Series)

Given:

1. The 1000-ton turbine driven centrifugal compressor in the figure below is supplied with steam at 30,00 lb/h at 125 psig. The turbine exhaust pressure is 15 psig. The temperature rise through the condenser is 10°F.
2. A 1500-ton lithium bromide water chiller uses exhaust steam at 12 psig from the steam turbine. It has a 4-pass evaporator with a pressure drop of 15 ft. The leaving temperature for the 4800 gpm condenser water is 105.3°F.
3. Water velocity for the condenser and chilled water piping is limited to 10 ft/s.
4. Chilled water supply temperature is 40°; chilled water return temperature is 60°F.
5. Cooling tower design data: 95°F dry bulb, 76°F wet bulb, 9°F approach.

Required:

1. Calculate the overall steam rate in pounds per hour per ton for the refrigeration plant.
2. Calculate the chilled water flow rate in gpm.
3. What is the temperature of water off the tower? What is the temperature of the water entering the cooling tower?
4. In the evaporator of the centrifugal compressor, what is the pressure drop and water velocity in the tubes?
5. In the condenser of the centrifugal compressor, what is the pressure drop and water velocity in the tubes?
6. Using Schedule 40 pipe, what size pipe would you use for the condenser water piping to each machine (a,b) the cooling tower (c), and the chilled water piping (d)?

2 Absorption Chiller Selection

A small college is to be built in the Santa Fe, New Mexico area (elevation 7000 ft). You have the assignment to design

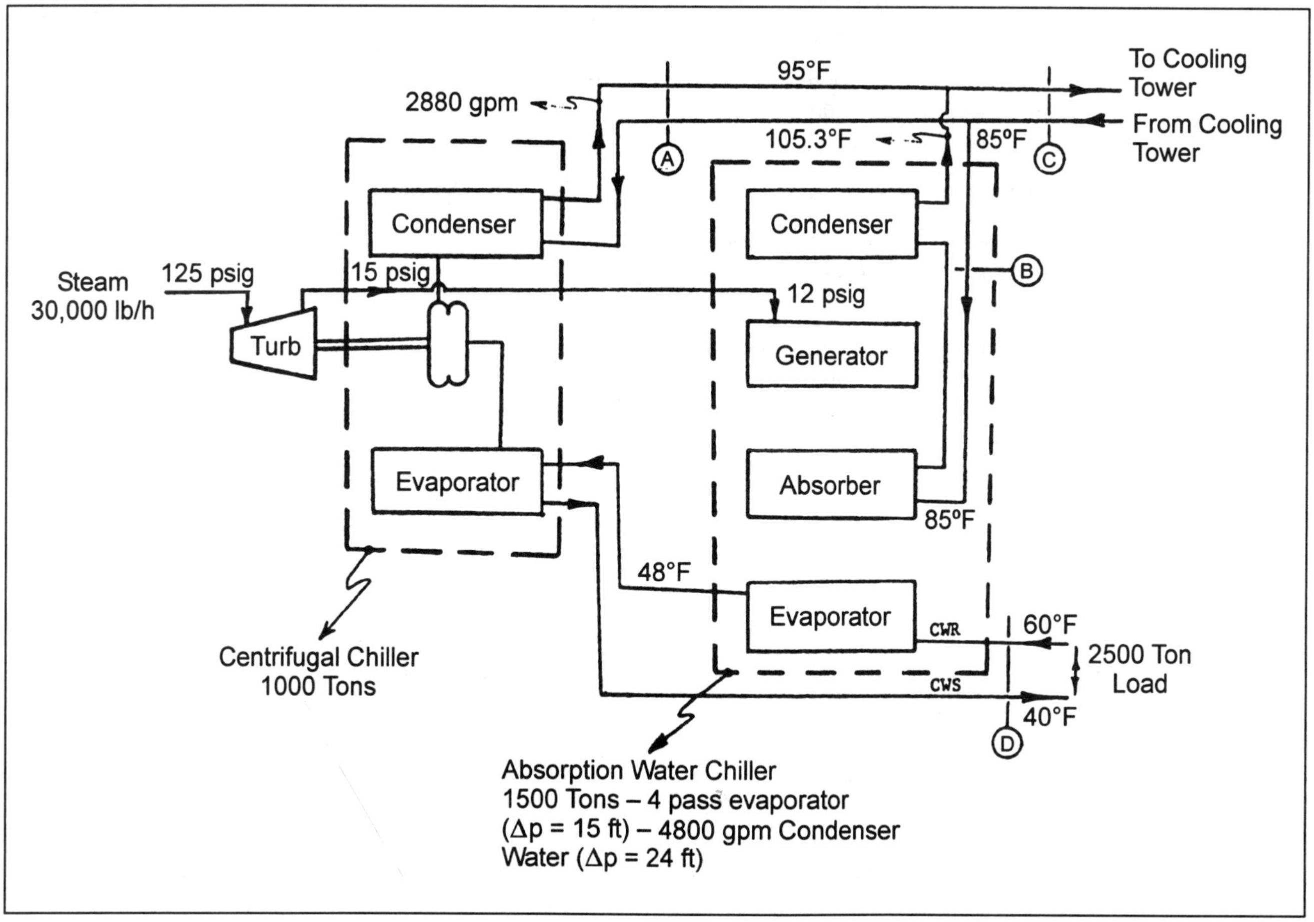

the mechanical systems for this project. You decide to recommend a central plant for both heating (steam) and cooling (chilled water). Since the available fuel is relatively inexpensive, you decide to use absorption refrigeration to keep the electrical demand as low as possible and to make use of the steam boilers which would otherwise be idle in the summertime.

Your preliminary analysis indicates that the first four buildings to be built will have the following characteristics:

Building	Area, ft^2	Estimated ft^2/ton	Estimated Total Tons
A	75,000	400	190
B	50,000	325	150
C	65,000	350	185
D	25,000	300	85

In addition, you decide to install sufficient additional capacity to handle 100,000 ft^2 of building (you do not know exactly what type of building it will be, so average and estimate). Also estimate a 5% loss in capacity in the piping and distribution system.

Steam is available at 30 psi and can be reduced to any pressure you desire. You decide to have 42°F to 58°F or a 16°F temperature difference (TDO as your chilled water design temperatures. Condensing water is available from the cooling tower at 80°F. The maximum allowable pressure drop through the chiller is 40 ft for the condenser-absorber and 20 ft for the evaporator. You want at least a 0.001 fouling factor on the condenser and a 0.0005 factor on the evaporator.

A. Select and specify an absorption chiller to handle the determined capacity. Indicate water and steam flow rates and unit pump motor horsepower requirements.

B. What is the rate of refrigerant flow at maximum load?

C. What is the theoretical pump horsepower required for the chilled water and condensing water due to the pressure drop through the unit?

D. What is the total hourly purchased energy requirement for this chiller (electrical + thermal)? How does this compare with an equivalent motor driven centrifugal machine? Which one is more economical to operate (assume electricity costs 5 times as mu as steam)?

E. What is the cooling tower requirement for the absorption machine compared with a centrifugal machine? How might this affect your answer to question D above?

3 Owning and Operating Costs

Management has decided to move a subsidiary of your company to Indianapolis, Indiana. This will necessitate a new office building. The chief engineer was asked to estimate the owning and operating cost for the refrigeration and summer air-conditioning services in the building. The chief just called you in this morning and now it is your estimate. Here is all the information available.

Building: Five-story, 160 ft by 300 ft gross with 90% of floor area air conditioned

Refrigeration: reciprocating compressors, R-12, 95°F condensing temperature, 40°F evaporator temperature

Power rate: $0.02 per kWh. Includes both demand and energy charge.

Water rate: $0.33 per 1000 gal

Water rate for condenser: 3.0 gpm per ton for full load operating hour

Operating hours for auxiliaries: 5 1/2 days per week

Power requirements:

Fan, air: 0.4 bhp per 1000 cfm
Fan, cooling tower: 0.05 bhp per ton
Pump, chilled water: 1.10 bhp per ton
Pump, cooling tower: 0.09 bhp per ton

Annual operating labor and maintenance: 4 1/2% of first cost (average for life of equipment).

Interest: 7%

Taxes: $2.00 per $100 of assessed valuation.

Assessed valuation: 25% of first cost.

4 Animal Rooms

Facilities to house laboratory animals control temperature, humidity, air motion, odor, and bacterial count. Design conditions vary widely depending on whether the animals are subjected to test environments or simply quartered. A general range of design temperatures and relateve humidity is tabulated in Table 1.

Table 1 Animal Room Temperature

Animal	Temp., °F	Relative Humidity, %
Mice	73 to 77	45 to 50
Rats	73 to 77	45 to 50
Guinea Pigs	72 to 74	45 to 50
Rabbits	70 to 72	45 to 50
Cats	75 to 77	45 to 50
Dogs	70 to 72	45 to 50
Monkeys	76 to 79	75

Recommended tolerances are +2°F dry bulb and ±5% rh at the point of control. Low temperature gradients are desirable. The maximum spread vertically and horizontally within the cage zones should be limited to within ±1.5°F of the control point. Air motion limits in the cage zone are 35 to 50 fpm for general applications and 25 to 35 fpm in quarters for mice. See the diagram on the following page.

The approximate amount of heat relaesed by laboratory animals at rest and during normal activity is shown in Table 2.

Conformance to temperature and humidity requirements requires control on a room basis and preferably on a module basis, because cage loading, occupancy distribution, and animal heat release are variable. A module constitutes two rows of cages with a working aisle separation. Temperature and

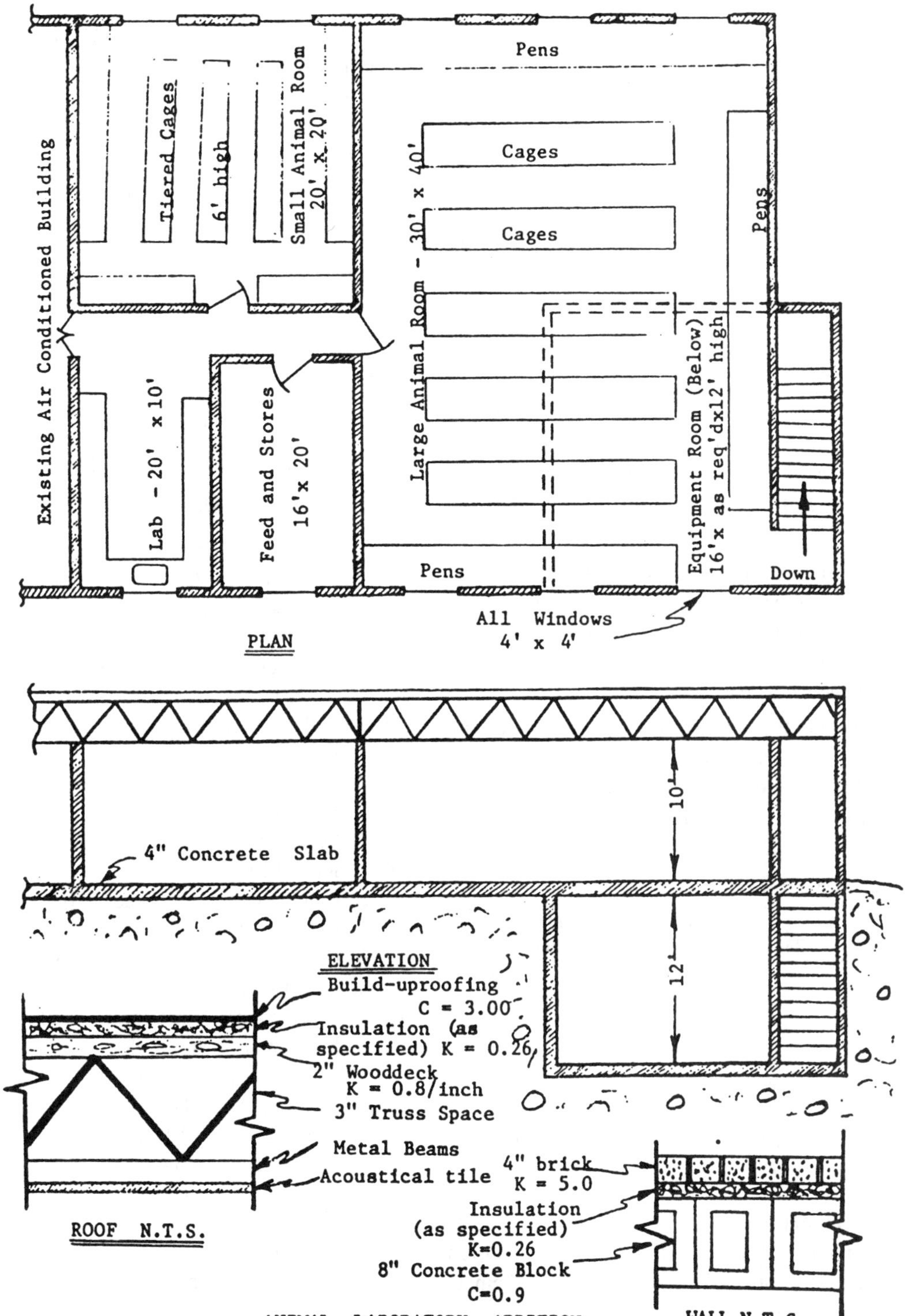

ANIMAL LABORATORY ADDITION

Table 2 Heat Generated by Laboratory Animals

		Heat Generation, Btu/h per Animal			
		Response (Basal)	Normally Active (est.)		
Animal	Mass, g	Total Heat	Sensible	Latent	Total
Mouse	21	0.6	3.3	1.7	5.0
Hamster	118	1.65	10	3	13
Pigeon	275	4.63	15	3	18
Rat	300	4.46	22	11	33
Guinea Pig	410	5.80	32	15	47
Chicken	2,100	18.8	64	12	76
Rabbit	2,600	19.3	61	18	79
Cat	3,000	25.1	75	25	100
Monkey	4,200	34.5	92	46	138
Dog	16,000	87.5	250	120	370
Goat	36,000	137.0	410	130	540
Sheep	45,000	192.0	560	190	750
Pig	250,000	718.0	2100	700	2800

velocity gradient control requires low supply air to room air temperature differential, overhead high induction diffusion, uniform horizontal and vertical air distribution, and low return outlets.

Odor control within animal rooms requires 100% outdoor air for odor removal from recirculated air. Unidirectional single pass airflow through the room is an aid for lowering odor levels. Air rates range from 10 to 20 air changes depending on the animal occupancy and density.

Odor-free air rates for various animal occupancies are listed in Table 3. Control of odor dissemination to adjoining spaces requires that the animal room be maintained under negative pressure or that air locks be employed. Bacterial control require high efficiency filtration or germicidal treatment.

Table 3 Average Odor-Free Requirements

Animal	Mass, g	Gross Space ft^3/animal	Odor-Free Air cfm/animal
Mice	21	1.0	0.10
Rats	200	3.5	0.75
Guinea pigs	410	6.0	1.5
Chickens	2,100	8.0	2.0
Rabbits	2,600	10.0	2.0
Cats	3,000	35.0	8.0
Monkeys	3,200	100.0	20.0
Dogs	14,000	150.0	50.0

Conditions in animal rooms must be continuously maintained, which requires year-round availability of refrigeration and, in some cases, dual air-conditioning facilities and emergency power for motor drives and control instrument energy.

An air-conditioning system is to be designed for an animal room for housing laboratory animals. The area is a separate wing of a research facility and is to have its own completely independent system to provide year-round temperature and humidity control. The large animal room will have a maximum of 80 dogs or their equivalent and the small animal room will contain mice, rats, rabbits and a few monkeys, with an equivalent heat release of 200 rabbits.

Insulation and window construction shall be selected as follows:

Design Temperature	Insulation	Windows (all sealed)
+30 °F and above	None	Single pane
+10 °F to +30°F	1 in.	Single pane
−20 °F to +10°F	2 in.	Two pane
below −20 °F	3 in.	Two pane

U for single pane = 1.13 Btu/h·ft^2·°F
U for double pane = 0.45 Btu/h·ft^2·°F

Lights:

In animal rooms: 1 W/ft^2
In feed room: 1 W/ft^2 (fluorescent)
In laboratory: 4 W/ft^2

For laboratory: 3 bunsen burners, one 1100 W sterilizer

For feed room: 1 hp electric food grinder

Perform the following:

(a) Calculate the heating loads for each room.
(b) Calculate the cooling loads for each room.
(c) 1. Calculate the air quantities (cfm) for each room.
    2. Make a schematic diagram of the apparatus required for air conditioning. (Heat air with hot water from hot water boiler).
(d) Calculate the areas of the cooling coil required and the face area (frontal area).
(e) 1. Make a single line duct layout.
    2. Size the ducts.
    3. Select the grilles, diffusers, and other components.
(f) 1. Select filter pressure loss.
    2. Calculate pressure losses in other parts of the air distributing system, coils, and outdoor louvers.
    3. Calculate the total pressure loss.
    4. Select fan, fans or units.
(g) 1. Select a refrigeration water chilling unit or units.
    2. Select a hot water boiler.
    3. Select pump or pumps for chilled water circulation.
(h) 1. Draw a plan of the building on 22 in. × 17 in. tracing paper (1/2 in. = 1 ft 0 in.).
    2. Draw the mechanical system designed on the plan. (Make sure mechanical system outline is heavier than building outline).
    3. Draw a plan and elevation of equipment room showing main items of equipment and ducts (1/2 in. = 1 ft 0 in.).

5 Greenhouse

An environmental control system is to be developed for a greenhouse located in the Lafayette, Indiana, area. This greenhouse is a rigid frame structure, 40 ft wide and 100 ft long with a roof slope of 6/12 and a sidewall height of 6 ft. The covering material is a single layer of polyethylene plastic.

Determine the following, listing your sources of data and assumptions used:

1. What is the maximum heat requirement for the house in Btu/h if the inside temperature is not to fall below 60°F?
2. On a clear winter day, January 21, with an outside noon temperature of 30°F and 65% rh, how much heat (Btu/h) or ventilation (cfm) is required to maintain an inside temperature somewhere between 60 and 70°F at 12 noon solar time? (consider sensible heat only).
3. Reconsider *Problem* 2 assuming that half of the solar radiation load is used to evaporate water from the plants, soil, and floor and manifests itself as a latent heat load. A further restriction of a maximum 50% inside rh is added to prevent condensation on the inside of the plastic covering. Under these conditions, what is the amount of heat (Btu/h) and/or ventilation (cfm) required to maintain an inside temperature of 75°F?
4. On a clear summer day, July 21, with an outside noon temperature of 85° and 50% rh, what is the minimum ventilation rate (cfm) required to prevent the inside temperature from exceeding 90°F? (Consider sensible heat only).
5. A pad evaporative cooler is to be considered for cooling the greenhouse on a clear day, August 21, with a noon temperature of 90°F and 40% rh. The entering air, after passing through the pad, has 90% rh. Using the ventilation rate from *Problem* 4, what is the exhaust air temperature? How many square feet of pad are required if the velocity through the pad is restricted to 150 fpm?

6 Drying Room

You are making a feasibility study for a 90,000 ft^3 drying room built inside a factory. An air conditioner is located outside the drying room. Air enters the conditioner from the plant at 82°F dry bulb, 50% rh and is distributed to the drying room at 82°F dry bulb, 10% rh. The air leaves the drying room at 112°F dry bulb, 90% rh and is exhausted from the factory through an exhaust system. Product passes through the drying room on a belt conveyor entering at 3600 lb/h at 128°F dry bulb, 40% moisture content.

Assume 10 air changes per hour through the drying room. Assume no heat or moisture flow through the drying room structure.

(a) What is the refrigeration load on the conditioning apparatus in tons?

(b) What is the moisture content of the product leaving the drying room?

You report the results to the product engineer who wants to know if you can dry the product to 20% moisture. The engineer says the 112°F leaving air is maximum; otherwise; the product will be too hot and will have to be cooled after it leaves the drying room to prevent checking.

You study the conveyor and feel it will be possible to modify the air distribution arrangement in the drying room. This will give more intimate contact between air and product and perhaps the same air volume flow rate can be used.

(c) What will be the humidity ratio of the air leaving the drying room for a 20% moisture content of the product? (You retain the 10 air changes per hour and the 112°F dry-bulb leaving air).

7 Air Washer

A chiller supplies water to a washer. The water leaves the chiller at 44°F and is returned at 54°F. Design conditions in the building are 78° dry bulb and 64.5°F wet bulb. A mixture of outdoor and recirculated air enters the washer at 88°F dry bulb and 72°F wet bulb. The total air circulated is 33,000 cfm. the washer has a performance factor of 0.85. The washer is a two-bank single-stage design.

1. What is the refrigeration load on the chiller?
2. What water quantity should it be handling in gpm?
3. What room SHR will these operating conditions exactly satisfty?
4. How many nozzles would you expect to find in the washer assuming 2 gpm per nozzle?
5. What should be the cross-sectional area of the washer assuming a velocity of 500 fpm?
6. Suppose the design engineer made a mistake in estimating the head on the chilled water circulating pump. The operating head was lower than the selection point for the pump. From the characteristic pump curve you estimate, the pump is now delivering 30% more water than in *Part* 2. Assuming the same performance factor, load, and air flow, what is your answer to *Part* 3? Discuss the effect of the conditions in the building.

8 Two-story Building

As both Architect and Chief Mechanical Engineer of your own consulting engineering firm, you are responsible for the design of the building and for the sizing and selection of the major components of the HVAC system for the building. A report on your design, analysis, and recommendations for the HVAC system must be prepared for the sponsor and his staff. Sizing and selection are to cover only the heating, cooling, and humidifying equipment with cost estimates. Estimates of annual HVAC energy use and cost are to be included.

Simple tables of design conditions, building data, results and recommended equipment should be included in the body of report. A cover letter is mandatory. Completely labeled sketches and diagrams should be included as appropriate. Detailed calculations and/or computer printouts are to be included as appended material.

The 24,000 sq ft, two floor office building is to be located in Louisville, Kentucky. There are to be six, separately thermostated zones; three on each floor. The east and north ends are the be combined into one zone; the west and south into a second, and a center portion into the third. The zones are each approximately the same size. The east and north zones are to contain a minimum of 70% glass in the exterior walls while the exterior walls of the west and south zones are to contain between 20 and 40% glass.

Since the owner will be picking up the utility bills, he or she is somewhat energy conscious. However, the owner is also very concerned about the first cost of the building and does not plan extreme departures from common building practices and materials. A rooftop installation is planned to conserve interior space.

As the engineer and architect hired by the owner-to-be of the building, you are to design the building, specifying the layout, wall and ceiling descriptions, types of glass, doors, etc, etc. Neglect details such as closets, room dividers, halls, etc. Items to be determined include:

Design heating load for each space.
Design cooling load for each space.
Projected energy requirements for heating and for cooling.
Sizing of major components (heating unit, cooling unit, fan, humidifier).
Sizing and layout of ducts.
Specific recommendations for equipment and fuels.
Estimated initial cost of HVAC equipment and annual operating cost.

9 Motel

As both Architect and Chief Mechanical Engineer of your own consulting engineering firm, you are responsible for the design of the building and for the sizing and selection of the major components of the HVAC system for the building. A report on your design, analysis, and recommendations for the HVAC system must be prepared for the sponsor and his staff.

Sizing and selection are to cover only the heating, cooling, and humidifying equipment with cost estimates. Estimates of annual HVAC energy use and cost are to be included.

Simple tables of design conditions, building data, results and recommended equipment should be included in the body of report. A cover letter is *mandatory*. Completely labeled sketches and diagrams should be included as appropriate. Detailed calculations are to be included as appended material.

The 24-unit (plus office) single building motel is to be located in St. Louis, Missouri, in the Lambert Airport area. Each unit is to be 12 ft by 24 ft with the office twice the size of a regular room. Two thirds of the units are to be non-smoking. Each unit will be conditioned with its own packaged terminal air conditioner (PTAC) or packaged terminal heat pump (PTHP).

Since the owner will be picking up the utility bills, he or she is somewhat energy conscious. However, the owner is also very concerned about the first cost of the building and does not plan extreme departures from common building practices and materials.

As the engineer and architect hired by the owner-to-be of the building, you are to design the building, specifying the layout, wall and ceiling descriptions, types of glass, doors, etc, etc. Items to be determined include:

Design heating load for each space.
Design cooling load for each space.
Projected energy requirements for heating and for cooling.
Sizing of major components (heating unit, cooling unit, fan, humidifier).
Specific recommendations for equipment and fuels.
Estimated initial cost of HVAC equipment and annual operating cost.

10 Building Renovation

As Chief Mechanical Engineer of a consulting engineering firm, you are responsible for the design, sizing and selection of the major components of the HVAC system for the building. A report on your design, analysis, and recommendations for the HVAC system must be prepared for the sponsor and his staff.

Sizing and selection are to cover the heating, cooling, and humidifying equipment with cost estimates. Estimates of annual HVAC energy use, *both before and after* the modifications, are to be included.

Simple tables of design conditions, building data, results and recommended equipment should be included in the body of report. A cover letter is *mandatory*.

Completely labeled sketches and diagrams should be included as appropriate.

Detailed calculations and/or computer printouts are to be included as appended material.

The project concerns the complete renovation of the office building located in St. Louis, Missouri and shown in the following sketch.

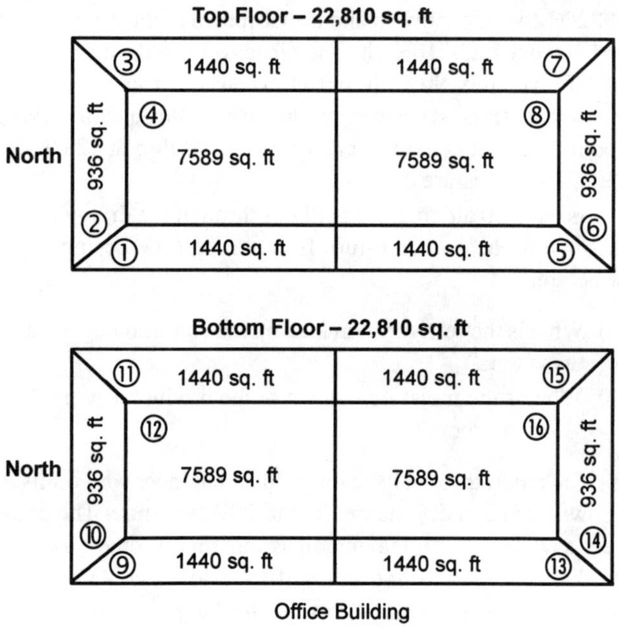

Sketch of Project 10 Building.

The building is divided into 16 separately thermostated zones. Physical description and building operation (base case) data are:

Building roof area: 22,810 ft^2
Building floor area: 45,620 ft^2
Ceiling height: 8.5 ft
Building exterior wall area: 9,460 ft^2 (net)
Building glass area: 7,536 ft^2
Building thermal mass: M (medium)
Uniform internal load density: 2.9 W/ft^2
Occupancy: 408 people (uniformly distributed)
Original U-factors:

Roof—0.25 Btu/h·ft^2·°F
Walls—0.20 Btu/h·ft^2·°F
Glass—1.0 Btu/h·ft^2·°F
Shading Coefficient for Glass: 0.6

Originally built in the late 1960s with an all-electric reheat HVAC system, the renovated building will replace the inefficient reheat system with all-electric packaged terminal air conditioners (PTACs) in each space. In the exterior zones, the PTACs will include provisions for ventilation air. For the interior zones, the PTACs will operate without outside air provisions and a separate rooftop make-up air system will be used for ventilation requirements. When renovated, all walls and ceilings will include an additional 2 inches of glass fiber, organic bonded rigid insulation, The windows will be upgraded to double pane, 1/4 inch air gap, aluminum frame with thermal break (non operable). The internal load density is estimated to have increased over the years from the original 2.9 W/ft^2 to 6.0 W/ft^2.

Items to be included:

Design heating load for each space.
Design cooling load for each space.
Projected annual energy requirements for heating and for cooling.
Sizing and selection of major components.
Sizing and layout of ducts for interior zones.
Estimated initial cost of HVAC equipment and annual operating cost.
Potential problem areas with this type of equipment.

11 Building with Neutral Deck Multizone

As the Chief Mechanical Engineer of your own consulting engineering firm, you are responsible for preliminary design of the HVAC system for the building shown in the accompanying figure. Selection of all major components is to be included. A report on your analysis and recommendations for the HVAC system must be prepared for the sponsor and his staff.

Sizing and selection will cover all heat exchangers (coils), fans, refrigeration units, boilers and/or other heating equipment, humidifiers, cooling towers, heat reclaim and/or air-to-air energy recovery equipment, and pumps. Piping, ducting, and related fittings need not be sized nor selected at this time.

Simple tables of design conditions, building data, results and recommended equipment should be included in the body of report. A cover letter is mandatory. Completely labeled sketches and diagrams should be included as appropriate. Detailed calculations and appropriate manufacturers' catalog data are to be included as appended material.

Building Location: Atlanta, GA

The ventilation requirements are to be in accordance with ASHRAE *Standard* 62. Anticipate occupany rate is 10 persons per 1000 ft^2 of floor space. Design pressure drop for the ducting system is 3.25 in. of water. The design loads are given in the following table.

Design Loads (Btu)

Zone	Heating (sensible)	Cooling (sensible)	Cooling (latent)
1	−95,000	164,000	47,000
2	+33,000	157,000	14,000
3	−98,000	199,000	40,000
4	−276,000	567,000	72,000

The winter latent load is negligible.

Type of HVAC System: Multizone with neutral deck

Primary Systems: R-22 condensing unit & DX coil, multiple gas fired boilers for steam coil

Auxiliary Equipment: Spray washer, heat pipe air-to-air energy recovery system, air-side economizer

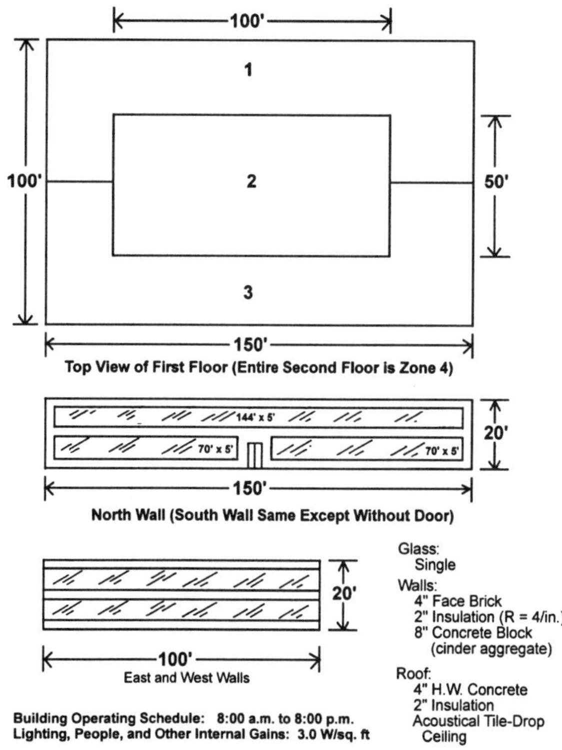

Figure for Project 11.

INDEX